BIOCHEMISTRY

BIOCHEMISTRY
EIGHTH EDITION

JAMES M. ORTEN, Ph.D.

Professor of Biochemistry, Wayne State University
School of Medicine, Detroit, Michigan

OTTO W. NEUHAUS, Ph.D.

Professor and Chairman of Biochemistry
University of South Dakota, School of Medicine
Vermillion, South Dakota

With 289 illustrations, including 3 in color,
and 2 color plates

The C. V. Mosby Company
SAINT LOUIS, 1970

DEDICATED TO ISRAEL SIMON KLEINER

(in memoriam)

inspiring teacher, meticulous investigator, author,

and progenitor of this book

PREFACE

The completion of the eighth edition of this book is both pleasant and sad. The sadness of the occasion is the reminder of the loss by death on June 10, 1966, of the original author, then coauthor, of the first seven editions, Dr. Israel Simon Kleiner. This edition is dedicated to his memory. He was indeed a talented and congenial coauthor as well as a friend and valued mentor. He is greatly missed.

The pleasant part of this occasion is the opportunity to welcome a new coauthor, Dr. Otto W. Neuhaus, a former colleague and longtime friend. Dr. Neuhaus brings to the book a point of view and a major interest complementary to that of the senior author. He is an experienced teacher with thorough, broad training in biochemistry under the late Professor Howard B. Lewis and Professor Lila Miller, both of the University of Michigan. Dr. Neuhaus also spent a valuable year as a NATO Research Fellow at the Laboratoire de Chimie Biologique, Université de Lille, Lille, France, studying with Professor G. Biserte.

In the present revision, we felt a reorganization of the text, with a somewhat different sequence of subject matter, was desirable. This need became urgent primarily because of the dramatic advances of the past decade in the biochemical-biologic sciences, specifically in molecular biology. The role of the nucleic acids in genetic phenomena, the genetic code, and the mechanism and control of the biosynthesis of proteins are three examples of the tremendous progress in this field. The entire second section of the present edition, therefore, deals with biochemical genetics and the role of nucleic acids and proteins in the process of transcription and translation of genetic information. Later sections are devoted to the chemistry and metabolism of cell constituents and of the various body tissues and fluids. Finally, the biochemistry of the nutrition of the living organism is considered. Thus the overall purpose is to correlate chemical subject matter with biologic processes in living matter. At the same time, every effort has been made to preserve proper consideration for the classic concepts of biochemistry and its relation to human problems as presented in earlier editions.

If preferred, the subject matter of the present edition is easily adaptable to the more traditional sequence of presentation. The chapters on the chemistry of the proteins, carbohydrates, and lipids (Chapters 5, 8, and 11) can be considered immediately after the introductory chapters (Section I), followed by those on metabolism, etc.

A number of chapters (1 through 7 and 14) have been completely rewritten because of extensive advances in these areas. Also, the other chapters have been partially rewritten and extensively revised to include important current developments. A number of new charts, tables, and illustrations have been added, and others have been deleted. Section V, on the vitamins and nutrition, has been almost completely redone.

Because of the vast expansion of biochemical literature during the past few years, increasing use of books, monographs, and reviews as general references at the end of each chapter has been made. The fewer special references to original papers in the literature are limited mainly to earlier classic papers describing original discoveries or concepts, or to current articles deemed of special significance. We offer regrets for any omission of important work not included because of space limitations or perhaps errors of human judgment.

Appendixes have been added to replace former text discussions dealing with physicochemical phenomena important in biochemistry and with newer techniques that have proved essential to recent progress in the field. The food tables of the Appendix of former editions have been discontinued, with references to other sources of this information being provided.

This edition has been designed with not only the needs of the medical student and students of other health-related sciences in mind but also those of the general biologist and chemist. Our hope is that it will prove of value to each.

The suggestions and comments, as well as assistance in other ways, of many colleagues and co-workers has greatly facilitated the preparation of this new edition. Special gratitude is due Dr. Ray K. Brown, for critically reading a number of chapters and making many helpful suggestions, and to Dr. Walter H. Seegers, who rewrote the entire section on the coagulation of blood. Deep appreciation is expressed to the following colleagues and friends for helpful suggestions and material: Drs. W. N. Arnold, G. J. Cox, Dana Dabich, Marilyn Doscher, M. F. Dunker, R. A. Hudson, A. C. Kuyper, R. A. Mitchell, F. C. Neuhaus, C. J. Parker, R. J. Peanasky, G. D. Small, E. H. Shaw, Jr., and S. N. Vinogradov. Gratitude is extended to fellow biochemists and journals who have generously permitted us to use illustrations, data, quotations, or concepts from their own publications. These have added greatly to the value of the book. Our thanks are also expressed to Louise Globke, Patricia Kosmyna, Maribel Andonian, and Evelyn Oden, for valued help in the preparation of the manuscript.

A special word of gratitude is reserved for our wives, for their constant support, aid, and understanding during the months required for the preparation of this manuscript. Dr. Aline U. Orten has read the final three chapters and offered many valuable suggestions and criticisms of these as well as of other chapters of the book. Special gratitude is also expressed to Dorothy E. Neuhaus for the preparation of numerous figures in Chapters 4 through 7 and 18 as well as for invaluable assistance in reading, organization, and correspondence.

Finally, and perhaps of greatest importance, gratitude is expressed to the users of this book. Their many helpful suggestions, comments, and criticisms have been invaluable in its continued revision and improvement. After all, the users of a book— postgraduate, graduate, and undergraduate students primarily, in this instance—are the *raison d'etre*, the very reason for its existence.

James M. Orten
Otto W. Neuhaus

CONTENTS

CONTENTS

APPENDIXES

APPENDIX A
PHYSICOCHEMICAL PHENOMENA OF IMPORTANCE IN BIOCHEMISTRY, 879

APPENDIX B
ANALYTIC TECHNIQUES FREQUENTLY USED IN BIOCHEMISTRY, 901

COLOR PLATES

SECTION **one**

PREFATORY

CHAPTER 1

BIOCHEMICAL CHARACTERISTICS OF LIVING MATTER

NATURE OF BIOCHEMISTRY

Biochemistry, according to a classic definition, is the study of the chemical composition of living matter and of the chemical changes that occur in it during life processes. In perhaps a broader sense, biochemistry may be defined as a discipline in which biologic phenomena are analyzed in terms of chemistry. Thus *biology*, including the medical and health sciences, poses the questions and, in this context, *chemistry* provides the intellectual and technical tools for their answer. Indeed, a working definition of a *biochemist*, adopted in 1965 by the American Society of Biological Chemists as a guideline for eligibility for membership in that society, is as follows: "A biochemist is an investigator who utilizes chemical, physical, or biological techniques to study the chemical nature and behavior of living matter."

Biochemistry, consequently, involves studies of the chemical constituents of the cell, the unit of living matter, and of the chemical mechanisms by which living material is formed, maintained, and eventually destroyed. The latter processes are conventionally termed *metabolism*. Hence, a major portion of biochemistry deals with this subject. The principal emphasis is properly on metabolism under normal, *physiologic*, conditions. However, deviations of metabolism under abnormal, *pathologic*, conditions will be considered too not only for so-called practical reasons but also because such deviations frequently aid in the elucidation of normal patterns. This will be evident as the subject is discussed in the ensuing pages.

DEVELOPMENT OF BIOCHEMISTRY

Biochemistry, as such, is a relatively young science, dating back only some 150 years. Indeed, the term *biochemistry* itself was not introduced until 1903 by the eminent German chemist Carl Neuberg. However, the beginnings of biochemistry date back much earlier than this and are intertwined with the development of the older sciences of organic chemistry (indeed of alchemy itself), physiology, biology, and medicine. The studies of the great Swedish chemist Karl Scheele, in the mid-1700's, on the chemical composition of plant and animal tissues contributed significantly to the founding of biochemistry as a separate discipline. Likewise, the classic investigations of Lavoisier (1785) on respiration, of Pasteur on fermentation, of Spallanzani, Reaumur, Beaumont, and Claude Bernard on digestion, and of Berzelius and Liebig in the first half of the 1800's on the quantitative analysis of naturally occurring substances served as a basis for later biochemical work and thought. Wöhler's chemical synthesis of urea in the 1820's permanently laid to rest the ancient belief that "vital forces" were required for the formation of biologically occurring organic compounds, thus placing biochemistry on a firm chemical foundation.

From these rather fragmentary beginnings, biochemistry emerged as a separate entity, sometimes termed "physiological chemistry" or "pathological chemistry," in the later 1800's. From this time into the early 1900's, high points in its development include Chevreul's pioneer work on the chemical nature of fats, Emil Fischer's classic studies on carbohydrates and amino acids, F. Miescher's discovery of the "nucleins" and nucleic acids, and E. Buchner's important observations on the fermentation of sugars by extracts of yeast, leading to the postulation of *enzymes* as organic catalysts.

The period of greatest progress in biochemistry, however, began in the 1920's with such classic investigations as those of Osborne and Mendel and of F. G. Hopkins on protein requirements for the animal organism; Hans Fischer's synthesis of heme; Funk, Mendel, and McCollum's pioneer discoveries on the vitamins; Sumner, Northrop, and Kunitz' studies on the chemical nature and functions of certain enzymes; and Harden and Young's and Embden and Meyerhof's work on the intermediary metabolism of carbohydrates. This period, into the 1930's, also included the brilliant discoveries of Steenbock, Elvehjem, and du Vigneaud in the vitamin field, and of Krebs, Szent-Györgyi, and others on the *citric acid cycle*, as well as W. C. Rose's now classic studies on the *essential amino acids*.

The post–World War II era witnessed the most remarkable period of progress in biochemistry. During this interval, and up to the present time, knowledge of the field has been estimated as *doubling every 8 years,* thus making biochemistry perhaps the most dynamic and productive area of human endeavor. This has been due to several fortunate occurrences in the early 1950's—the development of exquisitely sensitive and specific chromatographic methods for separating and identifying extremely small amounts of metabolites and other biologically active compounds, the availability of isotopes for "tagging" compounds and following their pathways in metabolism, and, of no less importance, the availability of sufficient funds for basic biochemical research. To illustrate the spectacular advances made in the past two decades, one needs only to mention such examples as the development of modern concepts of bioenergetics, the elucidation of the biosynthetic and degradative pathways for fatty acids, amino acids, and glucose, the details of the biosynthesis of cholesterol and certain steroid hormones and of heme, the determination of the primary, secondary, and tertiary structures of a number of biologically important proteins, and, of course, the elegant work on the structure of the nucleic acids with the concept of the role of deoxyribo-nucleic acid (DNA) and ribonucleic acid (RNA) in the genetic control of protein biosynthesis. A fuller discussion of these brilliant discoveries in modern biochemistry will make up a major portion of this book. It is safe to predict that the coming few decades will witness a similar, if not an even more dramatic, expansion of knowledge in this dynamic field.

CHEMICAL ORIGIN OF LIVING MATTER

We living things are a late outgrowth of the metabolism of our Galaxy. The carbon that enters so importantly into our composition was cooked in the remote past in a dying star. From it at lower temperatures nitrogen and oxygen were formed. These, our indispensable elements, were spewed out into space in the exhalations of red giants and such stellar catastrophes as super-novae, there to be mixed with hydrogen, to form eventually the substance of the sun and planets, and ourselves. The waters of ancient seas set the pattern of ions in our blood. The ancient atmos-pheres molded our metabolism.
                                                                                    G. Wald

This *vivid* statement expresses some of the highlights of current concepts of the chemical origin of living matter — a field that has developed significantly in the past few years. A somewhat more detailed proposition is that of Price,[1] summarized diagrammatically in Fig. 1-1. This scheme has been expressed similarly, in part at least, in a prevailing view that the chemical elements themselves *evolved* from nuclear reactions in stars, hydrogen being an early form of matter some 12 to 15 (or possibly even 70) billion years ago. Indeed, as Einstein once stated, "matter is energy congealed." From isotope-dating studies the age of the earth itself has been estimated as some 5 billion years.

There is now growing evidence to support the above concepts of the chemical origin of living matter. One of the fascinating developments in biochemistry during the past decade has been the beginning of some under-standing of the origin of living matter from simple chemical molecules.

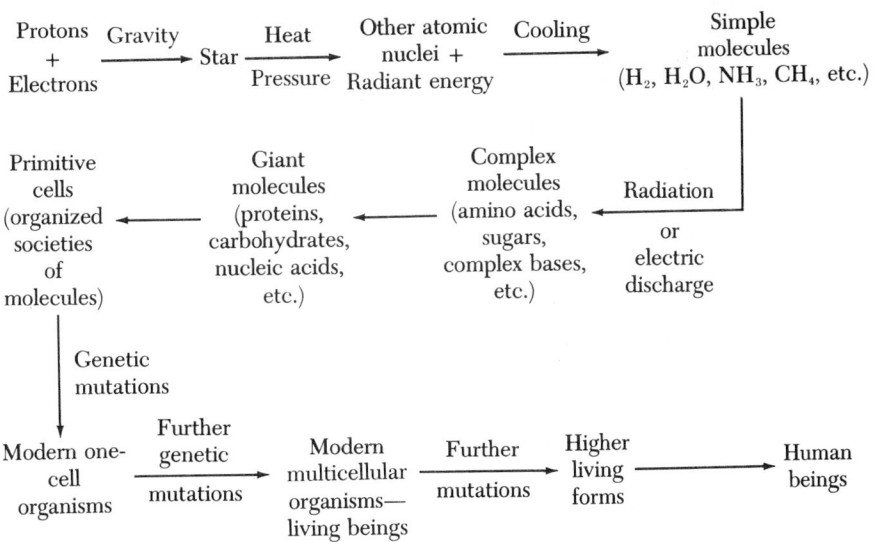

Fig. 1-1. Diagrammatic representation of the chemical origin of life. (From Price, C. C.: Sci. Res. 3:27, 1968.)

Primitive organic molecules such as hydrocyanic acid, acetic acid, formic acid, and formaldehyde began to be formed perhaps 3 to 4 billion years ago[2] from the primeval atmosphere composed of water, carbon dioxide, hydrogen, methane, and ammonia. The energy sources for these transformations were probably ultraviolet light from the sun, cosmic rays, and other types of radiation. Indeed, several scientists in the early 1950's found that the foregoing simple compounds, and even malic acid, aspartic acid, glycine, and alanine, could be formed in the laboratory from various mixtures of water, carbon dioxide, methane, ammonia, and hydrogen circulated past an energy source under conditions of temperature (150° C.) and pressure prevailing on earth at that time. More recently, methionine has been synthesized from ammonium thiocyanate in aqueous solution by ultraviolet irradiation under prebiotic conditions. Calvin and his co-workers[3] found that adenine can be formed from hydrocyanic acid under similar conditions. Other purine bases could have been formed from adenine, and pyrimidines undoubtedly could also have been produced similarly. Recent studies[4] have shown that the phosphorylation of one of the pyrimidine bases, uracil (as uridine), can occur in its aqueous solution under prebiotic conditions, with the resulting formation of 5'-uridine monophosphate (UMP), a constituent of nucleic acids. Ribose and other sugars could have arisen from the polymerization of formaldehyde. Likewise, the polymerization of amino acids into *proteinoids* has been accomplished by heating (180° to 200° C.) amino acid mixtures in nitrogen gas.[5] These proteinoids have many properties of typical proteins. Glycogen, starch, and perhaps other important polymers could also be formed by a similar *abiologic* process. Several amino acids have been identified in fossil dinosaur bones and clam shells 150 to 300 million years old.[6] Currently,[7] some 22 different amino acids have been identified in a sample of pre-Cambrian sedimentary rock that is at least 3.1 billion years old.

Thus, under primeval conditions, it has been possible to produce and identify the preformed "building stones" (monomers) of living matter — i.e., the sugars, fatty acids, and amino acids, as well as their polymers, the proteins, lipids, and starch and glycogen, and the purine and pyrimidine bases that are essential constituents of nucleic acids. The latter, as will be seen, form the transmissible "code" for the synthesis of protein and other essential constituents of living matter.

Undoubtedly, catalysts for the regulation of the preceding synthetic processes must have been necessary then as now. Enzymes, an important class of biocatalysts, could have evolved from the proteinoids just mentioned. It is interesting that porphyrin derivatives, which are present in a number of biocatalysts, have been synthesized by several groups of investigators[8] under simulated primordial conditions, using a mixture of ammonia, methane, and water through which was passed a 12,000-volt continuous electric arc between tungsten electrodes. Porphyrins also showed up quite early in the evolutionary scheme. A recent report[9] states that porphyrins have been found in microfossils dated about a billion years ago. Likewise, Margoliash and Smith[10] have estimated that the cytochrome molecule has existed some 2 billion years! Since that time, cytochrome-c, like the hemoglobin molecule and a number of other functionally important proteins (e.g., certain enzymes), has undergone chemical evolutionary changes, in terms of portions of its amino acid sequence, that parallel the biologic evolution of the various animal species. Undoubtedly, preceding changes occurred in the base sequence of DNA, which controls by way of the several types of RNA the biosynthesis of these proteins in vivo.[11]

With the chemical evolution of the porphyrin molecule, the synthesis of chlorophyl by plants became possible; and, in turn, with the cytochromes and necessary cofactors (vitamin K–like substances), the generation by *cyclic phosphorylation* of chemical energy (adenosine triphosphate, ATP) from light energy of the sun was made possible. Such chemical energy then became available for the photosynthesis of carbohydrates from carbon dioxide and water, and for other biosynthetic reactions.[12] Thus, current evidence indicates that photosynthetic organisms with suitable catalysts have existed for more than a billion years, affording conditions that would complete the requisites for the synthesis of living matter from simple organic compounds even at this early period of biochemical evolution. Of course, it is also possible that some living matter may have been derived from meteorites from outer space, as postulated in the "seeding" theory.

BIOCHEMISTRY OF LIVING MATTER

Living matter, or protoplasm, cannot be defined adequately. It differs from lifeless material in possessing the capabilities of growth, repair, and reproduction. These properties may not be apparent at all times in the same degree, but they are present to some extent in all living organisms. Moreover, the life processes go on at comparatively low temperature and with great rapidity, the synthesis of a complex protein molecule such as hemoglobin, for example, apparently requiring only a few seconds. Comparable reactions in the laboratory, even if possible, require high temperatures, often with increased pressure, or else they go on very slowly and quite incompletely. Many reactions of the living cell are of great complexity—intricate interwoven oxidations, disintegrations, and syntheses—in comparison with which the manifold simultaneous operations of an electronic computer are like simple mechanical toys. Some of these marvelous reactions are known and partly understood. Many others are appreciated only because of our awareness of the end products. We must be impressed by the orderly way in which all the chemical activities of the body coordinate. This may be another attribute of living matter, the orderliness of its chemical reactions.

Chemical composition Protoplasm is composed of water, inorganic salts, and organic compounds. Water is a most important compound in tissues and comprises some 75% to 85% of the weight of most cells. The water of the tissues and body fluids is mostly in the free state; i.e., substances may be dissolved in it and it may pass back and forth from blood to tissues, in and out of cells. A small fraction of the water is believed to be bound. In other words, some of the water in hydrophilic colloid systems is combined so that the activity of the water molecules is reduced considerably. Free water varies according to diet and physiologic activity, whereas bound water is a rather constant constituent of the tissues.

Recent studies[13] using deuterated water (D_2O) in dogs have shown that the average water content of the body as a whole is 61% of body weight, with a range of 55% to 67%. The water content of the human body apparently has about the same range, being less than average in fat individuals and somewhat greater in thin persons. The water content of individual tissues also varies considerably, as will be discussed later.

Water content There are several mechanisms for maintaining and controlling the water content of the tissues (Chapter 15). When these go wrong, a number of pathologic states may ensue. Dehydration is a condition not at all uncommon and is likely to have a fatal outcome if not recognized and combatted. Edema is another—a condition in which fluid leaves the bloodstream and accumulates in the tissues. Sometimes what appears to be a minor disturbance results in a major catastrophe.

Water is needed for many and varied reasons. It is the solvent, the agency that enables water-soluble, water-miscible, or emulsifiable substances to be transferred in the body, not only in the blood, which is more than four-fifths water, but also intercellularly and intracellularly. Ionization takes place in water, and ionization is a prerequisite to many biochemical reactions.

In the regulation of body heat, water is most important because of its peculiar physical properties. It possesses *high specific heat;* i.e., the amount of heat required to raise the temperature of a gram of water 1° C. is much higher than the amount of heat required to raise the temperature of a gram of some other substance 1° C. The specific heat of water is 1. The values for all other common substances are much smaller. This enables the body to store heat effectively without greatly raising its temperature. Water has *high heat conductivity.* This permits heat to be transferred readily from the interior of the body to the surface. Finally, water possesses *high latent heat of evaporation,* which causes a great deal of heat to be used in its evaporation and thus cools the surface of the body. These are physical properties useful to the body in the physiologic regulation of body temperature.

Inorganic and organic constituents At least 60 of the 102 or more elements believed to be present in the universe occur in biologic matter. Only some 20 to 22 of these are found consistently, however, and some are present only in extremely minute amounts. About 1% of the total weight of an average soft tissue is ash, or inorganic salts, chiefly of the cations Na^+, K^+, Mg^{++}, Ca^{++}, NH_4^+ and the anions Cl^-, $H_2PO_4^-$, $HPO_4^=$, HCO_3^-, $SO_4^=$. Some of these may be linked to organic radicals, as is also the case for Fe, I, Cu, Zn, and Mn. Other *trace elements* consistently found in nearly all forms of living matter include B, Cr, Co, F, and Si. Biochemical functions of Co, F, and probably Cr, are now known, as will be discussed later (Chapter 15). Other elements are found in small amounts in some species, but as yet no definite function for them has been established. These include Ag, Al, As, Ba, Be, Br, Cd, Cs, Ge, Li, Mo, Ni, Pb, Rb, Se, Sn, Sr, Ti, and V. A few other elements, which are regarded as contaminants or accidental constituents, may be found in living matter. These include Ar, Au, Bi, He, Hg, and Tl.

A number of elements occur in living matter as mixtures of the more common form with varying amounts of other forms of the same element. These have slightly different atomic structure and atomic weight from the more common form and are called *isotopes*. Thus ordinary chlorine, with an atomic weight of 35.457, has been found to be a mixture of two isotopes, the first and more abundant one having an atomic mass of 35 and the second, less abundant one, an atomic mass of 37. Since isotopes in general have the same chemical and biologic properties as the more abundant form, they have proved extremely valuable as *tracers* in biochemical research. Metabolites labeled with isotopic atoms can be followed through an organism and metabolic "pathways" can thus be determined, as will be repeatedly mentioned in the following pages. Also, it is possible by determining the amount of an isotope, e.g., ^{14}C, in a specimen of wood or fossil, to accurately estimate the age of the specimen, by the so-called *isotope dating* technique. The amount of the isotope present is determined by either its *radioactivity*, as in the case of ^{14}C, or its *mass* (in a mass spectrometer), as in the case of ^{13}C or ^{2}H (deuterium).

With the exception of water and small amounts of gases, e.g., oxygen and carbon dioxide, the remaining chemical constituents of living matter consist of organic compounds: carbohydrates, lipids, proteins, and many others. The various tissues differ in all of these constituents qualitatively and quantitatively. It is to be expected that a nerve cell will not have the same composition as a salivary gland cell. However, all cells resemble each other chemically to some extent.

References

GENERAL

Baldwin, E.: Dynamic aspects of biochemistry, ed. 5, New York, 1967, Cambridge University Press.

Calvin, M.: Chemical evolution, New York, 1969, Oxford University Press, Inc.

Chittenden, R. H.: The development of physiological chemistry in the United States, American Chemical Society monograph no. 54, New York, 1930, The Chemical Catalog Co., Inc.

Florkin, M., and Stotz, E., editors: Comprehensive biochemistry, New York, 1962–1967, American Elsevier Publishing Co., Inc.

Nobel Foundation, Nobel lectures. Chemistry (3 vols.), Physiology and medicine (3 vols.), 1901–1962, New York, 1966, American Elsevier Publishing Co., Inc.

Vogel, H. J., and Vogel, R. H.: Some chemical glimpses of evolution, Chem. Eng. News 45:88, 1967.

Williams, R. J., and Lansford, E. M., editors: Encyclopedia of biochemistry, New York, 1967, Reinhold Publishing Corp.

SPECIAL

1. Price, C. C.: Sci. Res. 3:27, 1968.
2. Calvin, M., and Calvin, G. J.: Amer. Sci. 52:163, 1964.
3. Calvin, M., et al.: Proc. Nat. Acad. Sci. 49:737, 1963.
4. Lohrmann, R., and Orgel, L. E.: Science 161:64, 1968.
5. Ponnamperuma, C., et al.: Science 143: 1449, 1964.
6. Abelson, P. H.: Sci. Amer. 195:83, 1956.
7. Schopf, J. W.: Chem. Eng. News 45:22, 1967.
8. Hodgson, G. W., and Ponnamperuma, C.: Proc. Nat. Acad. Sci. 59:22, 1968.
9. Meinschein, W. G., et al.: Science 145: 262, 1964.
10. Margoliash, E., and Smith, E. L.: Proc. 6th Int. Congr. Biochem. 32:206, 1964.
11. Hill, R. L., and Buettner-Janusch, J.: Fed. Proc. 23:1236, 1964.
12. Arnon, D. I.: Sci. Amer. 203:105, 1960.
13. Gaebler, O. H., and Choitz, H. C.: Clin. Chem. 10:13, 1964.

CHAPTER 2

BIOCHEMICAL MORPHOLOGY OF THE CELL

Since the structural unit of all living matter, plant as well as animal, is the cell, as recognized by Schwann and Schleiden some 130 years ago, a brief consideration should now be given to the structure of a typical cell and to the principal biochemical processes involved in its development, maintenance, and eventual senescence and destruction.

The typical animal cell consists of a cell membrane that surrounds and encloses the nucleus and the cytoplasm. Both of these, in turn, contain other structures, such as a nucleolus and mitochondria, respectively, as shown in Fig. 2-1. Excellent electron micrographs showing the ultrastructures of various types of cells are given in the monographs by Porter and Bonneville and by Threadgold listed at the end of this chapter.

Cells of different tissues are modified as to size and shape and in chemical composition to adapt them best to their function. For example, the muscle cell has an elongated spindle shape and contains relatively large amounts of the contractile protein actomyosin. The living cell and its components are in a dynamic state, undergoing constant physical as well as chemical changes during cellular activity. The cell is made up of a number of subunits, called *organelles*, that perform specific biochemical functions within the cell. Knowledge of the structure and functions of the cellular organelles has greatly expanded in recent years as a result of improved methodology, such as electron microscopy and more sensitive and specific histochemical techniques. *Gradient centrifugation* in solutions of controlled density (e.g., with sucrose) has permitted the isolation of cellular subunits (e.g., mitochondria, polysomes) in relatively pure form and thus has enabled detailed studies of their composition and biochemical characteristics to be performed.

CELL MEMBRANE

The typical cell membrane performs several vital functions: it holds the cell together mechanically; it permits, and in some instances even enhances, the absorption of essential nutrients into the cell while preventing the diffusion of needed metabolites; it excretes cellular waste products; it keeps out

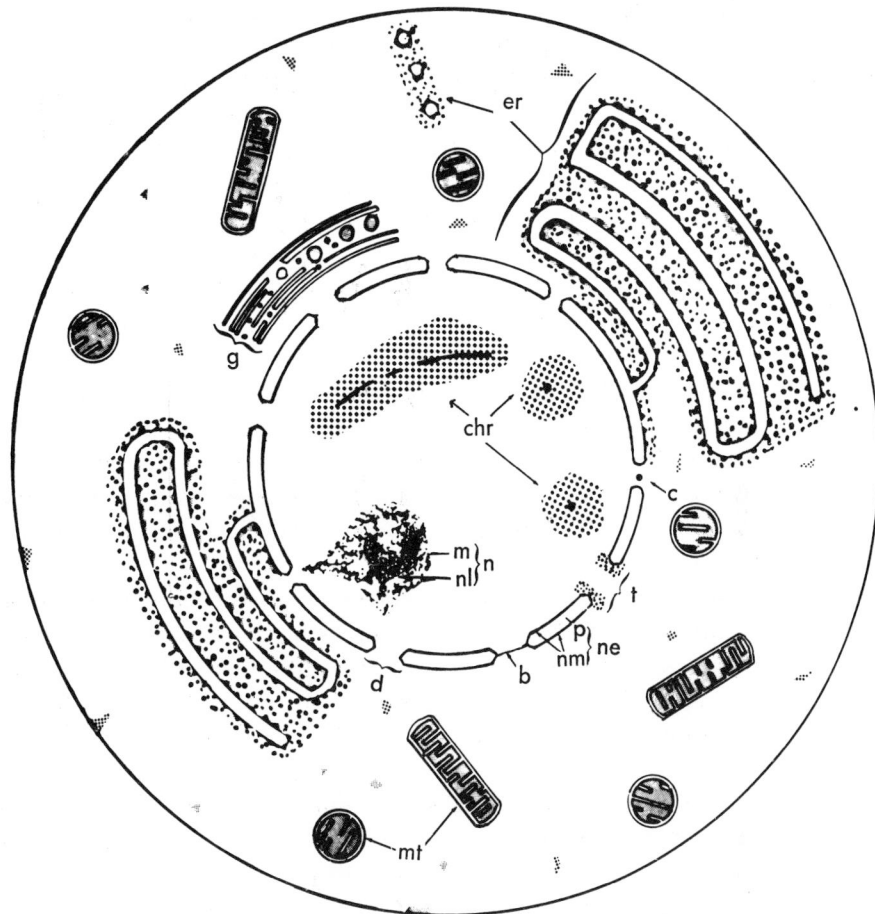

Fig. 2-1. Schematic representation of the structural components of a hypothetic cell as seen by means of the electron microscope. The cytoplasm contains the ergastoplasm, *er*, which is made of its two elements, the endoplasmic reticulum and its attached small particles, ribosomes, or microsomes. Near the nucleus are the Golgi apparatus, *g*, which are made up of closely packed and flattened cisternae and many small vesicles. Mitochondria, *mt*, seen in cross and longitudinal sections, are distributed throughout the cytosome. The nucleus is surrounded by its nuclear envelope, *ne*, which is made up of two membranes, *nm*, enclosing the intermembranous zone, *p*. At the places where the membranes unite, discontinuities, *d*, whose margins are sometimes evident as a band, *b*, are present. The discontinuities are associated with tubelike structures, *t*, and sometimes they are found to contain a central granule, *c*. The connection between the nuclear envelope and ergastoplasm is also illustrated. Within the nucleus, the nucleolus, *n*, is seen as being made up of two elements: a coiled nucleolonema, *nl*, and a finely granular matrix, *m*. Nucleolar material extends toward the discontinuities, which may be one of the mechanisms for nucleocytoplasmic exchange. The chromosomes, *chr*, each contain a linear density as their axis. (From Wischnitzer, S.: Int. Rev. Cytol. **10**:137, 1960.)

some toxic materials; and it binds certain cellular constituents, particularly enzymes, in a location apparently most advantageous for the performance of their specific biochemical functions. Obviously, a unique type of structure with a high degree of selectivity must be required to serve such manifold purposes as a support and a barrier.

Structure Chemical analyses of typical isolated cell membranes show that they are composed primarily of lipid (about 40%) and protein (about 60%) and that they are rich in certain enzymes, depending on the nature of the cell itself. Electron microscopy has revealed that the typical cell membrane is about 75 Å thick and is multilayered, as previously proposed by Danielli, Robertson, and others. The outer and inner layers are protein in nature and surround an inner double lipid layer, mainly phospholipid. The lipid layers are oriented with the fatty acid chains (hydrophobic) pointing toward the center and the polar end groups (hydrophilic) pointing out, with a layer of protein covering the polar ends. The protein and lipid layers are each about 25 Å thick. There is a central separating fluid space also of approximately 25 Å. At intervals, the protein-lipid layers are discontinuous, leaving "polar pores" about 8 Å in diameter. These apparently permit the free passage of water and potassium ions, but not sodium ions, and of some small molecules less than 8 Å in diameter.

Recent renewed interest, however, in the chemical composition of cell membranes, with extensive investigations using modern sophisticated chemical and physical techniques, has resulted in significant changes in concepts of membrane structure.[1] Currently, the importance of protein in membrane structure and function is emphasized, rather than of lipid as in the older theory described above. The diversity, rather than the uniformity, of the chemical composition of membranes from different cells, has become evident. Membranes are now regarded as aggregates of controlled, directional processes. For example, the membranes of the mitochondrion catalyze the complex integrated processes of electron transport and oxidative phosphorylation. Likewise, the intricate events of photosynthesis are performed by isolatable membranes of the chloroplast. A number of metabolic activities, including protein synthesis (p. 18), are characteristic of the membranous network, the endoplasmic reticulum. Thus the intracellular membrane must no longer be regarded solely as a structure for delineating cytoplasmic spaces and as a barrier for free diffusion but rather as a specific locus of many major reactions of intermediary metabolism and macromolecular biosynthesis.

The same is true of the *plasma membrane* of the cell. It also incorporates a number of enzymes and is the site of many metabolic reactions. Also, *transport proteins*, whose function is the active transfer of specific metabolites into the cell, appear to be incorporated into the cell membrane. As will be discussed later, a number of transport proteins have been isolated from membranes and purified. A few have been prepared in crystalline form.

There is some indication that proteins are the first membrane components to be synthesized and that lipids are then added in specific arrangements dictated by the structure of the proteins. The resultant lipoproteins then interact with each other to form the membrane. The entire membrane is thus a mosaic of such subunits, which themselves may differ in composition and structure depending upon their functions. The lipid component is still very important, for it ensures relative impermeability of the membrane to solutes for which specific transport mechanisms do not exist.

Recent analytic data for a number of purified membranes support the foregoing concept of cell membrane structure. Significant differences in the protein and lipid components of membranes have been found. The proteins of cell membranes appear to vary in type and quantity in different kinds of cells. The purified membrane of the human erythrocyte, for example, has been reported as containing at least five different proteins, two of which are glycoproteins; these have been separated by electrophoresis and by microcolumn chromatography and have been studied extensively. The lipid components also vary considerably from one type of membrane to another. Lipids found in varying proportions include phosphatidylcholine, phosphatidylserine, phosphatidylethanolamine, several other phosphatidylglycerol derivatives, cerebrosides, sphingomyelins, plasmalogens, sulfolipids, and cholesterol. The fatty acids appear to be mainly saturated acids with 16 and 18 carbons, although some oleic acid is present in the myelin membrane. In further studies, using the classic "divide and conquer" biochemical approach, membranes have been dissociated into fragments that are then examined by infrared spectroscopy, optical rotatory dispersion, and circular dichroism. High-resolution x-ray diffraction analysis and electron microscopy, with its limitations imposed by the drastic procedures involved in tissue preparation

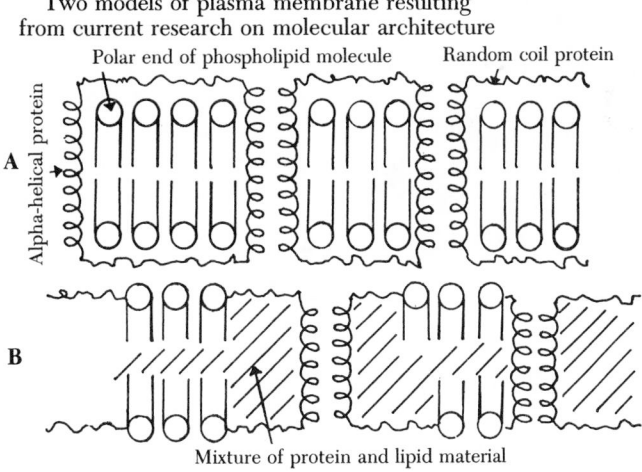

Fig. 2-2. Schematic representation of a typical cell membrane. **A** and **B** show protein in α-helix and random coil forms, with α-helical regions buried in hydrophobic environment of fatty acids. Both emphasize the lipoprotein nature of the membrane and its division into protein-coated globules, as opposed to the old theory of a continuous lipid bilayer to which protein is ionically bound. Neither model should be considered static in structure. The models may, in fact, be interchangeable. Protein is the fundamental determination of structure (lipid was under the old theory), and functional and structural proteins are one and the same. (From Korn, E. D., et al.: Chem. Eng. News **45**:60, 1967.)

and fixation, have also been used as a basis for a number of new membrane models. A schematic representation of one of these is shown in Fig. 2-1.

Present data indicate that the interactions between the lipids and proteins of a membrane are primarily hydrophilic in nature rather than ionic, as previously thought. Also, the α-helical sections of the membrane proteins are buried in the relatively hydrophobic internal region. This tends to orient the polar groups of both proteins and lipids at the aqueous interface, as shown in Fig. 2-2.

Thus current evidence does not support the older, classic, "paucimolecular unit" theory of membrane structure; rather, accumulating biochemical and biophysical data point to a major role of proteins in membrane structure as well as function. Furthermore, it now appears likely that membranes differ from one another to such an extent that they cannot be usefully described by *one* unifying model.

Function   As just stated, one of the characteristic features of the cell membrane is its *selective permeability,* by which it may accept or reject, retain or excrete substances. This is accomplished, in part at least, by *transport systems* incorporated in the membrane that serve as pumps. These may bring a metabolite from outside the cell into a higher concentration inside the cell or may force substances, e.g., sodium ions, out of the cell. In general, this is an energy-requiring process and is termed *active transport* to differentiate it from passive transport and facilitated diffusion, which do not require energy. *Passive transport* depends primarily on both diffusion and osmosis, probably through the alleged "pores" of the membrane. The molecular size, shape, charge, and solubility of the substance, as well as molecular concentration on the two sides of the membrane, are rate-limiting factors. *Facilitated diffusion,* on the other hand, requires the presence of a carrier but not energy. *Pinocytosis* is another possible method of transport into the cell. This process involves attachment of the substance to the cell membrane, invagination of the membrane engulfing the substance, and finally migration of the particle into the interior of the cell. One or perhaps all of these mechanisms may operate simultaneously.

The energy for active transport is usually provided by adenosine triphosphate (ATP) or other high-energy phosphate compounds. Apparently the purpose of ATP is to provide energy necessary for changing either the conformation or the chemical nature of the transport protein or that of the substance being transported. For example, it has been reported[2] that the transport of certain sugars by a bacterial transport protein entails the conversion of the protein to a phosphoprotein, in the presence of an enzyme and magnesium ions, and the phosphoprotein in turn converts the transported sugar into a 6-phosphate derivative. Any inhibitor or condition that limits the energy supply of the cell will correspondingly limit the active transport of the substance involved.

A considerable amount of recent work[3] indicates that a necessary feature of such active-transport systems, in addition to an energy supply, is a *transport protein,* as just mentioned, that is an integral part of the cell membrane. At the present time, at least eight different transport proteins have been pre-

Table 2-1. Properties of some membrane transport proteins*

| Source | Substance transported | Protein characteristic | | |
		Molecular weight ($\times 10^{-4}$)	Number of sites	Crystalline
Chick duodenum	Ca^{++}	2.8	1	No
Beef brain	Na^+, K^+	67	1	No
Salmonella typhosa	$SO_4^=$	3.2	1	Yes
Escherichia coli	β-Galactosides	3.1	—	No
Escherichia coli	Leucine	3.6	1	Yes
Escherichia coli	Leucine	3.6	1	Yes
Escherichia coli	Galactose	3.5	1	No
Escherichia coli	Phosphoenolpyruvate	0.9	1	No

* Adapted from Pardee, A. B.: Science **162**:632, 1968.

pared in chromatographically pure form from certain bacteria and from chick duodenum and beef brain, as shown in Table 2-1.

The transport proteins described in Table 2-1 appear to be traditional proteins in the sense of containing rather usual amounts of the 18 common amino acids. All thus far studied apparently have one active site, which accounts for the remarkable specificity of their transport ability—a specificity analogous to that of enzymes. Indeed, they are able to "recognize" such subtle features of the substrate being transported as the optical isomeric form. Like enzymes, too, the rate of transport is linearly dependent upon the concentration of the substrate up to the point of saturation of the active sites of the carrier protein. The two transport proteins for leucine, from *Escherichia coli*, are the same in the properties listed in the table but differ in other properties not included (dissociation constants, frictional coefficients).

There is evidence that, in many instances, the biosynthesis of transport proteins is under genetic control and can be induced or repressed. Interesting is the fact that the long–sought for mechanism of action of vitamin D (cholecalciferol) (p. 784) is apparently as an inducer of the synthesis of the transport protein for calcium ions in the mucosal cells of the intestine (p. 414).

The steps involved in active transport appear to include (1) "recognition" of the substance to be transported; (2) its translocation; (3) its release into the interior of the cell; and (4) recovery of the system to its original state. This sequence of events is shown diagrammatically in Fig. 2-3.

The above transport system is apparently reversible, depending on conditions such as concentration of the substance transported.

Allosteric transformation of the transport protein could be sufficient to account for the translocation of the protein-bound solute from one side of the membrane to the other. Inhibitors of the syntheses of RNA and protein, e.g., actinomycin-D and puromycin (p. 100), in general inhibit active transport

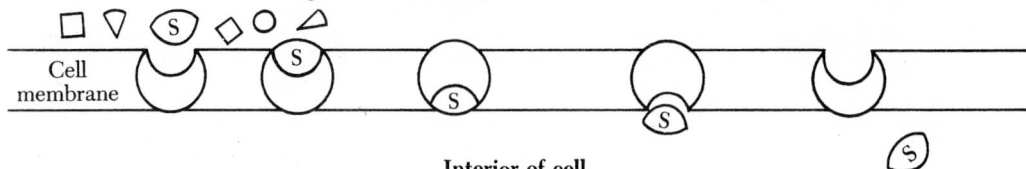

Fig. 2-3. Steps involved in active transport. S, Substance transported. (Adapted from Pardee, A. B.: Science **162**:632, 1968.)

by blocking the biosynthesis of transport proteins needed to replace those lost in the normal biologic turnover of proteins.

The problem of transport through the cell membrane is important in all cells but especially so in those of the gastrointestinal tract mucosal epithelial cell, the capillary endothelium, the renal tubule epithelium, and the blood-brain barrier.

It should be added at this point that in most bacteria an additional barrier to transport is the *cell wall*, which surrounds the cell membrane. The cell wall apparently excludes larger molecules by a "molecular sieve" action. Chemically it is entirely different from the cell membrane, as will be discussed in some detail later (p. 176).

THE NUCLEUS

The nucleus is the "information center" of the cell. It contains a comparatively large amount of nucleoprotein (p. 30) located in the chromosomes. The nucleoprotein consists of approximately 50% deoxyribonucleic acid (DNA) (p. 37) and 50% protein, primarily histones and protamines (p. 89). Some ribonucleic acid (RNA) is also found in the nucleus, as will be discussed in more detail later (p. 42). More than 95% of the nucleic acid of the cell is in the nucleus.

The nucleus has a relatively large size and high density and therefore is easily separated by centrifugation for chemical analysis. It is surrounded by a two-layered membrane that contains structured discontinuities, "nuclear pores." These pores permit the exchange of materials between the nucleus and the cytoplasm. The inner layer of the membrane encloses a deeply staining nuclear material, *chromatin*. Ribosomes (p. 18) are present on the outer layer of the membrane, which is in continuity with the endoplasmic reticulum, to be described later.

The DNA of the nucleus carries information in the sequence of its purine and pyrimidine bases (p. 31) for the synthesis of various proteins in the living organism. It also carries other hereditary information. Some of the proteins of the nucleus (histones) have been linked with the control of cellular specialization. Thus all cells of the body have the potential, as does the fertilized egg, of synthesizing all tissue proteins, but, of course, not all do so. *Histone repression* is one explanation for this fact. According to current concepts, genes (DNA, histones) are organized within chromosomes so that those having related functions and regulatory controls are grouped into clusters, called *operons*.[4] The structure and regulatory functions of the operon will be considered later (p. 105).

A wide variety of enzymes have been found in the nuclei of cells from various tissues. Among these are the enzymes concerned with the synthesis of the nucleic acids. Other chemical constituents of the nucleus include small amounts of free amino acids and lipids and the inorganic elements calcium and magnesium, with little potassium (most of the potassium is in the cytoplasm).

Nucleolus. The nucleolus is a small, round, dense body present within the nucleus. It is rich in RNA, containing 10% to 20% of the RNA of the entire cell. The RNA is chiefly *messenger RNA* (mRNA), which carries information from nuclear DNA to the protein-synthesizing particles, *polysomes*, in the cytoplasm (p. 97).

The nucleolus appears to serve as a storehouse for mRNA prior to the movement of the latter into the cytoplasm by way of the nuclear pores.

THE CYTOPLASM

The cytoplasm is the aqueous phase of the cell in which many particulate constituents (mitochondria, ribosomes, etc.) are suspended. It contains a wide variety of solutes, including proteins, RNA, metabolites for cellular utilization (e.g., glucose), waste products of cellular activity (urea, creatinine, uric acid), and a number of electrolytes. Many enzymes, including those of the glycolytic *Embden-Meyerhof pathway* (p. 186), are also found in the cytoplasm. *Microbodies*, some of which may consist of small particles of multienzyme complexes such as the *pyruvate oxidase system* (p. 203) and the complex involved in the biosynthesis of fatty acids, have been described in the cytoplasm.

Mitochondria. The mitochondria are the second largest organelle of the cell, measuring some 0.5μ to 1.0μ in diameter and from 1μ to 10μ in length. They are usually ellipsoidal in shape and are visible in the living cell; they may be stained with the dye Janus green. As shown in the idealized structure (Fig. 2-1), the mitochondrion has a double membrane structure, an outer and an inner. The inner membrane is convoluted to form shelves, termed *cristae*. A number of enzymes, especially those concerned with ATP generation by way of the *citric acid cycle* (p. 263) and the *electron-transport chain* (p. 249), are believed to be structural components of the inner membrane. The enzymes are apparently arranged in the precise order of their functional sequence to permit maximal efficiency.

Mitochondria are sometimes termed the "powerhouse" of the cell since ATP generation by oxidative phosphorylation (p. 252) is their prime function. As will be discussed in detail later (p. 254), the high-energy phosphate bond of ATP supplies the energy for such vital cellular functions as mechanical motility (flagellae, muscle contraction), active transport, and exergonic metabolic reactions — both anabolic (biosynthetic) and catabolic (degradative).

Mitochondria contain the remainder of the cell's DNA and therefore are independent; they apparently reproduce themselves. It has been suggested that mitochondria represent an early living form that entered a cell and established a symbiotic relationship. The hormone L-thyroxine (p. 477) is said to cause the swelling of the mitochondrion and thus increase its permeability.

Endoplasmic reticulum. By electron microscopy, the endoplasmic reticulum appears to be a system of interconnected tubules or canaliculi extending throughout the cell cytoplasm. It is continuous with the outer nuclear membrane. *Microsomes* are probably fragments of the endoplasmic reticulum formed during the homogenization of cells and isolation by differential centrifugation. There are two types of endoplasmic reticulum, smooth and rough. Smooth endoplasmic reticulum lacks ribosomes and appears to be involved in the biosynthesis of steroids, phospholipids, and complex polysaccharides. Rough endoplasmic reticulum, *ergastoplasm* (Fig. 2-1), is lined with a number of small (150 Å), spheric, electron-dense particles called *ribosomes* or, if in a cluster of several, *polysomes*. These are responsible for the rough appearance of this type of endoplasmic reticulum.

Ribosomes. Ribosomes consist of approximately 50% RNA and 50% protein. They are involved in protein synthesis in the cell and are sometimes called the "workbench" for protein synthesis, as will be described later (p. 96). Cells that produce a large amount of protein contain much rough endoplasmic reticulum.

Golgi apparatus. The Golgi apparatus are structures composed of flattened sacs with vesicles, probably continuous with the endoplasmic reticulum. They are organelles to which synthesized proteins are transported and temporarily stored (e.g., zymogen granules) before release from the cell. They are referred to as "packaging stations" and are particularly abundant in cells that produce much protein, especially enzymes.

Lysosomes. Lysosomes are the so-called "suicide bags" of the cell. They are membrane-bound organelles some 0.4μ to 0.8μ in diameter containing a variety of hydrolytic and degradative enzymes and having optimal acid pH values of about 5.0. Upon the death of the cell or its exposure to extreme environmental conditions, the membrane of the lysosome disintegrates, releasing its contents, which cause the digestion or *autolysis* of the cell constituents.

· · ·

Thus, from the standpoint of biochemical morphology, the cell represents a remarkably organized and efficient structural unit of living matter well adapted for its specific functions. Since its major chemical constituents include the various nucleic acids, proteins, carbohydrates, lipids, inorganic substances, and essential organic compounds (e.g., the vitamins and hormones), the subject of biochemistry properly must deal with the chemistry of these materials. Also, since various metabolic processes, both biosynthetic and degradative, are continually taking place in the cell, many of the following pages will be devoted to a consideration of the biochemical mechanisms involved. The various enzymes and cofactors that make metabolic reactions possible at the mild environmental conditions existing in living matter will be discussed. Likewise, the ways in which the cell derives energy, *bioenergetics,* for various cellular processes merits a full chapter. The biochemical mode of action of the hormones and the vitamins also will be considered in some detail, as acid-base, water, and electrolyte balance, and, finally, the biochemistry of specialized tissues.

References

GENERAL

Albert, R. W.: Biochemical aspects of active transport, Ann. Rev. Biochem. **36**:727, 1967.

Brachet, J.: Biochemical cytology, New York, 1957, Academic Press, Inc.

Brachet, J., and Mirsky, A. E., editors: The cell, biochemistry, physiology, morphology, New York, 1959–1961, Academic Press, Inc.

Dalton, A. J., and Haguenau, F., editors: Ultrastructure in biological systems, vols. 3, 4, New York, 1968, Academic Press, Inc.

Gran, F. C., editor: Structure and function of the endoplasmic reticulum in animal cells, New York, 1968, Academic Press, Inc.

Green, D. E., and Goldberger, R. F.: Molecular insights into the living process, New York, 1967, Academic Press, Inc.

Gross, P. R.: Biochemistry of differentiation, Ann. Rev. Biochem. **37**:631, 1968.

Kennedy, E. P.: Recent progress in the biochemistry of membranes, Proc. 7th Int. Congr. Biochem. **30**:51, 1968.

Korn, E. D.: Cell membranes: structure and synthesis, Ann. Rev. Biochem. **38**:263, 1969.

Lehninger, A.: The mitochondrion, New York, 1964, W. A. Benjamin, Inc.

Martin, H. H.: Biochemistry of bacterial cell walls, Ann. Rev. Biochem. **35**:457, 1966.

Palade, G. E.: The organization of living matter, Proc. Nat. Acad. Sci. **52**:613, 1964.

Porter, K. B., and Bonneville, M. A.: Introduction to the fine structure of cells and tissues, Philadelphia, 1964, Lea & Febiger.

Rich, A., and Davidson, N., editors: Structural chemistry and molecular biology, San Francisco, 1968, W. H. Freeman & Co., Publishers.

Rothfield, L., and Finkelstein, A.: Membrane biochemistry, Ann. Rev. Biochem. **37**:463, 1968.

Slater, E. C., Kaninga, Z., and Wojtezak, A., editors: Biochemistry of mitochondria, New York, 1967, Academic Press, Inc.

Stein, W. D.: The movement of molecules across cell membranes, New York, 1967, Academic Press, Inc.

Threadgold, L. T.: The ultrastructure of the animal cell, New York, 1968, Pergamon Press, Inc.

SPECIAL

1. Korn, E. D.: Science **153**:1491, 1966; J. Gen. Physiol. **52**:8257, 1968; Fed. Proc. Sympos. **28**:6, 1969.
2. Roseman, S., et al.: Proc. Nat. Acad. Sci. **58**:1963, 1967.
3. Pardee, A. B.: Science **162**:632, 1968.
4. Jacob, F., and Monod, J.: J. Molec. Biol. **3**:318, 1966.

CHAPTER 3

METABOLISM—AN OVERVIEW

DEFINITIONS

Metabolism in the classic sense is the "sum of the physical and chemical processes by which living matter is produced and maintained." The word *metabolism* itself is derived from the Greek, meaning "a turning about." Thus metabolism includes both the physical and the chemical aspects of life processes. For many years there was a tendency to distinguish between the two. Physical aspects were considered to be concerned more with energy production, "energy metabolism," and the degradation of substances in the organism, termed *catabolism* (from the Greek, "a tearing down"). Chemical aspects were believed to apply primarily to chemical reactions involved in the *anabolism* (Greek, "a building up") of body constituents. The latter process also has been termed "intermediary metabolism." However, with the tremendous increase in knowledge in this area of biochemistry in the past two decades, it has become obvious that no such arbitrary distinction can be made. Energy may be either required or produced in many metabolic reactions, both catabolic and anabolic. Thus, any distinction today between *intermediary* metabolism and *energy* metabolism is made primarily for reasons of convenience or of organization.

Since metabolism is concerned with the physicochemical reactions of life processes, a knowledge of the chemistry of the compounds participating in metabolic reactions, so-called "metabolism," is essential. Therefore in this book a discussion of the chemistry of the principal groups of metabolic reactants, carbohydrates, lipids, proteins, amino acids, will immediately precede consideration of their metabolism. Also, since these substances are supplied to the organism as complex macromolecules in foods, their digestion, absorption, and mechanism of transport to cells as nutrients for *intermediary metabolism* will be discussed. The latter will include not only the steps in the biosynthesis of body constituents from the various nutrients but also their degradation and final disposal as excretory waste products.

SPECIFIC ENZYMES AND COFACTORS REQUIRED

Nearly all metabolic reactions take place at extremely rapid rates. This is possible at the rather mild conditions of temperature, pH, and ion concentrations in living matter through catalysis by specific enzymes, frequently with the participation of essential coenzymes or cofactors. Their roles will be included, of course, in the discussion of each reaction. Today some 600 or more enzymes have been characterized in living matter and many have been prepared in crystalline form (Chapter 7). All are proteins. The primary, secondary, and tertiary structures for some are known and the amino acid sequence and essential chemical groups of the *active site* of a few have been established. This is an area of intensive research, with a resulting expansion of knowledge. For example, it is known today that a number of hereditary metabolic diseases (e.g., phenylketonuria [PKU], p. 375) are the result of deficiency of an enzyme required for a specific step in a metabolic reaction.

SEQUENCE OF METABOLIC REACTIONS

Modern biochemical research into metabolic processes has established the fact that the chemical reactions involved are not random and haphazard but occur in an orderly, logical, stepwise sequence. Indeed, the sequence apparently is that dictated by physical laws of the expenditure of minimal energy. Pertinent in this connection is the fact that the steps and sequence apparently used in the formation of porphyrins (p. 608) in the prebiotic era on earth several billion years ago were the same as those used by living organisms today. Thus, physical laws appear to dictate the sequence of individual metabolic reactions and follow the pattern most economical of energy expenditure from the initial step to the final product.

METABOLIC PATHWAYS

Since metabolic processes take place in a series of progressive, stepwise individual reactions, they can be described conveniently in the form of metabolic pathways as shown in Fig. 3-1. These may be outlined schematically, with only the chemical names of the intermediate reactants being shown, or they may be illustrated more completely, with the structures of the metabolites involved, the mechanisms of the reactions, and the roles of the specific enzymes and cofactors required all being delineated. Numerous examples of metabolic pathways will be presented in the ensuing pages.

Precursors   Another general parameter in anabolic, biosynthetic pathways in living organisms is the fact that the starting material, or precursor, used is invariably some rather simple, plentiful substance. For example, the biosynthesis of sterols (cholesterol) in the animal organism starts with acetic acid, as its

Precursor	Intermediates	Product

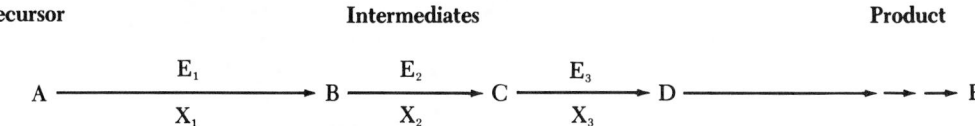

Fig. 3-1. Schematic representation of a typical metabolic pathway, showing the initial starting substance or precursor, A, intermediate compounds formed, B, C, and D, and the final product, P. The specific enzymes required for each step are E_1, E_2, and E_3. Cofactors, *if required*, are X_1, X_2, and X_3.

coenzyme-A derivative, acetyl-CoA. Acetyl-CoA is abundant since it is an end product in the metabolism of both carbohydrate (glucose) oxidation (p. 196) and fatty acid oxidation (p. 305). Further, the biosynthetic pathway of cholesterol in animal tissues entails some 28 or more progressive individual reactions, each catalyzed by a specific enzyme and cofactor (p. 326). The biosynthesis of heme (p. 608) in some nine or 10 separate steps from glycine, succinyl-CoA, and iron is another excellent example.

Reversibility of metabolic sequences   For a metabolic sequence to be effective in supplying a product, it must be essentially nonreversible. Reversibility usually occurs at one or sometimes more steps. However, it may be accomplished by a separate reaction and its corresponding enzyme at this step, as shown in Fig. 3-2. Important examples of the principle of reversibility are glycolysis (p. 205) and the synthesis and degradation of liver glycogen from or to glucose (p. 189). There is usually a large loss of free energy at an essentially irreversible step, which, of course, may account for the difficult reversibility of the reaction.

Branched metabolic sequences   Some metabolic sequences may have a common pathway for several steps then branch into two or more separate pathways (see Fig. 3-3). This is true, as will be seen later, in carbohydrate metabolism, in which glucose-6-phosphate derived from free glucose serves as a starting point for the biosynthesis of glycogen (p. 189), the *Embden-Meyerhof* pathway (p. 196), and the *pentose phosphate* pathway (p. 208). The first step after such a branch point is some-

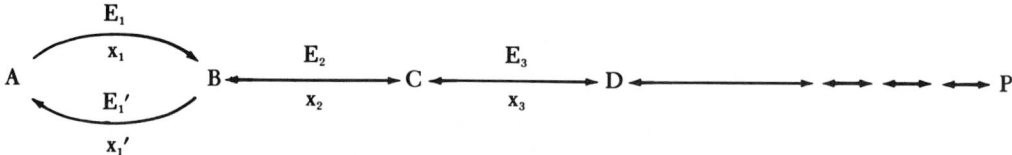

Fig. 3-2. Schematic representation of a typical nonreversible metabolic pathway, showing the point of irreversibility, A to B. For reversal to occur, different enzymes, E_1 and E_1', and usually different cofactors, x_1 and x_1', are required for the forward and backward reactions, respectively.

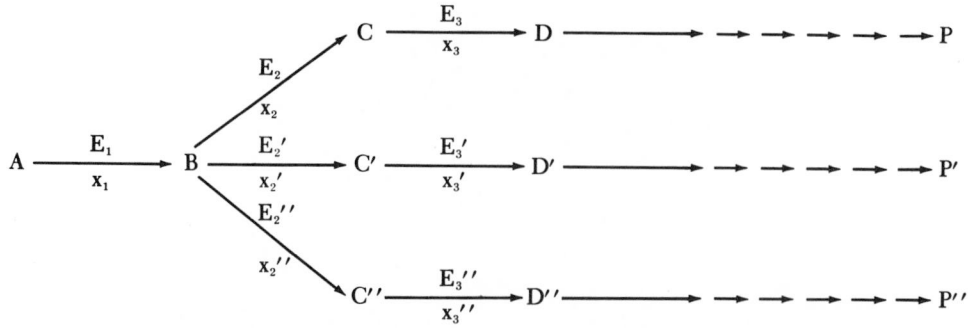

Fig. 3-3. Schematic representation of a branched metabolic pathway, using B as a common starting point. Deficiency of an enzyme, E_2, E_3, etc., or a cofactor x_2, x_3, etc., required for any of the pathways shown may result in a diversion of B into one or both of the other pathways. PKU is a classic example (see text).

times termed a *committed step* since its metabolite and succeeding ones have no role in metabolism other than the formation of the specific product of that pathway. Usually this step involves a large loss of free energy and hence is essentially irreversible, as noted above. Also, metabolic control is usually exerted at this point in the interest of economy of energy, as is discussed below.

Branched metabolic pathways are important in yet another way. If there is a block of one branch, e.g., due to a hereditary deficiency of an enzyme, the metabolism of the initial metabolite will be diverted into one or more of the other "alternate" pathways at the branch point. *PKU* is an example of this (p. 375). The diversion of phenylalanine into other pathways occurs, and there is formation of excessive amounts of phenylpyruvic acid and related metabolites. These are toxic in the increased amounts and apparently are responsible for some of the abnormalities seen in affected children.

Balance between metabolic pathways It has been estimated that a simple unicellular organism, e.g., a bacterium, may contain as many as 2000 or 3000 different proteins and as many as 1000 or more other different organic compounds. In a multicellular organism such as man, these figures undoubtedly are considerably greater. As well as indicating the numeric complexity of cellular metabolism, such figures emphasize the need for adequate control mechanisms for *regulating* metabolic pathways so that there is neither a lack nor an excess of any essential product. An excess as well as a deficiency of a metabolic product or even of its intermediate metabolites can be injurious to the cell. Thus, in the normal healthy individual, regulatory mechanisms maintain a balance between the various anabolic and catabolic pathways. This regulation occurs during most of man's adult life, and he may be said to be in a metabolic "steady state," as evidenced grossly by a rather constant body weight and body composition. In the infant and growing child, however, anabolic processes predominate, and weight gain, growth, and change in body composition result. In old age, the reverse is frequently true and catabolic processes with weight loss predominate. The same may be true in starvation and in many diseases in which aberrations in metabolism due to infection or other pathologic processes occur.

Regulation of metabolic pathways Metabolic pathways must be regulated so that the amount of the product formed will meet the needs of the organism and neither an excess nor a deficiency of the product will exist. The regulation of metabolic pathways is accomplished by several control mechanisms (Fig. 3-4). These may act di-

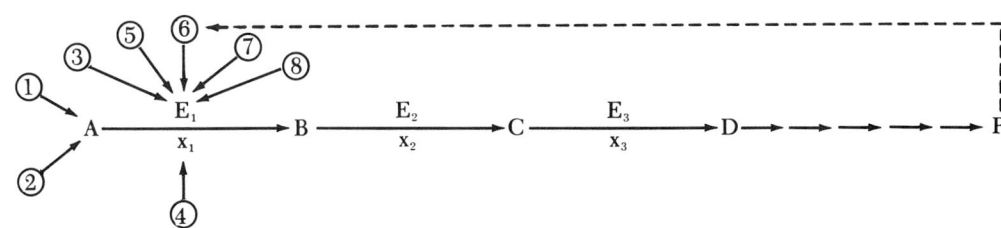

Fig. 3-4. Regulation of metabolic pathways. Numbers refer to mechanisms of regulation described in text.

rectly, at a local cellular or subcellular level, or indirectly, at an extracellular level, as will be shown.

1. Nutrient supply (precursor). Metabolic pathways tend to adapt quantitatively to the supply of a nutrient. This usually entails an increase (or decrease) in the amount of one or more enzymes involved in the metabolic pathway. An example is the presence of relatively large amounts of the milk-coagulating enzyme, rennin, in the gastric mucosa and gastric secretion of young, nursing animals and its virtual absence in the adult. A lack of appropriate metabolizing enzymes in the absence of its substrate may occur also. An example of this is the low tolerance of certain Asiatic populations to milk, due primarily to a lack of the enzyme lactase in their intestinal secretions (see also p. 183).

2. Nutrient transport. The nutrient or substrate supply into a cell can be regulated by controlling the transport of the nutrient across the cell membrane. One of the important ways that insulin regulates carbohydrate metabolism is by facilitating the transport of glucose into cells (p. 230).

3. Enzyme level or activity. The amount of enzyme available for a metabolic reaction may be controlled genetically by induction or repression (p. 104) (and is also involved in nutrient supply and transport mentioned above); or an enzyme's activity may be affected at the cellular level by its own inherent capacity for interconversion to inactive or active forms (p. 112), by allosteric effects (allosteric effectors or modifiers, which alter the conformation of the enzyme or its subunit structure, p. 129), or by inhibitors. The synthesis of a number of enzymes is either induced or repressed by certain specific hormones. For example, the adrenoglucocorticoid hormones are inducers for the formation of the gluconeogenic enzymes (p. 466), whereas insulin apparently serves as a repressor for the synthesis of these same enzymes but an inducer for the formation of key glycolytic enzymes (p. 231). Thyroxine apparently acts as an inducer for the synthesis of mitochondrial α-glycerophosphate dehydrogenase (p. 477).

An example of the regulatory control of an allosteric effector is the action of adenosine monophosphate (AMP) on phosphofructokinase in relieving the inhibition by ATP and citrate (p. 199). As the level of AMP increases due to an increased utilization of ATP, glycolysis is increased, with a resulting increase in ATP formation. Then, when the level of ATP satisfies cellular requirements, inhibition of glycolysis by ATP again occurs, shutting off further ATP formation. Glucose may then be diverted into glycogen formation or other pathways (Chapter 9).

4. Cofactor availability. Those steps in metabolic pathways requiring a cofactor as well as a specific enzyme will be affected by the amount of the cofactor available. An example is the relatively large requirement for nicotinamide adenine dinucleotide (NAD^+) as a cofactor for the metabolism of ethanol (p. 206). Thus, when significant amounts of alcohol are being metabolized, the amount of NAD^+ available may become the rate-limiting factor in its utilization. Also, less NAD^+ may then be available for other metabolic pathways also requiring NAD^+ as a cofactor. These pathways then may become partially or even completely blocked. However, metabolic reactions requiring $NADH_2$ (formed from NAD^+ during alcohol oxidation) as a cofactor may be stimulated, e.g., lactate formation from pyruvate (p. 203).

5. Product need. A demand for the product of a metabolic pathway may act as stimulation for the increased output of that product. This could conceivably result directly, from a *mass action* effect, or indirectly, by way of other regulatory mechanisms, e.g., hormonal or neural control. Stimulation of hepatic glycogenolysis by a low blood sugar level (p. 194) is a typical example, as is stimulation of the biosynthesis of hemoglobin in anemias by the hormone erythropoietin (p. 507).

6. Product inhibition. The product of a metabolic pathway may serve to inhibit further output of the product by a process known as *feedback inhibition*. Usually the sufficient supply of the product acts as a repressor to "shut off" synthesis of the enzyme when a sufficient amount of the product is formed. Normally the product's point of action is on the *first* enzyme of its particular pathway. This effect is, of course, advantageous from the standpoint of economy of energy, as stated previously. Also the accumulation of later metabolites in the sequence, which may be deleterious to the cell, is prevented. This could occur if a later enzyme in the sequence were the one repressed. Product inhibition appears to be a major mechanism for the regulation of metabolic pathways. A classic example is the feedback inhibition of porphyrin-heme biosynthesis by the end product, heme. The biosynthesis of the first enzyme in the metabolic sequence, δ-aminolevulinic acid synthetase, is repressed.

7. Endocrine control. Hormonal control of metabolic sequence is accomplished in several ways. Mentioned above are the regulation of transport through the cell membrane (e.g., insulin) and enzyme induction or repression. Other mechanisms include conversion of an inactive form of the enzyme to an active form, e.g., conversion of phosphorylase-b to active phosphorylase-a in hepatic glycogenolysis by epinephrine and glucagon via *cyclic-AMP* (p. 195).

8. Neural control. Effects of nerve stimulation on metabolic pathways are probably indirect by way of hormonal or other more direct regulatory mechanisms. For example, the effect of such psychologic factors as fright or anger on carbohydrate metabolism, specifically in increasing the blood sugar level, apparently results from an increased secretion of epinephrine, which, in turn, accelerates glycogenolysis by the mechanism cited under "Product Need" above. Neural effects by way of an increased secretion of *neurohormones* (p. 488) are still another indirect means of affecting metabolic pathways.

● ● ●

Thus it is evident that, while the above eight factors are involved in the regulation of metabolic pathways, the more fundamental control of these mechanisms is by way of three basic routes: (1) the amount of available precursor and cofactor; (2) the level and activity of enzymes involved as determined by induction, repression, or the action of various effectors or inhibitors; and (3) the level of the product of the pathway.

As stated earlier, a number of hereditary metabolic diseases are due to a lack of some specific enzyme in a vital metabolic pathway. PKU was cited as a classic example. A few diseases, e.g., acute intermittent porphyria (p. 611), apparently result from excessive formation (impaired regulation?) of a key enzyme in a metabolic sequence. Conceivably, hereditary metabolic disease could also result from the formation of a defective enzyme, perhaps having an abnormal amino acid sequence at its active site, due to genetic mutation, and hence being inactive. Reports of such abnormal enzymes have indeed appeared in the literature. Also, certain *isozymes* (p. 130) may be responsible for aberrations in metabolic pathways. For example, the presence of a hexokinase in place of glucokinase in certain tumor tissues may be responsible for the excessive glycolytic characteristic of this tissue. The isozyme may not be responsive to the same metabolic controls as glucokinase, hence the uncontrolled glycolysis with excessive lactic acid production (p. 570).

METHODS OF STUDY

The foregoing summary highlights the tremendous increase in understanding metabolic pathways and their regulation during recent years. These advances have been made possible, as has progress in all of biochemistry, by the development and application of superb, sophisticated methods of study. Improved techniques and equipment have made possible the graduation from early studies almost exclusively on blood, tissue, and excreta of whole intact animals to investigations into isolated organs, tissue slices and homogenates, intact cells, and indeed ultimately into isolated cellular organelles, cell-free extracts, and pure enzyme-metabolite solutions. The improved methodology employed includes chromatography—paper, column, and liquid-gas—the current availability of numerous isotopically labeled metabolites whose fate may be traced through suspected pathways, and more sensitive and accurate spectrophotometric and fluorometric methods for analysis. Likewise, as will be discussed briefly in Appendix B, newer sophisticated techniques such as scanning electron microscopy, x-ray analysis, optical rotatory dispersion, mass spectrometry, nuclear magnetic resonance, electron spin resonance, and circular dichroism, to mention only a few, are adding depth to the capabilities of the biochemist in determining and understanding heretofore unknown facets of cellular metabolism.

References

See lists at ends of Chapter 1 and Chapter 2.

BIOCHEMICAL GENETICS

Role of nucleic acids and proteins

CHAPTER 4

STRUCTURE AND BIOSYNTHESIS OF NUCLEIC ACIDS

Cellular metabolism comprises all the physical and chemical processes by which protoplasm is produced and maintained, as stated in the preceding chapter. It includes *anabolism*, the biosynthetic processes, and *catabolism*, the degradative processes. Both anabolism and catabolism require the presence of numerous organic catalysts or *enzymes*, which are produced by the living cell. The living cell is, therefore, a *multiple-enzyme system*, and the life process can be understood as a dynamic organization of enzymes. The interrelationship of enzymes, their substrates, and their products is fundamental to the biochemical control mechanisms that regulate cellular metabolism. Metabolic processes are often sequences of numerous enzyme-catalyzed steps or pathways. In such pathways, the first enzyme acts on the metabolite to produce a product, which in turn becomes the substrate for the second enzyme, and so on until an ultimate product evolves. A deficiency of a single enzyme in such a pathway can have a profound effect on the overall process, sometimes leading to the accumulation of undesired intermediary stages and an insufficient production of the final product. Many hereditary diseases are now known to be caused by an inability to produce a specific enzyme.

Since enzymes are protein in nature (Chapter 5), an understanding of cellular mechanisms should be sought at the level of the control of protein biosynthesis. It is thought that, for the cell to know which enzymes and how much of a given enzyme system is to be produced in response to a metabolic need or hormonal stimulus (Chapter 6), the essential information for protein synthesis must be selectively available on demand. According to our present knowledge, the location of this information-retrieval center is the genetic material, or chromosomes, of the cell nucleus.

With the recognition that *genetic information* is retained in the cell nucleus as the structure of chromosomal components (DNA), genetics became a molecular science. It is thought that all the information needed to produce a complete human being, comprising approximately 10^{13} individual cells, is present in the original fertilized or diploid egg. The amount of information that must be present staggers the imagination.

The process of human embryonic development is described in terms of morphologic stages in which the initial step is the duplication of a single cell. To produce an identical daughter cell presupposes the exact *replication* of the genetic information. This means that the composition of chromosomal material must be copied exactly so that all genetic information in the offspring will be identical. Errors in the replicative process would lead to genetic defects and possibly to disease.

Replication of DNA can now be understood in molecular terms involving the so-called Watson and Crick model and the principle of *base complementarity*. It is possible to visualize how the structure of DNA and consequently the genetic information can be duplicated exactly. This model yields an insight into the process of mutation and the concept of molecular disease.

NUCLEOPROTEINS

Treatment of tissues rich in nuclei (thymus gland, pus cells, salmon sperm) with strong neutral salt solutions (1M NaCl) leads to an extraction of the characteristic chromosomal component called *nucleoproteins*. Nucleoproteins are composed of a protein and a nonprotein moiety or *nucleic acid*. The protein is essentially cationic while the nucleic acid is anionic in character so that the binding force between these is the result of electrostatic attraction.

Proteins The cationic proteins are large–molecular weight polymers composed of fundamental subunits, the amino acids (see Chapter 5). Two proteins are frequently found in nucleoproteins, i.e., the *protamines* (certain fish sperm) and the *histones* of somatic cells. The molecular weight of histones is approximately 30,000. Many protein subunits combine with a nucleic acid to yield a final complex or nucleoprotein having molecular weights in the millions.

The histones probably function to hold the nucleic acids in the tightly wound configuration of the chromosome. It has been estimated that the nucleic acid of a chromosome, if stretched, would be 15 cm. long. Another function of histones may be in blocking or selecting the specific genetic messages for expression. Thus, this selectivity of genetic expression may be involved in the process of differentiation. It is likely that each of the 10^{13} cells of the human body possesses the same genetic machinery as the original diploid egg; yet, remarkably, only the β-cells of the pancreatic islets of Langerhans synthesize insulin. Muscle cells, nerve cells, connective tissue fibroblasts, leukocytes, etc. all must possess the same genetic information for producing insulin. However, the essential messages are locked in a repressed form possibly blocked by the histones.

Nucleic acids Nucleic acids are polyanionic molecules of high molecular weight. These polymers are composed of a sequence of subunits or *nucleotides* so that the whole is usually termed a *polynucleotide*.

The nucleic acids are of two main varieties, *ribonucleic* (RNA) and *deoxyribonucleic* (DNA). Although it was previously thought that the former occurred only in plants and the latter only in animals, this is known to be

Table 4-1. Hydrolytic products of RNA and DNA

	Ribonucleic acid		Deoxyribonucleic acid
Acid	Phosphoric acid		Phosphoric acid
Sugar	D-Ribose		D-2-Deoxyribose
Bases	Adenine	Purines	Adenine
	Guanine	|	Guanine
	Cytosine	Pyrimidines	Cytosine
	Uracil		Thymine

incorrect. DNA is found primarily in the chromatin of the cell nucleus, whereas 90% of RNA is present in the cell cytoplasm and 10% in the nucleolus. Upon total hydrolysis the two nucleic acids yield the constituents shown in Table 4-1.

The two classes of nucleic acids are distinguished primarily on the basis of the five-carbon atom sugar or *pentose* present. The structural differences of the two pentoses are apparent from the diagrams below.

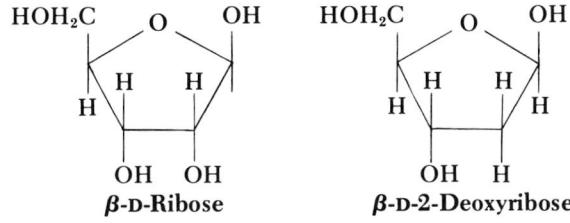

β-D-Ribose   *β*-D-2-Deoxyribose

In these structural formulas it should be noted that D-ribose is considered the parent sugar while D-2-deoxyribose is a derivative in which the hydroxyl group on carbon-2 has been replaced by hydrogen. A second feature is that the carbon-1 atom is asymmetric as a result of the five-membered furanose ring structure (Chapter 8). Consequently, the carbon-1 hydroxyl group may exist in either a right- or a left-handed orientation, i.e., α or β. The structural formulas shown above are for β-D-ribose and β-D-2-deoxyribose. The importance of this distinction to nucleic acid structure will become evident shortly.

Purines   Two general kinds of bases are found in all nucleic acids. One type is a derivative of the parent compound purine. Principal examples are *guanine* and *adenine*.

It may be noted that hydrogen atoms are omitted from several carbon atoms (nos. 2 and 8) in the structure of adenine and no. 8 in the structure of guanine. However, their presence is assumed, to complete the fourth valency of the carbon atom involved. This common practice will be followed throughout the text.

31

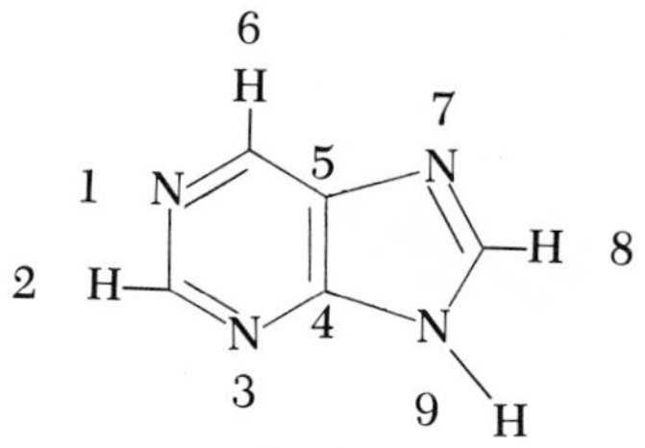

Purine

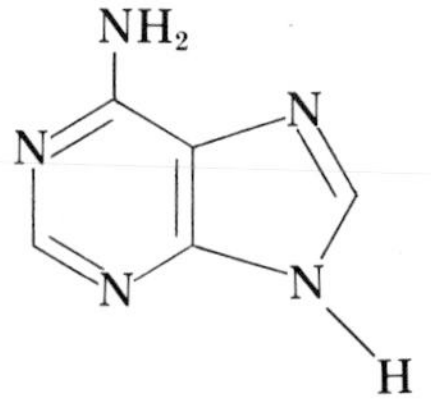

Adenine
(6-aminopurine)

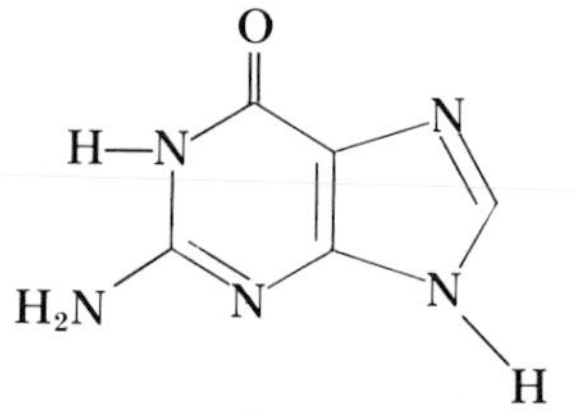

Guanine
(2-amino-6-oxypurine)

The oxypurines exist in enol-keto (lactim-lactam) forms that are in equilibrium, as shown below for xanthine. The enol (lactim) form for *uric acid* is weakly acidic; it forms mono- and disodium or potassium salts.

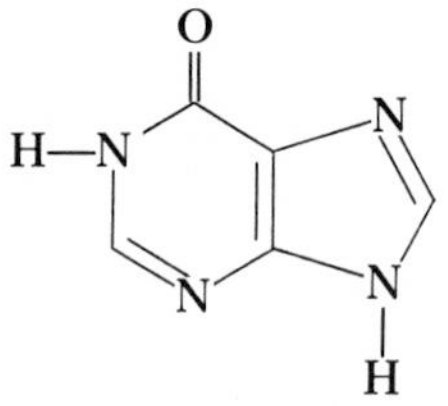

Hypoxanthine
(6-oxypurine)

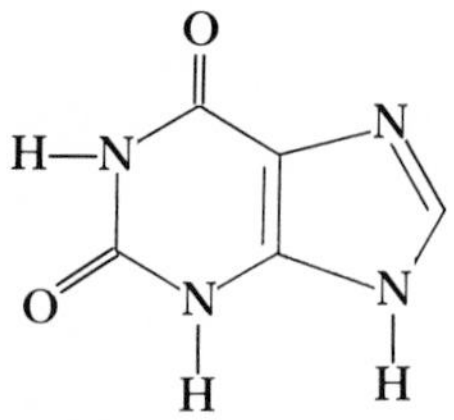

Xanthine
(keto)

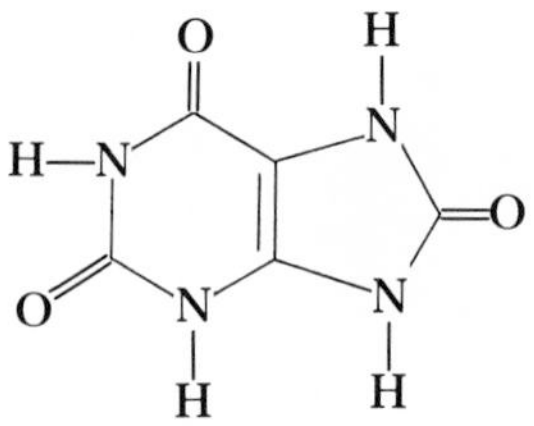

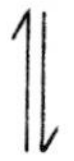

Uric acid
(2,6,8-trioxypurine)

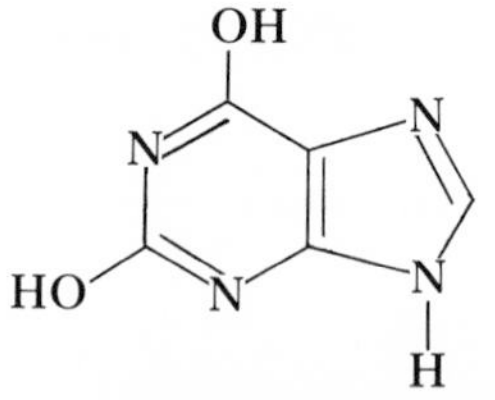

Xanthine (enol)
(2,6-dioxypurine)

Pyrimidines   The second class of bases found in all nucleic acids is derived from the parent compound pyrimidine. Principal examples are *cytosine, uracil,* and *thymine.*

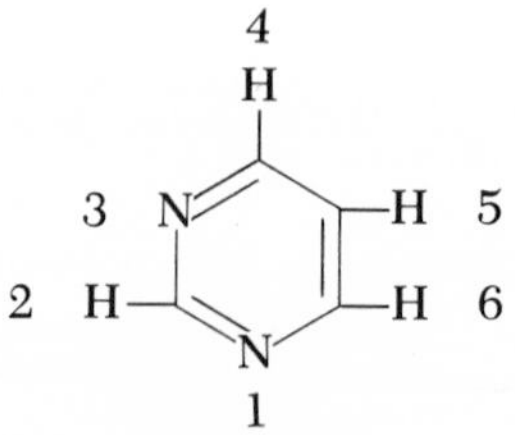

Pyrimidine

OH

Uracil
(lactim or enol form)

HO

NH₂

O

O

Cytosine
(2-oxy-4-aminopyrimidine)

Uracil
(lactam or keto form)
(2,4-dioxypyrimidine)

Thymine
(2,4-dioxy-5-methylpyrimidine)

The pyrimidines uracil and thymine, which differ only by a methyl group, also serve to distinguish DNA (thymine) from RNA (uracil). As do the purines, the pyrimidines exhibit tautomerism (above) and exist in lactim-lactam forms. At physiologic pH the lactam or keto form predominates.

Adenine, guanine, cytosine, thymine, and uracil are the purines and pyrimidines most prevalent in DNA and RNA. There are, however, a number of important exceptions that deserve mention. The DNA of bacteriophage contains a hydroxymethylcytosine instead of cytosine. Transfer RNA (tRNA, p. 43) is characterized by its content of methylated purines and pyrimidines as well as other derivatives. A number of examples follow:

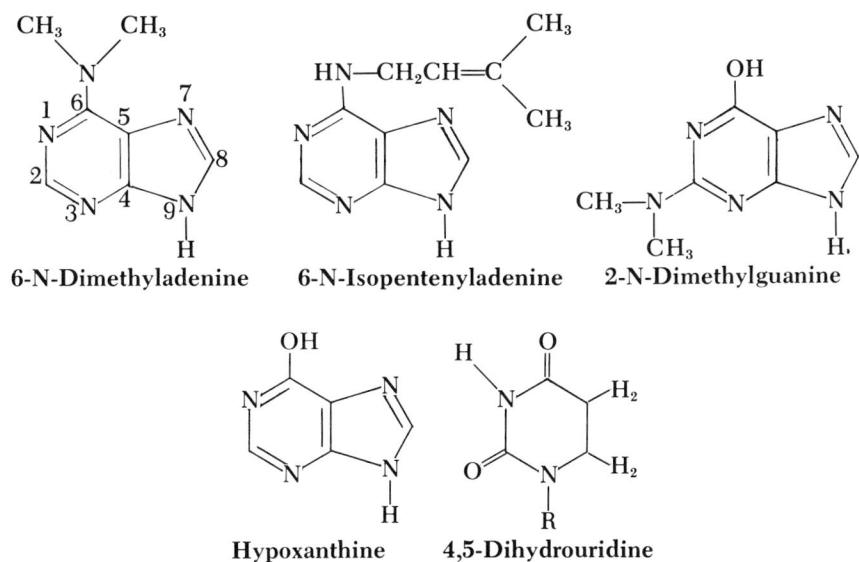

6-N-Dimethyladenine   **6-N-Isopentenyladenine**   **2-N-Dimethylguanine**

Hypoxanthine   **4,5-Dihydrouridine**

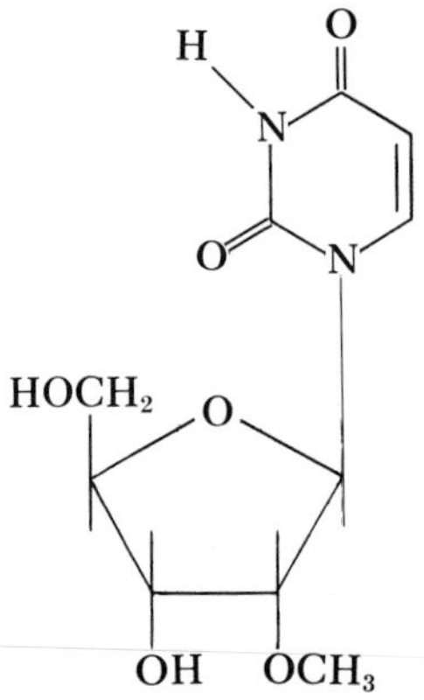

2'-O-Methyluridine 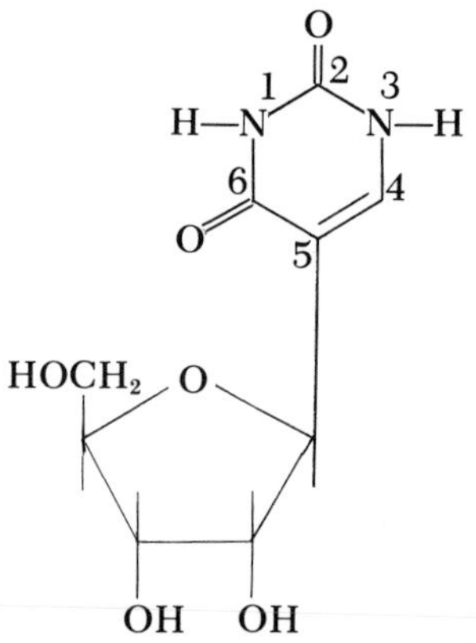   Pseudouridine 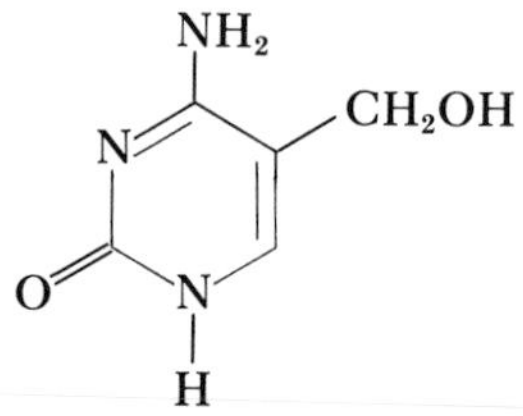   5-Hydroxymethylcytosine

Nucleosides   The purine and pyrimidine bases are attached to the appropriate pentose sugar by *glycosidic bonds* involving carbon-1 of the sugar:

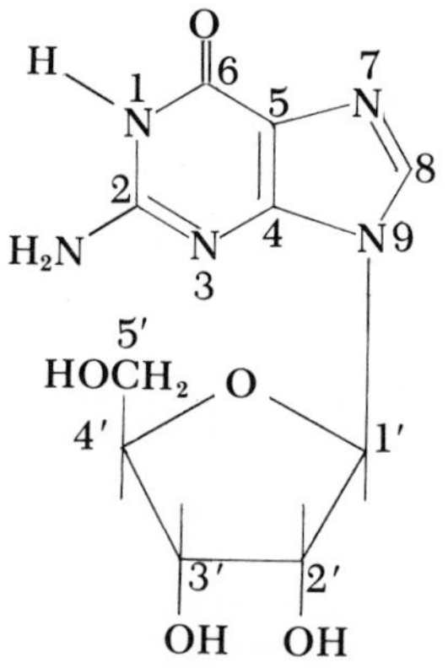

Guanosine

In these glycosidic bonds a molecule of water is eliminated between the hydrogen of N-9 for the purines, or N-1 for the pyrimidines, and the hydroxyl of C-1 of the pentose. The resulting compounds or glycosides are called nucleosides. In nucleosides, only the β-form of the sugars has been observed; the covalent bond is, therefore, specifically called a β-N-glycosidic linkage.

The atoms of the base in nucleosides are given cardinal numbers, whereas the carbon atoms of the sugars are given primed numbers as shown in the diagram.

Nucleosides are generally named for the particular purine or pyrimidine present:

Adenine nucleoside:	Adenosine
Guanine nucleoside:	Guanosine
Hypoxanthine nucleoside:	Inosine
Uracil nucleoside:	Uridine
Thymine nucleoside:	Thymidine
Cytosine nucleoside:	Cytidine

Each of these terms is associated with the sugar ribose. For the corresponding deoxyribosides, the prefix *deoxy* is added, e.g., deoxyadenosine, deoxycytidine.

Nucleotides   Nucleosides are found in nature primarily as 5'-phosphate esters, called nucleotides. These occur either in the free form or as subunits in nucleic acids.

**Guanosine monophosphate
(guanylic acid)**

Nucleotides are named as follows:

Adenine nucleotide or adenylic acid:	Adenosine monophosphate (AMP)
Guanine nucleotide or guanylic acid:	Guanosine monophosphate (GMP)
Hypoxanthine nucleotide or inosinic acid:	Inosine monophosphate (IMP)
Uracil nucleotide or uridylic acid:	Uridine monophosphate (UMP)
Cytidine nucleotide or cytidylic acid:	Cytidine monophosphate (CMP)
Thymine nucleotide or thymidylic acid:	Thymidine monophosphate (TMP)

As is apparent from this list, each of the nucleotides is usually referred to by its abbreviation, AMP, UMP, etc. All these examples are ribotides. When the sugar deoxyribose is involved (deoxyribotides), the prefix *deoxy* must be added to the name, e.g., deoxyadenosine monophosphate or dAMP.

Of particular importance in biosynthetic and other energy-requiring biologic processes are the nucleoside di- and triphosphates. In these compounds, additional units of phosphoric acid have been added to the nucleoside monophosphates by means of anhydride bonds. Although the triphosphates of all nucleosides are of importance in the biosynthesis of nucleic acids, *adenosine triphosphate* and *uridine triphosphate* assume roles of special significance in metabolism, as will be discussed later (Chapter 9).

Adenosine triphosphate (ATP)

Uridine triphosphate (UTP)

In these structures, a special designation is given two of the P-O bonds. This is not intended to mean that they are unique but rather that on hydrolysis of ATP to ADP, as also on the hydrolysis of ADP to AMP, a considerable amount of energy ($-\Delta F = 7000$ cal./mole) is released. Because of this high energy of hydrolysis, it is conventional to speak of *high-energy bonds* and to designate them with a special symbol, $\sim$. The nucleoside triphosphates, especially ATP and UTP, are important as carriers of usable energy (Chapter 9).

The 5'-nucleoside phosphates are not the only forms of nucleosides that are important in the cell. Evidence showing metabolic functions for the 3',5'-cyclic phosphate diester of adenosine continues to accumulate (p. 455).

3',5'-Cyclic adenylic acid (cyclic-AMP)

The preceding examples of nucleoside triphosphates are all ribotides. In those nucleotides associated with the biosynthesis of DNA, the presence of deoxyribose must be designated, with the prefix *deoxy*. The deoxynucleoside triphosphates are abbreviated dATP, dGTP, dCTP, etc. This designation is often omitted in the case of thymidine triphosphate since the nucleotide is found in nature only associated with DNA and, hence, with deoxyribose.

Polynucleotides   A nucleic acid may be visualized as a polymer of a nucleotide monomer, in other words, a polynucleotide.

$$(\text{base—deoxyribose—phosphate})_n$$

$$(\text{base—ribose—phosphate})_n$$

The constituent units are coupled by means of 3',5'-phosphodiester bonds.

3',5'-Phosphodiester bond

The nature, properties, and function of the nucleic acids (DNA, RNA) depend on the exact order of the purines and pyrimidines in the molecule. This sequence of specific bases is called the *primary structure*.

DEOXYRIBONUCLEIC ACID

The proportions of the nucleotide bases from complete hydrolysates of DNA's from various sources were first studied by Erwin Chargaff. On the basis of such chemical analyses, he postulated the following fundamental relationships:

1. The sum of the purines equals the sum of the pyrimidines.

Table 4-2. Base composition of representative types of DNA

			Moles per 100 moles			
	A°	G	C	MC	T	A + T/G + C + MC
Man	30.5	19.9	20.6	–	28.9	1.47
Rat						
(bone marrow)	28.6	21.4	20.4	1.1	28.4	1.33
Rainbow trout						
(sperm)	29.7	22.2	20.5	–	27.5	1.34
Wheat germ	28.1	–	16.8	5.9	27.4	1.25
Escherichia coli						
(K-12)	24.6	25.6	25.6	–	24.3	1.00

°A, adenine; G, guanine; C, cytosine; MC, methylcytosine; T, thymine.

2. The molar proportion of adenine equals that of thymine.

3. The molar proportion of guanine equals that of cytosine.

These principles are illustrated in Table 4-2.

The implications of Chargaff's principles with regard to the actual structure of DNA were not apparent until suitable x-ray diffraction studies (Appendix, p. 904) were completed. Thereafter it became possible to visualize the probable location of the constituent atoms in a three-dimensional pattern. On the basis of the x-ray diffraction studies of Wilkins and the analytic data of Chargaff, Watson and Crick proposed the now familiar three-dimensional model of DNA (Fig. 4-1). They suggested that DNA consists of two polynucleotide chains wound about a common axis in the form of a *double helix*.

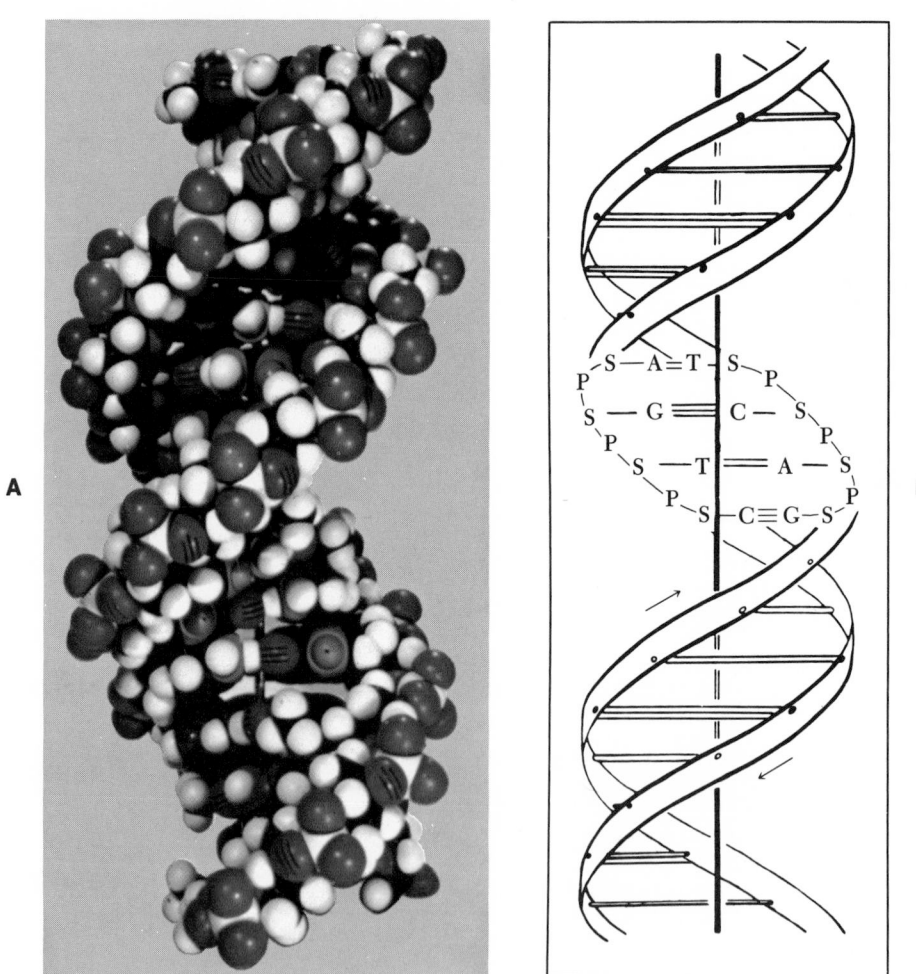

Fig. 4-1. A, Photograph of a Watson-Crick model of DNA produced from space-filling atomic models. **B,** Diagrammatic representation of the Watson-Crick model. *P* represents phosphate; *S,* sugar; *A,* adenine; *T,* thymine; *G,* guanine; *C,* cytosine. Horizontal parallel lines symbolize hydrogen bonding between complementary bases. (**A** courtesy F. Ferguson, Ealing Corp.; **B** from Beadle, G. W.: Missouri Agric. Exp. Station Res. Bull., p. 588, 1955.)

Fig. 4-1, showing a model of DNA, as well as the diagrammatic representation, illustrates how the two helices are wound so as to yield two interchain spacings or grooves. The figure shows a minor or narrow and a major or wide groove that form as when two wires are wound about a pencil or common axis. Such double helices cannot be pulled apart and can be separated only by an unwinding process. They are called *plectonemic coils*. The practical implications of this will be apparent in Chapter 6.

Base complementarity   Essential to the Watson-Crick hypothesis[1] is the concept of *base pairing* or *base complementarity*. Two of Chargaff's principles were interpreted to mean that the parallel polynucleotide chains were so oriented that an adenine was always located in the space opposite a thymine and a guanine was opposite a cytosine. This positioning of the bases is called base complementarity.

X-ray diffraction analysis showed that the complementary bases approach each other so that some of the hydrogen and nitrogen atoms are within a distance of 3 Å (Fig. 4-2). This means that in some instances the hydrogen atoms may be shared by a nitrogen of one base and the oxygen or nitrogen of another. The hydrogen bonds between adenine and thymine, guanine and cytosine are illustrated in Fig. 4-2. Although hydrogen bonds, taken individually, are weak in nature, the large numbers involved in a molecule of DNA assure that these contribute to the stability of the molecule. Fig. 4-1, *B*, shows that the base pairs are found in the center of the double helix with the phosphates on the periphery. The purine-pyrimidine pairs are planar structures and are arranged or stacked one above the other so that their sur-

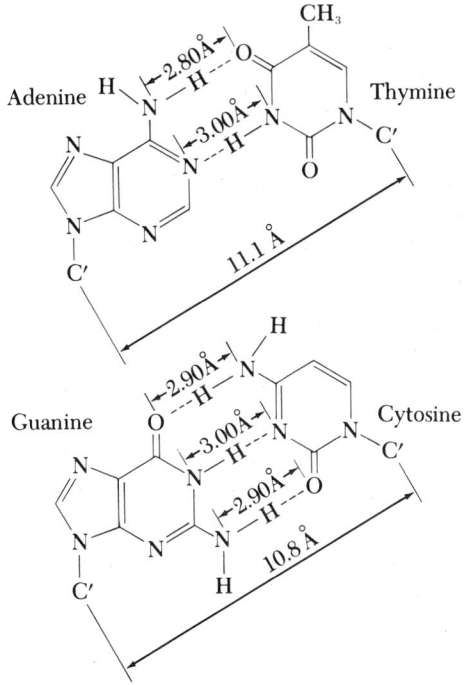

Fig. 4-2. Structure of an adenine-thymine base pair (upper) and guanine-cytosine base pair (lower).

faces are separated by 3.4 Å. It is now thought that the stability of the DNA is primarily a consequence of van der Waals forces between the stacked planes.

The existence of two hydrogen bonds between adenine and thymine (or uracil) and three between guanine and cytosine is fundamental to the principle of base complementarity. As we shall see, this principle is essential to an understanding not only of DNA and RNA structure but also of the process of DNA replication, RNA transcription, and the translation of genetic information into protein structure.

Further analysis of the primary structure of the two companion polynucleotide chains, involving a procedure called *nearest neighbor analysis*, shows that the two complementary chains are arranged in an *antiparallel* fashion. If we consider that one of the constituent chains has a directionality in terms of the 3',5'-phosphodiester bonds, then we note that the corresponding bonds of the complementary chain are 5',3'-. This feature is illustrated in the accompanying diagram.

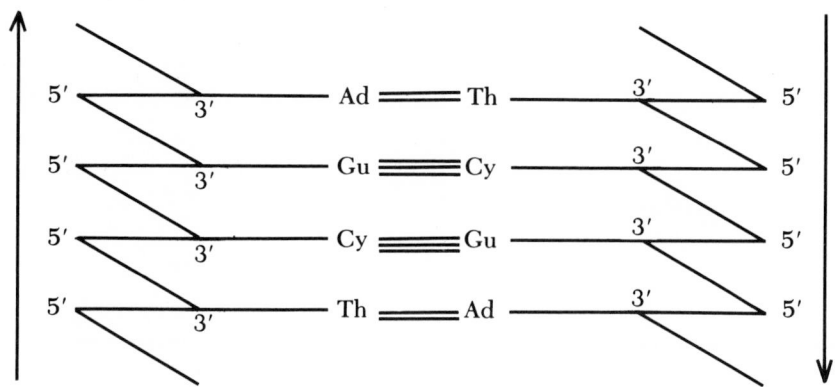

The two antiparallel chains are twisted about a common axis to create the effect of a right-handed screw, 20 Å in diameter and having 10 bases per turn. Fig. 4-1 shows the three-dimensional and secondary structure of the DNA double helix.

Although the DNA double helix is stabilized by hydrogen bonding, it can be denatured by heat. Denaturation is a rupturing of hydrogen bonds and a separation of the double helix into the two constituent polynucleotide chains. This occurs at a characteristic temperature called the *melting temperature* (T_m). A melting curve of DNA is obtained by measuring the absorbancy of light at a wavelength of 260 mμ of solutions heated to increasingly higher temperatures. Fig. 4-3 shows a number of such melting curves for various kinds of DNA. Nucleic acids absorb light at 260 mμ, a property of their purine and pyrimidine bases. Native DNA, however, does not absorb as much light as expected from its content of bases probably because of the interaction of the stacked bases in the secondary structure. If DNA is heated slowly, a T_m at which the light absorbancy increases is reached. At this point, the stable secondary structure of the DNA has been disrupted and the two constituent polynucleotide chains separated. If the denatured DNA is now cooled slowly

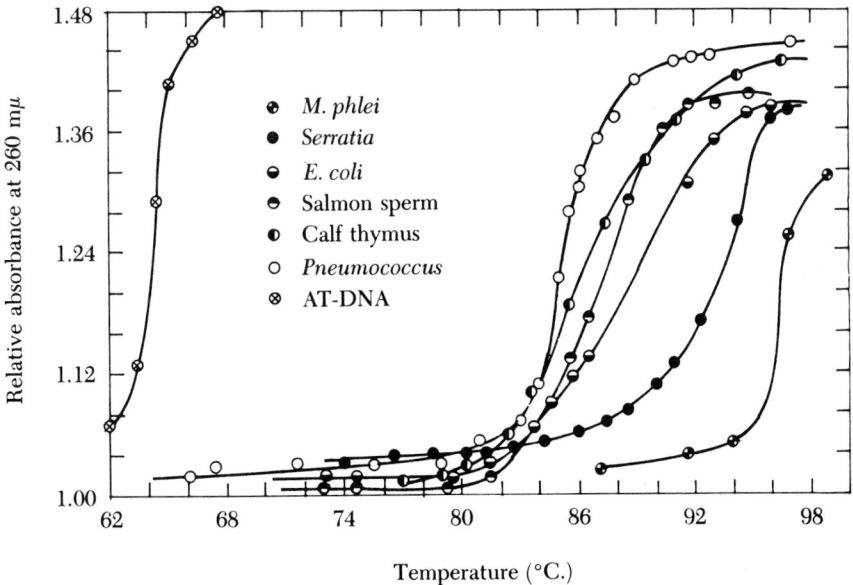

Fig. 4-3. Variation in absorbancy (260 mμ) as a function of the temperature of the DNA solution. (From Marmur, J., and Doty, P.: Nature **183**:1427, 1959.)

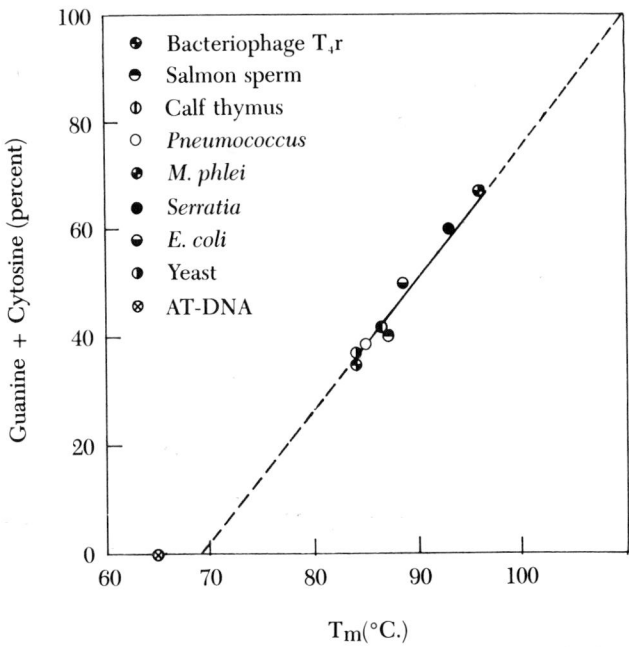

Fig. 4-4. Dependence of the denaturation temperature, T_m, on the guanine-cytosine content of various samples of DNA. (From Marmur, J., and Doty, P.: Nature **183**:1427, 1959.)

to room temperature, the original structure is often restored. The restoration occurs because the complementary bases again are hydrogen bonded and the double helix reforms.

Since the guanine-cytosine base pair has three hydrogen bonds compared with two for adenine-thymine, it follows that DNA's with high concentrations of guanine and cytosine might be more stable and have a higher T_m than those with high concentrations of adenine and thymine. This is illustrated by Fig. 4-4, in which the T_m of various DNA's is compared with their cytosine-guanine content.

RIBONUCLEIC ACID

Native RNA also consists of a polynucleotide structure involving 3',5'-phosphodiester bonds. It does not, however, exhibit the sharp melting temperatures and is usually believed to be a single-strand molecule.

There are in the living organism three fundamental classes of RNA. These can best be illustrated by the following experiment. Microorganisms, such as *Escherichia coli*, are radioactively labeled with a short exposure (20 seconds) or "pulse" of ^{14}C-uracil. The cells are ruptured and the RNA extracted. This mixture of RNA is then placed on a sucrose gradient in the tubes of a preparative ultracentrifuge (Appendix, p. 903). After the mixture has been submitted to high centrifugal forces for approximately 10 hours, the centrifuge tubes are punctured with a hypodermic needle and the sucrose solution

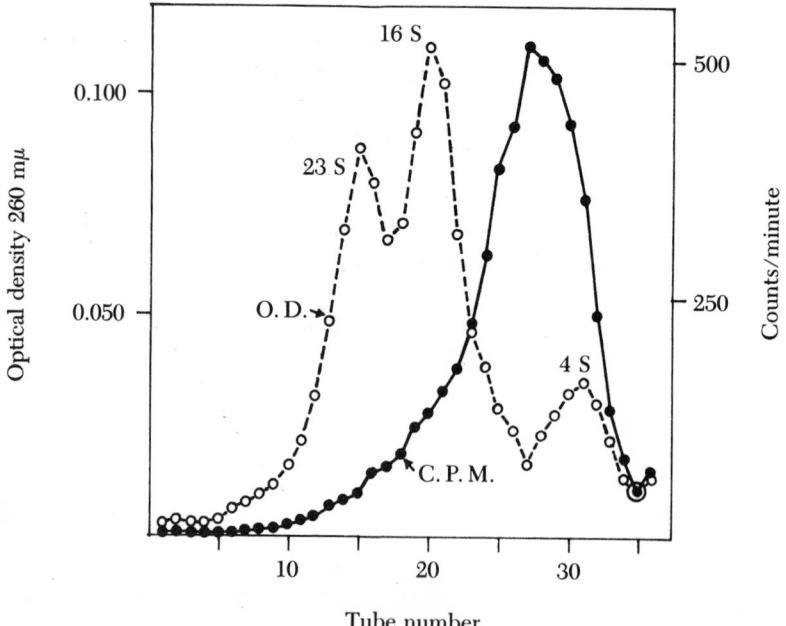

Fig. 4-5. Ultracentrifugal sedimentation of pulse-labeled RNA in a sucrose gradient. *C.P.M.* (counts per minute) represents the RNA with the highest rate of synthesis. (From Gros, F., Hiatt, H., Gilbert, W., Kurland, C. G., Risebrough, R. W., and Watson, J. D.: Nature 190:581, 1961.)

is collected in a series of fractions of equal size, e.g., 10 drops per tube. The light absorbancy at 260 mμ is then measured for each fraction in a spectrophotometer. This procedure yields a pattern or profile of the RNA as shown in Fig. 4-5.

The two major peaks appearing in the first 20 tubes represent the heaviest RNA's, 16 and 23 Svedberg units (S), and are called *ribosomal* RNA. This is the RNA of the cytoplasmic protein-synthesizing particles, the ribosomes (Chapter 6). In *E. coli* each ribosome is composed of two subunits, a 50 S and a 30 S particle. When the constituent RNA is extracted from these particles, RNA's sedimenting at 23 and 16 S are obtained in the sucrose gradient. Near the top of the profile, tube no. 30, is a single peak of relatively small RNA's with a sedimentation constant of 4 S. This region consists of the transfer RNA's and represents approximately 10% to 15% of the total. When the amount of radioactivity (^{14}C) is measured in the various tubes, a second profile consisting primarily of a peak between 8 and 14 S is obtained. Under these conditions, where only a short exposure or pulse of ^{14}C-uracil is used, the ribosomal and transfer RNA's are not labeled significantly. The highly radioactive 8 to 14 S RNA is called *messenger* RNA and represents approximately 5% of the total. Messenger RNA is considered to be the material that is transcribed from the DNA to carry the genetic information from the nucleus to the cytoplasm.

The properties of the three classes of RNA may be summarized as follows.

Ribosomal RNA In general, ribosomal RNA (rRNA) represents 75% to 80% of the total. The 23 S and 16 S RNA's, typical of bacterial ribosomes, have molecular weights of 1.1×10^6 and 0.55×10^6, respectively. In animals the ribosomes are 80 S particles with 60 S and 40 S subunits. The latter are composed of 28 S and 18 S RNA's. The 50 and 60 S subunits have a third kind of rRNA with a sedimentation constant of 5 S and containing only 115 nucleotides compared with 1000 or more for the larger RNA's. The small 5 S molecules, however, appear to be a structural entity in the 50 and 60 S subunits.

Messenger RNA Messenger RNA (mRNA) is a heterogeneous mixture of large–molecular weight RNA's of approximately 2×10^6. It represents 5% to 10% of the total cellular RNA. In bacteria, mRNA may be distinguished by its rapid turnover. This, however, is not a consistent characteristic since the mRNA for hemoglobin in rabbit reticulocytes appears to be fairly stable.

Transfer RNA Transfer RNA (tRNA) represents 10% to 15% of the total and is characterized by its small molecular weight, 25,000 (4 S). The function of tRNA is to bind the specific amino acids (p. 94); hence there must be at least one for each amino acid. Because of its small size, tRNA has lent itself more readily to isolation procedures and to studies of nucleotide sequence. Holley[2,3] first succeeded in determining the primary structure of tRNA specific for the amino acid alanine (Fig. 4-6). It now appears that all tRNA's are of approximately the same length, 90 nucleotides, and all terminate in the sequence cytosine-cytosine-adenine. Transfer RNA's are also characteristic in their content of unusual and methylated purines and pyrimidines (p. 33). These are 6-N-dimethyladenosine; 1-methyladenosine; 6-N-isopentenyladenosine; 5-methylcytidine; 6-N-acetylcytidine; 2'-O-methylcytidine; 2-N-

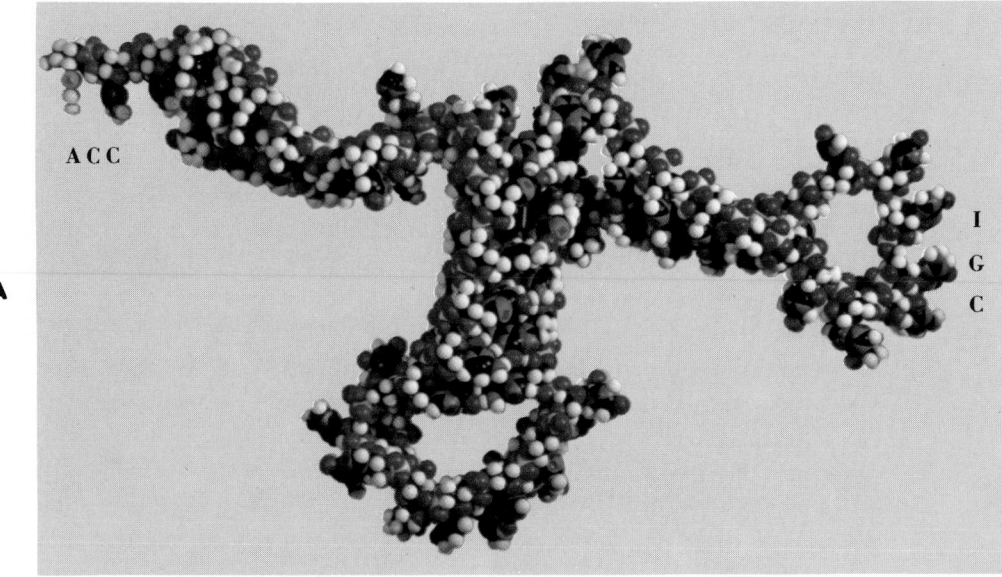

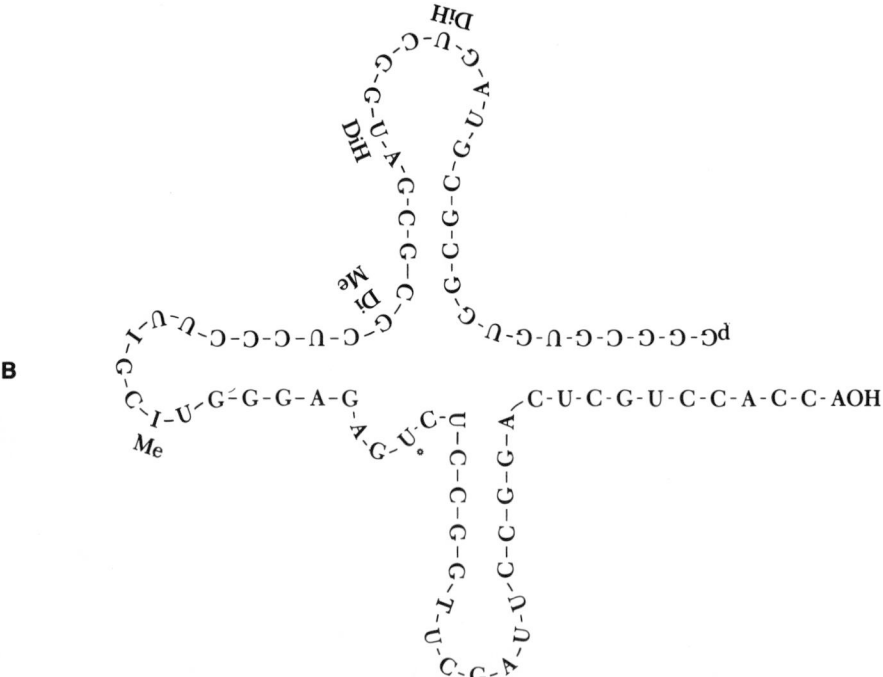

Fig. 4-6. **A,** Space-filling model of the tRNA molecule specific for the amino acid alanine. **B,** Primary structure of alanyl-tRNA. Alanine is attached to the terminal *CCA* sequence. *IGC* represents the sequence inosine, guanine, cytosine and is the anticodon for alanine (Chapter 6). (**A** courtesy R. W. Holley; **B** adapted from Madison, J. T., Everett, G. A., and King, H. K.: Sympos. Quant. Biol. **31**:409, 1966.)

methylguanosine; 1-methylguanosine; 2-N-methylguanosine; 2'-O-methyl-guanosine; 7-N-methylguanosine; inosine; 1-methylinosine, 4,5-dihydrouridine, 2'-O-methyluridine; and pseudouridine. All the tRNA's so far studied have a characteristic secondary structure shown in Fig. 4-6. The three loops are formed by regions of limited base complementarity.

BIOSYNTHESIS OF NUCLEIC ACIDS

The successful synthesis of nucleic acids in a cell-free system has made possible a much clearer concept of the process as it occurs in the living cell. The purification of the responsible enzyme, *DNA polymerase*, by Kornberg[4] in 1959, represented a major breakthrough in biologic science. This enzyme, first isolated from the microorganism *E. coli*, catalyzes the formation of 3',5'-phosphodiester linkages from nucleoside triphosphates.

$$\left.\begin{array}{l} dATP \\ dGTP \\ dTTP \\ dCTP \end{array}\right\} \xrightarrow[Mg^{++}]{Polymerase} (dAMP, dGMP, dCMP, dTMP)_n + PP_i$$

The reaction requires a suitable supply of nucleoside triphosphates in addition to the purified enzyme. Furthermore, a small quantity of primer DNA is needed to serve as the template onto which the new polynucleotide chains are built. The need for a primer is restricted in this instance to DNA. The polymerase enzyme itself does not seem to determine the nature of the final DNA product, although this issue is still contested. A polymerase from *E. coli* can be used to synthesize a variety of DNA's depending on the primer used. For example, an experimental system using microbial polymerase and a small amount of bovine thymus gland DNA,[5] yields a product similar to thymus gland DNA. The process of replication is dependent on the principle of *base complementarity*. When the primer DNA is first heated beyond its

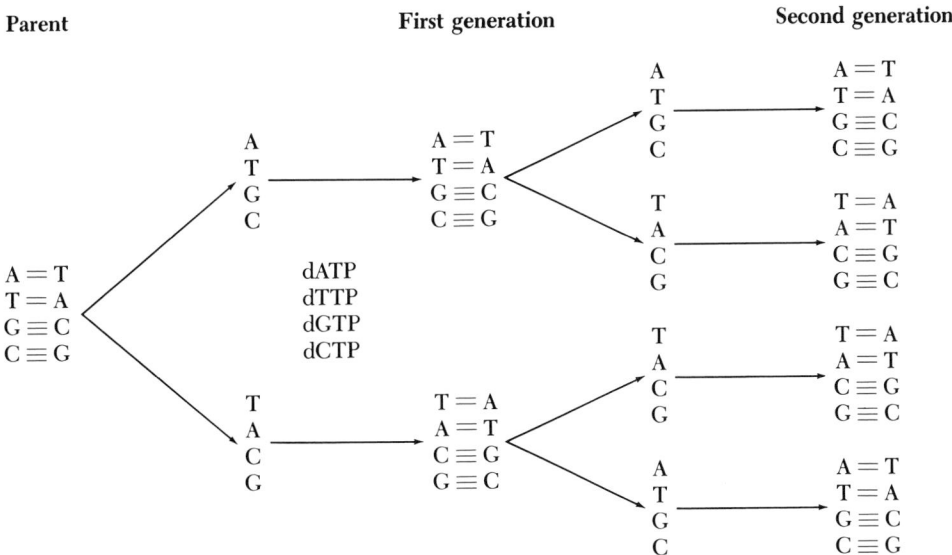

Fig. 4-7

T_m (p. 40), its effectiveness in the polymerase system is considerably enhanced. Therefore, it is thought that replication first requires an unwinding of the parent DNA. Deoxyribonucleoside triphosphates then line up to form A=T and G≡C base pairs. In the presence of the polymerase, the pyrophosphate is eliminated and 3',5'-phosphodiester bonds are formed. This model, based on the Watson-Crick structure of DNA, explains the manner in which the primary structure of each polynucleotide chain is copied. Not only are the base sequences copied exactly, but the new polynucleotide chain is antiparallel and forms a double helix with the parent template. In other words, in the double helices of the first generation, one chain is from the parent and one is newly synthesized. The principle of the replication of DNA is illustrated in Fig. 4-7.

The validity of this model was tested by using synthetic polynucleotides as primer molecules and determining the nature of the newly synthesized polynucleotide. A simple poly-A chain, made only of adenines, yielded, in the presence of polymerase from *E. coli* and the four deoxyribonucleoside triphosphates, a new chain of thymidine only (poly-T). Likewise, an alternating poly-AT chain yielded a complementary poly-TA product.

The chemical composition of a variety of enzymatically synthesized DNA produced from different natural primers and the microbial polymerase are compared in Table 4-3.

Despite the general agreement of analytic data with the model proposed, it is extremely difficult to conceive, on purely logistic grounds, how this

Table 4-3. Chemical composition of enzymatically synthesized DNA, synthesized with different primers*

DNA	A†	T	G	C	$\dfrac{A+G}{T+C}$	$\dfrac{A+T}{G+C}$
Mycobacterium phlei						
Primer	0.65	0.66	1.35	1.34	1.01	0.49
Product	0.66	0.65	1.34	1.37	0.99	0.48
Escherichia coli						
Primer	1.00	0.97	0.98	1.05	0.98	0.97
Product	1.04	1.00	0.97	0.98	1.01	1.02
Calf thymus						
Primer	1.14	1.05	0.90	0.85	1.05	1.25
Product	1.12	1.08	0.85	0.85	1.02	1.29
Bacteriophage T_2						
Primer	1.31	1.32	0.67	0.70	0.98	1.92
Product	1.33	1.29	0.69	0.70	1.02	1.90
AT copolymer	1.99	1.93	<0.05	<0.05	1.03	40

° From Kornberg, A.: Science **131**:1503, 1960.
† A, Adenine; T, thymine; G, guanine; C, cytosine. The numbers are molar proportions.

process of unwinding occurs in the nucleus of the intact cell. The staggering length of DNA in a nucleus is suggested in the electron micrograph[6] (Fig. 4-8) showing the DNA in a single bacteriophage.

Also, as was noted previously, the double helices of DNA are *plectonemic coils;* i.e., the two polynucleotide chains cannot be pulled apart except by an unwinding process. A system of local or general unwinding preceding the formation of new chains is illustrated in Fig. 4-9. Apart from the logistics of this process, the model is difficult to rationalize because of the antiparallel

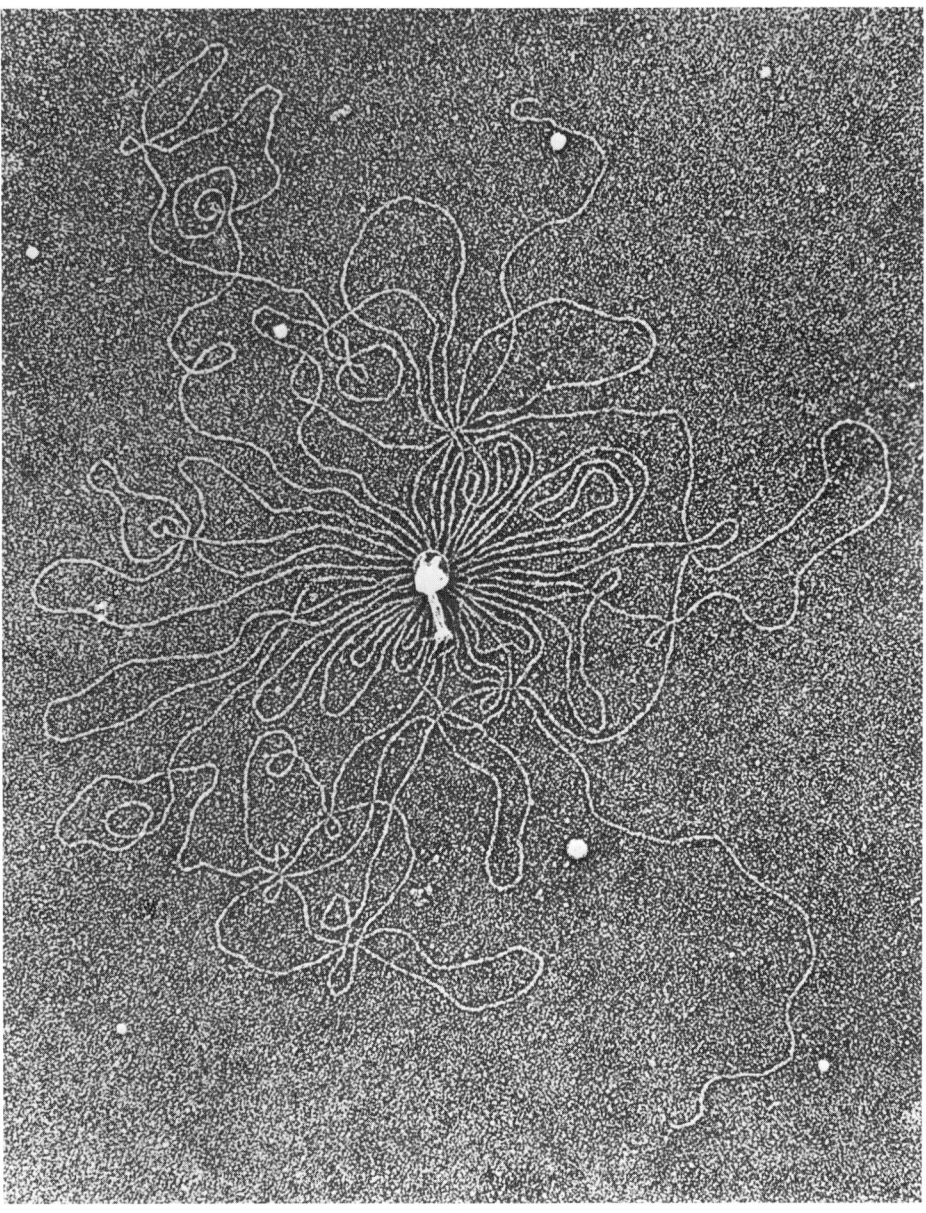

Fig. 4-8. Electron micrograph of T_2 DNA (×100,000). (From Kleinschmidt, A. K., Lang, D., and Zahn, R, K.: Biochim. Biophys. Acta **61**:857, 1962.)

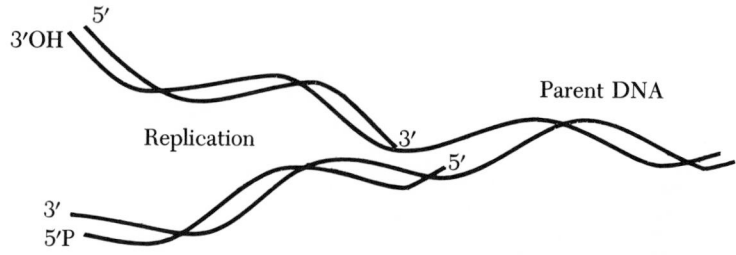

3'OH

5'

Replication

3'

5'

Parent DNA

3'

5'P

Fig. 4-9. Suggested model of DNA replication, showing the unwinding of the double helix. Each strand might serve as a template for the synthesis of a new polynucleotide chain.

nature of the two chains. If they unwind as illustrated, these chains would present both a 3'-terminal end and a 5'-terminal end to the enzyme. This might imply that the polymerase would be able to recognize two different points of attachment on the template molecule. Actually the enzyme can produce a chain only in a 5' to 3' direction so that it should be able to use the chain only with the 3'-hydroxyl terminal end as a template. The suggestion that the replicative process actually occurs in a piecemeal fashion has now been made. Short segments of 1000 or so nucleotides are produced, and all are synthesized in a 5' to 3' direction. These so-called *Okasaki fragments*, named for their discoverer, are then thought to be joined by a special enzyme.

The discovery of circular DNA in *E. coli*,[7] bacteriophage φX174, and mitochondria has led to another suggestion for the unwinding and replicatory process.

Fig. 4-10 shows such a strand of circular DNA visualized by radioautography. The newly synthesized chain incorporates ^{3}H-thymidine and therefore is radioactive. The radioactivity has been located by allowing it to "expose" a special photographic film. A model in which the parental double helix can unwind at a special point indicated by the fork marked X has been proposed. As each polynucleotide strand unwinds, it serves as a template for the replicative process. The growth of daughter DNA proceeds around the full periphery of the Y. When the growth point Y has completed the full circuit of parental DNA and reached point X, two daughter double helices, each having one parental and one new chain, result. Goulian, Kornberg, and Sinsheimer[8] subsequently showed that single-strand, circular DNA of φX174 phage could be used as a primer in a highly purified polymerase system to produce a synthetic, biologically active, circular DNA. Their studies also showed that a second enzyme, DNA ligase, is essential to complete the process. Although replication of circular DNA might help in some degree to understand how replication occurs in the confines of the chromosome, this form of the polynucleotide has been observed only in microorganisms and mitochondria.

DNA AND GENETIC INFORMATION

The in vitro synthesis of DNA has shown us how such a molecule can be duplicated without error and how genetic information may be passed from

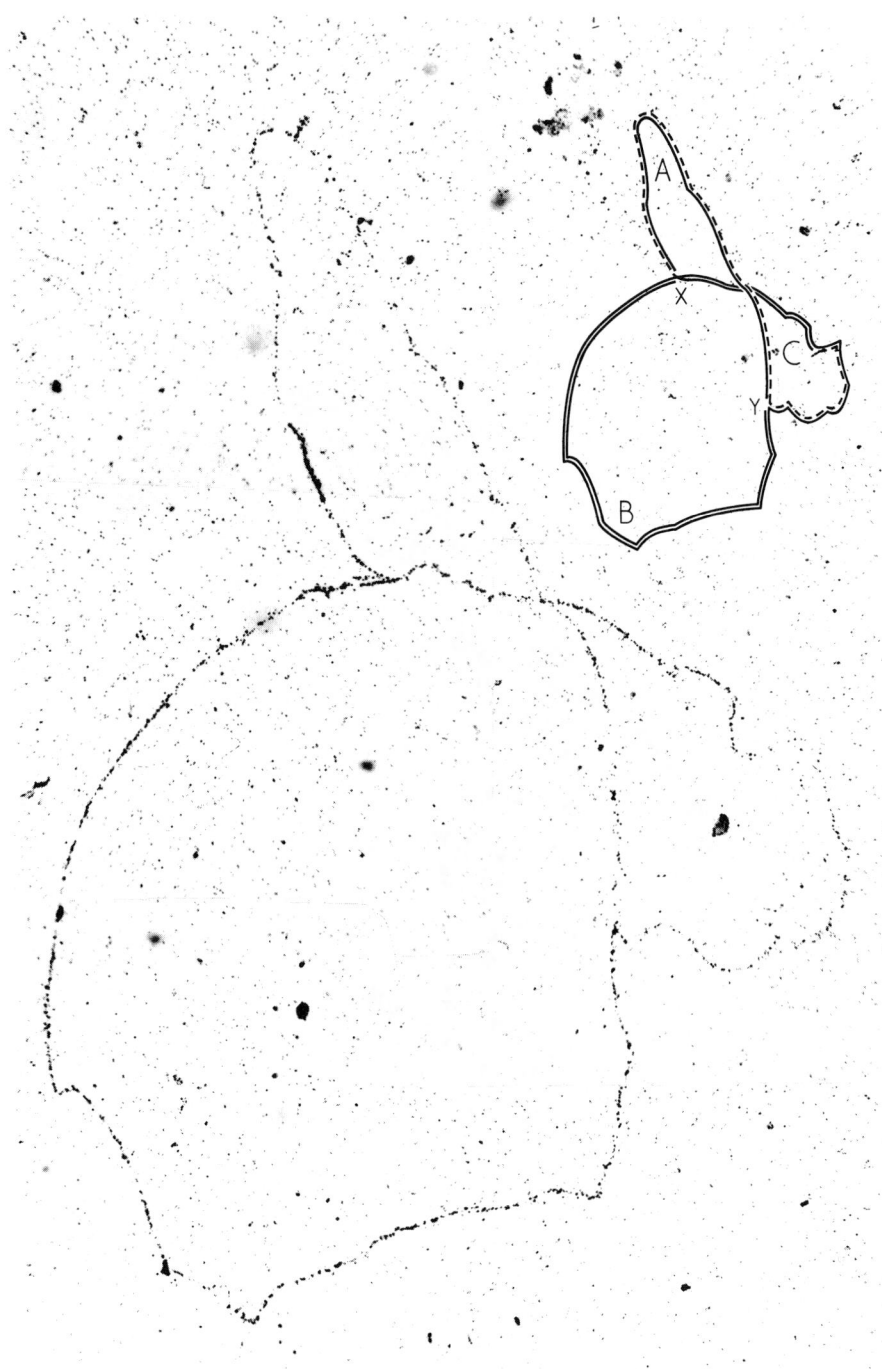

Fig. 4-10. Autoradiograph of the chromosome of *E. coli* labeled with tritiated thymidine for two generations and extracted with lysozyme. Exposure time 2 months. The scale shows 100μ. Inset, the same structure shown diagrammatically and divided into three sections (*A*, *B*, and *C*) that arise at the two forks *X* and *Y*. (From Cairns, J.: Sympos. Quant. Biol. **28**:43, 1963.)

parent to progeny. Inherent in this concept lies the understanding that genetic information must exist in the chromosomes as some sort of "language" made up perhaps in terms of the sequence of the four bases, i.e., guanine, adenine, cytosine, and thymine. Various combinations of these bases must exist in the polynucleotide chains in such a way as to spell out the genetic information.

That genetic information is part of the DNA molecule has been appreciated for some time; e.g., in 1928, Griffith studied the transmission of genetic traits in two strains of *Pneumococcus*, one having a polysaccharide cell wall, yielding colonies of smooth (S) appearance and the other, devoid of the polysaccharide coat, yielding colonies of rough (R) appearance. In other words, the R strain did not have the necessary genetic information to produce the polysaccharide cell wall. To determine whether the capacity to produce a cell wall could be transmitted from the S to the R strain, Griffith heated the S bacteria and then combined the dead organisms with a sample of living R strain. This mixture was injected into mice. Upon reisolation of the microorganisms, both living S and living R bacteria were observed. This meant that the genetic information in the dead S organisms was transmitted to the R organisms. The substance involved was called the *transforming factor*. In 1944, Avery extracted the transforming factor from a preparation of dead smooth pneumococci and demonstrated that this material was DNA. When DNA, purified from S bacteria, was injected into mice in combination with living R pneumococci, the subsequent generations of bacteria proved to be both S and R strains. This and similar studies have shown that the processes of genetic transformation involve the chemical substance, DNA.

SEMICONSERVATIVE REPLICATION

Fig. 4-7, which illustrates the transmission of base sequences from parent to daughter DNA molecules, shows that a single parent strand appears in the first generation daughter double helix. This phenomenon is called *semiconservative replication*. The principle is best illustrated by the experiment of Meselson and Stahl[9] (Fig. 4-11).

E. coli was grown in a medium containing ammonium sulfate labeled with the heavy isotope of nitrogen (^{15}N). After many generations the progeny DNA was saturated with ^{15}N. DNA from these bacteria was isolated and separated by ultracentrifugation on a cesium chloride density gradient (Appendix, p. 904). In the gradient, the ^{15}N-DNA sedimented further than ^{14}N-DNA because of its greater density. In other words, it was possible to separate ^{14}N- and ^{15}N-species because of differences in density. When *E. coli* saturated with ^{15}N was allowed to grow in the presence of ^{14}N–ammonium sulfate for a single new generation and this DNA was subsequently isolated and centrifuged in the cesium chloride gradient, an intermediate layer of hybrid ^{14,15}N-DNA was observed (Fig. 4-11). Subsequent generations of bacteria, grown in the presence of ^{14}N–ammonium sulfate, yielded a mixture of ^{14,15}N-DNA as well as ^{14}N-DNA. The existence of the hybrid showed that the DNA of the first generation consisted of one parent and one newly formed strand. Reconsideration of the diagram on p. 45 will show how replication based on the Watson

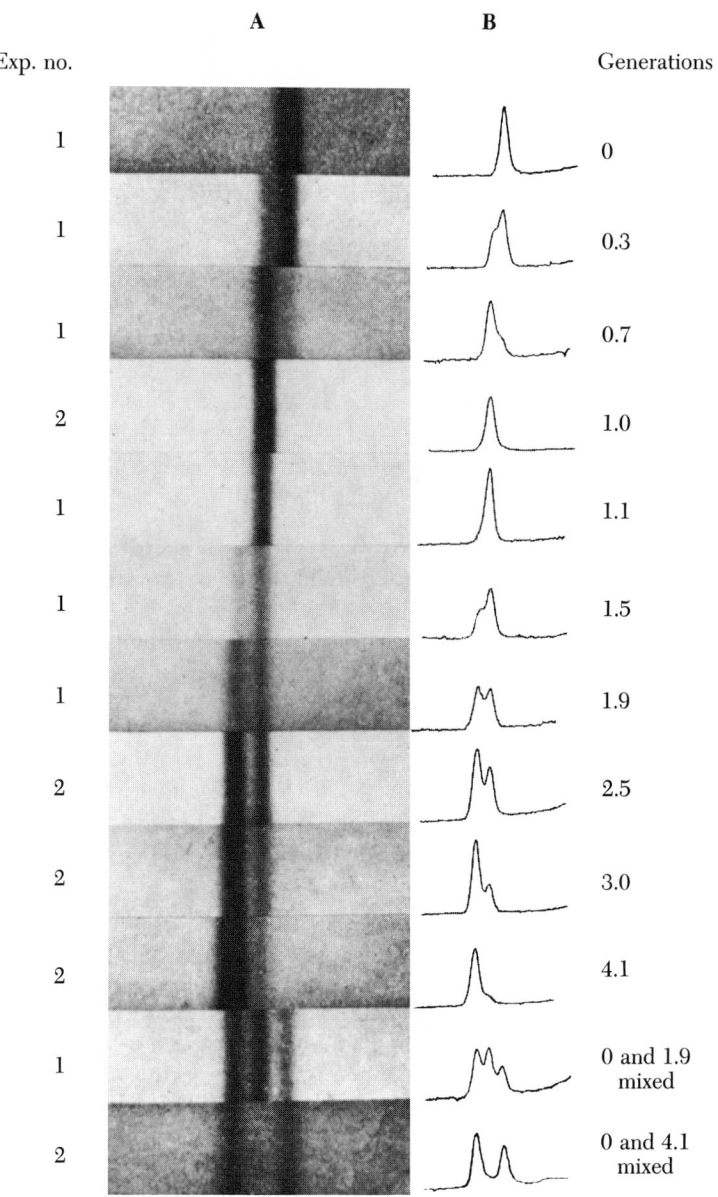

Fig 4-11. Photograph of the sedimentation of DNA in a CsCl density gradient in the experiment of Meselson and Stahl. At O, generation of the DNA is enriched in ^{15}N. The first generation consists of hybrid $^{14,15}N$-DNA while subsequent generations are mixtures of hybrid and ^{14}N-DNA. (From Meselson, M., and Stahl, F. W.: Proc. Nat. Acad. Sci. 44:671, 1958.)

and Crick model can explain the results of the experiment by Meselson and Stahl.

GENETIC REPAIR MECHANISMS

The accuracy of the replicative process is extraordinary. For example, a bacterial gene may be duplicated 1×10^8 times before there is a 50:50 chance that even a single gene is altered. In the face of this accuracy, one is inclined to wonder whether the cell possesses some sort of corrective machinery in the event of error possibly induced by the environment.[10] Ultraviolet light, which is lethal to bacteria, causes unwanted covalent bonds to form between neighboring pyrimidine bases of the same polynucleotide chain. A thymine dimer can form as shown in the following diagram:

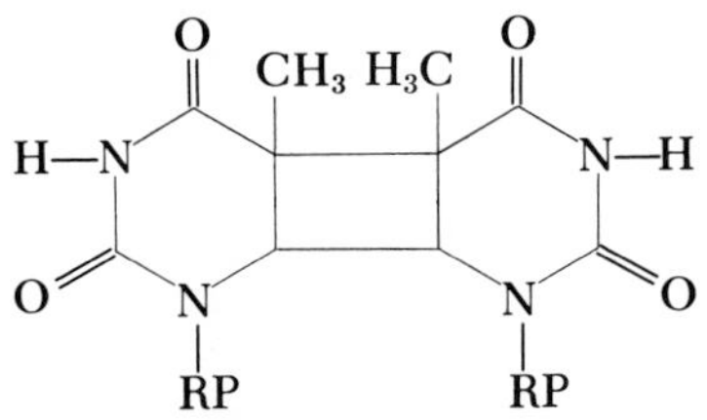

These "errors" distort or kink the DNA chain and prevent subsequent replication. The process of repair involves an initial enzymatic excision of the unwanted dimer by means of cellular endonuclease. The second step is a patching process in which DNA polymerase and ligase apparently catalyze the insertion of two new thymidine nucleotides. Once again the principle of base complementarity is fundamental because the adenine bases in the intact chain determine the insertion of new thymidine units. Although most evidence for such a repair mechanism is from studies using bacteria, some experiments show the presence of repair systems in mammalian cells. Such errors may be purposely induced in tumor cell DNA by treatment with X rays. If the cell's repair mechanisms could be inhibited chemically, the tumor cells might be made more sensitive to X rays, thereby increasing the therapeutic effectiveness of these radiations.

IN VITRO REPLICATION OF RNA

Much fundamental information regarding genetic transmission has been obtained from the studies of Spiegelman and co-workers[11] using a variety of bacteriophage ($Q\beta$). In this phage, RNA serves exclusively as the genetic material. Isolated viral RNA was combined in a test tube with the nucleoside triphosphates and the appropriate RNA polymerase previously isolated from infected *E. coli*. Since RNA in this instance serves as primer, the product is actually a replication and the enzyme has been called a *replicase*. The product RNA was isolated and in turn used as primer for the second generation. This test tube procedure was repeated 15 times or until no original or native phage RNA contaminated the product; all RNA was, in effect, synthetic. The final RNA was then tested for infectivity on the host *E. coli* and found to produce a perfectly normal phage. In other words, all the information needed to produce a normal phage, including the protein coat and various essential enzymes, was to be found in the information store of the synthetic RNA. It is challenging to speculate on the possibility of synthesizing the original RNA itself by methods of organic chemistry and thereby "create" a synthetic self-replicating system.

TRANSCRIPTION OF RNA

The principle whereby genetic messages in chromosomes are transmitted accurately from parent to progeny is base complementarity. This same principle explains how messages are transmitted from the DNA-containing genes to the protein-synthesizing mechanism present in the cytoplasm via the formation of RNA. The transfer of genetic information from DNA to its ultimate manifestation as proteins, is illustrated as follows:

$$DNA \xrightarrow{\text{Replication}} DNA \xrightarrow{\text{Transcription}} RNA \xrightarrow{\text{Translation}} Proteins$$

Whereas the duplication of DNA is called *replication*, the transmission of this information to cytoplasmic RNA is called *transcription*, and the final manifestation of genetic information as proteins is *translation*.

The manner in which genetic information is transcribed from the primary structure of DNA to the structure of RNA is illustrated by the experiments of Hurwitz and associates.[12] In these, a mixture of the four nucleoside triphosphates is combined with a purified preparation of a cytoplasmic polymerizing enzyme of *RNA polymerase* (or transcriptase) and the appropriate DNA primer (see Table 4-4).

$$\left.\begin{array}{l} ATP \\ GTP \\ UTP \\ CTP \end{array}\right\} \xrightarrow[Mg^{++}]{\begin{array}{c} DNA\text{-dependent} \\ RNA \\ polymerase \end{array}} (AMP, GMP, UMP, CMP)_n + PP_i$$

Unlike the DNA-replicating system, the use of heated or denatured DNA primer in the RNA-synthesizing system does not improve the amount of RNA produced. Apparently the primer retains its double helical configuration during the transcriptive process. It is thought that perhaps some local unwinding occurs and one of the two chains then acts as the effective template. This may be visualized in Fig. 4-12. The role of the second or untranscribed DNA chain is unknown; this chain may be required to release the newly formed RNA molecules.

Table 4-4. Genetic transcription

	DNA primer A + T/G + C	RNA product A + U/G + C
Calf thymus	1.35	1.50
E. coli	0.97	0.92
M. lysodeik	0.39	0.49

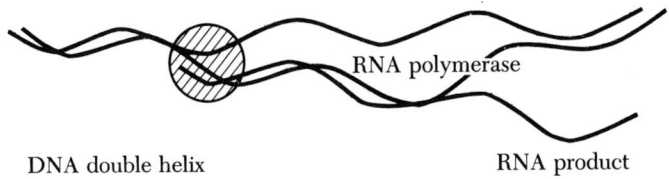

DNA double helix   RNA product

Fig. 4-12

The transcriptive process can be visualized using the giant multistrand or *polytenic* chromosomes of the salivary glands of the fruit fly, *Drosophila*, or midge, *Chironomus*. Histologic studies have demonstrated the formation of local bulges or "puffs" on the chromosomes.[13] These regions were found to be primarily RNA. When the salivary glands were exposed to radioactive uridine, the puffs became highly radioactive as shown by radioautograph *A* of Fig. 4-13.

In a similar experiment,[14] in which the antibiotic actinomycin-D was included, very little radioactivity was present in the puff region, showing that transcription had been inhibited. Actinomycin-D is known to block transcription by combining with DNA at the sites of the guanine residues.

When algae were grown in the presence of radioactive uridine for a very short time only (pulse labeled), radioautographs showed the location of RNA to be restricted to the nucleus and specifically to the region called the nucleolus.[15] Continued incubation of the labeled algae in a nonradioactive medium, i.e., a chaser, led to a migration of the radioactivity from the nucleus to the cytoplasm. Such experiments illustrate the sequence of events in which the genetic information residing in chromosomal DNA is transcribed into RNA and then transmitted to the cytoplasm.

As far as is known, each kind of RNA, whether messenger, ribosomal, or transfer, is transcribed from special genes by comparable processes. Mammalian ribosomal RNA (rRNA) is composed of 18 S and 28 S polynucleotides and appears to be derived from a single precursor and a single gene. The transcriptive process leads to the formation of 45 S chains that are broken by a stepwise process into the 28 and 18 S units. The assemblage of mammalian ribosomes composed of approximately 50% RNA and 50% protein occurs in the nucleoli. When toads (*Xenopus laevis*) are bred by crossing adults having recessive *anucleolate* traits, the resultant embryos are incapable of producing ribosomes and, therefore, never mature. This demonstrates the important role of the nucleolus in the formation of rRNA.

Ribosomal as well as transfer RNA (tRNA) are unique in being methylated. At some time during the transcriptive process, the 45 S rRNA is methylated principally at the 2'OH of the ribose, thereby forming 2'OCH$_3$. It has been suggested that methylation in this position of the ribose stabilizes the RNA by blocking ribonuclease activity. Ribonuclease requires the formation of an intermediate 2',3'-phosphodiester compound (p. 116), which is impossible in the methylated polynucleotide. Transfer RNA is methylated on the purine and pyrimidine bases. Examples of these derivatives are on p. 33. It appears that methylating enzymes, tRNA methylases, add methyl groups to the bases in a specific manner. Suggestions that these chemical changes "edit" the

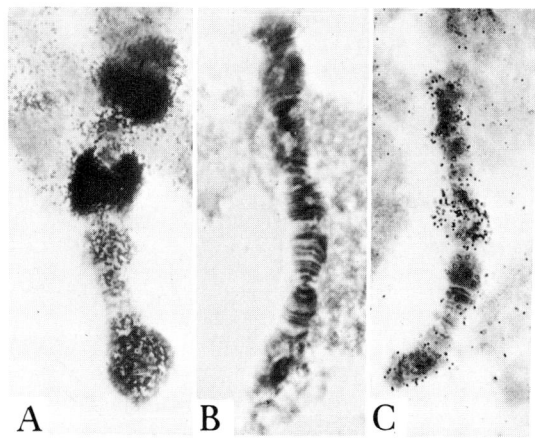

Fig. 4-13. **A,** Autoradiographs of the salivary gland chromosomes of *Chironomus tentans* after incubation of the glands in a medium containing ³H-uridine for 30 minutes. For **B** and **C,** the larvae were treated with actinomycin-D, 10 and 20 hours, respectively, before the salivary glands were incubated with ³H-uridine. (From Clever, U.: Science **146**:794, 1964.)

genetic information inherent in the polynucleotides have been made (p. 91). Currently a relationship between methylating activity and tumor formation is being sought, since tumors contain a higher proportion of methylated bases in their tRNA's than do normal cells.

The assemblage of ribosomes[16] from rRNA may be a spontaneous process in which the RNA and protein subunits combine to form the final structure. This process may be similar to the spontaneous combination of tobacco mosaic virus–RNA and the 2300 individual coat protein subunits that form a complete viral structure (Fig. 103).

In mammalian cells the three RNA's, formed by transcription of genetic information, find their way to the cytoplasm. This sequence of events is visualized in the "pulse-chase" experiments described above, using algae. In the cytoplasm these polynucleotides are fundamental to the final translation of genetic information into proteins, as will be described in detail in Chapter 6.

References

GENERAL

Busch, H.: Histones and other nuclear proteins, New York, 1965, Academic Press, Inc.

Chargaff, E., and Davidson, J. J.: The nucleic acids: chemistry and biology, New York, 1955–1960, Academic Press, Inc.

Ingram, V. M.: The biosynthesis of macromolecules, New York, 1965, W. A. Benjamin, Inc.

Watson, J. D.: Molecular biology of the gene, New York, 1965, W. A. Benjamin, Inc.

SPECIAL

1. Crick, F. H. C.: Proc. 6th Int. Congr. Biochem. **33**:109, 1964.

2. Holley, R. W.: Sci. Amer. **214**:30, 1966.

3. Burton, K.: In Burton, K., editor: Essays in biochemistry, New York, 1965, Academic Press, Inc., vol. 1. p. 57.

4. Richardson, C. C., et. al.: Sympos. Quant. Biol. **28**:9, 1963.

5. Bollum, F. J.: Sympos. Quant. Biol. **28**:21, 1963.

6. Kleinschmidt, O. K.: In Taylor, J. H., editor: Molecular genetics, New York, 1967, Academic Press, Inc., part 2, p. 47.

7. Cairns, J.: Sympos. Quant. Biol. **28**:43, 1963.

8. Goulian, M., et al.: Proc. Nat. Acad. Sci. **58**:2321, 1967.

9. Meselson, M., and Stahl, F. W.: Proc. Nat. Acad. Sci. **44**:671, 1958.

10. Sueoka, N.: In Taylor, J. H., editor: Molecular genetics, New York, 1967, Academic Press, Inc., part 2, p. 1.
11. Spiegelman, S., et al.: Sympos. Quant. Biol. 33:101, 1968.
12. Hurwitz, J., et al.: Sympos. Quant. Biol. 28:59, 1963.
13. Beermann, W., and Clever, U.: Sci. Amer. 210:50, 1964.
14. Clever, U.: Science 146:794, 1964.
15. Perry, R. P.: Progr. Nucl. Acid Res. 6:219, 1967.
16. Maden, B. E. H.: Nature 219:685, 1968.

CHAPTER 5

AMINO ACIDS AND PROTEINS

In Chapters 3 and 4 we learned that anabolic and catabolic processes require the presence of numerous organic catalysts or enzymes. These enzymes are examples of biologically active proteins. However, proteins generally assume a position of primary importance to the living cell and are essential in many other ways as well, e.g., (1) *in a structural sense*, for membranes or for musculature or connective tissue; (2) *for transport mechanisms*, as oxygen by hemoglobin; (3) *for maintenance of fluid balance*, by blood serum albumin; (4) *for regulation of metabolism*, by hormones; (5) *in genetics*, as by the nucleoproteins; and, finally, (6) *in defense mechanisms*, as by the γ-globulins of blood.

Proteins are polymeric molecules in which the subunits are *amino acids*. The composition of the protein in terms of these amino acids as well as their actual arrangement in the molecule is of great importance not only to the structure of the polymer but also to its biologic activity. In other words, biologic activity is to be understood in terms of protein structure. The actual sequence of amino acids, called the *primary structure*, is determined genetically and resides in the language of the DNA molecules.

In general, proteins have large molecular weights, usually ranging from 5×10^3 to 1×10^6, some as much as 25×10^6. Because of their large size, they form colloidal dispersions. Nevertheless, proteins are obtainable in crystalline form when sufficiently pure. Today crystallization is accepted as a criterion of purity.

Although a knowledge of the primary structure, or amino acid sequence, is essential to an understanding of the process of genetic expression, *primary* as well as *secondary, tertiary*, and *quaternary* structures must be understood to determine the nature of biologic activity.

Proteins are ubiquitous in nature and form a vast variety of substances. Their diverse physical, chemical, and biologic properties are dependent on the nature and arrangement of their constituent subunits, the *amino acids*. Consequently, it is necessary first to understand the nature and structures of amino acids before considering the properties of proteins themselves.

AMINO ACIDS

There are 20 amino acids commonly found in proteins. All are α-amino acids and have the general formula given below:

$$\underset{\underset{\displaystyle COO^-}{|}}{\overset{\overset{\displaystyle R}{|}}{H-C-NH_3^+}}$$

In accord with the nomenclature regarding aliphatic acids, the α-carbon is that carbon nearest the carboxyl; the β-carbon is second; the γ-carbon is third; the δ-carbon is fourth; the ϵ-carbon fifth, etc. Other examples of amino acids, e.g., β-alanine, not found in proteins, will be presented later.

Amino acids are obtained from proteins by *hydrolysis*, catalyzed by a proton (HCl, H_2SO_4), a hydroxyl (NaOH), or such enzymes as pepsin, trypsin, and chymotrypsin. If, after hydrolysis, the pH is adjusted to 5.5 and then the mixture of amino acids is separated by paper electrophoresis (Appendix, p. 903) at the same pH, the amino acids divide into three general groups.

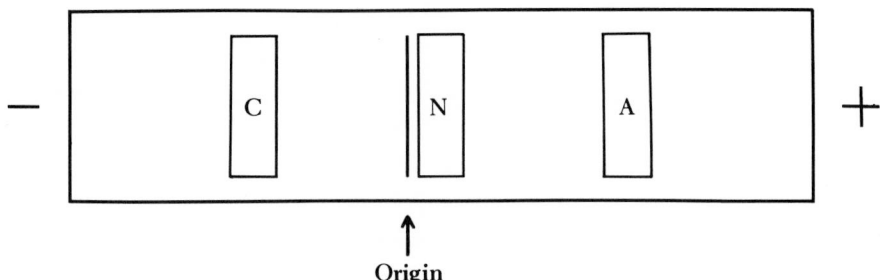

Origin

N represents a group of nonmigrating, neutral amino acids that have no net charge at pH 5.5 and, therefore, do not migrate from the origin. These are the *monoamino-monocarboxylic* acids. A second group, C, migrates cathodically and consists of those amino acids with a net positive charge. These have more than one nitrogen-containing group and are called *basic* amino acids. A third group, A, migrates anodically and consists of amino acids with more than one carboxyl group. They are called *acidic* amino acids.

The various structures of amino acids will be considered in accord with this classification, i.e., neutral, basic, and acidic.

NEUTRAL AMINO ACIDS

The neutral amino acids are monoamino-monocarboxylic acids and are characterized by the nature of their side chains. The accepted three-letter abbreviation of each amino acid is indicated in parentheses following the common and chemical names of the amino acid.

Aliphatic amino acids   Straight or branched chains of carbon atoms as well as other substituents distinguish these amino acids from each other.

Glycine, or aminoacetic acid (Gly).

$$\underset{\underset{H}{|}}{\overset{\overset{NH_2}{|}}{H-C}}-COOH$$

Alanine, α-aminopropionic acid (Ala). It is helpful to consider alanine as the basic structure for all the other amino acids. In other words, the other amino acids may be considered as derivatives of alanine, substitutions on the β-carbon.

$$\underset{\underset{H}{|}}{\overset{\overset{NH_2}{|}}{CH_3-C}}-COOH$$

Valine, α-aminoisovaleric acid (Val). Here two methyl groups have replaced two hydrogens on the β-carbon of alanine.

$$\overset{CH_3}{\underset{CH_3}{}}CH-\underset{\underset{H}{|}}{\overset{\overset{NH_2}{|}}{C}}-COOH$$

Leucine, α-aminoisocaproic acid (Leu). A three-carbon or isopropyl group is attached to alanine.

$$\overset{CH_3}{\underset{CH_3}{}}CH-CH_2-\underset{\underset{H}{|}}{\overset{\overset{NH_2}{|}}{C}}-COOH$$

Isoleucine, α-amino-β-methylvaleric acid (Ileu or Ile).

$$\overset{CH_3}{\underset{CH_3CH_2}{}}CH-\underset{\underset{H}{|}}{\overset{\overset{NH_2}{|}}{C}}-COOH$$

Serine, α-amino-β-hydroxypropionic acid (Ser).

$$HO-CH_2-\underset{\underset{H}{|}}{\overset{\overset{NH_2}{|}}{C}}-COOH$$

Threonine, α-amino-β-hydroxybutyric acid (Thr). Here both a hydroxyl group and a methyl group have been substituted on alanine.

$$HO-\underset{\underset{H_3C}{|}}{\overset{\overset{H}{|}}{C}}-\underset{\underset{H}{|}}{\overset{\overset{NH_2}{|}}{C}}-COOH$$

59

Aromatic amino acids These consist of amino acids with phenyl, hydroxyphenyl, or indole rings substituted on alanine.

Phenylalanine, α-amino-β-phenylpropionic acid (Phe).

$$\text{C}_6\text{H}_5-\text{CH}_2-\overset{\displaystyle \overset{\text{NH}_2}{|}}{\underset{\displaystyle \underset{\text{H}}{|}}{\text{C}}}-\text{COOH}$$

Tyrosine, α-amino-β-hydroxyphenylpropionic acid (Tyr).

$$\text{HO}-\text{C}_6\text{H}_4-\text{CH}_2-\overset{\displaystyle \overset{\text{NH}_2}{|}}{\underset{\displaystyle \underset{\text{H}}{|}}{\text{C}}}-\text{COOH}$$

Tryptophan, α-amino-β-indolylpropionic acid (Try or Trp).

$$\text{indolyl}-\text{CH}_2-\overset{\displaystyle \overset{\text{NH}_2}{|}}{\underset{\displaystyle \underset{\text{H}}{|}}{\text{C}}}-\text{COOH}$$

Sulfur-containing amino acids Two monoamino-monocarboxylic acids containing sulfur are cysteine and methionine. A third is cystine, which is actually dicysteine and is a diamino-dicarboxylic acid.

Cysteine, α-amino-β-mercaptopropionic acid (CySH).

$$\text{HS}-\text{CH}_2-\overset{\displaystyle \overset{\text{NH}_2}{|}}{\underset{\displaystyle \underset{\text{H}}{|}}{\text{C}}}-\text{COOH}$$

Methionine, α-amino-γ-methylthiobutyric acid (Met). Here the group CH_3-S-CH_2 may be considered to be substituted on alanine.

$$\text{CH}_3-\text{S}-\text{CH}_2-\text{CH}_2-\overset{\displaystyle \overset{\text{NH}_2}{|}}{\underset{\displaystyle \underset{\text{H}}{|}}{\text{C}}}-\text{COOH}$$

Cystine, di-(α-amino-β-thiopropionic acid) (CyS-SCy or Cys).

$$\text{HOOC}-\overset{\displaystyle \overset{\text{NH}_2}{|}}{\underset{\displaystyle \underset{\text{H}}{|}}{\text{C}}}-\text{CH}_2-\text{S}-\text{S}-\text{CH}_2-\overset{\displaystyle \overset{\text{NH}_2}{|}}{\underset{\displaystyle \underset{\text{H}}{|}}{\text{C}}}-\text{COOH}$$

BASIC AMINO ACIDS

There are three so-called basic amino acids, all of which have six carbon atoms.

Lysine, α,ε-diaminocaproic acid (Lys).

$$\underset{\displaystyle H}{\overset{\displaystyle NH_2}{H_2N-CH_2-CH_2-CH_2-CH_2-\overset{|}{\underset{|}{C}}-COOH}}$$

Arginine, α-amino-δ-guanidinovaleric acid (Arg).

$$\underset{\displaystyle NH}{\overset{\displaystyle }{H_2N-\overset{\|}{C}-NH-CH_2-CH_2-CH_2-\overset{NH_2}{\underset{H}{\overset{|}{C}}}-COOH}}$$

Histidine, α-amino-β-imidazolylpropionic acid (His). An imidazole ring is substituted on alanine.

$$H-\text{(imidazole ring)}-CH_2-\underset{\displaystyle H}{\overset{\displaystyle NH_2}{\overset{|}{\underset{|}{C}}}}-COOH$$

ACIDIC AMINO ACIDS

There are two acidic amino acids, aspartic and glutamic, each having two carboxyl groups.

Aspartic acid, aminosuccinic acid (Asp). A carboxyl group may be considered substituted on alanine.

$$HOOC-CH_2-\underset{\displaystyle H}{\overset{\displaystyle NH_2}{\overset{|}{\underset{|}{C}}}}-COOH$$

Glutamic acid, α-aminoglutaric acid (Glu). Here the element of acetic acid has been added to alanine.

$$HOOC-CH_2-CH_2-\underset{\displaystyle H}{\overset{\displaystyle NH_2}{\overset{|}{\underset{|}{C}}}}-COOH$$

Aspartic acid and glutamic acid occur in proteins largely as the corresponding acid amides, asparagine and glutamine.

Asparagine (Asn)   **Glutamine (Gln)**

61

IMINO ACIDS

There are two heterocyclic or pyrrolidine amino acids, in which the α-amino nitrogen is part of a ring structure.

Proline, pyrrolidine-2-carboxylic acid (Pro).

Hydroxyproline, 4-hydroxypyrrolidine-2-carboxylic acid (Hypro).

The foregoing 20 amino acids are found in most proteins. There are, however, other α-amino acids that either are found free in the cell or participate as substituents in factors other than proteins, e.g., citrulline and ornithine, monoiodo- and diiodotyrosine, and thyroxine.

COMPOSITION OF PROTEINS

Until relatively recently, efforts to understand the biologic activity of proteins were limited to studies of the protein contents of amino acids. Amino acid analysis of proteins usually begins with an acid hydrolysis of the sample. In the past, some amino acids were determined by their selectively forming certain insoluble salts, which could then be isolated and weighed. Others were determined by means of specific color reactions. Still others were identified by the special nutritive requirements of some strains of microorganisms, mutant bacteria, or fungi that could be used in their microbiologic analyses. Specific enzymes were at times of value in determining the amounts of some amino acids present. Today, however, the most valuable procedure is ion-exchange chromatography (Appendix B). A sulfonated polystyrene resin is used in a continuous and automated process whereby all amino acids, with the exception of tryptophan, can be analyzed quantitatively on a single sample. Tryptophan is destroyed during acid hydrolysis and must be determined by other means.

Peculiarities in amino acid distributions of various proteins were sought in such data as given in Table 5-1. Gliadin, of wheat and rye flour, gives to bread dough the tacky consistency needed to trap gas bubbles during the rising process. Curiously this protein is almost 50% glutamic acid. Pepsin, a digestive enzyme, is 12% glutamic acid, and 9% tyrosine, while insulin, a hormone, is 18% glutamic acid, 12% cystine, and 13% tyrosine. Salmine, a constituent of the nucleoproteins of salmon sperm, is 87% arginine while

Table 5-1. Amino acid composition of some typical proteins
(as grams per 100 gm. of protein)*

Protein	Gliadin	Elastin	Horse hemoglobin	Egg albumin	Insulin	Pepsin	Wool	Casein	Silk fibroin	Oxhide collagen
Nitrogen	17.7	17.1	16.7	15.5	15.7	15.4	16.0	15.6	18.7	18.6
Sulfur	1.24	0.17	0.58	1.83	3.33	0.94		0.8	0.0	
Arginine	2.7	0.9	3.7	5.9	3.1	1.0	10.1	4.1	1.1	8.2
Histidine	2.3	0.1	8.7	2.6	4.9	0.9	1.0	3.1	0.4	0.7
Lysine	1.1	0.5	8.5	6.5	2.5	1.6	3.1	8.2	0.7	4.0
Tyrosine	3.2	1.6	3.0	3.7	13.0	8.5	5.5	6.3	12.8	0.99
Tryptophan	0.6	0	1.7	1.2	0.3	2.4	1.5	1.2	0.0	
Phenylalanine	6.9	5.0	7.7	7.7	8.1	6.4	4.0	5.0	3.4	2.4
Cystine	2.6	0.6	1.0	2.8	12.5	2.1	13.6	0.35	0.0	
Methionine	1.7	0.3	1.0	5.3	0.3	1.7	0.7	3.4	0.0	0.97
Threonine	2.1	1.3	4.4	4.0	2.1	9.6	6.5	4.9	1.6	2.3
Leucine	6.5	8.7	15.2	9.9	13.2	10.4	8.6	9.2	0.9	3.7
Isoleucine	5.4	4.0	0.2	7.0	2.8	10.8	4.3	6.1	1.1	1.9
Valine	2.7	17.4	9.0	8.8	7.8	7.1	5.4	7.2	3.6	2.5
Glutamic acid	45.7	2.1	8.2	16.5	18.6	11.9	14.0	23.3	2.2	11.2
Aspartic acid	1.3	0.6	10.6	9.3	6.8	16.0	7.4	7.1	2.6	7.0
Glycine	<0.5	29.9	5.6	3.1	4.3	6.4	6.8	2.7	43.6	26.6
Alanine	2.1	18.9	7.4	6.7	4.5		4.0	3.0	29.7	10.3
Proline	13.4	17.0	8.5	3.8	2.5	5.0	8.0	11.3	0.7	14.4
Serine	4.9	0.8	5.8	8.2	5.2	12.2	7.4	7.7	16.2	4.3
Hydroxyproline		2.0								12.8

° Courtesy R. J. Block; from Bowes, J. H., Elliott, R. G., and Moss, J. A.: Biochem. J. **61**:143, 1955.

collagen, with a tensile strength of steel, contains 29% proline and 27% glycine. Although such considerations were all that was possible at one time, they did not yield much information concerning biologic activity. Present-day knowledge of primary, secondary, and higher orders of protein structure comes closer to yielding answers. Still we are unable to determine why one protein can hydrolyze another.

STEREOISOMERISM

Examination of the formulas of the amino acids will reveal that all, except glycine, have an asymmetric carbon atom. It is, therefore, possible to have a D-form and an L-form of each. Most of the naturally occurring α-amino acids are of the L-form; i.e., their configuration is similar to that of L-glyceraldehyde or more appropriately L-serine.

L-Glyceraldehyde   L-Serine

By convention the structure for L-glyceraldehyde (p. 146) is written with the hydroxyl group to the left, provided the functional group, i.e., the aldehyde, is placed uppermost. Likewise, when serine is written with the carboxyl group uppermost, the amino group in the two-dimensional structure appears to the left of the carbon chain.

The D- and L-stereoisomers are mirror images and the two structures cannot be superimposed. Although all amino acids in most proteins are L-isomers, there are situations where the D-isomers also exist in nature. Thus the antibiotic gramicidin and the cell walls of certain bacteria contain D-amino acids. The D- and L-nomenclature refers to stereoisomerism, not to dextro- or levo-optical rotation. Some amino acids, e.g., histidine, exhibit dextro- and levo-rotation, depending on the pH of the environment.

SOLUBILITY

Amino acids exhibit a wide range of solubilities. Proline, for example, is soluble to the extent of 162 gm. per 100 gm. of water (25°), whereas cystine is soluble only to the extent of 0.011 gm. per 100 gm. (25°). In general, amino acids are minimally soluble at their isoelectric points.

Table 5-2. Ionization constants and isoelectric points for amino acids*

Amino acid (25° C.)	pK_1† (COOH)	pK_2	pK_3	pI‡
Alanine	2.34	9.69	. . . . .	6.00
Arginine	2.17	9.04 (NH_3^+)	12.48 (guanidinium)	10.76
Aspartic acid	1.88	3.65 (COOH)	9.60 (NH_3^+)	2.77
Cysteine (30°)	1.96	8.18 (SH)	10.28 (NH_3^+)	5.07
Glutamic acid	2.19	4.25 (COOH)	9.67 (NH_3^+)	3.22
Glycine	2.34	9.60	. . . . .	5.97
Histidine	1.82	6.00 (imidazolium)	9.17 (NH_3^+)	7.59
Leucine	2.36	9.60	. . . . .	5.98
Lysine	2.18	8.95 (α-NH_3^+)	10.53 (ϵ-NH_3^+)	9.74
Phenylalanine	1.83	9.13	. . . . .	5.48
Proline	1.99	10.60	. . . . .	6.30
Serine	2.21	9.15	. . . . .	5.68
Tryptophan	2.38	9.39	. . . . .	5.89
Tyrosine	2.20	9.11 (NH_3^+)	10.07 (OH)	5.66
Valine	2.32	9.62	. . . . .	5.96

*From Cohn, E. J., and Edsall, J. T.: Proteins, amino acids and peptides as ions and dipolar ions, New York, 1943, Reinhold Publishing Corp.
†See Appendix A, p. 886.
‡pI = isoelectric point.

ISOELECTRIC POINT

In an electrophoretic system, amino acids migrate to the pole of opposite charge to that of the ionic state or species in solution. Since amino acids have both amino and carboxyl groups, they are ampholytes and may be either positively or negatively charged depending on the hydrogen ion concentration of the environment. There is a characteristic pH at which the amino acid has no net charge and is not attracted to either electrode of the electrophoretic system. This hydrogen ion concentration is called the *isoelectric point*. It may or may not be at the neutral figure, pH 7.0, as seen from Table 5-2.

Although at its isoelectric point a monoamino-monocarboxylic acid is completely ionized, the charges present on the two ions neutralize each other. This gives, in aqueous solutions, dipolar ions or *zwitterions*.

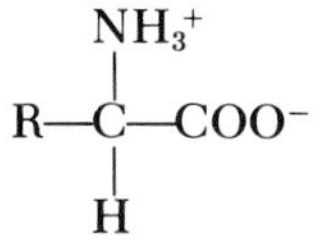

$$\begin{array}{c} NH_3^+ \\ | \\ R-C-COO^- \\ | \\ H \end{array}$$

If, now, an amino acid solution is titrated with an acid such as hydrochloric, the following reaction takes place:

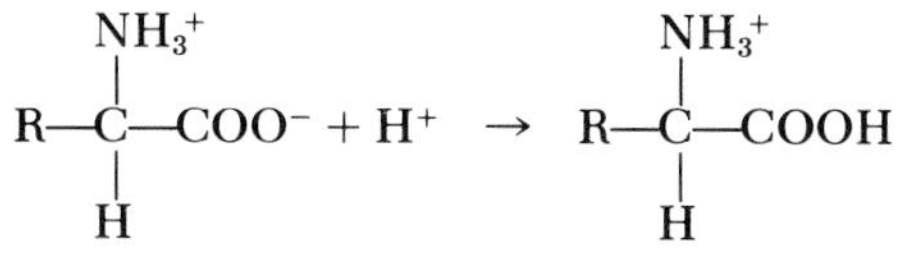

$$\begin{array}{c} NH_3^+ \\ | \\ R-C-COO^- + H^+ \\ | \\ H \end{array} \rightarrow \begin{array}{c} NH_3^+ \\ | \\ R-C-COOH \\ | \\ H \end{array}$$

The addition of an acid depresses the ionization of the carboxyl group, and the dipolar ion accepts the proton, thus placing a net positive charge on the amino acid molecule. In other words, in an electrophoretic system, this ionic species migrates toward the cathode. Its structure is more properly written in the salt form, i.e., as the amino acid hydrochloride.

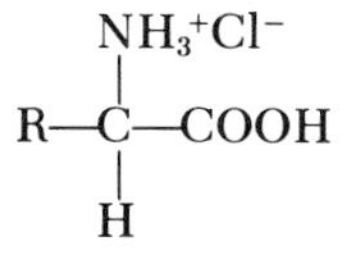

$$\begin{array}{c} NH_3^+Cl^- \\ | \\ R-C-COOH \\ | \\ H \end{array}$$

When the amino acid solution at its isoelectric point is titrated with an alkali, e.g., NaOH, the hydroxyl combines with the proton of the ammonium ion to form water. The amino acid then has a net negative charge from the carboxylate ion. The anionic amino acid species migrates anodically in an electrophoretic system.

Each carboxyl and amino group, as well as all other ionizable groups of an amino acid, has a characteristic pK value (Appendix A, p. 886), e.g., designated as pK_1, pK_2, etc., beginning with the most acidic group titrated. The pK values have been determined for all the common amino acids (Table 5-2).

TITRATION OF AMINO ACIDS

As shown above, each of the functional groups may be titrated either by acid or by alkali. This process follows a typical titration curve of weak acids and bases. Fig. 5-1 shows the curves for three amino acids, glycine, lysine,

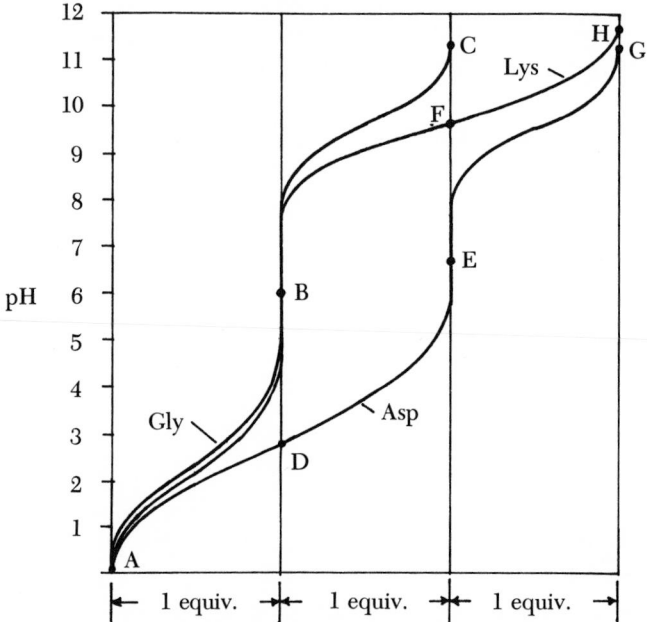

Fig. 5-1. Schematic titration curves for glycine, aspartic acid, and lysine. The following amino acid species exist in the solutions indicated by the lettered points on the graph.

Gly: *A.*
$$\underset{CH_2COOH}{\overset{NH_3^+}{|}}$$
B.
$$\underset{CH_2COO^-}{\overset{NH_3^+}{|}}$$
C.
$$\underset{CH_2COO^-}{\overset{NH_2}{|}}$$

Asp: *A.*
$$\begin{array}{c} COOH \\ | \\ CH_2 \\ | \\ CH-NH_3^+ \\ | \\ COOH \end{array}$$
D.
$$\begin{array}{c} COOH \\ | \\ CH_2 \\ | \\ CH-NH_3^+ \\ | \\ COO^- \end{array}$$
E.
$$\begin{array}{c} COO^- \\ | \\ CH_2 \\ | \\ CH-NH_3^+ \\ | \\ COO^- \end{array}$$
G.
$$\begin{array}{c} COO^- \\ | \\ CH_2 \\ | \\ CH-NH_2 \\ | \\ COO^- \end{array}$$

Lys: *A.*
$$\begin{array}{c} NH_3^+ \\ | \\ (CH_2)_4 \\ | \\ CH-NH_3^+ \\ | \\ COOH \end{array}$$
B.
$$\begin{array}{c} NH_3^+ \\ | \\ (CH_2)_4 \\ | \\ CH-NH_3^+ \\ | \\ COO^- \end{array}$$
F.
$$\begin{array}{c} NH_3^+ \\ | \\ (CH_2)_4 \\ | \\ CH-NH_2 \\ | \\ COO^- \end{array}$$
H.
$$\begin{array}{c} NH_2 \\ | \\ (CH_2)_4 \\ | \\ CH-NH_2 \\ | \\ COO^- \end{array}$$

and aspartic acid. In the curve for glycine, the isoelectric point occurs at a pH of 6.1 (*B*). Addition of hydrochloric acid equivalent to the amount of amino acid in solution results in the production of the hydrochloride or the cationic species (*A*), whereas the addition of an equivalent amount of sodium hydroxide results in the formation of the sodium salt or anionic species (*C*). When the carboxyl group is half neutralized by the addition of 0.5 equivalent of hydrochloric acid, the solution will contain an equal concentration of cationic and zwitterion species. In accord with the Henderson-Hasselbalch equation, at this point the pH will equal the pK. Since this is the pK for the carboxyl group, it is designated pK_1 and is 2.34 (Table 5-2). When alkali is added to the zwitterion species in an amount equal to half the glycine present, anionic glycine is formed equivalent to half the titratable ammonium or NH_3^+ groups. Since the solution now contains an equal amount of both zwitterion and anionic forms, the pH again equals the pK, but this time of the NH_3^+ group. The pK_2 of the NH_3^+ group is 9.60 (Table 5-2). The titration of each group, COOH and NH_3^+, follows the titration curve.

The location of these curves on the coordinates is determined by the various pK values. At each pH the amino acid solution contains a definable proportion of ionic species. If we titrate from pH 1 to 6, the solutions contain proportions of species *B* and *A*; from pH 6 to 11, the species are *C* and *B*. The proportions of species are defined by the Henderson-Haselbalch equation. One must keep in mind that the titratable groups are defined in accordance with the Brønsted definition of acid and base. In other words, a substance contributing protons to a solution, whether it is a COOH or NH_3^+ group, is called an acid; any group accepting protons is a base.

The titration of either group has been used as a means for the quantitative determination of an amino acid. Titration from a pH of 6 to 12, however, presents certain technical difficulties, which in the past were surmounted by resorting to the so-called *formol titration*. Neutralized formaldehyde solution added to a neutral amino acid solution results in a distinctly acidic mixture. Formaldehyde reacts only with the free amino group, not with the ammonium ion.

$$
\begin{array}{c}
\underset{H}{\overset{NH_2}{R-C-C}}\overset{O}{\underset{OH}{\diagdown}} + 2\ CH_2O \rightleftharpoons \underset{H}{\overset{\overset{HOH_2C\diagdown\ \diagup CH_2OH}{N}}{R-C-C}}\overset{O}{\underset{OH}{\diagdown}}
\end{array}
$$

The presence of the aldehyde diminishes the concentration of R—NH₂ species in the Henderson-Hasselbalch equation, thereby lowering the ratio of R—NH₂/R—NH₃⁺ and consequently lowering the pH. Despite the presence of the formaldehyde, the function of sodium hydroxide, used to titrate the amino acid, continues to be to strip protons from the R—NH₃⁺ species. The R—NH₂ forms are converted to the dimethylol derivative, thereby always reducing the RNH₂/RNH₃⁺ ratio. The effect is to produce a new titration curve in a more acidic range; the presence of the aldehyde leads to a new pK_2 value.

Table 5-3. pK Values of acidic and basic groups found in proteins[*]

Group	pK (25°)
α-Carboxyl	3.0– 3.2
β-Carboxyl (Asp)	3.0– 4.7
γ-Carboxyl (Glu)	About 4.4
Imidazolium	5.6– 7.0
α-Ammonium	7.6– 8.4
ε-Ammonium (Lys)	9.4–10.6
Sulfhydryl	9.1–10.8
Phenolic hydroxyl (Tyr)	9.8–10.4
Guanidinium (Arg)	11.6–12.6

[*] From Cohn, E. J., and Edsall, J. T.: Proteins, amino acids and peptides as ions and dipolar ions, New York, 1943, Reinhold Publishing Corp.

In the presence of formaldehyde, it is possible to titrate the amino acid with the aid of an ordinary indicator, e.g., phenolphthalein, since the entire titration curve for the amino group is complete between pH 6 and 8.

In proteins, the pK values of the various functional groups are somewhat modified from the values of free amino acids (compare Table 5-2 with Table 5-3). A consideration of the pK values in Table 5-3 shows that the maximal buffering capacity at a physiologic pH of 7.4 would depend upon α-ammonium and the imidazolium groups. Since, however, the α-ammonium groups occur only at terminal residues of the polypeptide chain, their quantity is too small to contribute significantly to the buffering action of proteins. The important buffering system (protein) $(H^+)/(protein\ H^+)$ is due largely to the ionization of the histidine (imidazolium) residues.

REACTIONS OF AMINO ACIDS

Amino acids yield a number of specific color reactions, which have been used traditionally for the purposes of identification. Today they are sometimes used to locate specific amino acids on paper chromatographs. Proteins containing the amino acids in question also yield the reaction. Some of the commonly used reactions are given in Table 5-4.

The following are general reactions of amino acids. In most instances, these are typical of reactions used in either the determination of structure or the synthesis of peptides:

1. All amino acids can be esterified.

$$CH_3-\underset{\underset{H}{|}}{\overset{\overset{NH_2}{|}}{C}}-C\overset{O}{\underset{OH}{\diagdown}} \xrightarrow{C_2H_5OH} CH_3-\underset{\underset{H}{|}}{\overset{\overset{NH_2}{|}}{C}}-C\overset{O}{\underset{OC_2H_5}{\diagdown}} + H_2O$$

Alanine ethyl ester

This property was used by Emil Fischer for the separation of amino acids by fractional distillation of their volatile esters.

Table 5-4. Amino acid reactions

Test	Conditions, reagents:	color	Amino acid
Xanthoproteic	Concentrated nitric acid:	yellow	Tyr and Trp
Millon	Mercurous nitrate in nitric acid:	red	Tyr
Hopkins-Cole	Glyoxylic acid in concentrated sulfuric acid	red	Trp
Sakaguchi	α-Naphthol and sodium hypochlorite:	red	Arg
Nitroprusside	Sodium nitroprusside in dilute ammonium hydroxide:	red	CySH
Pauly	Diazotized sulfanilic acid in alkaline medium:	red	His and Tyr

2. Amino acids can be acetylated and benzoylated.

Acetylation reactions are of general importance in the synthesis of peptides. In vivo, glycine is benzoylated to yield hippuric acid, which is of importance as a detoxication mechanism (p. 751).

3. Amino acids react with ninhydrin. If a solution of an α-amino acid is boiled with ninhydrin (triketohydrindene hydrate), carbon dioxide is split off and a color is produced. With the exception of proline and hydroxyproline, which give a yellow color, all α-amino acids, peptides, and proteins yield varying shades of purple.

The visualization of amino acids on paper chromatographs and the quantitative determination of amino acids following ion-exchange chromatography usually involve the ninhydrin reaction.

4. The free amino groups of amino acids or of peptides react with fluorodi-nitrobenzene to form the dinitrophenyl derivatives, which are yellow dyes. These can readily be separated by suitable procedures of paper chromatography.

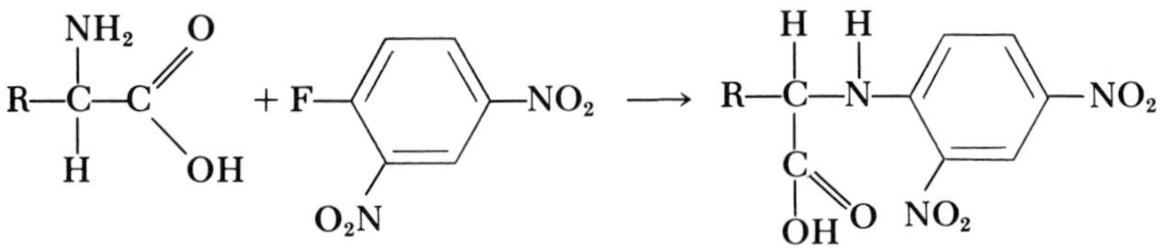

5. Amino acids also react with certain heavy metals by the process of chelation. Such ions as Cu^{++}, Co^{++}, Mn^{++}, and Ca^{++} react with amino acids to form chelates in the following manner:

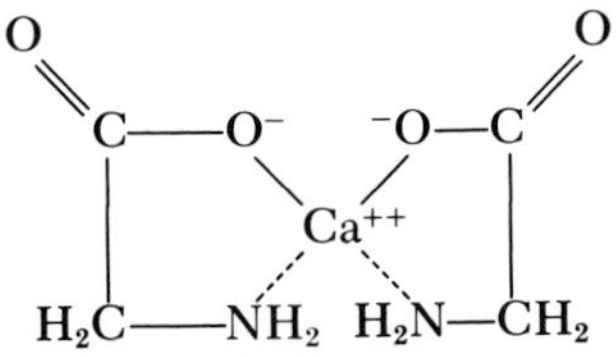

Calcium diglycinate

Chelation is the grasping of secondary valence bonds by the metallic ion. Chelates are non-ionic; therefore, amino acids and other chelate formers may be used to remove calcium from the bones and teeth. It is possible that dietary amino acids could, in this way, form soluble calcium complexes, causing a loss of calcium and the possible development of caries. Chelating agents have been used for removing calcium from the cornea in ocular lesions.

PEPTIDE LINKAGE

When two amino acids are joined by the union of a carboxyl and an amino group, with the elimination of a molecule of water, a *dipeptide* is formed.

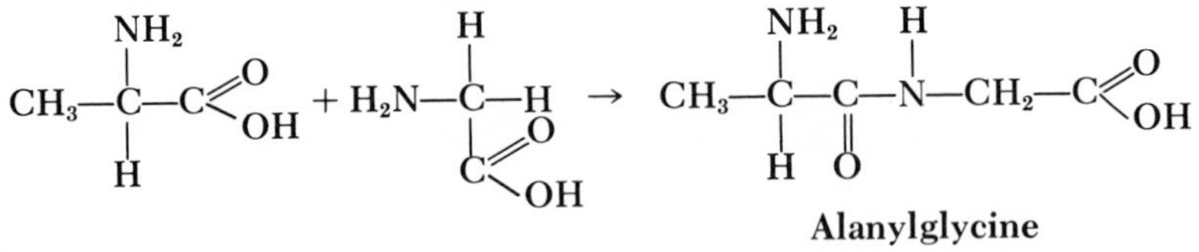

Alanylglycine

A third amino acid will form a *tripeptide* by being linked through its carboxyl to the amino of the first amino acid or through its amino group to the carboxyl of the second. The special amide link that joins the α-amino acids together is called the peptide bond.

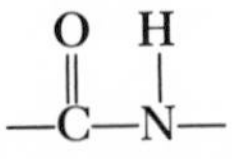

The convention used to name *peptides* or *polypeptides* is shown in the following example. Note that the amino acid contributing the free amino group (N-terminal) is named first and placed to the left in the sequence. The free carboxyl (C-terminal) is placed on the right side, and its amino acid is named last.

Alanyl-leucyl-cysteinyl-tyrosyl-glycine

The role of the peptide bond in protein structure was proposed in 1902, by Hofmeister, and also by Fischer. Numerous lines of evidence have been advanced in the ensuing years for the validity of this hypothesis. One test that demonstrates the specific presence of peptide bonds is the so-called *biuret test*. This reaction involves the addition of a very dilute solution of copper sulfate to an alkaline protein solution. The minimal presence of two neighboring peptide bonds, as in a tripeptide, results in the formation of a lavender color.

The successful synthesis of biologically active substances such as vasopressin, oxytocin, insulin, and ribonuclease leaves no doubt as to the central role of the peptide bond in the primary structure of proteins.

SYNTHESIS OF PEPTIDES

The process of producing a dipeptide of predictable structure was developed by Bergmann in 1935. For the purpose of illustration, a procedure for the synthesis of alanylglycine, but not glycylalanine, will be outlined. To do this, it is first necessary to block the free amino group of alanine so that it cannot enter into subsequent reactions. This must be accomplished by means of a reagent that forms a derivative of the amino acid and can later be removed without resorting to hydrolytic steps since hydrolysis would obviously result in splitting the dipeptide. Bergmann developed a process using the reagent carbobenzoxy chloride.

Benzyl alcohol   Phosgene   Carbobenzoxy chloride

Alanine plus carbobenzoxy chloride yields the carbobenzoxy derivative of alanine (abbreviated Cbz-Ala). The derivative is then treated with phosphorus pentachloride to form the corresponding acyl chloride of Cbz-Ala. The peptide bond may be formed by adding glycine.

The final product is the carbobenzoxy derivative of the alanylglycine. Treatment with hydrogen, in the presence of a platinum catalyst, leads to the release of a free amino group and the desired dipeptide.

This classic procedure serves to illustrate the two essential steps for the directed synthesis of peptides. These are the protection of amino acid groups not intended to participate in the reaction and the activation of the carboxyl group involved in the newly formed peptide bond. Numerous biologically active peptides have been synthesized using such procedures. Notable were the syntheses by du Vigneaud of vasopressin and oxytocin, two octapeptide hormones of the posterior pituitary gland. Other synthetic hormones are MSH or melanocyte-stimulating hormone (1960) and ACTH or corticotropin (1961). To advance from the synthesis of a large peptide, 23 amino acid residues in synthetic ACTH, to that of a protein was still a major step. The smallest protein is insulin, which is actually composed of two individual peptides of average size (p. 76). To produce insulin was comparable to synthesis of two peptide chains. Katsoyannis and co-workers succeeded in synthesizing the 21-residue A-chain of sheep insulin in 1963, while Zahn and his group in Germany synthesized the 30-residue B-chain. In 1965, a Chinese group of investigators succeeded in combining A- and B-chains and produced the first crystalline all-synthetic insulin.

Recently (1969) Denkwalter and co-workers completed the synthesis of the enzyme ribonuclease by means of classic procedures such as described above. At the same time Merrifield and his group also reported the synthesis of the 124-residue ribonuclease using the automatic *solid-phase* process. Both preparations were enzymatically active.

The automatic solid-phase synthesis of proteins[1] represents a major tech-

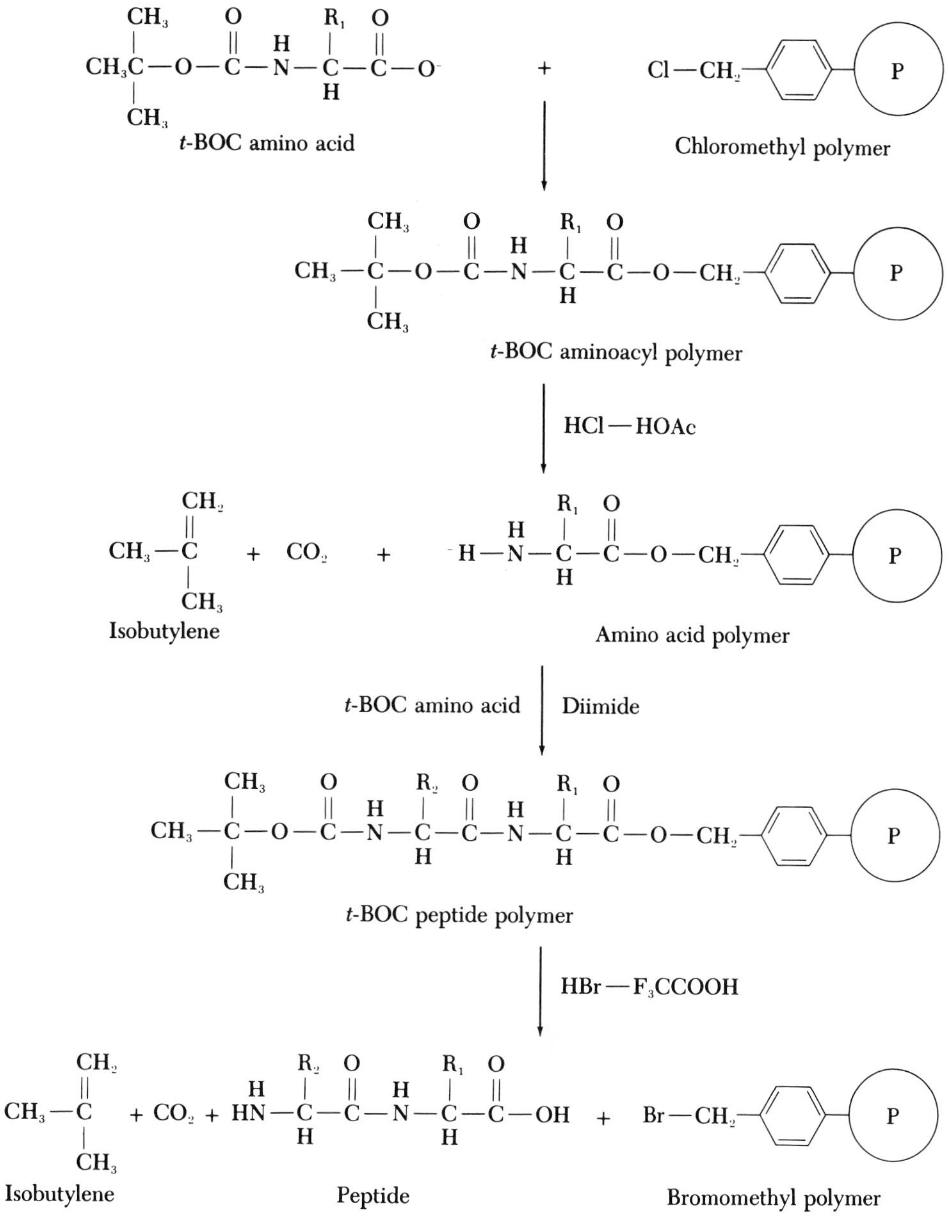

Fig. 5-2. General reaction scheme for solid-phase peptide synthesis. (From Merrifield, R. B.: Recent Progr. Hormone Res. 23:451, 1967.)

nologic breakthrough that will make possible the synthesis of many larger protein molecules. In this procedure, the peptide chains are assembled in a stepwise fashion, not in solution but while anchored chemically to small solid polystyrene beads. The carboxyl terminal amino acids of the peptide to be synthesized are attached to the polystyrene by means of a benzyl ester bond (Fig. 5-2).

The second amino acid, with its amino group protected by a tertiary butyl-oxycarbonyl group, is suitably activated. In the example of Fig. 5-2, the dicyclocarbodiimide (diimide) is used as the coupling agent. At the end of the synthesis of the polypeptide chain, the resin is suspended in anhydrous trifluoroacetic acid and dry hydrogen bromide is used to split the peptide from the polystyrene beads. This also removes many of the protecting groups. The entire procedure is accomplished in an automatic apparatus. One cycle of the synthesis requires about 4 hours, so it is possible to assemble six amino acids per day.

The automatic procedure has been used to synthesize such peptide hormones as bradykinin, angiotensin, and oxytocin as well as the antibiotics gramicidin S and tyrocidin. Insulin has also been synthesized in this apparatus. The road is now open to produce biologic analogues that differ from the parent proteins in precisely known ways. This procedure will also help produce hormones with greater or more prolonged activity than the natural ones. Studies of other protein analogues will make it possible to learn how the sequence of amino acids determines overall protein structure and biologic activity.

PRIMARY STRUCTURE

Obviously, before a protein such as insulin can be synthesized, it is necessary to determine the exact amino acid sequence or the primary structure. Insulin is the first protein for which a complete amino acid sequence was established (Sanger,[1a] 1956).

It is customary first to identify the N- and C-terminal amino acids. The N-terminal amino acid may be obtained by treating the protein with fluorodinitrobenzene. As mentioned previously (p. 70), this reagent will react with free amino groups and especially with those free α-amino groups found on the N-terminal end of the protein. The C-N bond formed between the amino group and the benzene ring is resistant to acid hydrolysis. Acid hydrolysis of the DNP-protein yields a mixture of all the constituent amino acids plus the DNP-derivative of the formerly N-terminal residue(s). The identity of these DNP–amino acids then may be established by paper chromatography. In the case of insulin, two DNP–amino acids were found in equal amounts, i.e., glycine and phenylalanine. Barring the possibility that some contaminant caused the second DNP-derivative, this observation was interpreted to mean that the protein insulin is composed of two polypeptide chains.

Another technique for the determination of N-terminal amino acids in a peptide chain involves the reaction with phenylisothiocyanate (Edman's reagent). In acid the phenylthiocarbamyl peptide (or protein) is degraded by a nonhydrolytic process yielding the phenylthiohydantoin (PTH) of the terminal amino acid. The PTH–amino acid is identified chromatographically. The reaction with phenylisothiocyanate is then repeated with the newly formed N-terminal amino acid.

Phenylisothiocyanate   **Peptide**

Phenylthiocarbamyl peptide

Phenylthiohydantoin   **Residual**
(PTH)   **peptide**

Determination of the amino acid sequence may be accomplished in this fashion. The process has been automated in an apparatus called the *protein sequenator*. With this apparatus it has been possible to establish the sequence of the first 60 amino acids of whale myoglobin.

The high concentration of sulfur and specifically the amino acid cystine lead to the suggestion that the two chains of insulin are held together by another bond that is important in protein structure, i.e., the disulfide linkage. Treatment of insulin with performic acid results in the oxidation of the disulfide link into sulfonic acid groups and the separation of the two chains. Once separated, the two chains can be isolated by chromatography. Further studies then may be performed on the N-terminal–glycyl A-chain, having 21 amino acids, and the N-terminal–phenylalanyl B-chain, with 30 residues.

It is also important to identify the C-terminal amino acids. This may be accomplished by treating the peptide with the enzyme carboxypeptidase, which attacks only the peptide bond joining the C-terminal amino acid to the chain. The amino acids released by this process can be identified and their

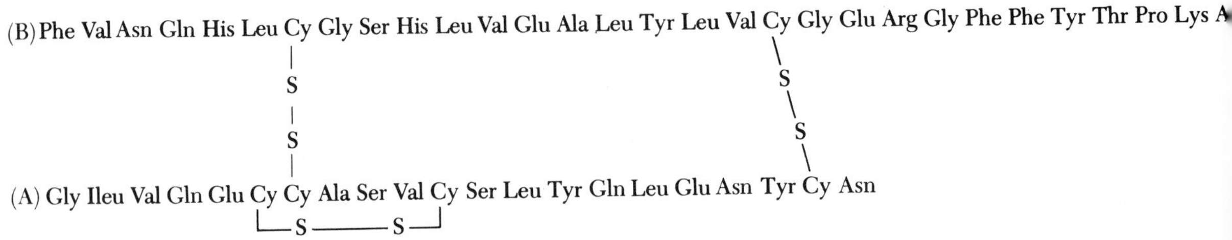

(B) Phe Val Asn Gln His Leu Cy Gly Ser His Leu Val Glu Ala Leu Tyr Leu Val Cy Gly Glu Arg Gly Phe Phe Tyr Thr Pro Lys A
S
S
S
S
(A) Gly Ileu Val Gln Glu Cy Cy Ala Ser Val Cy Ser Leu Tyr Gln Leu Glu Asn Tyr Cy Asn
S —— S

Fig. 5-3. Primary structure of beef insulin. (From Sanger, F.: Science **129**:1340, 1959.)

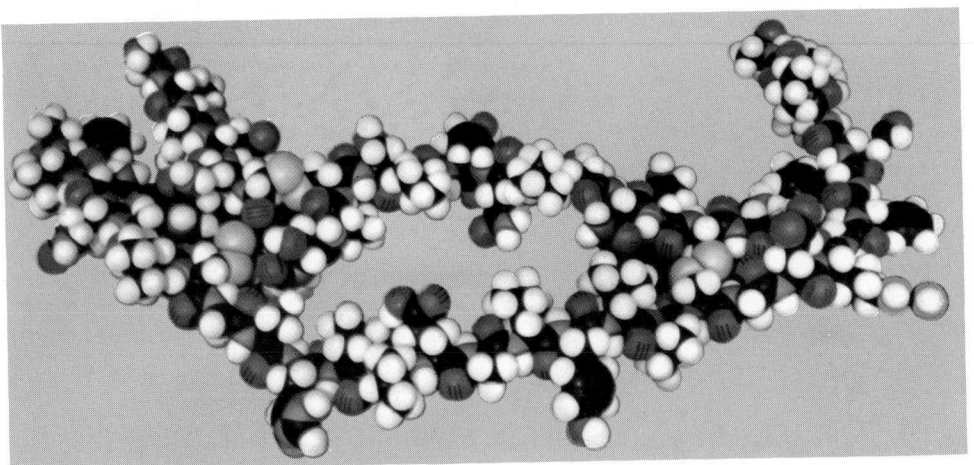

Fig. 5-4. Space-filling model of bovine insulin. (Courtesy R. A. Harte.)

Lys
Glu
Thr
Ala
NH2
Ala→Ala→Lys→Phe→Glu→Arg→Gln→His→Met→Asp→Ser→Ser→Thr→Ser→Ala→Ala
Ser
Ser
Ser
Asn
Tyr
Cys
Asn
Glu
Met
Met
Lys
Ser→Arg→Asn→Leu→Thr→Lys→Asp→Arg→Cys→Lys→Pro→Val→Asn→Thr→Phe→Val→His→Glu
Ser
Leu
Ala
Asp
Val
Gln→Ala→Val→Cys→Ser→Gln→Lys
Asn
Val
Ala→Cys→Lys→Asn
Gly
Gln
Thr→Asn→Cys→Tyr→Gln→Ser→Tyr→Ser→Thr→Met→Ser
Ileu
Thr
Asp
Cys
Arg
Glu
Thr
Gly
Ser
Ser→Lys→Tyr→Pro→Asn→Cys→Ala→Tyr→Lys→Thr→Thr→Gln→Ala→Asn→Lys
His
Ileu
Ileu
Val→Ala→Cys→Glu→Gly→Asn→Pro→Tyr→Val→Pro→Val→His→Phe→Asp→Ala→Ser→Val
COOH
I
II
III
IV
V
VI
VII
VIII

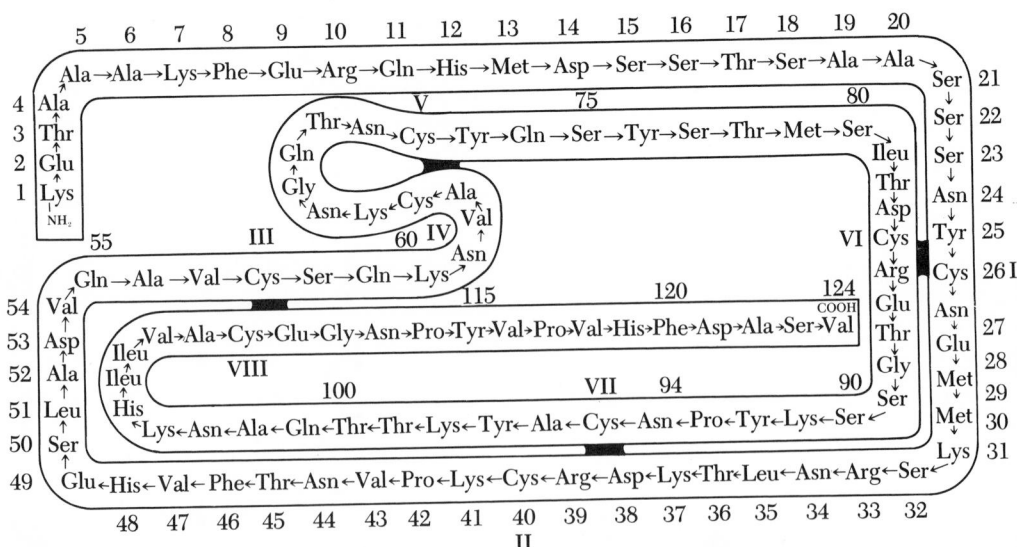

Fig. 5-5. Sequence of amino acid residues in bovine pancreatic ribonuclease-A, based on experiments of Hirs and associates, Spackman and associates, and Smyth and associates. (Modified from Smyth, D. G., Stein, W. H., and Moore, S.: J. Biol. Chem. **238**:227, 1963.)

rates of release measured by paper chromatography. For example, the C-terminal amino acids of insulin A- and B-chains are asparagine and alanine, respectively.

The polypeptide chains are usually partially hydrolyzed into a mixture of small peptide chains that can be separated by ion-exchange chromatography. The amino acid sequence of each peptide is then readily determined. This may be accomplished in part by identifying the N- and C-terminal residues of the amino acids. The principle whereby the amino acid sequence of the original polypeptide may be deduced from the individual sequences of the small peptides obtained by hydrolysis is illustrated below. This illustration utilizes the first eight amino acid residues of the A-chain of insulin. Eight small peptides are separated and their sequences determined to identify areas of overlapping amino acids. In this example, only one peptide contains glycine and, therefore, contributes the N-terminal sequence of the original A-chain.

Gly-Ileu-Val-Glu

Ileu-Val

Ileu-Val-Glu

Ileu-Val-Glu-Glu

Val-Glu

Glu-Glu

Glu-Cys

Glu-Cys-Cys-Ala

Cys-Cys-Ala

Thus the sequence of the first eight amino acids in the A-chain of insulin is Gly-Ileu-Val-Glu-Glu-Cys-Cys-Ala-. The complete primary structure for beef insulin is shown in Fig. 5-3, while a three-dimensional model of this protein is shown in Fig. 5-4. Insulin from other animals differs in three amino acids. Instead of Ala, Ser, and Val in positions 8 to 10 of the A-chain, human insulin has Thr, Ser, and Ileu, while sheep insulin has Ala, Gly, and Val.

Hirs, Moore, and Stein have determined the complete amino acid sequence of the enzyme ribonuclease, a much larger molecule than insulin (Fig. 5-5). Another enzyme for which we know the primary structure is lysozyme, with 129 amino acids. One of the longest single protein chains for which the complete sequence of amino acids is known is the enzyme subtilisin, of *Bacterium subtilis*, with 275 residues. This protein has an N-terminal alanine and a C-terminal glutamine. The structure of the first viral protein to be determined was that of tobacco mosaic virus. This protein is composed of 158 amino acid residues in a single chain. The N- and C-terminal residues are acetylserine and threonine, respectively.

SECONDARY STRUCTURE

Studies of model peptides using the x-ray diffraction method have shown the distance between the α-carbon and the peptide bond nitrogen to be 1.47 Å (Diagram A). This is longer than the interatomic distance of 1.32 Å between the carbonyl C and the peptide N. In other words, it is intermediate between

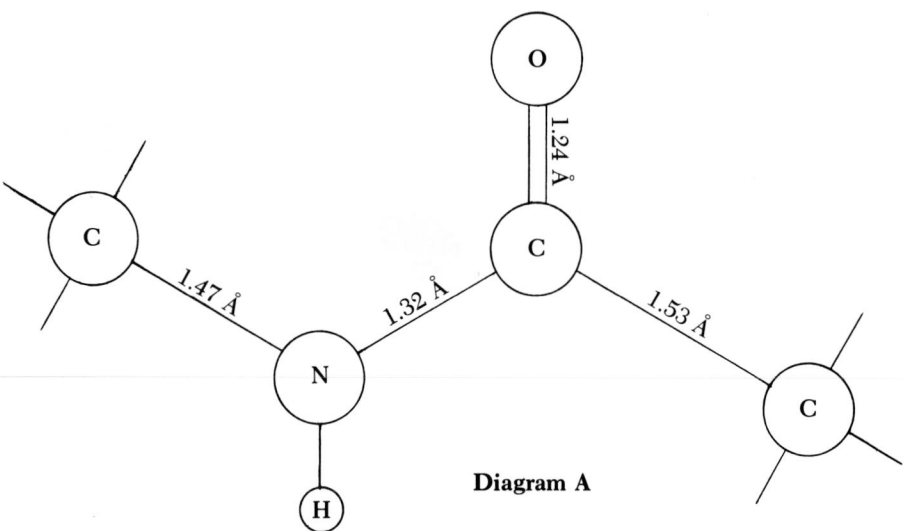

Diagram A

1.24 Å of the C=O and the regular C—N, suggesting that it is similar to the double bond. According to Pauling and his co-workers, the peptide bond actually exists in a resonance state between a single bond and a double bond (Diagram B).

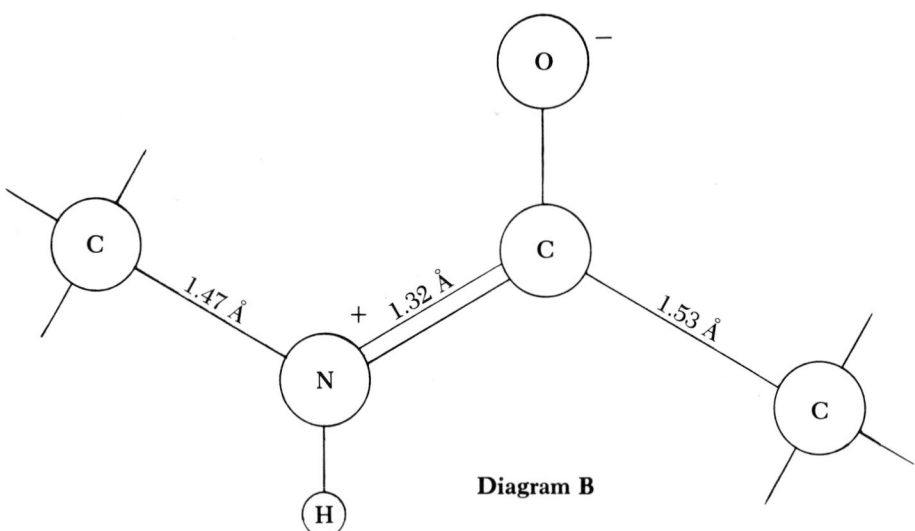

Diagram B

A direct consequence of the resonating state is that the otherwise tetrahedral carboxyl carbon and imino nitrogen lie in a plane. In other words, the carboxyl carbon, oxygen, nitrogen, and amide hydrogen all are part of a planar unit that is common to protein structures.

Two kinds of relationships between adjoining planar units are possible. One may be turned to either the right or the left of a reference plane (Fig. 5-6). If all subsequent planes are in the same direction, a helix results. Of the two possible helices, a right- or left-handed one, the right-handed appears to be the more stable, provided the amino acids are of the L- configuration. The α-helix model, which is in accord with x-ray diffraction data, has a total of 3.6

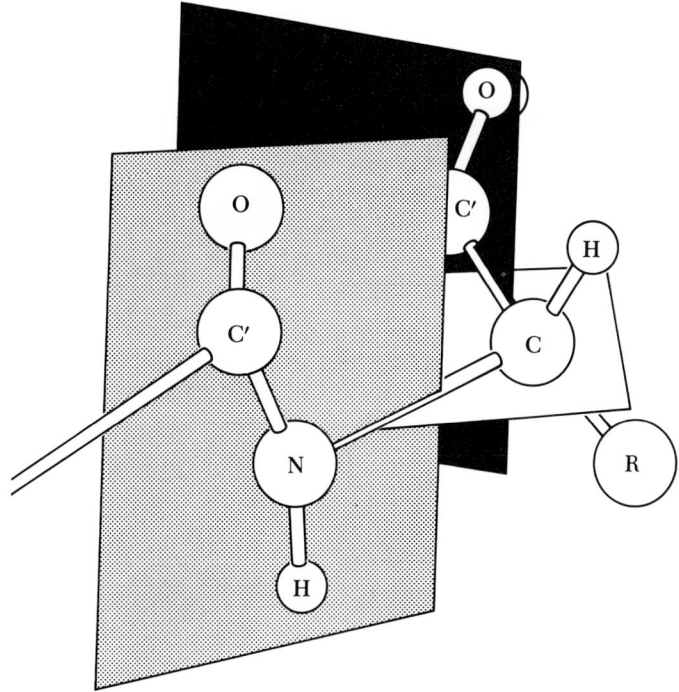

Fig. 5-6. Two planar peptide groups linked by an α-carbon, showing a segment of a right-handed helix of L-amino acids. (Modified from Schellman, J. A., and Schellman, C.: In Neurath, H., editor: The proteins—composition, structure and function, New York, 1964, Academic Press, Inc., vol. 2, p. 1.)

amino acid residues per turn and a pitch or spacing between turns of 5.4 Å (Fig. 5-7, A).

If neighboring planar peptide units have an alternate right-left arrangement, the structure is said to be of the "pleated sheet" or β-type. The pleated sheet form is commonly found in keratin and silk. In these proteins, the polypeptide units lie in parallel relation to one another and exhibit intermolecular hydrogen bonding (Fig. 5-7, B).

A third arrangement is the so-called random coil, in which there is no consistent relationship between planes and no stabilizing hydrogen bonds (Fig. 5-7, C).

The helical content may be determined by ultraviolet absorption and by *optical rotatory dispersion* (ORD) methods. The following list indicates approximately the variation in percentage of α-helix in several proteins.

Silk fibroin	12%
Ribonuclease	40%
Chymotrypsin	49%
Insulin	66%
Ovalbumin	81%
Myoglobin	82%

A procedure that is illustrative of the existence of hydrogen bonding in the secondary structure is the method of hydrogen-deuterium exchange. The principle of this method is that hydrogen atoms are free to exchange with those of the environment, i.e., H_2O, provided they are not involved in some form of bonding, as, for example, hydrogen bonds. In this procedure the protein in question is dissolved in deuterium-enriched water. The protein is allowed to equilibrate so that all exchangeable protons are replaced with deuterium. The protein is then lyophilized and redissolved in ordinary water. The rate of disappearance of deuterium into solution is a measure of readily exchangeable hydrogen. By such a method insulin contains 60% hard-to-exchange hydrogen, which presumably is that involved in intramolecular hydrogen bonding of the helical portion.

The α-helix is made rigid by intramolecular hydrogen bonds between carbonyl oxygens and amide nitrogens as indicated in Fig. 5-7, A.

Why certain regions of a protein are helical and others not is difficult to ascertain. In the case of insulin, we might reason that the helical portions are

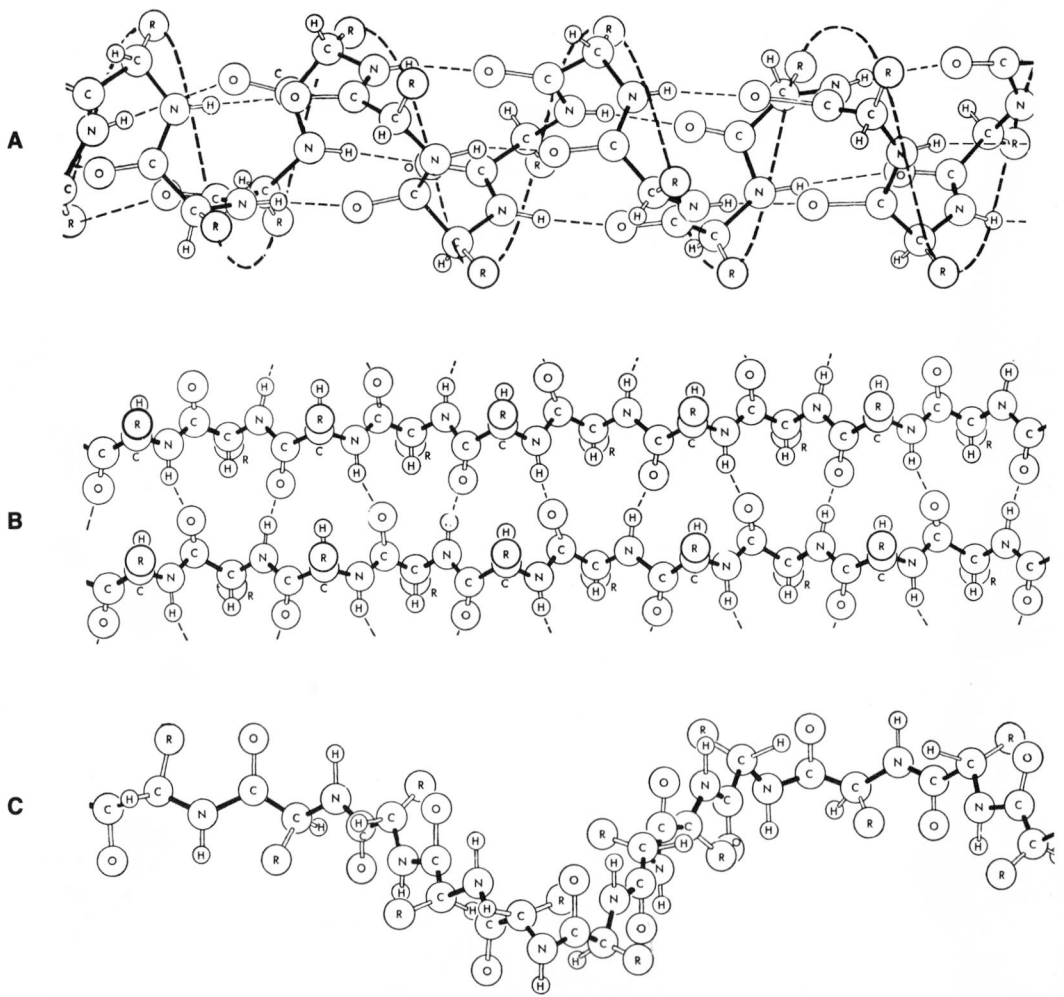

Fig. 5-7. For legend see opposite page.

maintained by the cross-linking disulfide bonds. Consideration of Fig. 5-7 suggests that random coiling would prevail "outside" the disulfide cross-links. This random coiled region would then be the location of areas of rapid hydrogen-deuterium exchange.

A departure from helical structure occurs at peptide bonds involving the amino acid proline or hydroxyproline. The nitrogens of these heterocyclic amino acids are incapable of forming a resonating peptide structure, so the peptide unit cannot exist in a planar arrangement.

A singular helical structure, not of the α-type, is observed in collagen, an important protein of connective tissues (Chapter 18). Collagen is unique in having 25% proline and hydroxyproline, which, as mentioned, excludes the α-helical form. Instead, this protein consists of three intertwined polypeptide chains each in a left-handed helical conformation (p. 78). The pitch of this structure is 9.4 Å, compared with 5.4 Å for the α-helix. There are three residues per turn instead of 3.6 as for the α-helix.

TERTIARY STRUCTURE

If a protein molecule, e.g., myoglobin, were simply an extended α-helical polypeptide chain, its length would be 20 times its width. X-ray diffraction data, however, have led to the following conclusions (see Fig. 5-8): First, the molecule is compact, with no more than five water molecules trapped inside the structure. Second, nearly all polar groups lie on the surface, whereas the interior is almost entirely nonpolar. Third, all surface polar groups, including free peptide carbonyl and amide groups, have bound water molecules. Thus we have the picture of a folded molecule so arranged as to give a football-like shape with dimensions of 43 × 35 × 25 Å. Kendrew[2] proposed the structure

---

Fig. 5-7. Configurations of polypeptide chains. A, Alpha helix gives a polypeptide chain a linear structure, shown here in three-dimensional perspective. The atoms in the repeating unit (CCONHC) lie in a plane; the change in angle between one unit and the next occurs at the C to which the side group R is attached. The helix is held rigid by the hydrogen bond (broken straight lines) between the H attached to the N in one group and the O attached to the C three groups along the chain. The curved wavy broken line traces the turns of the helix. B, Beta configuration ties two or more polypeptide chains to one another in crystalline structures. Here the hydrogen bonds do not contribute to the internal organization of the chain, as in the α-helix, but link the H's of one chain to the O's in the adjoining chain. The β-configuration is found in silk and a few other fibers. Polypeptide chains in muscle and other contractile fibers may make reversible transitions from α- to β-configuration when in action. C, Random chain is the configuration assumed by the polypeptide molecule in solution, when hydrogen bonds are not formed. The flat configuration of the repeating unit remains, but the chain rotates about the C's to which the side groups are attached. The random chain may be formed from an α-helix when hydrogen bonds are disrupted in solution. A polypeptide chain may make a reversible transition from the α-helix to random chain, depending on the acid-base balance of the solution. (From Doty, P.: Sci. Amer. **197**:173, 1957.)

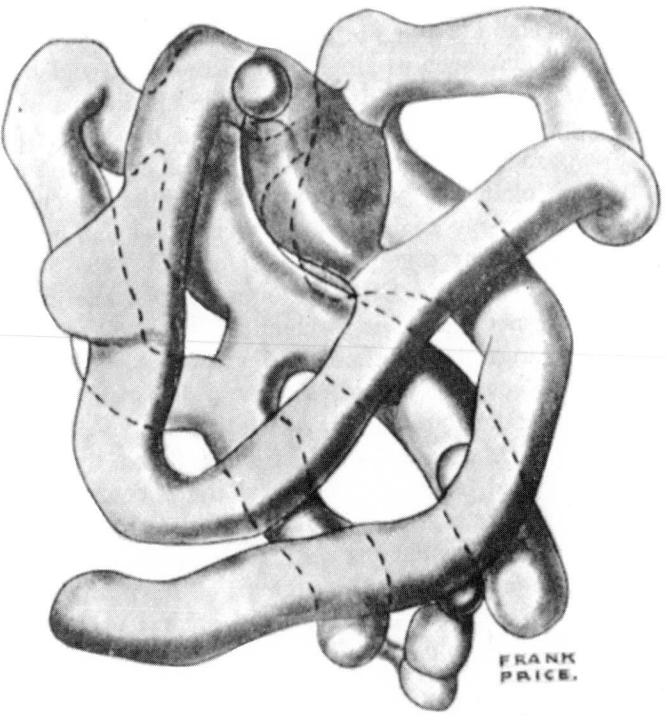

Fig. 5-8. Three-dimensional model of the myoglobin molecule obtained by x-ray analysis. (From Perlmann, G. E., and Diringer, R.: Ann. Rev. Biochem. 29:167, 1960; redrawn from Kendrew, J. C., et al.: Nature 181:662, 1958.)

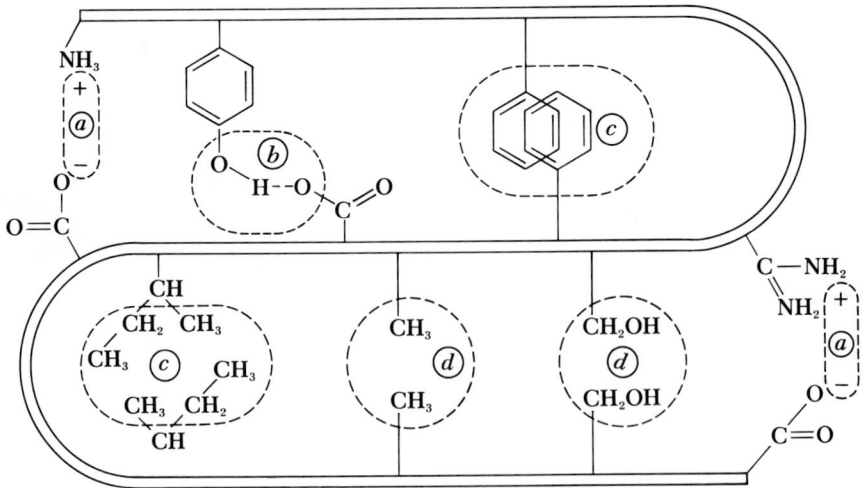

Fig. 5-9. Some noncovalent bonds that stabilize proteins. *a*, Electrostatic interaction; *b*, hydrogen bonding between tyrosine residues and carboxylate groups; *c*, interaction of nonpolar side chains caused by the mutual repulsion of solvent; *d*, van der Waals interactions. (From Anfinsen, C. B.: The molecular basis of evolution, New York, 1959, John Wiley & Sons, Inc.)

visualized in Fig. 5-8, in which the folded structure or tertiary conformation has seven α-helical regions. Although foldings may occur at proline residues, there are not enough proline-hydroxyproline residues to account for all regions of folding. The reason for nonproline folding and for the beginning and ending of α-helical regions is still unclear. Myoglobin has all hydrophobic (aliphatic, aromatic) residues turned inward and coming within van der Waals distances of one another. The attraction between hydrophobic residues, which represent an important factor in the tertiary conformation, is caused by an exclusion of solvent and by van der Waals forces (Fig. 5-9).

Tertiary structures may also be stabilized by other types of bonds, especially disulfide bonds. Pancreatic ribonuclease (Fig. 5-5) is a well-known example in which four disulfide bonds maintain the tertiary conformation.

Generally speaking, proteins have a three-dimensional structure or conformation.[3] Often proteins are classed as globular or fibrous, depending on whether the axial ratio (molecular length to width) is less or greater than 10. Proteins such as keratin, fibrinogen, and myosin are fibrous and have axial ratios greater than 10. Insulin, on the other hand, is almost spheric; other examples of globular proteins are albumin and plasma globulins, having axial ratios not over 3:1 or 4:1.

QUATERNARY STRUCTURE

Proteins have very large molecular weights, ranging between 5000 and several million. Some representative molecular weights are given in Table 5-5.

Molecular weights may be determined by physical and chemical means. For example, in hemoglobin the molecular weight may be calculated on the basis of the readily measured iron content of 0.34%. If we assume that there is at least one atom of iron per molecule, i.e., 1 gm. atom per molecular weight, then the molecular weight may be calculated as:

$$0.34/100 = 55.8/x$$

$$x = 16,400$$

This is known as the *minimal molecular weight*. Molecular weights may also be determined by ultracentrifugation (Appendix, p. 903) or by measure-

Table 5-5. Molecular weights of some proteins

Protein	Molecular weight	Protein	Molecular weight
Insulin	5,734	Ovalbumin	44,000
Ribonuclease	13,000	Hemoglobin	67,000
Trypsin	13,500	Serum albumin	69,000
Lactalbumin	17,400	Serum γ-globulin	96,000
Zein	40,000	Edestin	310,000
β-Lactoglobulin	42,000	Urease	370,000

ments of the osmotic pressure (Appendix, p. 895). Hemoglobin is then found to have a molecular weight of 68,000 by the former and 67,000 by the latter method. It appears, therefore, that one molecule of hemoglobin consists of four subunits (68,000/16,400 = 4), each containing an atom of iron. Such a grouping of four subunits in a molecule is called a *tetramer*.

Table 5-6. Amino acid sequences of the α-, β-, and γ-chains of human hemoglobin*

	1	2 3 4 5	10	15
α	Val-	-Leu-Ser-Pro-Ala-Asp-Lys-Thr-Asn-Val-Lys-Ala-Ala-Try-Gly-Lys-Val-Gly-Ala-
β	Val-His-Leu-Thr-Pro-Glu-Glu-Lys-Ser-Ala-Val-Thr-Ala-Leu-Try-Gly-Lys-Val-Asn-
γ	Gly-His-Phe-Thr-Glu-Glu-Asp-Lys-Ala-Thr-Ile-Thr-Ser-Leu-Try-Gly-Lys-Val-Asn-

1 2 3 4 5   10   15

	20	25	30	35
α	His-Ala-Gly-Glu-Tyr-Gly-Ala-Glu-Ala-Leu-Glu-Arg-Met-Phe-Leu-Ser-Phe-Pro-Thr-
β	-Val-Asp-Glu-Val-Gly-Gly-Glu-Ala-Leu-Gly-Arg-Leu-Leu-Val-Val-Tyr-Pro-Try
γ	-Val-Glu-Asp-Ala-Gly-Gly-Glu-Thr-Leu-Gly-Arg-Leu-Leu-Val-Val-Tyr-Pro-Try

20   25   29 30   35

	40	45	50	
α	Thr-Lys-Thr-Tyr-Phe-Pro-His-Phe- -Asp-Leu-Ser-His-Gly-Ser-Ala- - - -
β	Thr-Gln-Arg-Phe-Phe-Glu-Ser-Phe-Gly-Asp-Leu-Ser-Thr-Pro-Asp-Ala-Val-Met-Gly
γ	Thr-Gln-Arg-Phe-Phe-Asp-Ser-Phe-Gly-Asn-Leu-Ser-Ser-Ala-Ser-Ala-Ile-Met-Gly

40   45   50   55

	55	60	65	70
α	- -Gln-Val-Lys-Gly-His-Gly-Lys-Lys-Val-Ala-Asp-Ala-Leu-Thr-Asn-Ala-Val-Ala
β	Asn-Pro-Lys-Val-Lys-Ala-His-Gly-Lys-Lys-Val-Leu-Gly-Ala-Phe-Ser-Asp-Gly-Leu-Ala
γ	Asn-Pro-Lys-Val-Lys-Ala-His-Gly-Lys-Lys-Val-Leu-Thr-Ser-Leu-Gly-Asp-Ala-Ile-Lys

60   65   70   75

	75	80	85	90
α	His-Val-Asp-Asp-Met-Pro-Asn-Ala-Leu-Ser-Ala-Leu-Ser-Asp-Leu-His-Ala-His-Lys
β	His-Leu-Asp-Asn-Leu-Lys-Gly-Thr-Phe-Ala-Thr-Leu-Ser-Glu-Leu-His-Cys-Asp-Lys
γ	His-Leu-Asp-Asp-Leu-Lys-Gly-Thr-Phe-Ala-Gln-Leu-Ser-Glu-Leu-His-Cys-Asp-Lys

80   85   90   95

	95	100	105	
α	Leu-Arg-Val-Asp-Pro-Val-Asp-Phe-Lys-Leu-Leu-Ser-His-Cys-Leu-Leu-Val-Thr-Leu
β	Leu-His-Val-Asp-Pro-Glu-Asn-Phe-Arg-Leu-Leu-Gly-Asn-Val-Leu-Val-Cys-Val-Leu
γ	Leu-His-Val-Asp-Pro-Glu-Asn-Phe-Lys-Leu-Leu-Gly-Asn-Val-Leu-Val-Thr-Val-Leu

100   105   110

	110	115	120	125
α	Ala-Ala-His-Leu-Pro-Ala-Glu-Phe-Thr-Pro-Ala-Val-His-Ala-Ser-Leu-Asp-Lys-Phe-Leu
β	Ala-His-His-Phe-Gly-Lys-Glu-Phe-Thr-Pro-Pro-Val-Gln-Ala-Ala-Tyr-Gln-Lys-Val-Val
γ	Ala-Ile-His-Phe-Gly-Lys-Glu-Phe-Thr-Pro-Glu-Val-Gln-Ala-Ser-Try-Gln-Lys-Met-Val

115   120   125   130

	130	135	140 141	
α	Ala-Ser-Val-Ser-Thr-Val-Leu-Thr-Ser-Lys- Tyr- Arg
β	Ala-Gly-Val-Ala-Asp-Ala-Leu-Ala-His-Lys-Tyr-His
γ	Thr-Gly-Val-Ala-Ser-Ala-Leu-Ser-Ser-Arg-Tyr-His

135   140 141 142 143 144 145 146

* Gaps have been introduced into the sequences of the peptide chains in order to show the similarities in the sequences of the chains. These gaps do not actually exist in the hemoglobin molecule.

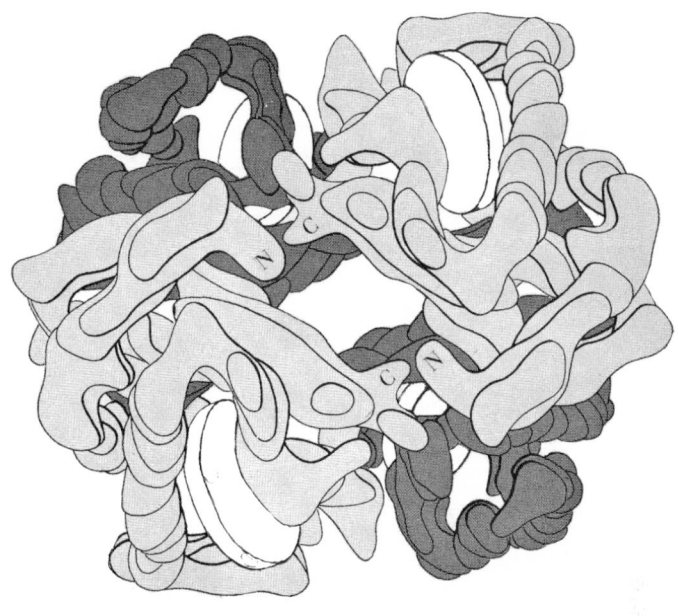

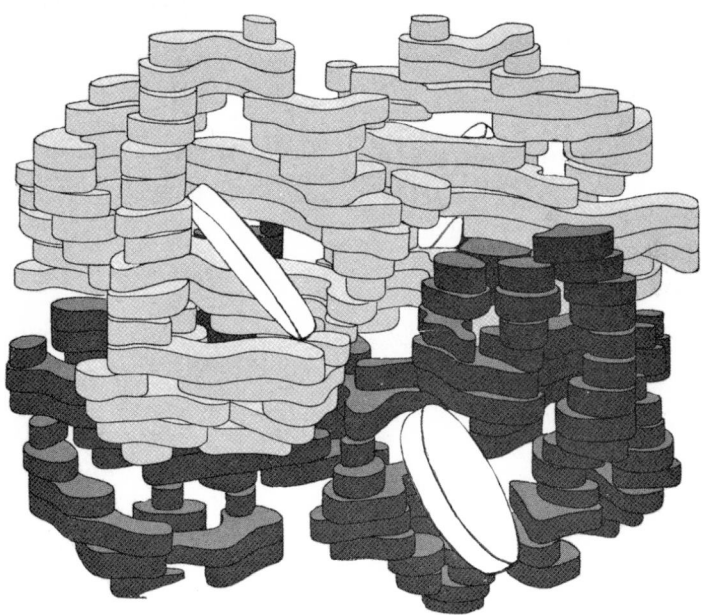

Fig. 5-10. Hemoglobin molecule, as deduced from x-ray diffraction studies, shown from above (top) and side (bottom). Drawings follow the representation scheme used in three-dimensional models built by Perutz and his co-workers. Irregular blocks represent electron-density patterns at various levels in the hemoglobin molecule. The molecule is built up from four subunits: two identical α-chains (light blocks) and two identical β-chains (dark blocks). *N* in the top view identifies the amino ends of the two α-chains; *C* identifies the carboxyl ends. Each chain enfolds a heme group (white discs), the Fe-containing structure that binds O to the molecule. (From Perutz, M. F.: Sci. Amer. **211**:64, 1964.)

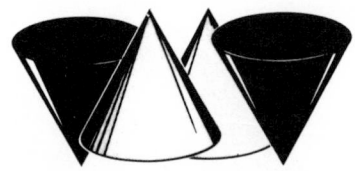

Fig. 5-11. Model illustrating the nesting of two α-chains (gray) and two β-chains (black) to form a molecule of hemoglobin.

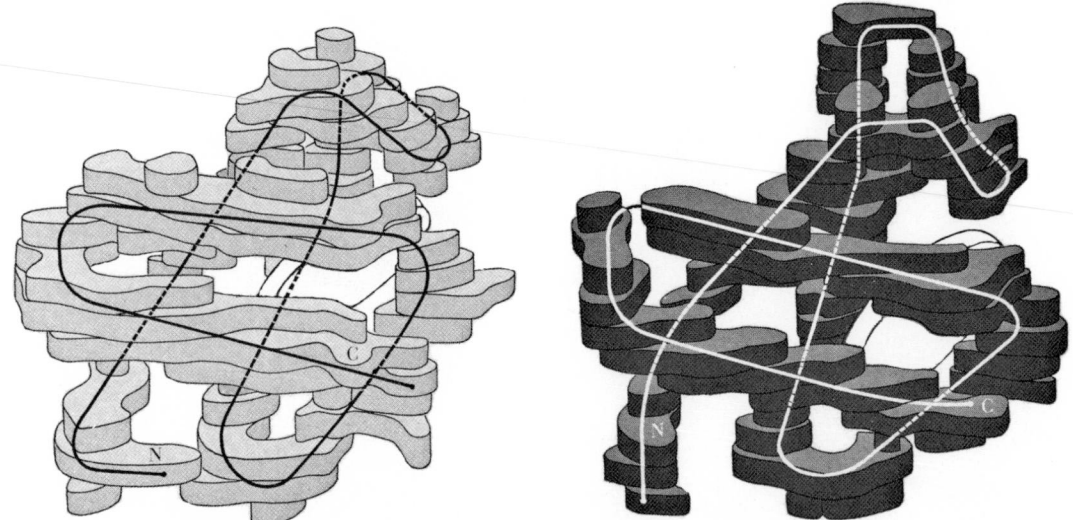

Fig. 5-12. Hemoglobin chains. Alpha at left and beta at right are redrawn from models built by Perutz and colleagues. Superposed lines show course of the central chain. A heme group (white disc) is partly visible, tucked in back of each model. (From Perutz, M. F.: Sci. Amer. **211**:64, 1964.)

Hemoglobin, in fact, possesses two kinds of subunits, each having a distinctive structure. Of the two subunits, called α- and β-chains, the α-chain consists of 141 residues, terminating with valine at the amino and arginine at the carboxyl end (see Table 5-6 for the primary structure). The β-chain has 146 residues, terminating with valine and histidine at the N- and C-terminals, respectively (Table 5-6). Although the primary structures of the α- and β-chains differ significantly from that of myoglobin, their secondary and tertiary conformations are remarkably similar (p. 82).

The aggregation of subunits in the final protein particle is called the quaternary structure. Fig. 5-10, top, shows that the two α-chains in gray are opposite the two β-chains in black. These units are actually nested as schematically illustrated in Fig. 5-11. Note that the two oppositely oriented gray, erect cones are nested with two "upside-down" cones (black).

This brings the positively charged N-terminal ammonium group of one α-chain close to the negatively charged C-terminal carboxylate of the second α-chain (Fig. 5-10). Electrostatic attraction is of considerable importance to the maintenance of the quaternary structure.

Increasing evidence points to a functional role of the quaternary structure in biologic activity of proteins. The classic example is afforded by the oxygen-binding of hemoglobin (p. 645).

A similar situation, involving a respiratory protein, is that of octopus hemocyanin, a copper-containing protein that is a decamer with a molecular weight of 2.8×10^6. Other examples of biologically active proteins having a quaternary structure are the enzymes lactic acid dehydrogenase (p. 130), aspartyl transcarbamylase (p. 129), and pyruvic acid dehydrogenase (p. 131).

Studies by Perutz[4] on horse hemoglobin have shown that the overall shape of the subunits is the same as that for myoglobin (Fig. 5-12). In other words, the nonpolar amino acids are internal and within van der Waals contact of one another. Amino acids that are ionized at neutral pH are at the surface of the molecule. This means that the typical protein is amphoteric in nature as a result of the polar amino acid side chains.

IONIZATION

In an acid environment, containing excess protons, the protein molecules assume a net positive charge, while in an alkaline medium the protein molecules have a net negative charge. As with the amino acids, there exists a pH at which the net charge is zero, the *isoelectric point*. This is illustrated by the following diagram:

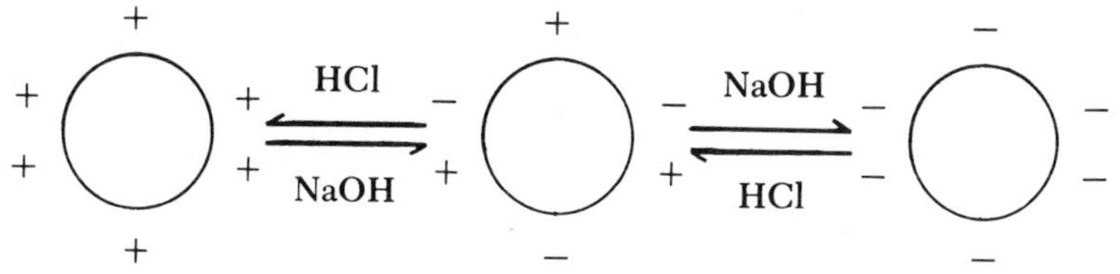

Although a protein is usually in solution at its isoelectric point, it is least soluble at this pH and consequently is most easily precipitated. Proteins differ greatly in their isoelectric points, as indicated in Table 5-7.

Actually proteins exist in the salt form on either side of the isoelectric point. Thus in acid solution, they may form soluble hydrochlorides or insoluble salts with such anions as salicylate, trichloroacetate, perchlorate, tungstate, picrate, and tannate. In an alkaline solution, proteins are found as sodium salts and are precipitated by such cations as Ag^+, Ca^{++}, Zn^{++}, Fe^{+++}, Cu^{++}, and Pb^{++}.

The insolubility of the various protein salts on either side of the isoelectric point is utilized in a number of practical ways. For example, picric acid hardens the skin around minor burns, tannic acid prepares and preserves leather, silver nitrate cauterizes wounds, and zinc combined with insulin affords a slow absorption of this vital hormone. In like manner, it is possible to use proteins, milk, egg white, etc. as antidotes in metal poisoning.

The diversity of physical and chemical properties of proteins is so great that the properties are difficult to correlate into neat, meaningful categories or classes. At best the most useful system of classification involves features of structure rather than function. The following classic separation of proteins

Table 5-7. Isoelectric points of some proteins*

Protein	Source	Isoelectric point pH
Recrystallized proteins		
Edestin	Hempseed	5.5–6.0
Egg albumin	Hen's egg	4.55–4.90
Hemocyanin	Snail blood	5.05
Hemoglobin, reduced	Horse blood	6.79–6.83
Hemoglobin, oxy-	Horse blood	6.7
Insulin	Beef pancreas	5.30–5.35
Lactoglobulin	Cow's milk	4.5–5.5
Serum albumin	Horse blood	4.88
Trypsin	Beef pancreas	5.0–8.0
Urease	Jack bean	5.0–5.1
Amorphous proteins		
Bence Jones	Human urine (pathologic)	5.20
Casein	Cow's milk	4.6
Gelatin	Calf's skin	4.80–4.85
Gliadin	Wheat (flour)	6.5
Myogen	Rabbit muscle	6.2–6.4
Myosin	Rabbit and cow muscle	6.2–6.6
Protamines	Fish sperm (from 9 different kinds of fish)	12.0–12.4
Protamine	Fish sperm (3 other varieties)	9.7, 10.0, 11.7
Serum globulin	Horse blood	5.4–5.5
Silk fibroin	Silk	2.0–2.4

* From Schmidt, C. L. A.: The chemistry of the amino acids and proteins, Springfield, Ill., 1938, Charles C Thomas, Publisher. (Corrected according to Addendum, 1943.)

into groups is intended to be instructive rather than rigorous. Two broad classes of proteins are usually accepted. These are (1) *simple proteins*, which are composed chiefly of amino acids, and (2) *conjugated* or *compound proteins*, which contain other components in addition to amino acids. The various subcategories and some of their properties are presented in Table 5-8.

DENATURATION

Numerous proteins are characterized by an unusual sensitivity to adverse changes in environment. Some are so sensitive to removal from their normal environment that they must be considered to be partially denatured upon purification. Since, in many instances, biologic activity is dependent on an appropriately ordered molecular conformation, it is not unusual that alterations in structure would lead to a loss of activity. This represents what is probably the most sensitive indication of change in structure. Alteration from the naturally ordered conformation to a randomly structured molecule is called *denaturation*. Although denaturation involves structural changes, there is no apparent hydrolysis. However, it includes many kinds of changes, some reversible, others not. Solubility has long been accepted as an index of this phenomenon. When heated to 50° C. or higher, most proteins become

Table 5-8. Classification of proteins

Classification	Distinctive constituents and properties	Examples
	Simple proteins	
Albumins	Soluble in H_2O, precipitated by saturated $(NH_4)_2SO_4$	Serum albumin, milk lactalbumin, egg ovalbumin
Globulins	Soluble in dilute NaCl solution, precipitated by 1/2 saturation with $(NH_4)_2SO_4$	Serum globulins plant seed globulins
Histones	Soluble in H_2O, insoluble in NH_4OH	Nucleoproteins (somatic cells)
Protamines	Soluble in H_2O, soluble in NH_4OH, 87% arginine	Nucleoproteins (germinal cells), salmine of salmon sperm
Prolamines	Soluble in 70% alcohol	Gliadin of wheat, zein of corn
Albuminoids	Insoluble in all solvents	Collagen and elastin of connective tissues, keratin
	Conjugated proteins	
Nucleoproteins	Nucleic acid prosthetic group, soluble in 1M NaCl solution	Nuclei in cells, viruses
Glycoproteins	Carbohydrate prosthetic group: mucopolysaccharides and smaller oligosaccharides	Ground substance of connective tissues, vitreous humor, salivary and cervical mucus
Lipoproteins	Lipid prosthetic group	Serum lipoproteins, proteins of egg yolk
Phosphoproteins	Phosphate ester	Casein of milk, vitellin of eggs
Chromoproteins	Fe: porphyrin prosthetic group	Hemoglobin, cytochromes
Metalloproteins	Fe, Cu, Zn	Plasma proteins: transferrin, ceruloplasmin, carbonic anhydrase

quite insoluble (coagulate). This is especially true if the pH of the solution of protein is first adjusted to the isoelectric point. Coagulation in all cases is preceded by denaturation. Denatured proteins may be soluble in dilute acid and alkali but insoluble at the isoelectric point. Precipitation at this point is called *flocculation*, and the flocculum is soluble on either side of the isoelectric point, if this is accomplished without delay. If there is delay or if heat is applied, the denatured protein coagulates and is no longer soluble.

The presence of some water is generally necessary for heat denaturation to occur, as can be shown by the fact that dry egg white can be heated to over 100° C. without loss of solubility.

Other methods of denaturation include extremes of pH, action of salts of heavy metals, light, mechanical agitation, alcohol, acetone, ether, urea, guanidine, and detergents.

References

GENERAL

Anfinson, C. B.: The molecular basis of evolution, New York, 1959, John Wiley & Sons, Inc.

Greenstein, J. P., and Winitz, M.: Chemistry of the amino acids, New York, 1961, John Wiley & Sons, Inc.

Neurath, H., editor: The proteins—composition, structure and function, New York, 1963-1966, Academic Press, Inc.

Perutz, M. F.: Proteins and nucleic acids: structure and function, New York, 1963, American Elsevier Publishing Co., Inc.

Ramachandran, G. N., editor: Aspects of protein structure, New York, 1963, Academic Press, Inc.

Sheraga, H. A.: Protein structure, New York, 1961, Academic Press, Inc.

SPECIAL

1. Merrifield, R. B.: Sci. Amer. 218:56, 1968.
1a. Sanger, F.: Science 129:1340, 1959.
2. Kendrew, J. C.: Sci. Amer. 205:96, 1961.
3. Schellman, J. A., and Schellman, C.: In Neurath, H., editor: The proteins—composition, structure and function, New York, 1964, Academic Press, Inc., vol. 2, p. 1.
4. Perutz, M. F.: Sci. Amer. 211:64, 1964.

CHAPTER 6

BIOSYNTHESIS OF PROTEIN: TRANSLATION OF GENETIC INFORMATION

A singular advance in modern medical sciences has been the recognition of *molecular disease*, first proposed, in 1949, by Linus Pauling. This concept was based on studies of the hemoglobin from persons having the genetic disease sickle-cell anemia. Approximately 25% of African natives inherit the recessive trait for this disease, which, for some unknown reason, bestows on the individual an increased resistance to malaria. The afflicted person's red blood cells collapse into sickle shape after releasing oxygen to the tissues. Such cells are destroyed quickly in the body, leading to a state of anemia. Pauling showed that the hemoglobin of these red cells is different from the normal in that the amino acid valine replaces glutamic acid as the sixth residue of the β-chain. This change in primary structure reduces the solubility of the hemoglobin.

If the gene A is needed for the formation of normal hemoglobin and a represents the sickling trait, a person with Aa has the sickle-cell trait and one with aa has sickle-cell disease and often dies in childhood. A mutation, perhaps a change of only one purine or pyrimidine base in the entire gene, may cause the substitution of the wrong amino acid into the hemoglobin molecule.

How is the sequence of nucleotide bases in DNA that is transcribed into a complementary sequence in RNA finally translated into the primary structure of proteins, and how can a mutation lead to the substitution of an incorrect amino acid?

GENETIC CODE

We have already seen in Chapter 4 that the primary structure of DNA is composed of a particular sequence of purine and pyrimidine nucleotides. If DNA is the repository of genetic information, it might contain a special code for amino acids dependent on the sequence of adenine, guanine, thymine, and cytosine. If each base were responsible for one amino acid, only four could be "read out." Since proteins are made up of some 20 amino acids, it is obvious that a combination of bases is needed for the code. Thus, if each amino acid is represented by a triplet of bases, then 4^3 or 64 different combinations are possible.

Table 6-1. Hypothetic nucleotide sequence

Number of bases deleted	
0	CAT CAT CAT CAT CAT CAT CAT
1	out-of-phase CAT C TC ATC ATC ATC ATC ATC A
2	out-of-phase CAT C TC A CA TCA TCA TCA TCA A T
3	out-of-phase in-phase CAT C TC A CA T AT CAT CAT CAT A T C

Table 6-2. Triplet code for amino acids

First letter		Second letter: U	Second letter: C	Second letter: A	Second letter: G	Third letter
U		Phe $\begin{cases} UUU \\ UUC \end{cases}$	Ser $\begin{cases} UCU \\ UCC \\ UCA \\ UCG \end{cases}$	Tyr $\begin{cases} UAU \\ UAC \end{cases}$	CySH $\begin{cases} UGU \\ UGC° \end{cases}$	U C
		Leu $\begin{cases} UUA \\ UUG \end{cases}$		Term. UAA°	Nonsense UGA	A
				Term. UAG°	Try UGG	G
C		Leu $\begin{cases} CUU \\ CUC \\ CUA \\ CUG \end{cases}$	Pro $\begin{cases} CCU \\ CCC \\ CCA \\ CCG \end{cases}$	His $\begin{cases} CAU \\ CAC \end{cases}$	Arg $\begin{cases} CGU \\ CGC \\ CGA \\ CGG \end{cases}$	U C A G
				Gln $\begin{cases} CAA \\ CAG \end{cases}$		
A		Ile $\begin{cases} AUU \\ AUC \\ AUA \end{cases}$	Thr $\begin{cases} ACU \\ ACC \\ ACA \\ ACG \end{cases}$	Asn $\begin{cases} AAU \\ AAC \end{cases}$	Ser $\begin{cases} AGU \\ AGC \end{cases}$	U C
		Met AUG°		Lys $\begin{cases} AAA \\ AAG \end{cases}$	Arg $\begin{cases} AGA \\ AGG \end{cases}$	A G
G		Val $\begin{cases} GUU \\ GUC \\ GUA \\ GUG° \end{cases}$	Ala $\begin{cases} GCU \\ GCC \\ GCA \\ GCG \end{cases}$	Asp $\begin{cases} GAU \\ GAC \end{cases}$	Gly $\begin{cases} GGU \\ GGC \\ GGA \\ GGG \end{cases}$	U C A G
				Glu $\begin{cases} GAA \\ GAG \end{cases}$		

° *Term.* codons can act as signals for chain termination; *AUG* and *GUG* signal chain initiation by coding N-formylmethionine.

After assuming that the genetic code must occur in the form of groupings of three bases, we must then establish how these groupings are actually read in the polynucleotide chain. In studies of T_4 bacteriophage, Crick and his co-workers[1] showed that messages in the DNA are read as triplets, starting from one end of the chain. This discovery was accomplished by using mutant bacteriophage from which one, two, or three bases were either deleted from or added to the DNA by the action of certain acridine dyes. The principle of the experiment is illustrated by the hypothetic phage DNA in the accompanying table.

From Table 6-1, it is apparent that deletion of any one base leads to nonsense information and, therefore, a nonfunctional gene. Two such deletions also yield an out-of-phase transcription of information. Deletion of three bases, however, at first yields nonsense information (out-of-phase), but then the process is once again in phase and consequently the gene is functional. Although this tells us that genetic information occurs in the gene as triplets of bases, read in an end-to-end sequence, it does not say what the triplet means in terms of amino acids.

**Breaking
the code**

In 1961, Nirenberg and Matthai performed experiments to determine the nature of this triplet code. These experiments utilized the earlier observations of Zamecnik showing that amino acids could be introduced into proteins in a cell-free (in vitro) system, provided certain constituents were included. Such an amino acid–incorporating system would include the following components:

> Microsomal fraction (ribosomes, mRNA)
> Cell sap (tRNA, amino acid–activating enzymes)
> Suitable buffer system, GTP, Mg^{++}
> ATP generating system
> Radioactively labeled amino acid

During incubation, the labeled amino acid was incorporated into protein by the formation of new peptide bonds. Nirenberg replaced the microsomal fraction with purified ribosomes and messenger RNA (mRNA). When the source of mRNA was omitted, little amino acid incorporation occurred. Natural mRNA could be replaced with synthetic polynucleotides such as poly-U. With poly-U (a uracil-containing synthetic polynucleotide), only phenylalanine was involved in peptide bond formation; the product was polyphenylalanine. This meant that poly-U was read by the system as a sequence of uracil triplets, *UUU UUU UUU*. Similarly, it was found that the triplet or *codon* AAA coded for lysine and that CCC coded for proline. Subsequent studies with synthetic mRNA polynucleotides allowed a complete designation of the codes[2,3] with their corresponding amino acids (Table 6-2). It should be clear that the codes presented in this table refer to the sequences of bases in mRNA.

The synthesis of the many polynucleotides of known triplet sequences needed for the complete determination of the amino acid code was accomplished by Khorana and co-workers.

The translation of triplet sequences might begin from either the 5′- or the 3′-end of the mRNA chain. To determine the direction of reading, similar amino acid–incorporating studies were performed using synthetic polynucleotides containing the sequences AAA and AAC:

```
                    NH₂
                     |
                    Lys—Lys—Lys—Lys—Lys--------COOH
         A   5'    AAC AAA AAA AAA AAA AAA..............3'

         B   5'    AAA AAC AAA AAA AAA AAA..............3'
                    Asn—Lys—Lys—Lys—Lys--------COOH
                     |
                    NH₂
```

AAC codes for asparagine, while AAA codes for lysine. In an experiment using A as mRNA, polylysine was obtained; when B was used, the product was polylysine with an N-terminal asparagine. Considering the manner in which polypeptide extention occurs (p. 98), these products could have formed only if the reading occurred from the 5'- to the 3'-end. The first triplet in the polynucleotide was not expressed as an amino acid in this instance.

TRANSLATION OF GENETIC CODE

The fact that the codon is a sequence of three bases in mRNA does not tell us how the individual amino acids "recognize" these triplets. The principle of code recognition is independent of the amino acid structure; rather it is dependent on base complementarity between polynucleotide molecules. In *translation*, the codon of mRNA is recognized by an anticodon (sometimes called *nodoc*) that is part of the primary structure of transfer RNA (tRNA). Thus the triplet UUU in mRNA is recognized by the anticodon AAA found at the recognition site of a tRNA specific for phenylalanine. The actual process of combining an amino acid with its proper tRNA is the function of the appropriate *aminoacyl synthetase* enzyme. There must be at least 20 specific synthetases, one for each amino acid. These enzymes appear to have two recognition sites, one for the amino acid and one for the tRNA.

Activation of amino acids The combination of an amino acid with its specific tRNA is a two-step process.

$$\text{Amino acid} + \text{ATP} + \text{Enzyme} \rightleftharpoons \text{Enzyme (aminoacyl adenylate)} + \text{Pyrophosphate}$$

$$\text{Enzyme (aminoacyl adenylate)} + \text{tRNA} \rightleftharpoons \text{Aminoacyl-tRNA} + \text{AMP} + \text{Enzyme}$$

In the first reaction the amino acid is activated by reacting with ATP to yield an aminoacyl adenylate. This involves the formation of a high-energy mixed anhydride bond between the carboxyl group of the amino acid and adenylic acid (AMP). Pyrophosphate is eliminated in this step. Apparently the adenylate remains attached to the synthetase for the second reaction, when the activated amino acid is transferred to the specific *tRNA*. The amino acid is bound to the 2'- or 3'-hydroxyl group of the terminal adenosine moiety (p. 44) of the tRNA by way of a high-energy ester bond. This ester linkage then supplies the energy required for peptide bond formation (p. 99). The nature of the overall activation process[4] and the role of the aminoacyl synthetases are best illustrated by Fig. 6-1.

The fact that the amino acid itself is not involved in decoding the message has been clearly demonstrated. In an experiment to prove this point, cysteine linked to its specific tRNA was isolated and treated with hydrogen in the presence of a nickel catalyst. In this way, the sulfhydryl group of the cysteine was replaced with hydrogen, thereby producing alanine. The alanine, however, was still attached to the cysteine-specific tRNA.

$$\text{CySH-tRNA}_{\text{CySH}} \xrightarrow[\text{Ni}]{\text{H}} \text{Ala-tRNA}_{\text{CySH}}$$

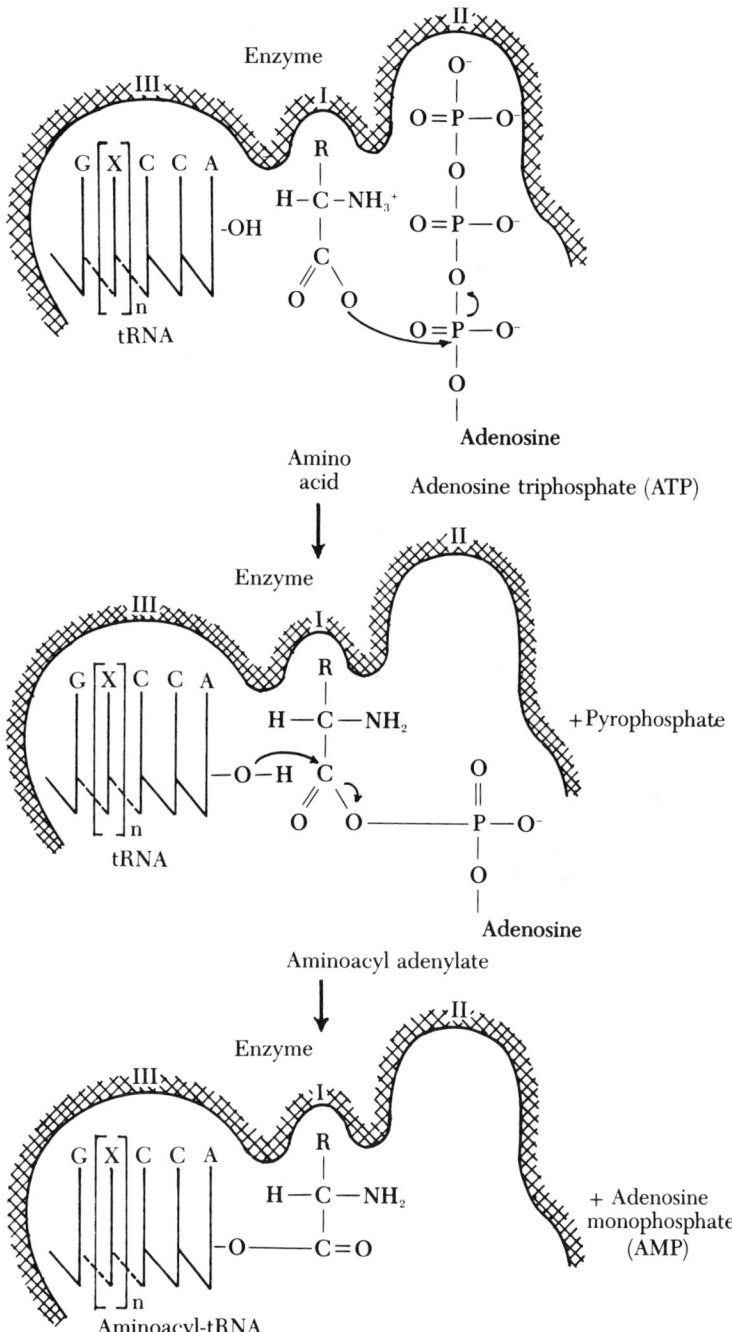

Fig. 6-1. Scheme showing amino acid activation and the biosynthesis of aminoacyl-tRNA. (From Arstein, H. R. V.: Brit. Med. Bull. **21**:217, 1965.)

The Ala-tRNA$_{CySH}$ was then used in an amino acid–incorporating system including a U and G–containing polynucleotide. The poly-UG supplied the triplet codons necessary for the incorporation of cysteine into peptide chains. Now, however, alanine was included in the peptide product instead of the cysteine. Furthermore, alanine-tRNA$_{Ala}$, i.e., alanine coupled to tRNA specific for alanine, was not incorporated by the U and G–containing polynucleotides. These experiments demonstrate that the translation of genetic messages into amino acid sequences depends on the principle of base complementarity.

In general the specificity of each aminoacyl synthetase is such as to preclude errors. There is the possibility that error in recognition might occur in the particular situation of valine by the isoleucine specific enzyme and isoleucine by the valine enzyme (Fig. 6-2). The erroneous formation of Val-tRNA$_{Ile}$ and Ile-tRNA$_{Val}$ is prevented by the spontaneous hydrolysis of the hybrid complex.

The aminoacyl-tRNA molecules translate the genetic information provided by the mRNA triplets into the appropriate sequence of amino acids. They do not, however, all attach themselves simultaneously to a single mRNA chain. This process is a stepwise one, resulting in a gradually growing peptide chain. The site at which the codon-anticodon recognition occurs, and the site of growth or peptide bond formation, is provided by the subcellular particles called the *ribosomes*.[5]

Single ribosomes obtained from such microorganisms as *E. coli*[6] have a sedimentation constant (Appendix, p. 903) in the ultracentrifuge of 70 S, while those from rat liver are 80 S. When the 70 S ribosomes are placed in an environment low in magnesium ions, two subunits, a 50 S and a 30 S particle, separate. Each contains its own kind of RNA, 23 S or 16 S (p. 43). In addition to a single strand of rRNA, ribosomes contain about 20 different kinds of proteins. It appears that some of these proteins are enzymes required for aminoacyl-tRNA binding, peptide bond formation, and ribosome movement relative to the mRNA.

Protein synthesis does not occur with a single ribosome-mRNA combination. Studies with sucrose density gradient ultracentrifugation (Appendix, p. 904) and electron microscopy have shown that the protein-synthesizing apparatus is composed of multiple ribosomes attached to a single mRNA (Fig. 6-3). Such a structure is called a polyribosome or simply *polysome*. A single ribosome occupies a length of mRNA equivalent to 80 nucleotides in a row. As an example of polysomal size, consider the mRNA specific for the

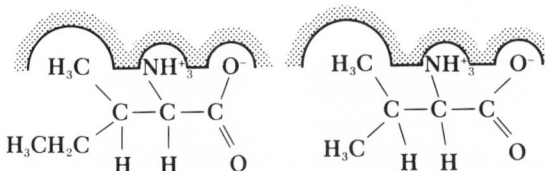

Fig. 6-2. Diagram showing a potential error in the recognition of valine by isoleucine-specific aminoacyl synthetase.

hemoglobin chain (150 amino acids). This would require a minimum of 450 nucleotides to supply the necessary information. Such a mRNA could accommodate four to six ribosomes; actually the average polysome is a pentamer. Electron microscopy (Fig. 6-3) shows that the individual ribosomes in a polysome are separated by a thin strand of material that is thought to be mRNA. The actual size of the polysome varies with the protein produced and even with the state of metabolism. Some polysomes involved in the biosynthesis of a protein of particularly high molecular weight, e.g., myosin, consist of 100 or more ribosomes. The number of ribosomes per polysome also may be variable and may actually serve as a level of *translational control*. When protein synthesis is stimulated, the average number of ribosomes per polysome may be increased, perhaps to make the translational process more efficient.

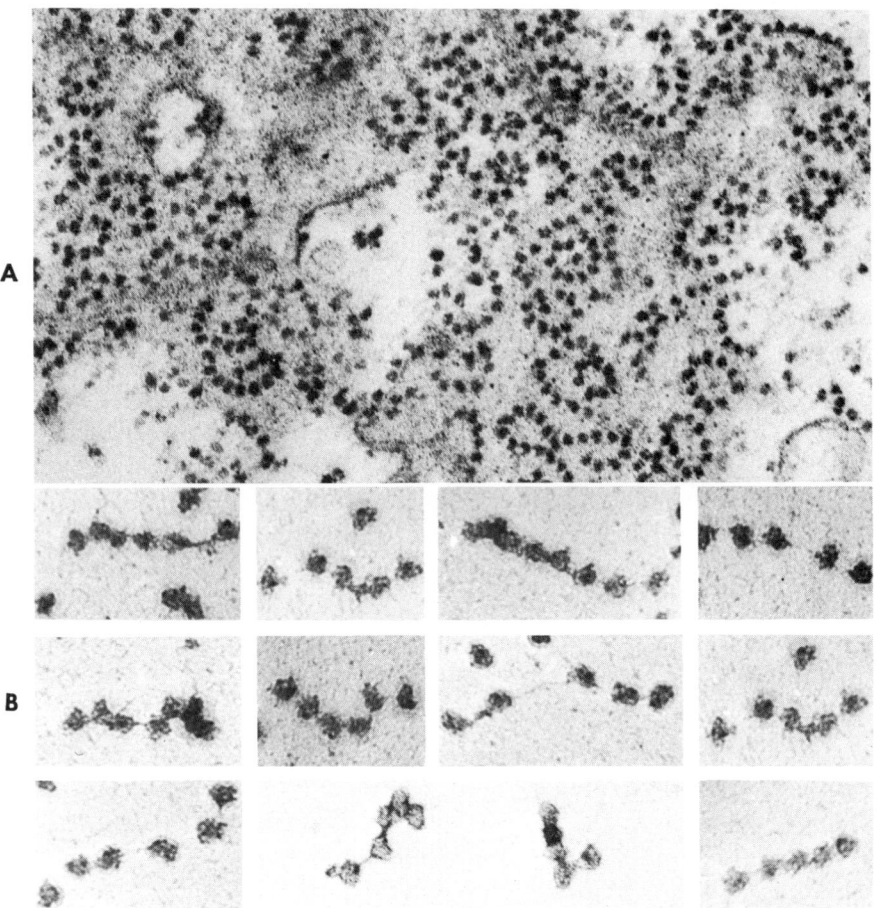

Fig. 6-3. A, Electron micrograph showing polysomes in root cells of the radish (×64,000). B, Representative polysomes from rabbit reticulocytes showing the connecting strands of RNA (×100,000). (A from Bonnett, H. R., and Newcomb, E. H.: J. Cell Biol. 27:423, 1965; B from Slayter, H. S., Warner, J. R., Rich, A., and Hall, C. E.: J. Molec. Biol. 7:652, 1963.)

Primary structure   In *E. coli,* the first step in protein synthesis is *chain initiation,* which requires a special derivative of methionine, N-formylmethionine.[7,8] It appears that the first codon at the 5′-end of the mRNA is AUG (Table 6-2), which signals the attachment to the ribosome of this amino acid. The binding of N-formylmethionyl–tRNA occurs at the *peptidyl binding* site. Binding takes place with the help of the enzyme *transferase I,* in accord with Fig. 6-4.

The next step in translation is the recognition of the second or "incoming" aminoacyl-tRNA, which binds to an *aminoacyl binding* site on the ribosome. Once again the selection of the specific amino acid depends on the principle of base complementarity between the mRNA codon and the anticodon of the tRNA. *Transferase II* then catalyzes the formation of a peptide bond utilizing the energy of the ester linkage in the N-formylmethionyl–tRNA. The first dipeptide bond is formed between the carboxyl group of the N-formyl-methionine on the peptidyl or donor site and the free amino group of the aminoacyl-tRNA on the aminoacyl or acceptor site. Once this peptide bond has formed, a *translocase* enzyme "rolls" or shifts the binding sites with respect to the mRNA. Now the dipeptidyl-tRNA is moved to the donor site formerly occupied by the N-formylmethionyl–tRNA. This exposes the aminoacyl or acceptor site for the next incoming aminoacyl-tRNA. It also brings the third codon (mRNA) into its position opposite the acceptor site. The system can now select and bind the third amino acid. In the meantime, the tRNA freed of its amino acid (N-formylmethionine) during peptide bond formation is released from the ribosome and returned to the environment, where it may once again engage in the amino acid–activating process. This sequence of events is repeated, thereby extending the peptide in a stepwise fashion. The growing polypeptide remains attached to the ribosome by the most recently introduced aminoacyl-tRNA. In a manner of speaking, there are two different kinds of tRNA's: one is the growing peptidyl-tRNA and the other is the new or incoming aminoacyl-tRNA. (See Fig. 6-5.)

In general, the growing peptide chain on the peptidyl site contributes the carboxyl group to the newly formed peptide bond while the nitrogen is the free amino group of the most recently bound aminoacyl-tRNA. In all cases

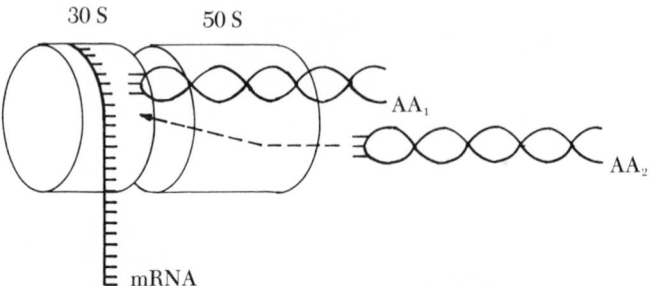

Fig. 6-4. Schematic diagram illustrating the two subunits, *50* S and *30* S, of a single ribosome. *mRNA* represents the messenger RNA specifically associated with the 30 S subunit. A tRNA specific for the amino acid *AA₁* is shown attached to the ribosome. A second aminoacyl (*AA₂*)-tRNA is shown approaching the codon.

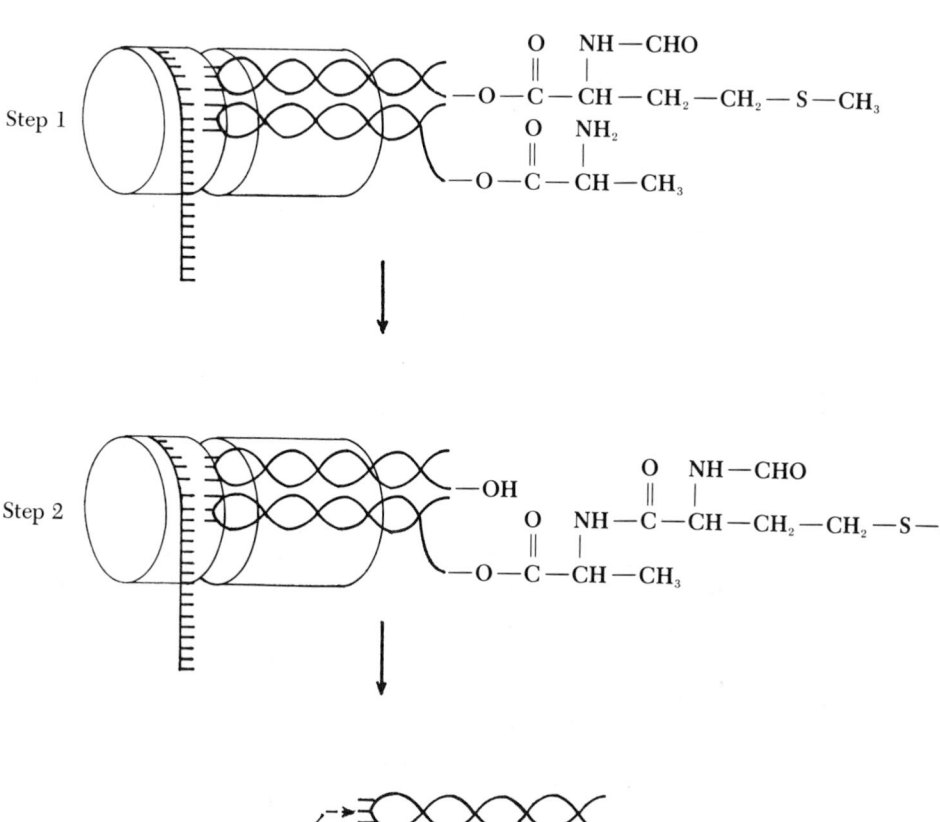

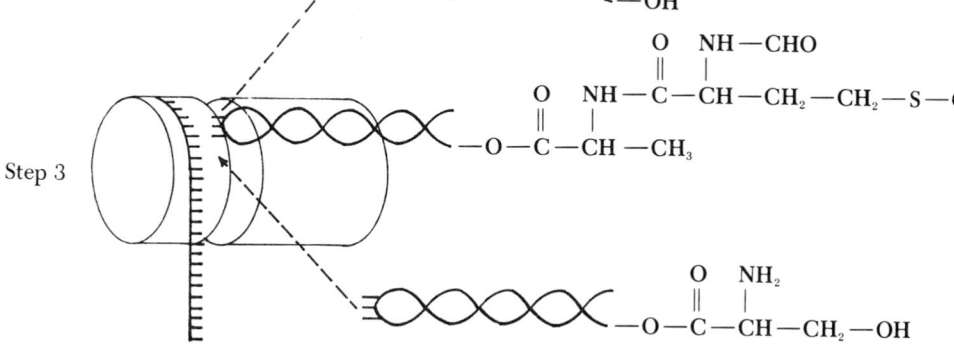

Fig. 6-5. Schematic diagram showing the sequence of events involved in peptide bond formation. *Step 1*, Initiating aminoacyl-tRNA (N-formylmethionine) in position on the peptidyl site and alanyl-tRNA in the aminoacyl binding site; *Step 2*, immediately after the formation of the dipeptide; *Step 3*, action of translocase has resulted in the transfer of the peptidyl-tRNA to the peptidyl binding site, thereby opening the aminoacyl site for the incoming seryl-tRNA. Notice that the tRNA formerly bound to the N-formylmethionine is now released.

the energy required for peptide bond formation is supplied by the high-energy ester linkage in the aminoacyl-tRNA. The N-terminal amino group in *E. coli* appears to be the N-formylmethionine residue. It is not yet known when this structure is eliminated from the polypeptide. This may occur at some point during or shortly after the peptide synthesis is complete, since proteins do not always terminate with this amino acid. The existence of such a chain-initiating step in mammalian systems has yet to be established.

As the peptide chain grows, sufficient mRNA "shifts" over the ribosomal structure so that a new ribosome may be accommodated. When this happens, chain initiation begins anew and a second polypeptide develops. This process continues with the acceptance of new free ribosomes so that protein synthesis may be viewed as involving a polysome supporting multiple peptide chains of increasing lengths. Ultimately the first ribosome reaches the end of the message or *cistron*. At this point a terminal codon, e.g., UAA, UAG, or UGA (Table 6-2), signals the termination of the translational process. The polypeptide is released and the ribosome is restored to the free pool for further use. The process of ribosomal migration and also of peptide chain release requires a supply of GTP. As far as is known, the nature of the protein synthesis is entirely a function of the specific mRNA. Ribosomes, on the other hand, are nonspecific and may be used in the synthesis of different kinds of proteins.

The mRNA may be used over again, in some instances approximately 15 times, before it is discarded and a new RNA takes its place. Protein synthesis is a reasonably rapid process, requiring approximately $2\frac{1}{2}$ minutes to synthesize the α-chain of hemoglobin. In bacteria the rate of protein synthesis is much faster; only 10 seconds are needed to produce a complete protein.

Considerable knowledge concerning translation comes from the ability to halt this process at will by aborting chain synthesis with the antibiotic *puromycin*. Puromycin is structurally an analogue for aminoacyl-tRNA. You will recall that the 3'-hydroxyl terminus for tRNA is pCpCpA (p. 44). Puro-

Puromycin

mycin is an analogue of the terminal adenosine unit. The amino acid portion, o-methyltyrosine, however, is bound to the ribose hydroxyl group by an amide, not by an ester bond. Puromycin is confused by the translating system for aminoacyl-tRNA and accepts the growing peptide at its free amino group. However, the newly formed puromycin peptide is released from the ribosome, thereby terminating chain growth. In this way all nascent or growing chains are released prematurely from the polysomes.

Other antibiotics also can block protein synthesis. Streptomycin, for example, binds to the ribosome and brings about a change in conformation. This distortion of the ribosome results in a change in reading of the codons and the insertion into the peptide chain of an incorrect amino acid, thus misreading the message. In addition, erythromycin, tetracycline, and chloramphenicol inhibit protein synthesis.

Mutation   It should now be apparent that any change in the identity of a single purine or pyrimidine base in the gene can affect the composition of the protein ultimately synthesized. An experiment illustrating this point involved treating tobacco mosaic virus (TMV)-RNA with nitrous acid. Nitrous acid replaces the primary amino groups of such bases as adenine and cytosine with a hydroxyl.

In this way the codon for proline, CCC, may be changed to UUU, CUU, CUC, etc. and may therefore code for another amino acid entirely, e.g., leucine (CUU, CUC). In this example, the *mutant* RNA leads to the formation of viral-coat proteins in which the C-terminal amino acid sequence is slightly altered; i.e., leucine replaces proline.

$$\text{Pro}-\text{Ala-Thr-COOH}\quad\text{(normal viral protein)}$$
$$\text{Leu}-\text{Ala-Thr-COOH}\quad\text{(mutant viral protein)}$$

The normal-coat protein is resistant to the action of the protease carboxypeptidase because this enzyme is unable to hydrolyze the proline-containing peptide bond. On the other hand, the mutant protein is readily digested so that this coat protein is not as effective as the normal one in protecting the all-important genetic material from the destructive action of the host cell. Therefore, this experiment also showed, on a molecular basis, how mutations more often than not are detrimental to the organism.

In sickle-cell anemia the primary structure of hemoglobin-S is different from that of normal hemoglobin-A only in the identity of the sixth amino acid residue of the β-chain.

Hb-A: H$_2$N-Val-His-Leu-Thr-Pro-Glu-Glu-Lys-

Hb-S: H$_2$N-Val-His-Leu-Thr-Pro-Val-Glu-Lys-

Table 6-3. Some molecular diseases

Hereditary disorder	Protein or enzyme involved
Afibrinogenemia	Fibrinogen
Albinism	Tyrosinase
Alkaptonuria	Homogentisic acid oxidase
Crigler-Najjar syndrome	Uridine diphosphate glucuronate transferase
Fructosuria	Fructokinase
Galactosemia	Galactose-1-phosphate uridyl transferase
Hartnup's disease	Tryptophan pyrrolase
Hemolytic anemia	Pyruvate kinase
Hemophilia	Antihemophilic factor
Histindinemia	Histidase
Maple syrup urine disease	Amino acid decarboxylase
Methemoglobinemia	Methemoglobin reductase
Orotic aciduria	Orotidine-5'-phosphate pyrophosphorylase
Pentosuria	L-Xylulose dehydrogenase
Phenylketonuria	Phenylalanine hydroxylase
Wilson's disease	Ceruloplasmin
Xanthinuria	Xanthine oxidase

Replacement of the polar glutamate residue with the nonpolar valine changes the solubility of this protein. More than 150 variations of hemoglobin are known to exist in man. These are all mutants involving only single amino acid changes. The so-called microheterogeneity of hemoglobin is discussed in Chapter 19. With the exception of Hb-M, or methemoglobinemia, these variations do not seem to impair the oxygen-carrying capacity of the blood.

Today many genetic defects or *inborn errors of metabolism* are recognized as molecular diseases (Table 6-3). In these, mutations lead to a deficiency of particular proteins, e.g., plasma proteins, enzymes. A replacement of a single amino acid by another might lead to the biosynthesis of an inactive enzyme.

Secondary-tertiary structure Once the primary structure has been assembled by the translational process, the secondary-tertiary conformation appears to occur automatically as a consequence of the formation of disulfide cross-linkages, hydrogen, electrostatic, and hydrophobic bonds. In other words, molecular conformation is determined by the side chains in the primary structure, not by special genetic information, a fact that has been shown for ribonuclease. When this enzyme is reduced so as to convert all disulfide linkages to sulfhydryl groups, the enzymatic activity is lost. Also when ribonuclease is synthesized by the *solid-phase process* (pp. 73–74), the polypeptide chain is extended and the protein is enzymatically inactive. Solutions of these reduced molecules spontaneously oxidize, with the formation of the four possible disulfide cross-linkages, and the enzyme becomes active.

The carbohydrate side chains of glycoproteins are attached to the poly-

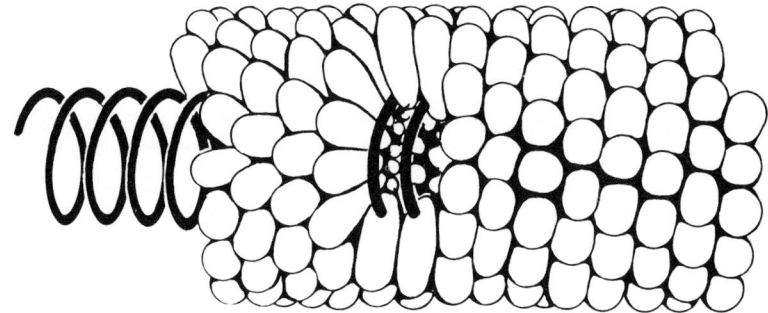

Fig. 6-6. Structure of tobacco mosaic virus. Inner helix represents RNA. Helically assembled ellipsoids of revolution represent protein subunits. (From Lauffer, M. A.: Advances Virus Res. 13:2, 1968.)

peptide "backbone" by enzymes found in the *endoplasmic reticulum.* It is thought that the Golgi apparatus are functional in this respect. As far as is known, the exact sequence of sugars in these oligosaccharide side chains is determined by the specificity of the enzymes involved, not by a mechanism related to a genetic code.

AGGREGATION OF SUBUNITS

The quaternary state of aggregation also occurs as a result of protein interaction and is not guided by a genetically determined process. The formation of hemoglobin tetramers is an automatic process and appears to depend on the existence of available subunits. In certain rare hemoglobin diseases in which there is no α-chain production, Hb-H tetramers of β-chains form instead. Likewise, in Hb-Bart's, tetramers of γ-chains form.

The formation of subcellular particles such as the ribosomes also appears to be a process of self-assembly. Since ribosomes are a combination of protein and RNA, much concerning the principles of self-assembly may be gathered from the formation of viruses. Tobacco mosaic virus (TMV), for example, has long been known to form spontaneously simply by mixing TMV-RNA and TMV-coat protein under suitable conditions of salt concentration and pH. This virus is 5% RNA and 95% protein. There are 2300 protein units of 18,000 molecular weight, having 158 amino acid residues each. These units arrange themselves about the RNA core as shown in Fig. 6-6. Similarly, in a more complex organism such as the T_4 bacteriophage, tail fibers, "heads," and stalks, when properly mixed, spontaneously combine to form a complete and active virus. It is now also possible to dissociate 30 S ribosomal subunits and recombine them spontaneously into active particles. These studies show that the assembly, at least of some subcellular structures, is probably spontaneous in vivo.

CONTROL OF PROTEIN SYNTHESIS

It is becoming increasingly evident that in many instances metabolism is regulated in the living organism through a process of controlling protein

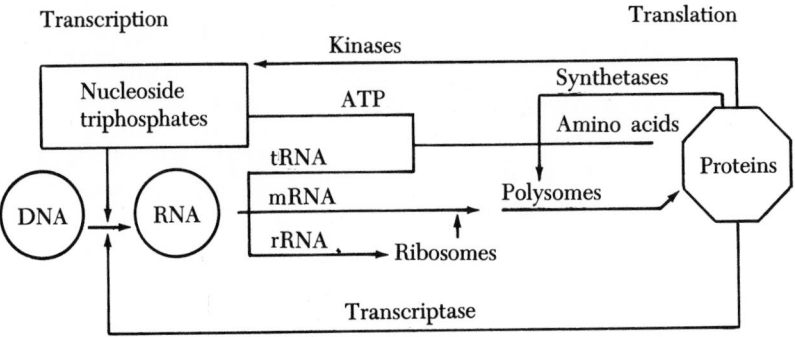

Fig. 6-7. Diagram showing the levels of control for the biosynthesis of proteins.

synthesis. Protein synthesis may be controlled at two levels, i.e., at the transcription of genetic information and at translation[9] (Fig. 6-7).

Transcription may well exert both a qualitative and a quantitative control over protein synthesis. The particular gene being transcribed determines the identity of the protein produced. In other words, a metabolic stimulus may well change the normal spectrum of proteins produced by first altering the complement of mRNA's. The actual amount of each mRNA transcribed may, in turn, also regulate the quantity of each protein synthesized. The amount of RNA may depend on such factors as the number of genes available for transcription, the activity of the transcriptase enzyme, and the availability of nucleoside triphosphates. Translation determines the amount of protein synthesized from the mRNA existing in the system. This, in turn, depends on the amount of mRNA, ATP, GTP, amino acids, polysomal aggregation, activating enzymes, etc.

Little is known concerning the manner in which genes are suppressed either permanently, as in differentiation, or temporarily. Each cell in the body, however, must contain all the information originally present in the fertilized egg. Yet, as is amply obvious, a fibroblast in the region of the big toe is incapable of producing insulin.

Presently the concept much quoted as an explanation of the genetic control of protein synthesis is that proposed in 1961 by Jacob and Monod. The theory originally was intended to explain the synthesis in *E. coli* of certain metabolically important enzymes.[10] At first these microorganisms grown on sucrose media are incapable of metabolizing the sugar lactose. Before metabolism, lactose must first be hydrolyzed into its component glucose and galactose monosaccharides (p. 163). This requires the action of *β-galactosidase*, an enzyme not found to any large degree in the cells grown on sucrose. When the *E. coli* cells are placed in a lactose-containing medium, the synthesis of the essential enzyme, *β*-galactosidase, is increased a thousandfold. This formation of the enzyme is called *induction* or *derepression*. In some way the lactose is transformed into a related compound that is thought to cause the expression of a latent gene, i.e., one existing in a repressed state. Derepression results in the formation of new mRNA specific for *β*-galactosidase as well as two other related enzymes.

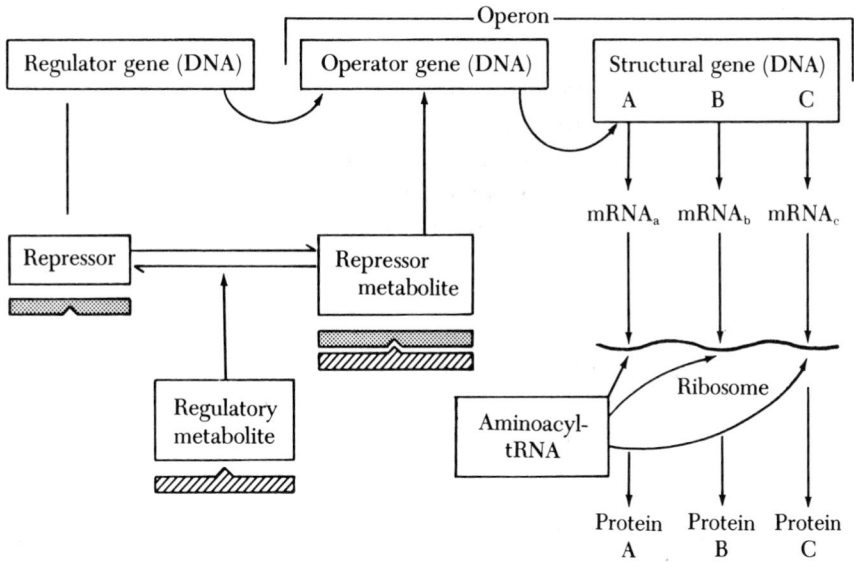

Fig. 6-8. Genetic control of protein biosynthesis — induction and repression.

Regulation by induction
According to the hypothesis of Jacob and Monod, the genes producing β-galactosidase as well as the permease and thioacetylase are part of a composite system called the *operon*. The operon is a series of structural genes or cistrons for several proteins that come under the control of an *operator gene*. The entire operon is then controlled by a *regulator gene* (Fig. 6-8). It is proposed that the regulator gene produces a protein, called the *repressor*, that has a great affinity for the operator gene. The combination repressor-operator gene is thought to "turn off," i.e., repress, the entire operon. The inducer, in this case a galactoside, is thought to combine with the repressor, thereby rendering it incapable of affecting the operator gene. This in effect "derepresses" the system, and the structural genes may be transcribed, leading to the formation of enzyme proteins such as β-galactosidase, permease, and thioacetylase.

Regulation by repression
Metabolism may also be regulated by the suppression of the biosynthesis of certain enzymes. As an example of this effect, *E. coli* growing in a glucose medium actively synthesizes isoleucine from threonine by a five-step process (p. 370), each step requiring a specific enzyme. If excess isoleucine is added to the medium, the cell no longer has to continue synthesizing its own isoleucine. In fact, isoleucine now halts further synthesis of itself by blocking the initial metabolic step, which is the deamination of threonine to α-ketobutyrate. The blocking of this step is called *feedback inhibition* and involves a process of allosteric binding (p. 129). Since it would now be wasteful for the cell to continue synthesizing the five enzymes required in this metabolic pathway, isoleucine serves to halt their biosynthesis by a process of genetic repression. Genetic repression also may be explained by the hypothesis of Jacob and Monod. In this system (Fig. 6-8) the regulator gene is thought to produce an inactive repressor protein, or *aporepressor*, that requires the addition of a metabolite, the *corepressor*, in this instance, isoleucine. The co-

repressor, together with the aporepressor, is now active or functional and binds the operator gene, thereby repressing the operon.

The hypothesis of Jacob and Monod serves to explain two opposing regulatory mechanisms: in one, the operon is normally repressed and must be induced for expression; in the other, the operon is usually functional and must be "turned off." Although there is no predisposing reason to think that regulation in the mammalian cell should be the same as that in microorganisms, the concept of Jacob and Monod does serve as a working hypothesis for understanding the functioning of such metabolic regulators as the hormones. It now appears possible that the hormone insulin controls the blood sugar level, partly by regulating the biosynthesis of certain enzymes such as pyruvate kinase, glucokinase, and phosphofructokinase. Other hormones are currently being studied in line with their effects on protein synthesis.

References

GENERAL

Campbell, P. N., and Sargent, J. R. editors: Techniques in protein biosynthesis, New York, 1966, Academic Press, Inc., vol. 1.

Cohen, N. R.: The control of protein biosynthesis, Biol. Rev. 41:503, 1966.

The genetic code, Sympos. Quant. Biol. 31:1, 1966.

Ingram, V. M.: The biosynthesis of macromolecules, New York, 1965, W. A. Benjamin, Inc.

Mechanism of protein synthesis, Sympos. Quant. Biol. 34:1, 1970.

Molecular biology comes of age, Nature 219:825, 1968.

Watson, J. D.: Molecular biology of the gene, New York, 1965, W. A. Benjamin, Inc.

SPECIAL

1. Crick, F. H. C., et al.: Sci. Amer. 215:55, 1966.

2. Speyer, J. F.: In Taylor, J. H., editor: Molecular genetics, New York, 1967, Academy Press, Inc., part 2, p. 137.

3. Yanofsky, C.: Sci. Amer. 216:80, 1967.

4. Arnstein, H. R. V.: Brit. Med. Bull. 21:217, 1965.

5. Osawa, S.: Ann. Rev. Biochem. 37:109, 1968.

6. Nomura, M., et al.: Nature 219:793, 1968.

7. Clark, F. C., and Marcker, K. S.: Sci. Amer. 218:36, 1968.

8. Lengyel, P.: In Taylor, J. H., editor: Molecular genetics, New York, 1967, Academic Press, Inc., part 2, p. 144.

9. Parker, W. C., and Bearn, A. G.: Amer. J. Med. 34:680, 1963.

10. McFall, E., and Maas, W. K.: In Taylor, J. H., editor: Molecular genetics, New York, 1967, Academic Press, Inc., part 2, p. 255.

CHAPTER 7

BIOLOGICALLY ACTIVE PROTEINS: THE ENZYMES

The nature of the biologic activity of such proteins as enzymes continues to be a mysterious phenomenon. What is the difference between two such proteins as egg albumin and pepsin that allows the latter to hydrolyze the former? At this time all we can do is describe structural requirements for enzyme activity and propose various mechanisms of action; yet the fundamental question remains unanswered. Enzymes must possess some unique arrangement of amino acids, special conformation, or quaternary structure. As will be seen in this chapter, the primary structure and conformation of enzyme proteins are important not only to biologic activity but in some cases also to metabolic control mechanisms.

Enzymes are defined as organic catalysts, produced by the living cell, that are not dependent on the intact cell for their activity. The enzymes act on one or more *substrates* and in many instances require a *coenzyme* or other *cofactors* for activity. It is apparent that in the metabolizing cell they are often part of a complicated, interrelated system. The product of one reaction becomes the substrate of the next and so on. Such interrelated pathways may be fundamental to the metabolic control mechanisms of the cell.

EARLY HISTORY OF ENZYME CHEMISTRY

Three concepts of enzymology, which are historical milestones, had already been expressed by Chittenden in 1894 and continue to be central to our thinking today: (1) Enzymes are proteins. (2) Catalytic activity is in some way related to protein structure. (3) Enzymes are not passive catalysts but function by forming an intermediary complex with the substrate.

Enzymes are proteins   At first, the conclusion that enzymes are proteins was a natural one since these substances were usually purified from complex mixtures of nonactive proteins. As technology improved, however, extremely active preparations that appeared to be devoid of proteins resulted. Willstätter, in 1922, proposed that the protein acted only as an inert carrier of the nonprotein catalytic substance. The crystallization of urease in 1926 by Sumner and pepsin in 1930 and trypsin in 1931 by Northrop showed that enzymes are in fact proteins. Many enzymes, however, are complex systems including certain nonprotein and nonenzymatic components. In 1904, for example, Harden and Young showed that a low–molecular weight, heat-stable substance, which they named cozymase (coenzyme-I or NAD$^+$), is essential to the activity of the enzymes responsible for fermentation.

Enzyme activity is related to protein structure   The concept of catalysis and of the catalytic activity of certain wheat enzymes was proposed in 1837 by Berzelius. Pasteur differentiated between "organized ferments," which he said required the intact cell for activity, and the "unorganized ferments," which could act apart from the living cell. Liebig contested this view and said that the catalytic activity was inherent in the structure of the enzyme molecule itself. In 1897, the Buchner brothers showed that cell-free extracts of yeast were capable of fermenting sugar. This observation made it clear that the intact cell or some related life process is not essential to enzymatic action. Kunitz and Northrop (1934) showed that a loss of proteolytic activity parallels the denaturation of trypsin. Treatment of pepsin with ultraviolet light and with β- and γ-rays from radium showed that proteolytic activity disappears as the protein molecules are destroyed or denatured. Subsequently, Herriott and Northrop (1934) demonstrated that blocking of certain functional groups, especially acetylation of phenolic hydroxyl, but not amino, groups causes a loss of activity that can be restored by deacetylation under mild conditions. Likewise, iodination of the phenolic hydroxyls of trypsin destroyed the activity.

Enzymes are not passive but form intermediate complex with substrate   Henri and Brown, in 1902, proposed the formation of an equilibrium between the enzyme, its substrate, and an enzyme-substrate complex. Later, in 1913, Michaelis and Menten extended this concept and derived the equation and constant that now bear their names (p. 124). In 1925, Briggs and Haldane reevaluated the Michaelis-Menten hypothesis and derived the equation applying the so-called *steady-state assumption*. Direct observations of the enzyme-substrate complexes were first made using horseradish peroxidase and its substrate, hydrogen peroxide (Chance, 1940).

PROTEIN STRUCTURE AND ENZYME ACTION

Some enzymes are entirely protein in composition; others contain metallic ions; still others are conjugated protein, the prosthetic group being involved

Table 7-1. Examples of enzymes containing coenzymes and cofactors

Enzyme	Cofactor	Coenzyme
Cytochrome oxidase	Fe, Cu	Porphyrin
Catalase	Fe	
Peroxidase	Fe	
Succinic dehydrogenase	Fe	FAD
Tyrosinase	Cu	
Lactase	Cu	
Ascorbic acid oxidase	Cu	
Carbonic anhdrase	Zn	
Carboxypeptidase	Zn	
Glucose oxidase		FAD
Phosphoglyceraldehyde dehydrogenase		NAD$^+$

in some way in the catalytic action. The protein or peptide portion, however, is always required for enzyme action. Certain amino acids appear to be required at the active center.

Examples of enzymes that are composed solely of amino acids are pepsin, trypsin, chymotrypsin, ribonuclease, urease, and most hydrolases. Many enzymes, however, are complex molecules containing nonprotein prosthetic groups and minerals. These enzymes are composed of a heat-labile, non-dialyzable protein component, the *apoenzyme*, plus a heat-stable organic prosthetic group, the *coenzyme*, and/or one of the numerous minerals, the *cofactors*. Examples of these enzymes are listed in Table 7-1.

The coenzymes are well-defined organic compounds and in many instances are structures related to the vitamins. Neither of the two components is active by itself, while together they form the active *holoenzyme*.

Nature of the active site A general statement of an enzymatic reaction, where E = enzyme, S = substrate, ES = enzyme-substrate complex, and P = product, is as follows:

$$E + S \ \rightleftharpoons \ ES \ \rightarrow \ E + P$$

The formation of the intermediary complex is based on the interpretation of the biphasic substrate-velocity curve (Fig. 7-8). The fact that increasing the substrate concentration leads to a maximal velocity or a saturation of the enzyme with substrate molecules indicates that there exist a finite number of sites at which catalysis can occur. These are the *active sites* or specific regions in the protein molecule responsible for the catalytic activity. The nature of the active site probably varies with the protein molecule or perhaps with the kind of reaction catalyzed by the enzyme. The active site is either a particular sequence or a special grouping of amino acids. It may be considered to have two functional parts. The first is a binding site, where the substrate adheres to the enzyme; the second is a catalytic site, composed of amino acids that bring about the formation or breakage of bonds in the substrate.

A reagent that has made possible the determination of some amino acid sequences at the active site is a World War II nerve gas called *diisopropyl-fluorophosphate*, DFP. This extremely poisonous compound reacts with the hydroxyl group of serine, thereby inactivating many enzymes. In chymotrypsin, only one of 28 possible serine residues (residue-195) reacts with the reagent, yielding an inactive enzyme. Apparently this serine is located at the active site. Since the covalent bond formed between the DFP and the serine is stable, the serine-containing peptide peculiar to the active site can be separated, after partial enzymatic hydrolysis of the protein derivative. This is particularly effective if the DFP contains the radioactive isotope ^{32}P. The amino acid sequence of the marked peptide is then determined.

Sequences in various enzymes can be compared and similarities between enzymes of like activities sought. This will help establish the existence of special arrangements of amino acids required for a particular catalytic mechanism and, therefore, increase our knowledge regarding the actual nature of enzyme reactions. A consideration of Table 7-2 suggests that some hydrolytic enzymes have in common an aspartyl-seryl-glycyl sequence at the active site. The fact that subtilisin does not fit this pattern shows that such generalizations may still be premature. However, these observations are also of interest from an evolutionary point of view.[1]

Kinetic studies, especially those showing variations of the Michaelis constant (K_M) or maximal velocity (V_{max}) (p. 124) with pH, allow predictions of the identity of other essential, functional groups. Usually it is necessary to confirm such predictions using reagents that either selectively react with or in some way destroy the suspected groups. In this way at least one of the two histidines (residue-57) in chymotrypsin can be shown to be requisite for activity. However, in the primary structure of this enzyme, residue-57 is a long way from serine-195. At this time there seems to be no compelling reason to conclude that the active site should be composed only of a sequence of special amino acids; rather, it might be better to speak of a special grouping of amino acids. These could be brought into the active site entirely by virtue of the conformation of the molecule. The primary structure of α-chymotrypsin has five disulfide bonds. These function to maintain the enzymatically active con-

Table 7-2. Sequences of serine-containing active sites*

Enzyme	Amino acid sequence
Proteolytic	
Bovine trypsin	···AsnSerCysGlnGlyAspSerGlyGlyProValVal···
Bovine chymotrypsin	···SerSerCysMetGlyAspSerGlyGlyProLeuVal···
Porcine elastase	···SerGlyCysGlnGlyAspSerGlyGlyProLeuHis···
Porcine thrombin	···AspSerGly···
Acetylcholine esterase	···GluSerAla···
Subtilisin (Carlsberg)	···AsnGlyThrSerMetAla···
Phosphorylating enzymes	
Alkaline phosphatase	AspSerAla
Phosphoglucomutase (*E. coli*)	ThrAlaSerHisAsp
Phosphorylase a (rabbit)	LysGlnIleSerValArg

*From Dayhoff, M. O., and Eck, R. V.: Atlas of protein sequence and structure, Washington, D. C., 1967–1968, National Biomedical Research Foundation.

formation. It is now also thought that the N-terminal isoleucine (α-ammonium group) is held by the β-carboxylate ion of aspartic acid (residue-194), the net effect being to bring histidine-57 into proximity with serine-195 (Fig. 7-2). In other words, the activity is dependent on the three-dimensional shape or conformation of the molecule.

Another example of the importance of protein conformation to enzyme activity is the enzyme ribonuclease. This protein is a single chain of 124 residues of which two, i.e., histidine-12 and histidine-119, are of special importance to catalytic activity. It is obvious that these two are located near the extreme ends of the chain. Four disulfide bonds (p. 76) are important in achieving the proper proximity of the histidines. Reduction of the disulfide linkages leads to a complete loss of activity. It should now be clear that ribo-

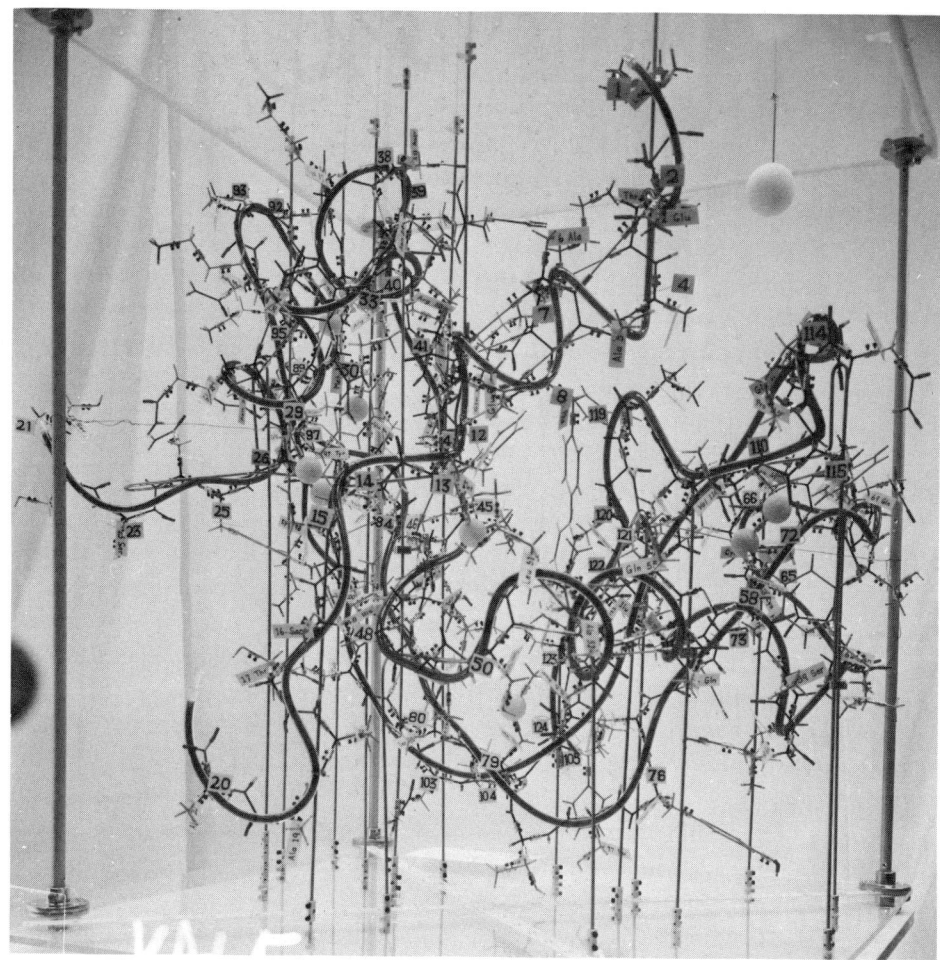

Fig. 7-1. Skeletal model of ribonuclease showing the three-dimensional conformation. Residues are labeled to show the proximity of histidines 12 and 119. (From Wyckoff, H. W., Hardman, K. D., Allewell, N. M., Inagami, T., Johnson, L. N., and Richards, F. M.: J. Biol. Chem. **242**:3984, 1967.)

nuclease is synthesized by its polysome (p. 102) as a single chain with its sulfur in the reduced form. These inactive chains are brought into their active conformation by oxidation of the sulfhydryl groups to disulfide cross-linkages. The proper relationship of residues to form the active site is inherent in the primary structure.

Treatment of the enzyme with fluorodinitrobenzene blocks lysine-41, with a loss of activity. This does not mean, however, that lysine is necessarily an essential part of the active site itself; but lysine does appear to be required in attaining the proper conformation. Fig. 7-1 is the three-dimensional structure of ribonuclease, showing how the two histidine residues are brought into proximity in space.

The importance of the three-dimensional structure of ribonuclease is also illustrated by an experiment in which the first 20 amino acids are removed as a single polypeptide following hydrolysis with the bacterial protease *subtilisin*. This inactivates the enzyme but does not destroy the conformation of the rest of the molecule, called ribonuclease S. The 20–amino acid polypeptide can be added to the ribonuclease S, with a restoration of activity. This means that the histidine-12 can be brought into proximity with histidine-119 even though the peptide bond that formerly held the chain to the rest of the molecule is not restored.

Activation Many proteolytic enzymes are produced by the cell in the form of inactive precursors called *zymogens*. It seems likely that a direct synthesis of active proteases would conceivably lead to the self-destruction of the cell. The zymogens are secreted into the gastrointestinal tract, where they are subsequently converted to their active forms. Activation involves a limited hydrolysis, which either allows the subsequent formation of the active site or removes an inhibitory peptide fragment.

Chymotrypsinogen (suffix *-ogen* is added to denote the zymogen) has a structure that is not conducive to the formation of the active site. Fig. 7-2 shows the location of the five disulfide bonds in the structure of this protein. Activation to α-chymotrypsin requires the hydrolysis of peptide bonds by trypsin and also active chymotrypsin. Since several bonds are split in this process, a number of distinguishable intermediary forms of the enzyme result. Trypsin hydrolyzes the peptide bond between arginine (15) and isoleucine (16). This yields the active π-form of chymotrypsin. The N-terminal isoleucine appears to be essential for activity. Further hydrolysis releases the dipeptide serylarginine, to form δ-chymotrypsin, while hydrolysis of bonds 146–147 and 148–149 releases threonylasparagine and forms α-chymotrypsin. Thus, there are three chains, the A-chain (residues 1–13), the B-chain (16–146), and the C-chain (149–245). All three are held together by the disulfide bonds (Fig. 7-2).

Bovine trypsinogen is a molecule composed of 229 amino acid residues. Activation is by removal of an N-terminal hexapeptide, Val-Asp-Asp-Asp-Asp-Leu, by an enzyme, *enterokinase*, or autocatalytically by trypsin. Removal of the peptide results in an active conformation in which serine-183 and histidine-29 are brought into proximity.

Pepsin, the proteolytic enzyme of the gastric juice, is synthesized and

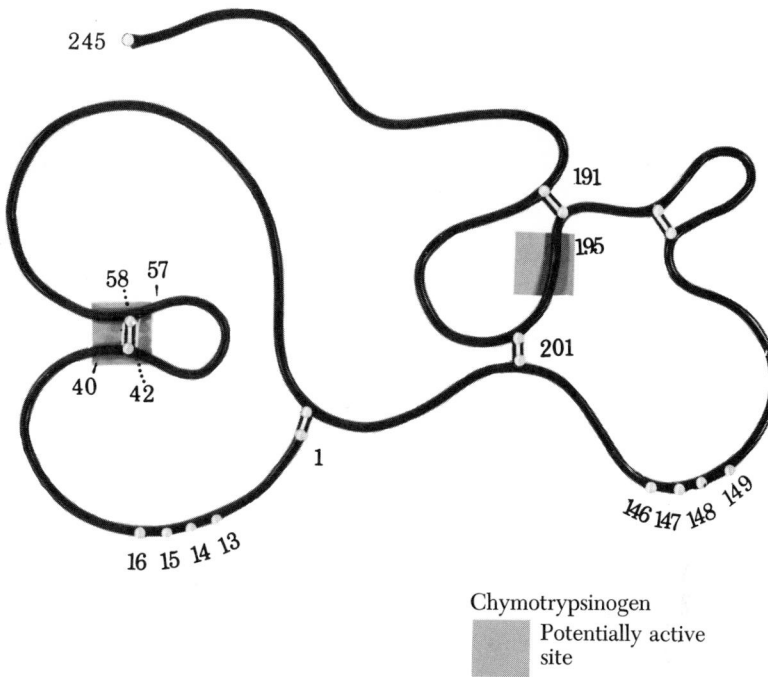

Chymotrypsinogen
Potentially active
site

Fig. 7-2. Model of the structure of chymotrypsinogen. Activation to chymotrypsin minimally requires hydrolysis between residues *15* (Arg) and *16* (Ile). Subsequent conformational changes bring residues *195* (Ser) and *57* (His) into proximity. Other residues labeled are *14* (Ser), *13* (Leu), *1* (Cys), *40* (His), *42* and *58* (Cys), *146* (Tyr), *147* (Thr), *148* (Asn), *149* (Ala), *191* (Cys), and *245* (Asn).

secreted as the zymogenic form, pepsinogen, which has a molecular weight of 38,900, with 362 amino acid residues. The enzyme is activated by the hydrogen ion concentration of the gastric juice. This involves the loss of 42 amino acids from the N-terminal portion of the zymogen. Of the peptides lost, one, having a molecular weight of 3242, is an inhibitor of the enzyme.

Enzyme specificity   Enzymes are unique as catalysts partly because of their specificity of action. Some act on a particular kind of covalent bond in closely related substrates and, therefore, exhibit a *relative* specificity; others appear to act only on one substrate and exhibit *absolute* specificity. Proteolytic enzymes hydrolyze the peptide bonds of polypeptides and, therefore, exhibit relative specificity. Likewise, glycosidases act on glycosidic bonds of carbohydrates; and esterases such as lipases split the ester bonds of lipids. Examples of absolute specificity are more restricted: urease, which acts only on urea; carbonic anhydrase, which acts only on carbonic acid; and fumarase, which acts only on fumaric acid. In addition, many enzymes exhibit stereospecificity. Arginase acts only on L-arginine, not on the D-isomer. Glucose oxidase converts only the β-D-anomer of glucose to gluconic acid, not the α-D-anomer.

Examples of specificity in proteolytic enzymes are shown on p. 114 for pepsin, chymotrypsin, and trypsin. All three hydrolyze peptide bonds, yet each has certain preferences regarding the participating amino acid.

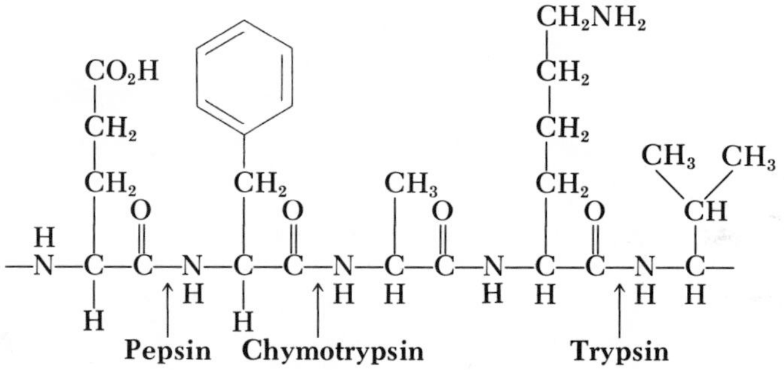

$$\begin{array}{c} \text{Pepsin} \quad \text{Chymotrypsin} \qquad\qquad \text{Trypsin} \end{array}$$

Although pepsin is not highly specific, it prefers those bonds involving the amino and carboxyl groups of aromatic and dicarboxylic amino acids, respectively. Since the bonds attached are usually located in the interior of the protein substrate, pepsin is called an *endopeptidase*. Trypsin likewise is an endopeptidase but hydrolyzes bonds in which the carboxyl group is contributed by either lysine or arginine. Chymotrypsin preferentially splits peptide bonds in which the carboxyl group is from an aromatic amino acid.

Specificity was explained by Emil Fisher on the basis of a template or *lock-and-key* mechanism. Only the proper substrate can fit into a complementary enzyme surface, as a key fits into its lock. Specificity, however, becomes complicated when we attempt to explain some examples of stereospecificity. In the action of the enzyme *glycerokinase* on glycerol to form glycerophosphate, only the L-isomer is formed:

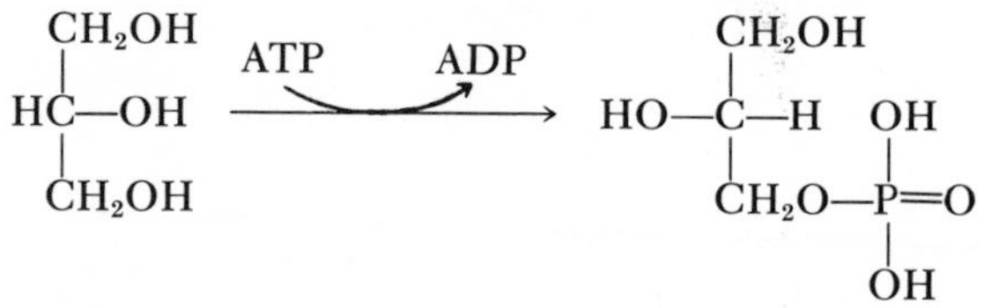

Glycerol does not possess an asymmetric carbon atom, so we cannot easily see how the enzyme distinguishes one hydroxymethyl group from the other. If the enzyme were not perceptive of these two groups, an equal mixture of D- and L-isomers would result. A similar situation of considerable importance to carbohydrate metabolism is the action of the enzyme *aconitase* on its substrate, citric acid (p. 264). Despite the fact that the two carboxymethyl groups of citric acid appear to be equivalent, as far as the enzyme is concerned, they are not. Ogston (1948) explained this phenomenon by invoking a three-point attachment of the substrate to the enzyme (Fig. 7-3). Three groups of the substrate attach in a specific way to the special binding sites on the glycerokinase molecule. Of these sites, only one is considered to be enzymatically active. Fig. 7-3 shows that there is only one way in which all three groups can bind to their corresponding sites. Thus only one of the two hydroxymethyl groups can be phosphorylated.

A rigid template concept does not explain all observations regarding enzyme specificity. In certain instances, substrate analogues bind to the enzyme but for some reason do not react. Our understanding of protein conformation and the importance of bringing specific amino acid side chains into proper

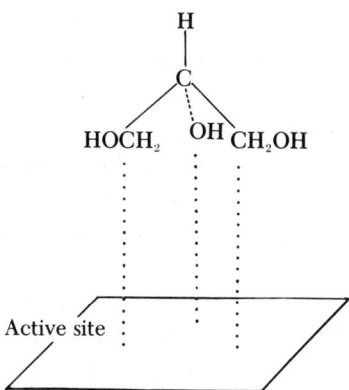

Fig. 7-3. Model showing three-point attachment of the substrate glycerol to the enzyme "surface." Note that each group would bind to a separate site only one of which is active as far as phosphorylation is concerned (active site). There is only one way in which the glycerol can bind in just this manner. Therefore, only one of the CH_2OH groups is phosphorylated by glycerokinase.

juxtaposition has led to another concept of specificity, i.e., the hypothesis of *induced fit* proposed by Koshland.[2] This is based on the idea that the active site is flexible; the protein may not have a proper proximity of reactive groups until the substrate binds to the enzyme. Only the appropriate substrate can cause the precise alignment of catalytic groups needed for enzyme action (Fig. 7-4).

Mechanism of action Kinetic studies and direct observations using spectrophotometric techniques show that an intermediate complex occurs as a step in enzyme-substrate reactions. It is desirable to determine the progression of events during catalysis and, where possible, identify the various responsible amino acid side chains. In the serine-requiring enzymes, this amino acid plays a central role in the catalytic process apparently by forming an ester bond with one of the products of the reaction. For example, when alkaline phosphatase is incubated with *p*-nitrophenyl phosphate (labeled with ^{32}P), the phosphate becomes covalently attached to the serine as serine phosphate, while at the same time releasing the first product, *p*-nitrophenol, as illustrated below. The phosphorylated enzyme is hydrolyzed to yield the second product, inorganic phosphate ($^{32}P_i$), with the simultaneous restoration of the serine hydroxyl.

$$EnOH + O_2N-\langle\rangle-O\overset{32}{\text{—}}P{=}O \longrightarrow EnO\overset{32}{\text{—}}P{=}O + HO-\langle\rangle-NO_2$$

$$^{32}P_i + EnOH$$

Another serine-requiring enzyme, chymotrypsin, also forms an intermediate acyl derivative. Fig. 7-5 shows the steps that have been proposed to explain the function of histidine-57 and serine-195 in the hydrolysis of the peptide bonds. In this scheme, apparently the first stage is the formation of

115

an ester bond between the serine hydroxyl and the peptide fragment contributing the carboxyl of the bond hydrolyzed (steps I to IV). Simultaneously the first product, $R'NH_2$, is released. This is the peptide fragment that contributes the amino nitrogen to the bond hydrolyzed. The acyl chymotrypsin is then hydrolyzed to yield the second product, RCOOH, and restore the serine hydroxyl (steps IV to VI).

An analogous mechanism has been proposed for pancreatic ribonuclease, which is also a hydrolytic enzyme. This enzyme hydrolyzes the 3′,5′-phosphodiester bonds in RNA. Its mechanism of action requires the formation of an intermediate, cyclic 2′,3′-phosphodiester compound (2′,3′-carbons of ribose). The specificity of this enzyme is such that its products are pyrimidine-3′-phosphomonoesters (Chapter 14). In ribonuclease, two histidine

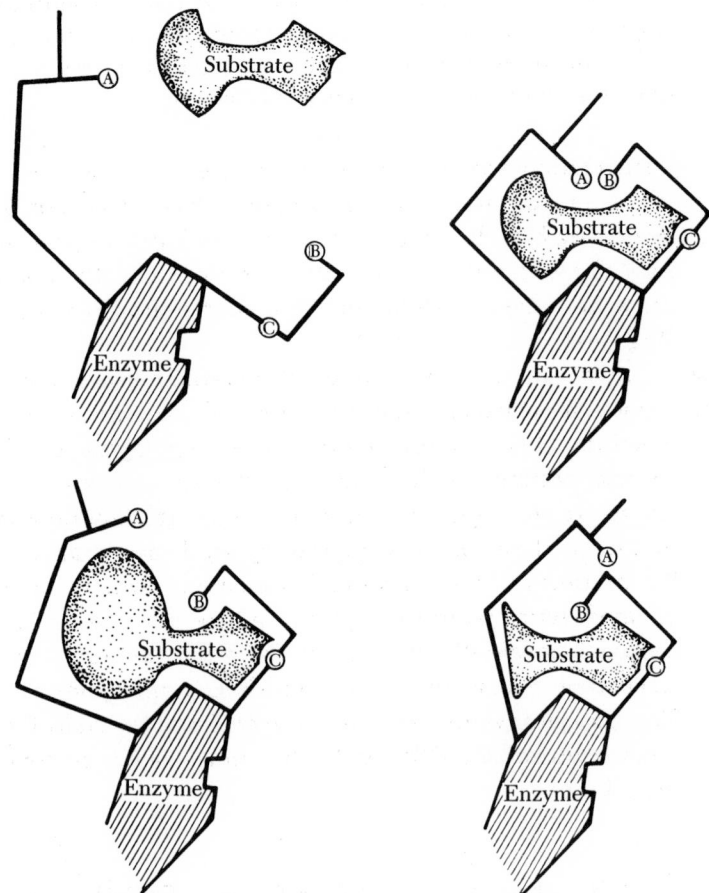

Fig. 7-4. Schematic model of flexible active site mechanism. Black lines indicate protein chains containing catalytic groups A and B and binding group C. Upper left: Substrate and enzyme dissociated. Upper right: Substrate with induced change of protein chains to bring A and B into proper alignment for reaction. Lower left: Bulky group added to substrate prevents proper alignment of A and B. Lower right: Deleted group eliminates buttressing action on chain containing A so that complex has incorrect alignment of A and B. (From Koshland, D. E., Jr.: Fed. Proc. **23**:719, 1964.)

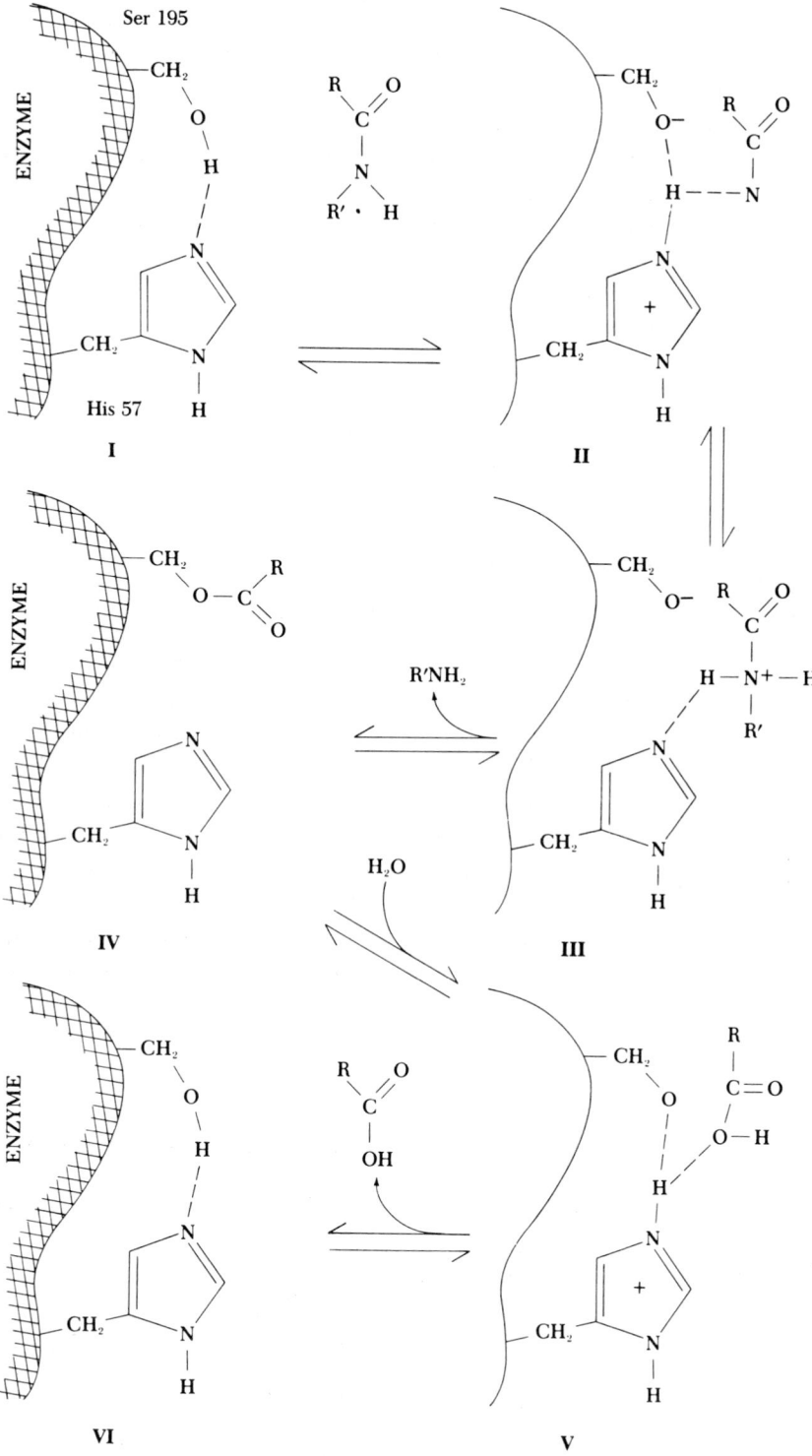

Fig. 7-5. Mechanism of the acylation step in the chymotrypsin-catalyzed hydrolysis of peptides. (Modified from Wang, J. H.: Science **161**:328, 1968.)

residues are functional instead of the combination histidine-serine described for chymotrypsin. The initial step in the mechanism of action is probably the formation of a hydrogen bond between one of the imidazole rings and the hydroxyl at the 2'-carbon of ribose. The second histidine residue, as an imidazolium ion, bonds with the phosphate group. Simultaneously, with the formation of the cyclic intermediate, the first product is released as the residual 5'-hydroxyl nucleotide. A water molecule then causes the formation of the pyrimidine-bearing nucleotide as the second product. In a manner of speaking, the covalent phosphodiester intermediate is analogous to the acyl intermediate of chymotrypsin.

The general mechanism by which the functional amino acids act as proton donors and acceptors is usually called *acid-base catalysis*.[3]

The overall process of catalysis is more complicated than suggested by a simple equilibrium:

$$E + S \rightleftharpoons ES \rightleftharpoons E + P$$

The reaction is more likely as follows:

$$E + S \rightleftharpoons ES \rightleftharpoons EP_2 + P_1$$
$$EP_2 \rightleftharpoons E + P_2$$

Even this is an oversimplification since *ES* may, in all likelihood, consist of several stages. These examples of mechanisms suggest how intermediate combinations of enzyme and substrate molecules can be formed and also how various amino acid side chains can be functional in the catalytic process. However, these mechanisms still do not really explain why or how the enzyme catalyzes a change in a covalent bond of the substrate molecule.

A catalyst acts to increase the rate of a normally slow reaction; it cannot initiate one. The reaction must be spontaneous in a thermodynamic sense. For example, peptide bonds can react with water spontaneously, but this re-

Table 7-3. Examples of activation energies of various catalyzed reactions

Reaction	Catalyst	Energy of activation (calories/mole)
Hydrogen peroxide decomposition	None	18,000
	Colloidal Pt	11,700
	Liver catalase	<2,000
Sucrose inversion	H^+	26,000
	Yeast invertase	11,500
Casein hydrolysis	H^+	20,600
	Trypsin	12,000
	Chymotrypsin	12,000
Ethyl butyrate hydrolysis	H^+	16,800
	OH^-	10,200
	Lipase	4,500

action is so slow that, for all intents and purposes, it is nonexistent. In the presence of peptidase, however, the reaction proceeds rapidly and can easily be measured. The peptide bond does not normally break down in water because of its *energy of activation*. This is an amount of energy, expressed in calories per mole, that must be supplied before there is sufficient interaction between reactants to form a product. A catalyst or enzyme reduces the necessary activation energy (Table 7-3) so that the energy in the system becomes sufficient for the reaction to proceed at a measurable rate.

Factors influencing enzyme action   Since enzymes are usually present in extremely small quantities in biologic systems and since often we are not able to measure the amount of enzyme in terms of quantity, we usually measure these proteins by their activity. A unit of activity is defined as the amount of enzyme that will produce 1 micromole of product per minute at 25° C. under standardized conditions.

A variety of factors influence the velocity of enzyme-catalyzed reactions. Among them are the following:

1. Hydrogen ion concentration
2. Temperature
3. Concentration of enzyme
4. Time
5. Concentration of substrate
6. Products of the reaction
7. Effects of light and other physical factors
8. Nature and concentration of various ions
9. Allosteric effects
10. Effects of hormones and other biochemical agents

To determine the effects of these factors on enzyme reactions, it is usual to study the velocity of the reaction under different conditions. It is possible to

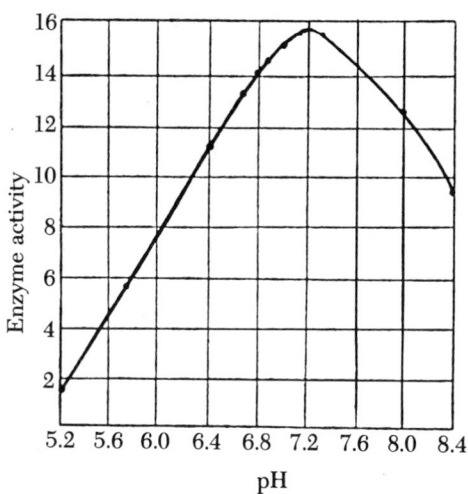

Fig. 7-6. Effect of pH on enzyme activity. These data were obtained by determining the number of milligrams of reducing sugar formed in reaction mixtures in which the amounts of enzyme (pancreatic amylase) and substrate (soluble starch) were constant. The pH was adjusted by using phosphate buffers (KH_2PO_4/Na_2HPO_4) in which the different H^+ concentrations were attained by using different ratios of the acid and alkaline salt. (From Myers, V. C., and Free, A. H.: Amer. J. Clin. Path. **13**:42, 1943.)

measure either the accumulation of product or the disappearance of substrate per unit of time. In any event, the activity of the enzyme is expressed in terms of velocity (V).

Hydrogen ion concentration. Enzyme reactions are influenced by varying the hydrogen ion concentration (Fig. 7-6). The *optimum pH* is that pH at which a certain enzyme causes a reaction to progress most rapidly. On either side of the optimum, the rate of reaction is lower and at certain pH's an enzyme may be inactivated or even destroyed. Therefore, in enzyme studies, buffers are used to keep the enzyme at an optimum or at least a favorable hydrogen ion concentration. The optimum pH is dependent on various conditions; the kind of buffer, the particular substrate, and the source of the enzyme may all have an influence. Table 7-4 shows, moreover, the wide range of optimal hydrogen ion concentrations for various enzymes.

Influence of temperature. The temperature coefficient of a reaction may be defined as the increase in the reaction rate for a 10° C. increase in temperature. It is designated Q_{10}. For enzymes this ranges mainly from 1.1 to 3; i.e., the velocity of an enzyme reaction is increased from 1.1 to 3 times for every 10° C. rise in temperature. An *optimum temperature* is usually reached at 40° to 50° C. for animal enzymes, whereas for plant enzymes it is higher, usually 50° to 60° C. Above this, the rate decreases because the enzyme is denatured at a rate faster then the increase in the reaction. Most enzymes are denatured above 60° C. Obviously the time of exposure is a factor also. An enzyme may withstand higher temperatures for short periods of time. Strictly

Table 7-4. Michaelis-Menten constants of some enymes and their optimum pH's*

Enzyme	Source	Substrate	K_M	Optimum pH
Sucrase	Intestine	Sucrose	0.016–0.04M	6.2
Amylase	Saliva, pancreas	Starch	0.8 –0.25%	5.6–7.2
α-Glucosidase	Yeast	Methyl-α-D-glucoside	0.037–0.075M	
β-Glucosidase	Almond	Methyl-β-D-glucoside	0.060–1.12M	
Lipase (esterase)	Pancreas	Ethyl butyrate	>0.03M	7.0
Dipeptidase	Intestine	Glycylleucine	0.02 –0.07M	7.3–8.1
Pepsin	Gastric mucosa	Ovalbumin	4.5%	1.5–2.5
Trypsin	Pancreas	Casein	2%	8 –11
Urease	Soybean	Urea	0.025M	7.2–7.9
Phosphatase	Bone	Glycerophosphate	<0.003M	8.4
Catalase	Liver	Hydrogen peroxide	0.025M	6.3–9.5
Xanthine oxidase	Milk	Xanthine	$3–4 \times 10^{-7}$M	5.5–8.5
Succinic dehydrogenase	Beef heart	Succinate	5×10^{-7}M	9

*These data have been obtained from a number of sources. Most of the enzymes are not pure preparations.

speaking, the optimal temperature has meaning only if the time of the reaction is also stipulated.

Concentration of enzyme. The velocity of an enzyme reaction is directly proportional to the concentration of the enzyme, provided the substrate is present in excess. This is particularly true at the beginning of the reaction, but it may not hold true as the reaction continues, especially as the substrate is used up (Fig. 7-7).

Influence of time. As we have already seen, the velocity of the reaction is the amount of product produced per unit of time. Sometimes one may need to increase the time during which an enzyme reaction is studied. For example, it might be assumed that after 1 hour 60 times as much product is formed as in 1 minute. Such extrapolation may be made only when it has clearly been shown that the formation of product is linear over a 1-hour period. To do this, the amount of product is plotted against the incubation time. Usually a curve in which the amount of product formed reaches a plateau is obtained. In other words, the amount of product becomes constant while the time factor increases; i.e., the velocity of the reaction (product over time) decreases. This slowing may be due to several causes: the amount of available substrate decreases; accumulation of product increases the reverse reaction; the product may have a deleterious effect on the reaction by denaturing the enzyme or changing the pH away from the optimum.

Concentration of substrate. For a given quantity of enzyme, the velocity of the reaction increases as the concentration of the substrate is increased. At first, this relationship is almost linear; but as seen from Fig. 7-8, the re-

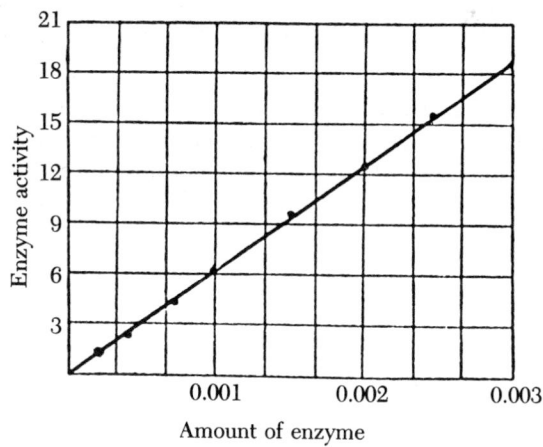

Fig. 7-7. Effect of enzyme concentration on enzyme activity. These data were obtained by determining the number of milligrams of reducing sugar formed in digestion mixtures containing different amounts of pancreatic amylase. The pancreatic amylase was supplied as duodenal contents, and the values of the abscissa indicate the number of milliliters of duodenal contents present in the digestion mixtures. The digestion mixture was buffered at an optimal pH and contained optimal amounts of chloride and substrate. (From Myers, V. C., and Free, A. H.: Amer. J. Clin. Path. **13**:42, 1943.)

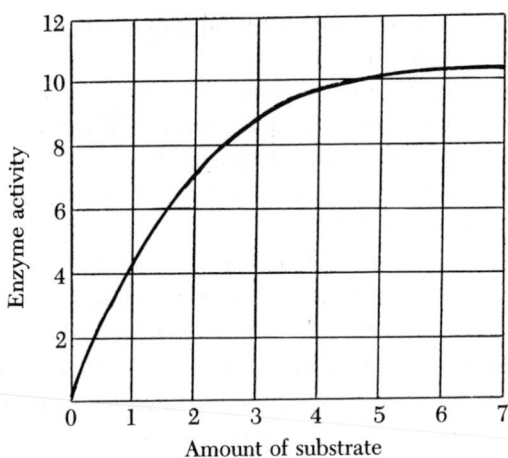

Fig. 7-8. Effect of substrate concentration on enzyme activity. These data were obtained by determining the number of milligrams of reducing sugar formed in reaction mixtures in which the amount of enzyme (pancreatic amylase) was constant. The amount of substrate indicates the number of milliliters of 1% soluble starch present in the reaction mixtures, all of which had the same total volume. (From Myers, V. C., and Free, A. H.: Amer. J. Clin. Path. **13**:42, 1943.)

action curve assumes a hyperbolic shape. This means that the reaction kinetics are biphasic. The reaction in the first, nearly linear, phase of the curve, in which the velocity is directly proportional to the concentration of substrate, follows *first-order* kinetics. In the second phase a plateau is reached in which the velocity is constant and the reaction is said to exhibit *zero-order* kinetics. This occurs at such a substrate concentration that further increases do not affect the velocity of the reaction; therefore the concentration is the amount of substrate that saturates the enzyme. Since the velocity-substrate curve is theoretically a hyperbola, the zero-order portion approaches a limiting or maximal velocity, usually termed V_{max} or V_m. The fact that a saturating concentration of substrate can be reached is suggestive not only of the formation of the ES-complex but also that there is a finite number of sites at which this interaction can occur. The ability to form an ES-complex is not unlimited.

An understanding of the kinetics of enzyme reaction as illustrated is essential in the design and use of methods for the quantitative determination of enzymes, a field assuming increasing clinical significance (p. 134). It is preferable to employ concentrations of substrate that will yield zero-order kinetics so that variations in substrate concentrations do not influence the measurements of the enzyme activity. It is only under the condition of zero-order kinetics that the velocity will vary with the enzyme concentration. Sometimes, however, substrates are expensive and it becomes necessary to consider the economics of the analysis. In this event the units of enzyme activity can be determined in the first-order part of the curve with the aid of the appropriate equation relating velocity to the substrate concentration.

Kinetics of enzyme reactions

As mentioned previously, a simplified statement of an enzyme reaction is the following:

$$E + S \underset{k_{-1}}{\overset{k_1}{\rightleftharpoons}} ES \underset{k_{-2}}{\overset{k_2}{\rightleftharpoons}} E + P$$

This equation illustrates the overall reversibility of the reaction. Each step of the reaction is characterized by a specific rate constant: the formation of ES from E and S by k_1; the dissociation of ES to E and S by k_{-1}; the formation of P and E from ES by k_2; the re-formation of ES from E and P by k_{-2}. Here ES may represent multiple steps or activated stages (p. 118), and actually more than one product may be produced. The amount of product formed depends on the concentration of the unstable ES-complex. (It should be remembered that all concentrations in this discussion are molar, not percentage.) Michaelis and Menten proposed a hypothesis relating the velocity at any given substrate concentration to the maximal velocity and the specified substrate concentration. Briggs and Haldane later modified this hypothesis to include the *steady-state* assumption. Soon after the enzymatic reaction begins, we assume that a state is reached in which the rate of change of ES-complex with time is practically zero. In other words, as soon as a molecule of ES breaks down to form product and enzyme, another enzyme molecule and another substrate molecule react to form more ES-complex. Stated algebraically:

$$\frac{d(ES)}{dt} = 0$$

The derivation of the Michaelis-Menten equation is simplified by assuming that all measurements of activity will be restricted to initial velocities when the concentration of product is negligible. Under this condition we may assume that no significant reversal of the reaction occurs; therefore, we can ignore the reaction described by the rate constant k_{-2}. The modified reaction becomes:

$$E + S \underset{k_{-1}}{\overset{k_1}{\rightleftharpoons}} ES \overset{k_2}{\longrightarrow} E + P$$

The velocity of ES-complex formation is

$$v_1 = k_1(E)(S)$$

where E and S are the molar concentrations of enzyme and substrate, respectively. The velocity of ES breakdown is:

$$v_{-1} = k_{-1}(ES) \quad \text{for the re-formation of E and S}$$

and

$$v_2 = k_2(ES) \quad \text{for the formation of P and E}$$

Under steady-state conditions the velocity of ES-complex formation must equal the sum of the velocities of breakdown.

$$v_1 = v_{-1} + v_2$$

or

$$\frac{d(ES)}{dt} = v_1 - v_{-1} - v_2 = 0$$

then

$$k_1(E)(S) = k_{-1}(ES) + k_2(ES)$$

$$\frac{(E)(S)}{ES} = \frac{k_{-1} + k_2}{k_1} = K_M \quad \text{(Michaelis-Menten constant)} \tag{1}$$

It is seldom possible to evaluate the concentration of free enzyme (E) or of the enzyme-substrate complex (ES). Therefore, E and ES must be eliminated from the equation. Recognizing that E is the concentration of free enzyme while the total enzyme $E_t = E_f + ES$ or $E_f = E_t - ES$, then:

$$K_M = \frac{(E_t - ES)(S)}{ES}$$

or

$$K_M(ES) = (E_t)(S) - (S)(ES)$$

$$K_M(ES) + (S)(ES) = (E_t)(S)$$

$$ES(K_M + S) = (E_t)(S)$$

$$ES = \frac{(E_t)(S)}{K_M + S} \tag{2}$$

The velocity of the forward reaction, v_2, is proportional to ES:

$$v_2 = k_2(ES)$$

or

$$ES = \frac{v_2}{k_2}$$

Then substituting in Equation 2:

$$\frac{v_2}{k_2} = \frac{(E_t)(S)}{K_M + S}$$

or

$$v_2 = \frac{(E_t)k_2(S)}{K_M + S} \tag{3}$$

When the system is saturated with substrate, all the enzyme, E_t, will exist as ES and the velocity will be maximal, V_{max}. Thus:

$$V_{max} = k_2(E_t)$$

Substituting in Equation 3:

$$v = \frac{V_{max}(S)}{K_M + S} \tag{4}$$

Equation 4 is the usual form of the Michaelis-Menten equation. To determine the nature of the constant, K_M, consideration of the equation will show that the constant is the substrate concentration that yields a velocity equal to one half the maximal velocity. In other words if we replace $V_{max}/2$ for v, then:

$$\frac{V_{max}}{2} = \frac{V_{max}(S)}{K_M + S}$$

and

$$S = K_M$$

This means that the Michaelis-Menten constant has the dimensions of moles/ liter. The relation of K_M to $V_{max}/2$ is apparent from Fig. 7-9, which shows how difficult it would be to determine V_{max} and hence K_M visually from the hyperbolic graph. To surmount this difficulty and to obtain an accurate value for K_M, the following linear form of Equation 4 was developed by Lineweaver and Burk. If we take the reciprocal form of Equation 4,

$$\frac{1}{v} = \frac{K_M + S}{V_{max}(S)}$$

or

$$\frac{1}{v} = \frac{K_M}{V_{max}} \cdot \frac{1}{S} + \frac{1}{V_{max}}$$

an equation yielding a straight line, i.e., $y = mx + b$, results. Here y and x are the ordinate and abscissa, respectively, and b is the y-intercept. In the Lineweaver-Burk plot the reciprocals $1/v$ and $1/S$ are plotted as shown in Fig. 7-10. The straight line has a slope of K_M/V_{max} and a y-intercept of $1/V_{max}$. If the line is extrapolated until $1/v = 0$ or when the line crosses the x-axis, this intercept of the abscissa equals $-1/K_M$; then $1/K_M = 1/S$.

The Michaelis-Menten equation is of great value in the study of enzymes,

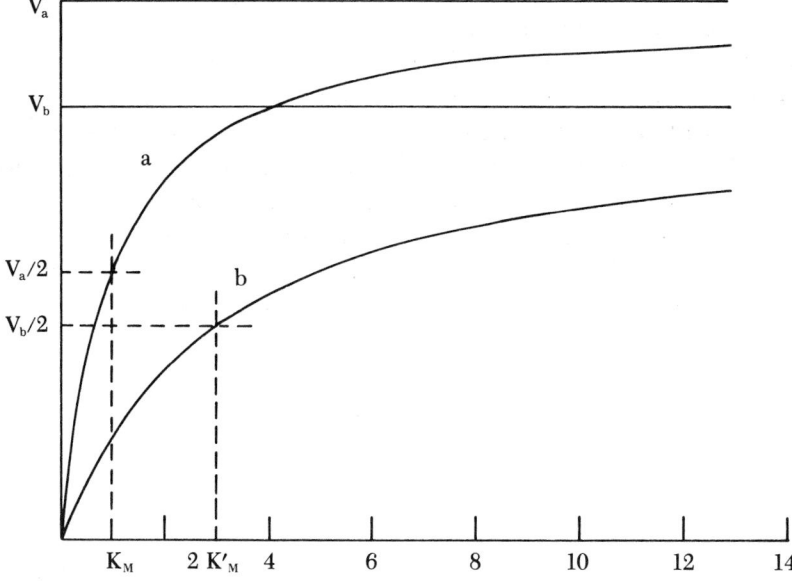

Fig. 7-9. Michaelis-Menten constants for a group-specific enzyme acting on two different substrates, a and b. The relations between reaction velocities, V_a and V_b, and substrate concentrations have been experimentally determined and the hyperbolic curves obtained. Ordinate: reaction velocity. Abscissa: molarity of substrates in arbitrary units. The maximum velocities are the asymptotic values to which the reaction velocities tend as the concentrations of the substrates increase. (From Baldwin, E.: Dynamic aspects of biochemistry, Cambridge, 1957, Cambridge University Press.)

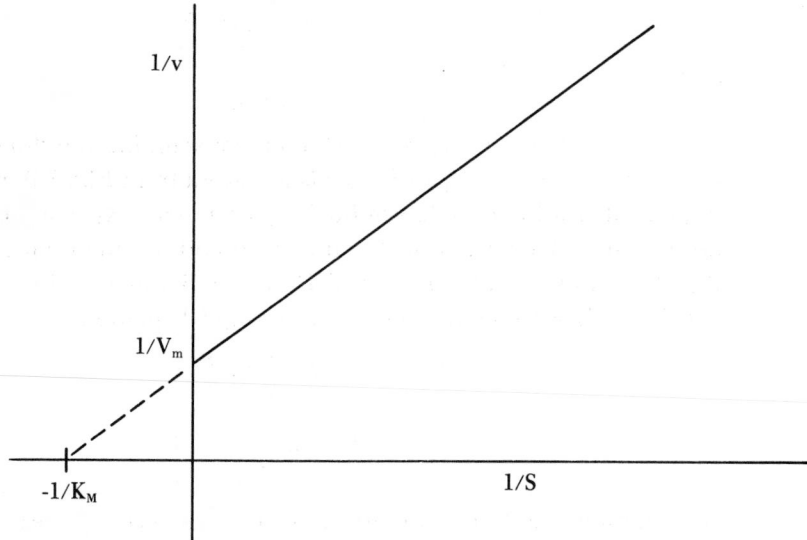

Fig. 7-10. Lineweaver-Burk plot showing the relation of the reciprocals of velocity of enzyme reaction to substrate concentration.

and the constants of many enzymes have been determined (Table 7-4). The range of values is from 1×10^{-8} to 1 or higher. It should be clear that this constant represents a ratio of rate constants $(k_{-1} + k_2)/k_1$ under conditions of constant pH, temperature, etc.

Enzyme inhibitors   Much can be learned concerning the nature of active sites and the reactions involved in ES-complex formation by studying the interaction of enzymes with substrate analogues and other inhibitors. Not only is this information of theoretic importance, but it also has practical applications in medicine.

One kind of inhibition involves the use of substrate analogues that are sufficiently like the true substrate in structure to combine with the enzyme at the active site. However, the formation of a product either may be much slower or may not occur at all, thereby slowing the rate of reaction. Since the substrate analogue competes with the substrate for the enzyme, this is termed *competitive inhibition*. Competitive inhibition is reversible, however, since the dissociation of enzyme-inhibitor complex is the same as the enzyme-substrate complex.

$$E + I \leftrightharpoons EI$$

The difference from the regular ES-reaction lies in the inability to continue the formation of the product. A classic example involves the enzyme succinic dehydrogenase (p. 264). This enzyme acts on its substrate, succinic acid, to remove two hydrogen atoms and form the product fumaric acid.

$$
\begin{array}{ccc}
\text{COOH} & & \text{COOH} \\
| & & | \\
\text{CH}_2 & & \text{CH} \\
| & \searrow & \| \\
\text{CH}_2 & & \text{CH} \\
| & & | \\
\text{COOH} & \text{2H} & \text{COOH}
\end{array}
$$

If malonic acid is added to the reaction mixture, this dicarboxylic acid competes with the succinic acid for the active site of the enzyme. However, two hydrogens cannot be removed from malonic acid.

$$\begin{array}{l} COOH \\ | \\ CH_2 \quad \nrightarrow \\ | \\ COOH \end{array}$$

If we now add an excess of succinic acid to the mixture containing the malonic acid, the binding of enzyme to inhibitor can be reversed because the frequency of the binding is diminished by the excess succinate. Thus the rate of product formation is increased even to the normal maximal velocity. In the presence of inhibitor, much more substrate must be added to the enzyme to reach the maximal velocity than is necessary in the absence of inhibitor. There are two logical conclusions: (1) the maximal velocity (V_m or V_{max}) in competitive inhibition is unchanged from normal; (2) the substrate concentration needed to reach $V_m/2$ is greater than normal. This means that K_M in the presence of inhibitor (apparent K_M) is greater than normal while V_m remains the same.

The reaction $E + I \rightleftharpoons EI$ allows the definition of a dissociation constant for this reaction, which is designated K_I. A modified Michaelis-Menten equation involving this constant can be derived:

$$v = \frac{V_m(S)}{K_M\left(1 + \frac{I}{K_I}\right) + S}$$

and

$$\frac{1}{v} = \frac{K_M\left(1 + \frac{I}{K_I}\right)}{V_m} \cdot \frac{1}{S} + \frac{1}{V_m}$$

The equation shows that a Lineweaver-Burk plot would have a slope greater than the normal by the factor $(1 + I/K_I)$. It also shows that the intercept is $1/V_m$, as is the case in the absence of inhibitor. These features of competitive inhibition can be seen graphically by the linear double reciprocal plot of Lineweaver and Burk (Fig. 7-11).

Another class of inhibition involves reaction with the enzyme in a *noncompetitive* fashion. Noncompetitive inhibition reactions are irreversible in the sense that an excess of substrate does not reverse the reaction between the enzyme and the inhibitor. In many instances these inhibitors may react with specific amino acid residues either at the active site itself or in such a way as to change the conformation of the molecule, thereby destroying or modifying the active form. Examples are the reaction of diisopropylfluorophosphate with the seryl residue of the active site and the reaction and inactivation of enzymes with iodoacetic acid. The latter combines with sulfhydryl groups of the cysteine residue. Likewise, mercury inactivates some enzymes also by combining at sulfhydryl groups. Under special circumstances these reactions are sometimes reversible by removing the reagent, e.g., mercury, by a chelating agent. Noncompetitive inhibition in effect removes active enzyme molecules from the system. This means that there is a lowered concentration of active molecules. The consequence is a reduction of the V_m. The amount of substrate needed to achieve $\frac{1}{2}V_m$, i.e., K_M, is the same since, for all intents and purposes, the reaction remains the same. The equation for noncompetitive inhibition:

$$\frac{1}{v} = \left(1 + \frac{I}{K_I}\right)\left(\frac{1}{V_m} + \frac{K_M}{V_m} \cdot \frac{1}{S}\right)$$

shows that both the slope and the intercept are increased by the factor $(1 +$

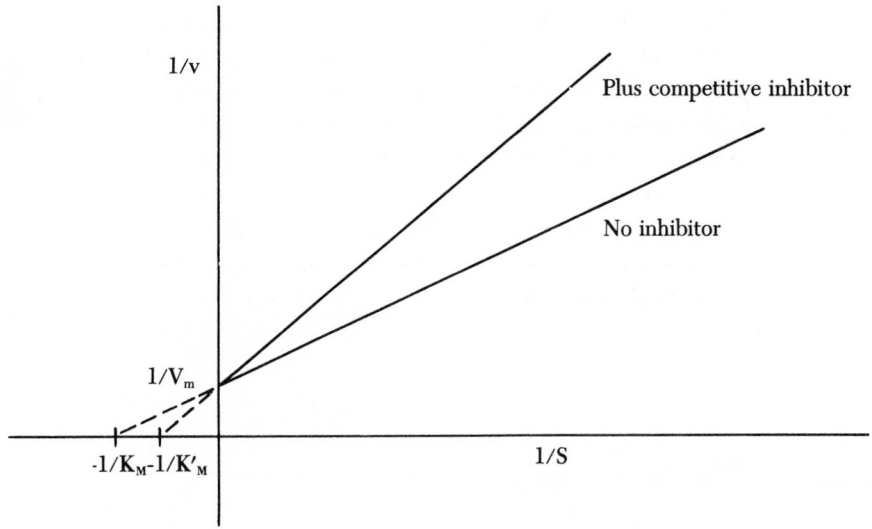

Fig. 7-11. Linear double reciprocal Lineweaver and Burk plot showing competitive inhibition.

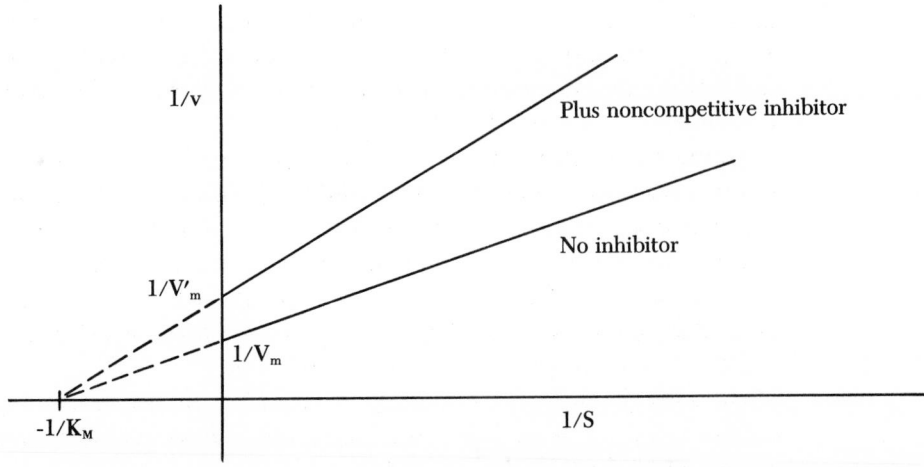

Fig. 7-12. Plot showing the effect of noncompetitive inhibitor.

I/K_I). Extrapolation of the reciprocal plot to $1/v = 0$ results in a value for $1/K_M$. However, the y-intercept is increased by $(1 + I/K_I)$. (See Fig. 7-12.)

Competitive inhibition finds its practical applications in medicine, especially in the use of certain antimetabolites such as the sulfanilamide derivatives. Sulfanilamide is a powerful inhibitor of bacterial growth (i.e., it is bacteriostatic). It is a competitive inhibitor for p-aminobenzoic acid, an essential metabolite for the bacterial cell. This action of sulfa drugs is reversed by p-aminobenzoic acid (p. 832).

Specific inhibitors of proteolytic enzymes exist in nature in the form of polypeptides or proteins of molecular weight 6000 to 25,000. For instance, the body wall of the parasitic worm *Ascaris lumbricoides* contains a peptide that specifically inhibits trypsin as well as one that inhibits chymotrypsin. These inhibitors make it possible for the parasite to thrive in the digestive environment of the host's intestinal tract.

Control mechanisms —allosterism Regulation of metabolic pathways is increasingly being related to a process called *feedback control*. Feedback control may be either positive (stimulation) or negative (inhibition). The manner in which substrates modify the activity of an enzyme is dependent on a phenomenon called the *allosteric effect*. Allosterism is usually defined as the action of a modifier on the activity of the enzyme by binding to a site, the allosteric site, that is topologically distinct from the active site. In this mechanism a small molecule, the *effector* (or modifier), can change the conformation of the enzyme. Changes in molecular conformation in allosterism usually involve systems having more than one protein subunit. The characteristics of allosterism can be illustrated by a system that actually is not an enzyme, i.e., hemoglobin. A consideration of the oxygen-saturation curve for hemoglobin and comparison with that of myoglobin (p. 646) will show one of the characteristics of allosteric binding. Both myoglobin and hemoglobin function physiologically by binding oxygen. Myoglobin molecules, however, remain free in solution while hemoglobin is actually a system of four subunits each capable of binding a molecule of oxygen. The degree of binding by the tetramer is not uniform for each subunit. Actually, after the first subunit has accepted its oxygen, it makes the binding of the second subunit simpler, and so on. The net effect is to yield a *sigmoid* oxygen saturation curve (Fig. 20-1). In the case of myoglobin, where there is no subunit interaction, the oxygen saturation curve is hyperbolic and, therefore, shows Michaelis-Menten kinetics. This indicates that the quaternary structure of some proteins plays an important role in the control of physiologic processes. Enzyme systems that show allosteric binding exhibit sigmoid velocity curves in much the same manner as does hemoglobin.

A classic example of allosteric control mechanism is the enzyme *aspartyl transcarbamylase* (p. 407). This enzyme catalyzes the first step in the biosynthesis of pyrimidines, namely, the combination of carbamyl phosphate and aspartic acid to form carbamyl aspartate. The ultimate accumulation of excess cytidine triphosphate (CTP) results in the inhibition of this enzyme. Aspartyl transcarbamylase has two kinds of subunits: one is the enzyme; the other is a regulatory unit that can bind the CTP. The overall enzyme possesses four enzyme subunits each having a molecular weight of 48,000; there

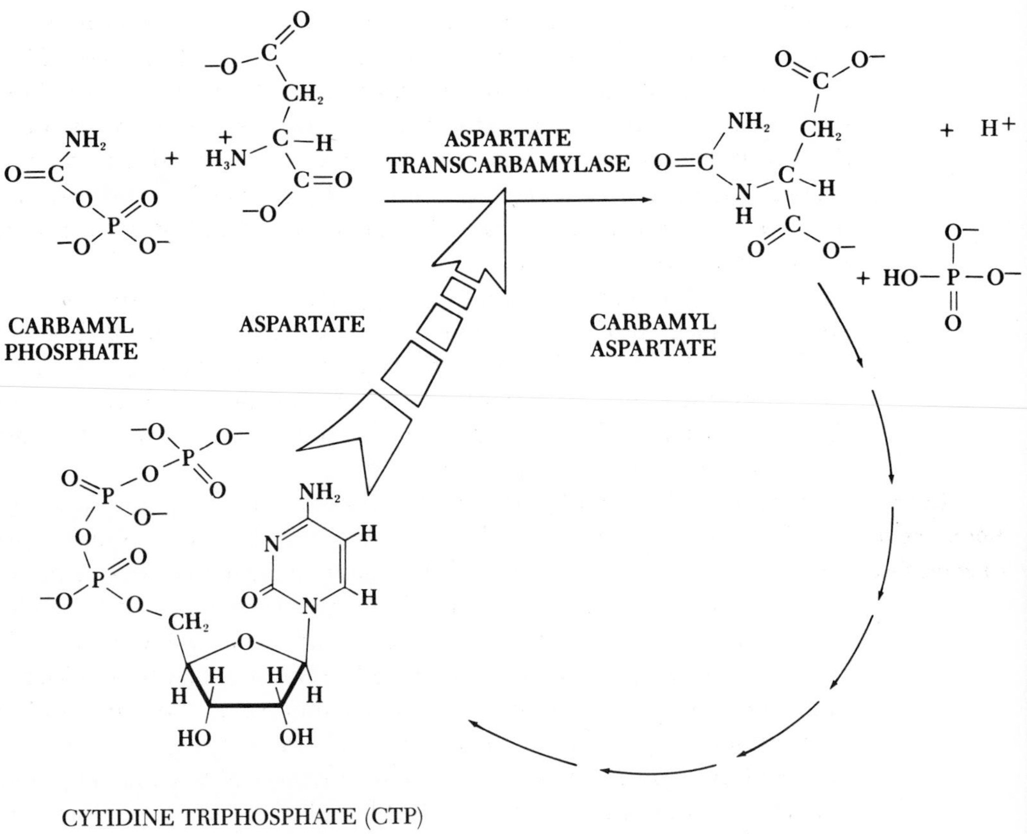

CYTIDINE TRIPHOSPHATE (CTP)

Fig. 7-13. Schematic diagram of feedback inhibition in the pyrimidine pathway of *E. coli.* (From Gerhart, J. C., and Pardee, A. B.: Sympos. Quant. Biol. **28**:491, 1963.)

are also four regulatory or CTP-binding subunits each with a molecular weight of 28,000 (Fig. 7-13). The subunits are held together by sulfhydryl groups supplied by the regulatory proteins. When the regulatory and enzymatic subunits are separated, as when the enzyme is treated with mercurials, the two kinds of proteins may be studied individually. The enzyme unit alone is still active but now exhibits typical Michaelis-Menten kinetics; i.e., the velocity-substrate curve is hyperbolic. The intact molecule, on the other hand, shows a sigmoid curve.

Isozymes   Another phenomenon that may have a role in control mechanisms and that depends on the quaternary structure of the enzyme protein is the formation of isozymes.[4] The classic example of this phenomenon involves the enzyme *lactic dehydrogenase.* Lactic dehydrogenase is a tetramer consisting of two distinct subunit molecules. Each subunit has enzymatic activity, yet the two proteins have an amino acid composition sufficiently different so that they are readily separated in an electrophoretic system. When the two subunits are mixed in equal proportions, a sequence of five bands is obtained by electrophoresis (Fig. 7-14). These bands represent a regular distribution of each subunit in the quaternary structure. Thus in Fig. 7-14, band *1* is a tetramer of

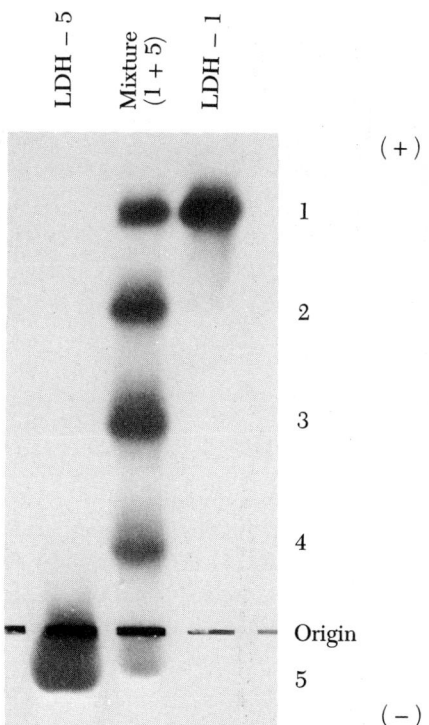

Fig. 7-14. Electrophoretic migration of purified ox heart LDH-1 and LDH-5. The two isozymes were separated by processes of chromatography and electrophoresis. The separation obtained in the central slot is that of an equal mixture of LDH-1 and LDH-5. (From Markert, C. L.: Ann. N.Y. Acad. Sci. **151**:14, 1968.)

LDH-1 only, band 2 contains three LDH-2 subunits and one of LDH-5, band 3 contains two LDH-1 and two LDH-5, band 4 contains one LDH-1 and three LDH-5, and band 5 contains only LDH-5.

MULTIENZYME SYSTEMS

Another level of enzyme structure is the highly organized multienzyme complex. A few examples of metabolic enzyme systems are known to exist, not as independent molecules but in a state of aggregation or architecture involving several different enzymes. Pyruvic acid dehydrogenase of *E. coli* is one that has received considerable attention.[5] This complex (molecular weight 4.8 million) consists of three enzymes, 24 molecules of pyruvate decarboxylase (90,000), 24 molecules of dihydrolipoic dehydrogenase (55,000), and eight subunits of lipoyl reductase transacetylase (120,000). Fig. 7-15 shows an electron micrograph of this enzyme as well as tentative models. The functions of the various coenzymes associated with this system are described in greater detail elsewhere (p. 203). Molecular organization provides a mosaic of enzymes in which each component is arranged so as to afford an efficient coupling of the individual reactions catalyzed by these enzymes. In other words, the product of the first enzyme becomes the substrate of the second, and so on.

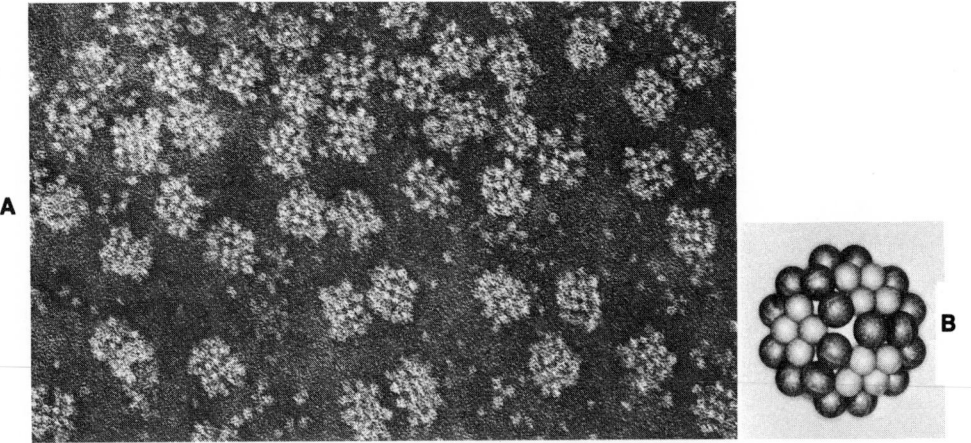

Fig. 7-15. **A,** Electron micrograph of the pyruvate dehydrogenase complex of *E. coli,* negatively stained with methylamine tungstate (×250,000). **B,** Interpretative model of the complex showing 24 dihydrolipoyl dehydrogenase subunits (white spheres) and 24 molecules of pyruvate decarboxylase (black spheres). (From Reed, L. J., and Oliver, R. M.: Brookhaven Sympos. Biol. **21:**397, 1968.)

CLASSIFICATION

The naming of enzymes has resulted in considerable confusion. Sometimes enzymes are named for the substrate, sometimes for the type of reaction, sometimes on other bases. As a result, one enzyme often was given several different names, and occasionally the same name was given to more than one enzyme. An international group of scientists was assigned the task of naming, classifying, and codifying the known enzymes and formulating rules that would indicate how newly discovered enzymes should be named and classified. Codifying meant assigning a series of numbers to each enzyme so that it would have its own identity. However, in many cases, in addition to a new scientific name, the old "trivial" name was permitted. About 700 enzymes were listed in the original publication; only a few representative examples are given here.

Six main groups of enzymes have been designated: (1) oxidoreductases, (2) transferases, (3) hydrolases, (4) lyases, (5) isomerases, and (6) ligases or synthetases.

A sample of the International Union of Biochemistry code is as follows:

1. Oxidoreductases—Concerned in biologic oxidations, a few of the many different oxido-reductases being the following:
   a. Dehydrogenases—Remove hydrogen from substrate, but only in the presence of suitable hydrogen acceptor; some of them called *reductases*
   b. Oxidases—Have O_2 as hydrogen acceptor, e.g., aldehyde oxidase

$$\text{Aldehyde } H_2O + O_2 \quad \rightleftarrows \quad \text{Acid} + H_2O_2$$

2. Transferases—Cause transfer of certain groups from one compound to another[9]
   a. Those transferring 1-carbon groups, e.g., methyl transferases

    b. Those transferring aldehydic or ketonic groups, e.g., transketolase

    c. Those transferring acyl groups, e.g., aminoacyl transferase

    d. Those transferring sugar groups, e.g., sucrose-1-fructosyl transferase, which converts sucrose into inulin and glucose

    e. Others – Those transferring alkyl, nitrogenous, phosphorus-containing, and sulfur-containing groups

3. Hydrolases – Bring about hydrolyses; i.e., they add water to substrate and simultaneously decompose it

    a. Simple esterases – Split esters of ethyl butyrate type, yielding monohydric alcohols and monocarboxylic acids

    b. Lipases – Convert fats into fatty acids and glycerol

    c. Phosphatases – Hydrolyze phosphoric acid esters into their main constituents; thus glycerophosphate is hydrolyzed to glycerol and phosphoric acid

    d. Cholinesterases – Hydrolyze esters of choline

    e. Peptide hydrolyses – Attack peptide linkages ($-\overset{\parallel}{\underset{O}{C}}-\overset{\mid}{\underset{H}{N}}-$) of proteins and peptides; some split off N-terminal residues, some the C-terminal residue, while others are very specific in attacking linkages joined to specific amino acids

    f. Nucleases, etc. – Hydrolyze nucleic acids to their constituents in several stages, each brought about by different enzyme; they include nucleases, nucleotidases, and nucleosidases

    g. Enzymes acting on carbohydrates

        (1) Amylases – Act on polysaccharides, starch, glycogen, and related compounds, yielding maltose and glucose

        (2) Cellulase – Acts on cellulose

        (3) Inulase – Acts on inulin, yielding fructose

        (4) Glucosidases – Attack glucosides, yielding an alcohol and D-glucose

    h. Enzymes attacking carbon-nitrogen linkages, splitting off amino-containing groups

        (1) Urease – Converts urea to CO_2 and NH_3

        (2) Asparaginase – Splits NH_2 from asparagine

        (3) Glutaminase – Splits NH_2 from glutamine

        (4) Nuclein deaminases – Split off NH_2 from substrate, which becomes oxidized in the process e.g., adenine deaminase

        (5) Arginase – Splits arginine into ornithine and urea

4. Lyases – Split groups from their substrate (not by hydrolysis), leaving double bonds, or, conversely, add groups to double bonds; formerly called *desmolases*

    a. Decarboxylases – Split off carboxyl groups, e.g., oxaloacetate carboxylase

$$\text{Oxaloacetate} \quad \rightarrow \quad \text{Pyruvate} + CO_2$$

    b. Carbonic anhydrase – Splits H_2CO_3 to $CO_2 + H_2O$

    c. Aspartate ammonia lyase – Splits aspartate to fumarate and ammonia; formerly called *aspartase*

    d. Cysteine desulfhydrase

$$\text{Cysteine} + H_2O \quad \rightarrow \quad \text{Pyruvate} + NH_3 + H_2S$$

5. Isomerases – Catalyze intramolecular rearrangements, e.g., glucose phosphate isomerase, or phosphohexoisomerase (p. 199), which changes glucose to fructose

    a. Racemases and epimerases – Change L-compounds to D-compounds, or α-compounds to β-compounds

    b. *Cis-trans* isomerases

    c. Intramolecular oxidoreductases – Convert aldehydes to ketones

    d. Intramolecular transferases – Transfer variety of groups from one carbon of a compound to another, e.g., phosphoglyceromutase, which changes 3-phosphoglycerate to 2-phosphoglycerate (p. 201)

6. Ligases or synthetases – Catalyze union of two molecules, coupled with breakdown of a pyrophosphate bond in ATP or similar triphosphate; may form C—O, C—S, C—N, or C—C bonds, e.g., pyruvate carboxylase, which carboxylates pyruvate (using ATP) to form oxaloacetate (p. 205)

CLINICAL ENZYMOLOGY

Enzymes are commonly used in medicine (1) as an analytic tool or reagent for measuring amounts of various constituents in biologic fluids; (2) as an index of pathology or disease; (3) as a therapeutic agent.

Enzymes as reagents There are a number of advantages to using enzymes as reagents for determining the levels of various substances in biologic fluids. Enzymes are highly specific, thus reducing to a minimum interference from other substances. Their reactions are extremely sensitive, thereby opening a wide potential for micromethods. Enzymatic reactions are rapid, thereby enabling a technician to do many analyses.

In general, enzyme technology requires a strict adherence to optimal environmental conditions as already discussed (p. 122). Where the purpose is to determine a substrate concentration, an excess of enzyme should be used. On the other hand, in measurements of enzyme concentration, zero-order kinetics should be used.

Some examples of clinical methods using enzymes as reagents are given below.

Urea. Urease is used to convert urea to carbon dioxide and ammonia. The ammonia is then measured colorimetrically by nesslerization (Nessler's reagent). A rapid micromethod uses a filter paper strip impregnated with urease. The ammonia released is absorbed in an area containing bromcresol green. The extent of color change is a measure of the concentration of urea.

Uric acid. Uricase converts uric acid to allantoin (p. 402). While uric acid absorbs light to 290 to 283 mμ, allantoin does not. The amount of uric acid is proportional to the decrease in optical density.

Glucose. Glucose is oxidized to gluconic acid in the presence of the enzyme glucose oxidase. A second product of this reaction is hydrogen peroxide. Methods involving this procedure include the enzyme peroxidase, which converts the peroxide into water and oxygen. The color resulting from the subsequent oxidation of o-dianisidine is a measure of the concentration of glucose. This procedure is also available in qualitative or semiquantitative form as filter paper strip tests.

Alcohol. Alcohol is converted to acetaldehyde by alcohol dehydrogenase. This system requires the presence of nicotinamide adenine dinucleotide (NAD$^+$), which is reduced to NADH$_2$, which absorbs light at 340 mμ whereas NAD$^+$ does not. The change in optical density can be related to concentration. There is also a colorimetric method in which a blue dye is reduced to its colorless form. Here again the change in optical density is related to the concentration of alcohol.

Diagnosis with enzymes The ultimate goal of clinical enzymology would be to determine an "organspecific" enzyme in body fluids. Presently this is impossible; however, certain enzymes or forms of enzymes (isozymes) are known to be derived primarily from predictable tissues. The primary purpose of clinical enzymology is confirmatory rather than diagnostic. The source of enzymes in body fluids as viewed from affects of pathology on levels of activity may be summarized according to the following diagram:

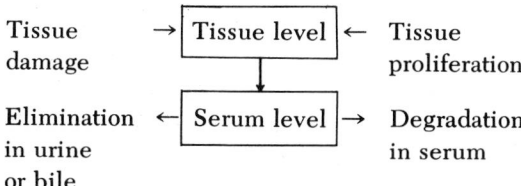

Normally, most serum enzymes are derived from the physiologic turnover of cells in various tissues, i.e., the "wear and tear" process. Most serum enzymes are, in fact, waste products. Tissue damage, as in myocardial infarction, and infection, as in hepatitis, cause a loss of tissue enzymes into the bloodstream. Proliferative processes, as in osteosarcoma or prostatic carcinoma, lead to an increased production of enzymes and then a spillage into the blood. Liver disease, leading to biliary obstruction, causes an increase in some serum enzymes by blocking their elimination into the bile.

Examples of clinically important enzymes are described below.

Amylase. The action of serum or urine on 0.1% starch solution is measured in terms of the disappearance of the blue starch iodine color. The normal level is markedly increased in pancreatitis.

Alkaline phosphatase. The method often used to detect alkaline phosphatases is that of Bessey-Lowry-Brock. It involves the hydrolysis of *p*-nitrophenyl phosphate to *p*-nitrophenol at a pH of 8.5 to 10. Levels of serum enzymes are elevated in osteologic diseases (e.g., osteogenic sarcoma, rickets) or biliary disorders (obstructive jaundice, cirrhosis).

Acid phosphatase. The method for detection of acid phosphatases is similar to that for alkaline phosphatases except that the pH optimum is 5. Levels are elevated in carcinoma of the prostate.

Serum transaminases. Two serum transaminases are used clinically. These are serum glutamate–oxaloacetate transaminase (SGOT) and serum glutamate–pyruvate transaminase (SGPT). The principle of transamination reactions is detailed elsewhere (p. 350). SGOT may be measured colorimetrically by forming the 2,4-dinitrophenylhydrazone of oxaloacetate:

$$\alpha\text{-Ketoglutarate} + \text{Aspartate} \rightleftharpoons \text{Oxaloacetate} + \text{Glutamate}$$

Oxaloacetate may also be measured by coupling the transamination reaction with malic dehydrogenase:

$$\text{Oxaloacetate} + \text{NADH}_2 \rightleftharpoons \text{Malate} + \text{NAD}^+$$

The reduction of NAD^+ is measured as the rate of increase in optical density at 340 mμ. Increased serum levels of SGOT are observed following myocardial infarction. The levels reach a maximum within the first 24 to 36 hours, rising to twice or even 20 times the normal range. This transaminase is also elevated in liver disease, e.g., viral hepatitis. On the other hand, SGPT is not elevated following myocardial infarction but is increased in liver disease. Thus the two conditions may be differentiated enzymatically.

Lactic acid dehydrogenase. The procedure used involves the dehydrogenation of lactic acid with a concomitant reduction of NAD^+. The increase in optical density at 340 mμ is measured. There is also a colorimetric modification of this method. LDH is increased in myocardial infarction but does not reach a maximum until 4 days after the episode. For this reason, in myocardial infarction occurring several days before diagnosis, the LDH is a more significant determination than the SGOT.

LDH-isozyme patterns are useful in distinguishing hepatitis or liver damage from cardiovascular disease. LDH-1 (p. 130) is derived principally from heart muscle, so serum from a patient suffering myocardial infarction has an increased level of the LDH-1 and LDH-2. Liver damage, as in viral hepatitis, leads to a decided elevation in LDH-5. Increases may also be seen in jaundice secondary to drug toxicity, hepatic contusions, and infectious mononucleosis.

Enzymatic debridement The material present in many infected or necrotic wounds, burns, or other lesions contains both fibrinous and purulent matter. The removal of such materials by enzymatic action is now being practiced clinically. Either profibrinolysin (p. 633) and an activator or the activated enzyme accomplish the lysis of fibrin, and deoxyribonuclease digests the pus. The latter enzyme is obtained from streptococci or from pancreatic tissue. The two enzymes are usually applied together, and it is essential that they remain in close contact with the area to be treated for several hours.

α-Chymotrypsin is used locally to digest the zonula threads in cataract operations. The intravenous injection of this enzyme has been found helpful in treating inflammation and thrombosis.

Many other clinical uses for enzymes have been recommended. Some of them are as follows: pancreatic dornase, for rendering purulent materials fluid; trypsin, for the proteolysis of blood clots; streptokinase and streptodornase, for both of the preceding uses; hyaluronidase, for increasing the spreading of injected fluids or of accumulated tissue fluids after trauma; pancreatic lipase, for reducing malabsorption of fats in steatorrhea; and penicillinase, to combat penicillin inactivators.

Lysozyme and hyaluronidase are examples of enzymes that act on highly polymerized mucopolysaccharides. These complex carbohydrates are found both in microorganisms and in animal tissues and are built up from hexosamines and uronic acids. Lysozyme occurs in egg white, tears, saliva, nasal secretions, and leukocytes. It is also found in some microorganisms. This enzyme is a muramidase and attacks the polysaccharide of bacterial cell walls. Under the influence of lysozyme,[6] the microorganisms swell to several times their normal size, the gram stain becomes negative, and nonprotein nitrogenous substances, inorganic phosphates, and the simple carbohydrates go into the surrounding medium. The enzyme is a basic protein, having a molecular weight of 14,600, and is unlike most other enzymes in being resistant to both heat and acid. Its primary and three-dimensional structures have been determined. The functions of lysozyme may relate to a protective action when tissues are in a weakened condition. The occurrence of lysozyme and similar enzymes in some microorganisms is explained by the assumption that these enzymes are involved in some metabolic process connected with the carbohydrate substrates in the membranes of these microbes. The membranes of microbes are sometimes very tough, and it is possible that the lysozyme softens them preliminary to cell division.

Sometimes large amounts of lysozyme may be harmful. Ulcerative conditions of the gastrointestinal canal have been linked with excessive levels of lysozyme. The enzyme is present in gastric mucosa and in the gastric juice of man. When the ulcers are brought under control, the lysozyme is diminished. Similarly, lysozyme has been found in excessive amounts in the stools of patients suffering from chronic ulcerative colitis. Lysozyme is thought to act on surface mucus, digesting it away. Then a proteolytic enzyme acts on the unprotected mucosal tissue, eroding it to produce an ulcer. Although grave doubt has been cast on an etiologic role for lysozyme, this enzyme appears to be an index of the severity of the disease process and a measure of functioning colonic tissue.

Hyaluronidase, a β-glucosaminidase, is often used clinically to depolymerize the mucopolysaccharides of connective tissue ground substance. A more detailed discussion of its clinical use is to be found in Chapter 18.

References

GENERAL

Batskis, J. G., and Briere, R. O.: Interpretive enzymology, Springfield, Ill., 1967, Charles C Thomas, Publisher.

Bernhard, S.: The structure and function of enzymes, New York, 1968, W. A. Benjamin, Inc.

Boyer, P. D., Lardy, H., and Myrbäck, K.: The enzymes, ed. 2, New York, 1958–1963, Academic Press, Inc.

Christensen, H. N., and Palmer, G. A.: Enzyme kinetics, Philadelphia, 1967, W. B. Saunders Co.

Dixon, M., and Webb, E. C.: Enzymes, ed. 2, New York, 1964, Academic Press, Inc.

Goodwin, T. W., Harris, J. I., and Hartley, B. S., editors: Structure and activity of enzymes, New York, 1964, Academic Press, Inc.

Hess, B.: Enzymes in blood plasma, New York, 1963, Academic Press, Inc.

Koshland, D. E., Jr., and Neet, K. E.: The catalytic and regulatory properties of enzymes, Ann. Rev. Biochem. 37:359, 1968.

Neilands, J. B., and Stumpf, P. K.: Outline of enzyme chemistry, ed. 2, New York, 1958, John Wiley & Sons, Inc.

Neurath, H.: The protein-digesting enzymes, Sci. Amer. 211:68, 1964.

SPECIAL

1. Watt, D. C.: In Munday, K. A., editor: Studies in comparative biochemistry, New York, 1965, Pergamon Press, Inc., p. 162.
2. Koshland, D. E., Jr.: Fed. Proc. 23:719, 1964.
3. Wang, J. H.: Science 161:328, 1968.
4. Vesell, E. S., editor: Ann. N. Y. Acad. Sci. 151:1, 1968.
5. Reed, L. J., and Oliver, R. M.: Brookhaven Sympos. Biol. 21:397, 1968.
6. Phillips, D. C.: Proc. 7th Int. Congr. Biochem. 34:63, 1967.

SECTION **three**

CHEMISTRY AND METABOLISM OF OTHER MAJOR CELL CONSTITUENTS

CHAPTER 8

CHEMISTRY OF THE CARBOHYDRATES

Carbohydrates, the second of the three major groups of organic substances occurring in living matter, are the most abundant compounds found in nature. Although they do occur as *simple sugars*, as will be discussed later, the largest portion is encountered in *bound* form, the *reducing* carbon atom of one simple sugar being attached to any of a great variety of organic or inorganic groups. The simple sugars may be attached to other like sugar molecules to form *polysaccharides*, e.g., starches, celluloses, inulin, etc. (p. 166); or certain simple sugars may be attached to purines, pyrimidines, and phosphate to form nucleic acids (p. 31); or they may be attached to proteins to form glycoproteins; or to lipids to form glycolipids; or to certain alcohols to form glycosides. These are a few outstanding examples of biologically important carbohydrates.

Carbohydrates serve many important purposes in living matter. As glucose and glycogen, they are the prime source of energy in the animal organism. As starch, they are the major form of stored energy produced by the process of photosynthesis (p. 219) in plants. As cellulose, they form part of the cell wall of plant cells. As complex polymers, they make up the protective outer cell wall of microorganisms (p. 177). As metabolites of glucose, they supply the precursors for the biosynthesis of many vital biologic substances, including the purines, pyrimidines, certain amino acids, porphyrins, cholesterol and its derivatives, mucopolysaccharides, glycoproteins, glycolipids, fats—both the glycerol and the fatty acid moieties—milk sugar (lactose), ascorbic acid, the Krebs citric acid cycle acids (p. 264), and many others.

DEFINITION

The carbohydrates are composed of carbon, hydrogen, and oxygen, the hydrogen and oxygen being present ordinarily in the same proportion as they are in water. The name *carbohydrate* indicates this usual composition. Examples are $C_5H_{10}O_5$, $C_6H_{12}O_6$, and $C_{12}H_{22}O_{11}$. Of course, compounds of quite different types have the same proportional molecular constitution, e.g., acetic acid and formaldehyde. Hence this is not a definition. A satisfactory definition of carbohydrates is as follows: polyhydroxy alcohols having potentially active aldehyde or ketone groups, and compounds yielding them on hydrolysis. *Hydrolysis* means the cleavage of a compound in the presence of water with the addition of water, or its ions, to the products.

The simplest carbohydrates are the sugars—water-soluble crystalline compounds, usually sweet in taste. The simplest sugars are glyceraldehyde and dihydroxyacetone.

$$
\begin{array}{ll}
\text{Glyceraldehyde} &
\begin{array}{c}
\mathrm{H{-}C{=}O} \\
\mathrm{H{-}\overset{|}{\underset{|}{C}}{-}OH} \\
\mathrm{H{-}\overset{|}{\underset{|}{C}}{-}OH} \\
\mathrm{H}
\end{array}
\qquad
\begin{array}{c}
\mathrm{H} \\
\mathrm{H{-}\overset{|}{\underset{|}{C}}{-}OH} \\
\mathrm{\overset{|}{\underset{|}{C}}{=}O} \\
\mathrm{H{-}\overset{|}{\underset{|}{C}}{-}OH} \\
\mathrm{H}
\end{array}
& \text{Dihydroxyacetone}
\end{array}
$$

Although these sugars do not enter into our food, they are formed in the body when the more complex carbohydrates are broken down. It is evident from the definition and from these two formulas that the simple sugars are of two general types, with aldehyde and ketone groups, respectively. Since the suffix -*ose* is used to designate a sugar, there are, accordingly, aldoses and ketoses.

CLASSIFICATION

Besides the simple sugars, there are more complex ones. On hydrolysis, the complex carbohydrates yield the simple sugars and sometimes other substances. The chief classification of carbohydrates is based on this relationship:

1. Monosaccharides: These are simple sugars, sometimes called *glycoses*.
2. Oligosaccharides: These are sugars of known structure composed of a few, usually two or three, monosaccharides. The disaccharides are composed of two simple sugars. There are also trisaccharides, composed of three monosaccharide molecules.
3. Polysaccharides: These are sugars formed by the polymerization of a number of molecules of simple sugars to form one molecule. These monosaccharides may form single chains of varying lengths, or the huge molecules may consist of such chains in branched arrangements. Polysaccharides that are polymers of a single monosaccharide are called *homopolysaccharides;* those that are polymers of sugars or sugar derivatives with other groups are called *heteropolysaccharides* (p. 172).

Monosaccharides The simple sugars $(CH_2O)_x$ are further classified according to (1) whether they are aldehyde or ketone derivatives and (2) the number of carbon atoms they contain. Thus there are (1) aldoses and ketoses and (2) trioses (3-C sugars), tetroses (4-C sugars), pentoses (5-C sugars), hexoses (6-C sugars), etc. Combining the two, we can more accurately describe a simple sugar as a ketopentose, an aldohexose, etc. The presence of a ketone group is usually indicated by using the ending *ulose*. Examples are as follows:

Trioses

$C_3H_6O_3$

Glyceraldehyde (an aldotriose)

Dihydroxyacetone (a ketotriose)

Tetroses

$C_4H_8O_4$

Erythrose (an aldotetrose)

Erythrulose (a ketotetrose or tetrulose)

Pentoses

$C_5H_{10}O_5$

Xylose (an aldopentose)

Xylulose (a ketopentose or pentulose)

Hexoses

$C_6H_{12}O_6$

Glucose (an aldohexose)

Fructose (a ketohexose or hexulose)

Heptoses

$C_7H_{14}O_7$

Sedoheptulose (a ketoheptose or heptulose)

Oligo-saccharides The most common oligosaccharides are the disaccharides. They are usually composed of hexoses, although theoretically any two monosaccharides could be joined to form such a compound. The most important sugars of this class are sucrose, lactose, and maltose. Sucrose yields one molecule of glucose and one of fructose, lactose yields glucose and galactose, whereas maltose gives rise to two molecules of glucose. Thus:

$$C_{12}H_{22}O_{11} + H_2O \rightarrow C_6H_{12}O_6 + C_6H_{12}O_6$$

Disaccharide   **Monosaccharides**

The disaccharides vary not only in their constituent simple sugars but also in the way these simple sugars are linked together. Indeed, there may be two distinct disaccharides, with different properties, each yielding the same two monosaccharides on hydrolysis. An example of such a relationship is sucrose and turanose. Turanose has reducing power, whereas sucrose has not. They have different melting points and are unlike in other respects as well. Yet on hydrolysis each yields one molecule of glucose and one of fructose. The reason for their dissimilarity is that the constituent monosaccharides are joined by different linkages.

Poly-saccharides The polysaccharide group includes the glycogens, starches, celluloses, and hemicelluloses. It also includes the intermediate products of hydrolysis of the higher polysaccharides, i.e., such compounds as the dextrins. There are many of these in the vegetable world, and some are to be found in animal tissues. In general, they hydrolyze thus:

$$(C_6H_{10}O_5)_n + (n-1)H_2O \rightarrow nC_6H_{12}O_6$$

Polysaccharide   **Monosaccharides**

MONOSACCHARIDES

Structure Most consideration will be given to the structure of glucose as typical of monosaccharides. Glucose is the chief physiologic sugar and will demand attention over and over again. Its chemistry and relationship to other physiologic compounds must be understood. Glucose is a monosaccharide, a hexose, and an aldose. Its molecular formula is $C_6H_{12}O_6$. Its structural formula, sometimes called a *Fischer projection structure,* may be written provisionally as

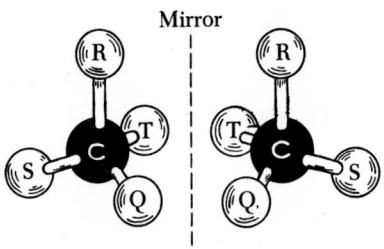

Fig. 8-1. Model of an asymmetric carbon atom and its mirror image.

shown below. Similarly ribose, an aldopentose, and fructose, a ketohexose, have the formulas shown:

Glucose	Ribose	Fructose
H—C=O	H—C=O	H—C—OH (with H above)
H—C—OH	H—C—OH	C=O
HO—C—H	H—C—OH	HO—C—H
H—C—OH	H—C—OH	H—C—OH
H—C—OH	H—C—OH	H—C—OH
H—C—OH	H	H—C—OH
H		H

There are two other physiologically important aldohexoses known, namely, galactose and mannose. Besides ribose, two aldopentoses, arabinose and xylose, are present in many plants. Moreover, certain derivatives of some of these sugars are of great interest, as we shall see. Glucose, galactose, and mannose all have six carbons, five hydroxyls, and an aldehyde group in their molecules. Since all differ from one another, they must have differences in the arrangement of the groups in the molecule.

Asymmetric carbon   These differences in arrangement are based on the fact that all sugars possess asymmetric carbon atoms. An asymmetric carbon is a carbon atom to which is attached *four different* atoms or groups. If a carbon atom can be pictured with four bonds projected into space in four different directions (as shown in Fig. 8-1) and each joined to a different atom or group (*Q,R, S, T*), we can see that a similar but not identical figure will be constructed, which is shown next to it. These two figures bear the same relation to each other as that of an object to its mirror image. They are not identical, which may actually be proved by attempting to superimpose one upon the other. Here are two compounds resembling each other, but they are different because the carbons are asymmetric. The two hypothetic compounds shown are geometric isomers, or *stereoisomers*, or *enantiomorphs*. The relation exhibited by such compounds is called *stereoisomerism*; i.e., their isomerism is explained on a basis of space relationships. Stereoisomers of this particular type are also called *optical* isomers, because compounds possessing asymmetric carbons have the power to turn the plane of a beam of polarized light.

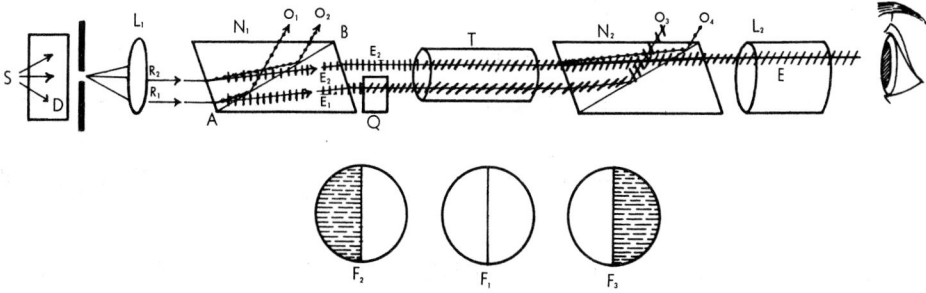

Fig. 8-2. Diagram of a polarimeter. *S*, Source of light; *D*, bichromate light filter, giving the effect of sodium light; L_1, collimator lens, from which the light emerges as a parallel beam, R_1, R_2; N_1, Nicol prism, polarizer; N_2, Nicol prism, analyzer—here the principal planes are parallel; *E*, eyepiece with lens, L_2. The courses of two rays are shown. R_1 is split into two rays, vibrating in planes at right angles to each other. O_1 is the ordinary ray, vibrating in a plane at right angles to the page and is reflected (by the surface *AB*) and eliminated. The extraordinary ray, E_1, passes out of the polarizer, vibrating in a plane parallel to the page. Similarly, O_2 is eliminated and E_2 passes out of the polarizer, vibrating in a plane parallel to that of E_1. A quartz plate, *Q*, covering half the field, is here interposed. Actually this covers the left or right half, but in the figure it is shown as covering the lower half. *Q* turns the plane of polarized light of E_1 at a small angle to E_2. Both now enter the tube, *T*, which contains the sugar solution. Here the planes of both E_1 and E_2 are again twisted. Now E_1 is vibrating in a plane at right angles to the plane of the page; hence, when it enters N_2, it becomes eliminated because the principal planes of N_1 and N_2 are parallel. Therefore all the light passing through *Q* is lost and half the field appears dark as shown at F_2 or F_3. E_2, although turned just as much as E_1, is vibrating in a different plane from E_1 and therefore can pass through N_2 to a slight extent. The analyzer may be rotated and thus permit E_1 and E_2 to pass through to an equal extent. The field, F_1, would then appear, and the amount of rotation necessary to produce this field, i.e., the compensation for the twisting due to the sugar solution in *T*, could be read off on a scale. (From Kleiner, I. S., and Dotti, L. B.: Laboratory instructions in biochemistry, St. Louis, 1966, The C. V. Mosby Co.; slightly modified with the aid of the staff of Bausch & Lomb.)

Ordinary light, vibrating in many planes, is passed through a Nicol prism in a polarimeter (Fig. 8-2). The light emerging is plane polarized; i.e., it vibrates in one plane. If a solution of an *optically active* compound is now placed in its path, the plane of the polarized light will be turned. To determine the direction and degree of rotation imparted to the polarized beam, a second prism is mounted between the solution and the eye of the observer. This prism may then be rotated in the opposite direction to compensate for the twisting produced by the solution.

Every optically active compound has a corresponding stereoisomer that rotates in an exactly opposite manner. Structurally, one is a mirror image of the other; if one compound rotates the plane of polarized light to the right, its mirror image will rotate the plane of polarized light to the left.

The sugars all contain asymmetric carbons. For instance, the simplest aldehyde sugar may be represented as shown at the top of p. 146 (the asymmetric carbon being shown in boldface type).

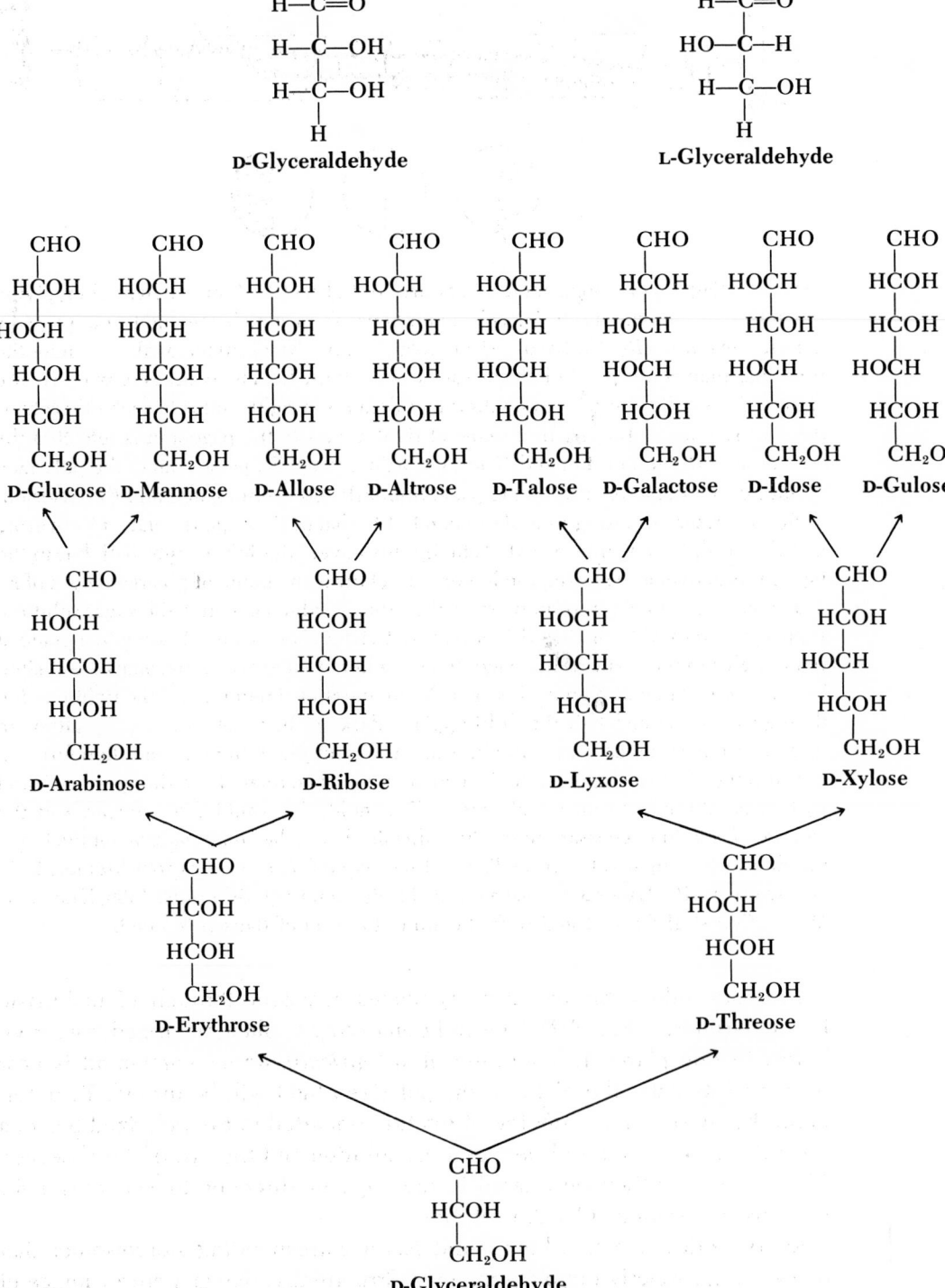

Relations of the D-aldoses. The L-aldoses can be similarly shown, with the hydrogens and hydroxyls of each asymmetric carbon reversed. (From Karrer, P.: Organic chemistry, New York, 1938, Nordeman Publishing Co., Inc.)

D-Glyceraldehyde rotates the plane of polarized light to the right, i.e., it is dextrorotatory, whereas L-glyceraldehyde is levorotatory. All simple sugars are regarded as derivatives of these two. For this reason, glyceraldehyde has been called the *reference sugar*. This means that all sugars with the same configuration as D-glyceraldehyde for the asymmetric carbon atom farthest from the (potential) aldehyde or ketone group are given the designation D, regardless of whether they are dextrorotatory or levorotatory. Those that are like L-glyceraldehyde in this respect are given the prefix L.

CHO	CHO	CH$_2$OH	CHO	CHO	CH$_2$OH
	R	C=O		R	C=O
		R			R
H—C—OH	H—C—OH	H—C—OH	HO—C—H	HO—C—H	HO—C—H
CH$_2$OH	CH$_2$OH	CH$_2$OH	CH$_2$OH	CH$_2$OH	CH$_2$OH
D-Glycer- **aldehyde**	**Type of** **D-aldoses**	**Type of** **D-ketoses**	**L-Glyceralde-** **hyde**	**Type of** **L-aldoses**	**Type of** **L-ketoses**

Glyceraldehyde has only one asymmetric carbon atom and there are only two steroisomers possible; and these two are known. If more than one asymmetric carbon atom is present in the molecule, the number of possible isomers is increased. Van't Hoff showed that this number would be 2^n, where n is the number of asymmetric carbons. From the formula for an aldohexose, it is evident that four asymmetric carbons are present; accordingly, there would be 2^4 or 16 possible isomers. Thus it can easily be seen why glucose, galactose, and mannose are all aldohexoses and are all different. It is also evident why fructose, which rotates the plane of polarized light to the left, is called D-fructose. A study of the formulas below will clarify this:

(1) C	CHO	CHO	CHO	CHO	CH$_2$OH
(2) C	H—C—OH	HO—C—H	HO—C—H	H—C—OH	C=O
(3) C	HO—C—H	H—C—OH	HO—C—H	HO—C—H	HO—C—H
(4) C	H—C—OH	HO—C—H	H—C—OH	HO—C—H	H—C—OH
(5) C	H—C—OH	HO—C—H	H—C—OH	H—C—OH	H—C—OH
(6) C	CH$_2$OH	CH$_2$OH	CH$_2$OH	CH$_2$OH	CH$_2$OH
	D-Glucose	**L-Glucose**	**D-Mannose**	**D-Galactose**	**D-Fructose**

Specific rotation These differences in structure are responsible for variations in physical, chemical, and physiologic properties of the sugars, e.g., degree of rotatory power, crystalline form, solubilities, reactions, sweetness, nutritive value. Their differences in degree of rotatory power are expressed as different "specific rotations." The specific rotation of a substance is that rotation, in angular degrees, produced by a solution containing 1 gm. of substance in 1 ml. of solution in a tube 1 dm. long. Dextrorotation is indicated by a plus sign, levo- by a minus sign. If $[\alpha]_D^{20°}$ is the symbol for specific rotation, using sodium light (D) at 20° C., and

$$\alpha = \text{observed rotation expressed in degrees}$$

147

l = length of the tube in decimeters

c = concentration in grams per 100 ml.

then

$$[\alpha]_D^{20°} = \frac{\alpha \times 100}{c \times 1}$$

By means of the polarimeter, sugars may be differentiated from one another if the concentration is known. Similarly, if the sugar is known, the concentration may be determined by ascertaining the rotation and using the following equation:

$$c = \frac{\alpha \times 100}{[\alpha]_D^{20°} \times 1}$$

It should be noted that if two or more optically active substances are present in the same solution each exerts its own rotatory power. The resulting rotation is the algebraic sum of the individual rotations. For example, if both D-glucose and D-fructose are in the same solution, the rotation might be dextro, levo, or zero, depending on the relative concentrations of the two sugars.

The specific rotation of sugars, and of certain other optically active substances (see Table 8-1), is determined by using sodium light (*D*-line of the spectrum, having a wavelength of approximately 585 mμ). The reason for this is that optical rotation varies as a function of the wavelength of the monochromatic light employed, a relation termed *optical rotatory dispersion*. Further, the *R* and *L* components of circularly polarized light are absorbed to varying degrees at different wavelengths by different substances, resulting in *circular dichroism*. Measurement of optical rotatory dispersion and circular dichroism have been extremely valuable in studies of the spatial arrangements of asymmetric molecules, especially in determining the secondary helical and nonhelical structure of proteins (p. 79).

Mutarotation   If some glucose is dissolved in water and observed in a polarimeter, it will be found to rotate the plane of polarized light to the right; but the amount of rotation will continually change until, after some time, it becomes con-

Table 8-1. Values of specific rotation of various carbohydrates at 20° C. (sodium light) (in degrees)

D-Glucose	+ 52.7	Lactose	+ 55.4
D-Fructose	− 92.4	Sucrose	+ 66.5
D-Galactose	+ 80.2	Maltose	+130.4
L-Arabinose	+104.5	Invert sugar	− 19.8
D-Mannose	+ 14.2	Dextrin	+195
D-Arabinose	−105.0	Starch	+196 or greater
D-Xylose	+ 18.8	Glycogen	+196 to +197

stant. Other sugars exhibit this same behavior. It is called *mutarotation*—changing rotation—and is explained by assuming that when the sugar is first dissolved it is largely in one form, but after solution some of it immediately changes to another form having a different specific rotation. At a certain stage, equilibrium is reached, and at this stage the rotation is stabilized. The mechanism of the reaction is explained by the fact that sugars can form hemiacetals as can other aldehydes:

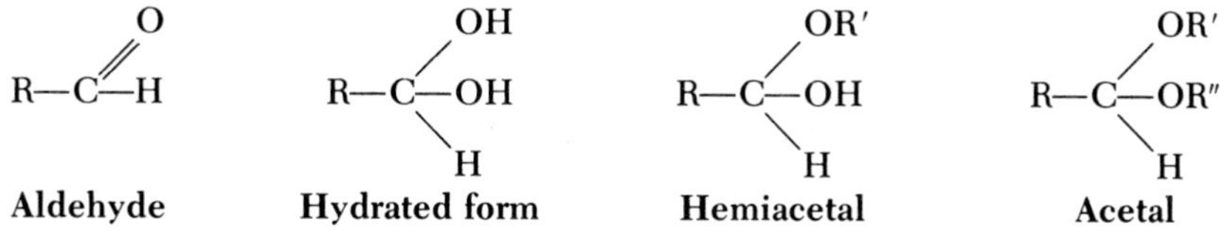

$$
\begin{array}{cccc}
\overset{\displaystyle O}{\underset{}{R-\overset{\parallel}{C}-H}} &
\overset{\displaystyle OH}{\underset{H}{R-\overset{|}{\underset{|}{C}}-OH}} &
\overset{\displaystyle OR'}{\underset{H}{R-\overset{|}{\underset{|}{C}}-OH}} &
\overset{\displaystyle OR'}{\underset{H}{R-\overset{|}{\underset{|}{C}}-OR''}}
\end{array}
$$

| Aldehyde | Hydrated form | Hemiacetal | Acetal |

Thus glucose, in solution, behaves as follows:

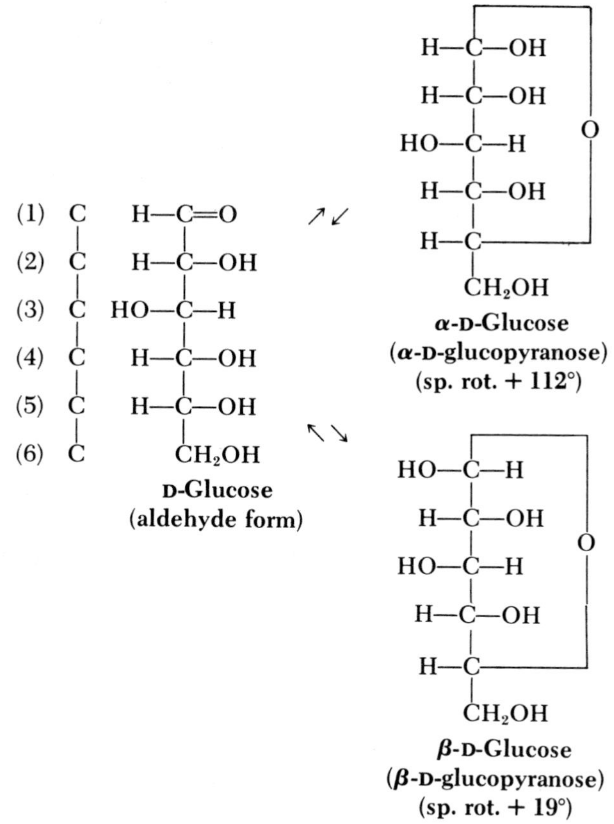

$$
\begin{array}{ll}
(1) \; C & H-C=O \\
(2) \; C & H-C-OH \\
(3) \; C & HO-C-H \\
(4) \; C & H-C-OH \\
(5) \; C & H-C-OH \\
(6) \; C & CH_2OH
\end{array}
$$

D-Glucose
(aldehyde form)

$$
\begin{array}{l}
H-C-OH \\
H-C-OH \\
HO-C-H \quad\; O \\
H-C-OH \\
H-C \\
CH_2OH
\end{array}
$$

α-D-Glucose
(**α-D-glucopyranose**)
(sp. rot. + 112°)

$$
\begin{array}{l}
HO-C-H \\
H-C-OH \\
HO-C-H \quad\; O \\
H-C-OH \\
H-C \\
CH_2OH
\end{array}
$$

β-D-Glucose
(**β-D-glucopyranose**)
(sp. rot. + 19°)

We can see, then, that carbon-1 now becomes asymmetric and is termed an *anomeric* carbon atom and that glucose really has five asymmetric carbons rather than four. This means that there are two new stereoisomers formed, called α- and β-*anomers,* when glucose is dissolved, with different specific rotations. When either pure isomer is dissolved in water, the rotation changes because some of the isomer is transformed into the other form, and this change continues until an equilibrium is reached. The equilibrium mixture contains about two thirds β-form and one third α-form and has a specific rotation of +52.7 degrees. The formulas do not show the presence of an aldehyde group. This harmonizes with the fact that the aldoses do not exhibit certain properties of true aldehydes. For example, they do not give a color with Schiff's aldehyde reagent. To account for the reducing action of sugars, we may assume that the two forms shown are in equilibrium, with a small amount of glucose in aldehyde form, and at room temperature the equilibrium favors the hemiacetal form. As the aldehyde form is used up in a reaction involving the aldehyde group, more and more is formed from the α- and β-types.

Ring structures of sugars These formulas indicate that glucose is a ring compound, a 1:5 ring as shown. The 1:5 ring structure is known as the *pyranose* form, i.e., as a derivative of pyran.

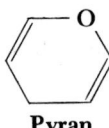

Pyran

The sugar formulas have also been pictured in perspective, as the so-called Haworth formulas, with a three-dimensional representation. The ring of five carbons and one oxygen is shown in one plane, at right angles to the plane of the paper, with the hydrogens, hydroxyls, and one primary alcohol group either above or below the plane. The bonds directed upward are above the plane and those directed downward are below the plane. "Up" corresponds to left in the straight chain, or Fischer formulas, and "down" corresponds to right.

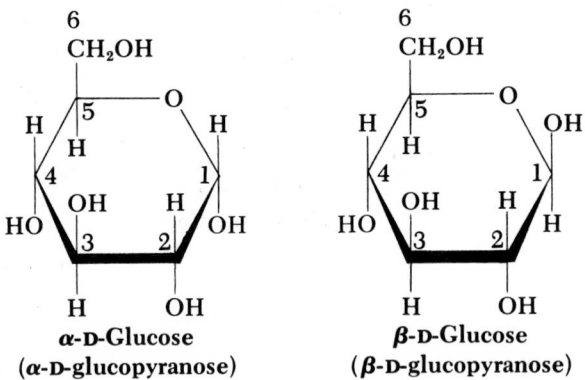

α-D-Glucose
(α-D-glucopyranose)

β-D-Glucose
(β-D-glucopyranose)

Other glycoses, likewise, exist in ring structures. The proof of these by methylation and periodate oxidation reactions has been accomplished by the brilliant work of Haworth, Hudson, Irvine, and others. Similarly, the precise structural configuration, i.e., spatial positions of the hydroxyl groups, of the various monosaccharides have been elucidated by the classic studies of Fischer and others. Details of the procedures used may be found in advanced treatises of organic chemistry.

Conformation of sugars Studies during the past decade or so, employing newer techniques of organic chemistry, particularly x-ray analysis, have elucidated still further the three-dimensional structures, or conformations, of a number of sugars. It now appears that the furanose ring forms of sugars, e.g., D-fructose (p. 160), D-ribose (p. 162), are coplanar whereas the pyranose ring forms, e.g., D-glucose (p. 150), are nonplanar and strainless. Previous studies of atomic models of cyclohexane had indicated that at least two types of spatial arrangements or conformations — the so-called *chair* form and the *boat* form — were possible. The pyranose ring, an analogous structure, likewise could exist in the same two forms. Of the two, the "chair" is more stable, with minimal torsional and van der Waals strain. Therefore, from energy considerations, this form is preferable. X-ray analysis of certain sugars has indeed shown this reasoning to be correct. The conformation of D-glucopyranose, for example, has been shown to be the chair form. Two subtypes, *c-1* and *1-c*, of the chair form may exist, depending on the location of the oxygen atom in the chair structure.

Further analogies between spatial configurations of models of organic compounds show that the hydrogen and hydroxyl groups of D-glucopyranose can exist as bonds either parallel to the axis of symmetry of the ring, termed *axial,* or radiating more or less in the plane of the ring, termed *equatorial.* The axial bonds are drawn as vertical lines and may extend *upward* from the ring, termed *beta* (β) and represented by a *solid* line; or they may extend *downward,* termed *alpha* (α) and represented by a *dotted* line. Thus, current conformational representations of α- and β-D-glucopyranose are as shown in Fig. 8-3.

The "bulkier" groups (hydroxymethyl, hydroxyl) occupy the "roomier" equatorial positions, as demonstrated by x-ray analysis. This is probably the reason that β-D-glucopyranose is present in a 2:1 ratio to α-D-glucopyranose in an aqueous equilibrium mixture and also that β-D-glucose is allegedly the most widely occurring organic group in nature.

Other common aldohexoses, β-D-mannopyranose, α-D-galactopyranose, and α-D-idopyranose, likewise exist in similar chair conformations. The spatial positions of the hydroxyl groups and hydrogen atoms would differ from those of D-glucopyranose. At least two common pentoses, D-xylose and D-arabinose, apparently also exist in the pyranose ring, chair conformation.

Three other important sugars, D-fructose (p. 160), D-ribose (p. 162), and D-deoxyribose occur in a furanose ring form that is coplanar in conformation.

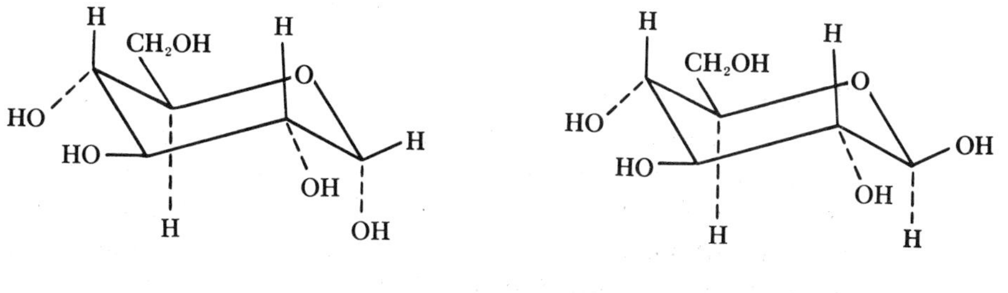

α-D-**Glucopyranose**   β-D-**Glucopyranose**

Fig. 8-3. Spatial conformation of α- and β-D-glucopyranose. α-Bonds, extending downward from plane of the ring, are represented by *dotted* lines; β-bonds, extending upward, are represented by solid lines.

The aldohexoses occurring in the common disaccharides (maltose, lactose, sucrose, p. 162) likewise appear to exist in chair conformation, as do the glucose units comprising the polysaccharides (amylose, amylopectin, glycogen, cellulose, p. 166).

The molecular shape, form, and symmetry of the various carbohydrates, as well as the conformations of other biologically important compounds (proteins, p. 81, sterols, p. 280, etc.) are vital in determining the biochemical reactions of these substances. The lock-and-key concept of the combination of enzyme with substrate (p. 114) is an excellent example of the importance of molecular conformation. For reasons of typography, however, the straight chain (stick) form or the Haworth ring form of carbohydrates will be used hereafter in this book, pending more widespread usage of conformational structures in the field of biochemistry.

Sugars as reducing agents The monosaccharides and most of the disaccharides are rather strong reducing agents, particularly at high pH's. Under suitable conditions they decompose to form fragments that reduce certain oxidizing reagents. The presence of the potential aldehyde or ketone group coincides with the great lability of the molecule when mixed with alkalies. Indeed, the aldehyde or ketone group is the most reactive of the functional groups present. Organic acids, together with a number of other products, result. The favorite type of reagent is an alkaline cupric solution, although other reagents, both acid and basic, metallic and nonmetallic, are used at times.

The fundamental reaction is shown very simply in Trommer's test. If to cupric sulfate solution is added a little sodium hydroxide, a bluish white precipitate of cupric hydroxide results. The addition of some glucose causes the solution of some, if not all, of this precipitate. Heating then leads to reduction of the cupric ions to cuprous ions and the formation of yellow to red precipitates.

$$CuSO_4 + 2\,NaOH \;\rightarrow\; \underset{\text{(bluish white)}}{Cu(OH)_2} + Na_2SO_4$$

$$2\,Cu(OH)_2 \xrightarrow[\text{+ Heat}]{\text{+ Reducing sugar}} \underset{\text{(yellow)}}{2\,CuOH} + H_2O + O \;\text{(taken up by the sugar}$$
$$\downarrow \qquad\qquad\qquad\qquad \text{and its products)}$$
$$\underset{\text{(red)}}{Cu_2O + H_2O}$$

Trommer's test is not a convenient method and is seldom used. Consequently, various mixtures of reagents with certain advantages have been prepared.

Benedict's qualitative solution is still almost universally used. It has the advantage of containing all the ingredients in a single solution. Cupric sulfate, sodium carbonate, and sodium citrate are the constituents, the citrate serving to keep cupric hydroxide in solution. Benedict's *quantitative* reagent contains, among other things, potassium thiocyanate, so that a white precipitate of cuprous thiocyanate is the end product. In the Folin-Wu quantitative method the cuprous oxide formed by the reducing action of glucose is reoxidized by phosphomolybdic acid, with the production of a dark blue phosphomolybdous acid, which can be measured colorimetrically.

Other alkaline metallic solutions can be used. An ammoniac silver nitrate solution may be reduced to metallic silver, producing a mirror. An alkaline bismuth solution, known as *Nylander's solution*, deposits black metallic bismuth on reduction. Picric acid in alkaline solution is reduced by reducing sugars to picramic acid. This reaction is shown by a change of color from a yellowish orange to a mahogany red. It is the basis for one of the quantitative blood sugar methods widely used for a time and still used to some extent. Ferricyanide may be reduced to ferrocyanide. In acid solution, the sugars reduce less vigorously. Barfoed's test utilizes this fact for distinguishing monosaccharides from reducing disaccharides. The former react, whereas the latter do not. The reason for this will be seen when the disaccharides are studied. Cupric acetate in weak acetic acid or, better, in lactic acid constitutes the reagent. There is also an enzyme method for both the qualitative and the quantitative determination of glucose. The qualitative method utilizes a test paper impregnated with glucose oxidase and a peroxidase. The former acts upon glucose (β-D-glucose anomer, specifically) to form hydrogen peroxide and gluconic acid, while the latter splits the peroxide. The oxygen liberated is detected by a color reaction with a suitable *chromogen,* such as *o*-toluidine or *o*-anisidine. In the quantitative procedure, the color produced by the oxidation of the chromogen is compared with that of a standard glucose solution similarly treated (p. 134).

Formation of osazones All sugars containing a potentially free aldehyde or ketone group form osazones when heated with an excess of phenylhydrazine ($C_6H_5NHNH_2$). Osazones are yellow crystalline compounds having characteristic forms (Fig. 8-4) and melting points. They are considerably less soluble than the sugars from which they are derived. This is an important reaction. Practically, it is one means of differentiating the various sugars. Thus it is an aid in distinguishing between lactose and glucose in the urine of lactating women. The reactions for glucose are as follows: In the first phase of the reaction, phenylhydrazine reacts with a carbonyl group to form a hydrazone; this then reacts with an excess of the reagent to produce the osazone.

$$
\begin{array}{lll}
\text{HC}\boxed{\text{O} + \text{H}_2}\text{NNHC}_6\text{H}_5 & \text{HC}=\text{NNHC}_6\text{H}_5 + \text{H}_2\text{O} & \text{HC}=\text{NNHC}_6\text{H}_5 \\
\text{HCOH} & \text{HCOH} & \text{C}=\text{NNHC}_6\text{H}_5 \\
\text{HOCH} & \text{HOCH} & \text{HOCH} \\
\text{HCOH} \longrightarrow & \text{HCOH} \xrightarrow{+\ 2\ \text{C}_6\text{H}_5\text{NHNH}_2} & \text{HCOH} \\
\text{HCOH} & \text{HCOH} & \text{HCOH} \\
\text{CH}_2\text{OH} & \text{CH}_2\text{OH} & \text{CH}_2\text{OH}
\end{array}
$$

D-Glucose   D-Glucose phenylhydrazone (soluble)   D-Glucosazone $+ C_6H_5NH_2$ Aniline $+ NH_3 + 2\ H_2O$

A study of the formulas on p. 155 will show that D-glucose, D-mannose, and D-fructose all yield the same osazone, because they have identical configuration for carbons numbered 3, 4, 5, and 6, whereas the other sugars shown form other osazones. The crystalline forms of the osazones of several of the more common sugars are shown in Fig. 8-4.

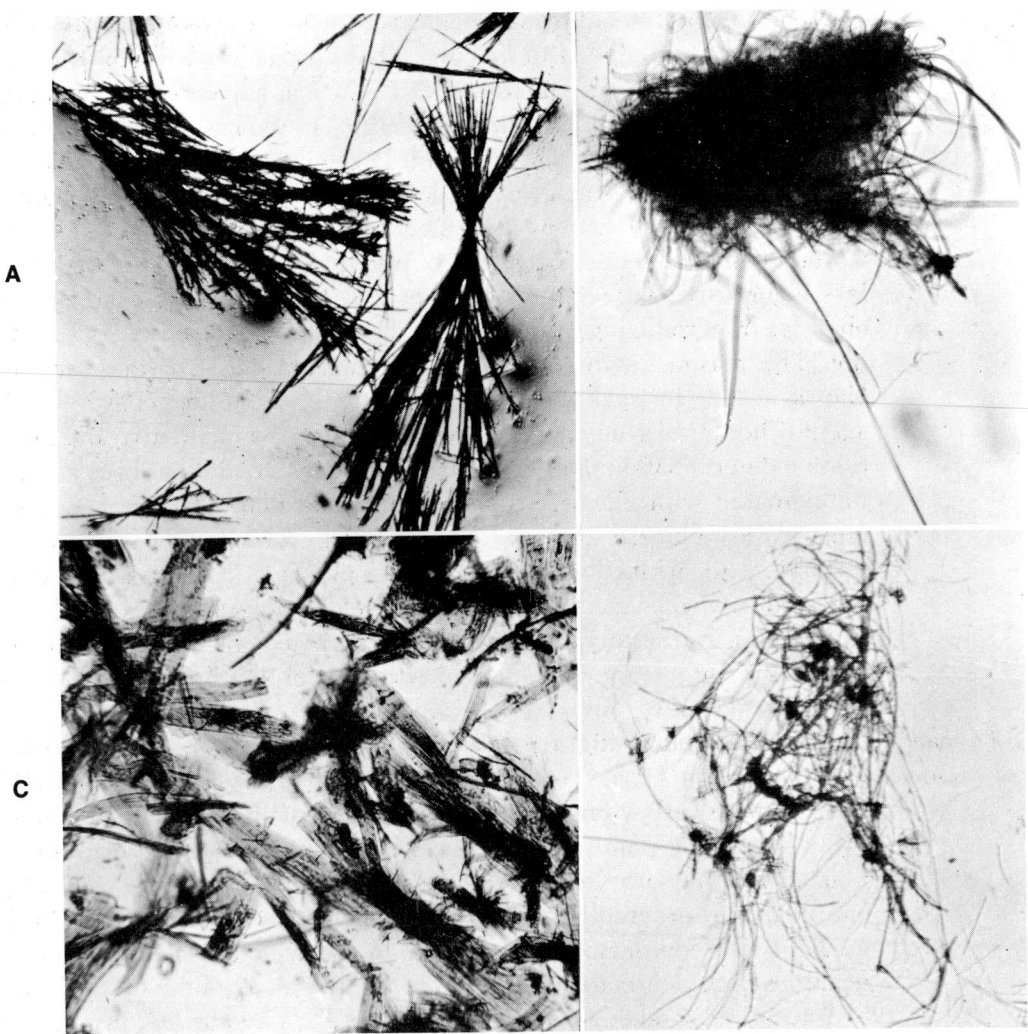

Fig. 8-4. Osazone crystals. **A**, Glucosazone. **B**, Lactosazone. **C**, Maltosazone. **D**, Arabinosazone. These are yellow in color.

Action of alkalies on sugars   One of the reactions common to all reducing sugars is Moore's test. When a reducing sugar solution to which has been added a small amount of sodium or potassium hydroxide is warmed, a yellow color is seen, changing to orange and then to dark brown. A faint odor of caramel, which is intensified on acidification, may be detected. Nonreducing sugars and polysaccharides do not give this test because the aldehyde or ketone groups are not free. The color is due to the polymerization of aldehydes liberated by the reaction, the final products being resins—probably similar to some of the products formed when almost any sugar is heated in the dry state to form caramel.

When treated with a weak alkali (e.g., barium hydroxide), glucose, fructose, or mannose is converted to a mixture of the three. Whichever sugar is used, the same proportion of all three is finally found at equilibrium. This is the Lobry de Bruyn–Alberda van Eckenstein transformation and is explained by the same relationship of these three sugars that accounts for their yielding the identical osazones. Remembering that carbons numbered 4, 5, and 6 have the same configuration in all three, we can show how this reaction proceeds by directing our attention to the first three carbon atoms:

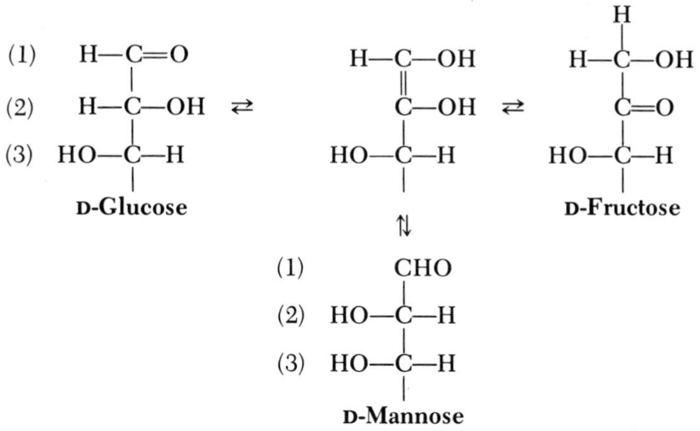

(1)   H—C=O   H—C—OH   H—C—OH
                                                                 |
(2)   H—C—OH ⇄   C—OH ⇄   C=O
                                                                 |
(3)   HO—C—H   HO—C—H   HO—C—H

   D-Glucose   **D-Fructose**

                          ⇅

(1)   CHO
(2)   HO—C—H
(3)   HO—C—H

      D-Mannose

It is assumed that an intermediate enol compound that readily changes to any of the three sugars is formed. Since this reaction easily occurs in the test tube, it may well be the mechanism whereby enzymes convert one hexose phosphate to another in the body. We know, for example, that all utilizable sugars can be converted to D-glucose or D-fructose and the transformation from D-glucose to D-fructose and vice versa seems to be going on continually.

Action of acids on sugars Strong acids react with monosaccharides to yield furfural derivatives. The pentoses are converted almost quantitatively into furfural itself, and this property is used in the estimation of pentoses. The reaction may be as follows:

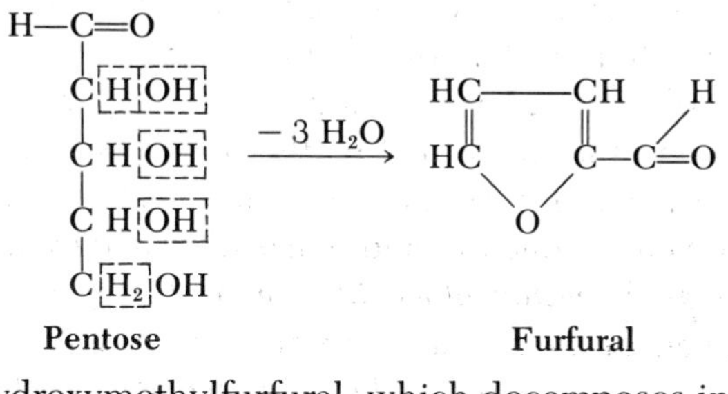

H—C=O
|
C H OH
|
C H OH $-3\,H_2O$ HC————CH   H
| ⟶   HC   C—C=O
C H OH   \ /
| O
C H₂ OH

      Pentose   **Furfural**

Hexoses yield hydroxymethylfurfural, which decomposes into levulinic acid and other products. Since furfural and its derivatives form colored compounds with a number of organic reagents, notably α-naphthol and thymol, the reaction can be used as a general test for carbohydrates. For example, if Molisch's reagent, an alcoholic solution of α-naphthol, is added to a carbohydrate and this is treated with concentrated sulfuric acid, a reddish violet color is produced.

Reduction of mono- saccharides The reduction of a simple sugar with hydrogen gas under pressure in the presence of a metal catalyst, or with certain other reducing agents, or enzymatically, converts the carbonyl group to an alcoholic hydroxyl group. For example, the reduction of D-glucose yields D-sorbitol (D-glucitol) as shown below. The reduction of L-sorbose also produces D-sorbitol. The structural relations between the two will become evident by rotating the formula of D-sorbitol through 180 degrees in the plane of the page.

The catalytic reduction of L-sorbose by hydrogen gas produces L-iditol (structure not shown) as well as D-sorbitol.

CHO		CH$_2$OH		CH$_2$OH
HCOH		HCOH		C=O
HOCH		HOCH		HOCH
HCOH	$\xrightarrow{+2\,H}$	HCOH	$\xleftarrow{+2\,H}$	HCOH
HCOH		HCOH		HOCH
CH$_2$OH		CH$_2$OH		CH$_2$OH
D-Glucose		**D-Sorbitol**		**L-Sorbose**

D-Sorbitol is an intermediate in the synthesis of fructose in the prostate gland (p. 214) and is sometimes used as a sweetening agent and as a diabetic food. L-Sorbose is used in the manufacture of ascorbic acid. Myoinositol, a cyclic hexahydroxy sugar, is formed by the reduction of D-glucose in vivo.

The chemical reduction of mannose and galactose yields mannitol and dulcitol, respectively. The reduction of the pentoses xylulose and ribose forms xylitol and ribitol, respectively. Xylitol is an intermediate in the glucuronate pathway of carbohydrate metabolism (p. 218). Ribitol is a component of certain bacterial cell walls (p. 177) and of flavin adenine dinucleotide (p. 246).

Deoxy sugars Sugars that have fewer oxygen atoms than carbon atoms are known as *deoxy* sugars. Several of them are of physiologic importance, particularly the pentose 2-deoxy-D-ribose ($C_5H_{10}O_4$). Its formula is given on p. 162. Since the carbon-2 does not bear a hydroxyl, this sugar cannot form an osazone. It will be recalled that deoxyribose is the pentose moiety in DNA (p. 31).

Glycosides If methyl alcohol and D-glucose are caused to react with each other, two new compounds are formed. These may be separated and purified, and it may then be shown that neither behaves as an aldehyde. The point of reaction is apparently at the aldehyde group, just as it was in the case of the mutarotation of glucose, and *glycoside linkages* are formed. These compounds are called *methyl glycosides* or, in this particular case, methyl glucosides. Here again are five asymmetric carbon atoms instead of four, since the first carbon is now seen to be asymmetric. The two methyl glucosides, which are named α- and β-, are represented thus:

Methyl α-D-glucopyranoside

$$
\begin{array}{l}
\text{H}_3\text{CO} - \text{C} - \text{H} \\
\text{H} - \text{C} - \text{OH} \\
\text{HO} - \text{C} - \text{H} \qquad \text{O} \\
\text{H} - \text{C} - \text{OH} \\
\text{H} - \text{C} \\
\text{CH}_2\text{OH}
\end{array}
\qquad \text{or}
$$

Methyl β-D-glucopyranoside

These two differ in rotatory power, in solubilities, and in other physical characteristics. They are hydrolyzed by different enzymes — maltase acts on the α-, and almond emulsin on the β-anomer.

The glycosides are widely distributed in the vegetable kingdom and are present in spices, vegetable dyes, and drugs. A large number are known. In plants they may have various functions, serving as reserve material, transport substances, coloring material, and poisonous and protective agents. The *aglycone*, or aglucone (the nonsugar residue of the glycoside), may be as simple as methyl alcohol or glycerol or as complex as the sterols. In between are the phenols, indoxyl, and the anthracene aglucones of rhubarb, aloes, and senna.

The *cardiac glycosides* are of prime importance in medicine. They are found in the leaves and seeds of *Digitalis,* the seeds of *Strophanthus,* the bulbs of squill, the flowers of lily of the valley, and in other plants. All the cardiac glycosides thus far studied are combinations of steroids and sugar molecules or chains of sugar molecules. Only a few sugars, i.e., D-glucose, rhamnose, digitoxose, cymarose, sarmentose, and digitalose, are present. However, recent work has shown that the 6-deoxy or the 2,6-dideoxy derivatives of D-galactose, L-gulose, L-talose, or D-allose are present in certain cardiac glycosides. The *Digitalis* glycosides include digitoxin, gitoxin, gitalin, and digoxin. From *Strophanthus* a number of glycosides have been isolated and identified. Among them are cymarin, strophanthin-K, and ouabain. Scillaren-A is one of the glycosides of squill.

Other pharmacologically active glycosides are phlorizin, which is found in the bark of the Rosaceae and has a marked influence on carbohydrate metabolism if injected into animals; salicin, found in willow bark; and amygdalin, found in the bitter almond. Among the glycosides found in spices and other plant products are sinigrin (in black mustard and horseradish), sinalbin (in white mustard), and saponin (in horse chestnuts).

The union between the monosaccharide constituents of disaccharides and polysaccharides is spoken of as a glycoside linkage, even though neither member is a nonsugar.

Glycosides were formerly called glucosides; but now any compound having glucose as one of its constituents is more correctly termed *glycoside*. Hence, if a glycoside has glucose as its sugar, it is both a glycoside and a glucoside.

157

Mono-saccharide phosphates Esters of phosphoric acid with sugars are formed in many biologic reactions; in fact, the formation of phosphates appears to be a prerequisite to many physiologic reactions. The hydroxyl radicals are esterified with phosphoric acid. Thus:

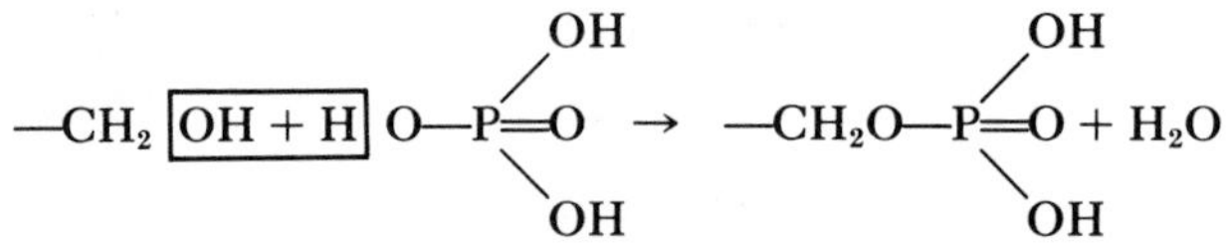

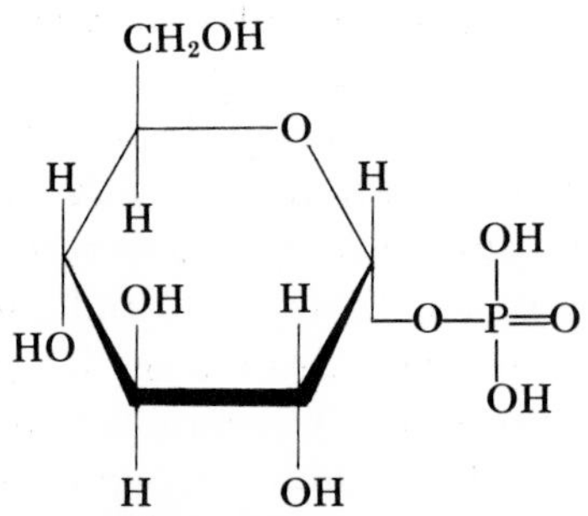

$$-CH_2 \boxed{OH + H} O\!-\!\underset{\overset{|}{OH}}{\overset{\overset{\displaystyle OH}{|}}{P}}\!=\!O \quad \rightarrow \quad -CH_2O\!-\!\underset{\overset{|}{OH}}{\overset{\overset{\displaystyle OH}{|}}{P}}\!=\!O + H_2O$$

α-D-Glucopyranose-
1-phosphoric acid
(Cori ester)

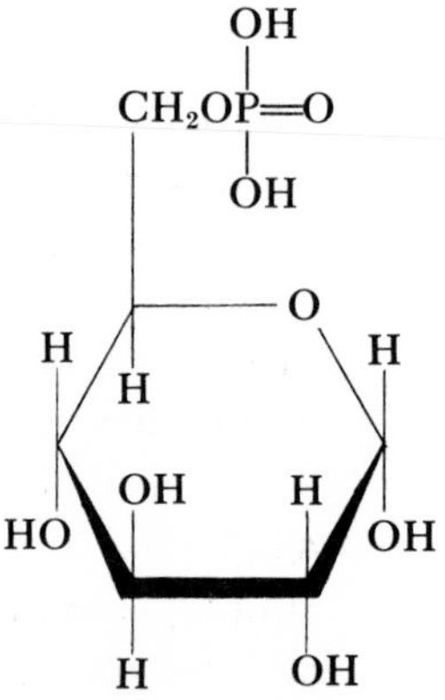

α-D-Glucopyranose-
6-phosphoric acid
(Robison ester)

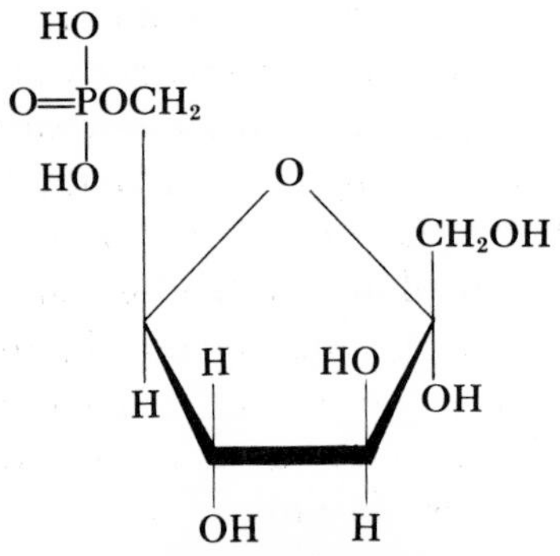

α-D-Fructofuranose-
6-phosphoric acid
(Neuberg ester)

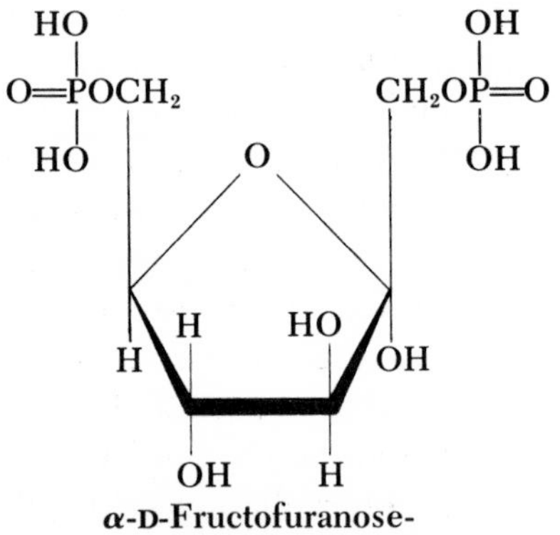

α-D-Fructofuranose-
1,6-diphosphoric acid
(Harden-Young ester)

The formation of such phosphate esters of sugars and their derivatives in the cells is called *phosphorylation*. Special enzymes and coenzymes are necessary to effect this, and these are quite specific, different enzymes being required to link the phosphate radicals to different positions, as will be described later (p. 189). Furthermore, as glucose is broken down either in fermentation or in carbohydrate utilization in animal tissues, the fragments are phosphorylated and the phosphate group is transferred from one part of the chain to another. Finally, the end products are obtained and the phosphate group is freed.

Fermentation When yeast is added to certain sugars, an evolution of carbon dioxide occurs and ethyl alcohol is formed. This reaction, which has been known and utilized since prebiblical times, is called *fermentation*. A fermentation is a decomposition of an organic substance, usually a carbohydrate, produced by the enzymes of a living organism. The term is often loosely used for any enzymic decomposition but is more properly restricted as stated. Until Buchner's time (1897) fermentation was believed to be dependent on the life of the yeast cells and could be brought about only by the growth, metabolism, and reproduction of such cells. Buchner, however, showed that the juice pressed out of yeast and containing no cells had the power to ferment sugars. He called the agent present *zymase*.

Ordinary baker's yeast ferments D-glucose, D-fructose, and D-mannose as well as sucrose and maltose. The latter two sugars, however, must first be split by another enzyme reaction into their constituent monosaccharides. Galactose may be fermented to some extent by baker's yeast. Other strains of yeast that are specific for other sugars are known. The reaction is commonly represented by the following equation:

$$C_6H_{12}O_6 \rightarrow 2\ C_2H_5OH + 2\ CO_2$$

However, it is not quantitative, and products other than carbon dioxide and ethyl alcohol are formed. Other microorganisms are capable of fermenting various sugars, and this specific ability is made use of in clinical diagnostic procedures.

Separation and identification of sugars Besides the methods customarily employed in organic chemistry, new techniques are available for the separation and identification of sugars from mixtures. In mixtures of aldoses and ketoses, the former may be oxidized to aldonic acids, which may then be retained on an ion-exchange resin. Sugar acids and amino sugars may also be exchanged on these resins. Column chromatography and paper chromatography are frequently used. For large amounts of material, column chromatography is the method of choice, and the individual sugars are adsorbed in bands on the column of adsorbent and may be eluted. Ion-exchange resins may be used here also since the carbohydrates form complexes with borate ions and then behave as anions. When only small amounts are at hand, paper chromatography is used to good advantage. The spots formed can be visualized and identified by color tests. Carbohydrates that can be converted to stable, volatile derivatives can also be separated and identified by gas-liquid chromatography. Bacteriologic methods can also be used for the identification of many sugars.

Occurrence and properties D-*Glucose.* D-Glucose is also called *dextrose*, because of its dextrorotation, and *grape sugar*, from one of its sources. It occurs widely in fruits and vegetables, frequently associated with other sugars. Linked with a second molecule of monosaccharide, it is a component of all the common disaccharides, and in the polymerized state it is a constituent of many polysaccharides. Thus digestion of these disaccharides and polysaccharides yields D-glucose for nutritive purposes. The syrup commonly named "glucose" commercially is chiefly D-glucose. It is produced by the hydrolysis of starch. These syrups, the so-called corn syrups, contain some dextrins and maltose besides glucose and are used to some extent to modify cow's milk for use in infant feeding.

D-Glucose is the chief physiologic sugar. It may be transformed into other monosaccharides for special uses. It is present in normal blood continually and at a fairly constant level, i.e., about 0.1% (100 mg. per 100 ml. blood). There are also minute traces normally in the urine, but these are too small to be detected by ordinary methods. Pathologically both blood sugar and urine sugar may increase considerably. The disease *diabetes mellitus* is a notable example.

D-*Fructose*. D-Fructose is a ketohexose. Its molecular formula is $C_6H_{12}O_6$, and its structural formula may be shown in three ways: (1) as a ketone (D-

α-D-Fructopyranose   **Keto-D-fructose**   **β-D-Fructopyranose**

α-D-Fructopyranose
(perspective formula)

β-D-Fructofuranose
(perspective formula)

fructose), (2) as α- and β-D-fructose, and (3) in the perspective formulas. It should be noted that the asymmetric carbon accounting for mutarotation, etc. is carbon-2 in the case of fructose. Fructose also occurs as fructofuranose, i.e., with a 2,5-oxygen bridge, as in furan.

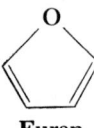

Furan

When combined in natural products, the sugar is always in the furanose modification. Fructose is commonly called *fruit sugar* because of its widespread occurrence free in fruits. It is one of the constituents of sucrose and of other sugars and also of the polysaccharide inulin. It is a very sweet sugar, much sweeter than sucrose, and more reactive than glucose. It rotates the plane of polarized light to the left, whence another name is derived, i.e., *levulose*. It also exhibits mutarotation. The letter D, which is prefixed in its exact scientific name, D-fructose, of course, refers to its configuration (p. 147). Thus, in the ketone formula it has the same configuration for carbon-5 as has D-glyceraldehyde, the reference sugar. Since carbons 3, 4, and 5 have the same arrangement of hydrogens and hydroxyls as those of D-glucose, the osazones of these two sugars are identical.

Fructose can further be distinguished from glucose by the Seliwanoff reaction. In this procedure a few drops of dilute sugar solution are heated with a reagent containing resorcinol in dilute hydrochloric acid (1:2) under carefully regulated conditions. There is formed hydroxymethylfurfural, which reacts with the resorcinol to give a red compound. Other ketoses and ketose-containing disaccharides, e.g., sucrose, give this test, and other sugars also if present in high concentrations or if the heating is continued beyond the prescribed period. A more decisive reaction is the formation of the fructose methylphenylosazone. This is specific for fructose and can be carried out in the presence of glucose or sucrose.

D-*Galactose*. D-Galactose is seldom found free in nature, but in combination it occurs in both plants and animals. In plants it appears in certain polysaccharides (e.g., in the seed coats of legumes) and in complex mixed carbohydrates. It apparently can be manufactured by the body, or, more probably, glucose is changed to galactose (p. 215). Among other sites of this transformation is the mammary gland, since *milk sugar* is made up of glucose and galactose. It is also a constituent of the glycolipids found in many tissues, particularly nervous tissue. Pathologically, it occurs in the urine of nursing infants having digestive difficulties. There is also an *inborn error of metabolism*, in which galactose occurs in the blood and urine (p. 216).

Galactose is not as sweet as glucose and is less soluble in water, but it has a higher specific dextrorotation. On oxidation by hot nitric acid, it yields mucic acid, which is less soluble than the corresponding saccharic acid, formed from glucose. This aids in its identification, since the crystals of mucic acid are not difficult to produce and detect. Another difference is that galactose is fermented much more slowly by yeasts than is glucose, and some yeasts do not ferment it at all.

D-*Mannose*. D-Mannose is not found free to any great extent, and the polysaccharides that yield it on hydrolysis are not very digestible. It is, therefore, of slight importance nutritionally in American dietaries. Baker's yeast ferments it. The two anomers of D-mannose differ physiologically, the α-anomer being sweet and the β-anomer being bitter.[1]

***Pentoses*.** Important pentoses—all having the molecular formula $C_5H_{10}O_5$— are L-arabinose, D-xylose, D-ribose, 2-deoxy-D-ribose ($C_5H_{10}O_4$), L-xylulose, and D-ribulose. The first four are aldoses and are not found free in nature. L-Arabinose results when gum arabic, cherry gum, and various other gums are hydrolyzed. D-Xylose is produced by the hydrolysis of straw and wood. β-D-Ribose and 2-deoxy-D-ribose are constituents of nucleic acids RNA and

DNA, respectively (p. 31). Deoxy sugars contain one oxygen atom less than the sugars from which they are derived. L-Xylulose is present in the urine in the condition known as *pentosuria*. D-Ribulose is important in carbohydrate metabolism (p. 209). The last two are ketoses. The structures of four of these pentoses are shown below. α-D-Ribose is given as a ring structure.

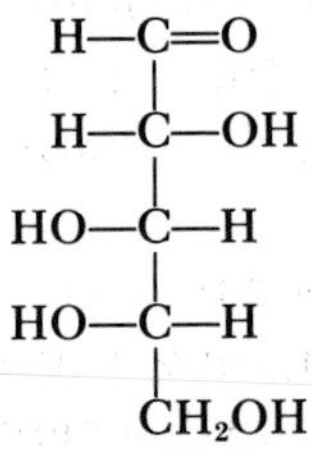

```
   H—C=O              H—C=O              CH₂OH
      |                  |                  |
   H—C—OH             H—C—H              C=O
      |                  |                  |
  HO—C—H              H—C—OH             H—C—OH
      |                  |                  |
  HO—C—H              H—C—OH            HO—C—H
      |                  |                  |
    CH₂OH              CH₂OH              CH₂OH
  L-Arabinose      2-Deoxy-D-ribose     L-Xylulose
```

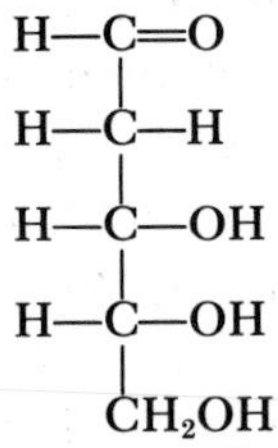

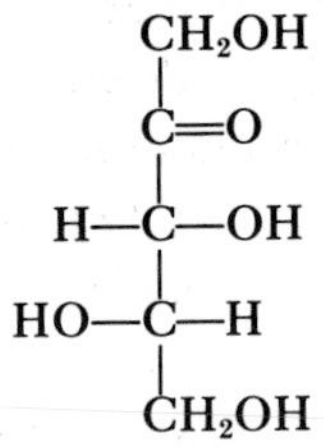

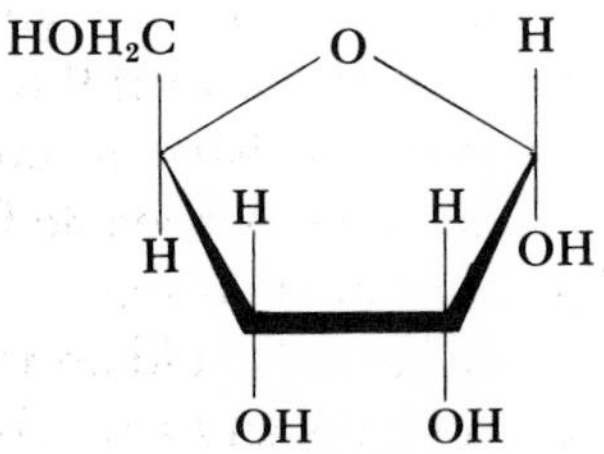

α-D-Ribose

The pentose pyranoses, D-arabinose and D-xylose, exist in the *chair* conformation (p. 151), whereas the pentose furanose, D-ribose, is coplanar in conformation (p. 151). As in the case of D-glucopyranose, α- and β-anomers of D-ribofuranose exist. The β-anomer of D-ribose exists exclusively in the nucleic acids (p. 31).

Other important sugars In the same metabolic pathway in which D-ribulose occurs (p. 209) are seen a tetrose, erythrose, and a seven-carbon sugar, sedoheptulose. The former is an aldose, and the latter a ketose.

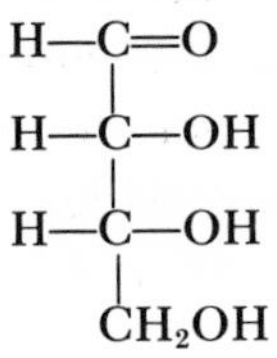

```
   H—C=O                  CH₂OH
      |                      |
   H—C—OH                 C=O
      |                      |
   H—C—OH              HO—C—H
      |                      |
    CH₂OH               H—C—OH
                            |
                         H—C—OH
                            |
                         H—C—OH
                            |
                          CH₂OH
  D-Erythrose           D-Sedoheptulose
```

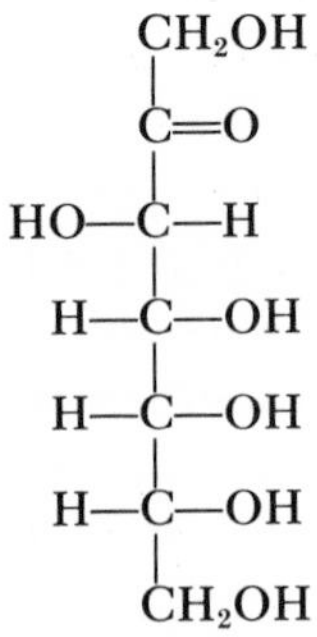

OLIGOSACCHARIDES

The three most common oligosaccharides are the disaccharides maltose, lactose, and sucrose. Each has the molecular formula $C_{12}H_{22}O_{11}$ and is hydrolyzed by hot acids and by appropriate enzymes according to the following equation:

162

$$C_{12}H_{22}O_{11} + H_2O \rightarrow C_6H_{12}O_6 + C_6H_{12}O_6$$

Maltose $\rightarrow$ D-Glucose + D-Glucose
Lactose $\rightarrow$ D-Glucose + D-Galactose
Sucrose $\rightarrow$ D-Glucose + D-Fructose

Structure   The disaccharides are formed by the union of two constituent monosaccharides, with the elimination of a molecule of water. The points of linkage vary, as does the manner of linking, and the properties of the disaccharide depend to a great extent upon them. If both of the two potential aldehyde or ketone groups are involved in the linkage, the sugar has no reducing properties and is not able to form an osazone. However, if one of the aldehyde or ketone groups is not bound in this way, the sugar has properties of both reduction and osazone formation. Sucrose is formed from D-glucose and D-fructose by union at the aldehyde and ketone carbons. Hence, it is nonreducing and does not form an osazone. Lactose and maltose both have an unlinked potential aldehyde and consequently are reducing sugars that form osazones.

A comparison of the formulas of the disaccharides with those for methyl α- and β-glucosides will show that maltose has an α-glucoside linkage and lactose a β-galactoside linkage. The constituents of sucrose are joined by an α-glucoside–β-fructoside linkage. It is also seen that in sucrose the oxygen bridge of the fructose portion is from carbon-2 to carbon-5. Upon hydrolysis this changes to the more stable carbon-2 to carbon-6 bridge.

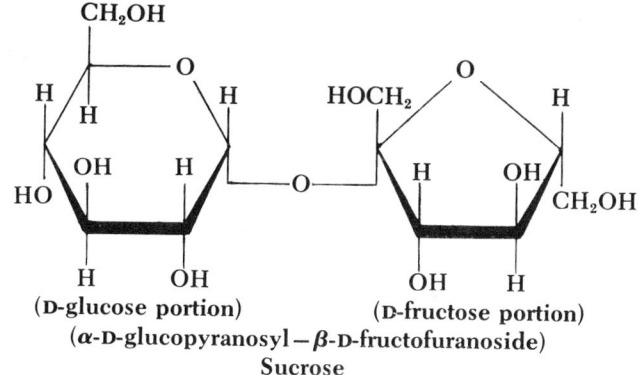

(D-glucose portion)   (D-fructose portion)
(α-D-glucopyranosyl – β-D-fructofuranoside)
Sucrose

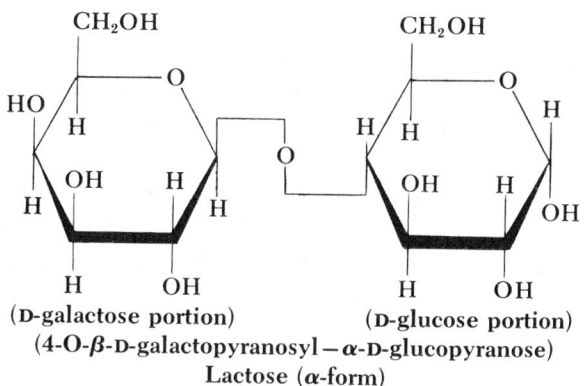

(D-galactose portion)   (D-glucose portion)
(4-O-β-D-galactopyranosyl – α-D-glucopyranose)
Lactose (α-form)

163

(D-glucose)   (D-glucose)
(4-O-α-D-glucopyranosyl — D-glucopyranose)
Maltose (β-form)

Maltose. Maltose or *malt sugar* is an intermediary in the acid hydrolysis of starch and can also be obtained by the enzymatic hydrolysis of starch. One of the time-honored methods utilizes the action of sprouting barley, which contains the enzyme diastase, on grain. This is the first step in the production of alcohol. Various food preparations, such as baby foods and invalid foods, produced by hydrolysis of grains, contain large amounts of maltose. Starch digestion in the body yields maltose, which requires only one further hydrolytic action to be converted to glucose. It is a rather sweet sugar, very soluble in water. Since one aldehyde is free, or potentially free, maltose has reducing properties and forms a characteristic osazone. It usually crystallizes in the β-form.

Lactose. Lactose is *milk sugar.* It is found in appreciable quantities only in milk and occurs at body temperature as an equilibrium mixture of the α- and β-anomers in a 2:3 ratio. However, lactose usually crystallizes in the α-form. It is, to be sure, found also in very low concentration in the blood and urine of lactating women, but this should be considered accidental and is by no means a constant occurrence. If the mammary gland produces an excess of lactose or if the milk is not removed rapidly enough, lactose enters into the circulation. The body cannot utilize unhydrolyzed disaccharides; therefore this "wandering" lactose is excreted by the kidneys. Lactose also has reducing properties and forms a characteristic osazone. It is not very soluble and is not as sweet as the other common sugars. This property may be made use of when it is desirable to force carbohydrate feeding in patients having a distaste for sweets. The sugar is dextrorotatory. Because it contains galactose as one of its constituents, it yields mucic acid when hydrolyzed and is subsequently oxidized by hot nitric acid. It is not fermented by baker's yeast, and its behavior toward other microorganisms is also noteworthy. It is fermented by the colon bacillus but not by the typhoid bacillus. This reaction is used by bacteriologists to distinguish between these two organisms, which resemble each other in many ways. Many organisms that are found in milk, e.g., *Bacillus coli, B. aerogenes, Streptococcus lactis,* convert lactose to lactic acid, thus causing the souring of milk. *Lactobacillus acidophilus* and *L. bulgaricus* are examples of other organisms that have the same action; these two are used to produce the therapeutic sour milks.

Sucrose. Ordinary table sugar is sucrose or *saccharose.* It is obtained from the sugar cane, the sugar beet, and, to a lesser extent, the sugar maple. It also occurs free in most fruits and vegetables, e.g., pineapples and carrots. It is very soluble and very sweet and on hydrolysis yields glucose and fructose. Sucrose is dextrorotatory, but its hydrolytic products are levorotatory because fructose has a greater specific levorotation than the dextrorotation of glucose. Since this hydrolysis therefore inverts the rotation, the resulting mixture of glucose and fructose is called *invert sugar* and the process is called *inversion.* Honey is largely invert sugar, and the presence of fructose accounts for the greater sweetness of honey. Sucrose does not reduce alkaline copper solutions, nor does it form osazones. The explanation for this is that the aldehyde and ketone groups of its constituent monosaccharides are linked together and consequently neither one is free to react. Sucrose is fermented by ordinary yeast but is first inverted by invertases present in, or secreted by, the yeast cell. Sucrose is easily inverted by invertases present in the intestinal tract and, together with D-glucose, is the most important sugar of our dietary. The monosaccharides formed—glucose and fructose—are readily absorbed and utilized by the body. However, it must be emphasized that this is true only of sucrose taken into the body per os. If introduced by any path other than the gastroenteric tract, i.e., *parenterally,* sucrose is hardly utilized at all. Disaccharides are unphysiologic substances when present in the bloodstream, as just mentioned in the case of lactose. Therefore, sucrose should not be injected intravenously if its nutritive properties are desired. Sometimes it is injected in this way, but the clinician uses it to change the osmotic pressure of the blood and to cause a flow of water from the tissues into the blood. Invert sugar, however, may be given intravenously as a nutrient fluid. If sucrose, or some other disaccharide, is not hydrolyzed in the intestinal tract, because of the absence of the appropriate enzyme, diarrhea is likely to occur.[2]

Table 8-2. Relative sweetness of sugars*

Sugar	Numeric rating (sucrose = 100)	Units of weight of sugar equivalent to 1 unit of sucrose
Lactose	16.0	6.3
Raffinose	22.6	4.4
Galactose	32.1	3.1
Rhamnose	32.5	3.1
Maltose	32.5 (?)	3.1 (?)
Xylose	40.0	2.5
Glucose	74.3	1.3
Sucrose	100.0	1.0
Invert sugar†	127.4	0.8
Invert sugar‡	130.0	0.8
Fructose	173.3	0.6

° From Biester, A., Wood, M. W., and Wahlin, C. S.: Amer. J. Physiol. 73:387, 1925; Willamen, J. J., Wahlin, C. S., and Biester, A.: Amer. J. Physiol. 73:397, 1925.
† Prepared by the action of invertase on sucrose.
‡ Equal parts of glucose and fructose mixed.

Sucrose is the principal sugar in carbohydrate transport in plants, as is glucose in animals. It is formed from or converted to stored carbohydrate, usually as starch in the roots. It is the transport sugar, as an approximately 20% solution, to and from metabolically active areas such as the leaf, where during the warmer seasons glucose is formed by photosynthesis (p. 219). The reason for the evolutionary survival of sucrose as the transport sugar of choice in plants, in contrast to glucose in animals, is not understood at this time. It may be related to the greater stability of sucrose or to some osmotic advantages.

Sweetness of sugars The relative sweetness of sugars cannot be determined with great accuracy. However, observations on a series of subjects have given the figures shown in Table 8-2. With sucrose as the standard, the relation of this sugar to other sugars was determined by observing the highest dilution at which the sweet taste was detectable.

POLYSACCHARIDES

The polysaccharides are much more complex substances than the other carbohydrates so far discussed. Some are polymers of a single monosaccharide (*homopolysaccharides*), and some contain other groups (*heteropolysaccharides*). Most are white amorphous compounds, of which starch is a typical example. They are not sweet and, when pure, do not reduce or give other characteristic aldose or ketose reactions. Since they are polymers of sugars, the molecules are, in general, very large. Consequently, polysaccharides that are not insoluble form colloidal solutions. The molecular weights of the celluloses probably range from 200,000 to 400,000; those of the starches, from 10,000 to 1,000,000; and glycogen from different sources is said to vary from

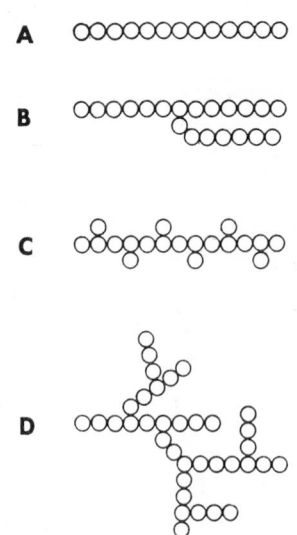

Fig. 8-5. Some types of structures of polysaccharides. Each circle represents a glycose unit. (From Whistler, R. L., and Corbett, W. M.: In Pigman, W., editor: The carbohydrates, New York, 1957, Academic Press, Inc.)

1,000,000 to 4,000,000. These polysaccharides are not all straight-chain compounds, although some of them are. Fig. 8-5 indicates some types of these structures. Each circle represents a glycose unit. They form linear, cyclic, or branched patterns. Some are helical, but none is netlike or cagelike.

The polysaccharides are given names ending in *an*, attached to the particular glycose making up the polymer. Thus a name for the polysaccharides in general is *glycans*, from *glycose*, a simple sugar, and the ending *an*, a sugar polymer. Particular ones are arabans, xylans, mannans, and galactans, which are polymers of arabinose, xylose, mannose, and galactose, respectively. The old term *pentosan* has not been shortened to pentan, nor have the names glycogen, starch, amylose, and amylopectin been changed. There are, in addition, other polysaccharides, chiefly animal in origin, that have names such as hyaluronic acid, heparin, etc. referring to their structure or origin.

Pentosans. Pentosans occur chiefly in vegetable gums, e.g., cherry gum, and in other vegetable materials such as straw. On hydrolysis they yield pentoses, but because pentosans are complex mixtures of polysaccharides, it is difficult to obtain pure sugars from such sources.

Hexans. The hexans yield hexoses on hydrolysis.

Starch. Starch occurs in many plants as storage foods. It may be found in the leaves and stems as well as in the roots, fruits, and seeds, where it is usually present in greater concentration. Granules of starch under the microscope appear as particles made up of concentric layers of material. They differ in shape, size, and markings according to the source (Fig. 8-6). In this way experts can identify starches that have been mixed with spices or other products as adulterants. Starchy foods are a mainstay of our diet. Large amounts are present in cereals (e.g., wheat, rye, corn, barley) and in potatoes, legumes, and nuts. In the ripening process of some plants (e.g., apples, bananas), starch is changed to sugar; in others (corn, peas) the change is in the opposite direction. Starches also are used in industry and in the household in many ways, e.g., in laundering, as adhesives, as sizes for textiles, and as thickening agents for puddings, etc.

The starch granule contains two polysaccharides, both polymers of glucose but differing in molecular architecture and in certain properties. One is called *amylose* and the other, *amylopectin*. There is usually 20% to 28% amylose and the rest amylopectin. The amylose aggregate consists of 250 to 300 D-glu-

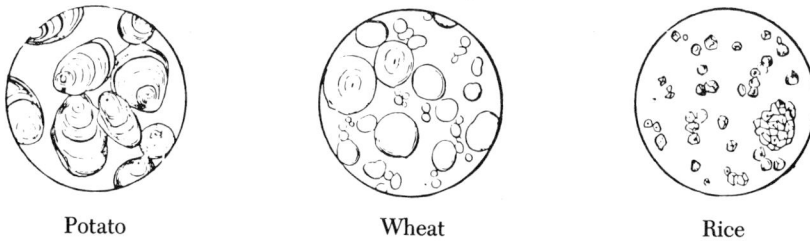

| Potato | Wheat | Rice |

Fig. 8-6. Starch granules (×200). (From Fearon, W. R.: An introduction to biochemistry, St. Louis, 1940, The C. V. Mosby Co.)

167

cose units linked by α-1,4-glucosidic bonds (see formula below). These tend to twist the chain into a helix. In amylopectin, the majority of the units are similarly connected by α-1,4-glucosidic bonds, but there are occasional α-1,6-glucosidic bonds. The structure is a branch-on-branch arrangement of perhaps a thousand D-glucopyranose units, like D, in Fig. 8-5, put together as shown in Fig. 8-7. Starch granules are insoluble in cold water, but when their suspension is heated, water is taken up and swelling occurs, at first to a slight degree but later to several hundred times their original volume. Viscosity increases, and starch gels or pastes result. Both the granules and the colloidal solutions react with iodine to give a blue color. This is chiefly due to the amylose, which forms a deep blue complex, whereas amylopectin solutions are colored blue-violet or purple.

Starches are capable of forming esters with either organic or inorganic acids. There is present in some starches a minute amount of phosphoric acid. This is linked by primary ester bonds to carbon-6. Some synthetic starch esters are useful as plastics, whereas starch nitrates are violent explosives.

The exact molecular structure of both amylose and amylopectin is not entirely settled, although the general pattern of each is known. Amylose consists of long chains of from 250 to 300 glucose units, uniformly linked by α-1,4-glucosidic bonds, which linkage tends to cause a spiraling of the molecule in a helixlike fashion. The α-D-glucopyranose units of amylose (and amylopectin) apparently exist in the chair form conformation (p. 151). Since the aldehyde-bearing carbon (C-1) is joined in each case to the next unit, its reducing action is nullified. A portion of such a structure is shown thus:

α-Linked glucose units in amylose

The amylopectin molecule is thought to be made up of a large number of branches, each consisting of about 25 glucose units. Each of these small branches resembles the larger amylose chains, but the molecules are joined together in such a way that the free-reducing group of a glucose unit at the end of one branch is glucosidically linked through the sixth carbon of a glucose unit (not an end one) in an adjoining chain. The resulting molecule is much larger than that of amylose (Fig. 8-7), with a thousand or more D-glucopyranose units.

Hydrolysis of starch yields a succession of polysaccharides of gradually diminishing molecular size. Simultaneously, glucose or maltose is split off and the color reaction with iodine changes.

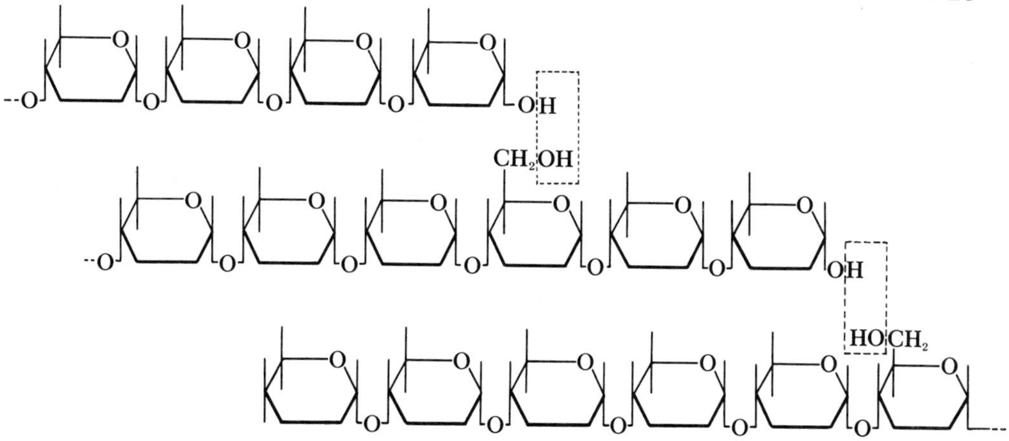

Fig. 8-7. Haworth and Hirst's diagrammatic formula for glycogen or amylopectin. Each chain (repeating unit) contains from six to 25 glucose residues.

Iodine reaction	Course of hydrolysis
Blue	Starch
	↓
Blue	Soluble starch
	↓
Purple	Amylodextrin
	↓
Red	Erythrodextrin
	↓
Colorless	Achroodextrin
	↓
	Maltose

Enzyme (amylase) hydrolysis ends at maltose and, of course, is not quantitative; traces of the dextrins remain. If a maltase is present or if the hydrolysis is accomplished by acid, much of the starch is converted to glucose.

Glycogen. Glycogen is often called *animal starch,* although now it is known to occur also in yeasts and in algae and fungi and a polysaccharide very similar to it is in golden bantam sweet corn. It is found in significant amounts in oysters and other shellfish, and the muscle of the scallop is particularly rich in it. Carbohydrates of a glycogenlike nature abound in tapeworms. In higher animals it is deposited in the liver as storage material and in the muscle as a more immediate source of energy.

Glycogen may be precipitated from its beautifully opalescent solution by ethyl alcohol and, on drying, forms a pure white powder. It is dextrorotatory with an $[\alpha]D^{20°} = +196$ to $+197$ degrees. It is not destroyed by a hot strong potassium hydroxide or sodium hydroxide solution. This property is made use of in the method for determining glycogen quantitatively in tissues. The weighed minced tissue, to which strong alkali has been added, is heated on a steam bath until the tissue disintegrates and dissolves; then the glycogen is precipitated out by alcohol and, after purification, is hydrolyzed to glucose, which may be determined by some standard quantitative procedure. With iodine, glycogen gives a deep red color. In this respect it resembles erythrodextrin, but it may be distinguished from erythrodextrin by its opalescence in solution and by certain other properties. The glycogen-iodine reaction requires a much stronger iodine reagent than does the starch- or dextrin-iodine test.

Glycogen on hydrolysis yields D-glucose:

$$(C_6H_{10}O_5)_n + (n-1)\ H_2O\ \rightarrow\ n(C_6H_{12}O_6)$$

An analogous reaction is constantly occurring in the body. However, in the body this is a reversible reaction and phosphoric acid is involved (Chapter 9). Glucose and other monosaccharides are transformed to glycogen in muscle and liver, and glycogen is rapidly converted to D-glucose as needed for physiologic requirements. Glycogen resembles amylopectin in structure in that it is made up of branched chains of glucose units. The individual glucose units are attached to each other by the same α-1,4-glucosidic linkages, but the chains are somewhat shorter, averaging 12 glucose units. These short chains are joined together in much the same way as those of amylopectin. Glycogen, as well as many other polysaccharides, does not exist in the form of homogeneous molecules all having the same molecular weight and possessing the same number of monosaccharide units. The glycogen units are collections of polymers, having the same general branching plan but a rather wide range of molecular weights, depending upon the animal from which it is derived, and varying even with tissue of the same animal. When prepared by the usual procedures, glycogen may have a molecular weight of several million. However, glycogen prepared by a mild, water extraction procedure may have a molecular weight as high as 900,000,000.

Dextrins. When starch is partially hydrolyzed by the action of acids or enzymes, it is broken down to a number of products of lower molecular weight known as dextrins. These include *soluble starch* and the other dextrins listed on p. 169. Soluble starch forms a clear colorless solution, not at all "starchy" in appearance but giving a blue iodine reaction. The other dextrins are water soluble and react to iodine as indicated. They resemble starch in being precipitable by alcohol, forming sticky, gummy masses. Dextrin solutions are often used as mucilages, e.g., mucilage on the back of a postage stamp. Starch hydrolysates, consisting largely of dextrins and maltose, are widely used in infant feeding. These carbohydrates not only are easily digested, but their physical properties are useful in preventing the formation of large heavy curds when the milk, with which they are mixed, clots in the baby's stomach. Many breakfast foods contain dextrins, as do the malt preparations used in soda fountain beverages. Most preparations of dextrins are mixtures. One well-defined dextrin is called *limit dextrin.* This is the product remaining after the enzyme β-amylase has acted on starch until no further action is observed.

Dextrans. Certain microorganisms, when grown on sugar media, produce polysaccharides known as dextrans. These constitute what was formerly called *slime;* they were discarded when they appeared in industrial operations. Dextrans differ from dextrins in structure. They are made up of units of a number of D-glucose molecules having α-1,6-; α-1,4-; or α-1,3-glycosidic linkages within each unit, and the units are joined together to form a network. Dextrans, synthesized by *Leuconostoc mesenteroides* in a sucrose medium, have been recommended as blood "extenders"; i.e., solutions of them may be injected intravenously, after blood loss, in order to increase the volume of the circulating blood (p. 636). Because of their high viscosity, low osmotic pressure, and slow disintegration and utilization, they remain in the blood for many hours. The fractions of dextrans having molecular weights ranging from 25,000 to 75,000 are most suitable for clinical use. If the injections are not repeated too frequently, the dextrans are eliminated and do very little damage to the tissues.

Cellulose. Cellulose is a *glucan* that makes up a large part of the framework of plant tissues. Its synthesis in the laboratory, using plant enzymes, has been achieved.[3] It is quite insoluble, except in certain special reagents. Cotton and paper are composed largely of cellulose. It is not hydrolyzed readily by dilute acids, but heating with fairly high concentrations of acids yields the disaccharide cellobiose and D-glucose. Cellobiose is made up of two molecules of D-glucose, linked together by β-glucosidic linkages between the first and fourth carbon atoms of adjacent glucose units. Hence cellulose is considered to be long chains of glucose units joined together in this way. No cellulose-splitting enzyme is secreted by the mucosa of the human gastrointestinal tract. However, some microorganisms are capable of digesting it, and if such are present in our intestinal canal there is the possibility of some slight nutritive value in cellulose. Even termites, which use wood and other cellulose-containing materials as food, do not do so directly; rather, a symbiosis exists between these insects and their intestinal protozoa. The teeming protozoa either digest the cellulose completely or play an important part in its digestion. Although cellulose cannot be considered of any particular value nutritionally, it does have a physiologic role. It is a part of the roughage or indigestible matter of the diet. This is swept along the gut by the intestinal peristaltic wave, and its mere bulk is of value in stimulating this movement. In the large intestine this bulk aids in the formation of normal stools. Often an increase in roughage will relieve constipation, but too great an amount is not desirable and is even likely to aggravate the condition.

Methylcellulose has also been suggested for certain intestinal conditions, including constipation, since it absorbs large quantities of water to form colloidal solutions and otherwise has properties similar to cellulose.

The oxidation of cellulose by nitrous oxide under appropriate conditions yields an oxidized cellulose that is soluble in slightly alkaline solutions. Probably primary hydroxyl groups are attacked, yielding oxidation products containing combined uronic acid units, i.e., polyglucuronides. These cellulose products retain their fibrous structure and will undoubtedly find uses in medicine. Already some applications have been suggested. Pledgets of this cotton, containing thrombin, the blood-clotting principle, have been applied to wounds and left there. The mass is more adherent than a clot alone would be and is eventually dissolved by the faintly alkaline body fluids and is then absorbed. Absorbable paper and gauze have also been tested in animal experiments. When left in contact with brain, muscle, joints, etc., they are also absorbed after serving their purpose of supporting or protecting injured surfaces where a smooth membrane is desired in the final healing.

Inulin. Inulin is a *fructan*. It is a polysaccharide that occurs in the tubers of the dahlia, in the roots of the Jerusalem artichoke, dandelion, and chickory, and in the bulbs of onion and garlic. It is a white tasteless powder that is levorotatory and gives no color with iodine. Acids hydrolyze it to D-fructose, as does inulase, the enzyme that accompanies it in plants. For a while, inulin was recommended in the dietary of individuals with diabetes, on the assumption that it would be digested to fructose, which was further assumed to be more easily utilized by persons suffering from diabetes. It is not certain whether inulin is digestible, although it is possible that fructose is handled better than glucose in diabetes. Fructans are being discovered continually in various plant materials. They are found in large amounts in grasses and in smaller amounts in cereals.

Heteropolysaccharides and related substances   Agar-agar, a product derived from certain seaweeds, contains a large amount of *galactan*. Agar is used in the preparation of culture media in bacteriology. It is not digested in the human alimentary tract and therefore is of value in treating certain forms of constipation, acting as a soft, nonirritating type of roughage. Mannans are also quite indigestible. Some mannan is found in the carob bean, or St. John's bread, and also in the ivory nut. Many plant polysaccharides found in gums, mucilage, wood, and other plant tissues are not made up of any one pure carbohydrate. For example, gum arabic contains a nucleus relatively resistant to acid hydrolysis. This is composed of galactose and glucuronic acid units. With them are combined, more loosely, arabinose and 6-deoxyhexose, which can be easily split off by mild treatment with acids. Slippery elm mucilage and flaxseed mucilage both appear to contain rhamnose and galacturonic acid, but other carbohydrates are probably admixed.

Such polysaccharides constitute the major part of the indigestible residue of plant foods and therefore also become a part of the roughage. Those polysaccharides not digested and not easily hydrolyzed by acid or alkali are designated as crude fiber in reports of food analyses. A number of them have been included in an ill-defined group known as *hemicelluloses*. These occur in cell walls along with cellulose and were so called because they were thought to be intermediates in the formation of cellulose. Included are the xylans, acidic hemicelluloses, mannans, and pectins.

Pectins are responsible for the gelling properties of fruits. A suitable concentration of acid, sucrose, and pectin is necessary to produce a jelly. Pectins appear to yield, on hydrolysis, arabinose, galactose, acetic acid, methyl alcohol, and galacturonic acid; and various hypotheses have been advanced to account for all these constituents. Recent work indicates, however, that the arabinose and galactose are derived from arabans and galactans associated with the pectin. The term "pectic substance" is now used as a group designation for these complex carbohydrate derivatives. They contain a large proportion of methylated galacturonic acid molecules, which are believed to exist in long chains.

Uronic acids. The uronic acids are constituents of a number of types of heteropolysaccharides, including many plant gums and pectins, as mentioned above, the mucopolysaccharides (p. 174), and a wide variety of cell wall polysaccharides of plants and microorganisms (p. 176). Oxidation of the monosaccharides yields, among others, three important types of acids. Using D-glucose as an example, these may be shown as follows:

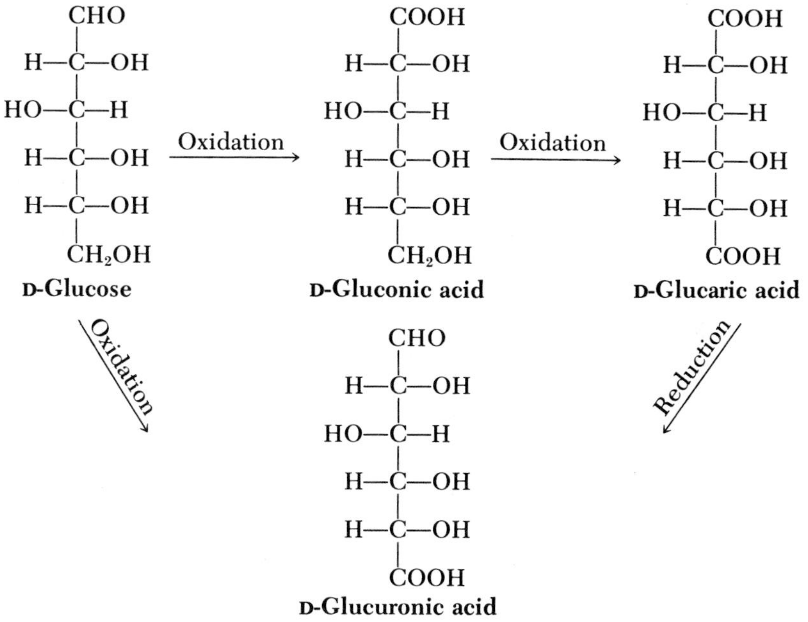

CHO	COOH	COOH
H—C—OH	H—C—OH	H—C—OH
HO—C—H	HO—C—H	HO—C—H
H—C—OH	H—C—OH	H—C—OH
H—C—OH	H—C—OH	H—C—OH
CH₂OH	CH₂OH	COOH
D-Glucose	D-Gluconic acid	D-Glucaric acid

Oxidation → Oxidation →

Oxidation ↓ Reduction ↙

CHO
H—C—OH
HO—C—H
H—C—OH
H—C—OH
COOH
D-Glucuronic acid

Glucaric acid is probably not formed in the body but is produced in vitro. It is the analogue of mucic acid, formed from galactose, but is soluble, whereas mucic acid is not very soluble. Gluconic and glucuronic acids are produced metabolically. Glucuronic acid is often found in urine in combination with various compounds. It unites in two ways, forming glucosides or esters.

Since these combining substances are often drugs or poisons and the resulting product is either less toxic or more easily excreted, the process is sometimes called *detoxication*, although innocuous substances are similarly treated by the body. The glucuronides do not reduce because the aldehyde groups are combined. However, glucuronic acid in the free form has reducing properties, is dextrorotatory, but cannot be fermented by ordinary yeast. With certain sex hormones it forms compounds that are much more soluble than the uncombined hormone in the aqueous body fluids. Acids of this type, possessing both aldehyde (or hemiacetal) and carboxyl groups, are called uronic acids.

Amino sugars. Amino sugars are essential parts of the molecules of mucosubstances. Mucosubstances are extremely important biologic compounds and include the *mucopolysaccharides*, the *mucoproteins*, and the *mucolipids*. They are diversified in their functions, in the ground substance of connective tissue, as a blood anticoagulant, as blood components, and as an energy source. In them the amino group replaces a hydroxyl group and, in most cases, is acetylated. There are three naturally occurring amino sugars, D-glucosamine, D-galactosamine, and D-mannosamine. In general, they enter into large carbohydrate polymers, alternating usually with a uronic acid, e.g., glucuronic. The special characteristics of these biologic entities are referable not only to the chemical makeup but also to the arrangement of the long chains, side chains, and hydrogen bonding. The formulas of two amino sugars are as follows:

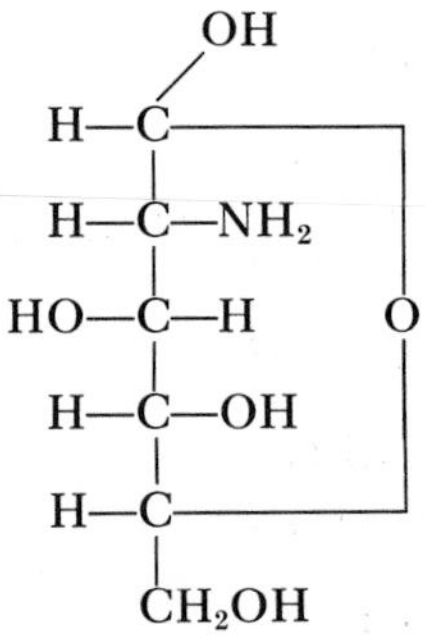

D-Glucosamine 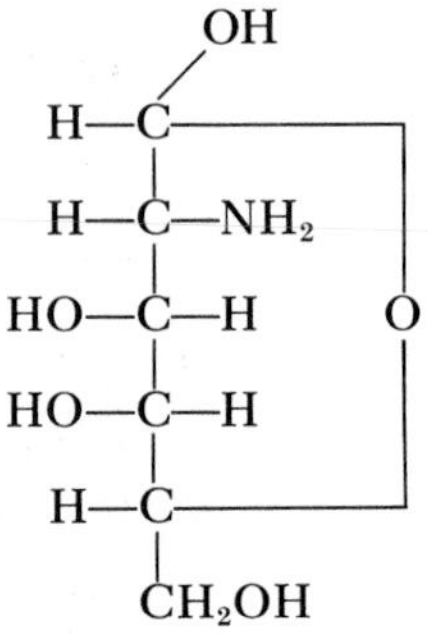   **D-Galactosamine**

These are constituents of various mucopolysaccharides, which will be discussed.

It is interesting to note that the antibiotic streptomycin contains N-methyl-L-glucosamine and that 3-deoxy-3-amino-D-ribose is present in puromycin. Other amino derivatives of sugars occur as parts of the molecules in still other antibiotics. N-Acetyl-D-glucosamine is one of the constituents of a tetrasaccharide occurring in human milk.

Mucopolysaccharides. The mucopolysaccharides are substances having hexosamines and a uronic acid as component parts of their molecules. In most cases they are combined with protein although some may occur free. Most of the mucopolysaccharides are long-chain polymers of repeating disaccharide units. Examples are chondroitin sulfates A, B, and C, heparin, hyaluronic acid, and keratosulfate. The chondroitin sulfates all contain N-acetylgalactosamine. The uronic acid of A and C is D-glucuronic, whereas that of B is L-iduronic, the uronic acid of idose. Chondroitin sulfate–A is the best characterized at the present time. The chondroitin sulfates are all tissue constituents. Heparin, a naturally occurring blood anticoagulant, contains a greater number of sulfate groups, the amino groups being sulfated instead of acetylated. It is a polymer of glucosamine and D-glucuronic acid. Hyaluronic acid is another compound of this general type and is distinguished from the two preceding ones by not containing sulfate. The repeating disaccharide unit here is glucuronic acid linked to acetylglucosamine. This compound is highly viscous and seems to be involved in maintaining the consistency of ground substance of connective tissue. Keratosulfate occurs in costal cartilage. It is a polymer composed of equimolar amounts of N-acetylglucosamine, galactose, and sulfate. The roles of chondroitin sulfate, heparin, and hyaluronic acid will be considered further in subsequent sections.

Repeating unit of chondroitin sulfate–A

Repeating unit of heparin (barium salt)

Repeating unit of hyaluronic acid

An interesting relation of the mucopolysaccharides of erythrocytes and hemagglutination by a globulin from the jackbean, concanavalin-A, has been described recently.[4] Concanavalin-A agglutinates erythrocytes from many species of animals, including man, by a unique type of antigen-antibody interaction. The specific sites of attraction between concanavalin-A and erythrocytes have been established as certain nonreducing terminal sugar residues on the red cell mucopolysaccharides. In further studies, it has been shown that almost any polysaccharide, including glycogen, with nonreducing terminal glucose, mannose, or fructose residues, will bind to concanavalin-A.

Pertinent in this connection is the fact that, although the stimulation of antibody production is usually observed with proteins (p. 583), certain polysaccharides, termed *immunopolysaccharides,* are also antigenic. These include the capsular polysaccharides of pneumococci and certain other microorganisms.

Sialic acids. The sialic acids are widely distributed in animal tissues and microorganisms as constitutents of a number of polysaccharides, muco- and glycoproteins (p. 89), and certain lipids. Chemically, they are N- or O-acyl derivatives of a nine-carbon, 3-deoxy-5-amino sugar called *neuraminic acid*. Neuraminic acid may be regarded as an aldol condensation product of mannosamine and pyruvic acid. The acyl groups attached to the 5-N- or to the 7- or 8-O-positions usually are acetyl, methyl, or glycolyl groups. The sialic acid moiety may be attached to the lysine residues of the protein portion of glyco- or mucoproteins by glycosidic covalent linkages, or they may be attached by the way of an oligosaccharide side chain. A sialic acid from a human plasma protein has the following structure:

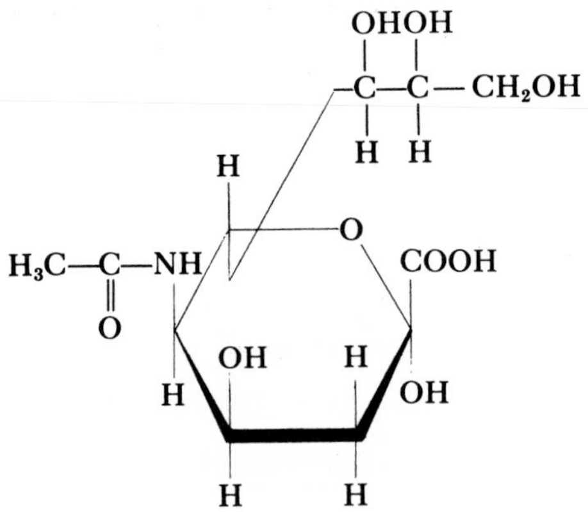

Sialic acid (N-acetylneuraminic acid) from human plasma

The sialic acids react directly with Ehrlich's reagent (*p*-dimethylaminobenzaldehyde) in hot acid solution to give a purple color.

Muramic acid. Muramic acid, like the sialic acids, is a derivative of an N-acyl sugar. It occurs in the mucopeptides, *mureins*, of bacterial cell walls (p. 177). It differs from the sialic acids, however, in that it contains an ether linkage between the three-carbon acid, in this case D-lactic, and the C-3 hydroxyl group of N-acetylglucosamine.

Teichoic acids. Biologically important compounds of a related type are the teichoic acids. These occur in the walls of many gram-positive bacteria in considerable amounts (up to 50% of their dry weight). They are water-soluble polymers composed of glycerol or ribitol (p. 156) units joined through phosphate diester linkages to form chains. To these polyol units are attached molecules of sugar and of an amino acid, D-alanine. The sugars present may be glucose, glucosamine, galactosamine, and probably disaccharides and trisaccharides.[5] In contrast, gram-negative organisms apparently contain little or no teichoic acid. The walls of gram-negative bacteria contain a considerable amount of a complex lipopolysaccharide, as well as protein and phospholipid.[6]

Cell wall poly-saccharides   The cell walls of plants and many types of microorganisms consist of a surprising diversity of substances that may be classed, in general, as homo- and heteropolysaccharides. Their principal functions are to protect the cell chemically from undesirable macromolecules and physically from severe mechanical and osmotic forces and stress. Plant cell walls consist primarily of densely packed cellulose fibers (p. 171) in a matrix of complex *hemicellulose* (xylans, which are polymers of D-xylose in β-1,4-linkages with side chains of 4-O-methylglucuronic acid and/or arabinose), *pectins* (polymers

176

of the methyl ester of galacturonic acid), and sometimes D-galactans, L-arabans, and various heteroglycans. The matrix of plant cell walls usually also contains about 5% of a protein, *extensin*, that is unique inasmuch as, like collagen, it is rich in hydroxyproline.

The cell walls of microorganisms, including algae, molds, fungi, yeasts, and bacteria, are composed of a wide variety of complex homo- and hetero-polysaccharides, some also containing various peptides. All are capable of withstanding great osmotic stress. The cell walls of algae contain relatively large amounts of polymannuronic acid. All fungi and most yeasts utilize chitin, a polymer of D-glucosamine, as the primary wall constituent. Some yeasts apparently employ highly branched polymannans.

The structure and composition of bacterial cell walls have been a topic of considerable study recently, particularly by Strominger and his co-workers,[7] using *Staph. aureus*. The primary component of most bacterial walls is a macromolecule, termed *murein*. This substance consists of a linear chain of polysaccharides composed of N-acetylglucosamine and N-acetylmuramic acid, with an attached phosphodiester of teichoic acid (p. 176). These linear polysaccharide chains are bridged by peptides to form the cell wall. The bridging peptides are unique, usually containing L-alanine, D-isoglutamine, L-lysine, and D-alanine. Replacement of L-lysine with L-hydroxyglycine, D- or L-ornithine, 2,4-diaminobutyric acid, or diaminopimelic acid occurs in some species. In some bacterial cell walls, the carboxyl group of D-alanine in the above peptide and the amino group of the diamino acid constituent are bridged by the peptide, pentaglycine, trialanylthreonine, or polyserine. This unique structure confers the important property of mechanical strength required for the survival of bacteria. A schematic representation of the cell wall of *S. aureus*[7] is shown in Fig. 8-8.

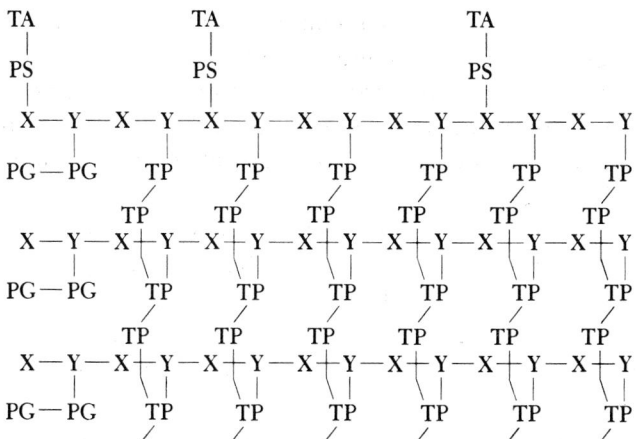

Fig. 8-8. Schematic representation of *S. aureus* cell wall. *X*, Acetylglucosamine; *Y*, acetylmuramic acid; *PG*, pentaglycine; *TP*, tetrapeptide of L-alanyl-D-isoglutaminyl-L-lysyl-D-alanine; *TA-PS*, teichoic acid attached to polysaccharide. (Adapted from Tipper, D. J., et al.: Biochemistry **6**:906, 1967; Tipper, D. J., et al.: Biochemistry **6**:921, 1967; Katz, W., and Strominger, J. L.: Biochemistry **6**:930, 1967.)

For further protection, most bacterial cell walls are coated with other macromolecular structures. In some bacteria this consists of a mucilaginous secretion of polysaccharides, varying from hyaluronic acid (p. 175) to complex highly branched structures containing several monosaccharide derivatives. The two major classes of substances found are the teichoic acids (p. 176), in gram-positive organisms, and the lipopolysaccharides, in gram-negative organisms.

Lipopolysaccharides. Lipopolysaccharides have been isolated from the cell walls of several species of gram-negative bacteria.[8] They are distinguished from glycolipids (p. 324) primarily on the basis of the size of the carbohydrate component. The lipopolysaccharide from one bacterium, *M. phlei,* has a molecular weight of approximately 3500. The structures are poorly defined as yet. The lipid components of the molecule (from *M. phlei*) include acetate, propionate, isobutyrate, and octanoate. The polysaccharide component apparently consists of a single chain of approximately 18 hexose units comprised of D-glucose and 6-O-methyl-D-glucose along with a terminal D-glyceric acid. Lipopolysaccharides from certain other bacteria apparently consist of long side chains of

$$\begin{bmatrix} \text{abequose} \\ | \\ \text{mannose—rhamnose—galactose} \end{bmatrix}$$

attached to a single unit of

$$\begin{bmatrix} & & & \text{glucose} \\ \text{N-acetylglucosamine—glucose—galactose} \dashv \\ & & & \text{galactose} \end{bmatrix},$$

which, in turn is attached to a "backbone" consisting of a repeating unit of two heptose molecules, an octulosonic acid, and lipid. The lipid fraction consists of an unknown combination of glucosamine, phosphate, acetyl residues, and β-hydroxymyristic acid.

The biologic functions of the lipopolysaccharides are poorly understood. Lipopolysaccharides are located on the cell surface and are effective antigens. Their antigenic property may be related to the more general phenomenon of *cell recognition.*

Other
derivatives It is beyond the scope of this book to discuss many other derivatives of carbohydrates. An example of the possibilities is the replacement of certain oxygen atoms by sulfur or another element. At least one sulfur derivative, 5-thio-α-D-glucopyranose, has bacteriostatic action, acting as a competitive inhibitor (p. 126) for natural D-glucose in fruitflies and *Escherichia coli.*[9] (See diagram at top of the following page.)

A gold derivative, gold thioglucose (1-AuS-D-glucopyranose), has the remarkable property of producing extreme obesity when given orally to experimental animals (rats, mice). Apparently this results from injury to the hypothalamic "feeding control center," which produces extreme polyphagia and the resulting obesity.

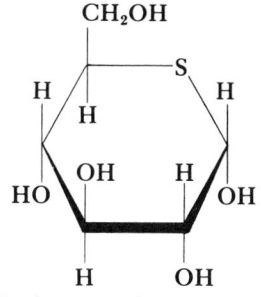

5-Thio-α-D-glucopyranose

As mentioned previously, compounds containing the radioactive or heavy isotope of one of the constituent elements of that compound are useful in biochemical studies. The synthetic preparation of carbohydrates containing radioactive carbon is, however, extremely difficult. A biologic method of producing starch, sucrose, glucose, or fructose so labeled has been described. Green leaves are placed in water in the dark to use up reserve carbohydrates. They are then exposed to light in an atmosphere containing carbon dioxide tagged with radioactive carbon. Photosynthesis results in the formation of one or more carbohydrates containing labeled carbon in the molecules. Different plant leaves produce different radioactive carbohydrates.

Parenteral administration of nutrients or medicines dissolved in sterile distilled water sometimes gives rise to febrile reactions that have been attributed to *pyrogens*. These are metabolic products of microorganisms that seem to be present as contaminants despite all precautions. They are heat stable, and, although their composition is not fully known, they seem to be polysaccharide complexes, containing some nitrogen, probably as amino sugars. These pyrogens should be distinguished from the one produced in inflammations, which is of a protein nature.

References

GENERAL

Hoffman, P., and Meyer, K.: Structural studies of mucopolysaccharides of connective tissues, Fed. Proc. **21**:1064, 1962.

Jeanloz, R. W., and Balazs, E. A., editors: The amino sugars: the chemistry and biology of compounds containing amino sugars, New York, 1965–1968, Academic Press, Inc.

Martin, H. H.: Biochemistry of bacterial cell walls, Ann. Rev. Biochem. **35**:457, 1966.

Mislow, K.: Introduction to stereochemistry, New York, 1966, W. A. Benjamin, Inc.

Morrison, R. T., and Boyd, R. N.: Organic chemistry, ed. 2, Boston, 1966, Allyn & Bacon, Inc.

Neufeld, E. F., and Ginsburg, V., editors: vol. 8, Complex carbohydrates. In Colowick, S. P., and Kaplan, N. O., editors: Methods in enzymology, New York, 1966, Academic Press, Inc.

Northcote, D. H.: Polysaccharides, Ann. Rev. Biochem. **33**:51, 1964.

Percival, E. G. V.: Structural carbohydrate chemistry, ed. 2, London, 1962, J. Garnet Miller, Ltd.

Pigman, W., editor: The carbohydrates, New York, 1957, Academic Press, Inc.

Quintarelli, G., editor: The chemical physiology of mucopolysaccharides, Boston, 1967, Little, Brown & Co.

Stacey, M., and Barker, S. A.: Carbohydrates of living tissues, Princeton, N. J., 1962, D. Van Nostrand Co., Inc.

Wolfram, M. L., and Tipson, R. S., editors: Advances in carbohydrate chemistry, New York, 1964, Academic Press, Inc., vol. 19.

Wolstenholme, G. E. W., and O'Connor, M., editors: Chemistry and biology of the mucopolysaccharides: Ciba Foundation symposium, Boston, 1958, Little, Brown & Co.

SPECIAL

1. Steinhardt, R. G., Jr., et al.: Science **135**: 367, 1962

2. Nutr. Rev. **22**:43, 1964.

3. Elbein, A., et al.: J. Amer. Chem. Soc. **86**:309, 1964.

4. Goldstein, I., et al.: Biochim. Biophys. Acta **121**:197, 1966; Arch. Biochem. **121**:88, 1967.

5. Baddiley, J.: Roy. Inst. Chem. J. **86**:366, 1962.

6. Osborn, M. J., et al.: Science **145**:783, 1964.

7. Tipper, D. J., et al.: Biochemistry **6**:906, 1967; Tipper, D. J., et al.: Biochemistry **6**:921, 1967; Katz, W., and Strominger, J. C.: Biochemistry **6**:930, 1967.

8. Ballou, C. E.: Accounts Chem. Res. **1**:366, 1968.

9. Whistler, R. L., et al.: J. Amer. Chem. Soc. **84**:122, 1962.

CHAPTER 9

CARBOHYDRATE METABOLISM

As stated previously (p. 141), carbohydrates form the chief source of energy in man and many animals. In adult man, carbohydrate supplies approximately 60% by weight of the total food intake and about 50% of the total daily caloric requirement. Thus one would expect the primary metabolic pathways of carbohydrate in the cell to involve *exergonic* reactions, yielding energy mainly in the form of adenosine triphosphate (ATP). This is the case, as will be seen. The major route of carbohydrate metabolism, primarily as glucose, entails the stepwise degradation of glucose through a series of phosphate intermediates via the Embden-Meyerhof pathway (p. 196), or the pentose phosphate pathway, and the Krebs citric acid cycle (p. 263) ultimately to carbon dioxide and water. ATP formation occurs in a number of the catabolic reactions involved.

The foundations of the study of carbohydrate metabolism were laid by Claude Bernard (1813–1878), the great French scientist, who perhaps may be called the first biochemist. Bernard's experiments began with an attempt to produce in animals a condition analogous to human diabetes mellitus. In this condition the outstanding symptom is the passage of glucose into the urine. At that time nothing whatever was known regarding its cause. In the course of his studies Bernard found that if the floor of the fourth ventricle of the medulla oblongata of rabbits was punctured a temporary diabetes resulted. This "piqûre," as it was called, could be produced only in animals that were in good nutritive condition—not in starving animals. His next step was to make a survey, so to speak, of the concentrations of glucose in the blood. This, under normal conditions, is about 0.1% (100 mg. per 100 ml.). However, he found that there were slight differences between venous and arterial blood; e.g., blood taken from the carotid artery had a concentration of about 120 mg.%, whereas that from the jugular vein nearby had 80 mg.%. Apparently the blood, in going from the arteries to the tissue capillaries and back to the veins, had left some of the glucose behind for use by the tissues.

By passing "sounds" (catheters) through the heart down the vena cava and withdrawing samples of blood at different levels, Bernard ascertained that the blood taken from a level opposite the kidneys contained about the same percentage of sugar as the venous blood in general. However, blood taken from a point near the opening of the hepatic vein contained more glucose (140 mg.%) than the arterial blood. Since the portal blood contained less sugar than the blood from the hepatic vein, the inference was that the sugar had been added while the blood was passing through the liver. Some substance present in the liver was being converted into glucose.

The next step was to find this source of glucose in the liver. A well-fed rabbit was killed instantly and the liver removed as rapidly as possible, plunged into boiling water, and cut up in it while the water was boiling. An opalescent solution resulted. This had very little reducing sugar in it, but it did contain a compound that yielded a reducing substance on hydrolysis. This was the material that caused the opalescence. Bernard called it the "glycogenous matter." It is what we now call *glycogen*. If the procedure described was not carried out with dispatch, little or no glycogen could be found but reducing sugars were present in abundance. This indicated the presence of a glycogen → glucose mechanism that could be regulated in the living organ and that was inhibited by boiling in the removed tissue. Today, we recognize this mechanism as an enzyme reaction. Bernard formulated the glycogenic theory, that glycogen is the form in which glucose is stored in the liver and that it can be changed to glucose, which is carried to the various organs and tissues for conversion to heat and energy or for reconversion to the glycogen of the tissues. Since Bernard's time, many additional facts have been gathered and many theories to explain the details of the various steps have been evolved. But the broad features of Claude Bernard's glycogenic theory remain just as true today as when they were first developed in the middle of the last century.

DIGESTION

From a quantitative standpoint, carbohydrate is the major group of chemical substances metabolized by man and most animals. Indeed, as stated above, approximately 60% by weight of the average American dietary, or some 400 to 500 gm. per day for the average adult male, is carbohydrate. This is in contrast to the approximately 100 gm. of protein and 200 gm. of fat consumed daily. As discussed in the preceding chapter, most of the food carbohydrate is in the form of polysaccharides. Extensive human dietary studies have shown that about 60% of the utilizable food carbohydrate is supplied by starches and dextrins, largely from the cereal grains and some vegetables (potatoes). Of the remaining food carbohydrate, about 30% is supplied by sucrose, 5% by lactose, and the remaining 5% by glucose, maltose, and other sugars. Cellulose is not utilizable by man or nonruminant animals and forms most of the *bulk* or nondigestible residue of foods. Obviously, the intestinal mucosal epithelium cannot absorb larger molecules, e.g., starches and oligosaccharides. Therefore, enzymatic cleavage of these polysaccharides and disaccharides to absorbable monosaccharides is a necessary first step in carbohydrate metabolism. The cleavage is effected by a series of carbohydrases secreted in different parts of the gastrointestinal tract. The first of these is *ptyalin*, an α-amylase, secreted in the saliva of man and some animals. This enzyme catalyzes the cleavage of α-1,4-glucosidic linkages of amylopectin (p. 168), which forms some 80% to 90% of dietary starches, and of amylose (p. 167) of starch. Salivary amylase, however, does not split α-1,6-glucosidic linkages[1] at the branching points in amylopectins, and it has little affinity for the adjacent α-1,4-linkages. Thus, the salivary digestion of starch results in a mixture of *limit dextrins,* the so-called amylo-, erythro-, and achro-dextrins (p. 169) (because of their color reaction with iodine), and some maltose. Salivary amylase has an optimum pH of 6 to 7, which is the approximate pH range of saliva. α-Amylases require the presence of chloride ions for activity. Bromide, iodide, nitrate, and several other anions have some slight activity.

Little digestion of carbohydrate, other than some limited acid hydrolysis, occurs in the stomach. A second α-amylase, pancreatic amylase or *amylopsin,* present in the secretion from the pancreas, continues the digestion of starch in the small intestine. Its action is much the same as that of salivary α-amylase. It has a similar optimum pH range (6.3 to 7.2) and also requires chloride ion for activity. Human pancreatic amylase has been crystallized and found to be indistinguishable from human salivary amylase. Pancreatic juice may also contain two disaccharidases, lactase and sucrase, that convert lactose and sucrose to their constituent monosaccharides. Apparently, no maltase is present in the pancreatic secretion.

The final digestion of the limit dextrins and oligosaccharides is accomplished by an α-dextrinase (*isomaltase* or *oligo-1,6-α-glucosidase*), an α-glucosidase (*maltase*), a β-galactosidase (*lactase*), and another α-glucosidase (*sucrase*) differing in specificity from maltase; these enzymes originate in the small intestinal mucosal cells[2] and are the *succus entericus* or intestinal juice. The end products of carbohydrate digestion are thus primarily glucose, fructose, and galactose, which are then ready for absorption. The removal of the end products of carbohydrate digestion by absorption, as described below, favors their continued digestion. Thus in the normal individual, the digestion and absorption of utilizable carbohydrates are 95% or more complete.

Interesting differences in intestinal disaccharidase activities are found with aging and between species and races. For example, lactase activity in newborn rats is high and decreases with age, whereas sucrase activity is low and rises with age. In contrast, intestinal disaccharidases in the newborn human being appear to be about the same as those in the normal adult. However, differences in intestinal disaccharidases may exist between several races of man. The Oriental is said to be less tolerant than the average American to lactose (milk).[3] Lactase deficiency is also reported to be common among Negroes. Thus it appears that the bulk of the world's population has a low tolerance to the lactose of milk. This may be an example of adaptation of enzyme formation to substrate (p. 105), the latter serving as an inducer of the biosynthesis of its specific enzyme, in this instance, lactase.

Hereditary deficiencies of the enzymes α-dextrinase, sucrase, and lactase have been described in infants and children with so-called disaccharide intolerance or *carbohydrate malabsorption.*[4,5] The failure to completely digest amylopectin, maltose, sucrose, or lactose, respectively, results in the bacterial decomposition of these carbohydrates in the lower intestine, with the production of glucose and other monosaccharides, organic acids, low pH (5.5 or less), and gases. This results in bloating, flatulence, and diarrhea from irritation to the bowel with ensuing increased motility. The reduction or elimination of the offending starch or disaccharide from the diet is necessary for the control of this condition. The problem usually disappears, partially at least, as the child matures.

ABSORPTION

Digestible carbohydrates are brought to the monosaccharide stage in the small intestine before they are absorbed, as previously stated. However, it is also known[2] that some disaccharides enter the cells lining the intestinal lumen and may be hydrolyzed within these cells. No carbohydrates higher than the monosaccharides can be absorbed directly into the bloodstream (except in minute amounts), and if administered parenterally, they are eliminated as foreign bodies. Probably all the monosaccharides are absorbed to some extent by simple diffusion. However, they are not all absorbed at the same rate—galactose is taken up most rapidly, glucose next, fructose still more slowly, then mannose, and finally the pentoses. In his now classic studies on the rat, Cori found the relative rates of absorption of different monosaccharides (taking glucose as 100) to be as follows: D-galactose, 110; D-glucose, 100; D-fructose, 43; D-mannose, 19; xylose, 15; and arabinose, 9. Galactose and glucose are therefore said to be *actively absorbed*, i.e., transported across the cell membrane by an energy-dependent mechanism.

The active absorption of D-glucose also requires the mediation of a specific transport protein[6] (p. 15) in the membrane of the brush border of the intestinal mucosal cell. Sodium ions are also required. It is believed[6] that sodium binding by the transport protein changes the conformation of the protein, enabling the binding to take place and thus the absorption of glucose to occur. Potassium and lithium ions are inhibitory to glucose absorption. Insulin, which enhances the transport of glucose across most cell membranes (p. 230), does not appear to be involved in the intestinal transport of glucose. Undoubtedly, an analogous transport protein for D-galactose exists, but as yet such a protein has not been identified.

Apparently D-fructose and D-mannose are absorbed by *facilitated transport* (p. 14) since their movement cross the mucosal membrane is more rapid than would be expected if simple diffusion were the sole mechanism.

It was formerly thought that the absorption of glucose and other utilizable monosaccharides involved their phosphorylation in the presence of ATP and a hexokinase. This "classic explanation" is no longer held.

Other sugars, including the common pentoses and, significantly, the L-isomers of glucose and galactose, are *passively absorbed* by simple diffusion.

The absorption of sugars occurs readily only in the small intestine and is most rapid from the upper portions.

The structural characteristics required for active transport have been extensively studied.[6] Sugars that are actively absorbed include D-glucose, D-galactose, 3-deoxy-D-glucose, and D-allose. Passively absorbed monosaccharides, i.e., those entering chiefly by physical means, include D-mannose,

D-talose, D-glucosamine, D-gulose, L-galactose, L-glucose, L-sorbose, D- and L-xylose, D-ribose, and D- and L-arabinose.

It has been shown that all the actively absorbed sugars have the following structural features:

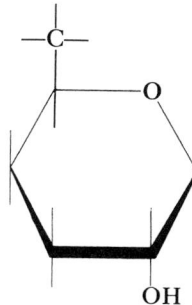

The 2-D-hydroxyl group and a 5-hydroxymethyl or methyl group on the pyranose ring thus appear to be essential structural requirements for the active transport mechanism. The transport system can be saturated by its substrate and shows typical Michaelis-Menten enzyme kinetics (p. 123).

Competitive interrelationships exist between the transport of glucose and the transport of galactose.[7] Recent studies of jejunal fistulas in dogs showed that glucose decreases the absorption rate of galactose and xylose. Similarly, galactose decreased the absorption rate of glucose; and xylose had no consistent effect on the absorption of glucose. This study suggests that glucose and galactose may share the same or a similar transport protein.

A number of compounds structurally related to glucose, e.g., phlorizin (p. 222), act as inhibitors of glucose (and galactose) transport. Phlorizin produces a glucosuria for this reason (p. 222). Likewise, 2,4-dinitrophenol is an inhibitor of the transport of both sugars.

HEPATIC INTERCONVERSIONS OF COMMON MONOSACCHARIDES

After their absorption from the small intestine, the common monosaccharides, primarily glucose, fructose, and galactose, with usually only small amounts of mannose and pentoses, pass mainly into the blood capillaries of the intestinal mucosa and thence into the portal vein and the liver. There, interconversions of the monosaccharides occur as shown schematically in Fig. 9-1. The monosaccharides are converted primarily to glucose-6-phosphate or glucose-1-phosphate in the hepatic cells. Thus, glucose-1- and -6-phosphates occupy a central position in the metabolism of carbohydrates. From these, other hexoses (p. 186) or their derivatives may be formed as required, or they may be converted to glycogen (p. 189). Some fructose may also be converted to glucose during its absorption in the intestinal mucosal cells.

Most of the pathways shown in Fig. 9-1 are reversible, either by the same enzyme systems (↔) or by different enzyme systems (⇄). This makes possible the interconversions of principal monosaccharides for use as metabolic needs dictate. The individual reactions and enzyme systems involved will be discussed in more detail later.

Pentoses as such are usually ingested in small amounts and are slowly

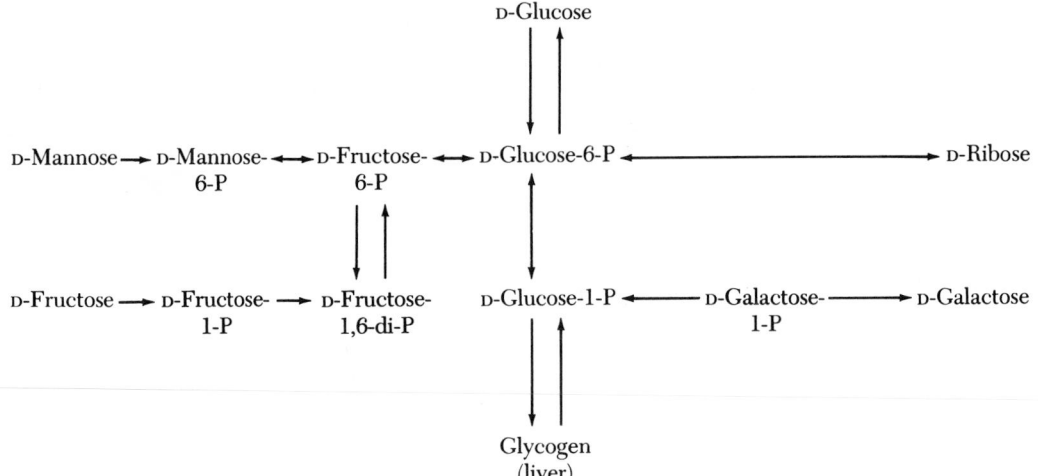

Fig. 9-1. Hepatic interconversions of common monosaccharides. Phosphate is indicated as *P*. Reactions that are reversible using different enzyme systems are indicated by double arrows ⇄. Reactions that are freely reversible are indicated by a single two-way arrow ↔.

absorbed and poorly utilized. They are largely excreted in the urine. However, the pentose D-ribose, which is an important constituent of nucleic acids (p. 31), nucleotides (ATP, etc.), and several other important biologic compounds (ribitol in riboflavin, certain coenzymes), can be formed readily from glucose as needed by way of the pentose pathway (p. 208).

GENERAL PATHWAYS OF CARBOHYDRATE METABOLISM

Free, α,β-D-glucose, either derived from dietary carbohydrate or formed in the liver from other hexoses, or from glucose phosphate esters, or from glycogen, passes into the systemic bloodstream as "blood sugar" and is transported to all cells of the body for utilization as energy or for other metabolic purposes. Hexose phosphate esters, as glucose-1- or -6-phosphate, cannot pass through cell membranes and are hence "locked" in the cell. If cellular needs for glucose are satisfied, the glucose may be converted to glycogen, principally in liver and muscle, and stored for subsequent use. If glucose is present in the blood in excessive amounts, either from the ingestion of large amounts of carbohydrate or because of impaired utilization, as in diabetes mellitus (p. 223), some may be excreted in the urine. The major pathways for the metabolic disposal of carbohydrates are shown schematically in Fig. 9-2. These and other pathways of carbohydrate metabolism will be discussed more fully later in this chapter. Details of the relations to fat (triglyceride) and protein metabolism are omitted from the figure but will be discussed elsewhere.

Liver glycogen may be converted back to blood glucose, whereas muscle glycogen cannot because muscle lacks the enzyme glucose-6-phosphatase. When muscle glycogen is used as a source of energy for muscle contraction (p. 564), some lactate is also formed. This is transported by the blood to the

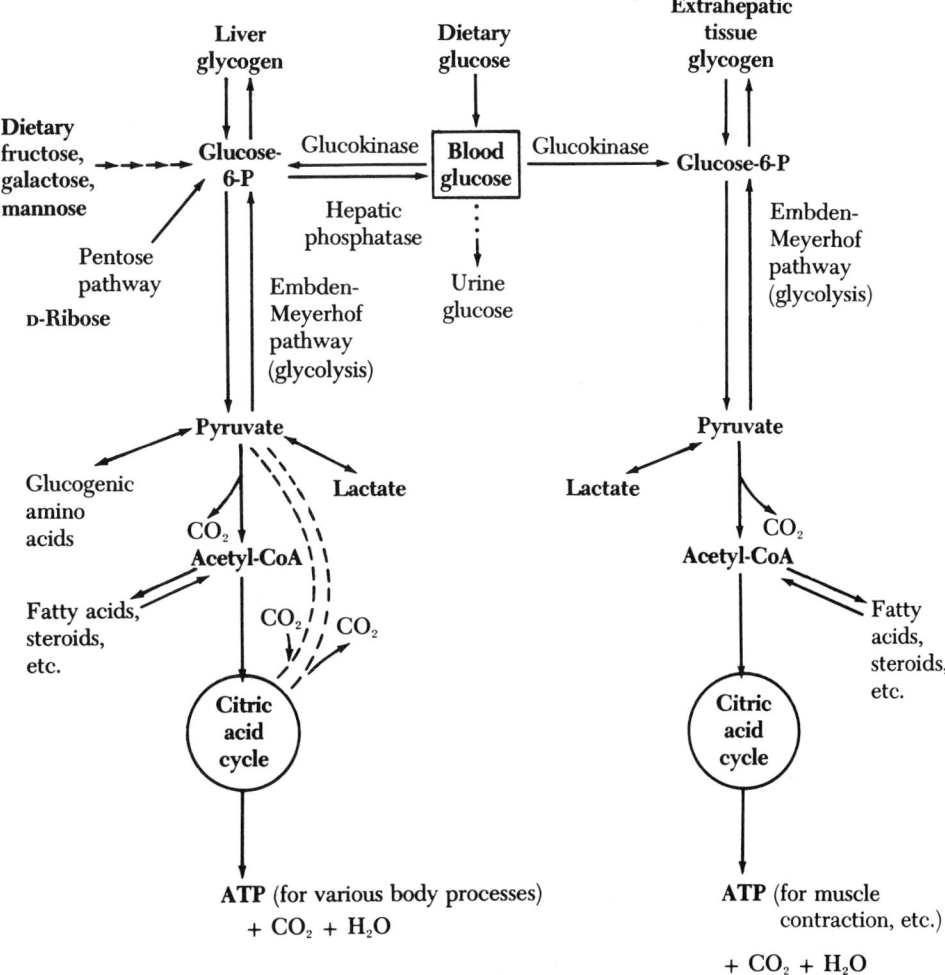

Fig. 9-2. Major pathways of carbohydrate metabolism, an overall representation. Phosphate group is indicated as *P*. Reactions that are reversible using different enzyme systems are indicated by double arrows ⇄. Reactions that are freely reversible using a single enzyme system are indicated by a single two-way arrow ↔.

liver for metabolic utilization by the pathways indicated. This process will be considered in more detail later (p. 203).

Blood sugar   It is generally accepted now that the sugar of the blood is mainly α,β-D-glucose, in addition to minor quantities of sugar phosphates, but there may be traces of the other hexoses, depending chiefly on the amounts in the diet. The concentration of blood glucose is normally fairly constant. Samples of blood taken before breakfast usually contain from 0.07% to 0.10% glucose, or, as generally stated, from 70 to 100 mg. per 100 ml. of blood. During the day the glucose concentration may range from 70 to 160 mg., although usually it seldom rises above 130 mg. After a meal there is a sharp rise followed by a gradual fall, so that in 1 or 2 hours the concentration is back to the 70 to 100 mg.% level. These figures refer to venous blood. Capillary blood and arterial blood usually are about 10 mg.% higher. During sleep the blood sugar reaches a low level, which is maintained usually until breakfast the next day. In Fig. 9-3 is shown approximately how the blood sugar varies with meals and with the time of day.

Constancy of blood sugar level. There are a number of factors influencing the level of blood sugar that are so delicately balanced the level ordinarily stays within limits from 70 to 130 mg.%. These include the following (see Figs. 9-3 and 9-4):

Glycogen ⇄ glucose reaction in the liver

Formation of glycogen in muscle and its utilization

Utilization of carbohydrate by other tissues

Conversion of carbohydrate to fat

Excretion of glucose

Indirectly a number of other factors operate, including gluconeogenesis, interconversion of fat and carbohydrate, and interplay of hormones (insulin,

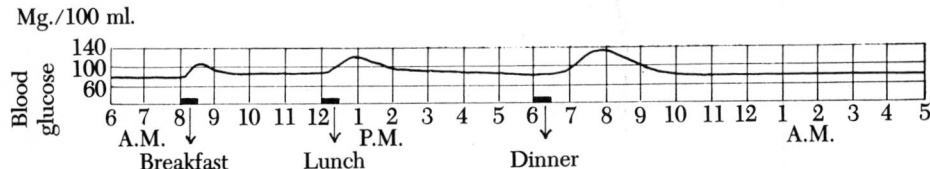

Fig. 9-3. Typical blood sugar variations in a normal young man throughout the day.

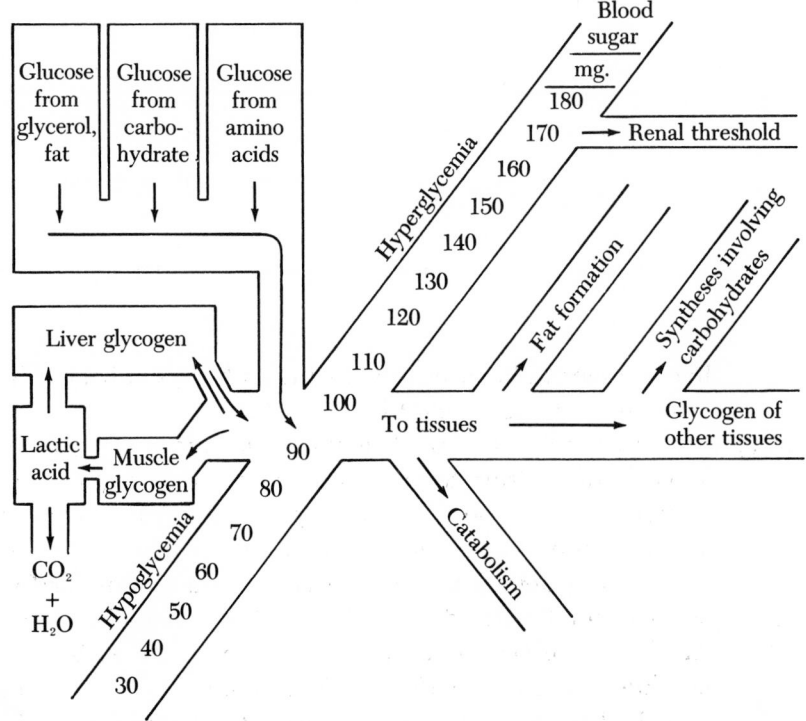

Fig. 9-4. Diagram showing the origin and disposition of blood sugar.

epinephrine, adrenocortical hormones, growth hormone, etc.). Blood sugar values above the normal range are termed *hyperglycemias,* those below it *hypoglycemias.* The hyperglycemia following an increased intake of carbohydrate in the diet is called an *alimentary hyperglycemia.* Galactose most easily produces this condition, with glucose next and fructose last. This is in harmony with the rates of absorption of these sugars.

Glycogen formation— glycogenesis *Phosphorylation.* The process of glycogen formation, called glycogenesis, occurs primarily in the liver and in muscle. Approximately 200 gm. of glycogen are stored in the entire body of a normal adult, about half in the liver and half in muscle.

The addition of a phosphate group to glucose is essential in converting glucose to glycogen. This is called *phosphorylation,* a term coined by Neuberg in 1910. As we shall see, the addition and removal of a phosphate group are necessary in many of the steps of carbohydrate metabolism, and accompanying them and bound up in them are the important transfers of energy.

For the phosphorylation of glucose, a hexokinase (in this case glucokinase), magnesium ions, and ATP are required. Phosphoric acid is attached at carbon-6. Thus:

CH_2OH $CH_2 \cdot O \cdot PO_3H_2$

Glucokinase, Mg^{++}
+ ATP $\longrightarrow$ + ADP

Glucose   **Glucose-6-phosphate**

The next step is a transfer of the phosphate group to carbon-1, which is brought about by phosphoglucomutase, in the presence of magnesium ions. Apparently this conversion is accomplished via glucose-1,6-diphosphate acting as an intermediate.

$CH_2 \cdot O \cdot PO_3H_2$ CH_2OH

Mg^{++}
Phosphoglucomutase $\longleftrightarrow$

Glucose-6-phosphate   **Glucose-1-phosphate**

Glucose is then ready for transformation to UDP-glucose (uridine diphosphate glucose) and glycogen (Fig. 9-5). Polysaccharide chains, already present, are lengthened by the addition of glucose from UDP-glucose, as

189

shown in Fig. 9-5, since the reaction does not occur in the absence of a small amount of polysaccharide primer. The formation of glycogen in liver and muscle occurs via a uridine pathway[8] (Figs. 9-5 and 9-6). UDP-glucose is apparently converted to glycogen in this pathway by means of UDPG-glycogen glucosyl transferase (glycogen synthetase), which produces its effect by synthesizing α-1,4-bonds (Fig. 9-6).

The primary linkage of the glucose units in glycogen is thus of a 1,4-glucosidic nature. In the formation of glycogen in the liver (or in muscle), glucose units are added to preexisting glycogen until a chain of about eight to 12 glucose units is formed. Units of this length are sometimes termed *amylose*. These amylose chains are then transferred to a branching point by the *branching enzyme*,[9] oligo-1,4- $\rightarrow$ -1,6-glucan transferase, and attached by a 1,6-linkage. The large glycogen molecule thus "grows" in a treelike manner.[10] It has a variable molecular weight that may reach a value as high as 50 million to 190 million. The entire process of glycogenesis, including the enzymes and cofactors involved, is summarized schematically in Fig. 9-7.

Glycogenesis occurs when the glycemia (i.e., level of blood sugar in the general circulation) rises above normal. The hexoses are not the only glycogen formers, or glycogenic substances. Proteins yield glucose approximately to the extent of 58% of their weight. This is because a nonnitrogenous fraction is left after deamination of certain of the amino acids. A good example is alanine. This is converted to pyruvic acid by oxidative deamination. Pyruvic acid, in turn, can be transformed to lactic acid. Both pyruvic acid and lactic acid are known glycogen formers.

The glycerol fraction of fats is also convertible to glucose and therefore to glycogen. The fatty acid portion is probably not changed directly to glucose.

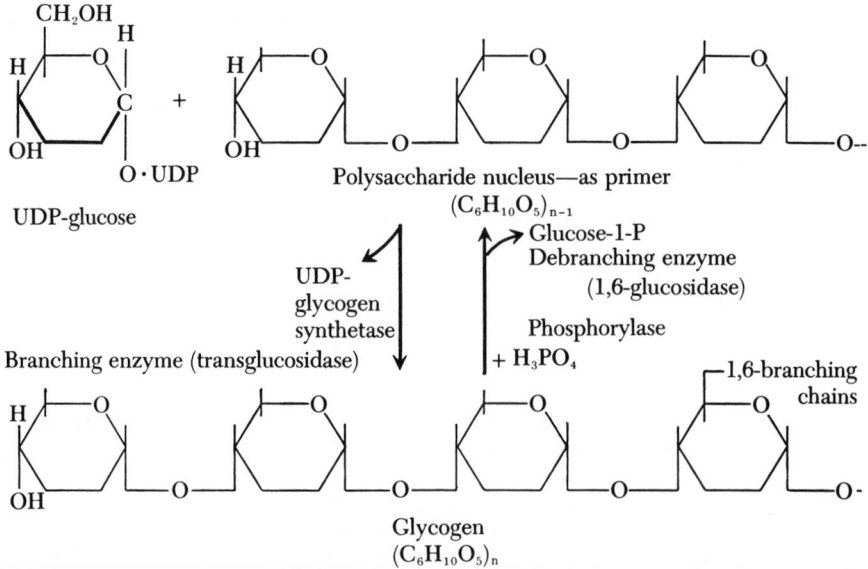

Fig. 9-5. Glycogenesis and glycogenolysis.

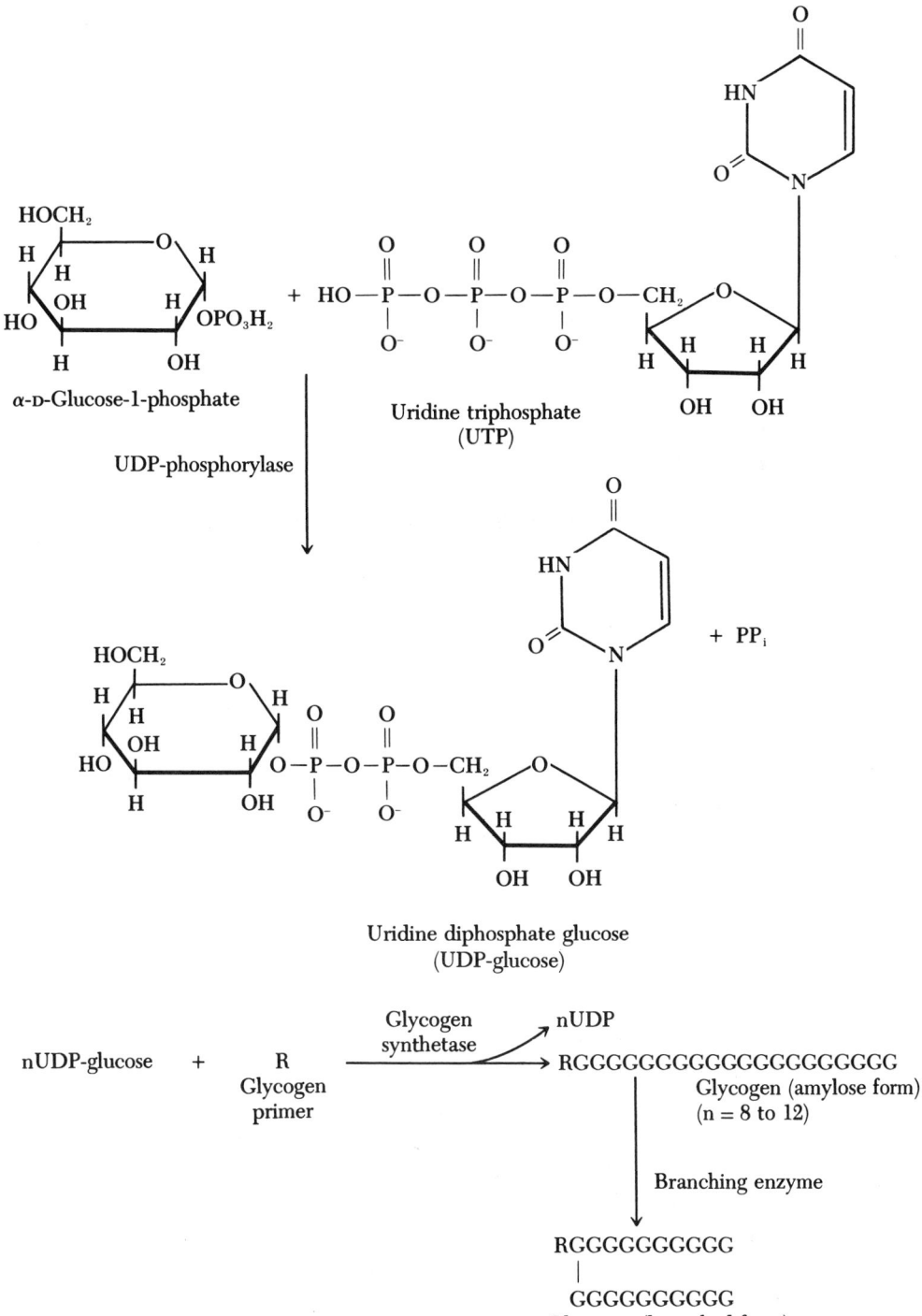

Fig. 9-6. Uridine pathway of glycogenesis.

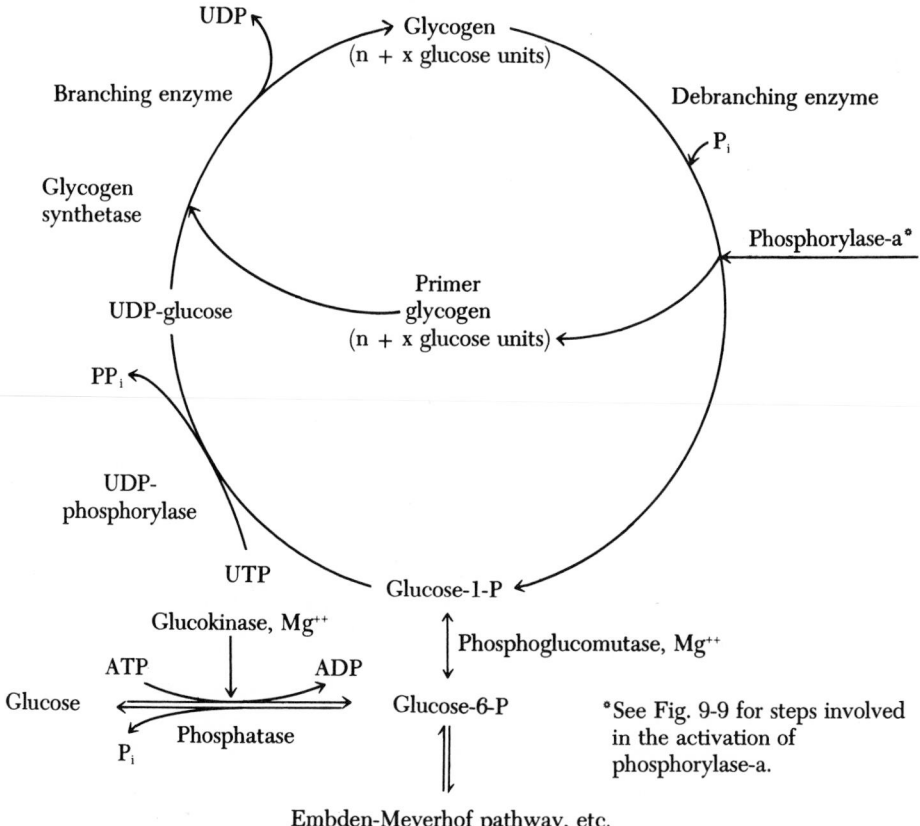

Fig. 9-7. Glycogenesis and glycogenolysis.

The formation of glucose from noncarbohydrate sources is given the term *gluconeogenesis*. Lactic acid, which is a product of carbohydrate catabolism, especially in muscle, has been found to be transported in the bloodstream back to the liver for reconversion to glycogen.

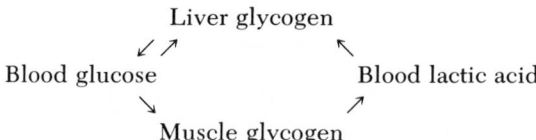

Experiments have brought forth some interesting facts concerning the conversion of lactic acid to glycogen. Lactate, containing radioactive carbon in the carboxyl group, was fed to rats, and the radioactivity of the liver glycogen and of the expired carbon dioxide was studied. Results indicated that only a small amount of the lactate is converted into glycogen as a three-carbon chain. Some of the carboxyl is split off and excreted as carbon dioxide in the expired air. Thus glycogen may be formed from two-carbon chains. It is even possible that carbon dioxide may enter into the formation of glycogen. When nonradioactive sodium lactate was fed and radioactive sodium bicarbonate was injected intraperitoneally, a small amount of the radioactive carbon appeared in the liver glycogen.

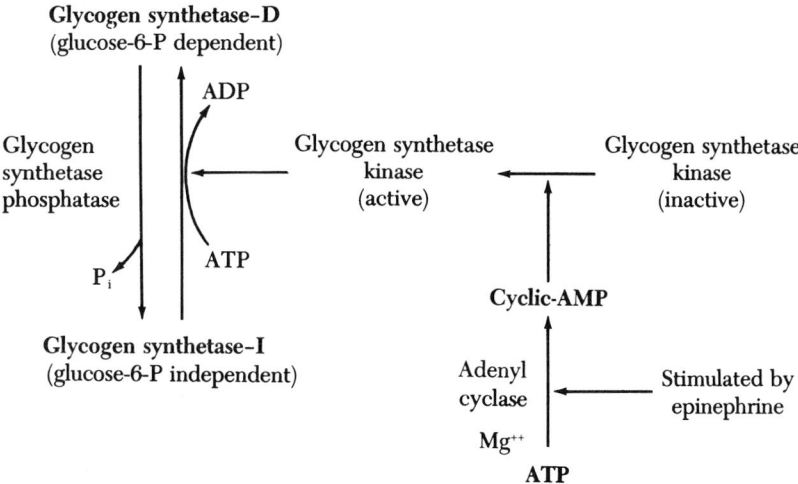

Fig. 9-8. Some factors affecting the activity of glycogen synthetase.

Control of glycogenesis. Both the synthesis and the degradation of glycogen are under the control of extremely effective regulatory mechanisms, as are all important metabolic pathways (Chapter 2). Glycogen synthetase now appears to be a key control point in glycogenesis, at least in muscle. Current evidence indicates that glycogen synthetase—like phosphorylase (p. 195)—exists in phosphorylated and dephosphorylated forms. The active dephospho-enzyme can be phosphorylated to a less active form by ATP and glycogen synthetase kinase. The activity of the phosphorylated form, however, can be markedly increased by glucose-6-phosphate. It is inhibited by free UDP, which could accumulate if the supply of glucose and ATP were limited. The two forms of muscle glycogen synthetase are termed *D* (dependent) and *I* (independent) because of the glucose-6-phosphate effect.

Glycogen synthetase kinase, like phosphorylase kinase (Fig. 9-9), also appears to exist in active and inactive forms, the latter being converted to the former by cyclic-AMP (p. 36), which, in turn, is formed from ATP in the presence of the enzyme adenyl cyclase and magnesium ions. The formation of cyclic-AMP is stimulated by epinephrine (glucagon, also in the liver) (p. 195). Apparently in muscle, glycogen synthetase kinase may also be activated by a *protein factor* in the presence of a sufficient level of calcium ions (increased during muscle contraction, p. 363). There is also current evidence that insulin has a direct stimulatory effect on glycogen synthetase activation in the liver. The precise action is not yet known, however.

The foregoing factors are important in regulating glycogen synthesis. During stress, for example, epinephrine increases the formation of cyclic-AMP, which converts glycogen synthetase kinase to an active form that, in turn, converts glycogen synthetase–I to the less active –D (glucose-6-phosphate dependent). The overall effect is to allow glycogen formation only if the level of glucose-6-phosphate is sufficient to activate glycogen synthetase and assure the formation of glucose-1-phosphate.

The conversion of glycogen synthetase–D back to the dephospho form –I is catalyzed by glycogen synthetase phosphatase. This enzyme is inhibited by glycogen itself, an example of product feedback inhibition (p. 129). In this sense, then, glycogen regulates its own level.

A schematic summary of factors affecting the activity of glycogen synthetase is given in Fig. 9-8.

Thus, a rather elaborate cascade-type control system, somewhat reminiscent of the blood coagulation control mechanisms (p. 623), exists for regulating glycogenesis. The overall purpose of the system is to limit glycogen formation to optimal levels so that undue amounts of glucose will not be drawn into this pathway and thus be diverted from other essential uses. Also, the excessive deposition of glycogen in the liver or muscles can lead to tissue damage and pathology, as is found in the so-called glycogen storage diseases (p. 195).

Glycogenesis is also profoundly affected by several hormonal factors, as will be discussed later (p. 224).

A somewhat analogous control system exists for regulating glycogenolysis, and this, too, will be considered later (p. 195).

Glycogenol-ysis — phosphorol-ysis The reverse of glycogenesis, glycogenolysis, is apparently not a simple reversal of the above steps (Fig. 9-7). First, successive outer 1,4-linked glucose units are phosphorylated by the action of the enzyme phosphorylase and split off as glucose-1-phosphate until 1,6-branching points are exposed. These linkages are then hydrolyzed by a different enzyme, the *debranching enzyme* — an amylo-1,6-glucosidase. Further splitting of the molecule can then proceed by the action of phosphorylase until another 1,6-branching point is reached, and the action of the debranching enzyme is repeated. The partial or even complete cleavage of the glycogen molecule can thus be accomplished, with the formation of glucose-1-phosphate, which, in turn, can be converted to glucose-6-phosphate and free glucose by the enzymes phosphoglucomutase and glucose-6-phosphatase, respectively. The complete process of glycogenolysis, including the enzymes involved, is summarized schematically in Fig. 9-7.

Phosphorylase is widely distributed in plants, microorganisms, and animals. In animals it is found in muscle, heart, liver, and brain. The debranching enzyme is also found in liver and muscle. Glycogenolysis occurs very rapidly and is the classic reaction described by Claude Bernard. The phosphorolysis of glycogen is accelerated when the body requires more glucose. Such is the case during muscular activity or exposure to cold, both of which tend to lower the blood sugar level. The glucose-6-phosphate, hydrolyzed by a phosphatase to glucose and phosphoric acid, raises the blood sugar to a normal level again.

Glycogenolysis is also under the control of epinephrine through the sympathetic nervous system. Stimulation of the sympathetic nerves causes the increased secretion of epinephrine, the hormone of the adrenal medulla. This augments glycogenolysis by stimulating the conversion of ATP into *cyclic-AMP*. This activates the enzyme phosphorylase kinase, which, in turn, converts inactive *phosphorylase-b* to *phosphorylase-a*. The latter progressively splits off glucose-1-phosphate units from glycogen, thus raising the blood sugar level. Glucagon, a hormone secreted by the α-cells of the pan-

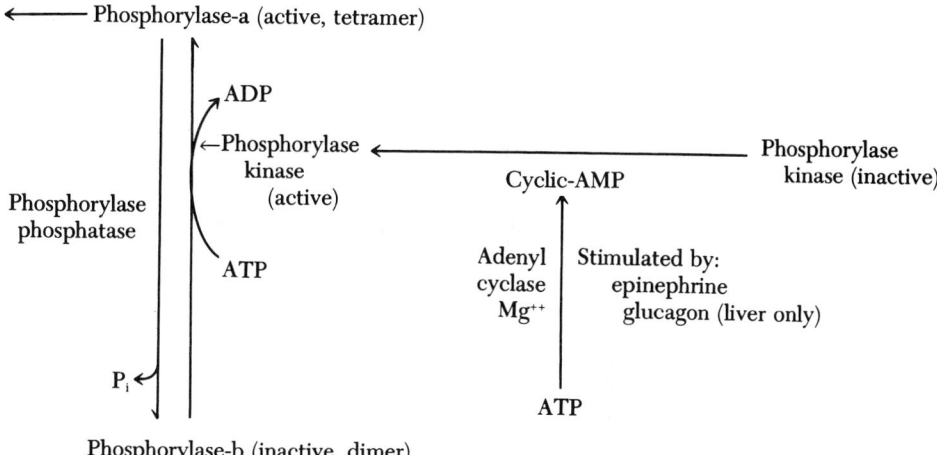

Fig. 9-9. Effect of epinephrine on glycogenolysis.

creas, has a similar action but in liver only. All the reactions mentioned are summarized in Fig. 9-9. Violent emotional reactions, e.g., fear and rage, lead to the formation of epinephrine, which in turn increases the blood sugar. This is an emergency reaction to furnish extra fuel to enable the animal or person to escape from danger or to fight, as the case may be. Insulin secretion has an opposite effect, tending to cause glycogenesis. Thus, these two hormones seem to counterbalance each other.

Glycogenolysis in muscle is essentially the same as in liver. However, there is one great difference. The phosphatase, which in liver converts glucose-6-phosphate to glucose and phosphate, is absent in muscle. Therefore glucose is not set free in muscle and is not sent into the blood to augment the blood sugar (Fig. 9-2). Evidence that muscle glycogen is not a source of blood sugar was furnished by experiments on hepatectomized dogs. When the liver was removed from a dog, the blood sugar concentration fell steadily to a very low level. The muscle, however, was found to still contain considerable amounts of glycogen. Evidently it was not available for conversion into blood sugar.

GLYCOGEN STORAGE DISEASES

During the past few years several types of derangements of glycogen metabolism in liver and muscle have been extensively studied in patients. One of these types, von Gierke's glycogen storage disease, has been known for a number of years. The absence of the specific phosphatase that converts glucose-6-phosphate to glucose and phosphate in the liver has been demonstrated in some cases of this type of glycogen storage disease; in others there seems to be a lack of the debranching enzyme. This is a rare congenital disorder of carbohydrate metabolism in which there is enlargement of the liver, due to the excessive storage of glycogen. There is usually hypoglycemia, hyperlacticemia,[11] and acidosis. It is a rather rare condition, but even more infrequent is the occurrence of a cardiac type (i.e., the glycogen is stored in the heart). This type is rapidly fatal.

195

Table 9-1. Types of glycogen storage disease

Disease	Organ distribution	Enzyme defect	Glycogen structure	Defect in glycogen metabolism
Type 1 (von Gierke's)	Liver, kidney	Glucose-6-phosphatase	Normal	Indirect
Type 2	Muscle	Lysosomal 1,4-glucosidase	Normal	Breakdown
Type 3	Generalized	Amylo-1,6-glucosidase	Abnormal or normal	Breakdown
Type 4 Type 5 Type 6	Generalized	Amylo-1,4→1,6-trans-glucosidase? (branching enzyme)	Abnormal	Synthesis
(McArdle)	Muscle	Phosphorylase	Normal	Breakdown
	Liver	Phosphorylase (?)	Normal	Breakdown
Type 7	Muscle	Phosphofructo-kinase (?)	Normal	Indirect (breakdown)

Certain other varieties of glycogen storage disease appear to be due to the deposition of abnormal forms of glycogen.[12] At the present time, at least seven different types of glycogen storage diseases have been characterized.[13] They are summarized in Table 9-1. Among the treatments recommended is administration of glucagon and synthetic androgen.

UTILIZATION OF GLUCOSE—GLYCOLYSIS—EMBDEN-MEYERHOF PATHWAY

A second major fate of blood glucose, along with its conversion to glycogen primarily in liver and muscle, is its utilization to form chemical energy as ATP, with carbon dioxide and water as by-products. Indeed, this is the principal fate of blood glucose under usual conditions. The broad reaction is as follows:

$$C_6H_{12}O_6 + 6\ O_2 \quad \rightarrow \quad 6\ CO_2 + 6\ H_2O + nATP$$

The number of moles of ATP formed vary from approximately 35 to 38 per mole of glucose metabolized, depending on the route by which it is metabolized, as will be discussed later.

The primary pathway for the utilization of glucose, probably as much as 80% to 90% of that metabolized, involves the conversion of glucose first to pyruvic and lactic acids in the cytoplasm of most types of cells but especially in liver and muscle. This is accomplished via a series of phosphorylated intermediates, with the formation of some ATP. The process is largely anaerobic and has been termed *glycolysis*. The reactions involved constitute the so-called Embden-Meyerhof pathway, in honor of these pioneer workers in the field, and still represents one of the greatest achievements in biochemistry. Other illustrious investigators who contributed significantly to the final elucidation of the glycolytic pathway include Parnas, Lipmann, Harden and Young, A. V. Hill, Neuberg, and the Coris. Remarkable is the fact that nearly all the details of glycolysis were worked out before the availability of isotopically labeled tracers and ultrasensitive and specific chromatographic procedures, which proved vital in the subsequent elucidation of other metabolic pathways.

The pyruvic acid and lactic acid formed in glycolysis are oxidized aerobically in cell mitochondria to carbon dioxide and water by way of acetyl-CoA and the citric acid cycle (p. 263), with associated oxidative phosphorylation and ATP formation (p. 252). The major portion of the ATP formed by the catabolism of glucose is produced in the aerobic oxidation of pyruvic acid (p. 267).

Glycolysis proceeds through a series of phosphorylated intermediates, which in mammalian tissues results in the net synthesis of two moles of ATP for each mole of glucose converted to lactic acid. The overall reaction is:

$$\text{Glucose} + 2\text{ ADP} + 2\text{ P}_i \;\rightarrow\; 2\text{ Lactic acid} + 2\text{ ATP}$$

Glycolysis apparently developed early in the evolutionary stages of living matter, when the earth's environment was largely anaerobic. Today many anaerobic organisms still form ATP in this manner. Lactic acid is not always the end product, however. In some species, propionic acid, acetone, or ethanol and carbon dioxide are the end products. Indeed, the earliest chemical studies of glycolysis were of alcoholic fermentation by grapes and brewer's yeast in the early nineteenth century by Lavoisier, Berzelius, Liebig, and Pasteur. Later, Buchner demonstrated the need for "enzymes" for fermentation, and Harden and Young showed the involvement of phosphate and a hexose diphosphate ester as intermediates in alcoholic fermentation:

$$2\text{ Glucose} + 2\text{ P}_i \;\rightarrow\; 1\text{ Hexose diphosphate} + 2\text{ Ethanol} + 2\text{ CO}_2$$

Since these pioneer studies, many investigations in the early part of this century by Meyerhof, Embden, Parnas, Neuberg, A. V. Hill, and the Coris elucidated the main steps involved in glycolysis. It was also shown that, except for the final steps, glycolysis and fermentation are strikingly similar.

The sequence of reactions and enzymes and cofactors involved as they are known today is shown schematically in Fig. 9-10.

As stated previously, the predominate fate of glucose is its oxidation to form ATP, carbon dioxide, and water. The main pathway is via anaerobic glycolysis to pyruvic and lactic acids, then final aerobic oxidation by way of the citric acid cycle. Probably as much as 80% of the glucose oxidized is by this metabolic route. Other alternate pathways are also available, as will be discussed later.

The individual reactions involved in glycolysis, as shown schematically in Fig. 9-10, will be summarized next.

Formation of glucose-6-phosphate. The first step in glycolysis is the conversion of glucose (actually an α,β-D-glucopyranose equilibrium mixture) taken up by the tissue cells (liver, muscle, brain, etc.) to glucose-6-phosphate by ATP. This is a nearly irreversible reaction catalyzed by the enzyme *hexokinase*, or more specifically in animal tissues by *glucokinase*, which has a higher specific activity for glucose. At least three different hexokinase isozymes have been identified by their electrophoretic mobilities in human

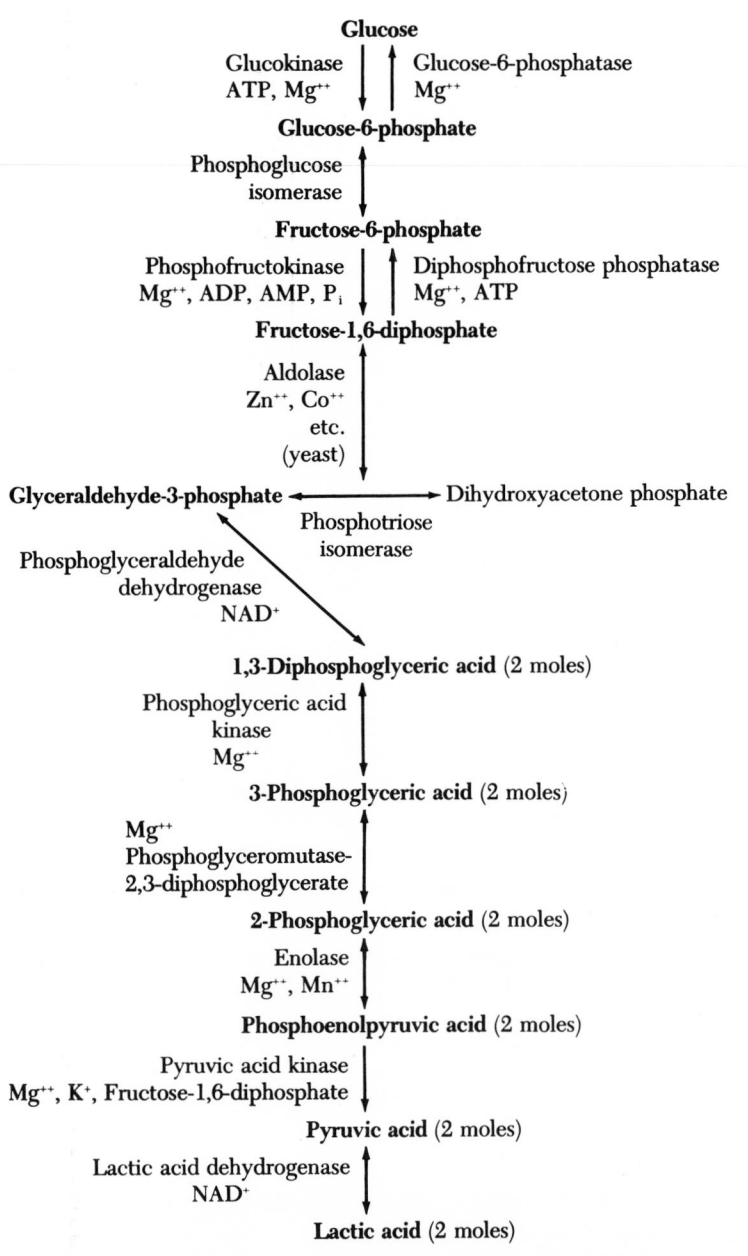

Fig. 9-10. Schematic representation of glycolysis (the Embden-Meyerhof pathway), showing enzymes and cofactors required. Reactions reversible by different enzyme systems are indicated by double arrows ⇄. Freely reversible reactions are indicated by a single two-way arrow ↔.

tissues and in tissues of other animal species. All three types are present in human liver and fat, and the first and third types are present in adult human erythrocytes. Magnesium ions are required as a cofactor. The equilibrium constant (6.30) highly favors the forward reaction. There is evidence that in some tissues product feedback inhibition (p. 129) by glucose-6-phosphate may occur at this step. Thus, the first step is extremely important in regulating the rate at which glucose is metabolized:

α-D-Glucose α-D-Glucose-6-phosphate

The reverse reaction requires a different enzyme, glucose-6-phosphatase, with magnesium ions as a cofactor. This reaction occurs in liver but *not* in muscle, which lacks glucose-6-phosphatase (pp. 186, 195). Citrate apparently inhibits the reaction, at least in liver.

Interconversion of glucose-6-phosphate and fructose-6-phosphate. Glucose-6-phosphate and fructose-6-phosphate are freely interconvertible, the reaction being catalyzed by the enzyme *phosphoglucose isomerase.* However, at equilibrium glucose-6-phosphate predominates, having a concentration somewhat over twice that of fructose-6-phosphate.

Conversion of fructose-6-phosphate to fructose-1, 6-diphosphate. This reaction is again essentially irreversible. ATP is used to form the diphosphate, sometimes called the *Harden-Young ester,* after its discoverers. The enzyme *phosphofructokinase* is the catalyst, with magnesium ions serving as a cofactor. The reaction is a key step in glycolysis. In addition to being a *committed step* (p. 23), it is an important control point. ATP with citrate inhibits phosphofructokinase activity by apparently binding at an allosteric site. The inhibition is relieved by *modifiers* (p. 129) such as ADP, AMP, inorganic phosphate (P_i), and fructose-1,6-diphosphate. The free energy change of this reaction is about -4500 calories, which explains the reaction's virtual irreversibility.

The conversion of fructose-1,6-diphosphate to fructose-6-phosphate requires a different enzyme, diphosphofructose phosphatase, with magnesium ion as a cofactor. However, in contrast to the above "forward" reaction, relatively high concentrations of ATP favor the "backward" reaction whereas AMP inhibits the reaction as a negative modifier. Thus, cellular concentrations of ATP, on the one hand, and ADP and AMP, on the other, serve as important *allosteric effectors* (p. 129) in regulating this key reaction of glycolysis.

$H_2O_3POCH_2$ O CH_2OH $H_2O_3POCH_2$ O $H_2COPO_3H_2$

H   OH   H   OH

H   OH   H   OH

OH   H   OH   H

Fructose-6-phosphate   **Fructose-1,6-diphosphate**

Formation of triose phosphates. The cleavage of fructose-1,6-diphosphate by the enzyme aldolase to form D-glyceraldehyde-3-phosphate and dihydroxyacetone phosphate is the next reaction in glycolysis. This is a reversible reaction. Aldolase has been crystallized from muscle and consists of four identical subunits. It has a molecular weight of approximately 150,000. Liver and yeast aldolases have properties similar to yet distinct from the muscle enzyme. Liver and muscle aldolases have no cofactor requirement, whereas yeast aldolases are activated by iron (II), cobalt (II), or zinc ions.

In the reverse reaction, isotopic studies have indicated that dihydroxyacetone combines with aldolase through the ϵ-amino group of a lysine residue to form a Schiff base, which by activating a hydrogen atom of the hydroxymethyl group facilitates the aldol condensation with glyceraldehyde-3-phosphate to form fructose-1,6-diphosphate.

Dihydroxyacetone phosphate and D-glyceraldehyde-3-phosphate are freely interconverted by *triose phosphate isomerase.* Thus, in effect, fructose-1,6-diphosphate may be cleaved to two molecules of D-glyceraldehyde-3-phosphate, as shown below, for further metabolism by way of the Embden-Meyerhof pathway.

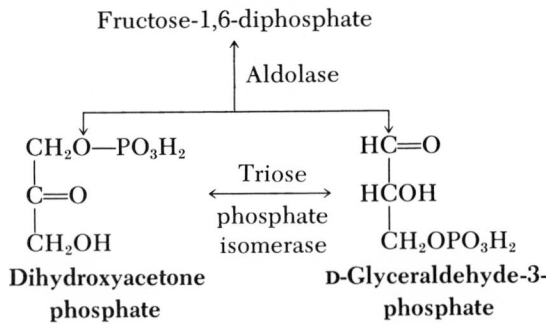

Fructose-1,6-diphosphate

Aldolase

$CH_2O-PO_3H_2$ $HC=O$

Triose

$C=O$ HCOH

phosphate

CH_2OH $CH_2OPO_3H_2$

isomerase

Dihydroxyacetone   **D-Glyceraldehyde-3-**

phosphate   **phosphate**

Dihydroxyacetone phosphate may also be converted by $NADH_2$ and a dehydrogenase to L-α-glycerophosphate for lipid synthesis (p. 314) and then by a phosphatase to glycerol.

The next step in glycolysis is the phosphorylation and oxidation of the two molecules of D-glyceraldehyde-3-phosphate to two molecules of 1,3-diphosphoglyceric acid, catalyzed by the enzyme *phosphoglyceraldehyde dehydrogenase.* NAD^+ is required as a coenzyme, and phosphate (P_i). Phosphoglyceraldehyde dehydrogenase has been prepared in crystalline form from muscle and yeast. It has a molecular weight of approximately 140,000 and contains two moles of NAD^+ in loosely bound combination per mole of enzyme. Iodoacetate inactivates the enzyme by reacting with the enzyme's sulf-hydryl groups.

The mechanism of the reactions involved has been studied rather exten-sively. Apparently an intermediate compound of the substrate with an oxi-dized enzyme-coenzyme complex is formed. The reduced coenzyme is then replaced by or oxidized to NAD^+, and the thioester bond is attacked by phos-phate to form 1,3-diphosphoglycerate and regenerate the sulfhydryl form of the enzyme-NAD^+ complex. The reduced $NADH_2$ apparently is reoxidized to NAD^+ by such metabolites as pyruvate, dihydroxyacetone phosphate, or oxaloacetate (p. 251), which themselves, in the presence of the appropriate enzyme, are reduced to lactate, α-glycerophosphate, or malate, respectively. The $NADH_2$ may also be oxidized by oxygen via the electron-transport chain, resulting in the formation of three moles of ATP per mole of triose phosphate metabolized.

The carboxyl phosphate of 1,3-diphosphoglyceric acid contains a high-energy bond (p. 254); and in the presence of an acceptor, ADP, magnesium ions, and the enzyme *phosphoglyceric acid kinase*, 3-phosphoglyceric acid and ATP are formed:

$$
\begin{array}{ccc}
\text{O=COPO}_3\text{H}_2 & & \text{COOH} \\
| & \xrightarrow[\text{ADP}\quad\text{ATP}]{\text{Mg}^{++}} & | \\
\text{HCOH} & & \text{HCOH} \\
| & & | \\
\text{H}_2\text{C—OPO}_3\text{H}_2 & & \text{H}_2\text{COPO}_3\text{H}_2 \\
\textbf{1,3-Diphosphoglyceric acid} & & \textbf{3-Phosphoglyceric acid}
\end{array}
$$

The equilibrium of the reaction is well to the right since the free energy of hydrolysis ($\Delta F'$) of 1,3-diphosphoglyceric acid is -11.8 kilocalories per mole whereas that of 3-phosphoglyceric acid is -8.0 kcal./mole. The reaction is therefore not easily reversible. It is further enhanced by the presence of an acceptor for the high-energy phosphate of ATP, e.g., glucose or creatine (p. 252). Increased levels of ATP tend to inhibit the reaction. The free energy changes in this reaction are such that the preceding aldolase and isomerase reactions are "pulled" to the right.

Apparently, 1,3-diphosphoglyceric acid may also be converted to 2,3-diphosphoglyceric acid by a *phosphoglyceromutase*. The latter may then be converted to 3-phosphoglyceric acid by the action of *phosphoglycerophos-phatase*. Relatively large amounts of 2,3-diphosphoglyceric acid accumulate in the normal erythrocyte and play an important role in oxygen release from hemoglobin in the tissues (p. 647).

The next phase of glycolysis is the conversion of 3-phosphoglyceric acid to 2-phosphoglyceric acid by the action of phosphoglyceromutase.

Formation of pyruvic acid. 2-Phosphoglyceric acid is then converted to phosphoenolpyruvic acid by dehydration in the presence of *enolase* and magnesium or manganese (II) ions as cofactors. The reaction is inhibited by fluoride, possibly because of the formation of a magnesium fluorophosphate complex. The reaction is freely reversible since there is little free energy change. However, there is a redistribution of energy so that a high-energy phosphate bond is formed in phosphoenolpyruvic acid. In the presence of

ADP and the enzyme *pyruvic acid kinase,* along with magnesium ions and potassium (in muscle) ions, ATP and enol pyruvic acid are formed. The latter rearrange to the common keto form of pyruvic acid.

$$
\begin{array}{ccc}
\text{COOH} & & \text{COOH} \\
| & & | \\
\text{HCOH} & \longleftrightarrow & \text{HC—OPO}_3\text{H}_2 \\
| & & | \\
\text{H}_2\text{COPO}_3\text{H}_2 & & \text{CH}_2\text{OH} \\
\textbf{3-Phosphoglyceric} & & \textbf{2-Phosphoglyceric} \\
\textbf{acid} & & \textbf{acid}
\end{array}
$$

Mg^{++} or Mn^{++} H$_2$O

$$
\begin{array}{cccc}
\text{COOH} & & \text{COOH} & \text{COOH} \\
| & & | & | \\
\text{COPO}_3\text{H}_2 & & \text{COH} & \text{C}=\text{O} \\
\| & & \| & | \\
\text{CH}_2 & & \text{CH}_2 & \text{CH}_3 \\
\textbf{Phosphoenolpyruvic} & & \textbf{Enolpyruvic} & \textbf{Pyruvic acid} \\
\textbf{acid} & & \textbf{acid}
\end{array}
$$

Mg^{++}, K$^+$ ADP   ATP

The free energy change in the reaction, $\Delta F'$, is about -6 kcal., so equilibrium is far to the right and there is formation of ATP (2 moles per mole of glucose glycolyzed).

The pyruvate kinase reaction is a second major control point in glycolysis, at least in yeast. Fructose diphosphate apparently accelerates the forward reaction some fiftyfold by a positive feedforward control. The reaction is inhibited by ATP and calcium ions.

Formation of lactic acid. As a final step in glycolysis, in the classic sense pyruvic acid may be converted to L-lactic acid by the enzyme *lactic acid dehydrogenase,* with NADH$_2$ as a cofactor. Again, the free energy change is some -6 kcal., therefore strongly favoring the production of lactic acid.

$$
\begin{array}{ccc}
\text{COOH} & & \text{COOH} \\
| & & | \\
\text{C}=\text{O} \quad + \text{NADH}_2 & \longleftrightarrow & \text{HOCH} \quad + \text{NAD}^+ \\
| & & | \\
\text{CH}_3 & & \text{CH}_3 \\
\textbf{Pyruvic acid} & & \textbf{L-Lactic acid}
\end{array}
$$

Energy production by anaerobic glycolysis and aerobic oxidation   Thus, in anaerobic glycolysis, each molecule of glucose forms two molecules of lactic acid and a total of four moles of ATP. However, two molecules of ATP are used in phosphorylation reactions (glucose → glucose-6-P, fructose-6-P → fructose-1,6-diP), leaving a net gain of two molecules of ATP per molecule of glucose in anaerobic glycolysis. This is equivalent to an estimated 15 kcal. (p. 254).

Since some 56 kcal. per mole are produced when glucose is degraded to lactic acid under standardized conditions, the overall efficiency of glycolysis is 15/56 × 100, or approximately 25% — a rather high figure!

The aerobic oxidation of pyruvic acid by way of acetyl-CoA and the citric acid cycle (p. 263) yields another 15 moles of ATP per mole of pyruvic acid or 30 moles at ATP per mole of glucose metabolized to carbon dioxide and water. Thus the net formation of ATP by anaerobic plus aerobic glycolysis is 38 moles of ATP per mole of glucose, or an equivalent of approximately 266 kilocalories of utilizable energy. Since the complete oxidation of glucose theoretically may yield some 686 kilocalories, the overall efficiency of the oxidation of glucose in the body is approximately 38%, indeed a remarkably high efficiency. The usual efficiency of machines, in contrast, is of the order of 20% to 25%.

The lactic acid and pyruvic acid, unlike their predecessor phosphated intermediates, readily diffuse from the cells in which they are produced (mainly muscle) into the general circulation for further metabolism, mainly in the liver.

No oxygen is consumed in the overall process of anaerobic glycolysis. Two steps involve oxidoreductions, the oxidation of 3-phosphoglyceraldehyde and the reduction of pyruvic to lactic acid. NAD^+ participates in both reactions; therefore, the two cancel out and there is no net oxidation or reduction.

It may be recalled (p. 130) that lactic dehydrogenase (LDH) is a tetramer consisting of four subunits each with a molecular weight of approximately 35,000. Two types of LDH subunits are distinguishable electrophoretically and are designated M (for skeletal muscle) and H (for heart muscle). Skeletal muscle LDH is mainly M_4 whereas heart LDH is largely H_4. However, various tissues contain all possible hybrids, M_1H_3, M_2H_2, M_3H_1. The M and H types of subunits differ in their susceptibility to inhibition by pyruvate. M_4 is not readily inhibited by pyruvate and hence is useful in a tissue in which a more anaerobic environment may predominate, e.g., skeletal muscle. In contrast, H_4 is readily inhibited by pyruvate and is better adapted for a more highly aerobic organ, which removes lactate and oxidizes it to pyruvate, largely in the mitochondria.

METABOLISM OF LACTIC ACID AND PYRUVIC ACID

Lactic acid is one of the few "dead-end streets" in metabolism. Its only metabolic pathway is reversal to form pyruvic acid. From this point a number of pathways are open. Perhaps the primary one is decarboxylation to form acetyl-CoA (p. 204), which may then be oxidized aerobically to carbon dioxide and water by way of the citric acid cycle (p. 263), or converted to fatty acids (p. 310) or sterols (p. 326). Other primary pathways of disposal include reconversion via phosphorylated intermediates to glucose and glycogen (Fig. 9-2) by a reversal of glycolysis to be described (p. 205), transamination to alanine (p. 351), and carboxylation to malic or oxaloacetic acid. These are shown diagrammatically in Fig. 9-11.

Formation of acetyl-CoA   The conversion of pyruvic acid to acetyl-CoA is one of the most complex reactions found in the metabolism of carbohydrates. It is catalyzed by the enzyme complex pyruvate oxidase and requires *five* cofactors—coenzyme-A, lipoic acid, NAD^+, thiamine pyrophosphate, and magnesium ions. As will be noted, the vitamins pantothenic acid, nicotinamide, lipoic acid, riboflavin, and thiamine, respectively, are involved as constituents of coenzymes in this single reaction—one of the major biochemical functions of vitamins in the body.

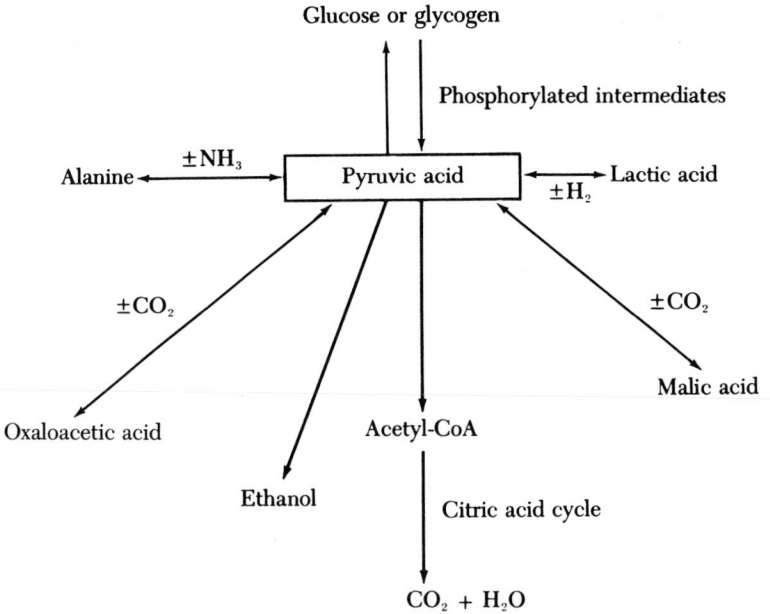

Fig. 9-11. Principal pathways for the metabolic disposal of pyruvic acid.

The sequence of reactions in the conversion of pyruvic acid to acetyl-CoA is as follows:

Pyruvic acid + Thiamine pyrophosphate → Active acetaldehyde + CO_2
CH_3—CO—COOH   (TPP) CH_3—CHOH—TPP
                                                (α-hydroxyethylthiamine
                                                     pyrophosphate)

CH_3—CHOH—TPP + Lipoic acid pyruvate oxidase → Lipoic acid pyruvate oxidase + TPP
                      ⌊—S—S—⌋ CH_3—COS ⌊—SH

Acetyllipoylpyruvate oxidase + CoASH → Acetyl-CoA + Lipoic acid
                                                    ⌊—SH ⌊—SH
                                                   (reduced form)

Lipoic acid + FAD → Lipoic acid + $FADH_2$
     ⎮⎮   ⌊—S—S—⌋
     S S
     H H   (oxidized form)
(reduced form)

Active acetaldehyde is:

![α-Hydroxyethylthiamine pyrophosphate structure]

α-Hydroxyethylthiamine pyrophosphate

Formation of oxaloacetate and malate Two other important metabolic routes of pyruvate disposal are conversion to (1) oxaloacetate and (2) malate by a carboxylation reaction (see Fig. 9-2). These two pathways represent mechanisms for the replacement of oxaloacetate, sometimes termed *anaplerosis,* or malate diverted from the citric acid cycle for other metabolic uses (p. 319). Since the reactions are reversible, by different enzyme systems, they also thus represent supplementary pathways for the reversal of glycolysis via the citric acid cycle (p. 263).

The conversions of pyruvate to malate and to oxaloacetate proceed as follows:

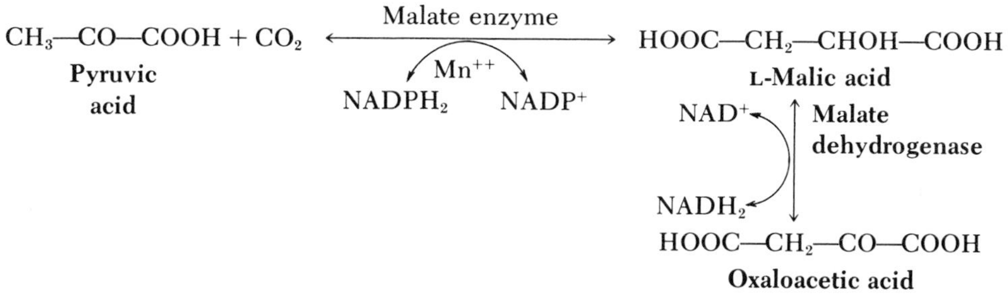

$$CH_3-CO-COOH + CO_2 \xrightleftharpoons[\underset{NADPH_2 \quad NADP^+}{Mn^{++}}]{\text{Malate enzyme}} HOOC-CH_2-CHOH-COOH$$

L-Malic acid

$$NAD^+ \quad \text{Malate dehydrogenase}$$

$$NADH_2$$

$$HOOC-CH_2-CO-COOH$$

Oxaloacetic acid

Oxaloacetic acid may also be formed in anaplerosis in animal tissues and yeast by the carboxylation of pyruvic acid in the presence of the mitochondrial enzyme pyruvate carboxylase, a biotin-containing protein (mol. wt. about 650,000). ATP and magnesium ions are required for this reaction and acetyl-CoA is needed as an allosteric effector (p. 129).

$$\text{Pyruvic acid} + ATP + CO_2 \xrightarrow[\underset{\text{carboxylase}}{\text{Pyruvate}}]{\overset{\text{Acetyl-CoA}}{Mg^{++}}} \text{Oxaloacetic acid} + ADP + P_i$$

Another route for the conversion of pyruvate to oxaloacetate, at least in plants, is via phosphoenolpyruvic acid.

$$\text{Phosphoenolpyruvic acid} + CO_2 \xrightarrow[\text{IDP (or GTP)}]{\text{Carboxykinase-}} \text{Oxaloacetic acid} + P_i$$

Reversal of glycolysis As stated earlier, certain of the above pathways of pyruvic acid may be important in the reversal of glycolysis. For example, in liver the conversion of oxaloacetate, formed from pyruvate by pyruvate carboxylase and ATP, to phosphoenolpyruvate by phosphoenolpyruvate carboxykinase and ITP (or GTP) appears to be a major route for the synthesis of glucose and glycogen from pyruvate (Figs. 9-2 and 9-7).

$$\text{Oxaloacetate} \xrightarrow[\underset{\text{(acetyl-CoA)}}{\text{ITP (or GTP)}}]{\overset{\text{Phosphoenolpyruvate}}{\text{carboxykinase}}} \text{Phosphoenolpyruvate} + CO_2$$

Some oxaloacetic acid is also decarboxylated directly by oxaloacetic decarboxylase and perhaps also, to a limited extent, spontaneously.

$$\text{Oxaloacetic acid} \xrightarrow{\text{Oxaloacetic decarboxylase}} \text{Pyruvic acid} + CO_2$$

The pyruvate → malate route could likewise be converted to phosphoenolpyruvate via oxaloacetate by means of malate dehydrogenase and NAD^+.

In muscle, however, there is apparently a direct conversion of pyruvic acid to phosphoenolpyruvic acid by pyruvic kinase, ATP, and magnesium ions in a limited reversal of glycolysis.

$$\text{Muscle pyruvate} \xrightarrow[\text{ATP, Mg}^{++}]{\text{Pyruvate kinase}} \text{Phosphoenolpyruvate} + ADP$$

In either case, then, but *primarily in liver*, the phosphoenolpyruvate formed could be converted to fructose-1,6-diphosphate by a reversal of the Embden-Meyerhof pathway and then to glucose (by substituting phosphatases for kinases in the first and third steps) and/or glycogen to complete the reversal of glycolysis. It may be noted that the overall conversion of two moles of pyruvate to one mole of glucose by a reversal of glycolysis entails the use of six moles of ATP whereas the conversion of one mole of glucose to two moles of pyruvate forms a net total of only two moles of ATP.

Yeast fermentation As stated earlier, in yeast and certain other microorganisms the breakdown of hexoses proceeds via pathways involving the same chemical reactions as does glycolysis in animal cells, forming pyruvic acid. However, in these microorganisms some pyruvic acid is converted to ethyl alcohol as a primary product as well as to acetyl-CoA. This was known as "fermentation" in the early classic literature—a term still used today.

The pathway involved is as follows:

$$CH_3-CO-COOH + \text{Thiamine pyrophosphate} \xrightarrow[\text{Mg}^{++}]{\substack{\text{Pyruvic} \\ \text{decarboxylase}}} CH_3-CHOH-TPP + CO_2$$

Pyruvic acid   **(TPP)**   **Active acetaldehyde**

$$CH_3-CHOH-TPP \xrightarrow{\text{TPP}} CH_3-CHO \xrightarrow[\text{NADH}_2 \quad \text{NAD}^+]{\substack{\text{Aldehyde} \\ \text{dehydrogenase}}} C_2H_5OH$$

Acetaldehyde   **Ethyl alcohol**

The NAD^+ formed serves to support the oxidation of 3-phosphoglyceraldehyde to 1,3-diphosphoglyceric acid and maintain anaerobic fermentation just as the conversion of pyruvic acid to lactic acid and NAD^+ serves to maintain glycolysis in muscle and other animal cells.

Metabolism of ethanol Ethyl alcohol is oxidized in animal cells (almost entirely in the liver) to yield ATP equivalent to approximately 7 kilocalories per gram of ethanol. Extensive studies have demonstrated that the reactions involved are as shown at the top of the following page.

The simultaneous metabolism of pyruvate or of glucose (carbohydrate) increases the rate of ethanol metabolism. Presumably this increase is due to the conversion of $NADH_2$, which may accumulate in the liver during alcohol metabolism, to NAD^+, the pyruvate being changed to lactate. The oxidation of $NADH_2$ frees more NAD^+ for further ethanol oxidation, thus increasing the

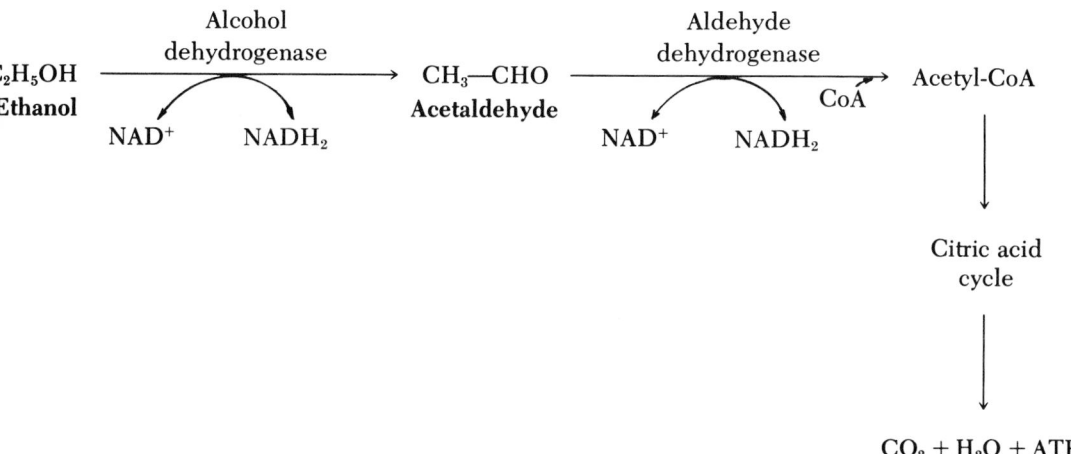

rate. Starvation or fasting decreases the rate of ethanol metabolism for the same reason, i.e., increasing the ratio of $NADH_2$ to NAD^+ in hepatic cells. There is a considerable amount of current evidence that many of the biochemical physiologic effects of ethanol result from the relatively high requirement of NAD^+ from other metabolic pathways. Also, the concomitant increase in $NADH_2$ could shift certain pathways into the formation of reduced metabolites. An accumulation or imbalance of such metabolites might be responsible for some of the biochemical and pharmacologic effects of alcohol in the body.[14]

Control of glycolysis   During the discussion of the various individual reactions of glycolysis, mention was made of the enzymes and various cofactors required. The levels of these as well as the levels of the substrate, on the one hand, and the product, on the other (p. 129), serve as key regulators of the separate reactions. However, a brief consideration of overall regulation is perhaps in order at this point.

When the need for chemical energy as ATP is high, e.g., during vigorous exercise, ATP is rapidly used and ADP plus inorganic phosphate (P_i) is formed. This increases the conversion of reserve energy stored in muscle as creatine phosphate (p. 566) to provide more ATP:

$$\text{Creatine phosphate} + \text{ADP} \leftrightarrow \text{ATP} + \text{Creatine}$$

Also an increase in ADP supplies an acceptor for the formation of more ATP. Likewise, P_i accelerates glycogenolysis to provide more glucose for glycolysis.

Further, ADP and P_i activate and thus increase the activities of at least two of the three rate-limiting enzymes of glycolysis, phosphofructokinase and pyruvate kinase. The increased fructose-1,6-diphosphate formed as a consequence also markedly accelerates the conversion of phosphoenolpyruvate to pyruvate, with the formation of one mole of ATP per mole of phosphoenolpyruvate. Conversely, elevated ATP levels inhibit several enzymes in the glycolytic pathway, as was brought out in the discussion of the individual reactions of Fig. 9-10.

Thus, although a number of control mechanisms operate in regulating the individual reaction of glycolysis, as indicated in Fig. 9-10, the overall control is the need for ATP as manifested by the conversion of ATP to ADP. This regulatory mechanism also operates to control *aerobic glycolysis* by way of the citric acid cycle, as will be discussed later (p. 260). Thus we have an excellent example of the principle (p. 25) that one of the basic controls in the regulation of metabolic pathways is the need for the product at the cellular level.

Pasteur effect. Pasteur observed that fermentation varies inversely with the oxygen concentration. Under anaerobic conditions yeasts ferment sugar, but upon the introduction of oxygen, fermentation ceases and oxidative reactions occur. This phenomenon has been seen to occur in most forms of life and is called the Pasteur effect. Although it has been extensively investigated, the basis of the reaction is still clouded in doubt. Likewise, in animal tissue preparations glycolysis, as measured by glucose utilization and lactic acid formation, is decreased in the presence of oxygen. At present, it appears that the chief cause of the effect is the competition between the glycolytic pathway and the citric acid cycle for ADP and P_i. Under anaerobic conditions, a sufficient level of ADP and P_i is available in the cell for a maximal rate of glycolysis. However, in the presence of oxygen, the aerobic citric acid cycle's greater demands for ADP and P_i for the higher level of aerobic ATP production (p. 267) decrease the supply for glycolysis and hence inhibition occurs.

Some investigators attribute the Pasteur effect to an inhibition of phosphofructokinase by the lessened availability of ADP, AMP, and P_i, which are needed to activate the enzyme (p. 199). Also, the increase in ATP, in the presence of oxygen, inhibits this enzyme.

The opposite of the Pasteur effect is the so-called *Crabtree effect*. This is the inhibition of cellular oxidations by high concentrations of glucose. The Crabtree effect is believed to be due to the competition of glycolytic reactions for P_i and NAD^+, leaving less for oxidative respiratory reactions.

ALTERNATE PATHWAYS—PENTOSE PHOSPHATE PATHWAY (PHOSPHOGLUCONATE SHUNT)

For a number of years, the classic Embden-Meyerhof scheme of glycolysis was considered to be the sole pathway for the conversion of glucose to pyruvic and lactic acids. Although it is still considered to be the major pathway, some 90% of the glucose normally utilized following this route, there is growing evidence that alternate channels exist. For example, various mammalian tissues can utilize glucose readily when anaerobic glycolysis is blocked by the specific inhibitor iodoacetic acid. Also, when aerobic oxidation by way of the citric acid cycle (p. 263) is impaired (ischemia or anoxia), glucose metabolism continues although at a reduced rate. Furthermore, the occurrence in tissues of such compounds as ribose, deoxyribose, galactose, glucosamine, the uronic acids, sialic and neuraminic acids, and sedoheptulose indicates that other pathways exist for the formation of these compounds, since their origin from any point in the classic pathway is not immediately evident. The discovery of glucose-6-phosphate dehydrogenase in yeast by Warburg in 1931 and of 6-phosphogluconate dehydrogenase a few years later led to the discovery of one such alternate pathway of glucose metabolism, the pentose phosphate pathway. This is sometimes also called the Warburg-

Dickens pathway, the phosphogluconate shunt, or the hexose monophosphate shunt. In addition to being a channel for the degradation of glucose to carbon dioxide, with the formation of $NADPH_2$ and possibly also ATP, this pathway appears to be a major route for the biosynthesis of pentoses, sedoheptulose, and erythrose. Other pathways have been described for the formation of galactose, the hexosamines, the uronic acids, neuraminic acid, and a few other carbohydrate derivatives. Certain of these will be described later.

The pentose phosphate pathway is summarized briefly in Fig. 9-12. The enzymes and intermediates involved have been adequately characterized. Several intermediary reactions have been omitted. For example, it has been

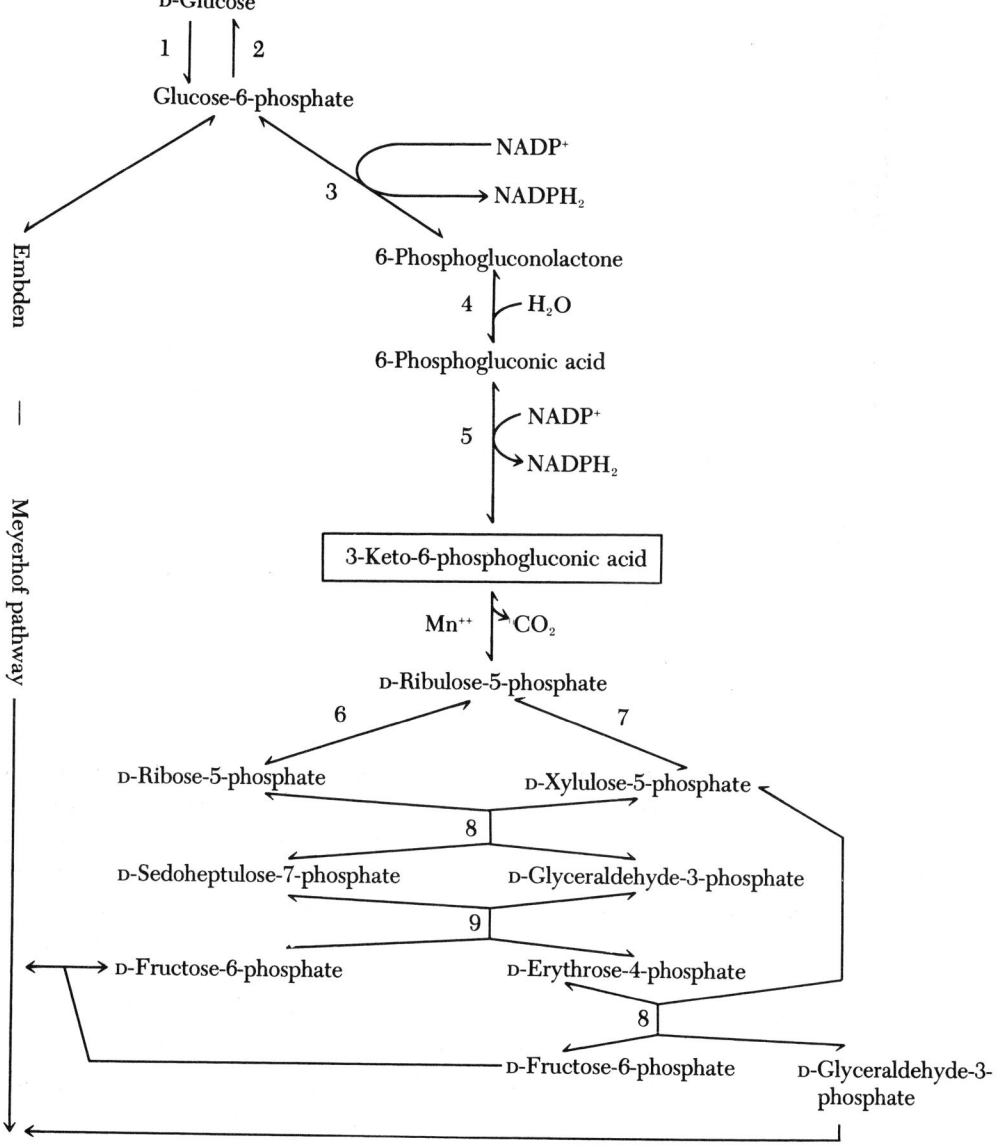

Fig. 9-12. Pentose phosphate pathway, or phosphogluconate shunt.

shown that xylulose is formed from ribulose and plays an important role in this series of reactions. It will be noted that for every two six-carbon molecules at the beginning, there are one six-carbon molecule, one three-carbon molecule, and three molecules of carbon dioxide at the end.

The enzymes involved in the pentose phosphate pathway are as follows (numbers refer to reactions in Fig. 9-12):

1. Glucokinase
2. Glucose-6-P-phosphatase
3. Glucose-6-P-dehydrogenase
4. Lactonase
5. 6-P-Gluconic acid dehydrogenase
6. P-Ribose isomerase
7. P-Ketopentose epimerase
8. Transketolase
9. Transaldolase

The cofactors required are ATP and magnesium ions (Reaction 1), $NADP^+$ (Reactions 2 and 3), manganese (II) ions (Reaction 5), and thiamine pyrophosphate and magnesium ions (Reaction 8). Thiamine pyrophosphate serves in the transfer of a two-carbon unit, *active glycolaldehyde*, in the transketolase reaction, similar to its role in the transfer of *active acetaldehyde* formed in the oxidative decarboxylation of pyruvate (p. 203).

The major importance of the pentose pathway, as stated above, is the formation of $NADPH_2$, D-ribose and other pentoses, sedoheptulose, and erythrose. As will be discussed later, $NADPH_2$ is required for a number of cellular anabolic reactions, particularly the biosynthesis of fatty acids (p. 310), the hydroxylation of steroids (p. 326), and the regeneration of sulfhydryl groups as in the reduction of methemoglobin by glutathione (p. 617).

An important feature of the pentose pathway is the fact that no ATP is required for its operation once glucose-6-phosphate has been formed. This means that the pathway may continue to function under relatively anaerobic conditions, as will be mentioned later.

The question of the formation of ATP by way of the pentose pathway is still unclear. Since the reactions all occur in the cytoplasm of the cell, the $NADPH_2$ formed apparently would need to react with NAD^+ in order to enter into oxidative phosphorylation and ATP formation (p. 252). This could occur by *transhydrogenation*, as described later (p. 252). If this indeed does occur, then each mole of $NADPH_2$ produced could form three moles of ATP. The complete oxidation of glucose could thus produce 35 moles of ATP. It is interesting that this amount is nearly the same as that formed by the oxidation of one mole of glucose by way of the classic Embden-Meyerhof pathway and the citric acid cycle (p. 263).

Apparently the pentose pathway is particularly active in those tissues that are active anabolic sites, such as in the biosynthesis of fatty acids and steroids, e.g., the liver, adipose tissue, mammary gland, adrenal cortex, and testis.

Some evidence[15] indicates that the pentose phosphate pathway is ordinarily a relatively minor pathway of glucose degradation. Liver slices from normal rats metabolized only 2% of glucose (^{14}C) by this route, and those from dia betic rats metabolized 6%. The shunt may be more important, however, in the biosynthesis of pentoses from hexoses, as will be described later (p. 216). There is much evidence for this belief.[16-18]

The pentose pathway is also important in the metabolism of the erythrocyte for maintaining its structural integrity. Individuals with a genetic defect resulting in a deficiency of the enzyme glucose-6-phosphate dehydrogenase develop a severe hemolytic anemia from the defective erythrocyte structure and excessive hemolysis (p. 595).

Apparently increased amounts of glucose may be metabolized by way of the pentose pathway in situations resulting from tissue anoxia. The mechanism involved appears to be that the lack of tissue oxygen decreases the metabolism of pyruvate by way of the citric acid cycle (p. 263). Intermediates of the anaerobic Embden-Meyerhof glycolytic pathway therefore accumulate, resulting in a diversion of glucose-6-phosphate into the pentose pathway. $NADPH_2$, an important product of the pentose pathway, accumulates. The excess $NADPH_2$ is therefore diverted to fatty acid synthesis (p. 310), thus accounting for the fatty infiltration or fatty degeneration of tissues subjected to anoxia for extended periods of time. This sequence of events has been demonstrated beautifully in infarcted myocardial tissue following coronary occlusion.[19] Using glucose-1-^{14}C, it was shown that glucose utilization by way of the pentose pathway (as measured by $^{14}CO_2$ produced by heart tissue slices) increases markedly in infarcted heart muscle of dogs as compared to normal heart tissue. An increase in $NADPH_2$ and fat formation was also found in the infarcted heart tissue.

It appears possible that aerobic oxidation of glucose might occur without phosphorylation. A D-glucose dehydrogenase has been shown to transform glucose into gluconic acid. Other carbohydrate derivatives, as well as pentoses, are oxidized by this enzyme, which may well be an alternate mechanism for the oxidation of sugar in mammalian liver.

CARBOHYDRATE METABOLISM IN STRIATED MUSCLE

The concept of muscle contraction held until recent years was that energy for the contraction is derived from the combustion of glycogen, resulting in the production of carbon dioxide and water. Although glycogen is eventually converted to these products and oxygen is utilized in the transformations, the process is by no means a direct oxidation. There is, in fact, at the moment of contraction no combustion of fuel by the muscle (i.e., no absorption of oxygen or production of CO_2). Contraction of an isolated muscle can occur in the complete absence of oxygen. This may continue for an appreciable length of time, during which the glycogen is changed to lactic acid (lactate), which accumulates. If this is continued too long, *rigor mortis* sets in. However, if the contractions occur in the presence of sufficient oxygen, part of the lactic acid is reconverted to glycogen and part is oxidized. Normal muscle contraction, therefore, may be divided into two phases: (1) contractile or anaerobic and (2) recovery or aerobic. Although the contractile phase is called *anaerobic* and oxygen is not needed for it, this phase can and ordinarily does occur in the presence of oxygen. For the recovery phase, oxygen is necessary and carbon dioxide is formed. Consequently, the energy for contraction cannot originate in an oxidation but must come from the sudden breakdown of some labile molecule.

At one time it was thought that energy for muscle contraction came from the breakdown of creatine phosphate. At present, however, ADP and ATP are considered the agents that actually release energy, although other compounds may be involved in the intricate process.

Creatine phosphate. In 1927 the Eggletons,[20] in England, discovered in muscle an organic phosphate that was easily hydrolyzed. They called this "phosphagen." The same year Fiske and SubbaRow,[21] in the United States, made the same discovery and were able to identify the substance as creatine phosphate. It is such an unstable compound that the muscle must be frozen before removal for analysis, and even under these conditions there is evidence that some of the compound has been hydrolyzed. Meyerhof[22] showed that the decomposition of creatine phosphate to creatine and phosphoric acid, whether accomplished by an enzyme or by an acid, is accompanied by the release of heat. Muscle extract contains this enzyme, but if the extract is dialyzed, the enzyme becomes inactive. In the dialysate, magnesium ions and ATP, which are needed for this enzymic reaction, can be found. Adenosine phosphates are required for all such transformations in which the transfer of phosphate is accompanied by a release of energy. Because of the presence of two energy-rich phosphate bonds (p. 254), each of these hydrolyses is accompanied by the transfer of a large amount of energy. This release of energy upon a suitable receptor in a muscle fiber enables ATP to do biologic work. The energy-rich phosphate bonds of ATP can, however, be used to phosphorylate creatine, giving creatine an energy-rich phosphate bond; or they can phosphorylate glucose or fructose. Thus we see why creatine phosphate was at first thought to be the source of muscle energy. It is now considered to be an active phosphate carrier, capable of transferring its phosphate to ADP to form ATP.

CARBOHYDRATE METABOLISM IN HEART MUSCLE

Since the heart is a muscular organ that must contract almost constantly, we would expect to find in it a rich store of glycogen. This is probably true, and the very low values reported in the literature are undoubtedly due to extremely rapid postmortem glycogenolysis. The creatine content in heart muscle is less than half the concentration of that compound in striated muscle. However, the mechanism of carbohydrate metabolism in the heart is believed to be very similar to that described for skeletal muscle except that heart muscle apparently utilizes lactic acid to a greater extent. This may indicate a different metabolic pathway at one stage. Creatine phosphate and ATP play important roles here as they do in striated muscle contractions. The left ventricle contains higher concentrations of creatine, phosphorus, potassium, and adenine than does the right. This means that creatine phosphate and ATP, as the dipotassium salts, are found in greater concentration in the stronger muscle. Furthermore, when cardiac hypertrophy begins, a slight increase in these constituents is seen; but with further hypertrophy they fall, and with extreme hypertrophy and heart failure they reach their lowest values. This points to the great need of creatine phosphate and ATP for efficient heart muscle action. The ATP is obtained partly by oxidation of fatty acids, acetoacetic acid, and lactic acid. The lactic acid is derived from that in the blood as a result of exercise of skeletal muscle.

CARBOHYDRATE METABOLISM IN NERVOUS TISSUE

From the studies of Himwich, it appears that carbohydrate, or a derivative, is the sole source of energy in the brain of dogs. The respiratory quotient is close to 1.0, which is the respiratory quotient for carbohydrate (p. 517). Furthermore, blood coming from the brain contains less glucose and lactic acid than does blood going to the brain. In resting nerves, the respiratory quotient indicates combustion of a mixture of protein, carbohydrate, and fat; but during activity, the respiratory quotient rises to such an extent that it indicates that the extra metabolism is entirely derived from carbohydrate. There is very little glycogen present in the brain, and probably not much glycogenesis or glycogenolysis there either. Glucose is the principal carbohydrate used by nervous tissue, and the exact path of decomposition is unknown. Under anaerobic conditions, brain tissue transforms glucose into lactic acid, but if oxygen is present, the amount of lactic acid formed is greatly diminished. This may mean that lactic acid is always formed from glucose but in the presence of oxygen it is immediately oxidized and thus removed. As mentioned before, pyruvic acid increases in nervous tissue in the absence of vitamin B_1. This would indicate that pyruvic acid is a normal intermediary in glucose utilization in nervous tissue.

We know that the brain requires both oxygen and glucose. If glucose or lactic acid is added to chopped brain tissue, there results an increased oxygen consumption. Evidently brain tissue takes up oxygen for carbohydrate utilization. When a hypoglycemia occurs, one of the striking symptoms is its effect on the brain. There are mental confusion, dizziness, and sometimes delirium. These also may occur after an overdose of insulin. In this connection the use of insulin-induced hypoglycemia in the treatment of schizophrenia may be pointed out.

CONVERSION OF CARBOHYDRATE TO FAT

Another physiologic mechanism that tends to keep the blood sugar at a constant level is the transformation of excess glucose into fat. This is such a well-known phenomenon that it scarcely needs emphasis. The fattening of hogs and the production of cream are instances known to every farmer. The European custom of feeding geese much bread or other starchy foods to produce the fatty goose liver is another example. In these cases glycogenesis in the liver and muscles occurs first. When these tissues are not capable of storing more glycogen, fat formation begins. The mechanism of this action and the metabolic pathways involved are described in Chapter 12. We may assume that the formation of fat from an excess of carbohydrate is a normal process ordinarily. In other words, fat production is a provision of nature to enable the individual to store large excesses of carbohydrate (in the form of fat, the high caloric food), which can be drawn upon when the more readily convertible storage food, glycogen, has been depleted. This would imply that simple cases of obesity result from a normal tendency to store food when the caloric intake exceeds caloric requirement. The fact that some individuals have great difficulty in putting on weight is probably just as abnormal as the fact that others become obese.

EXCRETION OF GLUCOSE

Ordinarily the amount of glucose in urine is negligible. The range has been shown to be from 0.01% to 0.10% and certainly is not in sufficient concentration to give a positive reaction with Benedict's qualitative solution. Normally the blood sugar passes through the glomeruli of the kidneys and, in aqueous solution, flows into the tubules. Here it is reabsorbed. If reabsorption cannot keep pace with glomerular secretion, glucose will, of course, find its way into the urine. This is called "glycosuria" or, more exactly, *glucosuria*. The chief reason for the occurrence of glucosuria is an increased excretion of sugar as a result of a high blood sugar. Reabsorption cannot keep pace with the filtration and the excess sugar flows into the urine. There is usually a fairly definite level of blood sugar for a given individual, above which sugar is excreted. This *renal threshold* is usually found to be between 140 and 180 mg.% glucose, averaging 160 mg.%. It frequently is higher with older persons or if the kidneys are damaged. For this reason an abnormally high blood sugar is sometimes found when the urine is quite free from reducing substances. This indicates a disturbed carbohydrate metabolism just as definitely as does glucosuria. If the renal threshold is found to be normal, an examination of the urine obviates the necessity of frequent blood analyses.

It might be added that the renal threshold for glucose is lower than normal in individuals with a relatively rare condition called *renal glucosuria* or "renal diabetes" (see also p. 222).

METABOLISM OF OTHER HEXOSES

Fructose. As stated previously (pp. 184, 189), fructose is phosphorylated both in the mucosal cells of the intestine and in the liver to form fructose-6-phosphate. This can be catabolized to carbon dioxide and water by the glycolytic pathway or can be converted to glycogen or to blood glucose as described earlier.

Fructose can also be metabolized by way of fructose-1-phosphate as summarized in Fig. 9-13. Fructose administered *intravenously* is utilized better by the diabetic patient than is glucose.

D-Fructose is present in significant amounts in seminal fluid. Apparently it is synthesized in the prostate gland by the following pathway:

$$\beta\text{-D-Glucose} \xrightarrow[\substack{\text{Aldose} \\ \text{reductase}}]{\text{NADPH}_2} \text{D-Sorbitol} \xrightarrow[\substack{\text{Ketose} \\ \text{reductase}}]{\text{NAD}^+} \beta\text{-D-Fructose}$$

A rare error in the metabolism of fructose is known as *essential fructosuria* (p. 739). This condition appears to be due to a lack of the enzyme needed for the conversion of fructose to glycogen. There is an interesting recent claim

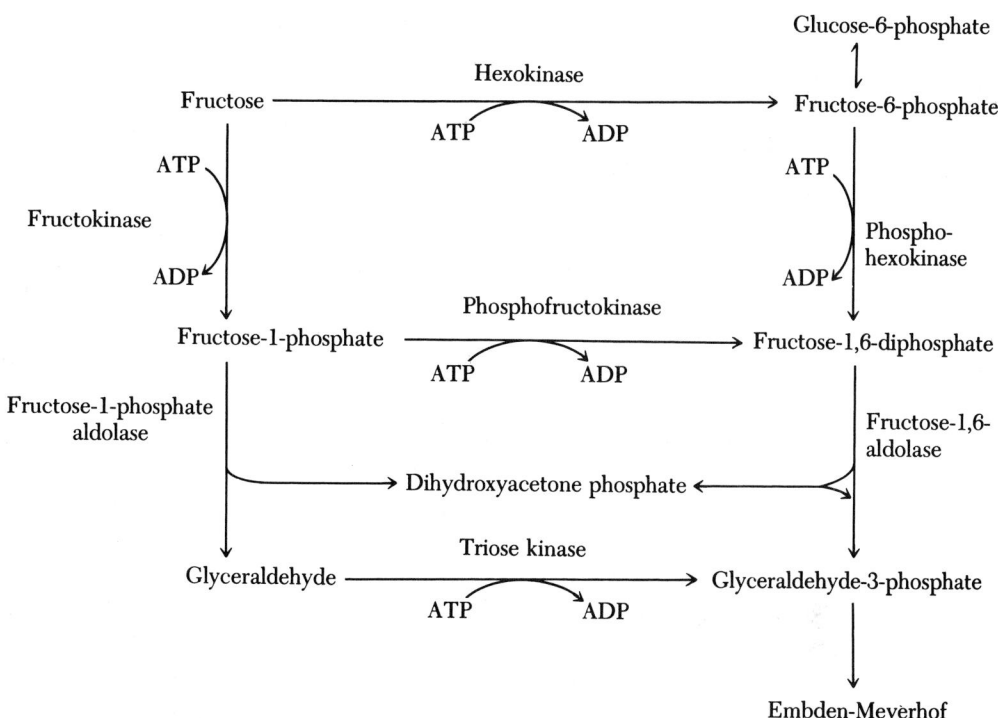

Fig. 9-13. Metabolism of fructose via fructose-1-phosphate.

that children with Tay-Sachs disease have a deficiency of fructose-1-phosphate aldolase.

Galactose. Galactose is derived chiefly from lactose of the diet. It is important in the body for the formation of certain glycolipids and glycoproteins and, of course, for the formation of lactose during lactation. As the first step in its metabolism, galactose is phosphorylated to form galactose-1-phosphate, which is then converted to glucose-1-phosphate by the formation of intermediary derivatives with uridine diphosphate.[23] The steps involved in the conversion are as follows:

(1)   Galactose + ATP $\xrightarrow[\text{Mg}^{++}]{\text{Galactokinase}}$ Galactose-1-phosphate + ADP

(2)   Galactose-1-phosphate + UDP-glucose $\xrightleftharpoons{\text{UDP-galactose transferase}}$ Glucose-1-phosphate + UDP-galactose

(3)   UDP-galactose $\xrightleftharpoons{\text{UDP-galactose-4-epimerase}}$ UDP-glucose

(4)   UDP-glucose + Pyrophosphate $\xrightleftharpoons{\text{Uridyl pyrophosphate transferase}}$ Glucose-1-phosphate + UTP

In this manner, then, galactose is phosphorylated and converted to glucose-1-phosphate, which can be metabolized by any of the routes previously described, including the formation of glycogen.[9]

It is interesting that galactose-1-phosphate can be synthesized in the mammary gland from glucose-1-phosphate presumably by the reverse of the above

215

steps. This was demonstrated[24] by the use of ^{14}C-labeled glucose-1-phosphate administered to guinea pigs. The galactose-1-phosphate thus formed is, of course, incorporated into lactose by the mammary gland, probably by way of UDP-galactose, as described previously, reacting with glucose-1-phosphate to form lactose-1-phosphate, which, in turn, forms lactose and inorganic phosphate.

An inborn error in the metabolism of galactose occurs in infants with congenital *galactosemia* or hereditary galactose disease, which may occur as frequently as once in 18,000 births.[25] If fed milk, these infants develop a high blood sugar due chiefly to galactose-1-phosphate, a galactosuria, and sometimes an aminoaciduria and a ketonuria. There is usually hepatomegaly, cataracts, and mental retardation. Removal of milk from the diet of the infant results in a decrease in blood sugar and a disappearance of the galactosemia. This condition is due to the congenital lack of one of the enzymes, UDP-galactose transferase (see Step 2 above), required for the metabolism of galactose. It may be noted that the feeding of large amounts of galactose produces cataracts in experimental animals.

Mannose. Mannose is of little practical importance since only small amounts appear in food carbohydrates. However, as stated before, this hexose appears to be well utilized. Apparently it is first phosphorylated to mannose-6-phosphate, then converted to fructose-6-phosphate by the enzyme phosphomannose isomerase. It is then metabolized by any of the pathways described previously.

Inositol. Inositol is hexahydroxybenzene and is sometimes considered as a sugar. It will be mentioned again (pp. 565, 566). It is essential to cell life for reasons not yet entirely clear.[26] It is necessary for the growth of mammalian cells in culture. It is a constituent of phosphatidylinositol (p. 286) and plays a role in active transport in brain tissue. One of its several isomers, *myoinositol*, has been shown to be converted to xylulose and catabolized by way of the pentose phosphate pathway in mammals. It is apparently synthesized from D-glucose in animal tissues.

METABOLISM OF PENTOSES

The pentoses in the food that we eat are not readily absorbed from the intestinal tract. They are not utilized as well as the hexoses when given by mouth. However, probably in physiologic combinations they are readily metabolized since it appears that the enzymes of various tissues can change the ribose group of purine nucleotides and nucleosides to some nonpentose form, probably a hexose. Another pentose, L-xylulose, may be synthesized by the body via glucuronic acid. In the condition known as *pentosuria*[27] it probably cannot be metabolized further. Pentoses arise in the body from hexoses, through gluconic acid. The enzyme system that accomplishes this reaction occurs not only in yeast, where it was first discovered, but also in the liver, muscle, and other tissues. Two interesting features of the reaction are a β-oxidation and the presence of a phosphopentose isomerase, which catalyzes the reversible conversion of D-ribulose-5-phosphate to D-ribose-5-phosphate. The following scheme represents the reactions:

```
   COOH                 COOH                      H₂COH                    HCO
   HCOH                 HCOH                       CO                      HCOH
          -2 H                         -CO₂
   HOCH   ⇌     CO      ⇌       CO            ⇌     HCOH
          +2 H                         +CO₂
   HCOH                 HCOH                       HCOH                    HCOH
   HCOH                 HCOH                       HCOH                    HCOH
   H₂COPO₃H₂            H₂COPO₃H₂                  H₂COPO₃H₂               H₂COPO₃H₂
6-Phosphogluconic      3-Keto-6-                  Ribulose-              Ribose-
     acid            phosphogluconic             5-phosphate           5-phosphate
                          acid
```

The reversibility of this reaction has been demonstrated by the fixation of $^{14}CO_2$ in 6-phosphogluconate.

It is possible that pentoses, e.g., ribose, may be converted to triose phosphate, as shown in Fig. 9-12, and then metabolized by the classic glycolytic pathway. It has also been claimed that deoxyribose, as its 3-phosphate ester, may be formed by the aldol condensation of acetaldehyde with glyceraldehyde-3-phosphate:

```
   CHO                CHO                               HCOH
   HCOH       +       CH₃      ─── Aldol ───→           CH₂
   H₂COPO₃H₂                    condensation            HCOH
D-Glyceraldehyde-3-    Acetaldehyde                     HCOH
   phosphate                                            H₂COPO₃H₂
                                                    2-Deoxy-D-ribose-5-
                                                        phosphate
```

The pentose phosphate shunt thus now appears to be an important pathway for pentose biosynthesis from hexoses and likewise for pentose degradation.

Biosynthesis of uronic acids Mention should be made of the pathway by which the uronic acids are formed. One of these substances, glucuronic acid, is extremely important for detoxication purposes (p. 754) as well as for the formation of such compounds as heparin, hyaluronic acid, and the mucopolysaccharides. The formation of glucuronic acid is believed to be as follows:

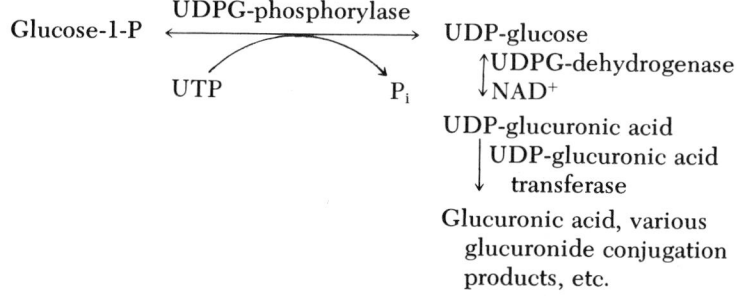

217

Other uronic acids, e.g., galacturonic acid, are presumably formed in a similar manner.

Interconversions of glucuronic acid. Glucuronic acid may be converted to D-xylulose and then further metabolized by way of the pentose phosphate pathway in the following manner:

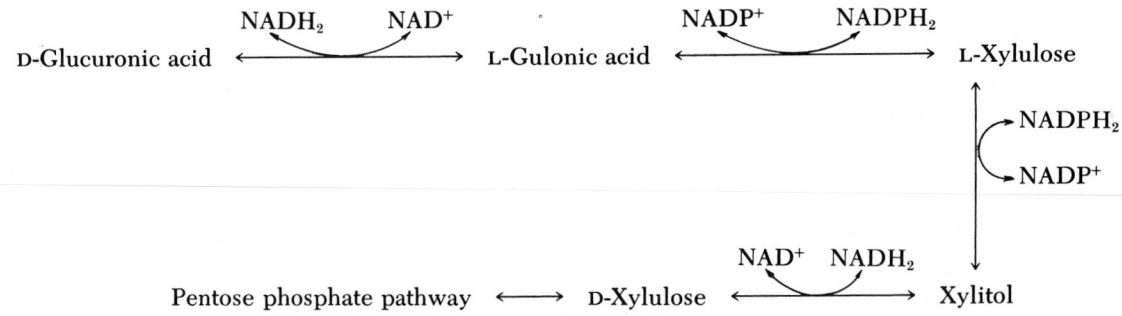

The reactions appear to be reversible, depending on substrate concentrations and other conditions. Appropriate enzymes are involved.

Biosynthesis of hexosamines Glucosamine appears to be formed from fructose-6-phosphate in the presence of glutamine and then converted in the presence of acetyl-CoA, ATP, and UTP to uridine diphosphate–N-acetylglucosamine. The UDP moiety is apparently split off when N-acetylglucosamine is incorporated into the mucopolysaccharides of connective tissue and other substances. N-acetylgalactosamine and N-acetylmannosamine are probably formed in a similar manner.

Abnormalities in the biosynthesis of mucopolysaccharides or in their association with proteins in connective tissue occur occasionally in man. For example, in gargoylism there appears to be a defect in the combination of mucopolysaccharides with protein, resulting in distortions of the skeleton and tissue defects. Large amounts of mucopolysaccharides may be excreted in the urine.

Biosynthesis of sialic acids and glycoproteins The sialic acids (p. 175) are present in a wide variety of mammalian glycoproteins (p. 89). The biosynthesis of these substances appears to occur by the following pathway:

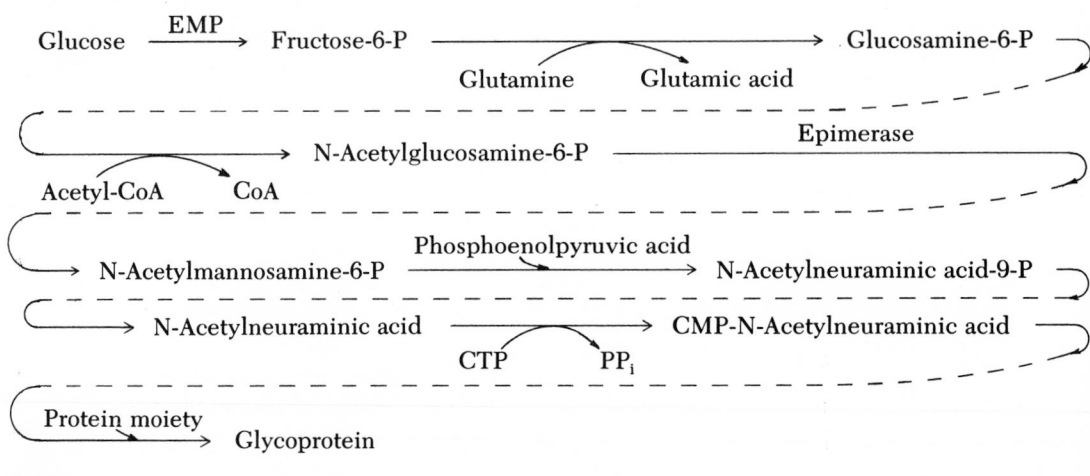

Note the unusual aldol condensation of N-acetylmannosamine-6-P with phosphoenolpyruvic acid to form the sialic acid derivative N-acetylneuraminic acid-9-P. The above biosynthetic pathway has been demonstrated in bacteria and, with slight modifications, in mammals.

PHOTOSYNTHESIS

It is appropriate next to have a brief study of photosynthesis in plants since this is the prime source of carbohydrates for the animal organism.

The primary function of photosynthesis[28,29] in the chloroplasts of green plants is to convert light energy into chemical energy (ATP and $NADPH_2$), which the cell can then use in various ways. One of these is the synthesis of carbohydrates from carbon dioxide. The overall reaction is:

$$6 \ CO_2 + 6 \ H_2O \xrightarrow{\text{Light}} C_6H_{12}O_6 + 6 \ O_2$$

Tiny subunits of the chloroplast membranes that transduce light energy into chemical energy have been called *quantasomes*. These particles are approximately 175 Å in diameter and are readily visualized by electron microscopy. Quantasomes form the well-known lamellae of chloroplasts and appear to be the "power units" of photosynthesis. They are probably also the site of oxygen evolution.

As shown in Fig. 9-14, the chlorophyl molecule plays a key role in photosynthesis by absorbing a photon of light, in the *light reaction*, thus sending an electron to a high-energy or excited state. This electron is captured by

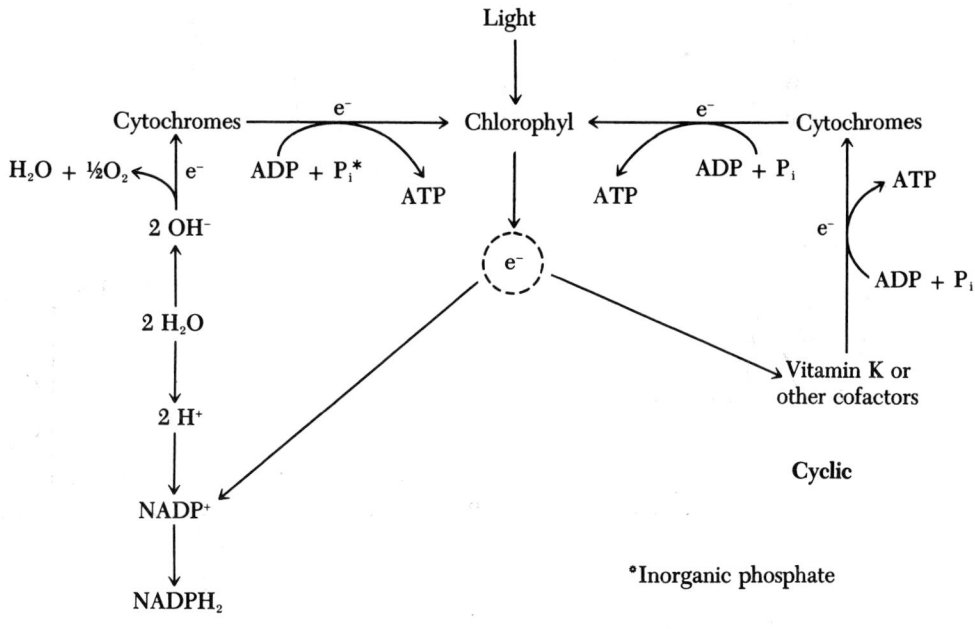

Fig. 9-14. Conversion of light energy to chemical energy (ATP and $NADPH_2$) by *cyclic* and *noncyclic* phosphorylation, the so-called light reaction.

vitamin K, or other cofactors (right side of diagram). The electron then may move to the cytochrome enzyme system, losing energy to a phosphorylating enzyme system, which, in turn, employs the energy to couple a phosphate group to ADP to form ATP. As the electron passes back to chlorophyl from the cytochromes, it again gives up energy to form another molecule of ATP. The chlorophyl molecule acquires a positive charge when the electron is ejected at the start of the cycle and thus is able to pull the returning electron from the cytochromes. This process has been termed cyclic photophosphorylation.

If the high-energy electron from chlorophyl is taken up by $NADP^+$, noncyclic photophosphorylation occurs, as shown on the left portion of Fig. 9-14. In this case, protons (H^+) from the dissociation of water are utilized to convert $NADP^+$ to $NADPH_2$, which can then be used in the biosynthesis of carbohydrate from carbon dioxide, by the *dark reaction*, as indicated in Fig. 9-15. Meanwhile, the hydroxyl groups left combine with each other to form water plus gaseous oxygen, characteristically evolved during photosynthesis. This process thus accounts for the major sequences occurring during photosynthesis, i.e., the conversion via chlorophyl of light energy to chemical energy as ATP, the formation of $NADPH_2$ to supply hydrogen atoms for carbohydrate formation, the conversion of carbon dioxide to carbohydrate, and the evolution of gaseous oxygen. The ATP and $NADPH_2$ can also be utilized, of course, for the biosynthesis of fat, certain amino acids, and other important biochemical substances in the plant.

It will be noted in Fig. 9-15 that carbon dioxide fixation in photosynthesis involves the addition of this molecule to ribulose-5-phosphate, formed by

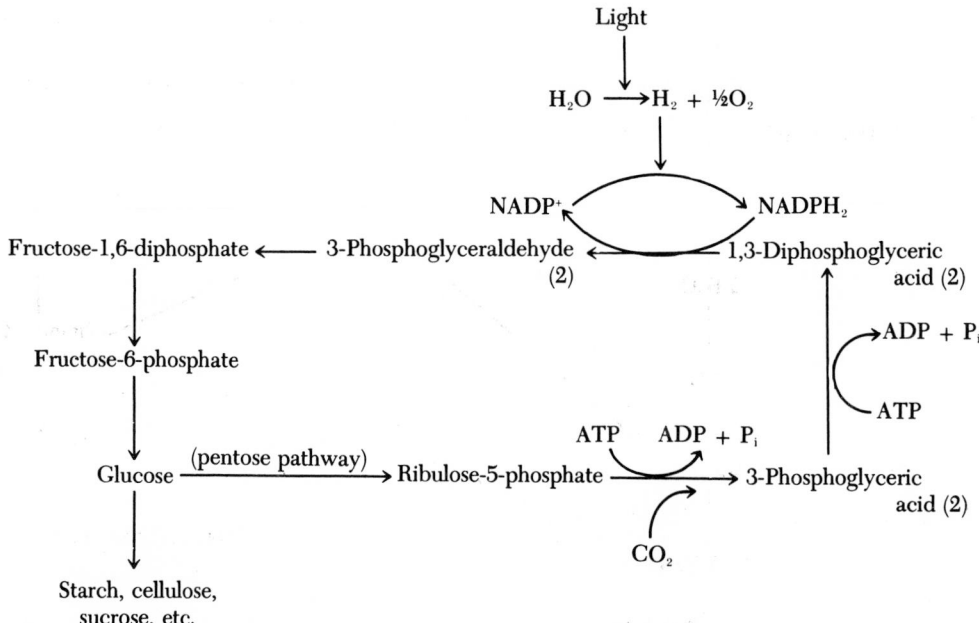

Fig. 9-15. Formation of carbohydrate by photosynthesis and CO_2 fixation, the so-called dark reaction.

way of the pentose pathway (p. 209). Actually, ribulose-5-phosphate is first converted by ATP to ribulose-1,5-diphosphate, which reacts with CO_2 to form an unstable derivative, probably a 2-carboxy derivative of the enol form. The reaction is catalyzed by the appropriate carboxylase enzyme. The unstable intermediate cleaves spontaneously in the presence of water to form two molecules of 3-phosphoglyceric acid. Using ATP formed in the light reaction, 3-phosphoglycerate is converted to 1,3-diphosphoglycerate and then to 3-phosphoglyceraldehyde with $NADPH_2$ (from the light reaction). The enzymes catalyzing the last two reactions are the appropriate kinase and dehydrogenase, respectively. Two molecules of 3-phosphoglyceraldehyde, in the presence of triose isomerase and aldolase, react to form one molecule of fructose-1,6-diphosphate. From this, fructose-6-phosphate and glucose can be formed by enzymatic reactions similar to those of the glycolytic pathway in animals (p. 198). Glucose can then be converted to sucrose, starch, cellulose, and other plant carbohydrates; or glucose can be converted back to ribulose-5-phosphate by way of a plant pentose pathway, again similar to that in animals (p. 209). Ribulose-5-phosphate can be converted by ATP and phosphoribulokinase to ribulose-1,5-diphosphate, and carbon dioxide fixation by the cycle can be repeated. The overall reaction is thus:

$$6 \text{ Ribulose-5-phosphate} + 6 \text{ } CO_2 + 18 \text{ ATP} + 12 \text{ } NADPH_2 + 6 \text{ } H_2O \rightarrow 1 \text{ Glucose}$$
$$+ 6 \text{ Ribulose-5-phosphate} + 18 \text{ ADP} + 18 \text{ } P_i + 12 \text{ } NADP^+$$

In summary, then, *six CO_2*, in the presence of *ribulose-5-phosphate, ATP, $NADPH_2$*, and *H_2O*, form *one glucose*, as stated earlier. Eventually, of course, photons of light would be required to replenish the supply of ATP and $NADPH_2$ by the light reaction.

There is recent evidence[30] for another, more direct, route for photosynthesis, at least in the photosynthetic bacterium *Chromatium*. This pathway involves carbon dioxide fixation into a two-carbon compound, acetyl-CoA, to form pyruvic acid. Hydrogen gas, the enzyme *pyruvate synthetase*, and the unique iron-protein complex ferredoxin are also required. Ferredoxin, called *photosynthetic pyridine nucleotide reductase*, is an electron acceptor. The mechanism involved appears to be as follows:

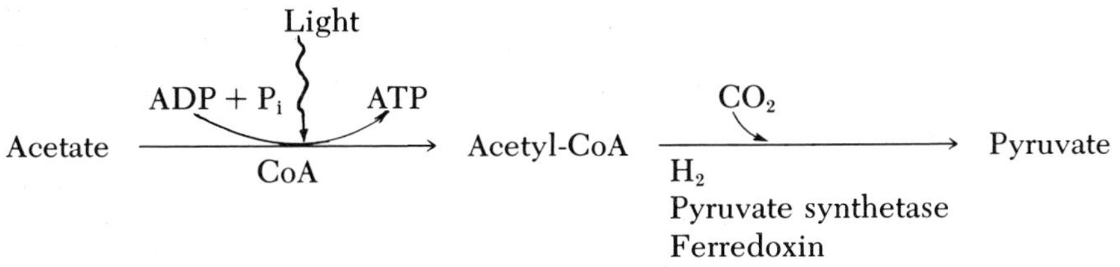

Pyruvate then can be converted to glucose and other carbohydrates by the usual pathways (p. 209). A number of other mechanisms for photosynthesis have been suggested.

ABNORMAL CARBOHYDRATE METABOLISM

The more common abnormalities of carbohydrate metabolism appear to be due to enzyme, hormone, dietary, or genetic deficiencies. The last, of course, may be manifested as enzyme or hormone deficiencies and are sometimes called "inborn errors of metabolism." Genetic deficiencies affecting the metabolism of carbohydrates may be classified into four main categories: (1) those involving the hexoses glucose, fructose, and galactose; (2) those involving the pentose L-xylulose (pentosuria); (3) those affecting glycogen metabolism; and (4) those related to abnormal glycolysis in the erythrocytes. Most of the conditions have already been discussed. However, further consideration of abnormalities in the metabolism of glucose is now pertinent.

An understanding of many of the phases of normal carbohydrate metabolism has come from a study of pathologic or experimental derangements. Most of these result in glucosuria. Glucosuria is merely a symptom of a metabolic disorder. The glucose appears in the urine either because the blood sugar is too high or the renal threshold is too low, and the real problem is why does either of these occur. The first to be considered is alimentary glucosuria. This is easy to understand. It occurs when large amounts of carbohydrate are available in the gastrointestinal tract and are absorbed more rapidly than they can be assimilated by the normal processes. The blood sugar rises above the renal threshold and glucosuria results. Individuals, however, vary in their power to utilize excessive quantities of carbohydrates, due in all probability to differences in their endocrine balance. Consequently alimentary glucosuria may be more easily provoked in some persons than in others.

The piqûre of Claude Bernard, i.e., an injury to the floor of the fourth ventricle, is an experimental method of inducing hyperglycemia with consequent glucosuria. It is probably a stimulation of the adrenal medulla, via the splanchnic nerves, causing an increased secretion of epinephrine, which is apparently the effective factor. Direct stimulation of the great splanchnic nerves or injection of epinephrine has the same result. The epinephrine increases glycogenolysis in the liver (p. 195) and the blood sugar rises. It has a similar action on muscle glycogen. All of these are temporary effects.

When phlorizin is administered to animals, glucosuria results. This was discovered by von Mering and has been developed and used in the United States by Lusk and others. The glucosuria continues as long as the drug is given, with results such as would be expected from a continued loss of sugar. The condition differs from true diabetes mellitus in that the glycemia is either normal or slightly below normal. The explanation[6] is that phlorizin interferes with the renal absorption of the glucose. The glomerulus permits glucose to filter through it into the tubules, from which normally it is reabsorbed. This reabsorption is blocked by phlorizin, and the glucose flows through the tubules into the urine. Thus, in phlorizin diabetes we have a low renal threshold due to a failure in absorption of glucose.

Nonhyperglycemic glucosuria occurs in man occasionally. Such a condition is "renal diabetes" or *renal glucosuria,* a rather rare state. The blood sugar is normal or below normal. Sugar is present in the urine at all times and is almost independent of the amount of carbohydrate ingested. There is no apparent disturbance of carbohydrate metabolism. This is evidenced by a normal respiratory quotient and no change in fat metabolism. It apparently never develops into diabetes mellitus and seems to be a harmless malady. The cause is unknown.

In a fairly large percentage of normal pregnant women glucosuria occurs. This is not a lactosuria, which is more likely to be found during the period of lactation. It is said to be due to a decreased carbohydrate tolerance resulting from physiologic hypertrophy of the pituitary gland that occurs during pregnancy. The blood sugar does not rise much above normal.

Glucosuria with hyperglycemia is known as *diabetes mellitus,* when it occurs in man. Among the symptoms of severe cases are excessive thirst and polyuria. If uncontrolled, there are muscular weakness and acidosis, with the possibility of diabetic coma and death. The excessive thirst and polyuria are due to the large amount of water needed to dissolve the glucose as it is excreted by the kidneys. The weakness is mostly due to the inability to utilize the requisite amount of food and often to dehydration due to the polyuria. The acidosis and coma result from excessive fat metabolism, which takes place concurrently with the disturbance in carbohydrate metabolism. Another effect is on protein metabolism. If the malady is not controlled, the patient goes into negative nitrogen balance. Thus diabetes is a disturbance of carbohydrate, fat, and protein metabolism.

For many years there was a suspicion that the pancreas was in some way related to diabetes. There was no proof of this until 1889-1891, when von Mering and Minkowski succeeded in completely removing the pancreas of a dog surgically. This was an exceptionally difficult feat since the pancreas is quite adherent to the duodenum. Moreover, the healing of the abdominal wound is difficult in the absence of the internal secretion of the pancreas. However, these workers did accomplish the feat and thereby ushered in a new era in the study of carbohydrate metabolism in general and of diabetes mellitus in particular. These depancreatized dogs developed a pathologic state that resembled severe human diabetes mellitus. They had hyperglycemia and glucosuria, became exceedingly thirsty and hungry, and passed large volumes of urine. In time, they grew weak and thin, had acetone bodies in blood and urine, and died in coma in from 2 to 6 weeks. If, instead of being removed, the pancreas was transplanted, with nerves and blood vessels intact, outside the peritoneal cavity and was left under the skin, diabetes did not result. This proved that the external secretion, i.e., the pancreatic juice, is not the factor involved in preventing diabetes. Subsequent removal of the transplanted pancreas caused glucosuria to occur.

Following the work of these pioneers, many experimenters attempted to determine the mechanism of this action. The explanation advanced by Lèpine was that the pancreas produces an internal secretion (besides its external digestive secretion) that is poured directly into the bloodstream and in some way regulates carbohydrate metabolism. A number of investigators planned various cross-transfusions between diabetic and normal animals and in vitro tissue and blood studies. Although not decisive, they indicated that the pancreas has an internal secretion that is effective only in the living animal. Carlson depancreatized a pregnant bitch and found that she did not become diabetic until after the pups were born. The fetal pancreases had protected the mother by their internal secretions.

The crucial experiment of injecting pancreatic extracts into diabetic animals was attempted many times, but the early work was indecisive. In 1908, Zuelzer prepared an alcoholic extract and noted reductions in the output of urinary sugar and acetone bodies in a diabetic dog and several patients. However, a decrease in urinary sugar is not a satisfactory criterion of improvement in this condition since it may result from a diminished intake of food, due to a loss of appetite resulting from treatment or to an influence on the kidneys. E. L. Scott used water extracts of pancreatic tissue that had previously been extracted with alcohol. Upon injection of these extracts into diabetic dogs, the sugar excretion was diminished and the glucose:nitrogen ratio also lowered (p. 363). This indicated that some of the glucose presumably arising from protein metabolism was being utilized, which discovery marked a distinct advance. In 1915, Kleiner and Meltzer[31] showed that a simple aqueous emulsion of pancreatic tissue, when injected very slowly intravenously into diabetic dogs, has an almost immediate effect in lowering the blood sugar and, of course, the excretion of glucose. This was considered definite evidence that the pancreas has an internal secretion that can be obtained from it by appropriate extraction methods, and they suggested that it might have possible therapeutic applications.

INSULIN

The climax of these many series of experiments came in 1922. Banting and Best conducted some brilliant researches that led to the discovery of insulin. The pancreas contains two types of cells, the acinar or glandular cells, which secrete the pancreatic juice and make up the bulk of pancreatic tissue, and groups of small, irregular, polygonal cells. The latter were discovered by Langerhans, in 1867, and have been called the *islets of Langerhans* or simply "islet tissue." It was suspected that here was the site of manufacture of the internal secretion of the pancreas. In fact D'Arnozan and Viaclard had shown that if the pancreatic ducts are tied off, so that pancreatic juice cannot flow into the duodenum, the acinar cells degenerate and disappear and nothing is left of the pancreas except islet tissue. Such animals do not develop diabetes. The idea occured to Banting,[32] "Ligate pancreatic ducts of dogs. Wait six to eight weeks for degeneration. Remove the residue and extract." After considerable difficulty, Banting and Best were able to perform this double experiment with results that bore out Banting's expectations.

The extract prepared from such islet tissue proved to have a potent effect in reducing the hyperglycemia of diabetic dogs, and, after careful purification, it was found to have similar effects on diabetic human beings. The best sources and methods of extracting, purifying, and concentrating insulin were sought. It has been known that in certain teleostean fishes the islets of Langerhans exist as organs separate from the acinar pancreatic cells. These furnished extracts having the same properties as those obtained from mammals, which gave added proof that the islets of Langerhans were the source of insulin.

Beef and hog pancreas are the commercial sources of insulin at present, and several methods of preparation have been devised. Insulin is soluble in water, in alcohol of a strength up to about 80%, in acids, and in alkalies. However, it is not stable in alkaline solution. Collip's method employs the principle of fractional precipitation with alcohol. Doisy, Somogyi, and Shaffer made use of the fact that insulin is least soluble at its isoelectric point, pH 5.3, and that impurities may be precipitated out of solution and thus be removed at pH's above or below 5.3. From preparations of insulin used therapeutically, Abel and collaborators obtained insulin in two different crystalline forms. However, it was undoubtedly one substance, i.e., a protein with a molecular weight of 5734. Its amino acid composition and structure have been described on p. 76. Cystine occurs in large amounts, and there is some evidence that the disulfide group is connected with its physiologic activity. Zinc is always found with this hormone but is not a part of the insulin molecule. The crystals are probably the zinc salt of insulin. Since insulin is a protein, it is, not surprisingly, digested and thus inactivated by the proteolytic enzymes pepsin and trypsin. Hence insulin has no effect when taken orally and must be administered parenterally. This constitutes one of the chief difficulties and objections to its use.

Alloxan diabetes. The injection of alloxan into animals is a chemical method of producing diabetes. It causes an initial hyperglycemia that is apparently due to a stimulation of the adrenal medulla. A transitory hypoglycemia, probably a result of liberation of insulin from the β-cells of the pancreas, is then seen. If glucose is now given to tide the animal over the hypoglycemic phase, hyperglycemia and other diabetic symptoms ensue.[33] The final effect is a necrosis of the β-cells, which produces the permanent diabetes. Alloxan is an oxidative product of uric acid:

Uric acid   Alloxan

The diabetes of these animals is characterized by very severe glycosuria with a high insulin requirement. However, the animals have a low ketone body excretion and if untreated with insulin live longer than depancreatized dogs under similar conditions. This is related to the fact that there are two types of cells in the islets of Langerhans, the α- and the β-cells, and their different functions have been strikingly shown experimentally. Dogs were made diabetic by the administration of alloxan, which destroyed their β-cells, and their insulin requirement was determined. They were then depancreatized, thus losing their α-cells as well as their β-cells. The insulin requirement was now found to be much *less* than before. The interpretation was as follows: Insulin is produced by the β-cells, and another hormone, *glucagon,* by the α-cells. The latter hormone has an opposite action to that of insulin, increasing blood sugar, and may also prevent the formation of excessive amounts of ketone bodies. Consequently an alloxan-diabetic dog not only lacks insulin because it lacks the β-cells, but it possesses a factor that still further acts in the same way that a deficiency of insulin does. Therefore the dog's blood sugar is higher than that of a depancreatized dog. Alloxan diabetes may be prevented if glutathione or cysteine is given along with the alloxan. It is possible that glutathione and cysteine reduce alloxan to dialuric acid, a substance that presumably has no diabetogenic effect. On the other hand, alloxan inactivates coenzyme-A, which, like cysteine and glutathione, has a sulfhydryl group. It is thought that the diabetogenic action of alloxan may, in part, be due to the inactivation of coenzyme-A within the β-cells of the islets of Langerhans, thus destroying those cells.

Whether these observations have any bearing on the etiology of the disease in man is still a matter of speculation, but it is interesting to note that the presence of alloxan in normal liver tissue has been reported.

In this connection it may be of interest to note that dehydroascorbic acid, dehydroisoascorbic acid, and dehydroglucoascorbic acid are all diabetogenic, and the explanation offered is that they act by destroying the sulfhydryl groups of enzymes essential to normal carbohydrate utilization. Evidently sulfhydryl and disulfide groups are quite important in carbohydrate metabolism. In fact, it has been shown that the sulfhydryl content of blood and tissues falls in depancreatized animals and that pretreatment with sulfhydryl compounds decreases the severity of the resultant diabetes. Among other compounds that have been shown to cause diabetes experimentally are β-hydroxybutyric acid and other intermediary products of fat metabolism.

Glucagon. Glucagon has been isolated and crystallized.[34] It is a protein but is quite different from insulin in its crystalline form and in having a low sulfur content. The small amount of sulfur present is in the form of methionine rather than cystine. The amino acid sequence of the 29 amino acids comprising the peptide chain has been determined. The pancreas of birds is very rich in this factor, and, since there is also present in bird pancreas a great number of cells resembling α-cells, this lends support to the concept that glucagon is formed by the α-cells of the pancreatic islets. The action of glucagon is manifested in the brief period of hyperglycemia that occurs after commercial insulin is injected intravenously into animals with adequate stores of liver glycogen. Glucagon is an impurity present in most brands of insulin. In fasted animals, glucagon has no effect. It thus appears to be a glycogenolytic agent but not a gluconeogenetic one. It causes hyperglycemia by accelerating liver glycogenolysis, but it has no effect on muscle glycogen. Pancreatectomy *decreases* the insulin requirement of the diabetic patient. Glucagon is believed to increase the activity of the enzyme phosphorylase as does epinephrine.

Besides its effect on carbohydrate metabolism, glucagon has other anti-insulin actions. It favors the production of ketogenic substances and inhibits the synthesis of fatty acids. It also increases protein metabolism, particularly in liver and muscle tissue.

Action of insulin When insulin is injected into a normal animal (rabbits are usually the species employed), the blood sugar falls to very low levels – 30 to 50 mg.%. "True" blood sugar (i.e., that due to glucose, apart from that due to non-sugars) is even lower and may fall to almost zero. Frequently convulsions ensue, with a possibly fatal outcome. They can be combatted if glucose is given soon after they begin. The effect of glucose under these circumstances is astonishing. In a very few minutes the animal, which has been lying on its side having violent convulsive movements, rights itself and hops around in a perfectly normal manner. This effect of insulin on the rabbit is utilized in standardizing commercial preparations (p. 463).

In diabetic animals and human beings the effect of insulin is the same. Insulin lowers blood sugar and thereby diminishes glucosuria. If ketonemia and acidosis are present, it tends to combat these conditions also. The effect, however, is temporary; the blood sugar eventually rises again and insulin must be administered at least once a day in order to keep the blood sugar at a normal level. The decrease in blood sugar is accompanied by glycogenesis in both liver and muscle. There is an increased consumption of oxygen and a consequent rise in the respiratory quotient, which indicates the utilization of glucose by the tissues. There is an inhibition of gluconeogenesis, i.e., the formation of glucose from proteins and fats. Last, insulin promotes the formation of fat.

Injection of epinephrine into normal animals at first causes glycogenolysis in both liver and muscle. The liver glycogen is converted to glucose and increases the blood sugar. The muscle glycogen forms lactic acid, which is carried back to the liver in the bloodstream to form liver glycogen, the level of which may eventually exceed that present before the epinephrine injection. Any insulin administered to a normal animal or person is an excess over the optimal amount already present. It prevents liver glycogenolysis at first and causes hypoglycemia. The blood sugar "lost" is deposited in the muscles as muscle glycogen. Now the hypoglycemia paradoxically opposes the effect of insulin on the hepatic glycogen because hypoglycemia causes the secretion of epinephrine. This is a normal physiologic result of hypoglycemia and is an emergency mechanism resulting in the epinephrine-glycogenolysis action; i.e., the effect of insulin here is to produce hypoglycemia; hypoglycemia causes the production of epinephrine; epinephrine results in glycogenolysis intended to counteract hypoglycemia. The sugar thus released is deposited in the muscles as glycogen and the blood sugar remains normal.

Glucose tolerance tests. A surprisingly large amount of glucose may be ingested by a normal person without any being excreted in the urine. At the same time there is only a moderate rise of blood sugar, and this for only a short time. If diabetes, even in the mildest degree, or renal diabetes, or certain other endocrine or renal disturbances exist, there is very likely to be glucosuria and an entirely different blood sugar picture. By a standard procedure known as a glucose tolerance test, more or less characteristic blood sugar curves are obtained. A solution of glucose supplying from 1.5 to 1.75 gm. per kilogram of body weight in a 50% solution, flavored with

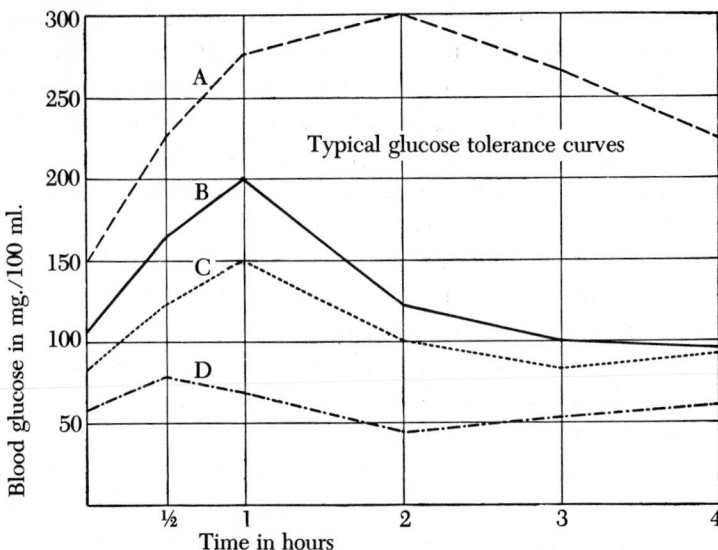

Fig. 9-16. Typical glucose tolerance curves. *A*, Diabetes mellitus; *B*, hyperthyroidism; *C*, normal; *D*, Addison's disease, or hypothyroidism, or hyperinsulinism. (From Andes, J. E., and Eaton, A. G.: Synopsis of applied pathological chemistry, St. Louis, 1941, The C. V. Mosby Co.)

lemon, is frequently used. Some workers favor other amounts; still others use a standard meal containing protein, carbohydrate, and fat. The blood is taken before the glucose or the meal is ingested and at regular intervals thereafter. Perhaps the most generally adopted plan is to take one sample at the half hour, then at the end of the first, second, and third hours. A normal curve is one that reaches its maximum (seldom over 160 mg.) at or before the end of the first hour, with a return to normal by the end of the second or, at most, third hour. Diminished tolerance is indicated by a more marked rise and a slower return to normal. The urine should be collected at about the same time each blood sample is taken. Normally there is little or no sugar excreted. A normal or subnormal curve *with glucosuria* is evidence of renal diabetes. A high curve (diminished tolerance), if accompanied by glucosuria, indicates diabetes mellitus, or a prediabetic state if the curve is not greatly accentuated. A high curve with no glucosuria may mean a renal condition with or without diabetes mellitus. Typical curves are shown in Fig. 9-16.

In the treatment of diabetes mellitus in human beings, the physician must estimate the correct amount of insulin to be given to enable the patient to utilize the carbohydrate needed for his activities. This will vary with the severity of the disease and the energy requirements of the patient. Insulin is given about a half hour before a meal in order to allow for proper absorption and distribution. An overdose is likely to have very unfortunate results. At first there may be hunger or a feeling of nervousness. This is followed by perspiration, alternate pallor and flushing, and dizziness. There may even be delirium, stupor, and convulsions. Many individuals who take insulin regularly wear identification tags stating that they are likely to have hypo-

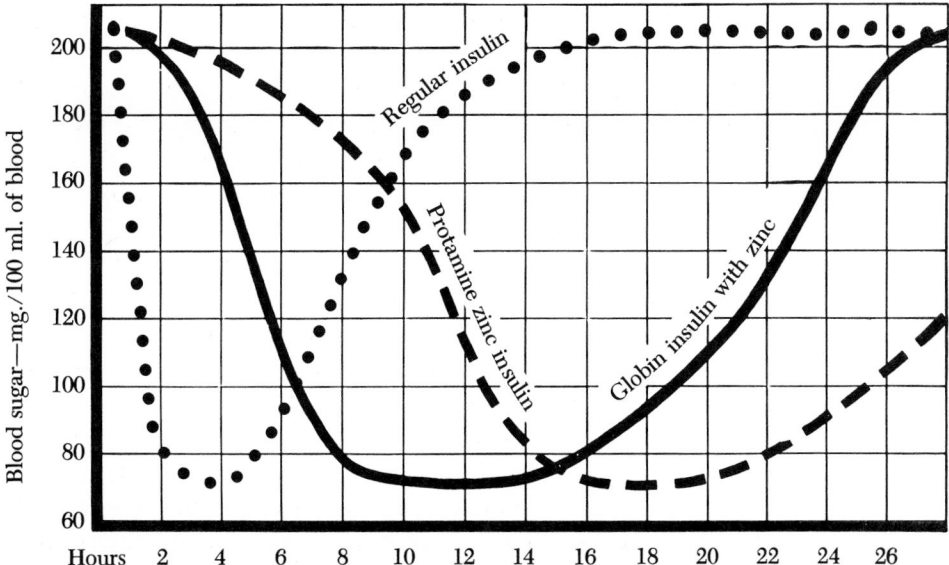

Fig. 9-17. General types of blood sugar curves following the administration of regular insulin, protamine-Zn insulin, and globin insulin. (Courtesy D. D. Searle, Burroughs Wellcome & Co., Inc.)

glycemic symptoms and giving instructions as to the treatment to be given them. A diabetic patient suffering from insulin shock should receive glucose intravenously but no additional insulin, whereas a patient in diabetic coma should be given insulin. Some diabetic patients can recognize the premonitory symptoms, whereupon they take some sugar or candy, which they must have with them at all times. Because of the inconveniences and possible dangers in the use of insulin, patients with mild cases are almost always treated by dietary regulation alone.

Since the effects of insulin wear off rather rapidly, several preparations that are absorbed slowly and therefore act over a longer period are now available. The first of these was produced by combining protamine with insulin, forming a sort of conjugated protein, protamine insulin. The addition of zinc to this gave protamine-zinc insulin, which is still more slowly absorbed. Globin insulin is a compound of globin, derived from hemoglobin, and insulin. This also contains added zinc. The onset of its effect is more rapid than the onset of the protamine-zinc insulin effect but not quite as rapid as the onset of the regular insulin effect. Its hypoglycemic action is not as prolonged as that of the protamine-zinc insulin. In Fig. 9-17 are shown the general types of blood sugar curves produced by the latter two in comparison with regular insulin. Another type of protamine insulin is called NPH (neutral protamine Hagedorn). Its action resembles that of globin insulin.

In the usual treatment of a diabetic patient, there is a nice adjustment of the diet and the insulin dosage. Often a mixture of regular and slow-acting insulin is prescribed, the regular for a quick effect and the slow-acting to sustain this effect. In severe cases the administration of insulin may have to be repeated in the course of the day. The total caloric and nitrogen requirements are calculated, and a diet carefully planned. There are several types of diet advocated by various authorities. The type, dosage, and timing of the insulin administration vary with the individual patient and with the experience of the physician. The aim is to keep the blood sugar level as near normal as possible, in order to accomplish the maximum utilization of carbohydrate, and also to prevent hyperglycemia, which is believed by some clinicians to have a harmful effect on tissues.

Another type of treatment should also be presented. This is called *clinical control* as contrasted with "chemical control," outlined above. Clinical control has the objectives of (1) elimination of the symptoms of the disease, (2) maintenance of or gain in weight, and (3) avoidance of ketonemia. Hyperglycemia and glucosuria are disregarded as long as no diabetic symptoms are present. The diet is not carefully computed; indeed the patient is allowed an almost normal diet. One daily dose of slow-acting insulin is given. The amount of insulin used depends on the severity of the condition. The rationale is that the insulin should permit of a sufficient utilization of carbohydrate for ordinary needs and the excess in the blood does no harm.

An approach from the nutritional side may also be mentioned. A study of a large number of diabetic patients gave evidence of some deficiency of the B vitamins in every case. It was pointed out that in diabetes there is an impairment of hepatic function. Therefore the administration of fairly large amounts of B vitamins and liver extract is advocated, and blood sugar levels and insulin requirements are usually reduced.

Mechanism of insulin action The points where some of the actions of insulin have been postulated are shown in Fig. 9-18. The first clue to the exact mechanism of insulin action was the discovery of its effect in the hexokinase or glucokinase reaction. Glucokinase is the enzyme that catalyzes the phosphorylation of glucose. ATP is the coenzyme or phosphate donor in this reaction. The formation of glucose-6-phosphate is a prerequisite for any further step in the utilization of glucose. Study of the scheme given in Fig. 9-18 will demonstrate the key position of glucose-6-phosphate both for the formation of glycogen from glucose and for the oxidation of glucose, whether derived from glycogen or from food. Utilization of glucose is inhibited by anterior pituitary extract, and this inhibition is abolished by insulin. Thus far no direct effect of insulin alone on the reaction has been discovered but only the indirect one described. Neither glucose nor fructose is converted to fatty acids by diabetic liver slices, although this process is accomplished by normal liver tissue. Insulin enables the diabetic tissue to make this conversion. This metabolic block has been localized at the point (3) where a two-carbon degradation product of the sugars is utilized in the formation of fatty acids. It has also been demonstrated[35] that the levels of the individual acids of the tricarboxylic acid cycle (4) are decreased in the livers of alloxan-diabetic rats and furthermore that little or no ^{14}C from labeled acetate is incorporated into the cycle acids in diabetic rat liver in contrast to the rapid incorporation in normal livers.

Another hypothesis involves the first step in the utilization of glucose.[36] This states that insulin facilitates the passage of glucose into the cell (1)

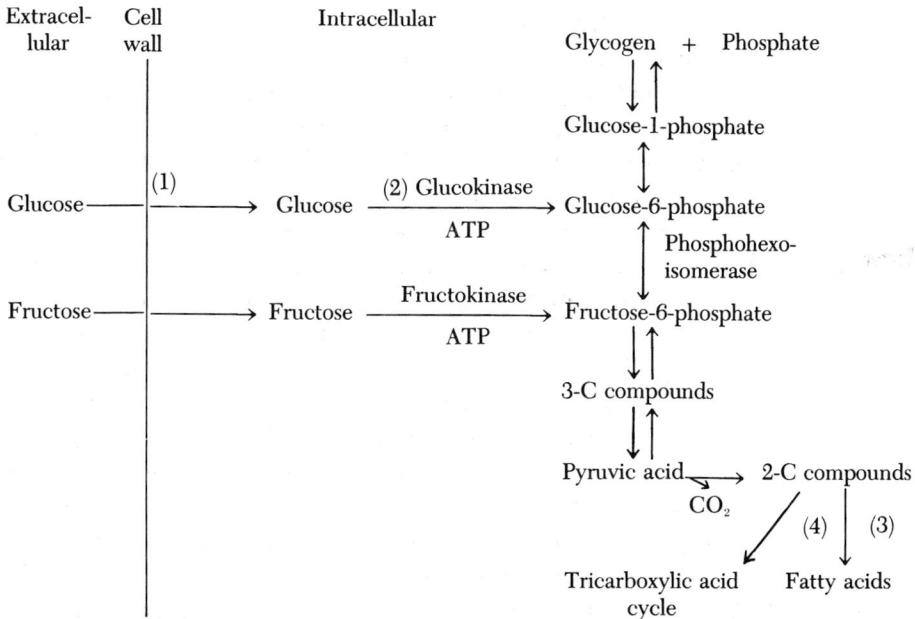

Fig. 9-18. Postulated locations of the action of insulin.

independently of the glucokinase reaction. Whether it has an effect on the permeability of the cell membrane is not definitely stated. Skeletal muscle does not have any galactokinase activity, but insulin facilitates the rate of distribution of D-galactose and does the same for L-arabinose and D-xylose. These three sugars, the only ones showing the same effect, have the same configuration of the first three carbons as has D-glucose. Stadie showed that insulin is combined at the surface of intact muscle fibers, a prerequisite for its action. Thus, the fixation of insulin may be related in some way to the phenomenon just described.

Current studies indicate still another possible explanation for the mechanism of insulin action—that insulin causes the *induction of certain enzymes* involved in carbohydrate metabolism. Specifically, insulin appears to induce the biosynthesis of hepatic pyruvate kinase,[37] perhaps by stimulating the production of a species of RNA involved in the formation of this enzyme. Insulin also affects the biosynthesis of glucokinase and phosphofructokinase, enzymes that apparently occupy the same functional genome unit.[38] If these indeed prove to be *direct* effects of insulin on subsequent studies, a new concept of the mode of action of at least this one hormone, insulin, may become established.

Insulin restores the ability of heart muscle to synthesize phosphocreatine, when this ability has been diminished by alloxan diabetes. This hormone has also been shown to have beneficial effects in carbohydrate metabolism in a number of in vitro experiments. For example, it increases the amount of pyruvate metabolized to carbon dioxide by diabetic muscle. This was ascertained by using pyruvate labeled with ^{14}C. It also stimulates the synthesis of fatty acids from acetate when pyruvate is also present. Indeed, some intracellular block or delay in glucose utilization at or below the level of pyruvate has been suggested[39] as a cause of diabetes. Furthermore, insulin has an effect on protein metabolism. It appears to be required for the nitrogen storage action of the growth hormone. The latter causes the secretion of extra insulin. The extra insulin then has a synergistic action with the growth hormone on protein anabolism.

Insulin antagonists It is known that most diabetics have a normal amount of insulin in the blood; and it has been suggested that a lack of endogenous insulin is not the sole cause of diabetes mellitus.[40] There may be a malfunction of the mechanism regulating insulin activity in the blood; i.e., insulin antagonists exist, and, indeed, three types have been discovered: (1) there are insulin antagonists in tissues; these "insulinases" act presumably as enzymes, destroying insulin; (2) some diabetics are resistant to insulin injections; this is due to the presence or formation of insulin antibodies, associated with plasma globulins; (3) other diabetics have antagonists preformed in the blood; these are part of the albumin fraction of the plasma proteins.[41] After incubation with adipose tissue extracts, the insulin activity is restored. Still another antagonist, a globulin, has been discovered in patients with severe diabetic acidosis.[42] The latter is thought to be responsible for the high insulin dosage often necessary for control of diabetic coma.

Oral hypoglycemic agents. Perhaps it should be mentioned at this point that insulin had scarcely been discovered before a search for oral insulin substitutes began. The reason is obvious since insulin must be administered by injection. A number of such substitutes have been described but have been discarded because of transient effect, toxic side reactions such as liver damage, etc.

Recently, interest in this field has been revived by the discovery that certain sulfonylurea derivatives are effective orally in reducing the blood sugar and glycosuria in certain types of diabetics. One of the most promising of these is tolbutamide (1-butyl-3-tolylsulfonylurea). With proper dosage it appears to be nontoxic, having first been studied in more than 13,000 patients for periods up to nearly 2 years. Animal studies also indicate a relatively low toxicity. The drug seems to be particularly effective in the control of milder cases of diabetes in adults, especially those over 40 years of age or those with associated overweight. Many patients were able to discontinue insulin therapy. It is not effective in the diabetes of young persons.

The mechanism of action of the sulfonylureas as hypoglycemic agents is not yet understood. There is some evidence that they may increase the secretion of insulin by the pancreas or may decrease the destruction of insulin by an "insulinase" in tissues,[43] or they may inhibit hepatic phosphatase or hepatic glycogenolysis. However, the most probable explanation seems to be that they release endogenous insulin from the β-cells of the pancreas. Oral hypoglycemic agents have no effect in pancreatectomized animals or in diabetic patients with functionally inactive islets of Langerhans.

Another group of oral hypoglycemic drugs are the biguanides, such as phenformin.[44] They apparently have a different mode of action from the sulfonylureas, not yet fully understood. They appear to interfere with insulin's potent lipogenic activity, thus reducing the diabetic's tendency to become obese.

Hypoglycemia. Before the advent of insulin, little was known of hypoglycemic conditions. The stimulation of the study of carbohydrate metabolism that this discovery brought about, and particularly the greatly increased number of blood sugar determinations that became almost routine hospital procedure, led to the realization that hypoglycemia is not a rare condition. Proliferation of islet tissue, i.e., tumor of the pancreas, frequently occurs; the increase in insulin secretion causes hypoglycemia. Administration of glucose tends to ameliorate the symptoms, and surgical removal often has a permanent beneficial result. Hypoglycemia also may be caused by a diminution in the secretion of those glands of internal secretion that have an opposite effect to the islets of Langerhans, namely, the anterior pituitary, the thyroid, and either the cortical or the medullary parts of the adrenal gland. An inhibited pituitary secretion, with hypoglycemia, is seen in Simmonds' disease. The adrenal cortex is affected in Addison's disease, with similar effect on the glycemia. In regard to the thyroid, there is increased susceptibility to insulin after surgical removal of that gland. In those pathologic conditions of the liver where there is a great liver damage, hypoglycemia is often discovered. Acute yellow atrophy and hepatitis are examples. Here the results may be attributed to the inability of the liver to take its usual part in carbohydrate transformations.

Another type of hypoglycemia, which Buehler[45] calls "relative hypoglycemia," is also a not uncommon condition. This appears to be due to some lesion of the central nervous system. Among the symptoms are headache, malaise, and nervousness. It is not relieved by administration of carbohydrate. Indeed, the treatment prescribes a high protein–low carbohydrate diet with heavy doses of vitamins, particularly niacinamide.

Of interest is the fact that certain chemical substances, e.g., diazoxide,[46] increase the blood sugar level, apparently by inhibiting the release of insulin from the pancreas. For this reason, diazoxide is being studied intensively as a therapeutic agent in certain hypoglycemic disease states.

INFLUENCE OF OTHER ENDOCRINE GLANDS ON CARBOHYDRATE METABOLISM

That the pancreas is not the only gland having an influence on carbohydrate metabolism has previously been mentioned. This might have been suspected from one curious fact that has been known for a long time. In experimental pancreatic diabetes almost the entire pancreas must be removed before diabetes ensues. Sometimes about one seventh may be left in connection with the pancreatic duct, to provide the digestive fluid, but that is the maximum. Yet many human diabetic cases that come to autopsy have apparently no destruction of pancreatic tissue whatever. It would seem that if the pancreas alone were involved more degenerative changes would be seen by the pathologist. It is known that some clinical disturbances of the adrenal and pituitary glands are associated with hypoglycemia or hyperglycemia. The effect of stimulation of the adrenal medulla and of injection of epinephrine has been mentioned before. This internal secretion has some control over both liver and muscle glycogenolysis. Moderate dosage first lowers liver glycogen and muscle glycogen and then raises liver glycogen, because muscle glycogen is changed to lactic acid, which is carried to the liver and enters into liver glycogenesis. A high dosage of epinephrine results in a decrease of both muscle and liver glycogen because of the loss of sugar in the urine.

Acromegaly is a hyperpituitary condition. It is often accompanied by hyperglycemia and glucosuria. It is an affection of the anterior pituitary gland (see Chapter 22). Thus, apparently the anterior pituitary secretion is antagonistic to the secretion of the islets of Langerhans. This is not an antagonism of a chemical nature: they do not neutralize each other in vitro but have opposing physiologic effects. An anterior pituitary extract accordingly causes hyperglycemia upon injection and opposes the effect of a simultaneous injection of insulin. Removal of the anterior pituitary gland (hypophysectomy) renders the animal hypersensitive to insulin. Houssay and Biasotti[47] showed that if a hypophysectomized animal is later depancreatized either no diabetes results or only a very mild form. Both the diabetes-preventive substance (insulin) and its antagonist formed by the pituitary are absent in such an animal. An animal having this double operation is known as the "Houssay animal." The active substance of the anterior pituitary may be termed the *insulin-antagonizing factor*. Its influence on hexokinase and the opposing action of insulin were mentioned on p. 230.

A second influence of this gland was discovered by Young and is called the *diabetogenic* action. If anterior pituitary extract is injected daily in large amounts into dogs, a permanent state of diabetes results in from 15 to 30 days. This seems to be due to a destruction of the β-cells and complete loss of insulin from the pancreas, similar to the action of alloxan. Both influences of the anterior pituitary are now considered to be due to the action of the growth hormone (p. 488).

In addition, the anterior pituitary gland influences carbohydrate metabolism indirectly by way of ACTH and TSH. The effects of ACTH and TSH are identical with those of the 11-oxycorticosteroids and thyroxine, respectively.

In Addison's disease, a pathologic condition of the adrenal cortex, the blood sugar is usually very low. This can be shown experimentally. Removal of both adrenal glands has the same effect, and it has been demonstrated to be due to the loss of the cortex rather than of the medulla. Furthermore, although adrenocortical extract by itself has no influence, it can intensify the inhibitory effect of anterior pituitary extract on the glucokinase phosphorylating reaction. This also demonstrates the antagonistic relation between the adrenal cortex function and the internal function of the pancreas. Long and associates[48] showed a relation similar to Houssay's for the adrenal gland and pancreas; i.e., adrenalectomy attenuates the diabetes resulting from depancreatization. In such "Long" animals, administration of the hormone of the adrenal cortex accentuates the diabetic condition. The 11-oxycorticosteroids apparently increase gluconeogenesis and increase liver glycogen and, to a lesser extent, muscle glycogen, and they may also inhibit glucose oxidation.

The thyroid, too, has an influence on carbohydrate metabolism. Hyperthyroidism, as exemplified by exophthalmic goiter, is often accompanied by slight hyperglycemia and glucosuria. At first glance this is paradoxic since an increased thyroid activity is associated with heightened metabolism, which would seem to require a greater utilization of blood sugar. However, the explanation seems to lie in an increased rate of hepatic gluconeogenesis or possibly glycogenolysis. The thyroid hormone also aids in absorption of glucose from the intestinal tract. At any rate, hyperthyroidism is usually accompanied by hyperglycemia, and hypothyroidism by hypoglycemia.

References

GENERAL

Cori, G. T.: Glycogen structure and enzyme deficiency in glycogen storage disease, Harvey Lect. **48**:145, 1952.

Dickens, F., Randle, P. J., and Whelan, W. J., editors: Carbohydrate metabolism and its disorders, New York, 1968, Academic Press, Inc.

Greenberg, D. M., editor: Metabolic pathways, ed. 3, New York, 1967, Academic Press, Inc., vol. 1.

Hsai, D. Y.: Inborn errors of metabolism, ed. 2, Chicago, 1966, Year Book Medical Publishers, Inc.

Kleiner, I. S.: Hypoglycemic agents—past and present, Clin. Chem. **5**:79, 1959.

Leloir, L. F.: The biosynthesis of polysaccharides, Proc. 6th Int. Congr. Biochem. **33**:15, 1964.

Levine, R., and Luft, R.: Advances in metabolic disorders, New York, 1964, Academic Press, Inc., vol. 1.

Renold, A. E.: Insulin biosynthesis and release—a still unsettled topic, New Eng. J. Med. **282**:173, 1970.

Soskin, S., and Levine, R.: Carbohydrate metabolism, ed. 2, Chicago, 1952, University of Chicago Press.

Umbreit, W. M.: Metabolic maps, Minneapolis, 1960, Burgess Publishing Co., vol. 2.

Whelan, W. J., editor: Control of glycogen metabolism, New York, 1968, Academic Press, Inc., vol. 5.

Wood, W. A., editor: vol. 9, Carbohydrate metabolism. In Colowick, S. P., and Kaplan, N. O., editors: Methods in enzymology, New York, 1966, Academic Press, Inc.

SPECIAL

1. Larner, J., and McNickle, C. M.: J. Biol. Chem. **215**:723, 1955.
2. Miller, D., and Crane, R. K.: Amer. J. Clin. Nutr. **12**:220, 1963.
3. Huang, S. S., and Bayless, T. M.: Science **160**:83, 1968.
4. Gray, G. M.: Fed. Proc. Sympos. **26**:1415, 1967.
5. Townley, R. R. W.: Borden Rev. Nutr. Res. **28**:33, 1967.
6. Crane, R. K.: Physiol. Rev. **40**:794, 1960.
7. Annegers, J. H.: Proc. Soc. Exp. Biol. Med. **127**:1071, 1968.
8. Villas-Palasi, C., and Larner, J.: Arch. Biochem. Biophys. **86**:270, 1960.
9. Cori, G. T., and Cori, C. F.: J. Biol. Chem. **151**:57, 1943.
10. Larner, J., et al.: J. Biol. Chem. **199**:641, 1952.
11. Lowe, C. U., et al.: Amer. J. Med. **33**:4, 1962.
12. Cori, C. F.: In Najjar, V. A., editor: Carbohydrate metabolism, Baltimore, 1952, Johns Hopkins University Press.
13. Larner, J.: Ann. N.Y. Acad. Sci. **29**:192, 1966.
14. Sardesai, V. M., editor: Biochemical and clinical aspects of alcohol metabolism, Springfield, Ill., 1969, Charles C Thomas, Publisher.
15. Ashmore, J., et al.: J. Biol. Chem. **224**:225, 1957.
16. Lipmann, F.: Nature **138**:588, 1936.
17. Dickens, F.: Nature **138**:1057, 1936.
18. Warburg, O., and Christian, W.: Biochem. Z. **242**:206, 1931.
19. Gudbjarnason, S., et al.: Amer. J. Cardiol. **22**:360, 1968.
20. Eggleton, P., and Eggleton, G. P.: Biochem. J. **21**:190, 1927.
21. Fiske, C. H., and SubbaRow, Y.: Science **65**:401, 1927; **67**:169, 1928.
22. Meyerhof, O.: Die chemische Vorgänge im Muskel, Berlin, 1930, Julius Springer Verlag.
23. Leloir, L. F.: Arch. Biochem. **33**:186, 1951.
24. Pazur, J. H., and Tipton, C. L.: J. Biol. Chem. **224**:381, 1957.
25. Ritter, J. A., and Cannon, E. J.: New Eng. J. Med. **252**:747, 1955; Kalckar, H. M.: Science **125**:105, 1957; Hansen, R. G., et al.: Proc. Soc. Exp. Biol. Med. **115**:560, 1964; Smetana, H. F., and Olen, E.: Amer. J. Clin. Path. **38**:3, 1962.
26. Bernhard, R.: Sci. Res. **3**:34, 1968.
27. Enklewitz, M., and Lasker, M.: J. Biol. Chem. **110**:443, 1935.
28. Arnon, D. I.: Sci. Amer. **203**:105, 1960.
29. Arnon, D. I.: Science **156**:535, 1967.

30. Arnon, D. I., et al.: Proc. Nat. Acad. Sci. **52**:839, 1964.
31. Kleiner, I. S., and Meltzer, S. J.: Proc. Nat. Acad. Sci. **1**:338, 1915; Kleiner, I. S.: J. Biol. Chem. **40**:1953, 1919.
32. Banting, F. G.: Edinburgh Med. J. **36**:1, 1929.
33. Dunn, J. S., et al.: Lancet **1**:484, 1943; Bailey, C. B., and Bailey, O. T.: J.A.M.A. **122**:1165, 1943.
34. Bromer, W. W., et al.: J. Amer. Chem. Soc. **79**:2807, 1957.
35. Frohman, C. F., and Orten, J. M.: J. Biol. Chem. **216**:795, 1955.
36. Levine, R., et al.: Amer. J. Physiol. **163**:70, 1950; Fed. Proc. **11**:56, 1952.
37. Weber, G., et al.: Science **149**:65, 1965.
38. Weinhouse, S.: Advances Enzym. Regulat. **2**:189, 1964.
39. Fry, I. K., and Butterfield, W. J. H.: Lancet **2**:66, 1962.
40. Antoniades, H. N., et al.: New Eng. J. Med. **267**:953, 1962.
41. Vallance-Owens, J., et al.: Lancet **2**:336, 1958.
42. Field, J. B., and Stetten, D.: Amer. J. Med. **47**:844, 1956.
43. Mirsky, I. A.: Metabolism **5**:138, 1956; Vaughn, M.: Diabetes **6**:16, 1957.
44. Danowski, T. S., editor.: Ann. N.Y. Acad. Sci. **148**:575, 1968.
45. Buehler, M. S.: Lancet **82**:289, 1962.
46. Smith, H. M., editor: Ann. N.Y. Acad. Sci. **150**:191, 1968.
47. Houssay, B. A., and Biasotti, A.: Endocrinology **15**:511, 1931.
48. Long, C. N. H., et al.: Endocrinology **26**:309, 1940.

CHAPTER 10

BIOLOGIC OXIDATIONS

One of the fundamental problems of biochemistry is the mechanism by which energy is transduced in living systems. It is common knowledge that "energy" is in some way obtained by the "burning" (oxidation) of food. Modern research has shown that the locus of this oxidation is in cellular organelles, the *mitochondria* (p. 17) — sometimes appropriately called the "powerhouse" of the cell. The mitochondrion thus serves in the transduction of oxidative energy into a special form of chemical energy, ATP. The chloroplast with its quantasomes serves a similar function in plants (p. 219).

As stated in the preceding chapter, carbohydrates form the chief source of energy in the animal organism, being converted ultimately to carbon dioxide and water with the formation of ATP. This is a stepwise process involving the degradation of glucose via glycolysis or alternate pathways to pyruvic acid and lactic acid and then to acetyl-CoA for final oxidation by way of the citric acid cycle and an electron-transport chain which will be discussed later in this chapter. Acetyl-CoA is also formed by the oxidation of the fatty acid moiety of fats and is likewise oxidized by way of the citric acid cycle and the electron-transport chain. Moreover, several amino acids are converted into keto acids, e.g., pyruvic, oxaloacetic, α-ketoglutaric, and enter into the same pathways for final oxidation, as will be described later. Hence, the citric acid cycle has been termed the "final common pathway" of metabolism.

Before discussing the citric acid cycle and the final oxidation of metabolites, however, a consideration of the mechanisms of oxidations in living matter, termed "biologic oxidations," is relevant.

OXIDATIONS

The term "oxidation" is applied to protoplasmic oxidations in the same senses as in nonvital oxidations — i.e., combination with oxygen or removal of hydrogen, in any case, *a loss of electrons.* In some of the complex reactions, the transfer of electrons may be difficult to express, particularly in our present state of knowledge. It is perhaps unnecessary to remark that every oxidation must be accompanied by a reduction. It might be more pertinent to note that biologic oxidation in itself cannot be a source of energy. Oxidation involves an increase in valence, i.e., a removal of electrons, which requires energy. Indeed, it is the oxidation-reduction reactions involved in the transfer of electrons from hydrogen through intermediary acceptors, to be described later, and ultimately to oxygen, that yield the energy released in cellular oxidations.

Although not all oxidations involve oxygen, nevertheless oxygen is a vital requirement. Anaerobic organisms may and do perform oxidative reactions in the absence of oxygen, and even aerobic organisms are able to do so under some circumstances. However, a human being cannot live in an oxygen-free atmosphere for more than about 3 minutes. It is probable that most, if not all, human tissues require oxygen for the completion of their vital oxidations, even though the intermediate stages may go on in its absence.

It must be remembered that molecular oxygen is incapable of oxidizing *biologic* substances outside the body at body temperature except to a very slight extent. Within the body such oxidations are occurring constantly. It is therefore evident that the body must possess means for making such reactions possible at such comparatively low temperatures. The two problems before us are (1) how the cell brings about oxidation of its substrates at the low temperature of the body and (2) how the energy derived from the oxidation of this substrate is utilized without being dissipated as heat. These are complicated reactions, many of them chain reactions, of such a nature that the oxidations are in small steps and are controlled. In this way the energy evolved may be used physiologically.

Energy relationships The degradation of biologic substrates in the living cell by the process of biologic oxidation involves changes in which compounds of higher levels of energy go to products having lower levels of energy. Not all the energy evolved is available for work. The thermodynamic function ΔF^0 is a measure of the maximum work available from a reaction occurring at constant pressure and constant temperature. ΔF^0 is also related to the equilibrium constant of a reaction as given in the following equation:

$$\Delta F^0 = -RT \ln K$$

where R is the gas constant, T is the absolute temperature, ln is the natural logarithm, and ΔF^0 is the standard free energy change.

Reactions that have a negative ΔF^0 are spontaneous, and reactions that yield energy are *exergonic*. However, a reaction, which may be thermodynamically spontaneous, may not occur by itself at any appreciable rate. In order for a reaction to occur, the energy that is needed to convert the reactants to the form in which they can actually react must be supplied. This is the so-called *energy of activation*. In biologic systems the function of enzymes may be to lower the activation energy and thus make possible the multitude of reactions at the rates that are seen in biologic systems. In other than biologic systems, many of these same reactions occur only at high temperatures.

Chemical reactions that require energy for their occurrence are termed *endergonic* and are representative of anabolic reactions. It should be kept in mind that the catabolism or breaking down of physiologic substrates has as its prime purpose the maintenance of anabolic reactions, as typified in growth and the performance of biologic work. Such endergonic reactions must, of course, be driven by the utilization of part of the energy of an exergonic reaction. The only mechanism available for such a transfer of chemical bond energy from one reaction to another is by the utilization of *a common reactant of both reactions.* Consider Reactions I and II below as being two steps in the overall reaction $A \rightleftharpoons C$, or $A \rightleftharpoons B \rightleftharpoons C$. K is the equilibrium constant, and ΔF^0 the free energy change between the initial compound and its product, both at standard concentrations.

$$\text{(I)} \quad A \quad \rightleftharpoons \quad B; \; (K = 0.01, \; \Delta F^0 = -RT, \ln K = +2470 \text{ cal.})$$
$$\text{(II)} \quad B \quad \rightleftharpoons \quad C; \; (K = 1000, \; \Delta F^0 = -RT, \ln K = -4110 \text{ cal.})$$

Since Reaction I is endergonic, it will proceed to the left unless the concentration of B is less than 1% of the concentration of A. However, since Reaction II is exergonic, it will proceed to the right until the concentration of B is less than 0.1% of C. Thus B will be removed from the coupled reactions as fast as it is formed from Reaction I. Consequently, Reaction I can proceed to the right. Energetically, the overall reaction $A \rightleftharpoons C$ may be considered in terms of its K and the ΔF^0 values.

$$K = K_1 K_2 = (0.01)(1000) = 10$$
$$\Delta F^0 = (2470 - 4110) = -1640 \text{ cal.}$$

Thus the reaction proceeds to the right until the concentration of C is 10 times that of A, and we have a net exergonic reaction. Another principle, demonstrated in this typical example, is the relationship between the endergonic or driven reaction and the exergonic or driving reaction. The driven reaction must precede the driving reaction.

In biologic systems, phosphate compounds occupy the unique position of being the common reactant in a multitude of reactions. Most particularly is this function seen in ATP and other so-called "high-energy" compounds. These will be discussed later in this chapter.

Terminology. The biochemical agents involved are *enzymes, coenzymes,* and *hydrogen acceptors* or *carriers.* Those enzymes that act on the substrate and make possible the removal of hydrogen from it are called *dehydrogenases;* those that act on oxygen and cause it to take part in an oxidative chain are termed *oxidases.* These enzymes are rather specific; there are many dehydrogenases and a number of oxidases. Hydrogen carriers or acceptors are defined as compounds that, by virtue of their ability to be oxidized and reduced, function in the transport of hydrogens or electrons from tissue metabolites to oxygen or some other oxidizer. In general, they are also of a complex protein nature but are characterized by particular prosthetic or active groups that make possible their specific functions. Certain coenzymes, i.e., NAD^+ and $NADP^+$, which will be discussed more fully later, are dissociable from their protein enzyme fractions but usually do not function independently as carriers.

Methods of study. Since the respiration of tissues involves the utilization of oxygen, either immediately or eventually, naturally the primary method of evaluation of such activity should involve a direct measurement of oxygen

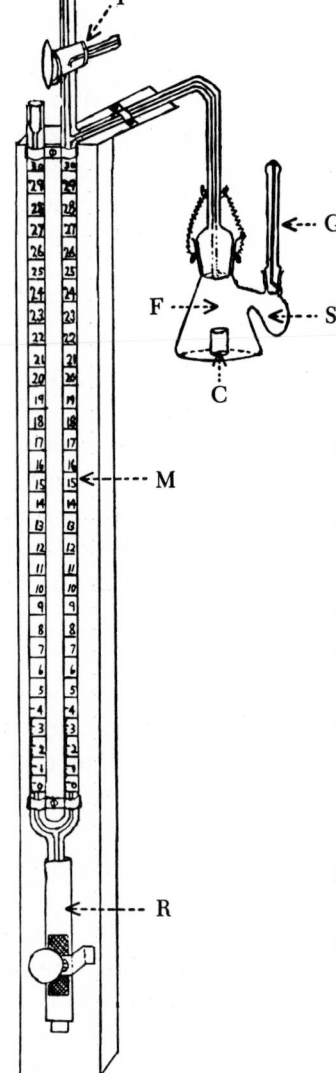

Fig. 10-1. Warburg constant-volume manometer. *F*, Flask; *S*, sidearm; *G*, sidearm stopper with gas vent; *C*, center well (for alkali); *M*, manometer proper containing a liquid of known density; *R*, fluid reservoir, which, by adjustment of the screw clamp, permits alteration of the level of the fluid in the manometer; *T*, three-way stopcock. The scale of the manometer is graduated in centimeters and millimeters. The principle involved is that, if the volume of a gas is held constant at constant temperature, any changes in the amount of gas can be measured by measuring changes in the pressure. In this apparatus, for example, if it is desired to determine the O_2 uptake of tissue, the tissue is placed in the flask, *F*. The sidearm, *S*, is provided so that a given reagent can be added during the course of the experiment. The flask has a center well, *C*, which contains alkali; this absorbs any CO_2 formed during the experiment. After introducing the tissue suspended in saline solution, and the special reagent, the entire system is filled with O_2, and the flask is immersed in a water bath at constant temperature. Readings are taken at regular intervals, and between readings the system is shaken to promote a rapid gas exchange between the fluid and the gas phase. As O_2 is absorbed by the tissue, the level of the fluid in the manometer changes and the amount can be determined by suitable calculations. (From Umbreit, W. W., Burris, R. H., and Stauffer, J. F.: Manometric techniques and related methods for the study of tissue metabolism, ed. 4, Minneapolis, 1964, Burgess Publishing Co.)

uptake. The development by Warburg of a microrespirometer provided the basic tool for investigation in this field. Although many variations of his apparatus have been devised, the techniques originally described by him are still widely used. Fig. 10-1 is a diagram of this apparatus.

Oxygen utilization in a system can also be determined by the use of an *oxygen electrode*. This device is somewhat similar to a pH electrode except that it detects and determines the concentration of free oxygen gas dissolved in the medium. In general, measurements can be made on four main types of test materials: (1) tissue slices, (2) tissue homogenates (fine minces), (3) subcellular fractions obtained by differential centrifugation, and (4) isolated components of the enzyme systems to be studied. Certain intrinsic limitations exist in each of these test materials. The purer the chemical system under study, the less may be inferred as to the direct participation of the system in intact tissues; the results obtained with tissue slices often fail to disclose the

240

complexity of the enzyme systems involved since only the end results are seen.

Investigation of the dehydrogenase activity of tissue slices, homogenates, or isolated enzyme systems has also been accomplished by means of the Thunberg technique. Here measurements are made of the rate of anaerobic decolorization of methylene blue. The methylene blue functions as a hydrogen acceptor, and the velocity of its reduction is thus a measure of the activity of the respiratory enzymes.

Tetrazolium salts have been employed to measure dehydrogenase activity of tissue slices and homogenates. The tetrazolium salts are water soluble and essentially colorless. By means of dehydrogenase or flavoprotein activity, they are reduced to colored water-insoluble formazans. The intensity of such enzymatic activity can be determined by the extraction and colorimetric measurement of the formazan, which give the amount of tetrazolium reduced per milligram of tissue. This procedure also permits a unique visualization of the intracellular localization of such activity by microscopic examination of frozen sections of the tissues.

Cellular localization of enzyme activity. Investigations in the field of enzyme activity have employed histochemical and ultracentrifugation techniques. The former demonstrate a cytoplasmic localization for cytochrome oxidase, peroxidase, and dehydrogenases. Further, in many instances, enzyme activity can be seen to be associated with the large granular or mitochondrial fractions of the cell. These findings are confirmed by the study of isolated cellular components obtained after centrifugation. In addition, it has been shown that the enzymes concerned with glycolysis are not associated with the particulate fraction but reside largely in the soluble cytoplasmic fraction. The particulate fraction is also the site of the enzymes of pyruvate and fatty acid oxidation, as well as of those concerned with phosphate esterification during biologic oxidation.

The mitochondria (Fig. 2-1) appear to be the major site of activity in the terminal stage of electron transport and oxygen activation. Indeed, Green[1] has isolated from mitochondria by ultracentrifugation an *electron-transport particle*, which contains all the enzymes and coenzymes needed for biologic oxidations. The particle has a molecular weight of about 1,560,000. It can be broken into several subunits that contain closely related members of the electron-transport chain. These particles apparently are attached to the inner membrane of the mitochondria, particularly on the cristae (p. 17). The enzymes of the citric acid cycle (p. 263) and for fatty acid oxidation are located nearby on particles in the matrix of the mitochondrion. In appreciation of their importance in cellular metabolism, Claude has described the mitochondria as "intracellular power plants." From the standpoint of chemical composition and structure, the mitochondria are asymmetric structures that, in the case of liver, contain about 10% of the nucleic acids of the cell. They show osmotic activity, but they are not simply small vacuolar osmometers since by electron microscopy they can be shown to possess an internal granular structure (see Fig. 2-1). They also contain a considerable amount of phospholipid. It should also be noted that factors of intracellular tonicity may influence

241

enzymatic activity associated with the mitochondria. Thus, the functional integrity of various enzyme systems, particularly the enzymes of the citric acid cycle, is facilitated by the structural organization of the mitochondria.

Synthetic (anabolic) as well as degradative reactions are also associated with mitochondrial enzymes. This occurrence of synthetic and oxidative enzymes in the same structural unit, where exothermic reactions are required to drive endothermic ones, is a remarkable phenomenon. A striking example of the significance of this organization is found in oxidative phosphorylation, which occurs in intact mitochondria and is decreased on disruption or isolation of the components of the reaction.

RESPIRATORY ENZYMES AND CARRIERS

The principal types of enzymes involved in biologic oxidations are the *oxidases* and *dehydrogenases*. Supplementing the action of the latter are several groups of hydrogen carriers, including NAD^+ (DPN^+) and $NADP^+$ (TPN^+) and the flavoproteins, and electron carriers, the cytochromes, to be considered later. The removal of carbon as carbon dioxide from metabolites being oxidized is catalyzed by a group of enzymes called *decarboxylases* (or *carboxylases*). The oxidation of the final two- to four-carbon fragments of metabolites from carbohydrates, fats, and proteins is accomplished by means of the Krebs citric acid cycle, also to be described later. Several other groups of enzymes, the *hydrases, peroxidases,* and *catalases,* have supplementary actions, as will be discussed.

Oxygen activation — the oxidases The oxidases utilize molecular oxygen as a hydrogen acceptor and thus bring about the oxidation of a metabolite.

$$\text{Metabolite-H}_2 + \tfrac{1}{2}\, O_2 \xrightarrow{\text{Oxidase}} \text{Oxidized metabolite} + H_2O$$

Oxidases are found in most animal tissues and also in plants and microorganisms. They are metalloproteins, usually containing iron or copper. Examples are cytochrome oxidase, tyrosine oxidase, and ascorbic oxidase. Cytochrome oxidase will be discussed in some detail later because of its general importance in cellular oxidations.

Some oxidases reduce molecular oxygen to a peroxide, which is then converted to water and a half molecule of oxygen by catalase or is utilized by way of a peroxidase. This group includes D- and L-amino acid oxidases, which are flavoproteins. The oxidases are not involved in ATP formation.

Hydroxylases (mixed-function oxidases) The hydroxylases are responsible for the introduction of a single atom of molecular oxygen into a substrate.

$$\text{Metabolite-H}_2 + O_2 + NADPH_2 \xrightarrow{\text{Hydroxylase}} \text{Metabolite-OH} + NADP^+ + H_2O$$

If isotopically labeled oxygen (^{18}O) is used, the label appears in both the metabolite and the water ($\text{M-}^{18}\text{OH} + H_2^{18}O$), thus proving the above reaction.

Mixed-function oxidases are found in the microsomes (smooth endoplasmic reticulum) of cells (p. 18), especially hepatic cells, and are involved in the metabolism of a number of drugs and various steroids. They are also concerned in the metabolism of tryptophan (p. 378).

NADPH$_2$ is the usual cofactor (cosubstrate), as indicated on p. 242; hence a frequent prosthetic group in the hydroxylases. Cytochrome P-450 (p. 248) serves as an important mixed-function oxidase.

Oxygenases (oxygen transferases) The oxygenases catalyze the introduction of both atoms of molecular oxygen into the substrate concerned, as shown by the use of ^{18}O.

$$\text{Metabolite-H}_2 + O_2 \xrightarrow{\text{Oxygenase}} \text{Metabolite-(OH)}_2$$

Ferrous ion (Fe^{++}) or *heme* is the usual prosthetic group. A number of the oxygenases are involved with the change of aromatic rings. An example is tryptophan oxygenase, which converts L-tryptophan into L-formylkynurenine (p. 378).

Hydrogen activation— the dehydrogenases We owe the advancement of the hypothesis of hydrogen activation to Wieland. In hydrogen activation, a very common phenomenon, the organic substance to be oxidized is acted on by a dehydrogenase in such a way that specific hydrogen atoms are removed. In other words, the metabolite is oxidized by dehydrogenation. The hydrogen removed is simultaneously taken up by a suitable oxidizing agent or by molecular oxygen. Another concept of dehydrogenation is that the metabolite together with the hydrogen acceptor combines with the dehydrogenase (protein) molecule in such a way that the hydrogen passes from the metabolite to the hydrogen acceptor. The oxidized metabolite and the reduced carrier then separate from the dehydrogenase and the process can be repeated with another set of metabolite and carrier molecules, the dehydrogenase being used over and over again.

There are many dehydrogenases, each apparently specific as to the substrate from which it removes hydrogen. For example, the oxidation of acetaldehyde to acetic acid may be accomplished in this manner:

Another instance:

243

Both illustrations show oxidation by dehydrogenation. It should also be noted that in both cases there is actually more oxygen in the end products, although neither molecular nor activated oxygen is introduced, the oxygen coming from water. Atmospheric oxygen is also eventually required because the hydrogen must at some stage be oxidized to water or hydrogen peroxide.

If a dehydrogenase transfers hydrogen from the metabolite directly to molecular oxygen to form hydrogen peroxide, it is called an *aerobic dehydrogenase*. An important example is L-amino acid dehydrogenase (usually called L-*amino acid oxidase*). If the hydrogen is passed to one or more hydrogen acceptors, the enzyme is termed an *anaerobic dehydrogenase*. The majority of dehydrogenases appear to be the latter type.

Hydrogen and electron carriers *Coenzymes.* By definition, coenzymes are dialyzable, heat-stable, organic compounds necessary for the functioning of enzymes. The coenzymes of importance in biologic oxidation reactions include the phosphopyridine nucleotides and coenzyme-A. The latter will be discussed later.

Coenzyme-I has two phosphoric acid molecules and is known now as NAD$^+$ (old name, DPN) (see p. 810), or cozymase. Its structural formula is given below. Coenzyme-II is the triphosphoric derivative and is often called TPN (for triphosphopyridine nucleotide), or, by the terminology preferred today, NADP$^+$. The position of the third phosphoric acid in NADP$^+$ is indicated by the asterisk (*) in the formula for NAD$^+$.

NAD$^+$ (nicotinamide adenine dinucleotide) or cozymase (coenzyme-I)

These nucleotides, then, consist of adenine, two molecules of D-ribose, two or three molecules of phosphoric acid, and nicotinamide (a vitamin). The nicotinamide imparts to the nucleotide the latter's important reversible oxidation-reduction activity; i.e., it is the hydrogen-carrier part of this large molecule, which may be shown in the following way:

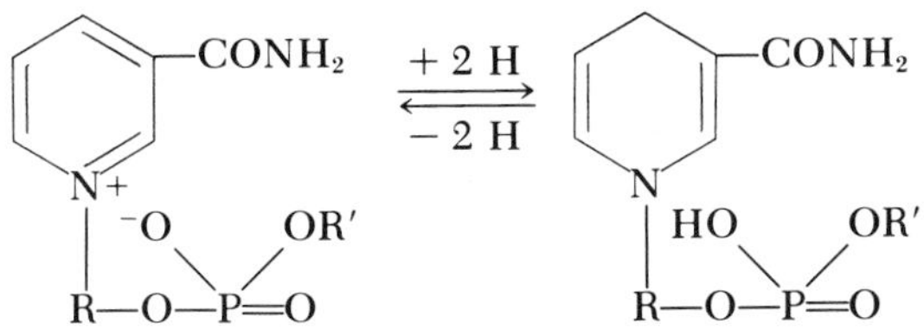

The *2 H* are transferred as a "reducing equivalent" from the metabolite being oxidized by its specific dehydrogenase to the NAD^+ as a hydride ion (H^-); $2\,H \rightarrow H^+ + H^-$. The hydride ion is transferred to position no. 4 of nicotinamide, as shown above. There is, of course, a corresponding shift of double bonds (electrons) in the ring and the loss of the positive charge on the nitrogen atom of the ring. The reaction thus may be shown schematically:

$$NAD^+ + 2\,H \;\rightleftharpoons\; NADH + H^+$$

Frequently the reaction is written indicating the transfer of the H^- only and the H^+ is omitted, or the reduced form may be written $NADH_2$, as recommended by the International Union of Biochemistry. This convention will be used throughout the book.

Among the metabolites requiring NAD^+ are lactic acid, malic acid, β-hydroxybutyric acid, ethyl alcohol, and glyceraldehyde-3-phosphate. Glucose and glutamate use either NAD^+ or $NADP^+$.

Functionally, the coenzyme oscillates between the oxidized and the reduced state, accepting the hydrogen (electrons) of the substrate (metabolite) and transferring it to a flavoprotein, e.g., the yellow enzyme. Certain barbiturates are known to block the transfer of hydrogen from $NADH_2$ to flavoprotein.[2]

Apparently the hydrogen atoms from metabolites requiring $NADP^+$ can be transferred along the regular electron-transfer chain by the conversion of $NADPH_2$ to $NADH_2$ by *transhydrogenases.* The process is termed transhydrogenation. There does not appear to be a direct mitochondrial path for electrons from $NADPH_2$ to oxygen, as there is for $NADH_2$ (p. 249).

$$NADPH_2 + NAD^+ \xrightarrow{\text{Transhydrogenase}} NADP^+ + NADH_2$$

Flavoproteins. Flavoproteins are an interesting group of compounds that act as dehydrogenases and hydrogen carriers. They have been called *yellow enzymes* because they contain a yellow compound, flavin, identical with riboflavin (a vitamin). Attention to this group of substances came with the discovery of a yellow oxidation enzyme by Warburg and Christian.[3] Since then, numerous other oxidative enzymes possessing flavin groups have been demonstrated. The list of such enzymes includes xanthine oxidase, diaphorase, D-amino acid oxidase, succinic dehydrogenase, and cytochrome-c reductase. Each of these is composed of a specific protein united with the prosthetic group, flavin. In the case of the "old" yellow enzyme and of cyto-chrome-c reductase, the flavin may exist as a mononucleotide (FMN), whereas in the others it is found as a dinucleotide (FAD). The mononucleotide form may be represented by the following structure, in which the phosphoric acid is linked to the specific protein that gives it its protein character. Note that the reactions with hydrogen occur via nitrogen atoms (arrows):

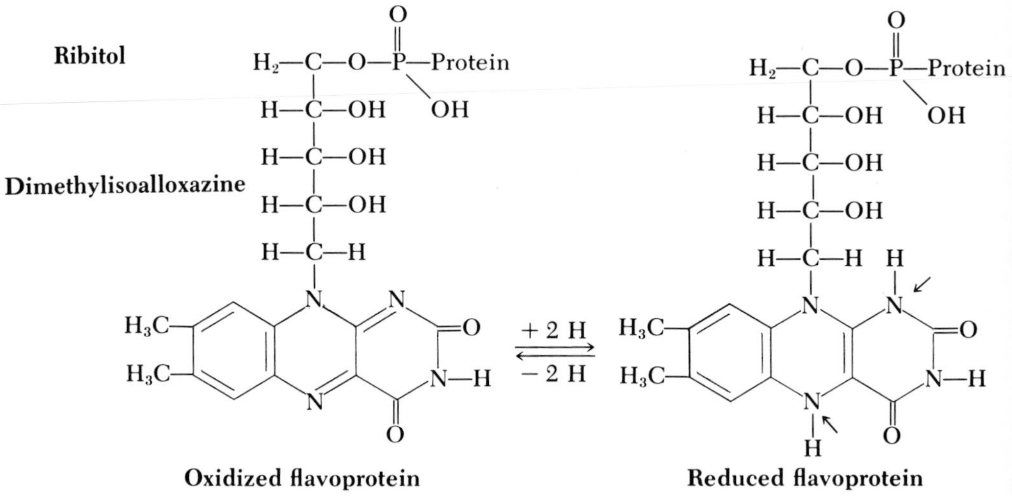

Oxidized flavoprotein　　　　**Reduced flavoprotein**

The dinucleotide may be represented as follows:

Dimethylisoalloxazine — D-Ribitol — Phosphate — Phosphate — D-Ribose — Adenine

An example of the functioning of these agents is as follows:

The dehydrogenase activates certain hydrogen atoms of the metabolite, and the NAD^+ accepts them:

$$\underset{\textbf{Metabolite}}{MH_2} \xrightarrow{\text{Dehydrogenase} + NAD^+} NADH_2 + M$$

The $NADH_2$ immediately transfers them to the flavoprotein, FAD:

$$NADH_2 + FAD \rightarrow NAD^+ + FADH_2$$

For regeneration of the reduced flavoprotein, in some instances only atmospheric oxygen is necessary:

$$FADH_2 + O_2 \rightarrow FAD + H_2O_2$$

It should be noted that the first reaction indicates the main oxidation, i.e., the oxidation of the substrate. However, this reaction cannot proceed in the absence of the second. The third reaction brings the flavoprotein back to its original state.

An example of oxidation by the flavoprotein system is to be found in the oxidation of hexose monophosphoric acid to phosphohexonic acid. Indicating only the reacting group, we have:

$$
R-C\overset{O}{\underset{H}{\big\langle}} + HOH \rightarrow R-\underset{[H]}{\overset{O[H]}{C}}-OH \xrightarrow[\substack{NAD^+ \quad NADH_2}]{\substack{FADH_2 \quad FAD}} R-C\overset{OH}{\underset{O}{\big\langle}}
$$

In this system two vitamins, as essential factors, nicotinamide and riboflavin, are parts of the molecules of the coenzyme and flavoprotein, respectively.

Metalloflavoproteins. During the past decade or so a group of metalloflavoproteins active in cellular oxidations have been identified. Molybdenum and iron are found in several of these enzymes. Copper or manganese is present in a few. Both molybdenum and iron are present in xanthine oxidase, which has been prepared in crystalline form and found to contain also 0.51% flavin adenine dinucleotide (FAD). As will be mentioned later, this enzyme is concerned with the oxidation of certain purines to uric acid. Aldehyde oxidase has likewise been shown to be a molybdenum flavoprotein. The metalloflavoproteins appear to function primarily in the linkage of hydrogen transport to electron transport. Several of the metalloflavoproteins apparently serve at the level just before cytochrome-c in the electron-transport chain. They are therefore sometimes called *cytochrome-c reductases.* The enzyme succinic dehydrogenase (p. 263) is an important example of this type of metalloflavoprotein. The flavin moiety of the molecule is apparently present as the mononucleotide (FMN).

Cytochromes. The third type of oxidation reaction is exemplified by the cytochrome systems. In 1925, Keilin[4] discovered that there were widely distributed in animal tissues certain hemochromogens, which he called cytochromes. These combinations of heme and proteins have characteristic absorption spectra differing from those of hemoglobin and its derivatives and are designated as a, b, c, and a_3. Cytochrome-c is the one that has been most carefully studied. It is present in largest amounts and has been isolated in a relatively pure state. The existence of the other cytochromes has been indicated by their characteristic absorption spectra. Chemically cytochrome-c is a heme-protein with the heme residue united to the protein by a thioether linkage. Characteristic absorption bands are found in the visible spectra at 550, 522, and 415 mμ for reduced cytochrome-c and at about 530 and 400 mμ for oxidized cytochrome-c.

Cytochrome-c's isoelectric point is pH 9.86; this hemochromogen contains between 0.34% and 0.43% iron. The iron is chelated to a porphyrin similar to the protoporphyrin of heme. Indeed, the porphyrin moiety is synthesized in cells by nearly the same pathway as that for heme. The amino acid sequence of the purified protein moiety of cytochrome-c has been studied extensively by E. L. Smith, Margoliash, and their associates in a number of species.

Another cytochrome, called cytochrome P-450, from its characteristic absorption spectrum, is an important mixed-function oxidase (p. 242). It plays a role in the oxidation of a number of drugs and steroids. $NADPH_2$ and flavoprotein are also involved. However, these constitute a *microsomal* system for biologic oxidations. The other cytochromes are part of the mitochondrial system, of course.

As described later (p. 601), the amino acid sequences of cytochrome-c preparations from a wide variety of species, from man through various fishes and even yeast, are practically identical in portions of the molecule having functional importance. Variations in sequences in other portions of the molecule occur, however, and have been shown to be evolutionarily significant (p. 601). The complete amino acid sequence of crystalline human heart cytochrome-c has been reported recently.[5] It contains 104 amino acid residues differing in only 12 positions from those of horse heart cytochrome-c. The heme moiety of cytochrome-c is attached to the protein part of the molecule by a thioether bridge with two cysteine residues at positions 14 and 17 in the polypeptide chain. This type of bonding permits the reversible shift of the iron of heme from ferrous to ferric, essential to the function of cytochrome-c in electron transport, as will be described.

Perhaps most significant from the point of view of the functioning of a typical oxidation-reduction chain is the fact that, from the cytochrome stage on, hydrogen is no longer transported but instead the changes involve electron transfer. Thus, whereas the electrons of the substrate are delivered to oxygen in a continuous chain, the hydrogen ion may enter or be withdrawn at several places in the chain. Furthermore, the components of the chain may be classified as to their ability to transfer electrons. The cytochromes can transfer but one electron per cycle of oxidation and reduction of their prosthetic group, whereas the flavoproteins and pyridine nucleotides can transport two electrons per cycle. The electrons are finally transferred to molecular oxygen to complete the oxidation of that portion of the metabolite involved. The process is repeated sequentially with succeeding intermediates, employing the specific dehydrogenases for each, until the metabolite is converted to a small fragment, usually acetyl-CoA, which is finally oxidized—usually by way of the citric acid cycle (p. 263).

Cytochrome oxidase. Cytochrome oxidase has been shown to be identical with cytochrome-a_3 or Warburg's respiratory enzyme. It is found in practically all forms of life, and the reduced form gives rise to water in its capacity of reducing oxygen so that the latter may combine with hydrogen atoms. It contains an iron atom, which can oscillate between the ferrous and ferric state with reduction and oxidation.

There is evidence that a copper-containing component of cytochrome oxidase exists. At least part of the copper is cuprous (Cu^{++}) and undergoes oxidation-reduction in the presence of an acceptor or substrate of the enzyme (molecular oxygen or reduced cytochrome-c). A study of the kinetics of the reaction[6] has shown that the copper of cytochrome oxidase reacts at a rate no less than that of the heme components of the electron-transport chain. This interesting work obviously raises questions as to the role of copper in cytochrome oxidase in electron transfer between cytochrome-c and molecular oxygen.

A dehydrogenase first *activates* specific hydrogen atoms in a metabolite. These are then accepted by a carrier, usually NAD^+, and then FAD (flavoprotein), as shown in Fig. 10-2. Coenzyme-Q may serve as the next hydrogen (electron) acceptor for certain metabolites, as will be discussed later. At this point electrons are passed sequentially from one cytochrome to another, in the order b, c, and a, finally to cytochrome oxidase. Here, two hydrogen ions react with oxygen ($\frac{1}{2} O_2$) plus two electrons to form the terminal product of biologic oxidations (H_2O). As shown in Fig. 10-2, each carrier is regenerated as it passes its hydrogen atoms or electrons to the next member of the electron-transport chain in a bucket brigade fashion. Thus the metabolite is oxidized by dehydrogenation, but ultimately oxygen is required for the consummation of this reaction. Several such chains are known and are being actively studied. An example of one such complete hydrogen-transport system, in which a number of the reactions already described will be recognized, is shown in Fig. 10-2. The significance of suggested factors X, Y, and Z in Fig. 10-2 and their role in the formation of high-energy phosphate, as ATP, will be discussed on p. 258.

The various types of oxidizing systems outlined should not be considered inflexible categories. For example, it is known that the oxidation of a number of metabolites does not require all the steps represented in the diagram. Some steps apparently may be bypassed. An important example of this is seen in the oxidation of succinic acid by succinic dehydrogenase. Two hydrogen atoms from succinate are taken up by a metalloflavoprotein (cytochrome-c reductase), bypassing the NAD^+ step, which is the first hydrogen acceptor for most other metabolites. The mitochondrial chain for the oxidation of succinate[7] was reconstituted recently from its individual components. The nec-

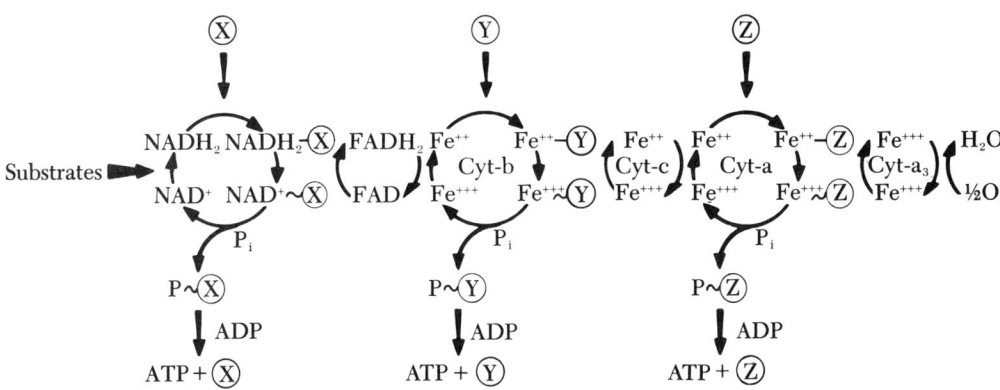

Fig. 10-2. Schematic representation of hydrogen transport-system and coupled oxidative phosphorylation. The H_2 liberated at the *FADH₂* step is changed to $2H^+$ by the loss of two electrons to cytochrome-b; it terminally reacts with $\frac{1}{2}O_2$ plus two electrons to form H_2O. This scheme is not a proved mechanism but a reasonable hypothesis based on current knowledge. (From Lehninger, A. L.: Fed. Proc. 19:954, 1960.)

essary constituents include succinate dehydrogenase, cytochromes b, c_1, c, cytochrome oxidase, coenzyme-Q_{10}, and phospholipids. The oxidation of xanthine by xanthine oxidase, actually a metalloflavoprotein, likewise by-passes the NAD^+ step. The two electrons are sent directly to cytochrome-c.

Also, as stated previously, coenzyme-Q may serve as a hydrogen (electron) acceptor between flavoprotein and cytochrome-b for certain metabolites. Similarly, it is unlikely that all three cytochromes, b, c, and a, are obligatory components of the electron-transport system for all metabolites. Cytochrome-c appears to be the major cytochrome, along with cytochrome oxidase. The other cytochromes, b and a, may be functional only for certain metabolites. Further changes in the current concept are likely as our knowledge increases. It is evident that all the molecular oxygen that enters any biologic oxidation appears as water.

Of interest in this connection is the fact that lipid-soluble vitamin K has been implicated in electron transport, as have coenzyme-Q and the ubi-quinones, to be discussed later.

Other possible agents. Mention should be made of certain compounds, e.g., glutathione, ascorbic acid, that possess the ability to be reversibly oxidized and reduced but have not been shown to have any direct reaction to the res-piratory chains. Interesting is the fact that *ferredoxin*, a nonheme, nonflavin-containing iron-protein complex, serves for electron transport in certain anaerobic bacteria. It also appears to be involved in photosynthesis[8] (p. 219).

Peroxidases and catalases. In the end reaction of some of the chains that have been described, the oxygen has been shown to unite with the hydrogen to form *hydrogen peroxide*. Peroxides thus might be expected to accumulate in large amounts in the tissues. Peroxides, being toxic, must be disposed of, and there are two enzymes capable of accomplishing this. The more impor-tant one is catalase. It is present in all animal cells but in varying concentra-tions. Its action is to decompose hydrogen peroxide, yielding gaseous oxygen:

$$2\ H_2O_2 \quad \rightarrow \quad 2\ H_2O + O_2$$

Other peroxides are not attacked.

Peroxidase, in the presence of hydrogen peroxide, catalyzes the oxidation of diverse phenols and aromatic amines. It has been pictured as forming "active" oxygen, which then may directly oxidize the substrate.

$$H_2O_2 \xrightarrow[\text{Peroxidase}]{} H_2O + \underset{\textbf{Active oxygen}}{O}$$

$$\underset{\textbf{Metabolite}}{M} + O \longrightarrow MO$$

It is extremely doubtful whether enough hydrogen peroxide to bring about such oxidations can occur in cells that contain catalase. There is also some doubt as to the occurrence of peroxidases in animal cells, because hemo-globin, cytochrome, and other substances react similarly and mask the pres-ence of peroxidase. A peroxidase is found in milk, however.

Interesting recent studies indicate that catalase and one or more hydrogen peroxide–producing oxidases are associated in cytoplasmic particles called *peroxisomes.* These particles have the morphologic features of *microbodies* and have been found in the cytoplasm of a number of animal and plant cells. Depending on the source, peroxisomes may contain a number of additional enzymes indicative of a variety of metabolic functions.

Hydrogen transfer between the cytoplasm and mitochondria Another important problem involved in biologic oxidations is the mechanism of transfer of hydrogen between the cytoplasm and mitochondria of the cell. The mitochondrial membrane is impermeable to $NADH_2$ and other members of the electron-transport chain; these are bound to the cristael membrane, as described previously, and are essentially "locked" inside the mitochondrion. The glycolytic enzymes, on the other hand, are located in the cytoplasm; hence any hydrogen (hydride ions) in the form of $NADH_2$ produced by them must enter the mitochondrion by some special mechanism. The same is true of $NADH_2$ found in the conversion of lactate to pyruvate and in the metabolism of ethanol and other metabolites. Conversely, $NADH_2$, or more generally $NADPH_2$, is required for many biosynthetic reactions in the cytoplasm (the biosynthesis of fatty acids, p. 310, of cholesterol, p. 326, etc.). Since the cytoplasmic formation of $NADH_2$ or $NADPH_2$ may not meet the needs of such anabolic reactions, a mechanism for their transfer from the mitochondrion is essential.

Current evidence indicates that this need is met, in mammalian cells at least, by a "shuttle mechanism" involving oxaloacetate and malate. The reaction apparently is catalyzed by malate dehydrogenase bound to the mitochondrial membrane. The reaction may be shown schematically as follows:

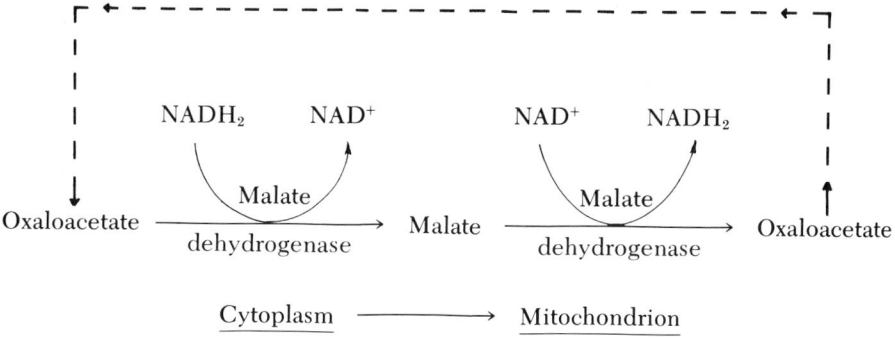

$NADH_2$ in the cytoplasm is oxidized by oxaloacetate to form malate in the presence of malate dehydrogenase. Malate enters the mitochondrion and is oxidized to oxaloacetate by mitochondrial malate dehydrogenase and mitochondrial bound NAD^+. The oxaloacetate may then reenter the cytoplasm for reduction by another molecule of $NADH_2$. The mitochondrial $NADH_2$ thus formed may then be oxidized by the electron-transport chain, with the formation of ATP.

Similar hydrogen-transport systems involving dihydroxyacetone phosphate–α-glycerophosphate and β-hydroxybutyric acid–acetoacetic acid may function in some species.

Although the principal metabolic function of cytoplasmic $NADPH_2$ is as a reductant in anabolic reactions, e.g., the synthesis of fatty acids, the hydroxylation of steroids, and the regeneration of sulfhydryl groups, $NADPH_2$ as well as mitochondrial $NADPH_2$ may form some ATP indirectly by transhydrogenation with NAD^+. There seems to be no direct mitochondrial path for electrons from $NADPH_2$ to oxygen. The oxidation of $NADPH_2$, therefore, requires the presence of NAD^+, and the reaction appears to be catalyzed by the enzyme *transhydrogenase*, as follows:

$$NADPH_2 + NAD^+ \xrightleftharpoons{\text{Transhydrogenase}} NADP^+ + NADH_2$$

The reverse reaction requires energy and has been observed in heart and liver mitochondria.

ENERGY PRODUCTION AND UTILIZATION — OXIDATIVE PHOSPHORYLATION

At the beginning of this chapter, it was stated that one of the two main problems in the field of biologic oxidations is how the energy derived from the oxidation of the substrate is utilized rather than dissipated as heat. An explanation that has been advanced for this phenomenon will now be considered.

The energy of biologic oxidations is derived from the transfer of the electrons obtained from the hydrogen atoms of metabolites through intermediary carriers ultimately to oxygen. It is now generally believed that ATP, or more specifically its labile so-called high-energy phosphate bonds, is the primary energy carrier or coupling agent between the foregoing energy-yielding, exergonic reactions and the energy-requiring, endergonic reactions. This concept is illustrated diagrammatically in Fig. 10-3. The process of energy production in this manner is termed oxidative phosphorylation.

The concept that ATP is a universal intracellular carrier of chemical energy is based on a number of classic investigations dating back to the pioneer

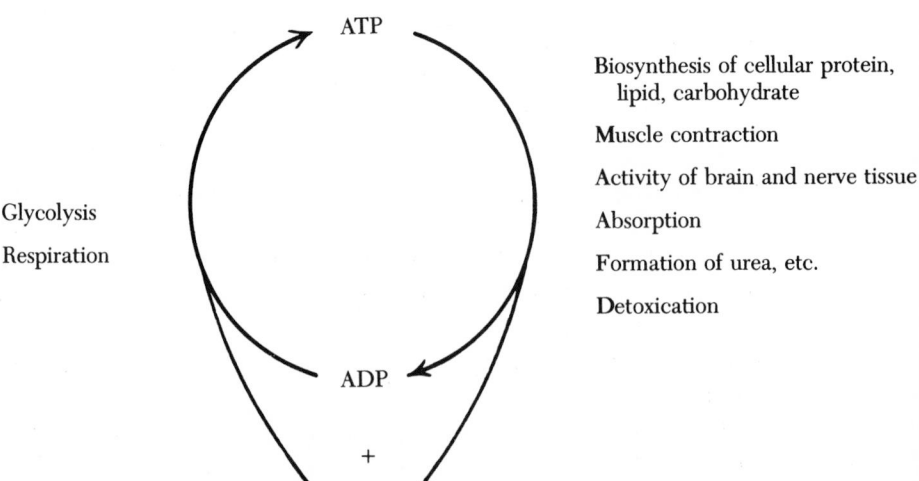

Fig. 10-3. Diagrammatic illustration of adenosine triphosphate (ATP) as a carrier or coupling agent in energy transfer.

studies of Meyerhof, Lohmann, and Kalckar, in the decade from the mid-1920's through the mid-1930's. The former two investigators described the high energy of the hydrolysis of ATP and the use of ATP (and reserve creatine phosphate) as energy for muscle contraction. Kalckar observed that phosphate ions disappeared as glucose was oxidized in muscle or kidney tissue and that organic phosphate, which he identified as ATP, concomitantly increased in concentration. These fundamental observations led to the conclusion that the energy of the oxidation of glucose was converted in some manner to ATP, which, in turn, could be utilized to carry out essential body processes, e.g., building new tissues, muscle contraction, active transport across cell membranes, and the synthesis of essential metabolites.

We will next consider the nature of high-energy phosphate and related compounds, the mechanism of their formation, and their functions. It must be stated at the outset, however, that this is a controversial subject at the present time. Some authorities contend that the term *energy-rich* phosphate bond, in the sense of yielding high free energies ($-\Delta F^\circ$) upon hydrolysis, is misleading because energy is required to break any bond, including the phosphate bond. The term actually refers to the free energy of hydrolysis of the bond. This free energy change is a function of the total hydrolytic reaction and cannot be ascribed to any one bond in the reactants. These compounds may serve as transfer agents or catalysts. In fact, it will be noted that every so-called high-energy or energy-rich bond gives rise to either acidic or basic products, which are immediately neutralized in buffered solutions, e.g., body fluids. This yields free energy. An exception is the change from the enol to the keto form, which, in itself, yields a large amount of free energy. The function of phosphorylation in metabolism may be to reduce the energies of activation by stabilizing the corresponding intermediate complexes through chelation and inductive effects. The energy of activation is the energy required to bring the reactants into the state or form in which they can react. When a reaction has a very high negative free energy, it probably does not occur in a finite length of time if it also has a high energy of activation. Further fundamental studies will be required to resolve these differences of opinion. With this reservation in mind, the concept of the role of energy-rich phosphate and related compounds in energy metabolism as it has developed in the past 30 years will be presented now.

Formation and utilization of energy-rich compounds It has long been known that the oxidation of triose and pyruvic acid occurs only in the presence of inorganic phosphate. These three-carbon molecules may be considered typical metabolic units prepared by the body for oxidation. Phosphorylation and oxidation seem to be definitely linked together in physiologic reactions. In the oxidation of the triose 3-phosphoglyceraldehyde, the first reaction supposed to occur is the addition of a second phosphoric acid to produce the hypothetic intermediary substance 1,3-diphosphoglyceraldehyde. In the presence of an enzyme and a carrier, this is oxidized to 1,3-diphosphoglyceric acid, which is the oxidation *proper*. Although the reaction as a whole has liberated a small amount of energy, a large proportion of the

---

$^\circ$ This carries the minus sign, $-\Delta F$, because the system is losing energy, i.e., is exergonic.

energy of oxidation is said to be stored in the pyrophosphate bond created. This is a labile phosphate bond and has been termed an "energy-rich" phosphate bond by Lipmann.[9]

The energy-rich phosphate bond represents 5000 to 12,000 calories of free energy per mole, depending on the nature of the compound involved,[10] as contrasted with about 3000 calories for the ester phosphate linkage. Numerous experiments[10] indicate that the breakdown of ATP to ADP yields about 7.6 to 7.8 kcal. per mole. The 5000 to 12,000 calories condensed in the energy-rich bond were, until recently, considered a *biologic energy unit*. Removal of a phosphate linked to an alcoholic hydroxyl group (ester phosphate) yields little free energy. Through metabolic reactions phosphate may, however, become linked with carboxyl or certain other groups and form energy-rich phosphate bonds. As stated before (p. 36), these bonds are indicated by the symbol $\sim$. Acetyl phosphate is:

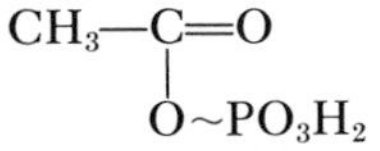

$$CH_3-C=O$$
$$|$$
$$O\sim PO_3H_2$$

with one energy-rich phosphate bond. The structure of ATP was given on p. 35. Other such bond types, with an example of a compound containing each, are as follows:

$$NH$$
$$\|$$
$$-N\sim PO_3H_2 \text{ as in } H-N-C-N-CH_2\cdot COOH$$
$$| \quad |$$
$$PO_3H_2 \quad CH_3$$

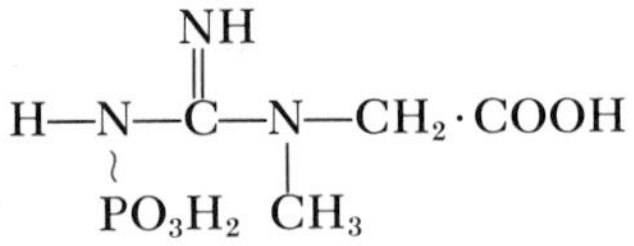

Creatine phosphate

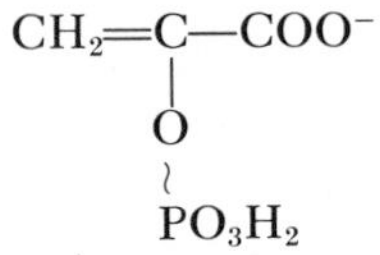

$$CH_2=C-COO^-$$
$$|$$
$$O$$
$$\wr$$
$$PO_3H_2$$

Phosphoenolpyruvate

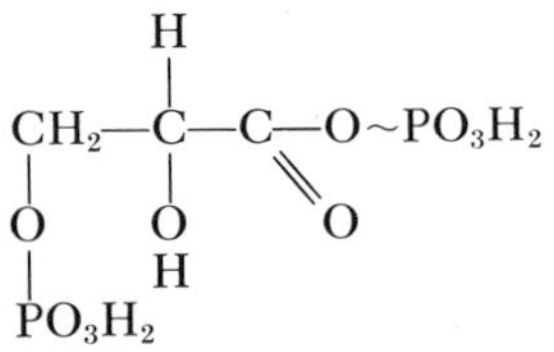

$$H$$
$$|$$
$$CH_2-C-C-O\sim PO_3H_2$$
$$| \quad | \quad \backslash\backslash$$
$$O \quad O \quad O$$
$$| \quad H$$
$$PO_3H_2$$

1,3-Diphosphoglyceric acid

In general, then, high-energy bonds are bonds in which resonance is hindered by the positive charge on the phosphorus atom, resulting in electrostatic repulsion, as in the case of ATP (p. 35); or there is similarly a decreased-resonance form in 1,3-diphosphoglyceric acid and creatine phosphate, or a change in free energy due to isomerization, as in the case of phosphoenolpyruvate.

In the reactions shown in Fig. 10-4 the energy-rich phosphate bond has been inserted where it is postulated to be present. In the further catabolism of triose, the energy-rich phosphate bond is transferred from 1,3-diphospho-

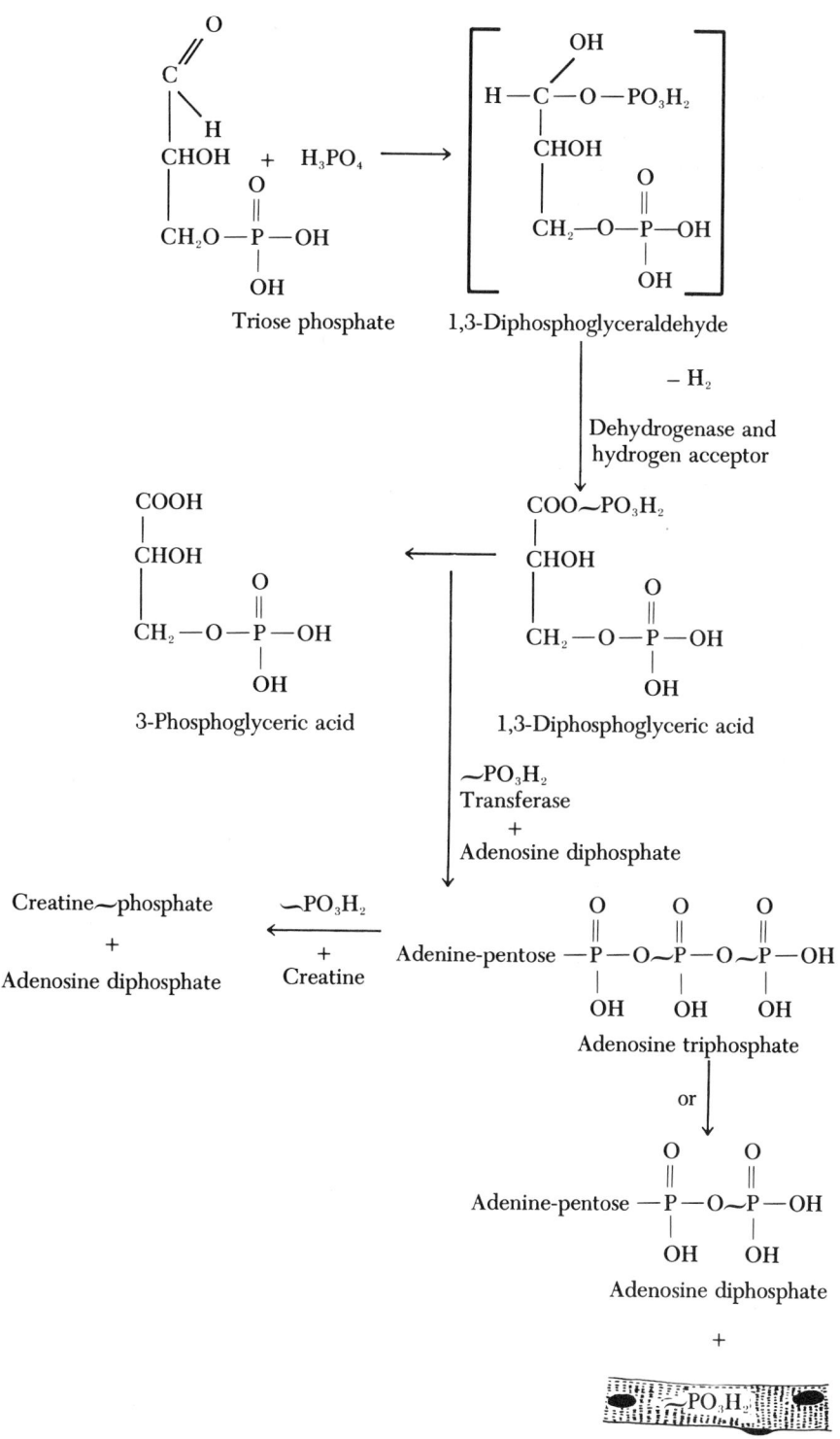

Fig. 10-4. Energy transfers during the catabolism of triose.

glyceric acid to adenylic acid or ADP by a specific enzyme, a transferase. At the same time this transfers about 5000 to 12,000 calories to the adenosine molecule, which, in turn, can discharge this energy upon cellular structures for the performance of biologic work, or it may transfer the energy to creatine. Most transphosphorylation reactions involve the adenyl pyrophosphate system, which acts as a phosphate acceptor from substances like phosphopyruvate, acetyl phosphate, and 1,3-diphosphoglyceric acid. The adenosine polyphosphates can then act as phosphate donors to such organic substances as glucose, creatine, etc. The energy is finally made available when the energy-rich phosphate bond is broken, yielding inorganic phosphate, the dephosphorylated compound (e.g., adenylic acid), and approximately 5000 to 12,000 calories. The further metabolic reactions in this series, with the formation of another energy-rich phosphate bond, are shown in Fig. 10-4.

We may thus classify phosphate carriers into three groups:

1. Relatively inert phosphate carriers, e.g., ester phosphates, such as triose phosphate and hexose phosphates

    On hydrolysis these yield only 3000 calories; i.e., the $\Delta F^0 = -3000$ calories.

2. Active phosphate carriers, e.g., creatine phosphate, 1,3-diphosphoglyceric acid, phosphoenolpyruvic acid

    These yield on hydrolysis about 5000 to 12,000 calories for each energy-rich phosphate bond. They possess the property of *transphosphorylation*, which means the transfer of these energy-rich groups to other active carriers or to the third class.

3. Active phosphate carriers and dischargers, e.g., adenosine diphosphate and triphosphate

    These possess the properties of group 2 but, in addition, function in the performance of biologic work, which includes muscle contraction, maintenance of cell potential, etc. They also phosphorylate organic molecules such as hexose and triose, thus creating inert and active carriers.

Thus, oxidative energy, from the oxidation of triose, is converted into phosphate bond energy and the adenylic system serves as the mediator of the transfers involved. When glucose is the phosphate acceptor, the system, once started, is self-perpetuating. The phosphorylation of glucose enables it to undergo oxidation by way of triose phosphate and pyruvate, and this oxidation causes further phosphorylation of glucose.

Electron-transport chain and ATP formation. The mechanism of formation of ATP during the transfer of electrons in the electron-transport chain, as shown in Fig. 10-2, has been clarified considerably during the past few years. In 1951, Lehninger[11] obtained evidence that ATP is formed at three different points along the electron-transport system. Subsequent work by the Lehninger, Green, and Chance groups[12] has led to the current concept of the mechanism of oxidative phosphorylation and its coupling with the electron-transport chain as depicted diagrammatically in Fig. 10-2.

At the stages immediately following NAD⁺, cytochrome-b, and cytochrome-a, three as yet unidentified substances, designated X, Y, and Z, respectively, transfer the energy released in the passage of electrons along the chain to ADP to form ATP. The details of the transfer are not completely understood but may involve the formation of a high-energy bond to the transfer enzyme, then a combination of the enzyme with a phosphate group, and finally the addition of the phosphate group to ADP to form ATP. The passage of two hydrogen atoms or their electron equivalents along the entire electron-transport chain (i.e., from NAD^+ to O_2) gives rise to the formation of three moles of *ATP*. If the first NAD^+ step in the electron-transport chain (Fig. 10-2) is bypassed, as in the case of the oxidation of succinate to fumarate via succinic dehydrogenase, only *two moles* of ATP will be formed. It should be emphasized that this is not a proved mechanism but a reasonable hypothesis based on current knowledge.

One of the significant recent discoveries in this field is that of Crane and his co-workers[13] and others demonstrating that coenzyme-Q and certain other *ubiquinones* (which are somewhat similar chemically to vitamin K) are components of mitochondrial lipids. Their evidence indicates that coenzyme-Q and related quinones serve as electron-transport agents and may be involved in the formation of ATP at the cytochrome-a stage. A suggested mechanism of their action is shown in Fig. 10-5.

Various homologues of coenzyme-Q, containing six to 10 isoprene units, have been isolated from different microorganisms, chloroplasts of green plants, and mitochondria of beef heart and other animal tissues. Apparently

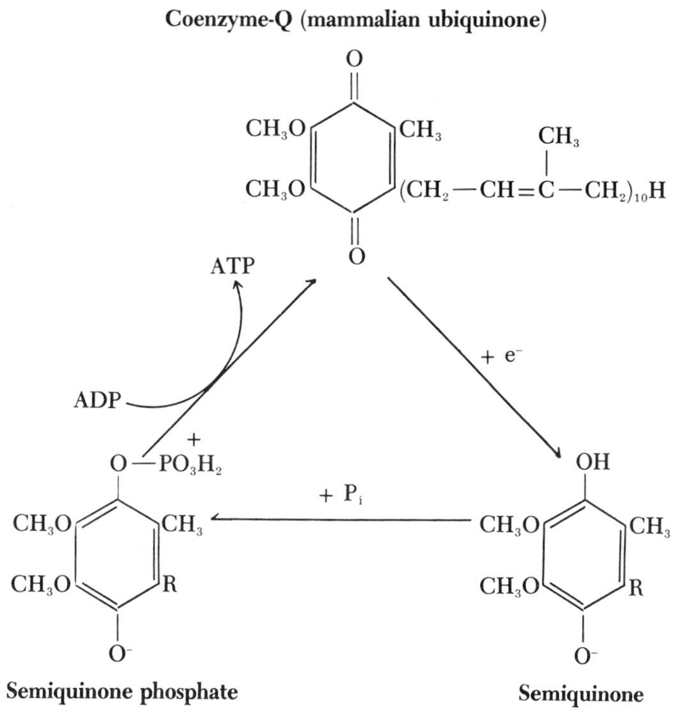

Fig. 10-5. Suggested mechanism of the role of coenzyme-Q in ATP formation.

these quinones, as well as vitamin K, serve a universal function in electron transport in most, if not all, types of cells. There is some evidence that vitamin E is also involved in some electron-transport systems.

Recent evidence, reviewed by Griffiths, is suggestive as to the chemical nature of substances X, Y, and Z (Fig. 10-2), serving as intermediates in the transfer of energy to ATP. It is possible that substance-X is the niacinamide moiety of NAD^+ itself. Phosphorylated intermediates, apparently with a high-energy bond formed at the carbon-6 atom of nicotinamide, have been suggested. This is transferred to ADP to form ATP, thus completing a *pyridine nucleotide cycle,* with a resultant transfer of two hydrogen atoms and the formation of one mole of ATP.

Similarly, substance-Y may be one of the respiratory chain quinones, ubiquinone (coenzyme-Q) plastoquinone, vitamin K, or vitamin E (α-tocopherol). Again, a high-energy phosphate bond is formed, as a semiquinone phosphate, which is transferred to ADP to form ATP (Fig. 10-5).

The nature of substance-Z is more speculative. A high-energy derivative of cytochrome-c has been proposed, but little is known as to its possible structure.

Boyer[14] has suggested that phosphohistidine may be a component of an intermediate in oxidative phosphorylation, but thus far no substantiative evidence has been reported.

A general mechanism of oxidative phosphorylation involving substances X, Y, and Z, as reviewed by Griffiths, is as follows:

$$
\begin{aligned}
&(1)\quad \text{X—OH} \xrightarrow{\;+\,P_i\;} \text{X—O-P} + H_2O \\
&(2)\quad \text{X—O-P} \xrightarrow{\;-2\,e^-\;} \text{X}^{++}\text{—O}{\sim}\text{P} \\
&(3)\quad \text{X}^{++}\text{—O}{\sim}\text{P} \xrightarrow{\;+\,ADP\;} \text{X}^{++}\text{—OH} + ATP \\
&(4)\quad \text{X}^{++}\text{—OH} \xrightarrow{\;+2\,e^-\;} \text{X—OH}
\end{aligned}
$$

Green and his co-workers[15] recently suggested still another explanation for the conversion of oxidative energy into chemical energy (ATP) and, in turn, to physiologic work. The oxidation of metabolites in the mitochondrion leads to the liberation of electrons of high reducing potential, "hot electrons," analogous to the high-energy electrons produced in photosynthesis by the action of photons of light on the chlorophyl of chloroplasts (p. 219). The high-energy electrons traverse the electron-transport chain, being transferred from one component to another, with a gradual fall in energy due to the energy's transfer to ADP plus inorganic phosphate to form ATP. Ultimately the electrons are passed to molecular oxygen ($\frac{1}{2}\,O_2$) as the final electron acceptor to form water in the presence of two hydrogen ions.

The problem of energy transduction is thus basically the question of how the released oxidative energy is utilized for the synthesis of ATP. While final answers probably are not yet possible, Green's current investigations suggest that conformational changes in repeating transducing units located in the inner membranes of the cristae of mitochondria (p. 17) are involved. The transducing unit, shown schematically from electron-microscopic examina-

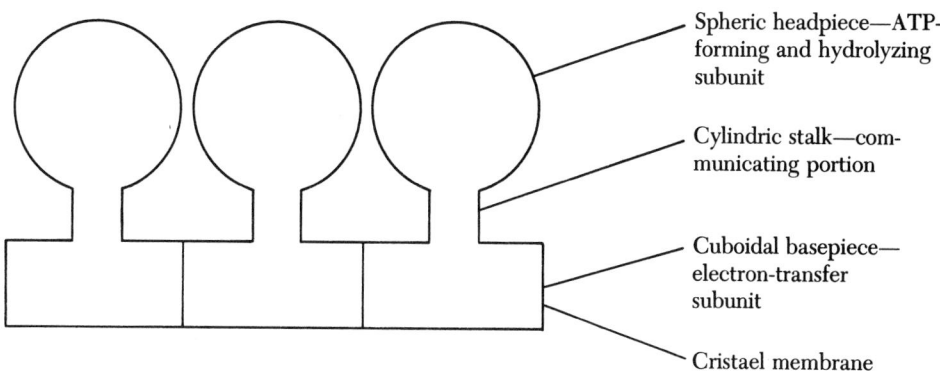

Spheric headpiece—ATP-forming and hydrolyzing subunit

Cylindric stalk—communicating portion

Cuboidal basepiece—electron-transfer subunit

Cristael membrane

Fig. 10-6. Schematic representation of the repeating units of energy-transducing elements of the cristael membranes of mitochondria. (Adapted from Penniston, J. T., et al., and Harris, R. A., et al.: Proc. Nat. Acad. Sci. **59**:624, 830, 1968; Green, D. E., et al.: Arch. Biochem. **125**:684, 1968.)

tions in Fig. 10-6, consists of a spheric headpiece, a connecting cylindric stalk, and a cuboidal base piece. The base piece of one unit nests into the base piece of the next, etc., forming the inner cristael membrane. The electron-transfer chain is localized in the base piece, and the ATP-forming or -hydrolyzing capacity is localized in the headpiece. The cylindric stalk serves as some kind of a communicating link between the two. Many thousands of these energy-transducing units then form the cristael membrane. Apparently the ultrastructure of the cristael membrane changes during the process of transducing oxidative energy into chemical energy, ATP, or the reverse— conversion of ATP energy into work performance, e.g., the translocation (active transport) of ions (p. 14) or the transfer of a hydride ion (H^-) from $NADH_2$ to $NADP^+$ (transhydrogenation). Green and co-workers,[15] on the basis of studies with agents that inhibit (cyanide) or uncouple (dinitrophenol) electron transfer or oxidative phosphorylation, respectively, postulated that the ultrastructural changes in the cristael membrane of beef and rat heart mitochondria, in vitro or in situ, respectively, are related to the formation or dissipation of the energized state of the cristael membrane. Three states of the membrane are recognizable by electron microscopy: (1) a tubular form; (2) a vesicular form; and (3) a zigzag form. Green and his group believe that this is a gross manifestation of molecular changes in the tiny repeating units themselves. Similar changes in the membrane ultrastructure of chloroplasts have been observed when chloroplasts are exposed to light. It appears, then, that energy transduction involves conformational changes in the cristael membrane, which then can be utilized to perform physiologic work as depicted diagrammatically in Fig. 10-7. The conformational change in the membrane is triggered by electron transfer or the hydrolysis of ATP. Electron transfer, these workers reasoned, leads to the generation of electrostatic energy by the delivery of two electrons to proximal molecular sites. The buildup of electrostatic energy leads to the transduction of this energy to conformational energy and this is what drives the synthesis of ATP from ADP and inorganic phosphate.

259

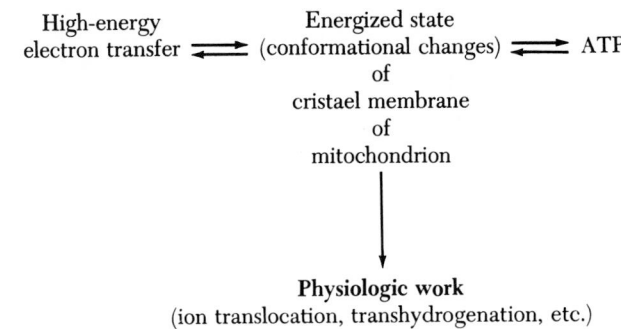

Fig. 10-7. Diagram showing how the energized state of the cristael membrane of the mitochondrion is generated and utilized to perform physiologic work. (Adapted from Penniston, J. T., et al., and Harris, R. A., et al.: Proc. Nat. Acad. Sci. **59**:624, 830, 1968; Green, D. E., et al.: Arch. Biochem. **125**:684, 1968.)

Estimates of the efficiency of the "trapping" of energy at ATP by the foregoing oxidative phosphorylation steps give the surprising values of some 40% to perhaps 50%.

In summary, the energy of biologic oxidations is produced by the flow of electrons from the hydrogen atoms of metabolites, along the electron-transport chain, to molecular oxygen. The current theory, however, is that the coupling of this flow of electrons with the formation of high-energy phosphate, ATP, and related compounds makes possible the utilization of this energy for biologic purposes. These purposes include (1) muscular contraction, (2) the biosynthesis of complex molecules from simpler ones and thus the storage of energy as glycogen, fat, etc., (3) the biosynthesis of tissue proteins and numerous substances of metabolic importance (enzymes, hormones, purines, pyrimidines, etc.), and (4) the transport of substances against concentration gradients, across cell membranes, etc. The problem of producing and utilizing energy in the living organism is thus currently one of fundamental importance.

Control mechanisms for biologic oxidations Although biologic oxidations in the cell are subject to most of the control mechanisms that regulate metabolic reactions in general (p. 23), the prime control is exerted by the cellular levels of ATP, on the one hand, and ADP and inorganic phosphate, on the other. When ATP is used for cellular processes, the levels of ADP and inorganic phosphate increase. This increase triggers an elevation of cellular oxidations to restore ATP to the original level. When such a level is reached, ATP decreases biologic oxidations in the cell by a sort of product feedback inhibition (p. 129) to maintain the appropriate level.

The rate of biologic oxidations ("respiration") in different tissues varies considerably, as measured by the milliliters of oxygen used per hour per milligram of tissue dry weight (QO_2). Values obtained by the use of the Warburg apparatus show that the respiratory rates of retina, kidney, liver, and other glandular tissues are notably high whereas those of skin, cornea, and resting muscle are relatively low. This undoubtedly is a reflection of the rate of utilization of, and hence requirement for, ATP.

Table 10-1. Agents dissociating oxidation-reductions from energy production

Agent	Stimulates	Inhibits
Dinitrophenol	Respiration and glycolysis	Maintenance of phosphocreatine
Dinitrophenol	Respiration and glycolysis	Assimilation of P_i
Dinitrophenol	Respiration and glycolysis	Sperm motility
Azide	Fermentation by yeast	Assimilation of P_i
Chloral hydrate	Respiration	Assimilation; luminescence
Gramicidin	Respiration	Assimilation; phosphate uptake

Applications. A detailed listing of the possible applications of the foregoing studies is beyond the scope of this volume. However, it might be well to mention a few of the applications and potentialities that are known.

1. There is a strong indication that the sulfonamide drugs and certain antibiotics act by affecting the activity of respiratory enzymes in the bacterial cell. Gramicidin has been shown to dissociate phosphate uptake from glycolysis so that energetic reactions are impossible.

2. Substances that uncouple oxidative phosphorylation and appear to dissociate cellular oxidations from energy production have been discovered. This provides an explanation of the mechanism of action of various compounds, from "weight reducers" to bacterial toxins. Table 10-1 lists a few of the agents affecting the coupling of oxidoreduction with energy (ATP) production.

   It is also interesting in this connection that the results of several studies have indicated that the thyroid hormone, thyroxine or triiodothyronine, may serve as a physiologic agent for controlling the coupling of oxidative phosphorylation with energy production from the respiratory chain. Indeed, the thyroid hormone may exert its characteristic effects on metabolic activity in this way.

   It thus appears that certain agents allow an exergonic step to occur without phosphorylation or that they catalyze the abnormal hydrolysis of phosphoric esters. This would account for the acceleration of oxidative and glycolytic processes and the failure of endergonic synthesis or work function.

3. Examination of malignant growths from the standpoint of their energetic and enzymatic constitution reveals unique features. It may be said that such malignancies exhibit very high values for both aerobic and anaerobic glycolysis and that they show deficiencies in their cytochrome–cytochrome oxidase systems. Based on these findings, chemotherapeutic methods of approach become possible.

4. Atabrine inhibits D-amino acid oxidase and also the oxidation of lactate, pyruvate, malate, or citrate. The site of action appears to be the inhibition of cytochrome reductase, glucose-6-phosphate dehydrogenase, and, to some extent, cytochrome oxidase. Addition of riboflavin overcomes the inhibition.

5. Certain sedative drugs (e.g., barbiturates) block the transfer of hydrogen (electrons) from $NADH_2$ to flavoprotein. Other similar drugs likewise appear to block some step in the electron-transport chain and interfere with ATP formation.

Three rare but extremely interesting cases of disease in man due to the uncoupling of oxidative phosphorylation in mitochondria have been reported recently. The original patient, with the *Luft syndrome*,[16] showed characteristic symptoms later seen in the other two cases. These included rapid respiratory and heart rates, fatigue, markedly increased appetite and thirst, and profuse, continuous sweating. Laboratory tests revealed an extremely high basal metabolic rate (+200 to +300) but normal serum thyroxin and protein-bound iodine levels. Other usual clinical laboratory tests were essentially negative. These clinical and laboratory findings suggested the possibility of an uncoupling of oxidative phosphorylation. Accordingly, a study using electron microscopy was made of muscle cell mitochondria taken by biopsy. Gross distortions of the shape and structure of the mitochondria were seen. The mitochondria were markedly increased in number and many contained dense inclusion bodies of unknown composition. Their oxygen uptake was much higher than that of normal mitochondria, but the conversion of inorganic phosphate to ATP was low. These observations thus supported the initial tentative diagnosis of hypermetabolism of nonthyroid origin with the indicated uncoupling of oxidative phosphorylation. The condition appears to be due to some mitochondrial defect of unknown nature resulting in a loss of respiratory control. The defect apparently involves a spontaneous mutation rather than a hereditary condition since neither parents nor siblings in the three cases were afflicted. This syndrome, then, presents a dramatic example of the practical importance of cellular-mitochondrial respiratory control mechanisms.

DEGRADATION OF CARBON CHAINS—DECARBOXYLATIONS

It is well known that the oxidation of metabolites in the body yields carbon dioxide as well as water and energy. In the preceding discussion, it was shown how oxidative reactions occur and oxygen enters into reaction in the respiratory chain of enzymes, appearing as water. Up to this point, however, the degradation of substrates to carbon dioxide has not been explained.

One of the principal mechanisms for the degradation of the carbon chains of metabolites is the decarboxylation of the corresponding organic acid, with the production of carbon dioxide. The successive dehydrogenation, hydration, and dehydrogenation of terminal carbon atoms of metabolites results in the formation of a carboxylic acid. The decarboxylation of these acid derivatives of metabolites is catalyzed by specific enzymes, the decarboxylases (sometimes called carboxylases). It is interesting that the vitamins thiamine pyrophosphate, pyridoxal phosphate, and possibly also lipothiamide pyrophosphate serve as coenzymes for certain of the decarboxylases. Decarboxylation by specific decarboxylases, for example, is particularly important in the degradation of the carbon chains of amino acids, as will be described in Chapter 13.

Citric acid cycle   The Krebs tricarboxylic acid cycle, or citric acid cycle, is a special mechanism for the final degradation of two-, three-, or possibly four-carbon fragments of metabolites by a combination of decarboxylation and dehydrogenation. Since these small fragments may arise from the metabolism of carbohydrates or from fats or proteins, as will be discussed in subsequent chapters, the citric acid cycle is sometimes called the "final common pathway" of metabolism.

An appreciation of the importance of this phase of intermediary metabolism is largely due to the pioneer work of Thunberg, Szent-Györgyi, and Krebs. Both Thunberg and Szent-Györgyi pointed out that there are no substances oxidized so rapidly by tissues as succinic, fumaric, and malic acids. Succinic acid has the unique property of possessing two carbon atoms that are both α- and β-carbons. The same is true of certain other four-carbon dicarboxylic acids. It is well known that such carbons are highly reactive and consequently would be expected to react rapidly under favorable conditions. A vast amount of experimentation led to the conclusion that there exist two four-carbon dicarboxylic acid systems, each reversibly oxidizable. These, when linked together, can transport hydrogen from the substrate metabolite to the cytochrome oxidase system.

Krebs and Johnson[17] pointed out that pyruvic acid, arising from carbohydrate metabolism, and oxaloacetic acid undergo a condensation to citric acid in order to bring about oxidation of the citric acid and the regeneration of four-carbon acids. The simultaneous observation, by Orten and Smith,[18] that the intravenous administration of four-carbon acids to dogs markedly increases the formation of citric acid in tissues likewise was indicative of some close metabolic interrelation between these substances. The formulation of the tricarboxylic acid cycle by Krebs resulted from these and other investigations. It is shown in Fig. 10-8. The enzymes and cofactors involved, indicated by numbers on the diagram, are as follows:

(1) Pyruvic dehydrogenase; NAD^+, thiamine pyrophosphate, FAD, CoA, Mg^{++}, and lipoic acid
(2) Citrate synthetase (condensing enzyme)
(3) Aconitase
(4) Aconitase
(5) Isocitric dehydrogenase; $NADP^+$
(6) Isocitric dehydrogenase; Mn^{++}
(7) α-Ketoglutaric dehydrogenase; thiamine pyrophosphate; lipoic acid; CoA, FAD, NAD^+, GDP, P_i
(8) Succinic dehydrogenase; Fe^{++} flavin
(9) Fumarase
(10) Malic dehydrogenase; NAD^+
(11) Oxaloacetic carboxylase; Mg^{++}
(12) Citrate-cleavage enzyme

Decarboxylation and oxidation of pyruvic acid (p. 204) constitute the first step and involve an enzyme, pyruvic dehydrogenase, together with NAD^+, cocarboxylase (thiamine pyrophosphate), coenzyme-A, magnesium ions, and lipoic acid.

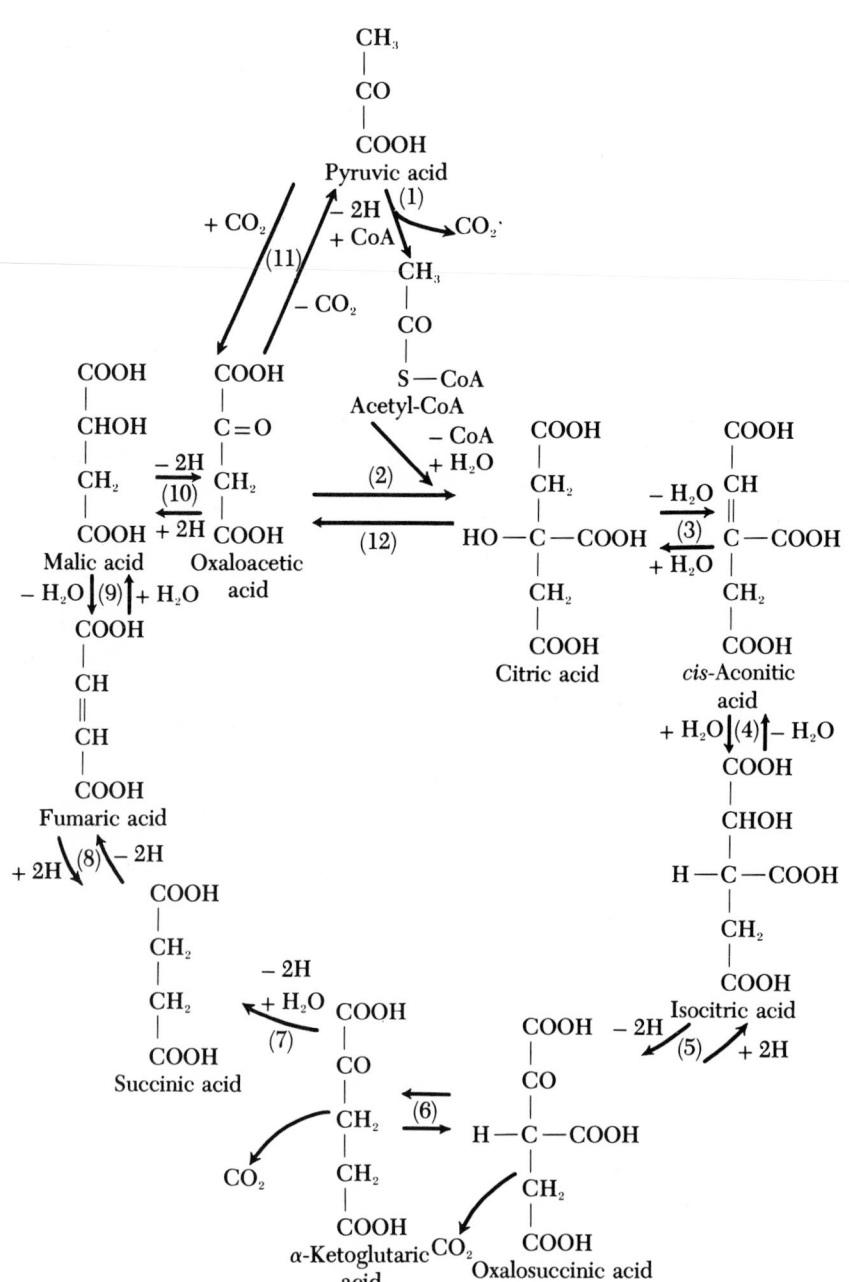

Fig. 10-8. Citric acid cycle.

$$\begin{array}{ccc} \underset{|}{CH_3} & & \underset{|}{CH_3} \\ \underset{|}{CO} & + \ CoA—SH + NAD^+ \ \rightarrow & \underset{|}{CO} & + \ NADH_2 + CO_2 \\ COOH & & S—CoA \end{array}$$

Pyruvic   **Acetyl-CoA**
acid

Citrate synthetase then catalyzes the addition of the acetyl group of acetyl-CoA to oxaloacetic acid, but note that the methyl group is attached to the oxaloacetic acid. Thus:

$$\underset{\text{Acetyl-CoA}}{CH_3—CO—S—CoA} + \underset{\text{Oxaloacetic acid}}{\overset{\displaystyle CO—COOH}{\underset{\displaystyle CH_2—COOH}{|}}} + H_2O \xrightarrow{\text{Citrate synthetase}} \underset{\text{Citric acid}}{\overset{\displaystyle CH_2COOH}{\underset{\displaystyle CH_2COOH}{HO—C—COOH}}} + CoA—SH$$

A series of reactions follows, resulting in the formation of three other tricarboxylic acids: *cis*-aconitic, isocitric, and oxalosuccinic. The last named is decarboxylated, yielding α-ketoglutaric acid and carbon dioxide. Another carbon dioxide is then released, producing succinic acid. A dehydrogenation yields fumaric acid, which is then hydrated to form malic acid. Another dehydrogenation results in oxaloacetic acid. In this manner, oxaloacetic acid is, in a sense, regenerated so that it can combine with another molecule of acetyl-CoA. This cycle thus continually oxidizes pyruvic acid.

The conversion of succinyl-CoA to succinate in Reaction 7 is rather unusual in that it requires GDP and inorganic phosphate, GTP being formed as follows:

$$\text{Succinyl-CoA} + \text{GDP} + P_i \xrightarrow{\text{Succinic thiokinase}} \text{Succinate} + \text{GTP} + \text{CoA}$$

Thus the energy of the thioester is conserved by the formation of GTP, which is equivalent to ATP as an energy source. Also, GTP can be converted to ATP by the following reaction:

$$\text{GTP} + \text{ADP} \xrightleftharpoons{\text{Nucleoside diphosphokinase}} \text{GDP} + \text{ATP}$$

UTP and CTP, which are involved in carbohydrate (p. 189) and lipid metabolism (p. 322), respectively, are interconvertible to ATP in an analogous manner.

Note that Reactions 1 and 7 of the citric acid cycle, which are nonreversible, involve oxidative decarboxylations, which are complex reactions involving six essential agents: (1) the specific dehydrogenase, (2) diphosphothiamine, and (3) magnesium ions, for the decarboxylation, thus creating an aldehyde intermediate, (4) lipoic acid, and (5) NAD$^+$, for the oxidation of the aldehyde to an acyl compound, which is then accepted by (6) coenzyme-A:

$$\text{Pyruvate} + \text{NAD}^+ + \text{CoA} \ \rightarrow \ \text{Acetyl-CoA} + \text{NADH}_2 + \text{CO}_2$$

Similar reactions hold for α-ketoglutarate decarboxylation wherein succinyl-CoA is formed.

One other step of the citric acid cycle, Reaction 6, merits some added comment. Oxalosuccinic acid is so unstable that its spontaneous decarboxylation may occur. However, the apoenzyme of isocitric dehydrogenase, as well as manganese(II) ions, is believed to be involved, thus increasing the rate of loss of carbon dioxide, with the formation of α-ketoglutaric acid.

It is clear now how carbon dioxide arises in biologic oxidations. The three carbon dioxide molecules, of course, are the oxidation products of the three carbons of pyruvic acid, whereas the water comes from the oxidation of the hydrogens. It will be shown subsequently how the products of protein and lipid metabolism enter into the tricarboxylic acid cycle.

Most of the enzymes involved in the various steps of the citric acid cycle have been prepared in highly purified form and the physical and chemical properties and kinetics have been extensively studied. Several have been prepared in crystalline form. Succinic dehydrogenase, for example, has been crystallized from heart muscle and has been found to be a ferriflavoprotein with a molecular weight of about 200,000. It contains four atoms of nonhemin iron and one molecule of flavin per molecule of enzyme. It forms the *trans* isomer, fumaric acid, only. The *cis* isomer, maleic acid, is not produced and is extremely toxic in the animal organism.[18] Malonic acid is a specific competitive inhibitor of the oxidation of succinic acid. Its administration results in the accumulation of citrate[18] and other preceding acids of the citric acid cycle.

Fumarase has been crystallized from pig heart. It has a molecular weight of about 200,000. It forms L-malic acid from fumaric acid and apparently requires a sulfhydryl compound as a cofactor. Further detailed information regarding other enzymes of the citric acid cycle may be found in the general references cited at the end of the chapter.

It should be noted that, according to present knowledge, Reactions 1 and 7 in the diagram of the citric acid cycle (Fig. 10-8) are *not* reversible. Step 2, the formation of citrate by the condensing enzyme, is also essentially nonreversible, the reaction being highly in favor of citrate formation. However, in the past few years a different enzyme, the citrate-cleavage enzyme, has been described in chicken liver, mammary gland, and certain other tissues.[19] This enzyme catalyzes the reaction:

$$\text{Citrate} + \text{ATP} + \text{CoA} \xrightarrow[\text{Mg}^{++}]{\text{Citrate-cleavage enzyme}} \text{Acetyl-CoA} + \text{Oxaloacetate} + \text{ADP} + \text{P}_i$$

Citryl-CoA is apparently the actual substrate for the enzyme. The enzyme has been purified a hundredfold from chicken liver. It has the same stereospecificity as citrate synthetase, the acetyl-CoA coming from carbon-1 of citrate, and oxaloacetate from carbon-4. The acetyl-CoA formed may be readily used for the biosynthesis of fatty acids by the cytoplasmic malonyl-CoA system, as will be described later. Apparently, citrate readily passes through the mitochondrial membrane into the cytoplasm for such biosynthetic use. Other studies[20] have shown that as much as 20% to 30% of ^{14}C-glutamate can be converted to fatty acids by way of citrate in mammary gland tissue. From labeling data, it was evident that the glutamate must have been converted to citrate by a "backward reaction" of the citric acid cycle, then to acetyl-CoA by means of the citrate-cleavage enzyme, and finally to fatty acids. Studies such as these emphasize the importance of the citric acid cycle in anabolic biosynthetic reactions as well as in the degradation (catabolism) of carbon chains.

In recent investigations[21] the citrate-cleavage enzyme has been prepared in purified form from rat liver. Kinetic studies, including the apparent K_M value of the purified material, were reported. Magnesium citrate appears to be the actual substrate. The enzyme is present in the extramitochondrial cell sap of chicken liver as well as in the mitochondrion itself apparently.

Current evidence thus indicates that citrate is the primary carbon source for fatty acid biosynthesis (p. 310) and that the amount of this enzyme in liver parallels fatty acid formation.

It may be recalled that oxaloacetate may be enzymatically decarboxylated to form pyruvate (p. 205) and also that pyruvate may be carboxylated by a different enzyme system to form oxalacetate. This serves as a means of replenishing the acids of the citric acid cycle to replace those lost by excretion, conversion, or other metabolic routes.

The oxidation of pyruvate by way of the citric acid cycle and the resulting oxidative phosphorylation yield about 15 high-energy phosphate bonds. These arise as follows:

Pyruvate	→	Acetate + CO_2 yields	3 ~P bonds
Isocitrate	→	Oxalosuccinate yields	3 ~P bonds
α-Ketoglutarate	→	Succinate yields	4 ~P bonds
Succinate	→	Fumarate yields	2 ~P bonds
Malate	→	Oxaloacetate yields	3 ~P bonds

From an energetic standpoint, it is significant to note that the creation of the 15 high-energy phosphate groups is possible since the ratio of phosphate to oxygen $\left(\dfrac{\text{Micromoles of phosphate taken up}}{\text{Microatoms of oxygen utilized}}\right)$ may be 2:4 as contrasted with oxidative phosphorylation in glycolysis, where the ratio is only 1:1.

The catalytic activity of the citric acid cycle thus brings about the oxidation to carbon dioxide and water of (1) pyruvic acid and members of the citric acid cycle, (2) fatty acids, and (3) L-proline, L-alanine, L-glutamate, and L-asparate. The citric acid cycle is thus indeed the "final common pathway" for the metabolism of carbohydrates, fats, and proteins. The common feature in these reactions is the participation of the citric acid cycle of reactions.

A recent investigation[22] demonstrated that all the acids of the citric acid cycle are present in the urine of normal human subjects. In several types of alkalosis, a significant increase was found in the urinary excretion of one of these acids, citric acid. In an acidosis the urinary citric acid concentration decreased. These observations, with others, suggest that citric acid may function as a physiologic acid in the maintenance of acid-base balance in man, as well as serving as a key member of the citric acid cycle.

In summary, it may be said that, although much remains to be explained, biochemistry is entering an era in which philosophic considerations of energy metabolism are opening new vistas in our understanding of the basic mechanics of the cell and the organism.

References

GENERAL

Chance, B., Estabrook, R. W., and Williamson, J. R., editors: Control of energy metabolism, New York, 1965, Academic Press, Inc.

Florkin, M., and Stotz, E., editors: Comprehensive biochemistry, vol. 22, Bioenergetics, New York, 1967, American Elsevier Publishing Corp.

Goodwin, T. W., editor: Metabolic roles of citrate, New York, 1968, Academic Press, Inc.

Green, D. E., and Goldberger, R. F.: Molecular insights into the living process, New York, 1967, Academic Press, Inc.

Green, D. E., and MacLennan, D. H.: The mitochondrial system of enzymes. In Greenberg, D. M., editor: Metabolic pathways, ed. 3, New York, 1967, Academic Press, Inc., vol. 1.

Griffiths, D. E.: Oxidative phosphorylation, Essays in Biochemistry 1:91, 1965.

Ingraham, L. L., and Pardee, A. B.: Free energy and entropy in metabolism. In Greenberg, D. M., editor: Metabolic pathways, ed. 3, New York, 1967, Academic Press, Inc., vol. 1.

Kaplan, N. O., and Kennedy, E. P.: Current aspects of biochemical energetics, New York, 1966, Academic Press, Inc.

Keilin, D.: The history of cell respiration and the cytochromes, New York, 1968, Cambridge University Press.

Klotz, I. M.: Energy changes in biochemical reactions, New York, 1967, Academic Press, Inc.

Lehninger, A. L.: The mitochondrion—structure and function, New York, 1964, W. A. Benjamin, Inc.

Lehninger, A. L.: Bioenergetics, New York, 1965, W. A. Benjamin, Inc.

Lehninger, A. L., Racker E., Chance, B., Lardy, H. A., Jagendorf, A. T., and Mitchell, P.: Energy coupling in electron transport, Fed. Proc. Sympos. 26:1333, 1967.

Lowenstein, J. M., editor: vol. 13, Citric acid cycle. In Colowick, S. P., and Kaplan, N. O., editors: Methods in enzymology, New York, 1969, Academic Press, Inc.

Racker, E.: Mechanisms in bioenergetics, New York, 1965, Academic Press, Inc.

Singer, T. P., editor: Biological oxidations, New York, 1968, John Wiley & Sons, Inc.

Slater, E. C., Kaniuga, Z., and Wojtczak, L., editors: Biochemistry of mitochondria, New York, 1967, Academic Press, Inc.

SPECIAL

1. Green, D. E.: Sci. Amer. 210:63, 1964.
2. Chance, B., et al.: Proc. Nat. Acad. Sci. 57:498, 1967.
3. Warburg, O., and Christian, W.: Biochem. Z. 254:438, 1932.
4. Keilin, D.: Proc. Roy. Soc. 98B:312, 1925.
5. Matsubara, H., and Smith, E. L.: J. Biol. Chem. 238:2732, 1963.
6. Beinert, H., and Palmer, G.: J. Biol. Chem. 239:1221, 1964.
7. Yamashita, S., and Racker, E.: J. Biol. Chem. 243:2446, 1968.
8. Arnon, D. I., et al.: Science 146:422, 1964.
9. Lipmann, F.: Advances Enzym. 1:99, 1941.
10. Podolsky, R. J., and Morales, M. F.: J. Biol. Chem. 218:945, 1956; Robins, E. A., and Boyer, P. D.: J. Biol. Chem. 224:121, 1957.
11. Lehninger, A. L.: J. Biol. Chem. 190:345, 1951; Burton, K.: Nature 181:1594, 1958.
12. Lehninger, A. L., et al.: Science 128:450, 1958; Sci. Amer. 202:102, 1960.
13. Crane, F. L., et al.: Biochim. Biophys. Acta 31:476, 1959.
14. Boyer, P. D.: Science 141:1147, 1963.
15. Penniston, J. T., et al.: Proc. Nat. Acad. Sci. 59:624, 1968; Harris, R. A., et al.: Proc. Nat. Acad. Sci. 59:830, 1968; Green, D. E., et al.: Arch. Biochem. 125:684, 1968; Harris, R. A., et al.: Science 165:700, 1969.
16. Luft, R., et. al.: J. Clin. Invest. 41:1776, 1962.
17. Krebs, H. A., and Johnson, W. A.: Enzymologia 4:148, 1937.
18. Orten, J. M., and Smith, A. H.: Proc. Soc. Exp. Biol. Med. 36:555, 1937.
19. Srere, P. A., and Bhaduri, A.: J. Biol. Chem. 239:714, 1964.
20. Abraham, S., et al.: J. Biol. Chem. 239:855, 1964.
21. Plowman, K. M., and Cleland, W. W.: J. Biol. Chem. 242:4239, 1967.
22. Gamble, W., et al.: J. Appl. Physiol. 16:593, 1961.

CHAPTER 11

CHEMISTRY OF LIPIDS

The lipids constitute a very important group of organic substances in plant and animal tissues, a group that is difficult to characterize clearly. Its members have certain solubilities and properties in common but are rather diverse in their chemical constitution. Lipids include the fats and other compounds that resemble them in physical properties. The terminology in this field is rather confusing, and various names other than lipid, e.g., lipoid and lipin, have been suggested for this group of compounds. *Lipid* seems to be the term preferred by most biochemists and was suggested by Bloor. It was also recommended by the International Congress of Pure and Applied Chemistry. According to Bloor, lipids are compounds having the following characteristics: (1) insolubility in water and solubility in one or more organic solvents (ether, chloroform, benzene, acetone—the so-called "fat solvents"); (2) some relation to fatty acids as esters, either actual or potential; (3) possibility of utilization by living organisms.

Bloor's classification is quite generally adopted in the United States and, with a few modifications, is as follows:

A. Simple lipids—esters of fatty acids with various alcohols
   1. Neutral fats and oils—triglycerides: triesters of fatty acids with glycerol
   2. Waxes: esters of fatty acids with monohydroxy aliphatic alcohols higher than glycerol
      (a) True waxes: products of both animal and vegetable origin in which esters are composed of palmitic, stearic, oleic, or other higher fatty acid esters of cetyl alcohol ($CH_3[CH_2]_{14}CH_2OH$) or other higher straight-chain alcohols
      (b) Cholesterol esters: esters of fatty acids with cholesterol
      (c) Vitamin A esters: palmitic or stearic acid esters of vitamin A
      (d) Vitamin D esters
B. Compound lipids—esters of fatty acids with alcohols plus other groups
   1. Phospholipids: lipids containing phosphoric acid and, in most cases, a nitrogenous base
   2. Glycolipids or cerebrosides: lipids containing a carbohydrate and also nitrogen but no phosphate and no glycerol
   3. Sulfolipids: lipids characterized by possessing sulfate groups
   4. Lipoproteins: lipids attached to plasma or other proteins
   5. Lipopolysaccharides: lipids attached to polysaccharides
C. Derived lipids—derivatives obtained by hydrolysis of those given in groups A and B that still possess general physical characteristics of lipids
   1. Saturated and unsaturated fatty acids
   2. Monoglycerides and diglycerides

3. Alcohols
   (a) Straight-chain alcohols: water-insoluble alcohols of higher molecular weight obtained on hydrolysis of waxes
   (b) Sterols and other steroids, including vitamin D
   (c) Alcohols containing β-ionone ring (vitamin A, certain carotenoids)
D. Miscellaneous lipids
   1. Aliphatic hydrocarbons: include iso-octadecane found in liver fat and certain hydrocarbons found in beeswax and plant waxes
   2. Carotenoids
   3. Squalene: a hydrocarbon found in shark and mammalian liver and in human sebum; also an important intermediate in biosynthesis of cholesterol
   4. Vitamins E and K

FATS AND OILS—TRIGLYCERIDES

As stated in the classification, fats and vegetable types of oils are all triesters of the trihydric alcohol glycerol and various fatty acids. In general, vegetable oils are triglycerides that are liquid at room temperature due to their higher unsaturated or shorter length carbon chain–fatty acids, as will be discussed later. Triglycerides are the most abundant naturally occurring lipid.

The type formula for a fat (or oil) is as follows:

$$
\begin{array}{c}
\text{H} \quad\quad \text{O} \\
| \qu\quad\quad || \\
\text{H--C--O--C--R}_1 \\
| \qu\quad\quad \text{O} \\
\text{H--C--O--C--R}_2 \\
| \qu\quad\quad \text{O} \\
\text{H--C--O--C--R}_3 \\
| \\
\text{H}
\end{array}
$$

R_1, R_2, and R_3 represent fatty acid chains that may or may not all be the same. Usually R_1 and R_3 are saturated fatty acids and R_2 is unsaturated. Since all three of the glycerol alcohol groups are esterified, fats are termed "triglycerides." Naturally occurring fats have apparently the D-structural configuration. Some typical fats are:

$$
\begin{array}{ccc}
\text{CH}_2\text{--O--C--C}_{15}\text{H}_{31} & \text{CH}_2\text{--O--C--C}_{17}\text{H}_{33} & \text{CH}_2\text{--O--C--C}_{15}\text{H}_{31} \\
\text{CH--O--C--C}_{15}\text{H}_{31} & \text{CH--O--C--C}_{17}\text{H}_{35} & \text{CH--O--C--C}_{17}\text{H}_{33} \\
\text{CH}_2\text{--O--C--C}_{15}\text{H}_{31} & \text{CH}_2\text{--O--C--C}_{17}\text{H}_{33} & \text{CH}_2\text{--O--C--C}_{17}\text{H}_{35} \\
\textbf{Tripalmitin} & \textbf{Stearodiolein} & \textbf{Palmitoleostearin}
\end{array}
$$

No naturally occurring fat consists solely of one simple triglyceride (i.e., having three identical fatty acid residues), such as tripalmitin or triolein. Indeed, it is questionable whether natural fats consist of mixtures of two or more simple triglycerides. It is more probable that they are mixtures of glycerides, e.g., stearodiolein and palmitoleostearin, in which the fatty acid residues are all different or there are at least two different residues to the molecule. A small amount of simple triglyceride is, of course, to be expected. Thus, a large number of triglycerides are possible and are found in nature.

Table 11-1. Common fatty acids

		Formula	Melting (or solidifying) point
Saturated	Butyric	C_3H_7COOH	$-7.9°$ (m)
	Caproic	$C_5H_{11}COOH$	$-3.9°$ (m)
	Palmitic	$C_{15}H_{31}COOH$	$63°-64°$ (m)
	Stearic	$C_{17}H_{35}COOH$	$70°$ (m)
Unsaturated	Oleic	$C_{17}H_{33}COOH$	$4°$ (s)
	Linoleic	$C_{17}H_{31}COOH$	$-12°$ (m)
	Linolenic	$C_{17}H_{29}COOH$	Liquid at very low temperature

Fatty acids   A fatty acid may be defined as an acid that occurs in a natural triglyceride and is a monocarboxylic acid ranging in chain length from four to about 24 carbon atoms and including, with a few exceptions, only the even-numbered members of the series. Some are saturated and some unsaturated, and certain ones contain substituent groups, such as hydroxyl or keto groups. Certain fatty acids apparently do not fit this definition because they have methyl and other groups, which may give them a branched effect; and some have an odd number of carbons. A few cyclic fatty acids are known. The most common fatty acids occurring in the fats and oils are shown in Table 11-1.

Many other fatty acids of both series are found in the naturally occurring fats. Capric, lauric, myristic, and arachidic acids may be included in the group of saturated fatty acids, and clupanodonic and arachidonic acids in the group of unsaturated fatty acids. Two hydroxy acids, ricinoleic and dihydroxystearic, are constituents of fats in castor oil. Another, cerebronic acid ($C_{23}H_{46}$[OH] COOH, 2-hydroxytetracosanoic acid), is a constituent of cerebrosides found in animal tissues (p. 289). Two cyclic acids, hydnocarpic and chaulmoogric, are of interest because chaulmoogra oil, in which they are combined, has been used in the treatment of leprosy.

Isomerism of fatty acids may be of several types. The saturated chains may be straight or branched. Thus there is normal butyric acid:

$$CH_3 \cdot CH_2 \cdot CH_2 \cdot COOH$$

and its isomer, isobutyric acid:

$$\begin{array}{c} CH_3 \\ \diagdown \\ CH_3 \diagup \end{array}\!\!CH \cdot COOH$$

In unsaturated fatty acids, isomerism may be due to the position of the double bond in the chain. This is usually indicated by the Greek letter *delta*, Δ, followed by the number position in the fatty acid chain of the first carbon atom of the double bond. For example, oleic acid is Δ^9; linoleic acid is $\Delta^{9,12}$; γ-linolenic (the isomer occurring in animal tissues) is $\Delta^{6,9,12}$; arachidonic acid is $\Delta^{5,8,11,14}$.

271

Still another type of isomerism depends on the spatial arrangement. The double bond limits the free rotation of the carbon atoms at this linkage, and therefore two forms are possible. If R_1 and R_2 represent the two ends of the molecular structure, we have two forms, termed *cis* and *trans*:

$$R_1—C—H$$
$$R_2—C—H$$
Cis

$$R_1—C—H$$
$$H—C—R_2$$
Trans

Oleic acid has a *trans* isomer, elaidic acid, that is useful in physiologic experiments because the body apparently does not distinguish it from the *cis* isomer. However, elaidic acid has characteristic differences that permit its separate isolation and analysis. Therefore, if elaidic acid is administered to an animal, the acid's path can be followed and we can infer how oleic acid is handled under the same conditions.

$$CH_3 \cdot (CH_2)_7 \cdot C \cdot H$$
$$HOOC \cdot (CH_2)_7 \cdot C \cdot H$$
cis
Oleic acid

$$CH_3 \cdot (CH_2)_7 \cdot C \cdot H$$
$$H \cdot C \cdot (CH_2)_7 \cdot COOH$$
trans
Elaidic acid

The naturally occurring unsaturated fatty acids, apparently without exception, are all *cis* isomers. Their formulas may be written also in the schematic form shown below for linoleic acid.

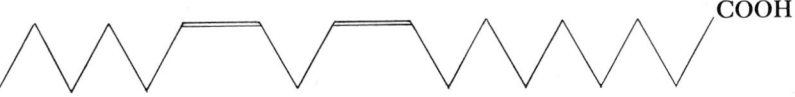

The amounts of the common fatty acids present in a number of fats have been determined. The older, classic methods, however, are laborious and none too accurate and have now been largely replaced by column chromatography on silica gel, especially *thin-layer chromatography,* and by the technique of *gas-liquid* chromatography. In the latter procedure, the methyl esters of the fatty acids are separated by passage through a chromatograph column containing a finely divided, inert material treated with a nonvolatile oil. The fatty acid esters pass through the column at different rates and may be measured quantitatively as they emerge by their thermal conductance or by other physical properties. This procedure permits the separation and accurate determination of even closely related fatty acids, e.g., *cis-trans* isomers, from complex mixtures.

Fatty aldehydes Fatty aldehydes, mainly of longer carbon chain length (16,18), occur in small amounts in blood and various tissues (beef heart, etc.). They are present normally in a ratio of about 1:100 to the corresponding fatty acid. Like free fatty acids (p. 271), they are associated with the albumin fraction of plasma proteins. Their function, if any, is unknown.

Physical properties The hardness or consistency of fats is related to the melting points of these fats, which are not sharp, because natural fats are mixtures rather than pure substances. The solidification points are considerably lower than the melting points. Glycerides of the lower fatty acids melt at lower temperatures than do glycerides of the higher fatty acids, and glycerides of the unsaturated fatty acids still lower. These are reflections, in part at least, of the melting points of the fatty acids (Table 11-1) present in fat. Many fats, e.g., triolein, are liquid at room temperatures and are commonly called *oils*. The term "oil" is rather confusing because it is often used for substances having no relation to the lipids, e.g., mineral oil (which is a mixture of hydrocarbons), oil of vitriol (which is concentrated sulfuric acid), and the volatile oils, such as oil of wintergreen and oil of peppermint (which are mixtures of volatile esters, aldehydes, etc. and are used as flavoring agents). We should therefore understand that the word "oil" indicates the physical state of a substance, rather than the chemical nature of that substance. The hardness of common fats depends largely on the relative amounts of fats present containing long-chain saturated fatty acids, like palmitic and stearic, and those containing unsaturated fatty acids, like oleic and linoleic. The former are solid, and the latter liquid at room temperature. There are larger proportions of soft fats in cold-blooded animals than in warm-blooded animals. This facilitates motility at low temperatures. Likewise, within a species of animals, the subcutaneous fat tends to be "softer" than that serving as a protective pad for the internal organs, e.g., the kidneys.

The specific gravity of all fats is less than 1.0. Consequently, all fats float on water. They are not soluble in water, at least not to any appreciable extent.

Emulsions of fats may be made by shaking vigorously in water, but, of course, emulsifying agents such as gums, soaps, and proteins produce more stable emulsions. The emulsification of fats in the intestinal tract is a prerequisite for digestion and absorption. All fats are soluble in ether, chloroform, and benzene, as well as in hot ethyl alcohol and hot acetone.

The flavor of food fats is attributed to foreign substances absorbed by the fat either from its natural environment or from materials produced during processing. For example, in the manufacture of butter, the bacterial flora are carefully controlled in order to impart a distinctive flavor to the butter.

The color of human body fat, as well as that of human milk fat, is derived from carotene and xanthophyll present in the diet. The amount of these plant pigments is very small, only 5 or 6 mg. being present in a kilogram of fat.

Hydrolysis   The fats may be hydrolyzed by superheated steam, by alkalies, or by the specific fat-splitting enzymes, lipases. They yield glycerol and the constituent fatty acids:

$$
\begin{array}{ll}
CH_2-O-\overset{\displaystyle O}{\overset{\displaystyle \parallel}{C}}-C_{17}H_{33} & CH_2OH \\[2mm]
CH-O-\overset{\displaystyle O}{\overset{\displaystyle \parallel}{C}}-C_{17}H_{33} \quad \xrightarrow{+\,3\,H_2O} & CHOH \; + 3\,C_{17}H_{33}COOH \\[2mm]
CH_2-O-\overset{\displaystyle O}{\overset{\displaystyle \parallel}{C}}-C_{17}H_{33} & CH_2OH
\end{array}
$$

Triolein   **Oleic acid** / Glycerol

If alkali is the agent used, the alkali salts or soaps are formed.

$$\text{Triolein} + 3\ NaOH \rightarrow \text{Glycerol} + 3\ C_{17}H_{33}COONa$$
$$\text{Sodium oleate (a soap)}$$

In this type of reaction, the hydrolysis is called a *saponification*. Soaps can, of course, also be formed by causing alkali to react with the fatty acid. Both products of saponification are of interest from several aspects.

Glycerol   Glycerol, commonly called glycerin, is the simplest trihydric alcohol. It is a colorless, oily fluid with a sweetish taste. Besides being a by-product in soap manufacture, it is also obtainable in the fermentation of glucose by changing conditions in such a way as to decrease the formation of carbon dioxide and alcohol. Considerable amounts are also obtained synthetically from products of petroleum cracking. It is miscible with water and alcohol in all proportions but is almost insoluble in ether. With dehydrating agents, acrylaldehyde, or "acrolein," is formed.

$$
\begin{array}{ccc}
CH_2OH & & CH_2 \\
| & & \| \\
CHOH & \rightarrow 2\ H_2O + & CH \quad O \\
| & & C \\
CH_2OH & & \diagdown H \\
\end{array}
$$

Glycerol   Acrylaldehyde

Acrolein has a very acrid odor and therefore is easily detected. Any compound containing glycerol, including the fats and oils, gives an acrolein test.

Glycerol finds many uses in industry as a result of its solubility, its solvent action, and its hygroscopic nature. Many pharmaceutic and cosmetic preparations have glycerol in their formulas. When treated with nitric acid, glycerol forms glyceryl trinitrate, or nitroglycerin.

$$
\begin{array}{c}
CH_2ONO_2 \\
| \\
CHONO_2 \\
| \\
CH_2ONO_2 \\
\end{array}
$$

This is an important explosive either alone or as a constituent of dynamite and smokeless powders. In medicine, nitroglycerin is a vasodilator of great value in certain types of circulatory disorders.

Physiologically, glycerol, a product of fat digestion, has a definite nutritive value. It has about the same caloric value as the sugars and follows a similar course when utilized by the cells of the body (p. 314).

Soaps   Soaps are salts of the nonvolatile fatty acids whose esters form the fats. However, the common soaps are those of sodium and potassium. Sodium soaps are the ordinary hard soaps, whereas potassium soaps are soft. When potash was cheaper than soda, soft soap was a common household article; now there is no advantage to using the less convenient and more expensive potassium soap.

The floating soaps are made light by beating air bubbles into the hot melted soap and then chilling it and trapping the air. Most household soap has sodium carbonate or sodium silicate added to overcome the hardness of water. Scouring soap has an abrasive added, and laundry soap may have naphtha or other special ingredients. Most toilet and household soaps have perfume added to give a pleasing aroma. Transparent soap acquires this property by the incorporation of sugar. Shaving soaps are in part potassium soaps of coconut and palm oils. Castile soap is a sodium olive oil soap, and green soap is sodium and potassium linseed oil soaps mixed. Many household soaps contain a certain amount of soap prepared from rosin mixed with the ordinary type derived from fats.

In general, soaps have a slightly alkaline reaction because of hydrolysis.

$$R \cdot COO^- + H \cdot OH \; \rightleftarrows \; R \cdot COOH + OH^-$$
$$Na^+ \qquad\qquad\qquad\qquad Na^+$$

In order to prevent irritation of the skin as a result of this alkalinity, toilet soaps sometimes are modified by adding an excess of fatty acids or a larger proportion of sodium oleate. The latter is not as readily hydrolyzed as most of the other sodium soaps.

The heavy metals produce insoluble soaps that are of relatively little importance. Zinc stearate is an exception. This is a white powder having a greasy feel. It is soft, water repellent, and mildly antiseptic and astringent and is used as a dusting powder, particularly for babies.

The cleansing action of soaps is probably due to the fact that soaps are effective emulsifying agents. Most dirt is held to surfaces by greasy substances. Soaps emulsify and wash away the grease, thus causing the dirt to be carried away. Soapy solutions also can wet and penetrate an oily texture because of their low surface tension. This is an additional aid in the cleansing action.

Insoluble soaps and hard water. Ordinary sodium soaps are not very soluble, although we usually consider them so. They are easily precipitated by strong salt solutions, which is one reason why the common soaps are useless in seawater. The calcium and magnesium soaps are even less soluble; and if sodium soap is added to water containing these ions, the soap is immediately precipitated as the insoluble calcium or magnesium soaps, which, of course, do not lather or cleanse. Water containing either or both calcium and magnesium ions is called hard water. Hard water is not harmful for drinking purposes; if it contains more than ordinary amounts of salts, it may have a slightly salty flavor, which some people like. The main objection to hard water arises from its precipitation of soap. This continues until all the calcium and magnesium ions are combined. Additional soap will then permit lathering, but this means that more soap will be required. Second, the precipitated calcium and magnesium soaps cling to washed materials and cause them to be harsh and irritating to sensitive skin. Hardness may be temporary or permanent. Temporary hardness is due to the bicarbonates of calcium or magnesium and is so called because the water may be softened by boiling. The bicarbonate is decomposed and the carbonate thus formed is precipitated.

$$Ca(HCO_3)_2 \rightarrow \underline{CaCO_3} + H_2O + CO_2$$

Permanent hardness is caused by the presence of such salts as are not changed by boiling, e.g., the chlorides. Temporary hardness is more conveniently abolished by the use of slaked lime.

$$Ca(HCO_3)_2 + Ca(OH)_2 \rightarrow \underline{2\ CaCO_3} + 2H_2O$$

There are several salts that soften permanent hard water, among them sodium carbonate, borax, and trisodium phosphate.

$$CaCl_2 + Na_2CO_3 \rightarrow \underline{CaCO_3} + 2\ NaCl$$

A combination of lime and sodium carbonate is utilized industrially (the Porter-Clark process). The resulting insoluble calcium and magnesium compounds are filtered off. Another method is more adaptable to homes, laundries, and hospitals. It is the *permutit* process. Permutit is an artificial zeolite —sodium aluminum silicate, $Na_2Al_2Si_2O_3$—which we may represent as Na_2Zeo. In contact with hard water, an exchange of the calcium or magnesium for the sodium occurs, and the water is thereby softened.

$$Na_2Zeo + CaCl_2 \rightarrow CaZeo + 2\ NaCl$$

This is accomplished by permitting the hard water to filter through a column of zeolite. Eventually the zeolite becomes depleted of all its sodium. It is then regenerated by allowing a sodium chloride solution to filter through it.

$$CaZeo + 2\ NaCl \rightarrow Na_2Zeo + CaCl_2$$

Detergents. The use of nonsoap detergents has found rather wide application in the home, in industry, and in medicine. Most of the detergents fall into three groups: (1) The *anionic:* These are exemplified by certain alkyl sulfates, e.g., the sodium salt of laurylsulfuric acid; sulfated esters, e.g., the sulfated lauryl monoglyceride; sulfated amines; and various sulfonates. (2) The *cationic:* These contain quaternary ammonium salts with a long aliphatic chain. (3) The *nonionic:* Among these detergents are esters and ethers, e.g., the palmitic acid ester of a sorbitan polyethylene derivative. These are all good wetting agents and emulsifiers and are therefore good cleansers. Since they are not soaps, they are independent of the hardness of water and are being used with increasing fequency in the home. Furthermore, soaps sometimes cause dermatitis, or they may be irritating to diseased skin and a nonsoap detergent may be desirable. However, there are some people who are sensitive to these nonsoap detergents and others who are sensitive to both soaps and nonsoap detergents. Some detergents are nontoxic when taken by mouth and have been used as agents to bring into solution or emulsion difficulty soluble foods or remedial substances. Sucrose monostearate is an example of the latter group.

Unsaturation Fatty acids that contain one or more double bonds in their chains are said to be unsaturated. In the oleic acid series there is only one such unsaturated linkage. Oleic acid is the most widely distributed acid of this or any other fatty acid series. Its double bond (—CH=CH—) occurs exactly in the middle of the chain, at Δ^9. By adding hydrogen, the unsaturated acids are converted to saturated.

$$CH_3(CH_2)_7\!-\!\overset{\displaystyle H}{\underset{\displaystyle |}{C}}\!=\!\overset{\displaystyle H}{\underset{\displaystyle |}{C}}\!-\!(CH_2)_7COOH \qquad \text{Oleic acid}$$
$$\downarrow + H_2$$
$$CH_3(CH_2)_7\!-\!CH_2\!-\!CH_2\!-\!(CH_2)_7COOH \qquad \text{Stearic acid}$$

Hydrogenation changes the liquid oleic acid, which solidifies at about 3° C., to solid stearic acid, which melts at 65° to 70° C. In this way soft fats containing large proportions of triolein are converted to hard fats. The hydrogenation is catalyzed by finely divided nickel. This transformation of soft fats of vegetable or animal origin to more savory cooking fats and margarines is a large industry.

Unsaturated fatty acids are also oxidizable at the point of unsaturation. They form hydroperoxide derivatives:

$$-\!\overset{\displaystyle H}{\underset{\displaystyle |}{C}}\!=\!\overset{\displaystyle H}{\underset{\displaystyle |}{C}}\!- \quad\xrightarrow{\ O_2\ }\quad -\!\overset{}{\underset{\displaystyle |}{C}}H \overset{\displaystyle O}{\diagdown\!\diagup} CH\!- \quad\xrightarrow{\ H_2O\ }\quad -\!\overset{}{\underset{\displaystyle \|}{C}}H + HC\!-$$
$$\hspace{6.5cm} \underset{\displaystyle O\!-\!O}{} \hspace{3cm} O \qquad O$$

Hydroperoxides hydrolyze to form shorter-chain keto acids. The drying oils used in paints owe their peculiar property to the fact that they contain highly unsaturated oils that on atmospheric oxidation are converted to hard films. Linseed oil is a familiar example.

Rancidity Most fats on exposure to air develop an unpleasant odor and flavor. This results from a slight hydrolysis of the fat, leading to the liberation of volatile fatty acids having rather unpleasant odors. It is known as rancidity. Simultaneous oxidation of the unsaturated acid occurs with the formation of the oxidation products just mentioned. Light, heat, moisture, and bacterial action are all factors that tend to bring about rancidity. Besides their disagreeable properties, the rancid fats and oils may have distinctly unphysiologic effects by oxidizing a number of essential dietary substances, e.g., vitamin A, carotene, vitamin E, linoleic acid. The rate of production of rancidity varies with the individual fat, as well as being influenced by bacterial growth, etc. There are present in the nonsaponifiable fraction substances that inhibit the autoxidation of fats. These are called antioxidants and occur in different concentrations in the various natural fats. The occurrence of antioxidants explains why some fats keep better than others. Compounds possessing this property include certain phenols, naphthols, and quinones. The most common natural antioxidant is perhaps vitamin E. It is often added to foods and other materials to prevent the production of rancidity.

IDENTIFICATION OF FATS AND OILS

It is frequently necessary to identify a pure fat or to determine the proportions of different types of fat in a mixture. Besides the melting and congealing points, several other values may be ascertained. These depend on certain chemical, physical, and structural characteristics of the fatty acid fraction.

The more important are the iodine number, the saponification number, the Reichert-Meissl number, and the acetyl number.[*]

Iodine number. The unsaturated fatty acids take up iodine and other halogens at the point of unsaturation, yielding saturated halogen derivatives. Consequently, the degree of unsaturation of fats may be determined by ascertaining how much iodine a given quantity will absorb. The result is called the iodine number, which is defined as the *number of grams of iodine absorbed by 100 gm. of fat.* The determination of the iodine number is useful to the chemist in assaying the quality of an oil or its freedom from adulteration. For example, the iodine number of cottonseed oil varies from 103 to 111; that of olive oil, from 79 to 88; and that of linseed oil, from 175 to 202. A commercial lot of olive oil having an iodine number somewhat higher than 88 might have been adulterated with cottonseed oil. Again, a shipment of linseed oil with an iodine number lower than 175 might also have been adulterated with the same oil. A slight modification of the iodine number has replaced this determination to a considerable extent. This is the *iodine-containing value,* i.e., the total amount of iodine present in the fat after mixing with iodine by a standardized procedure. The principle is the same as for the iodine number.

Saponification number. Since each carboxyl group of a fatty acid reacts with one molecule of sodium hydroxide or potassium hydroxide in a saponification, evidently the amount of alkali needed to saponify a given quantity of fat depends on the number of carboxyls present. Fats containing short-chain acids have more carboxyls per gram than long-chain acids and take up more alkali. The saponification number therefore becomes another criterion of value, giving a clue as to the average size of the fatty acid chain in the fat under investigation. It is defined as the number of milligrams of potassium hydroxide necessary to neutralize the fatty acids in 1 gm. of fat. Butter, containing a larger proportion of short-chain fatty acids, e.g., butyric, caproic, has the relatively high saponification number of 220 to 230. Oleomargarine, with more long-chain fatty acids, has a saponification number of 195 or less.

Reichert-Meissl number. The Reichert-Meissl number measures the amount of volatile soluble fatty acids. By saponification of the fat, acidification, and steam distillation, the volatile soluble acids can be separated and determined quantitatively. The Reichert-Meissl number is the *number of milliliters of 0.1N alkali required to neutralize the soluble fatty acids distilled from 5 gm. of fat.* Butterfat is the only common fat with a high Reichert-Meissl number, and this determination therefore is of interest in that it aids the food chemist in detecting butter substitutes in food products.

Acetyl number. Some of the fatty acid residues in fat contain hydroxyl groups. In order to determine the proportion of these, the fatty acids are acetylated by means of acetic anhydride. Thus an acetyl group is introduced wherever a free hydroxyl is present. After the excess anhydride has been

---

[*] The procedures for these as well as many other quantitative methods in food analysis will be found in Official and Tentative Methods of Analysis of the Association of Official Agricultural Chemists, ed. 9, Washington, 1960, Association of Official Agricultural Chemists.

Table 11-2. Acetyl numbers

Castor oil	146–150	Olive oil	10.5
Cod-liver oil	1.1	Peanut oil	3.5
Cottonseed oil	21–25		

washed out and the acid liberated, the acetylated fat can be dried and weighed and the acetic acid in combination determined by titration with standard alkali after it has been set free. The acetyl number, which is thus a measure of the hydroxyl groups present, is the *number of milligrams of potassium hydroxide needed to neutralize the acetic acid of 1 gm. of acetylated fat.* Examples of the values for certain oils are given in Table 11-2. The applications to adulteration are evident.

ESSENTIAL FATTY ACIDS

As will be seen later, the fats have a very high value as sources of energy to the body. Besides this, certain fatty acids appear to have specific nutritional importance. Burr[1] showed that skin lesions occur in rats fed a fat-deficient diet and that these may be cured by the addition of linolenic, linoleic, and arachidonic acids or of fats containing these polyunsaturated acids.

Linoleic acid is $CH_3 \cdot (CH_2)_4 \cdot CH{:}CH \cdot CH_2 \cdot CH{:}CH \cdot (CH_2)_7 \cdot COOH$

Linolenic acid is $CH_3 \cdot (CH_2 \cdot CH{:}CH)_3 \cdot (CH_2) \cdot (CH_2)_6 \cdot COOH$

Arachidonic (eicosatetraenoic) acid is $CH_3 \cdot CH{:}CH \cdot (CH_2)_2 \cdot CH{:}CH \cdot (CH_2)_2 \cdot CH{:}CH \cdot$
$$(CH_2)_2 \cdot CH{:}CH \cdot (CH_2)_4 \cdot COOH$$

Animals are capable of desaturating fatty acids, and thus producing certain unsaturated acids, e.g., oleic, but they do not seem to be able to form these particular ones, although linoleic acid can be converted to arachidonic acid in man (p. 320). These fatty acids are called essential or indispensable. Steenbock reported that these same fatty acids have curative properties for the skin affections caused by lack of vitamin B_6, which can, of course, also be cured by administration of the vitamin. This does not mean that the unsaturated fatty acids are vitamins; but they undoubtedly do play some important role, as yet undetermined, in metabolism (p. 320).

WAXES

Waxes are esters of fatty acids with certain alcohols—not glycerol. They are insoluble in water but are soluble in the fat solvents. They are not as easily hydrolyzed as the fats and are not digested by the fat-splitting enzymes. Therefore they are of no value from a nutritional standpoint. Examples are beeswax, spermaceti, Chinese wax, and carnauba wax.

Beeswax is secreted by the honeybee to form the comb. It is a mixture of waxes, the chief ingredient being myricyl palmitate. Spermaceti is likewise a mixture. It is found in the skull of certain whales and dolphins. It is chiefly cetyl palmitate and was formerly used in the manufacture of candles. Chinese wax and carnauba wax are derived from the cuticle of leaves. These and other vegetable waxes are of value from an industrial standpoint as ingredients of shoe polish, floor waxes, varnishes, candles, etc.

STEROLS

Sterols are complex monohydroxy alcohols found in both plant and animal tissues. They belong to the group of compounds known as cyclopentanoper-hydrophenanthrenes, which are steroids. These have a four-ring structure, which is shown below with the rings lettered and the carbon positions numbered. *R* indicates an aliphatic side chain.

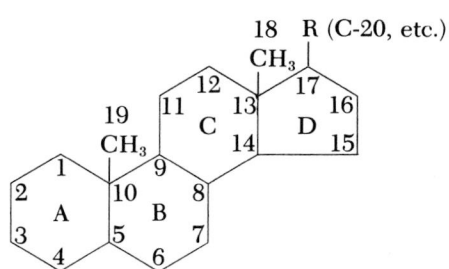

Steroid nucleus – conventional form

The steroid nucleus may also be shown as the conformational structure (*chair form*):

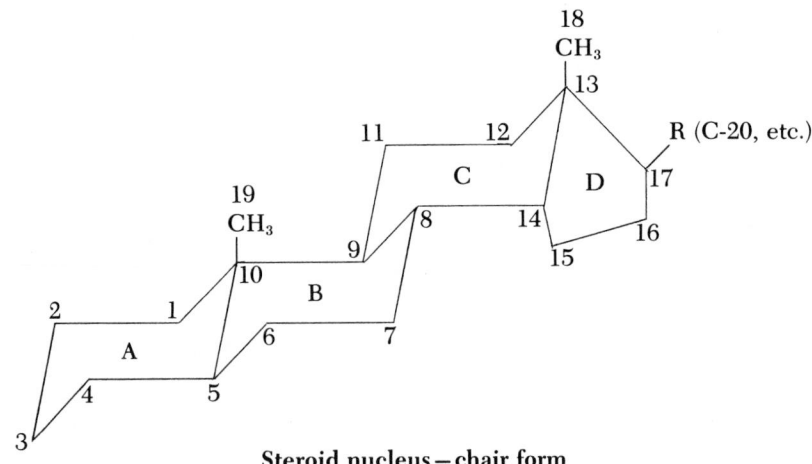

Steroid nucleus – chair form

Those carbons numbered above 17 are not present in every steroid compound. The steroids differ from each other in the arrangement of double bonds in the rings and in the presence of oxygen or of hydroxyl or other groups; and, in certain cases, there may even be a break in one of the rings. This numbering system is frequently referred to in biochemical and clinical literature. Among the steroids are the sterols, bile acids, sex hormones, adrenocortical hormones, cardiac aglycones, and D vitamins.

Many of the steroids are known by common or trivial names that do not

indicate their structure but are retained because of long usage, e.g., androsterone, progesterone, estrone. They, as well as the other steroids, can be given
more exact designations describing their formulas rather clearly. The system
of nomenclature now generally accepted is as follows.[2,3]

Nomenclature There are a number of hydrocarbons that are the parent substances of
different series of steroids. The ending of their names is *ane*, and the most
important ones follow:

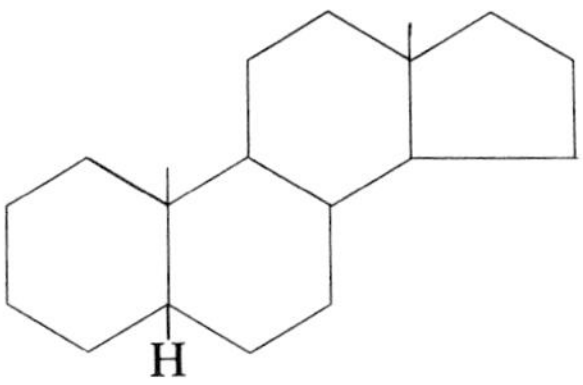

Etiocholane

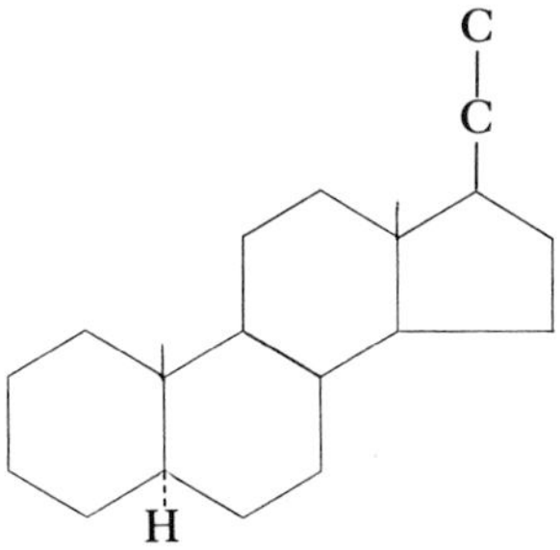

Allopregnane

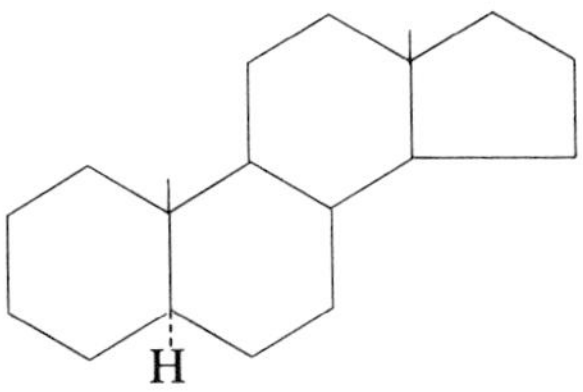

Androstane

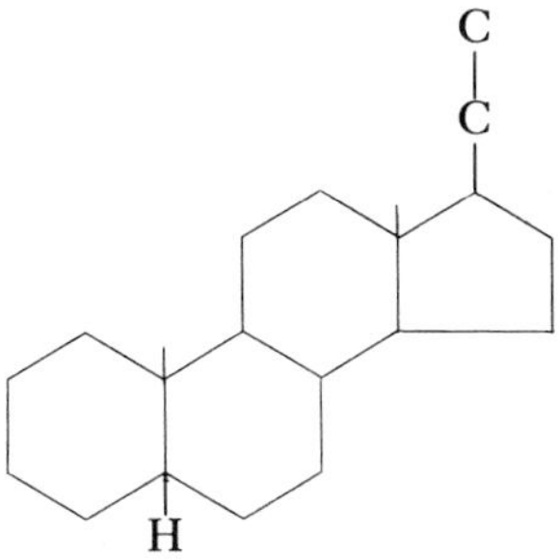

Pregnane

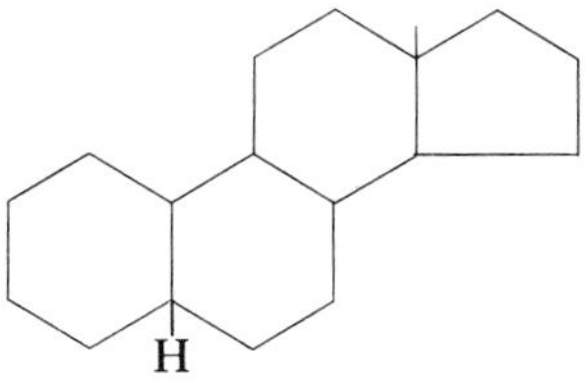

Estrane

The vertical bonds at positions 10 and 13 indicate methyl groups with
carbon-19 and carbon-18, respectively.

An unsaturated bond changes the name of the hydrocarbon to -*ene;* two
such bonds make it -*diene,* etc. The exact position of the double bond is indicated by the Greek letter Δ with a superscript numeral to indicate where
the double bond starts, e.g., Δ^5-androstene. The number of the carbon at the
end of the double bond is also given if it is not the next higher number (e.g.,
$\Delta^{7,9,11}$-androstadiene means that the second double bond in this case goes
from C-9 to C-11 [not from C-9 to C-10], while $\Delta^{7,\ 14}$-androstadiene indicates
that the two double bonds go from C-7 to C-8 and from C-14 to C-15).

If an oxygen atom is introduced in place of two hydrogens, the suffix is
changed to -*one,* or the syllable *one* is added, with a number to indicate its

position. Similarly, -ol is used for a hydroxyl (e.g., $\Delta^{1,3,5}$-estratriene-3-ol-17-one indicates that the compound has the estrane configuration but with three double bonds, from C-1 to C-2, C-3 to C-4, and C-5 to C-6; it also has a hydroxyl at C-3 and an oxygen at C-17). An aldehyde group is indicated by -al.

It is obvious that there are many asymmetric carbons in the steroid molecule and that in some cases it might be necessary to show precisely how a given substituent is oriented. Configurations relative to the molecule as a whole are designated β if the orientation of the hydrogen or group corresponds to that of the two methyl groups (C-18 and C-19, which are presumed to be above the plane of the page). A full line bond is used for such an orientation. If the orientation is opposite the carbon-18 and carbon-19 groups, i.e., below the plane of the page, it is called α, and a dotted line bond is used. The terms *trans* and *cis* are also applied to α and β, respectively.

The principles just presented will be understood if the following structures are compared with the names beneath them.

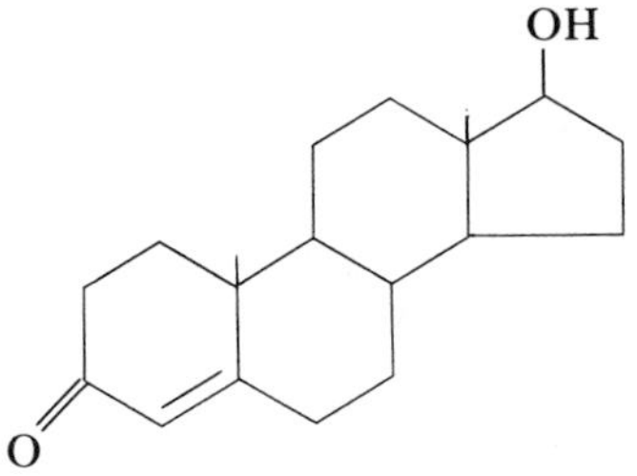

Testosterone
Δ^4-Androstene-3-one-17(β)ol

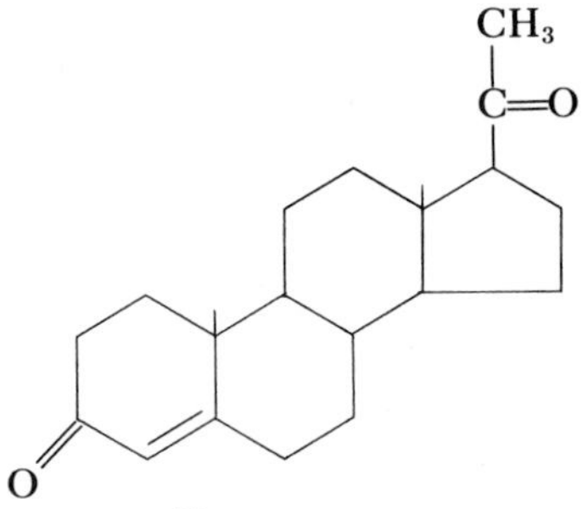

Progesterone
Δ^4-Pregnene-3,20-dione

Cholesterol   Cholesterol is perhaps the most important sterol; it is widely distributed and has been known and studied for many years. Its structural formula is as follows:

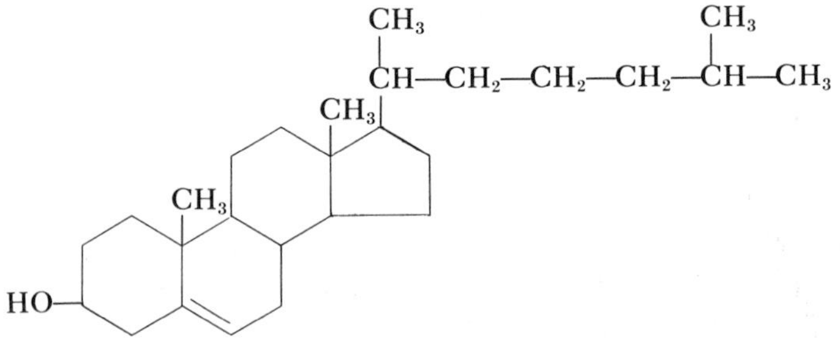

Cholesterol

Since there are eight asymmetric carbons, theoretically 256 stereoisomers are possible. The hydroxyl group on carbon-3 is in the β-position; therefore it is shown with a *solid* line bond. Cholesterol is probably a constituent of all animal cells; the corpus luteum and the adrenal cortex are particularly rich in this lipid. The adrenosteroid hormones and probably other steroid hormones and the bile acids appear to be formed from cholesterol in the animal organism (p. 331). Cholesterol is present in blood and bile and is usually a major constituent of gallstones, from which it was first isolated. The name is

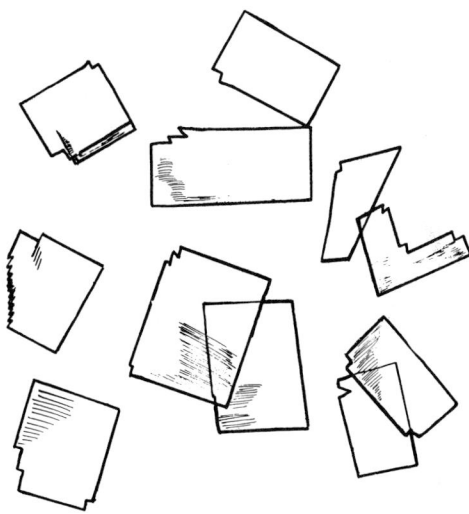

Fig. 11-1. Cholesterol crystals.

from the Greek words meaning "solid bile." For study it may be readily obtained from gallstones or from nervous tissue, where it is also found in high concentration. It is soluble in many fat solvents, e.g., ether, chloroform, benzene, and hot alcohol, and easily crystallizes from such solutions in colorless rhombic plates with one or more characteristic notches in the corners (Fig. 11-1). Since it has an unsaturated bond, it will take up two halogen atoms. It is not saponifiable. Cholesterol has also been found in some higher plants.[4]

Cholesterol gives a number of color reactions. These enable one to test for it both qualitatively and quantitatively. A beautiful series of colors is obtained by the Salkowski reaction. The chloroform solution of cholesterol is stratified over concentrated sulfuric acid. The acid assumes a yellowish color with a green fluorescence, whereas the chloroform layer becomes first bluish red, then gradually violet-red. If the chloroform solution is poured into a porcelain evaporating dish, it changes to violet to green to yellow. If to a chloroform solution of cholesterol are added acetic anhydride and concentrated sulfuric acid (under as nearly anhydrous conditions as possible), a blue to violet color, changing to emerald green, appears. Under carefully controlled conditions the green color produced is proportional to the amount of cholesterol present. Consequently, this reaction, known as the Liebermann-Burchard reaction, has become the basis for the quantitative estimation of cholesterol in blood and other biologic materials. In clinical work sometimes free cholesterol and cholesterol esters must be determined separately. In order to accomplish this, advantage is taken of the fact that free cholesterol unites with digitonin to form cholesterol digitonide. This is insoluble in petroleum ether, in which the cholesterol esters are freely soluble.

Other important sterols There is present in the skin an important sterol, 7-dehydrocholesterol. This differs from cholesterol only in having a second double bond (namely, between C-7 and C-8) and therefore only one hydrogen at carbon-7 and none at carbon-8. It is found in other tissues as well as the skin, probably along with cholesterol, but its special interest lies in the fact that when the skin is irradiated with ultraviolet light this sterol is converted to one of the D vitamins (p. 778). This explains the value of sunshine in preventing rickets.

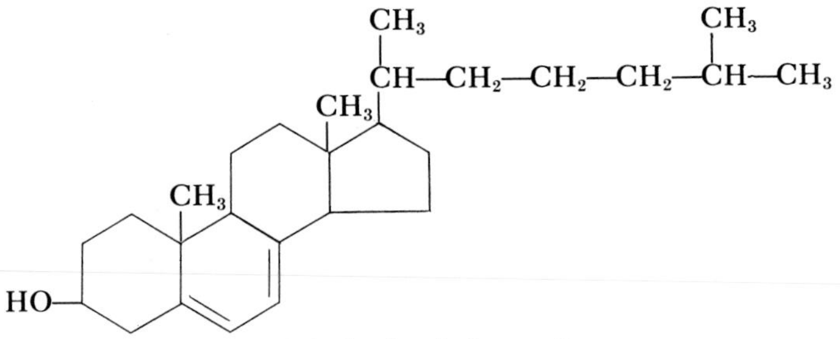

7-Dehydrocholesterol

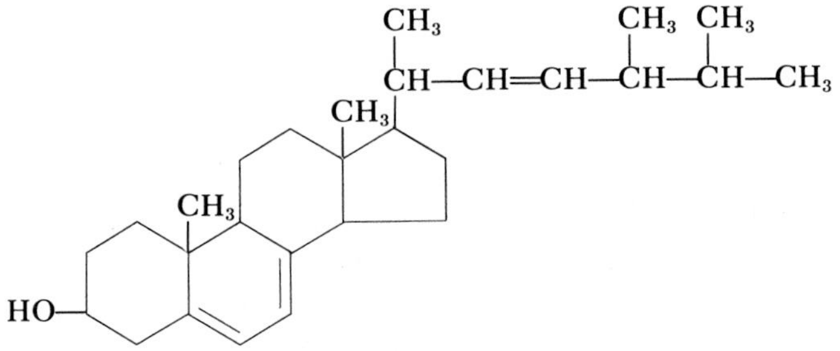

Ergosterol

In this connection, mention should be made of ergosterol. This sterol has the same nucleus as 7-dehydrocholesterol but differs slightly in its side chain. It may also be converted to a vitamin D by irradiation with ultraviolet light. Each of these sterols, therefore, is called a *provitamin D*. Ergosterol was first isolated from ergot, a fungus of rye, and later from yeast and certain mushrooms. Stigmasterol and sitosterol are among the other sterols occurring in the higher plants, but there is at present no evidence that they have any nutritional value for man. Indeed, the plant sterol, sitosterol, appears to *decrease* the intestinal absorption of both exogenous and endogenous cholesterol, lowering the blood cholesterol level. It has been sold on the pharmaceutic market for this purpose for some 10 years. On the other hand, the sterols of animal origin, notably cholesterol, are probably absorbed from the intestinal tract and utilized. However, all animals, herbivorous as well as carnivorous, can synthesize cholesterol from other dietary factors. This must occur to a considerable degree, because whether or not cholesterol is in the diet, it is continually being excreted by way of the bile. No doubt some of this is reabsorbed, but some continues down the intestinal tract and is largely converted to coprosterol. Coprosterol is formed by the hydrogenation of the double bond of cholesterol. This is probably brought about by bacterial action. Thus feces contain coprosterol, cholesterol, and the plant sterols. Coprosterol is soluble in chloroform and gives similar, but not identical, color tests to those given by cholesterol. Of course, it does not take up halogens.

As mentioned earlier (p. 157), sterol derivatives form an important part (the so-called *aglycone* portion) of the structure of certain cardiac glycosides, e.g., digitoxigenin, gitoxigenin, and oleonobrigenin.

PHOSPHOLIPIDS

The phospholipids, like the sterols, are present in all cells, plant as well as animal, and are the second most abundant naturally occurring lipid. They are also known as phosphorized fats, phospholipins, and phosphatides. Most of them are composed of fatty acids, a nitrogenous base, phosphoric acid, and glycerol, inositol, or sphingosine. They appear to have an L-structural configuration on the center asymmetric carbon atom. Five types are of special interest—phosphatidic acids, lecithins, cephalins, plasmalogens, and sphingomyelins. The lecithins predominate in animal tissues.

Phosphatidic acids The phosphatidic acids are the simplest type of phospholipids. They are derived from glycerophosphoric acid by esterification of the two remaining hydroxyl groups with fatty acids.

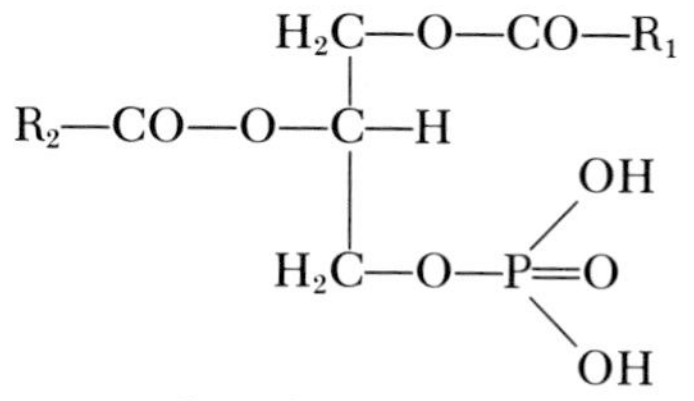

$$H_2C—O—CO—R_1$$
$$R_2—CO—O—\overset{|}{\underset{|}{C}}—H$$
$$H_2C—O—P{=}O$$

Phosphatidic acid

These substances occur in many plant and animal tissues. Since calcium phosphatidate has been found in blood, it has been suggested as the possible precursor of the other blood phosphatides.

Lecithins On hydrolysis, a molecule of lecithin yields two molecules of fatty acid and one molecule each of glycerol, phosphoric acid, and choline. Usually one of the fatty acids is saturated and one is unsaturated. The latter is usually on the center (β) carbon atom. Choline is ethanoltrimethylammonium hydroxide, or trimethylhydroxyethylammonium hydroxide. The following formula shows a typical lecithin.

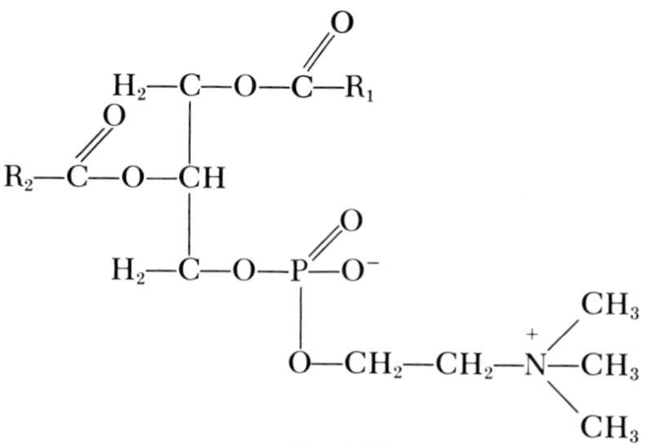

L-α-Lecithin

The R_1 and R_2 represent such fatty acid chains as stearic, oleic, etc. There are, accordingly, many different lecithins. The lecithins are soluble in fat solvents, including ether, chloroform, benzene, and hot alcohol. *They are not soluble in acetone*; this property is used in separating them (and other phospholipids) from cholesterol and fats. Although insoluble in water, they readily emulsify in it and have a great affinity for it. When first prepared, they are white waxy solids but are quickly oxidized and become very dark in color. The lecithins may be saponified by alkalies, which completely cleave the molecule, yielding glycerol, soaps, choline, and phosphate. They may also be hydrolyzed by lecithinases, specific enzymes that attack the lecithins. A lecithinase in cobra venom can split off an unsaturated fatty acid, producing lysolecithin, a substance with the power to hemolyze red blood corpuscles. This explains the toxicity of cobra venom, as well as of that of certain poisonous spiders and other stinging insects. Another lecithinase can split off both fatty acids; another enzyme, a phosphatase, can hydrolyze off the phosphoric acid, and still another can remove choline from the molecule (p. 324).

Cephalins and other phospholipids The cephalins resemble the lecithins in structure except for the component corresponding to choline. This was formerly thought to be ethanolamine in all cases. However, Folch[5] showed that brain cephalin is a mixture of phosphatides containing ethanolamine, serine (α-amino-β-hydroxypropionic acid), and inositol. The serine-containing phosphatides seem to be much less in amount than the other phosphatides.[6] They can be separated from one another because of marked differences in solubility in mixtures of chloroform and alcohol. Typical cephalins follow.

Phosphatidylethanolamine   Phosphatidylserine

A cephalin is probably concerned in blood clotting. The cephalins have practically the same solubilities as the lecithins, with one important exception: cephalins are insoluble in either ethyl or methyl alcohol. They are always associated with lecithins in tissues; and most lecithin preparations are really mixtures of these phospholipids.

The inositol phosphatides comprise lipositol and diphosphoinositide. Lipositol was obtained from soybeans. There is much doubt as to the composition of the pure lipid, but the crude product contains galactose, arabinose, D-tartaric acid, ethanolamine, and, of course, fatty acids. The presence of sugars would seem to relate lipositol also to the glycolipids (p. 288). Diphosphoinositide appears to be made up of equimolecular proportions of inositol-metadiphosphate, glycerol, and fatty acid. A possible formula for this lipid is as follows:

$$H_2C-O-\overset{\overset{\displaystyle O}{\|}}{C}-R$$

$$R'-\overset{\overset{\displaystyle O}{\|}}{C}-O-CH$$

Diphosphoinositide

Plasmalogens   Plasmalogens are a naturally occurring, widely distributed type of phospholipid in which an α,β-unsaturated fatty aldehyde replaces the fatty acid in the α-position. They were discovered in 1924 by Feulgen through the reddish purple color produced in the cytoplasm of cells treated with fuchsin-sulfurous acid. The three principal types of plasmalogens have been termed phosphatidalethanolamine, phosphatidalcholine, and phosphatidalserine. They all appear to be of the L-structural configuration. They all, of course, also contain a fatty acid, glycerol, and phosphate, in addition to the nitrogenous base and unsaturated fatty aldehyde. Stearic and palmitic aldehydes have also been identified as constituents of certain plasmalogens.

$$CH_2-O-CH=CH-R$$

$$R'COO-CH$$

$$CH_2O-\overset{\overset{\displaystyle O}{\|}}{\underset{\underset{\displaystyle O^-}{|}}{P}}-OCH_2CH_2\overset{+}{N}H_3$$

Phosphatidalethanolamine

Plasmalogens have been found in cardiac and skeletal muscle, brain, liver, and egg. Their function or functions are not known.

Sphingomyelins   A sphingomyelin was first prepared from brain by Thudichum, in 1884. The following scheme and formula show the probable structure of a sphingomyelin.

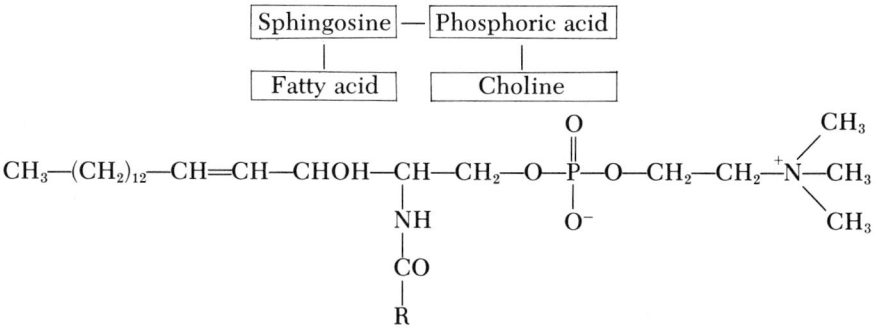

$$CH_3-(CH_2)_{12}-CH=CH-CHOH-\underset{\underset{\underset{\displaystyle R}{|}}{\underset{\displaystyle CO}{|}}}{\underset{\displaystyle NH}{|}}{CH}-CH_2-O-\overset{\overset{\displaystyle O}{\|}}{\underset{\underset{\displaystyle O^-}{|}}{P}}-O-CH_2-CH_2-\overset{+}{N}-CH_3$$

287

Sphingosine is an 18-carbon amine containing two hydroxyl groups:

$$CH_3—(CH_2)_{12}—CH{=}CH—CHOH—CHNH_2—CH_2OH$$

Dihydrosphingosine, which is present in some cases, is the fully saturated compound. Therefore, the sphingomyelins contain two nitrogenous bases, one fatty acid, and one phosphoric acid in each molecule. The fatty acids found in the sphingomyelins of nervous tissue appear to be limited to stearic, lignoceric, and nervonic acids, whereas spleen and lung sphingomyelins contain only palmitic and lignoceric acids. These lipids are more stable than the other phospholipids. They are not soluble in ether or in cold alcohol but are soluble in chloroform, benzene, and hot alcohol. From hot alcohol they crystallize out on cooling. They rotate the plane of polarized light to the right. Sphingomyelins occur in nervous tissue and also in other tissues.

Cardiolipids (polyglycerol phospholipids) Cardiolipids are present in a number of plant and animal tissues. They are present in largest amount in heart muscle, accounting for about 15% of the total lipid phosphorus content. They make up about 3% of the lipid phosphorus in liver and about 1% in brain. They appear to be mixtures that vary as to the fatty acid present, although unsaturated fatty acids (mainly linoleic) apparently predominate.[7] The structure probably consists of a chain of two or three phosphatidic acids joined together by glycerol, as shown schematically below:

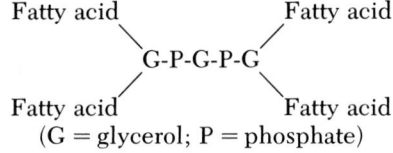

(G = glycerol; P = phosphate)

The biosynthesis of cardiolipids has been accomplished, as will be discussed later (p. 322).

Apparently the cardiolipids occur exclusively in cell membranes. Recent work indicates that they may serve to attach cytochrome-c of the electron-transport chain (p. 249) to the structural protein of the mitochondrial membrane, probably by way of hydrophobic bonds. Cardiolipids are also unique in that they are the only lipid known to be antigenic. Cardiolipid preparations are used in the serologic test for syphilis.

GLYCOLIPIDS

The glycolipids on hydrolysis yield a sugar (usually galactose), sphingosine, or dihydrosphingosine, and fatty acid. Thus they contain nitrogen but no phosphorus, unless the inositol phospholipids (p. 286) are included in this group. Like sphingomyelin, the glycolipids are almost insoluble in ether but they are more soluble in acetone than are the phospholipids and are also soluble in hot alcohol, benzene, and chloroform. The glycolipids are hydrolyzed by boiling with acids but are more resistant to action by alkalies. No enzymes capable of splitting them have been found.

The glycolipids occur in large amounts in the medullary sheaths of nerves and in brain tissue, particularly in the white matter of the brain, and are often called *cerebrosides*. They are not found in embryonic brain but develop as medullation progresses. Three glycolipids have been isolated from brain: kerasin, phrenosin, and nervon. They differ only in the individual fatty acids present.

By long hydrolysis with barium hydroxide, any cerebroside yields psychosin, which in turn can be hydrolyzed to sphingosine and galactose. Psychosin contains a free amino group and does not reduce alkaline copper solutions. Therefore galactose is probably linked to sphingosine through its aldehyde group. Since the cerebroside itself does not act as an acid or base and has no free amino group, it is evident that the carboxyl of the fatty acid is attached to the amino group of sphingosine.

Cerebrosides   A cerebroside or glycolipid is built on this plan:

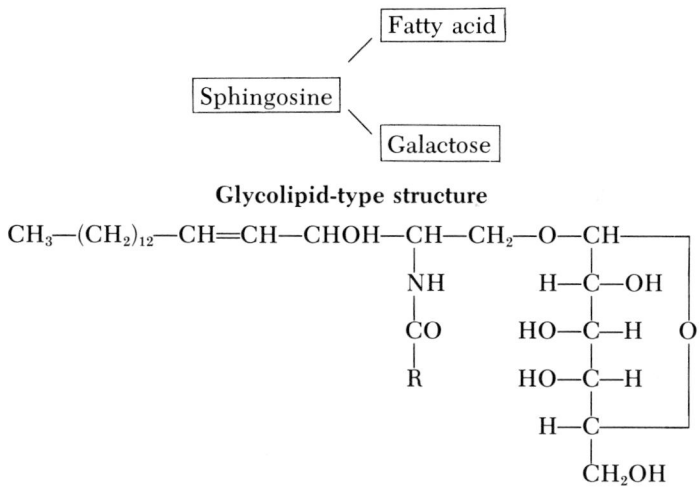

Glycolipid-type structure

Cerebroside

In Gaucher's disease, a congenital and familial derangement, kerasin is deposited, along with other lipids, in the spleen and liver. As much as 10% to 14% of the dry weight of the spleen has been found to be kerasin in this condition, and glucose appears to be present in one or more of the cerebrosides isolated. Only traces of glucose-containing cerebrosides are present in normal human spleen.

Gangliosides   The gangliosides are a group of glycolipids found in ganglion cells by Klenk, in 1940. They are also present in spleen and in erythrocytes. They are large complex lipids, their molecular weights varying from 180,000 to 250,000. Although the exact structures of the gangliosides are not definitely established at the present time, these compounds are known to contain a fatty acid (usually C-18 to C-24) combined with sphingosine, as a ceramide, and a carbohydrate moiety. The last contains, in addition to glucose and/or galactose, one mole of N-acetylgalactosamine and at least one mole of N-acetylneuraminic acid, a sialic acid (p. 175). Interesting is the fact that the ganglioside prepared from the stroma of horse erythrocytes contains N-glycolylneuraminic acid as the sialic acid moiety of the molecule.[8] The amount of gangliosides in brain and nervous tissue increases in the unusual hereditary disorder Tay-Sachs disease and in gargoylism, as will be discussed later (p. 335).

Sulfolipids   Several types of sulfur-containing lipids have been isolated from brain and other tissues. In general, they appear to be sulfate esters of glycolipids, the sulfate group being present on the hexose moiety of the molecule. Their exact structures and functions are still not definitely established.

LIPOPROTEINS AND LIPOPOLYSACCHARIDES

The lipoproteins are an extremely important type of lipid because of their vital role in the solubilization and transport of water-insoluble lipids in the plasma and other aqueous fluids of the body (p. 298). The lipid moiety of the lipoproteins consists mainly of triglycerides, phospholipids, and cholesterol. At least two binding or carrier proteins have been described and are termed α- and β-proteins. The weak association complexes with lipids are called α-lipoproteins and β-lipoproteins. They migrate electrophoretically as α- and β-globulins (p. 589). There is some evidence for a third transport protein in the plasma for lipids, termed the c-protein. The lipoproteins are usually also classified as conjugated proteins (p. 89).

The fact that the α- and β-lipoproteins contain different amounts of triglyceride, phospholipid, and cholesterol results in their having different physical properties, including density, electric charge, particle size, and adsorption characteristics. This, in turn, makes possible their separation and classification (p. 333). The two procedures most frequently used for this purpose are ultracentrifugation and electrophoresis. The rates of flotation of different lipoproteins upon ultracentrifugation are expressed as *Svedberg flotation units* (S_f). These differing rates are particularly useful for characterizing the several lipoproteins found in blood plasma, as will be discussed later (p. 333). Electrophoresis is also valuable in distinguishing the plasma lipoproteins (p. 333).

Association complexes of free fatty acids with plasma albumin also occur and are important in the transport of the free fatty acids.

Similarly, association complexes of lipids with certain polysaccharides, the lipopolysaccharides, have been described. They are formed in the cell walls of some microorganisms. Their chemical composition is uncertain at the present time, although the lipid moiety of some is known to contain glucosamine, acetyl residues, phosphate, and β-hydroxymyristic acid.

References

GENERAL

Bloor, W. R.: Biochemistry of the fatty acids and their compounds, the lipids, New York, 1943, Reinhold Publishing Corp.

Brady, R. D., and Trams, E. G.: The chemistry of lipids, Ann. Rev. Biochem. 33: 75, 1964.

Carter, H. E., Johnson, P., and Weber, E.: Glycolipids, Ann. Rev. Biochem. 34:109, 1965.

Deuel, H. J., Jr.: The lipids. Their chemistry and biochemistry; vol. 1, Chemistry, vol. 2, Biochemistry, New York, 1951, 1955, Interscience Publishers, Inc.

Fieser, L. F., and Fieser, M.: Steroids, New York, 1959, Reinhold Publishing Corp.

Gunstone, F. D.: An introduction to the chemistry and biochemistry of fatty acids and their glycerides, London, 1967, Chapman Hall, Ltd.

Hanahan, D. J.: Lipide chemistry, New York, 1960, John Wiley & Sons, Inc.

Holman, R. T.: Progress in the chemistry of fats and other lipids, New York, 1967, Pergamon Press, Inc.

King, H. K.: The chemistry of lipids in health and disease, Springfield, Ill., 1960, Charles C Thomas, Publisher.

SPECIAL

1. Burr, G. O.: Fed. Proc. 1:224, 1942.
2. Dorfman, R. I., and Ungar, F.: Metabolism of steroid hormones, Minneapolis, 1953, Burgess Publishing Co.
3. Fieser, L. F., and Fieser, M.: Steroids, New York, 1959, Reinhold Publishing Corp.
4. Johnson, D. F., et al.: Science 140:198, 1963.
5. Folch, J.: J. Biol. Chem. 177:497, 505, 1949; Folch, J., and Schneider, H. A.: J. Biol. Chem. 137:51, 1941.
6. Artom, C.: J. Biol. Chem. 157:595, 1945.
7. Rice, F. A. H.: Science 127:339, 1958.
8. Klenk, E., and Padberg, F.: Z. Physiol. Chem. 327:249, 1962.

CHAPTER 12

LIPID METABOLISM

Although lipid metabolism embraces the metabolism of all types of lipids, most of this chapter will be devoted to the fats. The major part of the lipids in our diet is made up of fats, and our knowledge of the biochemistry and physiology of these compounds is greater than that concerning other lipids. Much of our basic knowledge of the metabolism and transport of fats we owe to the studies of Bloor and his students. Recently, however, there has been a tremendous increase in experimental work on all lipids, not only the fats but also the phospholipids, sterols, lipoproteins, and other lipids.

BIOCHEMICAL SIGNIFICANCE OF FATS

Since the lipids are, in general, poor conductors of heat, their presence in the subcutaneous tissues tends to prevent loss of heat from the body. The greater the amount of fat, the more effective is this heat insulation. This is one very good reason why persons who have an exceptionally thick layer of fat are more comfortable in winter and less comfortable in summer than thinner people.

Chemically, fats are the best heat producers of the three chief classes of foodstuffs. Carbohydrates and proteins each yield about 4 kilocalories (4 kcal.) of heat for every gram oxidized in the body, whereas fats yield 9 kcal. —more than twice as much. This is because there is relatively more carbon and hydrogen in relation to oxygen in fats than in proteins or carbohydrates. In other words, the fats are compounds that are less completely oxidized to begin with and therefore can be oxidized further and yield more energy.

At one time, fats were considered optional constituents of the diet; after protein needs had been taken care of, the remaining caloric requirements could come from fat or carbohydrate, and whether any fat at all was needed was doubtful. Today, however, it is known that fat is a necessary part of the diet. This is partly because of the essential unsaturated fatty acids that must be present.

A quota of 20% to 40% of fat by weight in the diet improves the rate of growth of the young. This is not due entirely to a high caloric intake but also to a greater efficiency of utilization. There is an increase in the amount of calories retained when a higher proportion of fat is fed, because fewer calories are lost from the body. Sex maturation, pregnancy, and lactation are all said to be favorably influenced by a greater proportion of fats in the diet, particularly those fats containing essential unsaturated fatty acids. However, an excessive intake of fat and other lipids, especially those with a high saturated fatty acid and cholesterol content, is undesirable because of the suspected relation of this type of lipid to coronary heart disease, as will be discussed later (p. 331). Excessive fat intake should be avoided also by obese or obese-prone individuals.

Fats have several other noncaloric functions in addition to those mentioned above. These include the carrying by dietary fats of essential fat-soluble factors such as vitamins A, D, E, and K; the high satiety value of fat (p. 856); and the importance of fat in supporting vital organs and in protecting them mechanically from injury.

Digestion of fat The digestion of fats and other lipids poses a special problem because of the insolubility of fats in water and because lipolytic enzymes, like other enzymes, are soluble in an aqueous medium. The problem is solved by the emulsification of fats, particularly by bile salts, as will be discussed later (p. 294). The breaking of large fat or oil globules into fine particles increases the surface exposed to interaction with lipases and the rate of digestion is proportionally increased.

Little or no fat digestion occurs in the mouth or stomach since no significant amount of lipase is present in the secretions of these organs and no mechanism for the emulsifying of fatty material exists. There is some evidence for small amounts of a gastric lipase, but its minimal action, if any at all, is confined to highly emulsified fats, e.g., those of milk or egg yolk, or to fats with short-chain fatty acids since these are somewhat more water soluble. Furthermore, the acid pH of gastric secretions is not conducive to fat digestion.

Fats do play one important role in the stomach, however. They delay the rate of emptying of the stomach, presumably by way of the hormone *enterogastrone* (p. 458), which inhibits gastric motility and retards the discharge of foods from the stomach. Fats thus have a "high satiety value."

The major site of fat digestion is the small intestine. This is due to the presence of a powerful lipase, *steapsin*, in the pancreatic juice and bile salts (p. 294) that acts as an effective emulsifying agent for fats. Pancreatic juice and bile enter the upper small intestine, the *duodenum*, by way of the pancreatic and bile ducts, respectively. Secretion of pancreatic juice is stimulated by the passage of the acid gastric contents (chyme) into the duodenum by the hormones *secretin* and *pancreozymin* (p. 457). Secretin increases the secretion of electrolyte and fluid components of pancreatic juice, whereas pancreozymin stimulates the secretion of pancreatic enzymes. Fat in the acid chyme stimulates the secretion of the hormone *cholecystokinin* (p. 457), which, in turn, causes contraction of the gallbladder and discharge of the bile into the duodenum. These events thus prepare the small intestine for the digestion of fat.

Pancreatic lipase, steapsin, is an α-lipase specifically attacking the ester linkages at the 1- and 3-positions in the triglycerides, leaving a monoglyceride with the fatty acid esterified at the carbon-2 atom of glycerol.[1] This linkage may then be cleaved by an esterase to release the third fatty acid molecule and glycerol. There is some evidence that steapsin is secreted in an inactive zymogen form, steapsinogen, that is converted to active steapsin rather non-specifically by calcium salts, soaps, bile salts, etc.

Recent investigations[2] in which ^{14}C-labeled mono-, di-, and triolein was administered to rats with cannulated thoracic ducts indicated that there was digestive cleavage of *all* the fatty acids in the 1- and 3-positions (α- and α'-) stated above. There was hydrolysis of only 22% of the fatty acids in the 2-position (β), however. Thus about 75% of the fatty acids of this particular dietary fat were split and absorbed as *free* fatty acids. The remainder were absorbed primarily as a β-monoglyceride.

Monoglycerides, along with bile salts, play an important role in stabilizing and further increasing the emulsification of fat in the small intestine. The emulsified fat droplets are reduced in size to *micelles*, 0.1μ to 0.5μ in diameter. This further enhances the digestion of fats and other lipids solubilized in the micellar particle.

Thus 50% to 75% of dietary fat is split by steapsin to free fatty acids, which are absorbed as such. A smaller amount is partially digested to and absorbed as β-monoglycerides, and still less as di- and triglycerides. Some estimates are that the final digestion and absorption of usual dietary fats are about 95% complete in normal individuals.

Several other enzymes secreted in the pancreatic juices are involved in the digestion (hydrolysis) of certain lipids. For example, phospholipases hydrolyze the carbon-2 (β) fatty acid from lecithin, forming *lysolecithin*. Phosphatases and esterases, with α-lipases, complete the hydrolysis. Cholesterol esters are hydrolyzed to cholesterol plus fatty acids by cholesterol esterase.

Absorption of fats and other lipids Absorption of the digestion products of fats, primarily free fatty acids (70%) and β-monoglycerides (25%), occurs from the micelles in the microvilli (*brush border*) of the epithelial cells of the small intestinal mucosa. Bile salts of the micelle apparently are not absorbed at this point but are redissolved in other emulsoid particles, which solubilize them into micelles for absorption into the microvilli. Bile salts, however, are reabsorbed later in the lower part of the small intestine and return to the liver via the portal vein for resecretion into the bile. This is known as the *enterohepatic circulation* of the bile salts.

Current evidence,[3,4] based on electron microscopic studies, indicates that the products of fat digestion, free fatty acids and β-monoglycerides mainly, enter the microvilli and the apical pole of the absorptive mucosal epithelial cell by *simple* diffusion through the cell membrane. The short to medium–chain (6 to 10 carbons) and unsaturated fatty acids are more readily absorbed than the long-chain fatty acids (12 to 18 carbons). Also the short-chain fatty acids appear to enhance the absorption of fats in general, whereas long-chain fatty acids tend to impair the process. Furthermore, the monoglycerides of the less well-absorbed, long-chain fatty acids (e.g., stearic) are better absorbed than the corresponding free fatty acids.

Differences in the rates of digestion and absorption of the individual fatty acids are reflected in the overall rates of digestion and absorption of the dietary fats from which they are derived. Fats and oils with lower melting points (i.e., below 50° C.) are more rapidly and completely digested and absorbed than are those with higher melting points. Animal and vegetable triglycerides having similar melting points seem to be equally well digested and absorbed. Likewise, human milk fat is absorbed better than cow's milk fat because it contains a higher percent of unsaturated fatty acids and more palmitate in the carbon-2 position.

Pinocytosis does not appear to play a significant role in fat absorption as was formerly believed.[3]

The products of digestion next appear to be taken up by the smooth endoplasmic reticulum and resynthesized into triglycerides by enzymes present in the membranes or cavities of the reticulum. The rapid removal of fatty acids and monoglycerides, by their resynthesis into triglycerides, maintains a sharp gradient of concentration within the mucosal cell that favors the continued, rapid diffusion of the triglycerides into the cell from the intestinal lumen. There is a merging of the smooth endoplasmic reticulum into rough endoplasmic reticulum (p. 18) in which probably enzymes for triglyceride resynthesis are formed as well as the protein component of the chylomicron

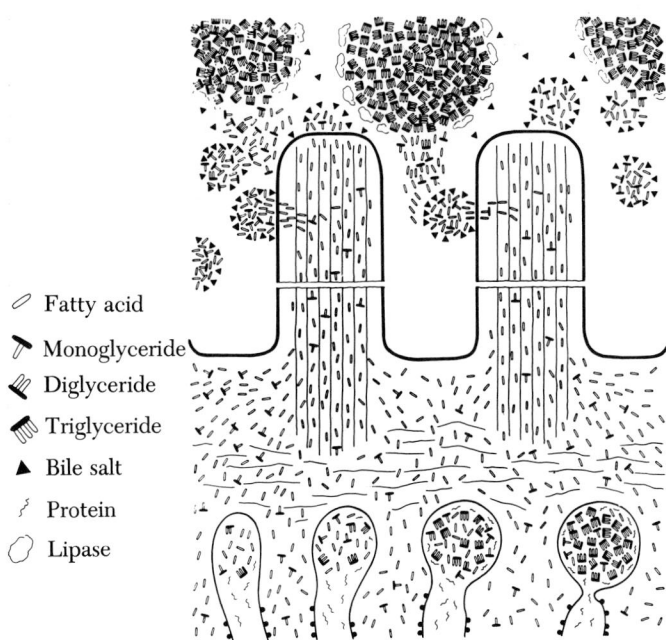

Fatty acid
Monoglyceride
Diglyceride
Triglyceride
Bile salt
Protein
Lipase

Fig. 12-1. Biochemical events in the digestion and absorption of fat. (From Porter, K. R.: Fed. Proc. Sympos. 28:35, 1969.)

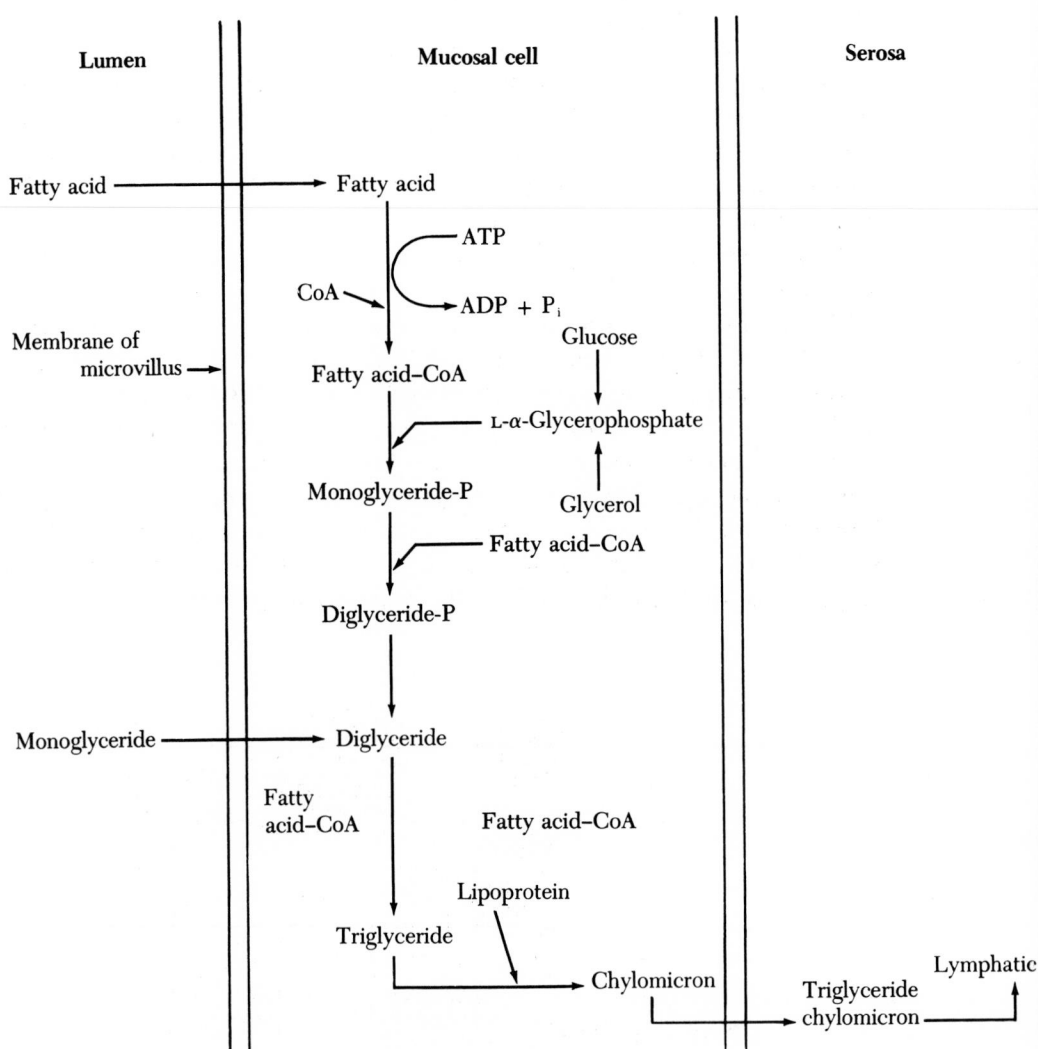

Fig. 12-2. Schematic representation of principal biochemical reactions during the intestinal absorption of long-chain fatty acids and monoglycerides. (Adapted from Isselbacher, K. J.: Fed. Proc. Sympos. **26**:1420, 1967.)

coat of the minute fat globules. The resynthesized triglycerides, in the form of chylomicrons, are discharged from the mucosal cell into the lymph and thence into the lacteals of the small intestine for transport into the lymphatic system and finally into the bloodstream for metabolic utilization. These biochemical events are shown schematically in Fig. 12-1.

The resynthesis of triglycerides from free fatty acids or monoglycerides in the mucosal cells entails the same reactions as those occurring in other cells, as will be discussed later (p. 314). Briefly summarized, these are (1) conversion of the free fatty acid to the fatty acid–CoA derivative by ATP and CoA; (2) conversion of the fatty acid–CoA derivative to monoglyceride phosphate in the presence of L-α-glycerophosphate; and (3) successive conversions, in the presence of two moles, of fatty acid–CoA to diglyceride phosphate, diglyceride, and finally triglyceride. Aggregates of triglycerides, plus small amounts of extraneous phospholipids, cholesterol, etc., are then "coated" with lipoprotein and secreted from the mucosal cell into the intracellular fluid, thence into the lacteals and lymphatics, and finally into the general circulation for metabolic disposal. These events are shown schematically in Fig. 12-2.

The foregoing discussion of the absorption of fatty acids and their resynthesis into triglycerides applies to long-chain fatty acids (12 to 18 carbons). The lower-molecular weight free fatty acids (6 to 10 carbons), representing less than 30% of the absorbed fat, are distributed, according to Frazer's *partition theory*,[5] bound to plasma albumin mainly via the blood capillaries, into portal blood and thence directly to the liver for oxidation or lengthening into long-chain fatty acids, as will be discussed later (p. 313).

Lipid malabsorption Impaired intestinal absorption of lipids occurs not infrequently in man, sometimes with serious consequences. Basically this may result[6] from (1) *defective lipolysis in the lumen of the small intestine:* this may stem from bile salt deficiency due to impaired hepatic formation or obstruction of the bile duct or from excessive bile salt loss; it may also result from pancreatic lipase deficiency due to pancreatic tissue damage or obstruction of the duct; (2) *defective mucosal cell metabolism:* this may be due to impaired resynthesis of triglycerides resulting from mucosal cell disorders, as in nontropical sprue or adrenocortical hormone deficiency (p. 466).

Defective mucosal cell function may also result in impaired lipoprotein synthesis for chylomicron formation. This, in turn, could stem from genetic defects, as in the synthesis of α,β-lipoproteins, or from the administration of certain drugs, e.g., puromycin, that inhibit protein synthesis.

Impaired fat absorption can decrease the absorption of other lipids, e.g., fat-soluble vitamins (p. 768), if prolonged, resulting in characteristic deficiency symptoms of vitamins A, D, or K.

There can be, of course, excessive loss of fat and other lipids in the stool (steatorrhea), as may be determined by clinical laboratory examination. In the normal individual, approximately 10% of the wet weight of feces is lipid. The lipids are equally distributed between triglycerides, soaps of calcium and magnesium ions, and sterols. The lipids represent unabsorbed dietary and bacterial lipids derived from the bacterial flora of the large intestine.

TRANSPORT OF FAT

After an average meal containing fat, there is a characteristic *alimentary hyperlipemia*. The peak usually occurs after about $2\frac{1}{2}$ to 3 hours, and the blood fat level returns to normal in from 5 to 6 hours. The fat transported in the blood appears to be in at least three forms: (1) microscopic particles of fat, about 1μ in diameter, termed *chylomicrons*; (2) invisible particulate fatty material, lipoproteins; and (3) unesterified fatty acid, bound to albumin. The first form, chylomicron, is responsible for the turbid or even milky appearance of the plasma after meals, particularly if the meal was rich in fat.

Since both fats and fatty acids are insoluble in water, it is obvious that the foregoing three special mechanisms for their transport are necessary. The chylomicrons appear to be microscopic particles of fat stabilized by the presence of about 2% protein, 7% phospholipid, and 9% cholesterol. The remaining 81% to 82% is triglyceride. The second form, invisible particulate fatty material, appears to consist largely of the low-density, β-lipoprotein ($S_f > 10$) and contains about 7% protein, 52% triglyceride, and 20% phospholipid and cholesterol. As stated above, the third form, nonesterified fatty acids (NEFA), is transported in combination with plasma albumin.

One of the rate-limiting steps in the transport of triglycerides may be their conversion to chylomicrons in the mucosal cell and their secretion into the lymph.[6] Thus, in congenital β-lipoprotein deficiency the transport of lipid into the lymphatics is markedly impaired. Triglycerides accumulate in the mucosal cell, presumably as a result of a deficiency of β-lipoprotein synthesis. An almost identical biochemical and morphologic picture has been produced experimentally in rats by inhibitors of protein synthesis, e.g., puromycin.

It is possible that cholesterol transports some fatty acid as cholesterol esters, but phospholipid is apparently not important in fat transport. When ^{14}C-labeled palmitic acid was fed to rats, 96% of the tagged acid recovered from blood was in forms other than phospholipid.

After the ingestion of fat-containing foods, the turbid, hyperlipemic plasma clears as it passes through various organs and tissues. This is apparently due to hydrolysis of the triglyceride portion of the transport protein complexes by the enzyme *lipoprotein lipase*,[7] also known as the clearing factor. Heparin appears to be closely associated with lipoprotein lipase, possibly serving as a cofactor for the enzyme. It has been known for a number of years that injection of heparin results in the rapid clearing of the opalescent plasma of dogs fed a fat-rich meal. Lipoprotein lipase is present in most tissues and in relatively large amounts in adipose tissue and heart muscle. The hydrolytic action of the enzyme thus releases free fatty acids for storage in fat depots or perhaps for other metabolic purposes.

Current investigations using labeled fatty acids indicate that the nonesterified fatty acids, transported by the plasma albumin, have an exceedingly high turnover rate to ^{14}C–carbon dioxide, the T/2 (half-life) being only 2 to 3 minutes, and thus they apparently represent the transport form used primarily for oxidation to meet energy needs. The unesterified fatty acids, of course, can be derived from storage depot fat, as will be discussed later, and from absorbed dietary fat.

Table 12-1. Plasma lipids of normal young adults

	Milligrams percent
Total lipid	590
Neutral fat	150
Total fatty acid (iodine number, 88.5)	350
Phospholipid fatty acid (iodine number, 124)	130
Cholesterol ester fatty acid	75
Neutral fat fatty acid	150
Nonesterified (free) fatty acids	20
Total cholesterol	160
Combined cholesterol	115
Free cholesterol	45
Phospholipid	200

The plasma nonesterified fatty acid (NEFA) level is affected by a number of hormones, particularly epinephrine and norepinephrine, that increase the level significantly.[8] This is due to an increase in the rate of release of NEFA from adipose tissue and may be another stress effect of epinephrine, analogous to its production of hyperglycemia by enhancing the breakdown of liver glycogen. Insulin, as well as glucose, decreases NEFA levels, whereas growth hormone, thyroxine, and ACTH appear to elevate the values. The mechanisms involved are not fully understood at present.

From Table 12-1, it can be seen that the phospholipids are present in blood plasma in greater amount than either cholesterol or neutral fat.

CHANGES OCCURRING IN LIVER

A large proportion of absorbed fat is carried to the liver, the chief site for its metabolic disposal. This includes not only fat that may go by way of the portal circulation but also fat circulating in the systemic circulation. Here a part is transformed to phospholipid, in which form it may be sent into the bloodstream for distribution to the organs and tissues. If this transformation to phospholipid is prevented, there is a deposition of fat in the liver, i.e., *fatty liver,* which is an abnormal and serious condition. For the building of lecithin, of course, choline is needed, or the constituents from which choline can be produced. Therefore choline or its precursors prevent, or cure, fatty livers.

The liver plays other important roles in fat metabolism; these will be considered later in this chapter.

FAT FROM CARBOHYDRATES AND PROTEINS

In addition to the fat derived from food fat, body fat may come from carbohydrate and protein. This has been discussed under carbohydrate metabolism (Chapter 9). The nonnitrogenous portion of some amino acids is converted to glucose, and this glucose, as well as other utilizable sugars, may be changed to fat. Proof that carbohydrates are changed to fatty acids was first supplied by the studies of Rittenberg and Schoenheimer.[9] To the drinking water of mice was added heavy water so that the concentration of heavy water in all the body fluids became constant. The animals were on a high-carbohydrate diet. The deuterium content of the fatty acids rose rapidly. Since all synthetic reactions involving tissue fluids were using a proportional amount of heavy water, this result indicates that carbohydrate and water were entering into the synthesis of fatty acids.

Chaikoff[10] fed glucose labeled with ^{14}C to mice. The isotope was subsequently found in tissue palmitic acid. This occurred largely in the liver but also in other organs. On a high-carbohydrate diet palmitic acid formation exceeds glycogenesis.

Positive demonstration of the synthesis of fat from protein has been obtained. A diet containing casein, salts, and yeast, i.e., almost no carbohydrate or lipid, was fed to rats that had been fasted to deplete them of their stores of fat. They regained their original weight on this diet, and analysis of the tissues showed that a large percentage of the new tissue was fat.

Since these early classic studies, a large number of investigations have elucidated the many interconnecting pathways of lipid, carbohydrate, and protein metabolism. These will be discussed in some detail in appropriate chapters.

FATE OF FATS IN BODY

Fats and other lipids are (1) oxidized to provide heat and energy, (2) stored for future utilization, (3) secreted in milk, (4) excreted in the feces, or (5) eliminated via the skin. Much of the milk fat originates in the neutral fat of blood, which in turn comes most readily from food fat. Feeding large quantities of cottonseed oil to cows changes the properties of the butterfat considerably. Although fat can be derived from carbohydrate and from protein, a lactating animal cannot produce milk of high fat content if the diet is too low in fat; i.e., synthesis cannot quite keep pace with the demand for fat.

The total lipids of the feces make up about one tenth of the fecal weight, of which about 7% to 25% is fatty acid and fatty acid derivatives. Very little, if any, fat is secreted by the intestinal mucosa under normal conditions, although sterols and other lipids may be so secreted. However, a significant amount of lipid is excreted into the intestine from the liver by way of the bile (p. 681). The bile lipids include neutral fat, phospholipids, and relatively considerable amounts of cholesterol. Fecal lipids are discussed further on p. 692. Very little lipid is excreted in the urine in the normal individual.

Storage of fats The fats and other lipids are deposited in various tissues of the body. If an animal is starved for a long time, lipids will still be found in the tissues. This is not fat but primarily phospholipid, along with smaller amounts of other lipids, including cholesterol (p. 282). This basic tissue lipid is called *élément constant* and is independent of previous feeding. It is necessary for the life of the cell, comprising the structural or functional material essential to the framework of the cell or to its proper activities. Lipid that is stored in excess of this is termed *élément variable*, which indicates that the amount fluctuates.

This represents the excess of intake over immediate utilization and when deposited in large masses is called *depot fat*, in which case it is the true adipose tissue. It is stored primarily for its fuel value but secondarily has other uses. Thus it is an insulator against heat loss; it serves to pad joints, nerves, and organs against shock; it may support kidneys or other organs. In visceroptosis the abdominal viscera drop because of too little support. This may occur when rapid loss of weight in obese individuals removes the supporting adipose tissue. Other functions include transformation into milk fat or into other lipids, e.g., phospholipids, sterol esters, cerebrosides, or for use as fat for the fetus.

Each species of animal tends to store a characteristic mixture of fats. Merely to mention lard, mutton fat, chicken fat, and fish oils indicates how true this is; and yet this characteristic fat can be modified by feeding large enough quantities of some unusual lipid. Unsaturated fats, low–molecular weight fats not synthesized by the animal, and halogenated fatty acids are examples of lipids that have been found to modify the body fats of animals to which they were fed. Feeding mutton fat, with a high melting point, to a dog raised the melting point of the animal's fat from about 20° to about 40° C., whereas linseed oil lowered it to 0° C. This is unusual and is due to forcing the "foreign" fatty acid. Under normal conditions the animal deposits fat having a melting point not far from its own body temperature. Therefore, in order to deposit its own peculiar fat under ordinary circumstances, the organism must oxidize unwanted fatty acids, retain those that are suitable, alter others, and even synthesize some.

Formerly it was the general opinion that the body used or oxidized as much fat as it needed and stored the rest and that these fat deposits remained, like hoarded gold, inactive until withdrawn for use. This is not the case. The experiments of Rittenberg and Schoenheimer,[9] and of others, are responsible for this change in scientific opinion. Using fats containing fatty acids tagged with deuterium, the following facts were brought out: Even small amounts of tagged fatty acids in the diet are first incorporated into body fat before they are oxidized. Since no changes in body weight or in total body fat occurred in these experiments, it is evident that there must have been a simultaneous removal of fatty acids from the body fat to make room for the dietary (new) fat. This is further shown by the fact that the deuterium rapidly disappeared from the body fat as soon as the dietary fat was changed to untagged fat. Apparently before fatty acids, long-chain ones at least, can be oxidized, they must be incorporated into body fats. The body fat, therefore, is not an inert mass but is part of a dynamic system, the fatty acids being continually deposited and withdrawn. This deposition of marked fatty acids occurs only when the fatty acids are of rather high molecular weight (above 10 carbons). Those of low molecular weight apparently may be either lengthened to 12 to 16 carbons or directly oxidized for energy.

There is considerable evidence that hormonal factors may regulate the mobilization of depot fat as it is needed for energy or for other metabolic purposes. Among the hormones involved may be epinephrine and norepinephrine. Still another factor, called *adipokinin*, secreted by the anterior pituitary, has been reported. This fat-mobilizing factor was found in human and rabbit urine.[11] It appears to be a peptide with a molecular weight of about 18,000 and is not related to the growth hormone or to corticotropin. It increases the plasma unesterified fatty acid level at the expense of depot fat.

Brown storage fat   In addition to the usual "white" storage fat, another type of pigmented, "brown" fat is stored in some species. It occurs most abundantly in neonatal animals and in hibernators, although it is present in the rat throughout life. It is located particularly in the thoracic regions. Its brown color is related to a relatively high cytochrome content. It also is relatively rich in carnitine, which is significant in fatty acid oxidation, as will be discussed later (p. 309).

Brown adipose tissue is unique for its relatively high rate of oxygen consumption and the short half-life (rapid turnover rate) of the fatty acids of its triglycerides. Brown storage fat has a somewhat higher temperature than other tissues. It has been suggested as playing a role in *heat production* for vital organs, serving as a sort of "heating pad" or "furnace" for the local application of its heat to the vital organs of the thorax, the upper spinal cord, and the autonomic sympathetic chain.[12] The amount of brown fat increases in animals subjected to cold stress. Indeed, direct measurements of heat production during cold stress in rats showed that brown adipose tissue accounts for 82% of the total heat production. The higher temperature and high rate of oxygen consumption may be due to a decreased coupling of oxidative phosphorylation and ATP production.[13] The energy of oxidation is therefore dissipated as heat in increased amounts. Heat energy is thus produced in animals having significant stores of brown fat without the necessity of shivering.

Fatty livers   Excessive amounts of fat in the liver have been seen by pathologists at autopsy for many years. *Fatty degeneration* and *fatty infiltration* are terms for some of these conditions. Consequently, the experimental study of fatty livers must be of more than passing interest. Fatty degeneration is a physical change in the cell and does not necessarily involve a change in the amount of fat. In fatty infiltration there is an increase in the fat intracellularly. Most of the fatty livers to be discussed under this heading are instances of fatty infiltration.

Depancreatized dogs, in addition to becoming diabetic, develop fatty livers. This occurs even if the animals are treated with insulin to control the hyperglycemia. Feeding raw pancreas can prevent this condition. The explanation first offered was that raw pancreas furnishes the pancreatic enzymes that are absent in a depancreatized animal. Later it was shown that lecithin has just as good an effect as pancreas, and finally that one component of lecithin, namely, choline, has this effect.[14] Other substances that affect this type of fatty liver are betaine and triethylcholine. Such substances are called *lipotropic*, which simply means that they prevent or cure fatty livers. Certain proteins, notably casein, are also lipotropic. This was shown to be related to their high content of methionine. Cystine, however, if fed together with a low-choline diet, tends to cause fatty livers; and there are a number of other methods of inducing this condition.

In attempting to account for some of these phenomena, the diagram in Fig. 12-3 may be of assistance. It indicates the source and fates of liver fatty

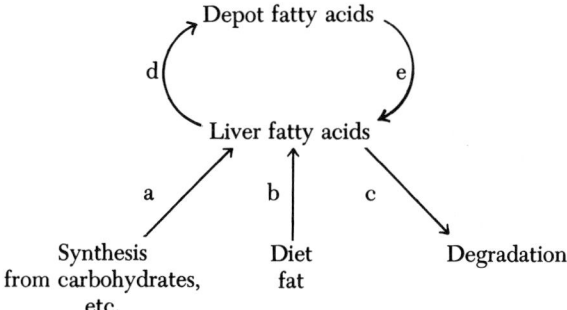

Fig. 12-3. Sources and fates of liver fatty acids. (After Stetten and Salcedo, 1943.)

acids and their relations to depot fatty acids. Part of the explanation lies in the fact that a great deal of the fatty acid is converted to phospholipid, mainly lecithin, in the liver, and choline is required for this formation. As was mentioned earlier, most of the triglycerides are converted to phospholipids in the liver before they are used by the tissues. If choline or the "makings" of choline are not present, the fats accumulate in the liver. The animal organism cannot readily synthesize methyl groups, as will be discussed later (p. 352). These are mostly obtained by transmethylation, i.e., the transfer of labile methyl groups from appropriate donor compounds to acceptors. Methionine, betaine, etc. are lipotropic because they can transfer their methyl groups to ensure the synthesis of choline. Then choline unites with phosphoric acid, fatty acids, and glycerol to form lecithin in the liver and replace the neutral fat with this phospholipid. A low-choline diet, therefore, produces fatty livers because of impaired transportation of fatty acids from liver to the fat depots via route *d* (in Fig. 12-3).

This seems a simple and logical explanation. It is not, however, the whole story. In treating a depancreatized dog with choline, at least 1 gm. per day is needed. The effective amount of raw pancreas supplies only about 6% of this requirement. Dragstedt prepared an extract of the pancreas, which he considered an internal secretion (in addition to insulin), and named it *lipocaic*. This was effective in preventing or curing fatty liver. There has been a great deal of controversy regarding lipocaic, some supporting Dragstedt's contention, others stating that it owes its efficacy entirely to choline, and still others maintaining that pancreatic juice is just as effective as the pancreatic tissue extract. McHenry suggested that the fatty liver of the depancreatized dog is due to a failure of digestion that prevents the liberation of a lipotropic factor, from protein, mainly methionine. Pancreatic extracts contain the free lipotropic factor, which is absorbed and tends to prevent fat deposition. This factor may possibly be inositol. The diet usually contains choline and protein (with its methionine), which are also lipotropic. If raw pancreas is fed, it aids in the digestion and liberation of the lipotropic factor, methionine.

Elvehjem and his co-workers[15] found that the amounts of several other amino acids in the diet, notably threonine, tryptophan, serine, and glycine, may affect the deposition of fat in the livers of rats fed a diet low in protein but adequate in choline. They believe that threonine and possibly other essential amino acids may be required for the formation of enzymes needed for normal fat metabolism in the liver. Glycine and serine may serve in a non-specific manner by sparing other essential compounds. Thus a *balance* of amino acids from dietary protein is important in maintaining normal fat metabolism in the liver.

Fatty livers may also be induced by feeding an excess of cholesterol or an excess of fat. This would appear to be an increased rate of fatty acid formation along route *b* (Fig. 12-3). In both cases, choline only diminishes the deposition of that fraction of lipid consisting of neutral fats. It has little or no effect on the cholesterol fraction. Inositol, another lipotropic agent, has a marked effect in reducing the amount of cholesterol in the liver. Choline also has no inhibiting action on the fatty livers produced by phosphorus poisoning or certain other specific hepatic poisons. It is interesting to note that diets which produce fatty livers fail to do so unless thiamine is present; i.e., diets low in choline, whether high or low in fat, will not result in fatty livers in the absence of vitamin B_1. The vitamin is essential for the conversion of carbohydrate to fat, and route *a* in Fig. 12-3 indicates this line of action. Riboflavin has a similar effect. The feeding of cystine also seems to result in increased synthesis (route *a*), as well as in antagonism to choline. Deficiencies of pyridoxine, pantothenic acid, folic acid, or vitamin B_{12} are also asserted to produce fatty livers by some mechanism not as yet clear. Both vitamin B_{12} and folic acid are involved in the biosynthesis of methyl groups (p. 352).

When anterior pituitary substance or the *ketogenic* fractions of anterior pituitary extract are administered to animals, fatty livers result. This is caused by excessive mobilization of depot fat and its migration to the liver, a stimulation of process *e* that cannot be prevented by choline. To summarize:

1. Fatty livers caused by depancreatization are prevented by (a) large amounts of choline or labile methyl donors or (b) lipocaic. The labile methyl donors produce choline, which is needed for lecithin formation. Lipocaic may owe its action to a vitamin, inositol. Raw pancreas is also effective because it aids in the digestion of food and liberation of inositol and methionine.
2. The same treatment is effective in fatty livers resulting from a low-choline diet, high fat feeding, and, with respect to neutral fats deposited, high-cholesterol diets.
3. Choline or lecithin feeding does not affect fatty livers that are due to phosphorus poisoning or anterior pituitary administration, since in both cases the accumulation of liver fat is derived from the fat depots of the body.

Obesity. Obesity is "that state in which the accumulation of reserve fat becomes so extreme that the functions of the organism are interfered with." It may arise from (1) overeating or (2) diminished utilization, or a combination of both. Various theories have been proposed to explain how this occurs. Among them is the hypothesis that the basal metabolic rate is low and, therefore, with a normal intake of food, an excess of calories is available. As we all know, the basal metabolic rate diminishes slightly as the individual grows older. Often the food consumption is not decreased proportionally, and as a consequence obesity may result. Otherwise, obesity cannot be accounted for by a diminution in the basal metabolic rate. In fact, the heat production of obese individuals is usually above normal, except when the obesity is associated with hypothyroidism. It has also been claimed that obese individuals show lower specific dynamic effects of food than do normal persons. This, too, has been proved incorrect. Nevertheless, persons afflicted with extreme obesity frequently cannot lose weight in spite of most rigorous undernutrition. Since the laws of conservation of matter and energy operate under all circumstances, it is possible that the answer to this problem may be found in a study of the water balance (p. 439). The obese person's tissues retain water more tenaciously than normal, and, perhaps, water takes the place of the fat that is lost. Just how the endocrine glands fit into the picture is difficult to explain. They may control water balance; they may influence the patient's "urge" for work. It is fairly definitely established that they do not directly cause the formation of adipose tissue, although they do seem to influence the *pattern* of the distribution of such tissue.

Another facet of the problem that is receiving considerable attention today is the relation of obesity to diabetes mellitus and insulin.[16] It is well known that obesity exerts a *diabetogenic* effect and leads to excess plasma levels of insulin (p. 463) in response to glucose or food loads. The excess of insulin either leads to an increased lipogenesis or exerts an antilipolytic effect, or it does both, thus increasing further the excessive deposition of body fat.

Thus, obesity remains an enigma today as it has for many centuries—the earliest recorded case of human obesity dating back to the Willendorf Stone Age Venus of about 22,000 B.C. While obesity is basically a result of a usually prolonged imbalance between caloric intake, on the one hand, and caloric needs, on the other, many factors may modify the balance in favor of calorie retention. These include environmental and hereditary factors as well as acquired emotional or neurologic, endocrine, or metabolic disorders.[17] Lack of sufficient physical activity (exercise) is a most common factor in many cases of obesity. Successful treatment must include nutritionally adequate diets of acceptable common foods with controlled caloric content and emphasis on regular physical exercise. The development of new interests, hobbies, or social activities as a replacement for excessive eating is usually of value. Fad diets for weight reduction, e.g., the low-carbohydrate diet, are not satisfactory on a long-term basis as is essential in these cases. Since obesity often develops in childhood and persists through adult life, early prevention is perhaps the best approach to the problem.

OXIDATION OF FATTY ACIDS

It is usually assumed that the glycerol fraction of fat is handled in much the same way as the carbohydrates. We have seen that three-carbon chains arise from a splitting of the hexoses and are oxidized eventually to carbon dioxide and water; and there is no reason why glycerol from fat should not follow a similar path. There is first a phosphorylation and an oxidation to 3-phosphoglyceraldehyde or to some similar derivative. The path illustrated on p. 314 shows the probable further route. That glycerol can enter into synthetic carbohydrate reactions is seen in the fact that when glycerol is fed to diabetic animals it is excreted as glucose. Studies with ^{14}C-glycerol likewise show the same conversion to glucose and its metabolites.

The oxidation of long-chain fatty acids has been the subject of many investigations. Leathes and Meyer-Wedell[18] formulated the hypothesis that the first step in the breakdown of a long-chain fatty acid is its desaturation in the liver. The evidence for this lay in the fact that the liver fatty acids are more unsaturated than those present in other tissues. Direct proof that desaturation occurs (although not necessarily in liver) has come from isotope experiments. Saturated fatty acids containing deuterium, when fed to experimental animals, were isolated as unsaturated acids. Saturation of unsaturated acids also occurs, as well as lengthening or shortening of the chains.[9] Apparently desaturation is limited to the formation of a single double bond, usually oleic acid. Thus the essential fatty acids linoleic and linolenic cannot be formed in the animal body. At the present time it is definitely known that desaturation does indeed occur in the β-oxidation of fatty acids, as will be described next.

Beta oxidation The most generally accepted hypothesis of fatty acid oxidation is one called β-oxidation. When fatty acids of different lengths are fed to man or animals, no derivatives can be isolated from blood or urine to throw any light on the mechanism whereby fatty acids are broken down. Consequently, in 1904, Knoop[19] conceived the idea of tagging the fatty acids. Isotope experiments were not possible at this time. His method was to feed the phenyl derivatives and isolate the compound containing the benzene ring from the urine. Benzoic acid is not oxidized by the body but combines with glycine to form hippuric acid. The next higher acid, phenylacetic acid, was eliminated as phenaceturic acid, a combination of phenylacetic acid and the same amino acid, glycine. On feeding the third in the series, phenylpropionic acid, the next higher homologue to phenaceturic acid was not formed but hippuric acid was formed instead. On the next higher step, phenylbutyric acid was transformed to phenaceturic acid. Thus the following sequence of steps occurred:

$C_6H_5 \cdot COOH$	eliminated as	$C_6H_5 \cdot CO \cdot NH \cdot CH_2 \cdot COOH$
$C_6H_5CH_2 \cdot COOH$	eliminated as	$C_6H_5 \cdot CH_2 \cdot CO \cdot NH \cdot CH_2 \cdot COOH$
$C_6H_5CH_2CH_2 \cdot COOH$	eliminated as	$C_6H_5 \cdot CO \cdot NH \cdot CH_2 \cdot COOH$
$C_6H_5CH_2CH_2CH_2 \cdot COOH$	eliminated as	$C_6H_5 \cdot CH_2 \cdot CO \cdot NH \cdot CH_2 \cdot COOH$

Inspection of this series shows that the first and third sets have the same decomposition product. In order to accomplish this, phenylpropionic acid must lose two carbons. The same relation exists between the second and fourth sets. The conclusion was reached that the fatty acid chain loses two carbon atoms at a time, i.e., that oxidation starts at the β-carbon, and when this results in the loss of two carbons the new β-carbon is attacked, and so on.

With a long-chain fatty acid, we would have, on the basis of this hypothesis, a chain of reactions somewhat as follows:

```
  R          R          R          R          R          CH₃        CH₃
  |          |          |          |          |          |          |
  CH₂        CH₂        CH₂        CH₂        CH₂         CH₂        C=O
  |          |          |          |          |          |          |
  CH₂        CH₂        CH₂        C=O        COOH        CH₂        CH₂
  |          |          |          |       ---------      |          |
  CH₂   →    CH₂        CH₂        CH₂   →  CH₃    →    CH₂    →    COOH
  |          |          |          |          |          |
  CH₂        C=O        COOH       COOH       COOH       COOH    Acetoacetic
  |          |       ---------                         Butyric      acid
  CH₂        CH₂        CH₃  →     COOH                   acid
  |          |          |
  COOH       COOH       COOH
```

```
                        CH₃              CH₃          2 CO₂
                        |                |        →     +
                        CHOH             COOH         2 H₂O
                   ⇌    |          →     |        -----------
                        CH₂              CH₃          2 CO₂
                        |                |        →     +
                        COOH             COOH         2 H₂O
                  β-Hydroxybutyric
                        acid
```

Apparently β-oxidation is at least the first step in fatty acid oxidation. Under most circumstances four-carbon chains seem to result from fatty acid degradation. Perfusion of isolated livers with blood containing fatty acids results in the formation of acetoacetic acid. Similar results have been obtained by the oxidation of fatty acids in vitro. Rittenberg and Schoenheimer[9] demonstrated that tagged stearic acid (18 carbons) when fed could be isolated as palmitic acid (16 carbons). The reverse also occurred.

During the past decade or so, other theories of the pathway of fatty acid oxidation have been proposed, e.g., the multiple alternate oxidation and β-oxidation-condensation theories. There also is some evidence that ω-oxidation occurs to a limited extent, forming dicarboxylic acid derivatives of the fatty acids. However, these hypotheses have been proved to be either incorrect or of minor importance.

The discovery that coenzyme-A is involved in the oxidation of fatty acids led Lynen,[20] Mahler,[21] Green, and others to suggest a modified, cyclic form of β-oxidation of fatty acids, a *fatty acid spiral* as shown diagrammatically in Fig. 12-4. The enzymes and cofactors involved in this fatty acid cycle or spiral are as follows:

1. Fatty acid–activating enzyme; CoASH; ATP; Mg^{++}
2. Acyl-CoA dehydrogenase; FAD → $FADH_2$
3. Acyl-CoA hydrase (crotonase)
4. β-Hydroxyacyl-CoA dehydrogenase; NAD^+ → $NADH_2$
5. β-Ketothiolase; CoASH
6. Continued repetition of Reactions 1 to 5 until finally only acetyl-CoA remains

Interesting is the fact that the above enzymes and cofactors are present in the mitochondria of liver and certain other tissue cells. Each has been pre-

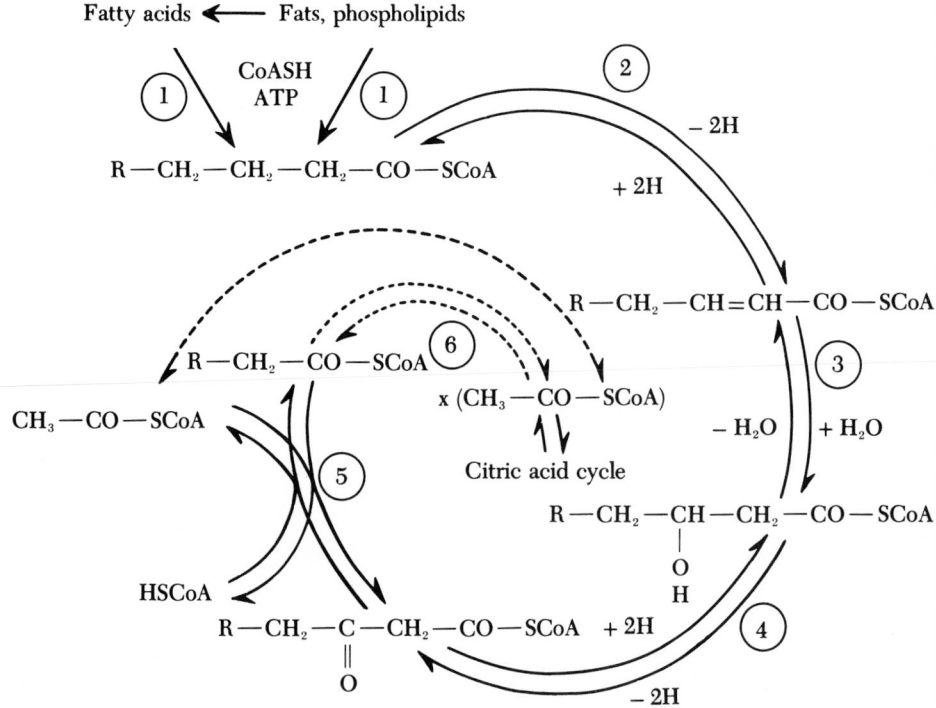

Fig. 12-4. Fatty acid spiral (Modified from Lynen, F.: Ann. Rev. Biochem. 24:653, 1955.)

pared in purified form and acyl-CoA hydrase has been crystallized. Perhaps it should be emphasized that the action of the fatty acid spiral is reversible, to a limited extent at least, so that some biosynthesis of fatty acids from acetyl-CoA as well as fatty acid oxidation can be accomplished. This has been confirmed in vitro by the use of cell-free mitochondrial preparations—one of the most significant achievements in the field of intermediary metabolism in recent years.

Thus, when β-oxidation occurs, the fatty acid loses two carbons. The process may be repeated again and again, two carbons being cut off each time. It should be pointed out at this time that acetoacetic acid, as acetoacetyl-CoA, is a *normal intermediate* in the final turn of the fatty acid cycle. It is formed from butyryl-CoA and finally converted to two moles of acetyl-CoA. Acetoacetic acid may be formed in considerable amounts by the condensation of two molecules of acetyl-CoA, resulting from the above series of reactions, as follows:

$$2 \text{ Acetyl-CoA} \rightleftarrows \text{Acetoacetyl-CoA} + \text{CoA}$$

In the liver there is an enzyme that hydrolyzes acetoacetyl-CoA, liberating acetoacetic acid:

$$\text{Acetoacetyl-CoA} + H_2O \xrightleftharpoons[\hphantom{xxxxx}]{\text{Deacylase}} \text{Acetoacetic acid} + \text{CoA}$$

Acetoacetic acid is one of the ketone bodies and will be discussed further on p. 315. Acetyl-CoA, you will remember, is the form in which two-carbon fragments enter the citric acid cycle for final oxidation.

A further problem involved in the oxidation of fatty acids is the mechanism by which fatty acids gain access to the mitochondrion, the cellular site of β-oxidation. The mitochondrial membrane is impermeable to fatty acids as such. The answer to this question seems to have been supplied by the discovery that *carnitine* (p. 566) serves as a transport agent,[22] "ferrying" the fatty acid across the mitochondrial membrane. Subsequent work has supported this concept. The entire process, including the activation of the free fatty acid in the cytoplasm, is shown schematically as follows:

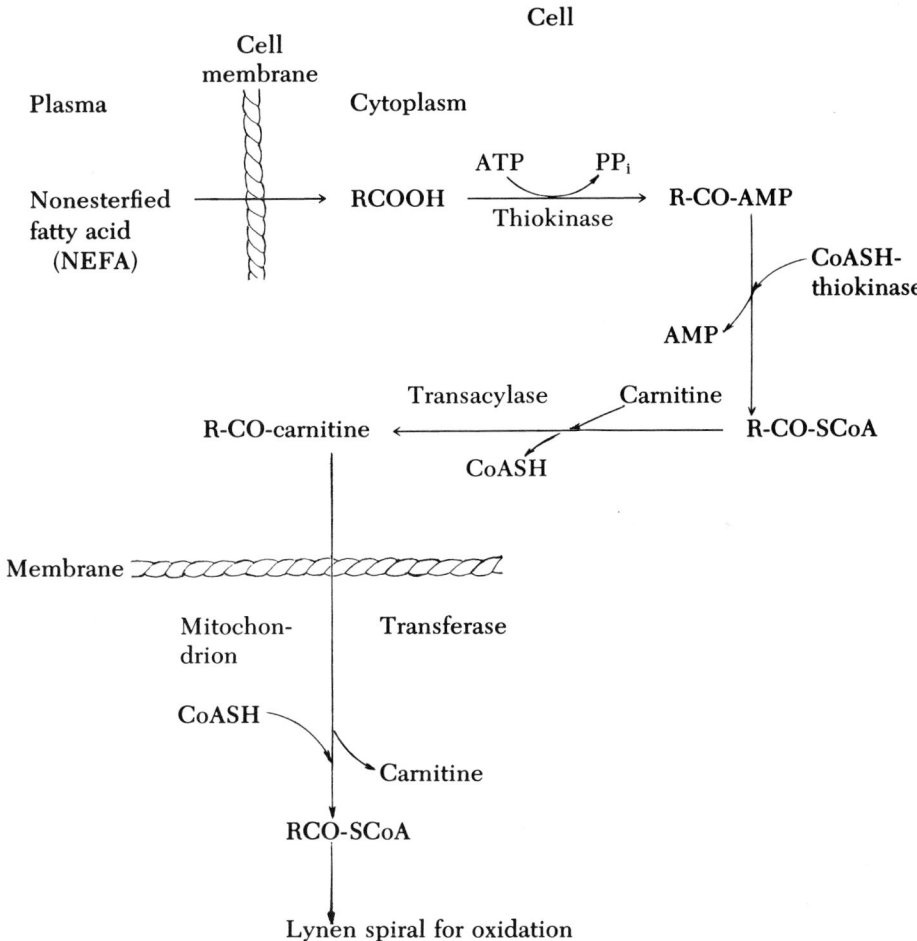

Lynen spiral for oxidation

The same mechanism may serve to transport acetyl-CoA in the reverse direction (mitochondrion → cytoplasm) as an intermediate acetylcarnitine for the cytoplasmic biosynthesis of fatty acids (p. 311).

Energy nsiderations   It may be noted that for each two-carbon atom removed from a fatty acid by β-oxidation, two moles of ATP are required to activate the fatty acid to its CoA derivative and five moles of ATP are formed, leaving a net gain of three moles of ATP. Then each two-carbon fragment formed (acetyl-CoA) yields another 12 moles of ATP in its final oxidation by way of the citric acid cycle.

This makes a total 15 moles ATP per two-carbon atom oxidized. Thus, for a 16-carbon fatty acid a grand total of 120 moles of ATP would be produced. This would be equivalent to approximately 900 kilocalories. The complete oxidation of palmitic acid theoretically yields 2340 kcal./mole. Therefore, the efficiency of the in vivo oxidation of fatty acids is roughly 38% — a surprisingly high figure.

Control of fatty acid oxidation   The control of the oxidation of fatty acids is by way of the usual mechanisms discussed earlier (p. 23). The immediate regulation is undoubtedly by way of product need (ATP) and substrate and cofactor availability. Longer-range control, of course, would be by way of enzyme induction or repression. However, more studies in the area are needed.

Oxidation of odd-carbon atom–chain fatty acids   Although most fatty acids metabolized by the animal organism are composed of an even number of carbon atoms, small amounts of fatty acids containing an odd number are utilized. β-Oxidation of these chains takes place by the preceding steps to form acetyl-CoA until propionyl-CoA is left, which is metabolized by the following steps:

$$\text{Propionyl-CoA} \xrightarrow[\text{CO}_2]{\text{ATP} \quad \text{Propionyl-CoA carboxylase}} \text{D-Methylmalonyl-CoA} \quad (\text{ADP} + \text{P}_i)$$

$$\begin{array}{c} \text{H} \\ | \\ \text{HOOC—C—CO—SCoA} \\ | \\ \text{CH}_3 \end{array}$$

Methylmalonyl-CoA racemase

$$\text{Succinyl-CoA} \xleftarrow[\text{mutase}]{\text{Methylmalonyl-CoA}} \text{L-Methylmalonyl-CoA}$$

The succinyl-CoA thus formed may be metabolized by way of the citric acid cycle. Propionyl-CoA carboxylase has been crystallized from pig heart. It contains four moles of biotin per mole of enzyme. Propionic acid is also produced in the oxidation of branched-chain amino acids (p. 370).

An interesting finding is the fact that patients with vitamin B_{12} deficiency excrete relatively large amounts of propionic acid and methylmalonate in the urine. Vitamin B_{12} is a constituent of the enzyme methylmalonyl-CoA mutase (p. 827).

BIOSYNTHESIS OF FATTY ACIDS

At the present time, it is believed that there are two systems (in liver cells at least) capable of synthesizing fatty acids from simple precursors, principally acetyl-CoA, together with the essential enzymes and cofactors. One of these may be termed a *mitochondrial* system, and the other a *cytoplasmic* system.

The first system apparently forms fatty acids by the simple reversal of the fatty acid cycle, shown in Fig. 12-4. This was initially demonstrated in Gurin's laboratory,[23] using a cell-free system from pigeon liver, and subsequently confirmed by the Lynen group and others. The primary function of the mitochondrial system now appears to be to lengthen shorter-chain fatty acids.

The second system, localized primarily in the nonparticulate cytoplasm of the cell, catalyzes the synthesis of palmitic acid from acetyl-CoA, derived primarily from citrate by the action of the citrate-cleavage enzyme (p. 266), without participation of the mitochondrial fatty acid oxidative enzymes. Evidence for the existence of this second system came from observations on fatty acid synthesis in the particle-free supernatant of avian liver. It soon became apparent that factors not required by the mitochondrial system are essential in the cytoplasmic system. These included the presence of carbon dioxide or bicarbonate, manganese (II) ions, $NADP^+$, and a biotin-containing enzyme called *acetyl carboxylase*. Then followed the significant discovery that malonyl-CoA is an intermediate in the synthetic reaction.

Apparently the enzymes involved in fatty acid synthesis by the cytoplasmic system, along with an acyl carrier protein (ACP), exist in a multienzyme complex called *fatty acid synthetase*. This multienzyme macromolecule was crystallized recently from yeast by Lynen and his co-workers. It has a molecular weight of about 2.3 million and appears to consist of some 21 subunits. Lynen and his group believe that the seven enzymes required for fatty acid synthesis are contained in this particle.

The fatty acid synthetase multienzyme complex is believed to consist of a central "core" molecule of ACP surrounded by subunits that include at least seven of the enzymes involved in fatty acid biosynthesis: an ACP-transacylase, the acetyl carboxylase–biotin complex, an acetyl transacylase, a keto reductase, an enoyl dehydrase, a crotonyl reductase, and probably a hydrolase. The citrate-cleavage enzyme may or may not also be loosely attached.

The ACP component of the multienzyme complex is apparently tightly bound in mammalian cells but can be separated and has been isolated by Vagelos and his co-workers[24] from *E. coli* and certain other bacteria. Its role in fatty acid biosynthesis appears to be as a carrier (implied in the name) of the fatty acid as an acyl thioester derivative. Purification of the synthetase that introduces CoA into apo-ACP has been accomplished also from *E. coli*.[25] ACP is a heat-stable protein with a molecular weight of about 9500. The prosthetic group is 4'-phosphopantetheine. Apparently all the reactions of fatty acid biosynthesis, at least in *E. coli*, occur with substrates bound as thioesters to ACP. The complete amino acid sequence of the ACP of *E. coli* has recently been determined.[26] The molecule is made up of 77 amino acid residues, apparently containing no cysteine. The pantotheine prosthetic group is attached covalently.

The significant discovery[27] that malonyl-CoA is an intermediate in the cytoplasmic biosynthesis of fatty acids added further clarification to this process. The major events in fatty acid biosynthesis as currently known in liver cell cytoplasm are summarized schematically as shown at the top of p. 312.

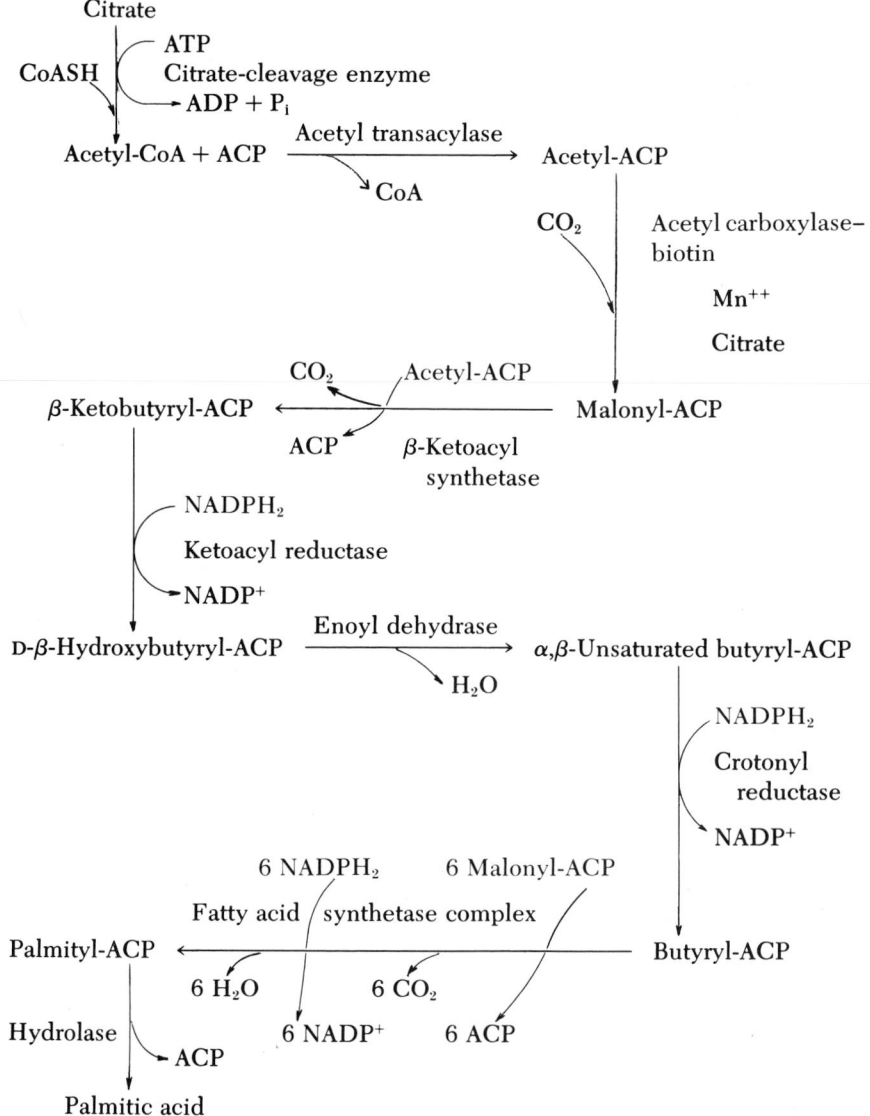

As shown, the carbon source for fatty acid biosynthesis is acetyl-CoA, derived from citrate by the action of the citrate-cleavage enzyme (p. 266) in the cytoplasm. Citrate diffuses freely through the mitochondrial membrane.

The structure of the carboxyacetyl carboxylase–biotin enzyme intermediate involved in malonyl-ACP formation has been shown by Lynen and co-workers to have the following structure:

N-Carboxybiotin enzyme complex

It may be noted that the end product of the cytoplasmic system for fatty acid formation is shown as palmitic acid. Conversion of palmitate to stearate or other longer-chain fatty acids is by elongation by the mitochondrial or microsomal system, described below.

A third system for the biosynthesis of fatty acids, a *microsomal* enzyme system, is apparently used exclusively for the elongation of 16-carbon fatty acids, both saturated and unsaturated. Unlike the cytoplasmic system, but like the mitochondrial system, fatty acyl–CoA derivatives, rather than fatty acyl–ACP derivatives, are used. Malonyl-CoA is employed as the elongating carbon source and $NADPH_2$ is the cofactor. The overall reaction is:

$$R\text{-COCoA} + \text{Malonyl-CoA} + 2 \text{ NADPH}_2 \rightarrow R\text{-(CH}_2)_2\text{-COCoA} + 2 \text{ NADP} + CO_2 + \text{CoA}$$

Regulation of the biosynthesis of fatty acids Apparently the factors controlling metabolic pathways in general (p. 23) apply also to the formation of fatty acids. Earlier claims that the citrate-cleavage enzyme plays a primary regulatory role have not been supported by recent studies.[28] However, the activity of acetyl carboxylase, which appears to be the rate-limiting reaction in fatty acid biosynthesis, is significantly increased by citrate and several related citric acid cycle acids, particularly α-ketoglutaric and isocitric acids. Citrate seems to stimulate the activity of acetyl carboxylase from liver by changing its conformation, apparently producing aggregation of an inactive monomer into an active polymer of some 10 or more subunits. The control by citrate is logical because citrate is the primary carbon source, via acetyl-CoA, for fatty acid synthesis.

The activity of acetyl carboxylase is also stimulated by the presence of long-chain fatty acid–carnitine derivatives. Long-chain fatty acid–CoA derivatives, on the other hand, inhibit the enzyme.

Biosynthesis of unsaturated fatty acids The mechanism of the biosynthesis of unsaturated fatty acids was studied extensively by Bloch and his co-workers.[29] In man and apparently most animals, this process is limited to the formation of only a single double-bond fatty acid, oleic and possibly palmitoleic. Hence, unsaturated fatty acids with two, or possibly more, double bonds must be supplied preformed by foods and are termed *essential* fatty acids (p. 279).

The biosynthesis of so-called "polyunsaturated" fatty acids with two, three, four, or possibly more double bonds occurs readily in microorganisms such as *E. coli* and certain yeasts and fungi. Two mechanisms of synthesis appear possible: (1) oxidative dehydrogenation and (2) oxidation of the β-carbon atom to a hydroxyl group, then dehydration of the resulting β-hydroxy acids.

By the first mechanism, oleic acid could be formed from stearic acid as follows:

$$\text{Stearic acid} \xrightarrow[\frac{1}{2} O_2 \quad H_2O]{NAD^+ \quad NADH_2} \text{Oleic acid } (cis)$$

$$C_{17}H_{35}\text{—COOH} \qquad\qquad CH_3(CH_2)_7\text{—}\overset{H}{C}\text{=}\overset{H}{C}\text{—}(CH_2)_7\text{—COOH}$$

The second mechanism apparently involves the following steps: The precursor, probably a 10-carbon acid, decanoic, is oxidized on the β-carbon atom to form a hydroxyl group, $-\overset{\displaystyle \underset{O \atop H}{H}}{C}-\overset{H}{C}-COOH$. Dehydration then occurs by way

of an appropriate dehydrase to form $-\overset{H}{C}=\overset{H}{C}-COOH$, an α,β-unsaturated fatty acid. The same enzyme, even when purified a thousandfold, also serves as a racemase, shifting the double bond to the β,γ-position. By chain elongation, two-carbon atoms at a time (reversal of the mitochondrial system) to add eight-carbon atoms, oleic acid is formed.

The second, third, and fourth double bonds of linoleic ($\Delta^{9,12}$), linolenic ($\Delta^{6,9,12}$), and arachidonic ($\Delta^{5,8,11,14}$) acids, respectively, are believed to be added by some variation of this mechanism, i.e., desaturation by oxidation and then dehydration, followed by chain elongation.

It may be recalled that the pentose pathway (p. 209) serves as an important source of $NADPH_2$ for fatty acid synthesis in the above systems. The citric acid cycle (p. 263) and glycolysis (p. 196) may also serve as sources for NAD^+. Carbohydrate, of course, is the major precursor of fatty acids (and fat) because of its conversion to acetyl-CoA and citrate by way of the glycolytic pathways.

SYNTHESIS OF TRIGLYCERIDES

Fatty acids synthesized by either of the mechanisms just described are, for the most part, converted to triglycerides by the following steps:

(1) Glycerol + ATP $\rightarrow$ L-α-Glycerophosphate

or

Dihydroxyacetone phosphate $\xrightarrow[\substack{\text{L-}\alpha\text{-Glycerophos-}\\ \text{phate dehydrogenase}}]{\overset{\text{NADH}_2 \qquad \text{NAD}^+}{}}$ L-α-Glycerophosphate

(2) L-α-Glycerophosphate + Fatty acid–CoA (2 moles) $\longrightarrow$ L-α-Phosphatidic acid

$$
\begin{array}{c}
H_2COH \\
| \\
HO-CH \\
| \\
H_2CO-PO_3H_2
\end{array}
\quad + \quad
\begin{array}{c}
2\ R-C-SCoA \\
\| \\
O
\end{array}
\quad \xrightarrow{\text{Acyl transferase}} \quad
\begin{array}{c}
\ \ \ \ \ \ \ \ H_2C-O-C-R_1 \\
O \qquad \qquad \| \\
\| \qquad \qquad O \\
R_2-C-O-C-H \\
| \\
H_2C-O-PO_3H_2
\end{array}
$$

(3) L-α-Phosphatidic acid $\xrightarrow[\text{+ H}_2\text{O}]{\text{Phosphatase}}$ D-1,2-Diglyceride + P_i

(4) D-1,2-Diglyceride + $R_3-\overset{\|}{\underset{O}{C}}-SCoA$ $\xrightarrow{\text{Acyl transferase}}$ Triglyceride + CoASH

$$
\begin{array}{c}
H_2C-O-C-R_1 \\
| \qquad \quad \| \\
\ \ \ \ \ \ O \\
H-C-O-C-R_2 \\
| \qquad \quad \| \\
\ \ \ \ \ \ O \\
H_2C-O-C-R_3 \\
\| \\
O
\end{array}
$$

The biosynthesis of triglycerides apparently occurs primarily in the liver and adipose tissue, but the epithelial cells of the intestinal mucosa are also active in this respect (p. 295). The fatty acids involved are primarily 16- and 18-carbon acids saturated and unsaturated. The L-glycerophosphate is derived preferentially from dihydroxyacetone phosphate but may come from glycerol, as indicated. The 1,2-diglyceride formed is designated D because of its stereochemical relation to D-glyceraldehyde.

KETOGENESIS

The term "ketogenesis" means formation of ketone bodies. The ketone bodies include acetoacetic acid, β-hydroxybutyric acid, and acetone. Acetone, however, is merely a breakdown product of either of the other two, which actually are the important substances concerned. Attention should therefore be centered entirely on acetoacetic acid (diacetic acid) and β-hydroxybutyric acid. Ketosis is the production of ketone bodies in excess of the ability of the body to utilize them. It occurs in severe diabetes, in starvation, in the acidosis of childhood, and during anesthesia, and it can be precipitated by feeding an unbalanced diet, namely, high fat–low carbohydrate. The appearance of these compounds in the urine is a danger sign, indicating usually an acidosis and warning the clinician of impending coma. As has been seen, they are normal degradation products of the fatty acids, or acetoacetic acid may be formed by a side reaction from two molecules of acetyl-CoA if the latter is produced more rapidly than it can be utilized.

Recent evidence indicates, however, that the major pathway of ketone body formation in the liver from acetyl-CoA and fatty acid oxidation (acetoacetyl-CoA) involves β-hydroxy-β-methylglutaryl-CoA (HMG-CoA) as an obligatory intermediate. The steps are as follows:

$$\text{Acetyl-CoA} + \text{Acetoacetyl-CoA} \rightleftarrows \text{HMG-CoA} \rightleftarrows \text{Acetoacetate} + \text{Acetyl-CoA}$$

CH_3	$COSCoA$	$COOH$	$COOH$	CH_3
$COSCoA$	CH_2	CH_2	CH_2	$COSCoA$
	$C{=}O$	$HO{-}C{-}CH_3$	$C{=}O$	
	CH_3	CH_2	CH_3	
		$COSCoA$		

You will recall that HMG-CoA is also an intermediate in the catabolism of leucine (p. 369) and that it is an obligatory intermediate in the biosynthesis of cholesterol (p. 327). Since the reaction is reversible as indicated, HMG-CoA serves as an interlink between the metabolism of fatty acids, ketone bodies, cholesterol, and leucine. It should be mentioned, however, that different enzymes apparently are involved in the forward and backward steps of the above reversible reaction. The enzymes involved are present mainly in the liver.

It appears quite likely that the high incidence of atherosclerosis in the diabetic may result from extra amounts of HMG-CoA being formed by the preceding reaction as a result of fatty acid catabolism and being converted to cholesterol as well as to ketone bodies.

On the basis of work done on liver slices in vitro, it is now accepted that HMG-CoA is formed chiefly in the liver. This has been corroborated for the intact animal. The blood flowing from the liver has a higher concentration of ketone bodies than that flowing toward it. Chaikoff and Soskin[30] demonstrated that the removal of the liver from a diabetic dog results in a drop in the ketone bodies of the blood. Although other tissues are capable of producing small amounts of these compounds, the liver is by far the chief ketogenic organ. It can, in fact, be regarded as practically the only site of ketone production. The formation of ketone bodies is regulated by one of the anterior pituitary hormones and also, possibly, by glucagon, secreted by the α-cells of the islets of Langerhans (p. 226).

Under normal conditions the liver breaks down the fatty acids to the ketone bodies and sends them into the bloodstream for distribution to the rest of the body. It is in the extrahepatic tissues that they are oxidized further; the liver does not use them to any appreciable extent. This oxidation occurs by way of acetyl-CoA and the citric acid cycle. Kidney, muscle, heart, brain, and testes all have been shown to utilize these substances. The end products are carbon dioxide and water. It has been found that the injection of the products of intermediary fat metabolism can produce pancreatic cellular changes of such a nature that a diabetic condition may result.

Ketosis Knowing that the ketone bodies are produced by the liver and utilized by the tissues, we should see how a ketosis might be caused by (1) increased production of ketone bodies by the liver or (2) decreased utilization by the extrahepatic tissues. The most common conditions associated with ketosis are starvation and diabetes. If the tissues of animals suffering from experimental ketosis are tested, they are invariably found to be ketolytic; i.e., they utilize the ketone bodies and are just as active in this respect as tissues of normal animals.

It is therefore apparent that in ketosis the liver must produce ketone bodies at a rate exceeding the *normal* capacity of the extrahepatic tissues to oxidize them. Why should this happen? Let us first study some of the observations made when ketone bodies were assumed to be abnormal products of fatty acid oxidation. It was known that they occur in diabetes mellitus, starvation, and in other conditions in which carbohydrate reserves are depleted. Furthermore, if the carbohydrate metabolism could be improved, the ketone production was diminished. This seemed to indicate that the combustion of sugar is necessary for the normal utilization of fats. The concept was fancifully summed up in the statement, "Fats burn only in the flame of carbohydrate."

In 1921, Shaffer[31] showed that the oxidation of acetoacetic acid in vitro is catalyzed by the presence of glucose. He grouped foodstuffs into two classes, ketogenic and antiketogenic, and stated that in order to prevent ketosis, there must be a definite ratio between the two classes actually being metabolized in the body; i.e. a certain amount of glucose and other antiketogenic factors must be used in order to oxidize completely the fatty acids and other ketogenic foods. The combustion of glucose was believed to be increased in the diabetic patient under the influence of insulin and its antiketogenic effect could thereby become effective. Dietitians planned diets so that the keto-genic:antiketogenic ratio would be correct. These mathematically planned diets usually were efficacious, but it now appears that their success was a happy coincidence because the hypothesis on which they were based is now generally held to be incorrect. This was proved by Mirsky[32] when he showed that glucose has no influence on the rate of ketone body utilization by the muscles. It was first demonstrated on eviscerated hepatectomized animals under various conditions and was corroborated by other types of experiments. The conclusion was that the utilization of ketone bodies is not affected by the concomitant consumption of glucose or by the presence of insulin. How-ever, insulin will diminish the ketosis of diabetes, and carbohydrates will do the same for the ketosis of starvation.

It was stated that ketosis must be due to an overproduction of ketone bodies by the liver rather than to a diminished utilization by the extrahepatic tis-sues. Now it is seen that the consumption of glucose does not cause the body tissues to use more ketone bodies. In fact, they can metabolize only a certain quota of these substances. Stadie has said, "Up to a certain level fat metabo-lism is complete and there is no ketonuria. Beyond this level fat metabolism is incomplete and part of the fat is excreted in the form of ketone bodies." The reason for the occurrence of ketosis in diabetes is that the body must make up the deficit in carbohydrate calories by burning more fat and more protein. Fat is ketogenic and so are some of the amino acids. The rate of ketogenesis exceeds that of the utilization of ketone bodies by the extra-hepatic tissues, and therefore ketone bodies accumulate in the blood and are excreted in the urine. In starvation the glycogen reserves are depleted first, and then body fat and body protein are called upon for the energy require-ment. Again ketogenesis exceeds the ability of the extrahepatic tissues to burn the ketone bodies, and ketosis results. Weinhouse and associates[33] suggested that carbohydrate may exert its effect at the two-carbon level of fatty acid breakdown. Pyruvic acid from carbohydrate may be carboxylated to oxaloacetate, which then combines with the two-carbon derivative formed by β-oxidation of fatty acids to form citrate, which is oxidized by way of the citric acid cycle.

In diabetes mellitus, ketosis can be alleviated by the administration of insulin, usually with carbohydrate, which improves carbohydrate metabo-lism. The ketosis of childhood is now ascribed to the fact that the young child does not retain glycogen as readily as the adult. Feeding sugar brings about a glycogenesis and relieves the condition.

Ketogenic and antiketogenic substances. The ketogenic substances are, of course, all the fatty acids. In addition, at least three amino acids belong to this group: leucine, phenylalanine, and tyrosine. Antiketogenic substances, in the sense of preventing the accumulation of ketone bodies, are the carbo-hydrates, the glycerol fraction of fat, and the following amino acids: glycine, alanine, serine, valine, cysteine, methionine, aspartic acid, glutamic acid, proline, ornithine, arginine, histidine, and threonine. These are antiketogenic because their nonnitrogenous residues are convertible to glucose.

COMMON PATHWAYS OF PROTEIN, CARBOHYDRATE, AND FAT METABOLISMS

The conversion of protein and fat to carbohydrate has been discussed previously (p. 190). The conversion of carbohydrate to fat has been demonstrated experimentally. When mice were fed glucose labeled with ^{14}C, palmitic acid subsequently recovered from liver and other organs contained the labeled carbon. On a high-carbohydrate diet, fatty acid formation may exceed glycogenesis.[10] The question of the transformation of fatty acids to carbohydrates

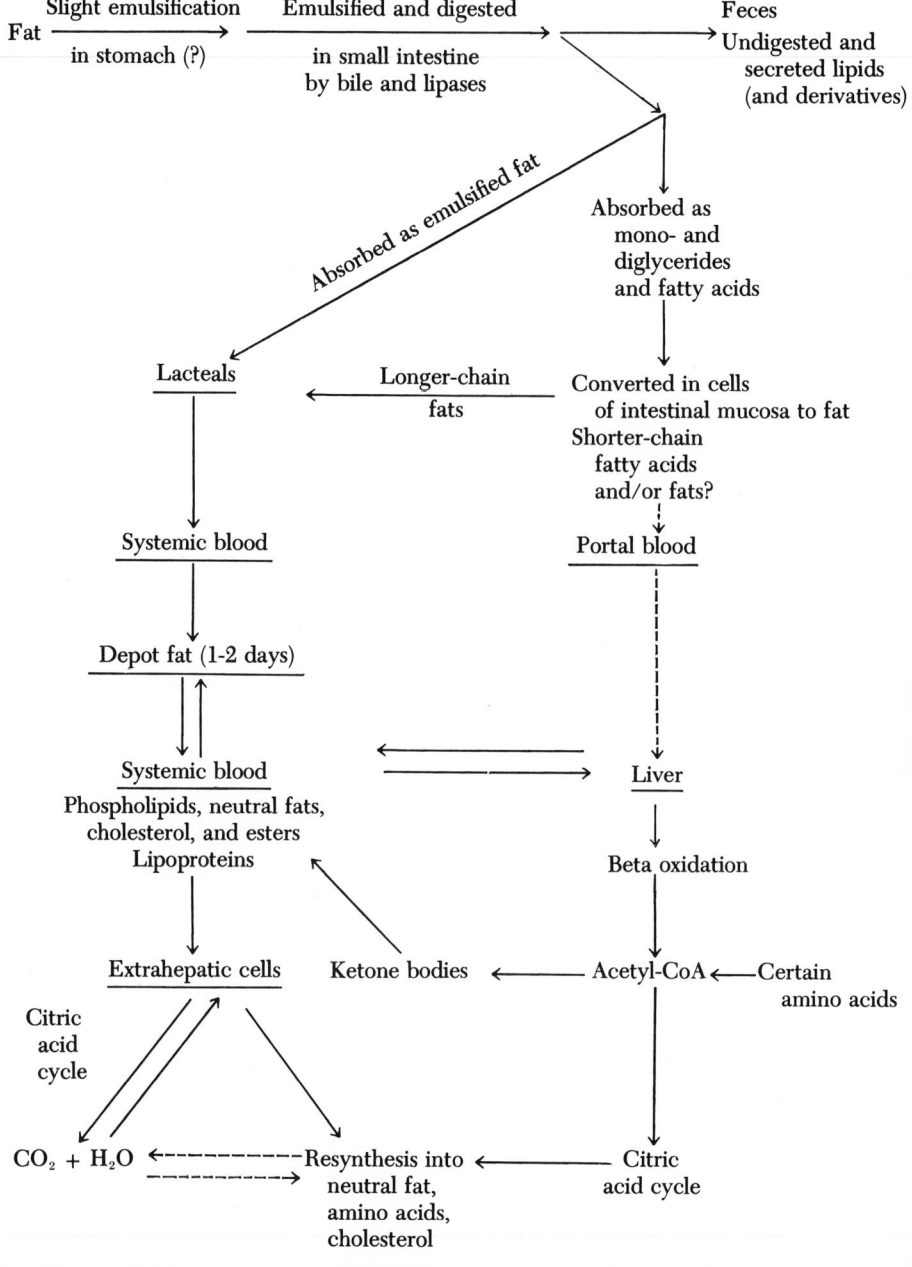

Fig. 12-5. Outline of fat metabolism (broken lines indicate possible routes).

has been a much-debated one for many years. However, the question is no longer significant in view of the fact that fatty acids are largely catabolized to a two-carbon stage. As acetyl-CoA these may condense with oxaloacetic acid and thus enter the citric acid cycle. Moreover, the conversion of fat to carbohydrate has been directly demonstrated. Palmitic acid-6-^{14}C was injected into a diabetic dog. The urinary glucose contained ^{14}C.

In Fig. 12-5 are shown the pathways of fat and its metabolites, as well as the relationship of the citric acid cycle.

Since many amino acids are glucose formers and others are acetoacetic acid formers, it follows that they also can be metabolized in the same cycle. Glutamic acid may also be converted to a α-ketoglutaric acid and thus enter the cycle at that point. The citric acid cycle therefore is a common pathway of metabolism of all three classes of foodstuffs and thus the question of interconvertibility becomes of no moment (Fig. 12-6).

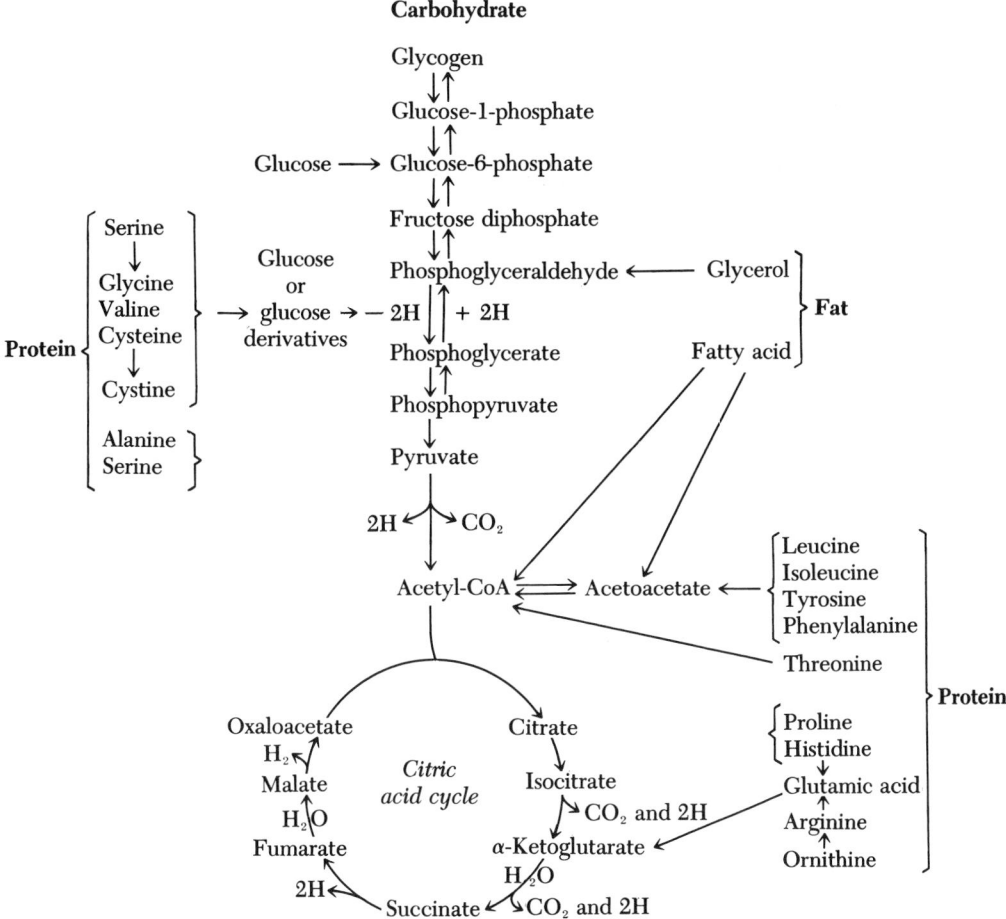

Fig. 12-6. Integration of protein, carbohydrate, and fat metabolisms. The scheme indicates various points at which the products of protein, carbohydrate, and fat metabolisms enter into common pathways. Most of these are discussed or mentioned in the text in Chapters 9, 10, 12, and 13.

319

ESSENTIAL FATTY ACIDS

If fat is entirely excluded from the diet of rats, there develops a condition characterized chiefly by retarded growth, scaly skin, necrosis of the tail, kidney lesions with bloody urine, and early death. This was studied carefully by Burr,[34] who found that certain unsaturated fatty acids are effective in bringing about a cure of the condition. These are linoleic, linolenic, and arachidonic. Strictly speaking, only linoleic acid is essential and cannot be synthesized by the body, and the others may replace it or spare it to some extent. However, interconversions between several of the polyunsaturated fatty acids may occur. A study[35] with rats demonstrated, for example, that ^{14}C-labeled linoleic acid is converted to arachidonic acid. The pathway is linoleic acid $\rightarrow$ γ-linolenic acid ($\Delta^{6,9,12}$) $\rightarrow$ $\Delta^{8,11,14}$-eicosatrienoic acid $\rightarrow$ arachidonic acid. Arachidonic acid is a 20-carbon chain acid with four unsaturated linkages ($\Delta^{5,8,11,14}$). Linoleic and linolenic each have 18 carbons, the former having two and the latter three double bonds.

Vertebrates apparently lack an enzyme required to convert oleic acid to linoleic acid, in contrast to plants and certain microorganisms.[36] Hence, linoleic acid is an essential fatty acid for vertebrates. Interesting is the fact that α-linolenic acid ($\Delta^{6,12,15}$), the plant isomer, is slightly active in promoting

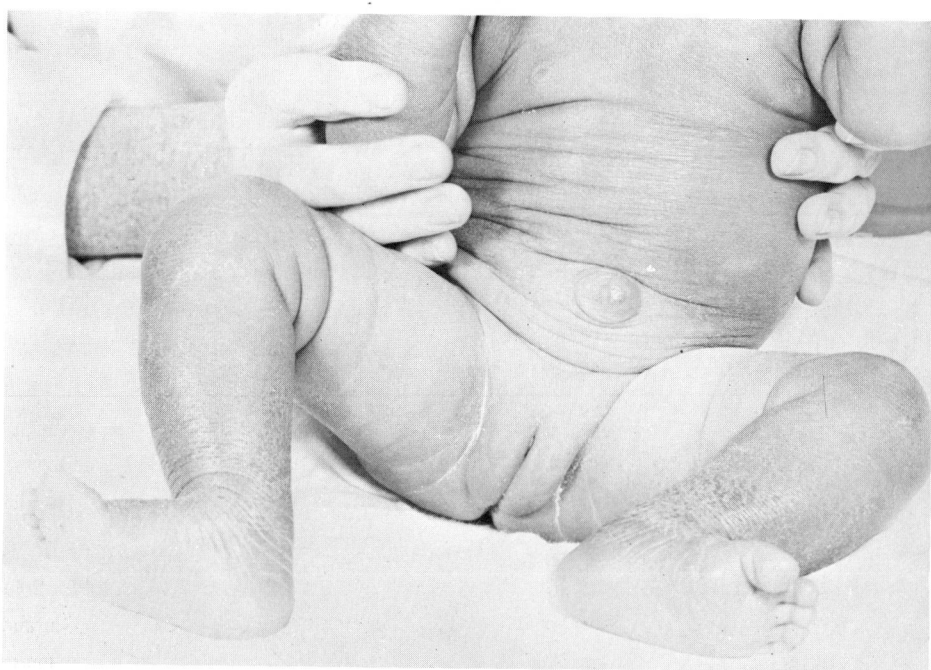

Fig. 12-7. Essential fatty deficiency in an infant, 3 months of age, who had been on a low-fat diet since birth. The skin changes appeared when the child was about 4 weeks of age. The addition of linoleic acid as trilinolein equal to 2% of the caloric intake or a milk mixture containing linoleic acid was found to effect complete clearing of the rough, desquamating skin and diaper region irritation within 2 weeks. (Courtesy A. E. Hansen; presented at the Conference on Essential Fatty Acids, Oxford, England, August, 1957.)

growth in animals deficient in linoleic acid but is ineffective in curing the dermal lesions. γ-Linolenic acid ($\Delta^{6,9,12}$), the animal form, is effective in both respects.

Investigation of this condition led to the discovery that, in rats suffering from a lack of essential fatty acids, the serum lipids have a low iodine number. It was soon found that children with eczema likewise have serum lipids with a low content of unsaturated fatty acids. The administration of suitable fats cleared up the skin lesions in many of these cases (Fig. 12-7). Evidently some individuals require a greater than average amount of these essential fatty acids in their diet.

Another deficiency disease with symptoms closely resembling those described above can be produced in rats by withdrawal of pyridoxine from the diet. Apparently there is a relation between the essential fatty acids and pyridoxine, because animals deprived of both the vitamin and the linoleic acid can be relieved by the administration of either. The nature of this relationship is at present uncertain.

It is now known that some of the physiologic properties of fats are due to the fats' content of essential fatty acids. These include favorable effects upon sex maturation, pregnancy, and lactation. The essential fatty acids protect against the harmful action of x-ray irradiation. Fat-deficient rats have a high capillary permeability and low capillary resistance, which can be remedied by diets containing linseed oil or linoleic acid. The essential fatty acids also are involved in cholesterol metabolism (p. 325).

METABOLISM OF PHOSPHOLIPIDS

As discussed in Chapter 11, the phospholipids are a class of *compound* lipids containing phosphate and in most cases a nitrogenous base along with, of course, esters of fatty acids with an alcohol. They are constituents of all cells and play vital roles as constituents of cell membranes and factors in regulating membrane permeability. They are present in the myelin sheath of nerve cells and in electron-transport particles. They serve as biologic detergents, aiding in the solubilization of the less polar lipids, e.g., triglycerides, cholesterol, in the aqueous fluids of the body. They play some role in blood clotting (p. 619). The five most important types of phospholipids are the phosphatidic acids, lecithins, cephalins, sphingomyelins, and plasmalogens.

Some phospholipids are extremely active metabolically, as evidenced by their rapid turnover rate in tissues, measured by means of ^{32}P labeling. The half-life of hepatic lecithin as thus determined is less than 24 hours. Phospholipids that serve a structural purpose, however, e.g., brain cephalin, have a much longer half-life, up to several months.

Whether or not food lecithin is digested is a question. None of the required enzymes is present in any digestive fluid, except perhaps as a contaminant because of disintegrating leukocytes or other cells. However, lecithins and other phospholipids get into the circulation even if they are not ordinarily digested in the gastrointestinal tract. During fat absorption the lecithin of the blood increases as the blood fat increases, and as a rule the high lecithin values persist longer. The lecithins are synthesized by the body.

Many lecithins are possible, of course, depending on the chain length and unsaturation of the R_1– and R_2–fatty acid moieties and their various possible combinations and permutations.

Radioactive phosphate fed to animals was found to be present in the tissue phospholipid fraction, more particularly as lecithin and cephalin, with very little as sphingomyelin. The rate of production of phospholipid, under these conditions, was found to be liver > intestine > kidney > muscle > brain. The slow production (and disappearance) in brain is interesting, in view of the high content of phospholipid in this tissue (p. 558). Most of the phospholipids of plasma are produced by the liver. This was shown when radioactive phosphate was injected into hepatectomized dogs. Almost no radioactive phospholipid was found in the blood plasma. Normal amounts appeared in the kidneys and small intestine, indicating that these organs can synthesize phospholipids for their own use.

Interesting studies have shown that if rats are fasted then refed a high-carbohydrate diet the fatty acids of the liver lecithins show a marked lowering of their unsaturated fatty acid content, particularly arachidonic acid. This is reminiscent of the classic "soft pork problem" in the earlier literature, in which it was found that feeding high-carbohydrate foodstuff (corn) to hogs resulted in the deposition of a firm "hard" fat in the subcutaneous tissues (i.e., bacon) in contrast to the "soft" fat deposited when a high intake of peanuts was allowed. The economic implications of this finding are evident.

Biosynthesis As a result of the beautiful work of Kennedy and his group[37] and their discovery, in 1955, of the key role of cytidine derivatives in the biosynthesis of certain phospholipids, the pathways of formation of most of these substances are rather well known at the present time. The biosynthetic pathway of the phosphatidic acids has been discussed earlier in this chapter (p. 314). That of lecithin may be shown schematically from D-1,2-diglyceride (p. 314) as follows:

$$\text{D-1,2-Diglyceride} + \text{CDP-choline} \xrightarrow[\text{Mg}^{++}]{\text{Transferase}} \alpha\text{-Lecithin} + \text{CMP}$$

$$
\begin{array}{l}
\text{CH}_2\text{—OOC—R}_1 \\
\quad | \\
\text{R}_2\text{COO—CH} \quad \text{O} \\
\quad\quad\quad | \quad\quad \| \\
\text{H}_2\text{C—O —P—O—CH}_2\text{—CH}_2\text{—N}\equiv(\text{CH}_3)_3 \\
\quad\quad\quad\quad | \quad\quad\quad\quad\quad\quad\quad + \\
\quad\quad\quad\quad \text{O}^-
\end{array}
$$

CDP-choline is formed as follows:

$$\text{Choline} \xrightarrow[\text{ATP} \quad \text{ADP}]{} \text{Phosphorylcholine} \xrightarrow{\text{CTP}} \text{CDP-choline}$$

The cephalins are formed in a similar manner from D-1,2-diglyceride plus CDP-ethanolamine as shown schematically in Fig. 12-8. The biosyntheses of phosphatidylserine and phosphatidylinositol are somewhat different, apparently requiring CDP-diglyceride and L-serine or L-myoinositol, respectively (Fig. 12-8). The mechanism of the formation of the plasmalogens and cardiolipids appears to be uncertain as yet.

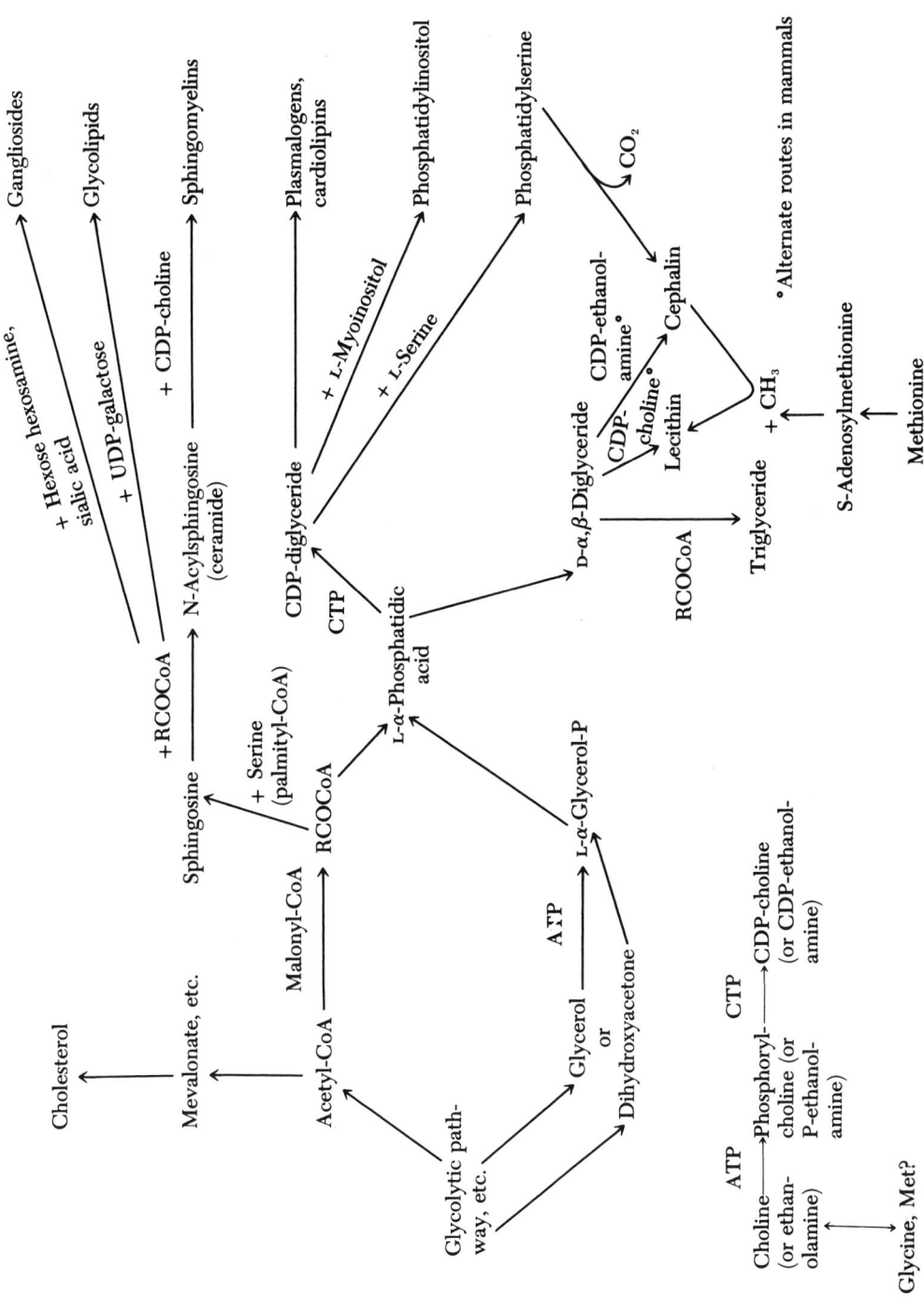

Fig. 12-8. Interrelations between the biosynthesis of triglycerides and various other lipids (liver, brain).

The biosynthesis of the sphingomyelins may be shown schematically:

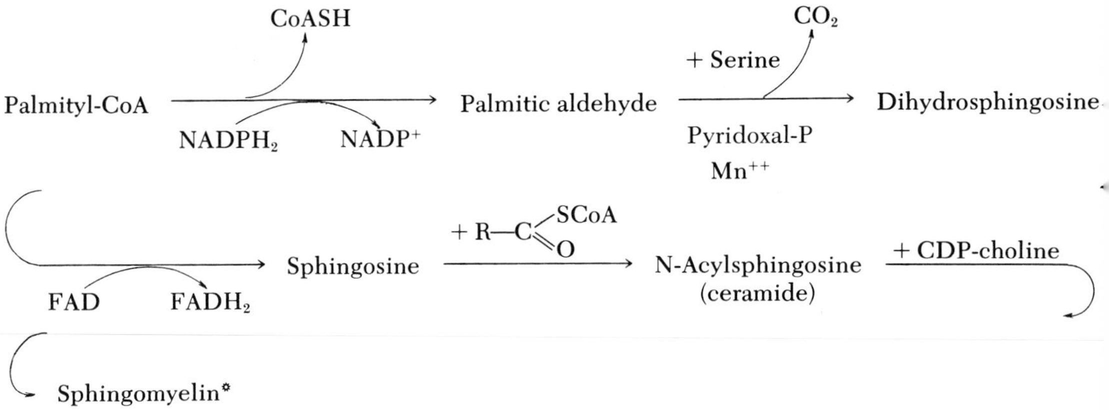

Palmityl-CoA $\longrightarrow$ Palmitic aldehyde $\longrightarrow$ Dihydrosphingosine

CoASH

NADPH$_2$ NADP$^+$

CO$_2$

+ Serine

Pyridoxal-P
Mn^{++}

$\longrightarrow$ Sphingosine $\longrightarrow$ N-Acylsphingosine
(ceramide)

FAD   FADH$_2$

+ R—C$\overset{\text{SCoA}}{\underset{\text{O}}{}}$

+ CDP-choline

Sphingomyelin*

The chemical and physical properties of enzymes involved in the biosynthesis of the foregoing phospholipids and various cofactors required are subjects of extensive investigations at the present time.

Degradation   Lecithin can be attacked by four different enzymes in the following manner:

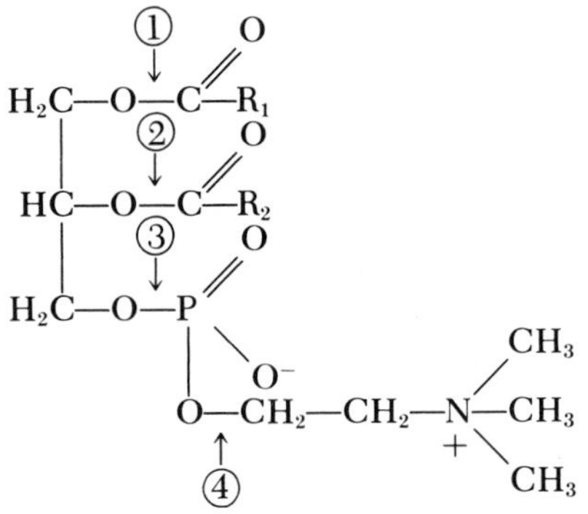

Lecithinase-A attacks at point 2, splitting off one fatty acid and forming lysolecithin, a hemolytic agent. This enzyme is found in animal tissues as well as in some snake venoms, etc. Lecithinase-B takes off two fatty acid molecules at points 1 and 2, leaving glycerocholine phosphate. It is found more generally in animal tissues. Point 3 is the spot where glycerophosphatase acts, and at point 4 choline phosphatase strikes phosphoric acid in another way. Phosphatases are also found in many tissues.

Presumably other phospholipids are catabolized similarly by means of appropriate enzymes.

METABOLISM OF GLYCOLIPIDS

The glycolipids, like the phospholipids, are compound lipids. They contain in the molecule a sugar (usually galactose), sphingosine, and a fatty acid.[38] Their structure was discussed earlier (p. 288). They are present in relatively large amounts in the myelin sheath of brain and nerve cells. Smaller amounts are found in liver and other tissues. Three types are known (kerasin, phren-

---

* See p. 287 for structure.

osin, nervon), differing only with respect to the type of fatty acid present (lignoceric or nervonic).

The biosynthetic pathway of the glycolipids may be shown schematically as follows:

$$\text{Sphingosine} + \text{UDP-galactose} \xrightarrow{\overset{\displaystyle \text{CoA}}{\underset{}{\nearrow}} + \text{R}-\text{C}=\text{O}} \text{Glycolipid}$$

The gangliosides are similar to the glycolipids but contain two hexoses, galactosamine, and a sialic acid in addition to sphingosine and a fatty acid in the molecule (p. 289). The pathway of their biosynthesis is uncertain.

A diagram summarizing schematically the major steps in the biosynthetic pathways of various lipids and their interrelationship is given in Fig. 12-8.

METABOLISM OF CHOLESTEROL

Cholesterol is absorbed from the intestinal tract provided there is fat absorption at the same time. Usually food containing cholesterol also contains enough fat for this purpose. Bile is necessary for cholesterol absorption, as it is for fatty acid absorption. When a neutral fat is fed to dogs or rabbits, its absorption is followed by an increase in the cholesterol esters of the blood but not in the total cholesterol. This seems to indicate that the fatty acids are partly combined with cholesterol during absorption. In man the same rise is not seen, or it is not so marked. The cholesterol and cholesterol esters then enter the lacteals and follow the same route as the neutral fats. It is interesting to note that a highly active cholesterol esterase is present in dog serum, but in human serum esterification goes on very slowly on incubation and is either catalyzed by an enzyme of very low activity or is nonenzymatic.

If there is an excess of cholesterol in the blood, part of it is excreted by the intestine and part via the bile. Reduction in the intestine to dihydrocholesterol and then to coprosterol by bacterial action prevents the reabsorption of this excess lipid. Plant sterols are not absorbed.

The importance of thyroid function in the regulation of cholesterol metabolism has long been known. Hypothyroidism is associated with a hypercholesterolemia, while administration of thyroid hormone lowers the serum cholesterol level both normally and in the hypothyroid state. The reason for this relationship is not understood at the present time. However, possibly the thyroid hormone increases the catabolism of cholesterol, thus lowering its blood and tissue levels; or possibly the hypercholesterolemia seen in hypothyroidism is merely coincidental to the hyperlipidemia seen in this condition.

After absorption, cholesterol is converted to a variety of substances, the main one from a quantitative standpoint being the bile acids, as will be discussed later (p. 687). This has been demonstrated by following the course of ^{14}C-cholesterol and ^{3}H-cholesterol in rats. Ring-labeled cholesterol has been shown to be transformed to the various steroid hormones (Chapter 16). Some radioactive carbon dioxide is formed in a relatively short time, particularly if the terminal carbons are labeled. However, some carbon dioxide is also derived from other parts of the molecule. Radioactive fatty acids were recovered from adrenals, liver, carcass, and feces. Some cholesterol was found to be converted to liver phospholipid and liver glycogen, and a variable amount of activity was seen in the urine. More than half was not degraded, since it was discovered in the nonsaponifiable fraction in the feces and in the liver. In the latter case, storage of cholesterol is indicated.

Cholesterol content of tissues. Cholesterol is found in largest amounts, in normal human adults, in the liver (about 0.3%), skin (0.3%), brain and nervous tissue (2.0%), intestine (0.2%), and certain endocrine glands, the adrenal gland containing some 10%. The relatively high content of cholesterol in skin may be related to vitamin D formation by ultraviolet light (p. 778), and that in the adrenal gland to steroid hormone synthesis (p. 469).

The total cholesterol content of an average 70 kg. man is about 140 gm. On a weight basis per entire tissue, the distribution is greatest in brain and nervous tissue, followed by connective and adipose tissue, muscle, skin, bone marrow, blood, and liver in that order.

Biosynthesis of cholesterol. Cholesterol is essential to life, but, if absent from the diet, it can be synthesized by the animal. A number of investigations have demonstrated acetate to be the carbon source for both the steroid nucleus and the octyl side chain. From the experiments of Bloch and his co-workers,[39] it appears that both carbons of acetate are used for cholesterol synthesis. The methyl carbon is the source of carbons 17, 18, 19, 21, 22, 24, 26, and 27, and the carboxyl carbon gives rise to carbons 10, 20, 23, and 25.

One of the most important developments in biochemistry in the past decade has been the elucidation of the main steps in the pathway of the biogenesis of cholesterol. This has been due to the work of a number of investigators.

Fig. 12-9. Biosynthesis of cholesterol. Summary of principal steps in the biogenesis of cholesterol from the prime precursor, acetyl-CoA. Cofactor requirements are indicated. The enzymes involved in the individual reactions, as presently known, are as follows:

Reaction ① Acetoacetyl kinase

② HMG-CoA (β-hydroxy-β-methylglutaryl-CoA) Condensing enzyme

③ HMG-CoA reductase

④ Mevalonic kinase

⑤ Phosphomevalonic kinase

⑥ Pyrophosphorylmevalonic kinase

⑦ Isopentenyl pyrophosphate synthetase

⑧ Isopentenyl pyrophosphate isomerase

⑨ Geranyl pyrophosphate synthetase

⑩ Farnesyl pyrophosphate synthetase

⑪ Squalene synthetase

⑫ Squalene oxidocyclase

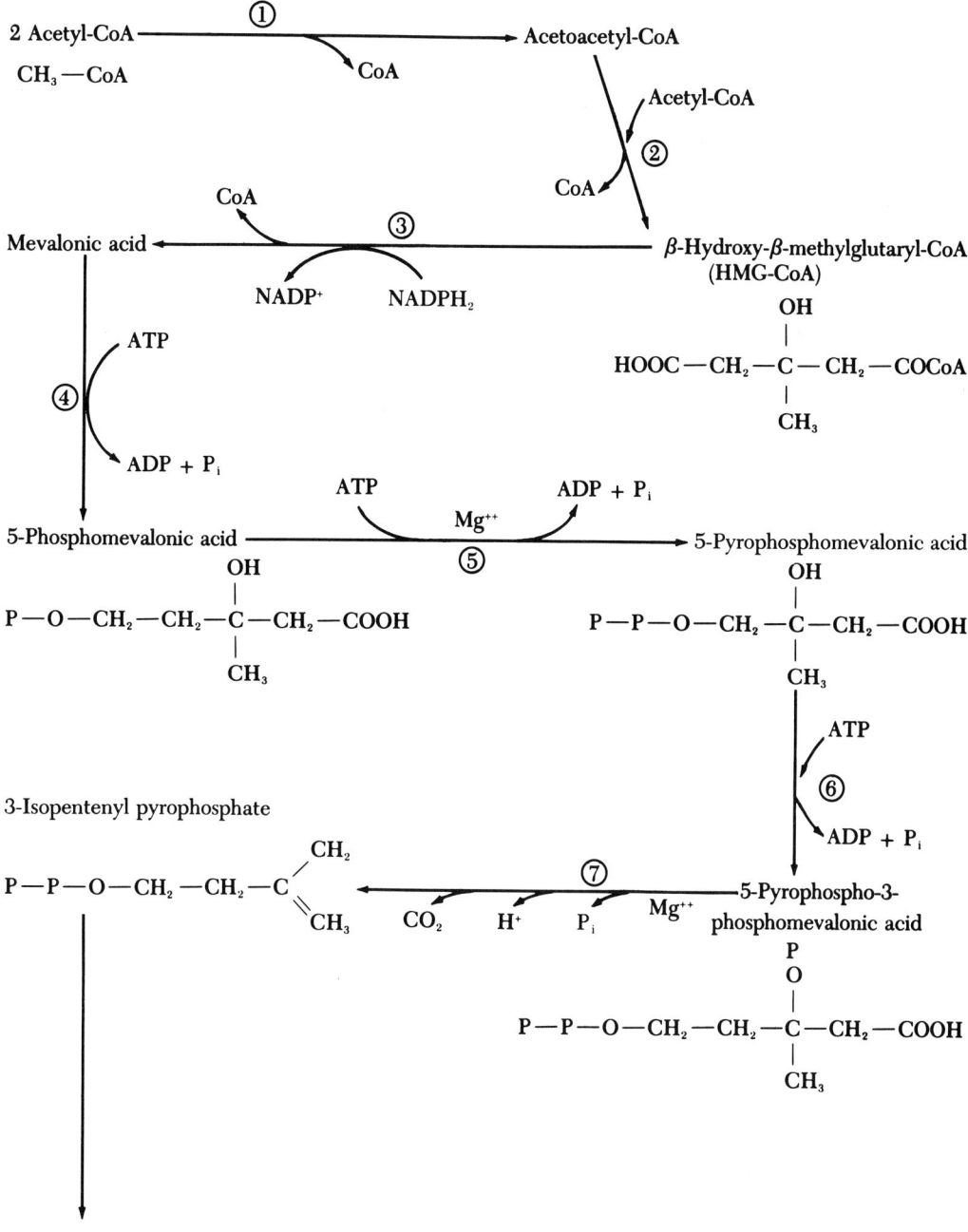

Fig. 12-9. For legend see opposite page.

Continued.

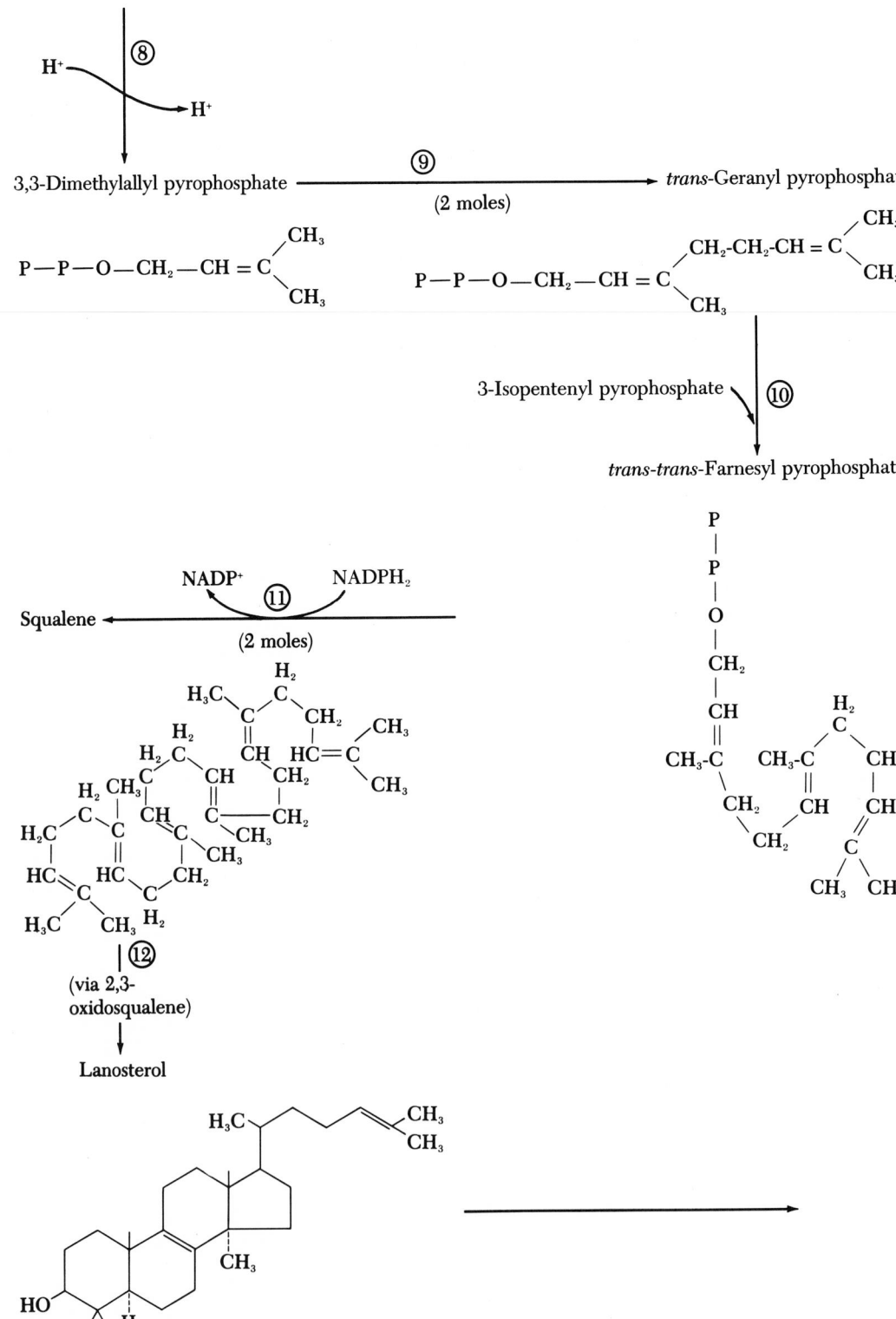

Fig. 12-9, cont'd. For legend see p. 326.

Details of these studies are given in excellent recent reviews.[40] A summary diagram is presented in Fig. 12-9. This diagram shows the major intermediates in cholesterol biosynthesis. There are apparently some 21 steps (not shown) involved in the conversion of lanosterol to zymosterol, desmosterol, and finally cholesterol. Most of these are still under investigation. The enzymes and cofactors involved sequentially in the biosynthetic pathway are given in Fig. 12-9.

The steps in the biosynthesis of cholesterol up to HMG-CoA are reversible. The formation of mevalonic acid, however, in the next reaction is irreversible and is the "committed step" (p. 23) of the pathway. The early steps of cholesterol biosynthesis are facilitated by the marked electron–withdrawing property of the coenzyme-A group. This results in the development

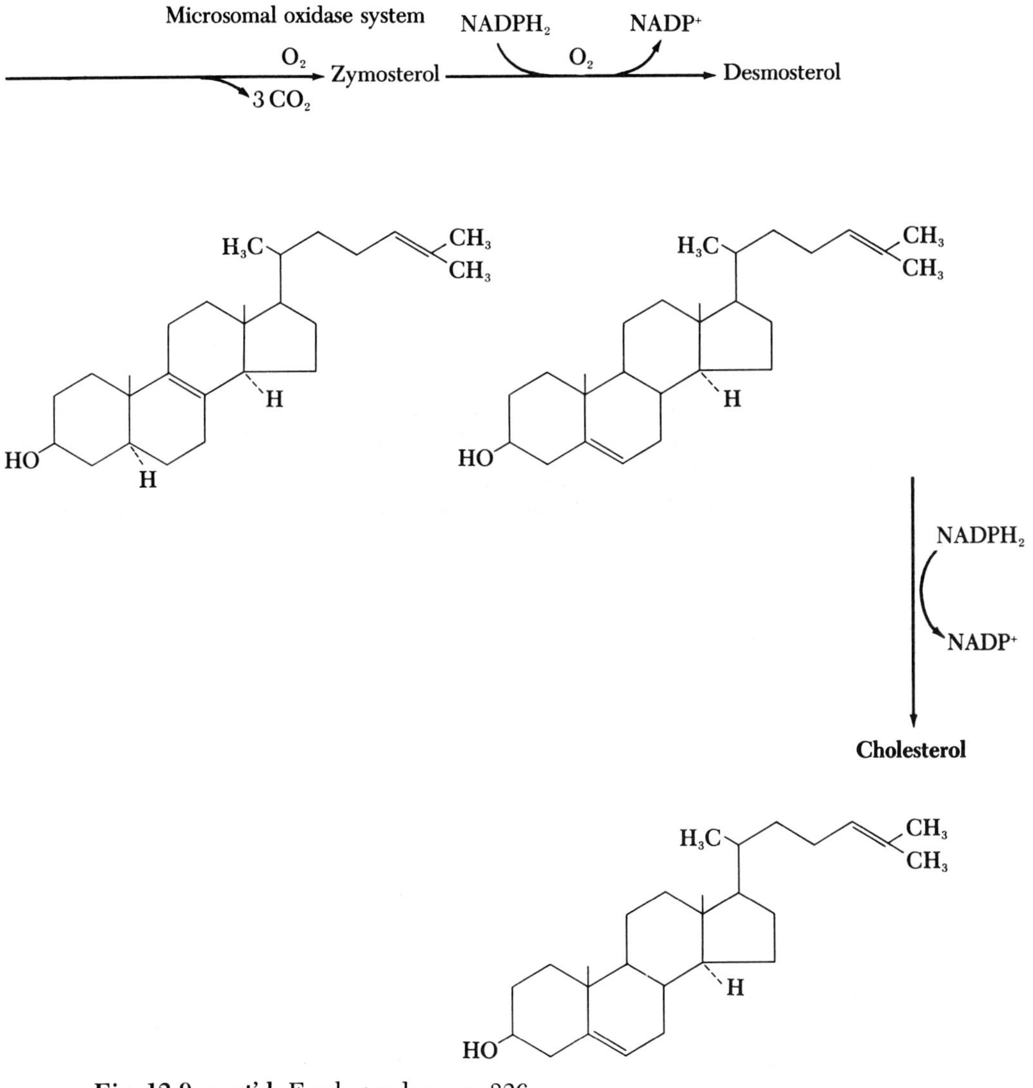

Fig. 12-9, cont'd. For legend see p. 326.

of charges on the carbon atoms of the acetyl moiety with the resulting head-to-tail condensation to form acetoacetyl-CoA, then HMG-CoA. Electron shifts are likewise involved in the head-to-tail condensation of two isoprenoid units to form the 10-carbon atom–geranyl pyrophosphate and the 15-carbon atom–farnesyl pyrophosphate. Additional electron shifts occur in the tail-to-tail condensation of two farnesyl pyrophosphate molecules to form squalene.

The reactions through the formation of squalene do not require oxygen and, therefore, may be performed by anaerobic organisms. Steps beyond squalene, however, require oxygen. They occur in the liver microsomes and require mixed-function oxidases (p. 242).

The conversion of lanosterol to zymosterol entails the oxidation of three methyl groups (positions 4 and 14) to hydroxymethyl and finally to carbon dioxide.

Saturation of the double bond in the side chain of desmosterol by means of $NADPH_2$ completes the conversion of desmosterol to cholesterol. The enzyme requirement for these later steps is under current investigation.

Alternate pathways and sequences that are tissue dependent exist for the biosynthesis of cholesterol from lanosterol. One such pathway is schematically shown as follows:

Lanosterol → 24,25-Dihydrolanosterol → α-4-Methyl-Δ^8-cholestenol → α-4-Methyl-Δ^7-cholestenol → Δ^7-Cholestenol → 7-Dehydrocholesterol → Cholesterol.

Other specific examples will be mentioned later.

It is interesting that the biosynthesis of cholesterol begins with acetyl-CoA, as does that of fatty acids. There is some current evidence that higher available $NADH_2$ (or $NADPH_2$) to NAD^+ ($NADP^+$) ratios favor fatty acid synthesis whereas lower ratios favor cholesterol formation. The discovery of mevalonic acid as a precursor of cholesterol,[41] in 1956, was an important step in the elucidation of the pathway.

Control of the biosynthesis of cholesterol. The rate-limiting step in the biosynthesis of cholesterol is the conversion of HMG-CoA to mevalonic acid. Cholesterol itself inhibits this step, providing an effective product feedback (p. 129) inhibition for controlling its formation. A second control point appears to be at the cyclization of squalene into lanosterol. Details of the regulation are not clear as yet. Fasting diverts HMG-CoA to ketone body formation, hence decreases cholesterol formation. Higher intakes of saturated fatty acids seem to augment the serum cholesterol level. An explanation of the relation is uncertain.

Analogues of mevalonic acid have a similar effect as competitive inhibitors. The compound triparanol inhibits the conversion of desmosterol to cholesterol, diverting the former into bile acids, which are excreted in the bile. This results in a lowering of the plasma cholesterol level. Nicotinic acid, in large doses, but not nicotinamide, also lowers the plasma cholesterol level, apparently by inhibiting the release of cholesterol from the fat stores of the body.

Functions of cholesterol. The esters of cholesterol with fatty acids are normally present in the blood in a more or less definite ratio to free cholesterol. Furthermore, the fatty acids so combined are the most unsaturated of all in the blood plasma. This suggests that cholesterol acts as a special transport agent for the unsaturated acids.

Another function of cholesterol is its role as a precursor of the bile acids (p. 325). One estimate is that 80% of the cholesterol utilized per day is converted to cholic acid (bile salts). This was shown by experiments on a dog. The gallbladder was anastomosed to the pelvis of one kidney in such a way that all the bile flowed into the urine. Cholesterol containing deuterium was injected intravenously. That some of this had been changed to cholic acid was indicated by the fact that the cholic acid isolated from the "urine" contained deuterium. The organs were also analyzed, and the administered cholesterol was found in highest concentration in the lungs, next in the liver, and in smaller amounts in all other organs except the nervous system. This again emphasizes the fact that brain and nervous tissue have a slow rate of general metabolism. The cholesterol in nervous tissue does not interchange with dietary cholesterol at appreciable rates. The cholesterol present in the "urinary" bile of this animal also contained deuterium, which shows that the liver removes some cholesterol from the blood.

Cholesterol also serves as a precursor of various steroid hormones, as will be discussed in Chapter 22. Cholesterol is convertible to vitamin D by irradiation (p. 778). Still another important function of cholesterol is as insulation for nerve fibers in the brain and nervous tissue. This is undoubtedly related to its high dielectric constant. Cholesterol is also a constituent of a number of types of cell membranes.

One type of arteriosclerosis, "hardening of the arteries," is atherosclerosis. This is a common ailment in man, and its treatment has completely baffled clinicians. In this condition there are an abnormal deposition of cholesterol and other lipids and a hardening or sclerosis due to calcification. Feeding cholesterol to rabbits produces this condition experimentally, and it is well known that a high concentration of cholesterol in the blood usually occurs in patients suffering from atherosclerosis, although many individuals with hypercholesterolemia have no evident arteriosclerosis, and not all arteriosclerotic persons have elevated blood cholesterol. Consequently there is a difference of opinion among clinicians as to whether low cholesterol–low animal fat diets should be advised in atherosclerosis. Unfortunately such diets are of little value unless carried out extremely rigorously. It must be remembered that the body is capable of synthesizing a considerable amount of this lipid. Keys[42] showed that the ordinary variations in cholesterol content of the diet have no influence on blood cholesterol; and moderately low cholesterol diets similarly do not reduce the blood level. Only on diets that are almost quantitatively devoid of cholesterol do patients experience a fall in blood cholesterol, and then it is quite dramatic.

The blood cholesterol level, however, does vary directly with the amount and possibly the type of fat in the diet. Extensive survey studies by Keys and others[43] showed conclusively that populations that traditionally ingest a low-fat diet, e.g., South African Bantus, certain Orientals, have significantly lower blood cholesterol levels than do Americans. The incidence of atherosclerosis in these populations is considerably lower too. An interesting current study by Trulson and co-workers[44] made biochemical and dietary comparisons between Irish-born Americans living in Boston and their brothers living in Ireland. The Boston brothers were heavier and fatter, had higher levels of serum cholesterol, exhibited a greater incidence of hypertension, were less active physically, but ate less, when compared with their brothers in Ireland. The Irish brothers consumed more calories and ate more animal fat and starches. The American Irish were heavier smokers. Some statistics show that the death rates from coronary heart disease are higher in the United States than in Ireland for men 45 to 65 years of age.

Another view is that it is not the actual cholesterol content of the diet that produces atherosclerosis, perhaps not even the hypercholesterolemia itself; rather, it is the physical condition of the lipids in the blood. Hueper was able to produce atherosclerotic lesions by introducing large colloidal particles of foreign substances (pectin, gum arabic, etc.) into the bloodstream of animals. In harmony with this is the work of Gofman, who has studied the occurrence in the plasma or giant molecules composed of cholesterol, its esters, fatty acids, lecithin, and protein. The ultracentrifuge is used to separate blood lipoproteins into classes, depending on the particle size and fat content. The density of these particles varies inversely with the rate of flotation (S_f). Normal lipoproteins have a slow flotation rate, $S_f 10$ and below. When lipid metabolism is deranged, as in atherosclerosis, the lipoproteins have a higher S_f. Figures of $S_f 12$ to $S_f 100$ seem to be associated with atherosclerosis or some other cardiovascular disturbance. The amount of the lipoproteins must be taken into account, as well as their S_f values. Only 10% to 15% of cholesterol is contained in particles of the $S_f 12$ to $S_f 100$ class in human beings. These particles may often be decreased in amount by restricting dietary fat and cholesterol.

Another method of shifting the lipoprotein pattern in human beings is by the parenteral administration of heparin, or *treburon*, a synthetic substance with heparin-like action. Hahn was the first to realize that after heparin administration there is an increase in the translucence of plasma, rendered hyperlipemic by high fat feeding. This clearing effect does not occur in vitro. If, however, such turbid plasma is treated in vitro with plasma from another animal that has been heparinized, the clearing phenomenon occurs. This may indicate that a deficiency of heparin is, in part, related to atherosclerosis. The clearing effect is also accompanied by an increase in lipolytic activity of the plasma, which may be responsible for the phenomenon, and is followed by the rapid removal of solubilized lipid from the bloodstream.

Another approach to this problem is indicated by the observation of Rinehart, who found that an arteriosclerosis develops in rhesus monkeys subjected to a prolonged pyridoxine deficiency. There is also current evidence that the amount of sugar,[45] or the amount and type of carbohydrate[46] or of pectin, or the amount of saturated fatty acid, myristic, in the diet may significantly affect the blood cholesterol level in man or experimental animals and hence presumably bear some relation to the atherosclerosis problem.

The question of the etiology of atherosclerosis is still unresolved. Undoubtedly multiple causative factors are involved, the following six being most important: (1) heredity—a family history of coronary heart disease; (2) high blood pressure; (3) obesity; (4) high serum cholesterol; (5) lack of regular exercise; and (6) excessive cigarette smoking. Persons with two or more of these characteristics are classed by some authorities as having a "coronary profile" and are potential heart attack victims.

LIPOPROTEINS

As stated in the preceding chapter (p. 290), the lipoproteins are association complexes of varying proportions of triglyceride, phospholipid, and cholesterol with α- and β-proteins as carriers. The lipoproteins are important in the transport of lipids in the plasma, practically all of the plasma lipids being transported in this manner. The protein moieties are formed primarily in the liver and to some extent in intestinal mucosal cells (p. 295).

There are four major types of lipoproteins found in the blood plasma as determined by electrophoresis on paper or cellulose acetate. They and their primary characteristics are as follows:

α-Lipoproteins — High density   pre-β-Lipoproteins — S_f 21 to 400

β-Lipoproteins — S_f 0 to 20   Chylomicrons — S_f greater than 400

Because of their low densities, the chylomicrons and pre-β-lipoproteins rise to the surface most rapidly upon ultracentrifugation and hence have the relatively high S_f values shown. The typical average composition of the four types of lipoproteins, expressed as percent dry weight, is shown in Table 12-2.

It is evident from the data in Table 12-2 that the pre-β-lipoproteins and chylomicrons are the primary transport substances for triglycerides. Pre-β-lipoprotein is apparently concerned mainly with the transport of endogenous triglycerides, whereas chylomicrons transport primarily exogenous triglycerides. Both are relatively low in protein, phospholipid, and cholesterol content. β-Lipoprotein appears to be the major transport medium for cholesterol.

The electrophoretic patterns of the plasma lipoproteins and their variations in disturbance of lipid metabolism are a subject of vigorous current research.

Table 12-2. Typical composition of major lipoproteins (expressed as percent of dry weight)[*]

Lipoprotein	Protein	Triglyceride	Phospholipid	Cholesterol
α-	50±5	7±2	30	18
β-	23±3	10±2	22	43
Pre-β-	7±5	65±15	18±8	16±7
Chylomicrons	1.5±1.0	87±7	9±6	7±5

[*] Adapted from data in Masoro, E. J.: Physiological chemistry of lipids in mammals, Philadelphia, 1968, W. B. Saunders Co., vol. I.

Table 12-3. Primary hyperlipoproteinemias (Fredrickson classification)*

Type	Sensitive to Exogenous	Lipoprotein elevated or altered	Plasma lipids	
			Triglyceride	Cholesterol
I	Fat	Chylomicrons	Elevated	Normal
II	Fat	β-Lipoprotein	Normal	Elevated
III	Carbohydrate & fat	Abnormal β-lipo-protein	Elevated	Elevated
IV	Carbohydrate	Pre-β-lipoprotein	Elevated	Normal (or elevated)
V	Carbohydrate & fat	Pre-β-lipoprotein & chylomicrons	Elevated	Elevated

*Adapted from Fredrickson, D. S., et al.: New Eng. J. Med. **276**:34, 94, 148, 215, 273, 1967.

This is partly due to the value of these proteins in the diagnosis and control of the lipidoses. During the past few years, Fredrickson and his co-workers[46a] have extensively studied such conditions and have suggested a classification of the primary hyperlipoproteinemias into five categories. These, together with their characteristics, are listed in Table 12-3.

The plasma obtained from patients with either type I or type V hyperlipoproteinemias is characterized by a creamy layer separating over a clear (type I) or turbid (type V) plasma. Types II, III, and IV are characterized by a turbid plasma.

It will be noted that types I and II are induced by the feeding of fat whereas type IV is carbohydrate induced. Types III and V are induced by feeding both carbohydrate and fat.

Clinical studies such as these are aiding greatly in the understanding of heretofore poorly characterized disorders of lipid metabolism, formerly termed *familial hyperlipidemias,* and in the detection of proneness of individuals to cardiovascular disease.

There are at least two known hereditary diseases of lipid metabolism involving deficiencies in plasma lipoproteins and concomitantly in lipid transport. One of these is *Tangier disease,* which is due to a hereditary deficiency of α-lipoproteins. As a result, there is a massive deposition of cholesterol esters in the liver, spleen, and other tissues. Hepatosplenomegaly is usually found. Plasma cholesterol and phospholipid levels are markedly reduced, whereas triglyceride values are normal or elevated.

The other hereditary disorder results from a deficiency of β-lipoproteins and is termed a-beta-lipoproteinemia, or sometimes *acanthocytosis.* The transport of triglycerides is impaired. Weakness and wasting of tissues occur. The patient's erythrocytes are distorted, becoming spheric with numerous projecting spines and spicules, hence the term acanthocytosis (from the Greek *akantha,* "thorn"). Plasma lipids are characteristically lower than normal. There is also extensive demyelinization of nerves.

Other abnormalities of lipid metabolism   The most common abnormality of lipid metabolism is obesity. However, obesity may be and often is a normal storage of fat and is related primarily to an excess of caloric intake over caloric requirement (p. 304). Its relation to endocrine disturbances will be considered later (Chapter 22). The formation of biliary calculi, containing varying proportions of cholesterol, is discussed on p. 688, atherosclerosis in the section just preceding this, and the fatty liver syndromes, which may be considered abnormalities of lipid metabolism, on p. 302.

There are several other pathologic conditions hereditary in nature in each of which lipids are deposited in the cells of certain tissues. Not much is known about the causes of any of them and it is quite possible that several may have a common etiologic factor.

Xanthoma is a disease in which yellow nodules or flat plaques appear in the skin, especially in the eyelids. The nodules may also be formed in tendon sheaths, bone, blood vessels, and elsewhere. They vary in size from that of a pinhead to that of a bean. Xanthoma is sometimes a complication of diabetes. Many xanthomatous deposits have been analyzed. The results indicate that the deposits are a mixture of various lipids, with cholesterol frequently predominating. The blood lipid level in these cases is often elevated. Sometimes the condition occurs in the absence of diabetes, jaundice, lipoid nephrosis, or any other disease that might be the cause of it. *Hand-Schüller-Christian disease* is considered a form of xanthoma. The yellow nodules are found in the cranial and other bones. The nodules contain large amounts of cholesterol and cholesterol esters. This rather rare disease occurs mainly in children.

Gaucher's disease is a congenital condition that sometimes affects several children of the same family. It is characterized by an enlargement of the spleen and liver (splenohepatomegaly) as well as by other symptoms. Although the lipids deposited in the spleen and liver are mixed, the outstanding feature of this abnormality is the presence of a large amount of kerasin, a cerebroside, in them. The sugar present in those lipids peculiar to Gaucher's disease may be glucose rather than galactose, normally found in glycolipids, which may result in a decreased catabolism of this abnormal cerebroside and hence its accumulation in tissues. The bone and marrow are also involved. Although ordinarily the onset is in childhood, the patient may live for many years.

Another familial and congenital disorder is *Niemann-Pick disease*. The liver and spleen are again the site of lipid deposits and are tremendously enlarged, but here the predominant constituent is a mixture of phospholipids, chiefly lecithin and sphingomyelin. It occurs in infancy and causes death within a few months.

Several other hereditary diseases of lipid metabolism have been described, e.g., idiopathic hyperlipemia (*Buerger-Grütz disease*), essential hypercholesteremic xanthomatosis, amaurotic familial idiocy (*Tay-Sachs disease*), and lipochondrodystrophy (*gargoylism*).

In amaurotic familial idiocy, large amounts of gangliosides are deposited in the brain and in nerve tissue. Apparently this interferes with normal cell function and results in the mental defects and neurologic manifestations observed. The gangliosides deposited in the brain may be an abnormal type having an altered carbohydrate moiety. This could impair their catabolism in nerve cells and result in their accumulation. An interesting recent study[47] indicated that there is a deficiency of fructose-1-phosphate aldolase in children with Tay-Sachs disease. This deficiency may be related to the alteration in the composition of the gangliosides found in these cases.

A recent report[48] indicated a marked deficiency of β-galactosidase occurring in liver, spleen, kidney, and brain of some patients with generalized gangliosidosis. This could result in a decreased catabolism of gangliosides in these tissues and hence an accumulation of gangliosides.

Current investigations[49] also indicate that a genetic deficiency of the key enzyme, hexosaminidase-A, may be an etiologic factor in Tay-Sachs disease in children. This enzyme is required in the catabolism of gangliosides. A deficiency thus results in an accumulation of this glycolipid in the brain, usually with a fatal outcome.

Current evidence[50] further indicates a hereditary deficiency of catabolic enzyme is responsible for the accumulation of tissue lipids in at least six different types of sphingolipidoses. The specific enzyme deficiency and the disease resulting are summarized in Table 12-4.

Table 12-4. Hereditary deficiencies of catabolic enzymes in certain sphingolipidoses*

Condition	Catabolic enzyme deficient
Gaucher's disease	Glucocerebrosidase
Metachromatic leukodystrophy	Aryl sulfatase–A (sulfatidase)
Niemann-Pick disease	Sphingomyelinase
Fabry's disease†	Ceramide trihexosidase (α-galactosidase)
Generalized gangliosidosis	β-Galactosidase
Tay-Sachs disease‡	N-Acetyl galactosaminidase

* From Brady, R. O.: Med. Clin. N. Amer. **53**:827, 1969.
† From Kint, J. A.: Science **167**:1268, 1970.
‡ From Okada, S., and O'Brien, J. S.: Science **165**:698, 1969.

References

GENERAL

Bloch, K., editor: Lipid metabolism, New York, 1960, John Wiley & Sons, Inc.

Blondy, P. K., and Rosenberg, L. E., editors: Duncan's diseases of metabolism. Genetics and metabolism, ed. 6, Philadelphia, 1969, W. B. Saunders Co.

Bloor, W. R.: Biochemistry of the fatty acids and their compounds, the lipids, New York, 1943, Reinhold Publishing Corp.

Brodoff, B. N., editor: Adipose tissue metabolism and obesity, Ann. N. Y. Acad. Sci. **131**:1, 1965.

Deuel, H. J., Jr.: The lipids. Their chemistry and biochemistry; vol. 1, Chemistry, vol. 2, Biochemistry, New York, 1951, 1955, Interscience Publishers, Inc.

Fieser, L. F., and Fieser, M.: Steroids, New York, 1959, Reinhold Publishing Corp.

Grau, F. C., editor: Cellular compartmentation and control of fatty acid metabolism, New York, 1968, Academic Press, Inc., vol. 4.

Greenberg, D. M., editor: Metabolic pathways, ed. 3, New York, 1967, Academic Press, Inc., vol. 2.

Hsai, D. Y.: Inborn errors of metabolism, ed. 2, Chicago, 1966, Year Book Medical Publishers, Inc., part 1.

Katz, L. N.: Nutrition and atherosclerosis, Philadelphia, 1958, Lea & Febiger.

Kennedy, E. P.: The metabolism and function of complex lipids, Harvey Lect. **57**:143, 1962.

Krebs, H. A.: The regulation and release of ketone bodies by the liver. In Weber, G., editor: Advances in enzyme reactons, New York, 1966, Pergamon Press, Inc. vol. 4.

Masoro, E. J.: Physiological chemistry of lipids in mammals, Philadelphia, 1968, W. B. Saunders Co., vol. 1.

Popjàk, G., and Grant, J. K., editors: The control of lipid metabolism, New York, 1963, Academic Press, Inc.

Sinclair, H. M., editor: The essential fatty acids, New York, 1958, Academic Press, Inc.

Stanbury, J. B., Wyngaarden, J. B., and Fredrickson, D. S., editors: The metabolic basis of inherited disease, ed. 2, New York, 1966, McGraw-Hill Book Co.

Symposium: Ketosis, Ann. N. Y. Acad. Sci. **104**:735, 1963.

Umbreit, W. W.: Metabolic maps, Minneapolis, 1960, Burgess Publishing Co., vol. 2.

SPECIAL

1. Nutr. Rev. **27**:18, 1969.
2. Mattson, F. H., and Volpenhein, R. A.: J. Biol. Chem. **234**:2792, 1964.
3. Porter, K. B.: Fed. Proc. Sympos. **28**:35, 1969.
4. Senior, J. R.: J. Lipid Res. **5**:495, 1964.
5. Frazer, A. C.: Fed. Proc. **20**:146, 161, 1961.
6. Isselbacher, K. J.: Fed. Proc. Sympos. **26**:1420, 1967.
7. Korn, E. D.: J. Biol. Chem. **215**:1, 1955.
8. Gordon, R. S.: Fed. Proc. **19**:120, 1960.
9. Rittenberg, D., and Schoenheimer, R.: J. Biol. Chem. **121**:235, 1937; Schoenheimer, R., and Rittenberg, D.: J. Biol. Chem. **114**:381, 1936.
10. Chaikoff, I. L.: Harvey Lect. **47**:99, 1953.
11. Chalmers, T. M., et al.: Lancet **2**:6, 1960.
12. Joel, C. D.: In Renold, A. E. and Cahill, G. F., Jr., editors: Handbook of physiology, section 5, Baltimore, 1965, The Williams & Wilkins Co., p. 59.
13. Kornacker, M. S., and Ball, E. G.: J. Biol. Chem. **243**:1638, 1968.
14. Best, C. H., et al.: J. Physiol. **79**:94, 1933
15. Harper, A. E., et al.: J. Biol. Chem. **206**:151, 1954.
16. Danowski, T. S., editor: Ann. N.Y. Acad. Sci. **148**:573, 1968.
17. Mayer, J., and Thomas, D. W.: Science **156**:328, 1967.
18. Leathes, J. B., and Meyer-Wedell, L.: J. Physiol. **38**:xxxviii, 1909.

19. Knoop, F.: Beitr. Chem. Phys. Path. **6**:150, 1904.
20. Lynen, F.: Fed. Proc. **12**:683, 1953; Harvey Lect. **48**:210, 1954.
21. Mahler, H. R.: Fed. Proc. **12**:694, 1953.
22. Fritz, I. B., and McEwen, B.: Science **129**:334, 1958.
23. Gurin, S.: Trans. N.Y. Acad. Sci. **15**:92, 1953.
24. Vagelos, P. R., et al.: Ann. N.Y. Acad. Sci. **18**:10, 1967; Science **154**:428, 1968.
25. Elvoson, J., and Vagelos, P. R.: J. Biol. Chem. **243**:3603, 1968.
26. Vanaman, T. C., et al.: J. Biol. Chem. **243**:6420, 1968.
27. Wakil, S. J.: J. Amer. Chem. Soc. **80**:2908, 6465, 1958.
28. Foster, D. W., and Srere, P. A.: J. Biol. Chem. **243**:1926, 1968.
29. Bloch, K., et al.: Science **143**:1006, 1964.
30. Chaikoff, I. L., and Soskin, S.: Amer. J. Physiol. **87**:58, 1929.
31. Shaffer, P. A.: J. Biol. Chem. **47**:433, 1921.
32. Mirsky, I. A.: J.A.M.A. **118**:690, 1942.
33. Weinhouse, S., et al.: J. Biol. Chem. **181**:489, 1949.
34. Burr, G. O.: Fed. Proc. **1**:224, 1942.
35. Howton, D. R., and Mead, J. F.: J. Biol. Chem. **235**:3385, 1960.
36. Erwin, J., and Bloch, K.: Science **143**:1006, 1964.
37. Kennedy, E. P., et al.: Harvey Lect. **57**:143, 1962; Fed. Proc. **20**:934, 1961.
38. Carter, H. E.: Ann. Rev. Biochem. **34**:109, 1965.
39. Wüersch, J., et al.: J. Biol. Chem. **195**:439, 1952.
40. Tchen, T. T.: In Greenberg, D. M., editor: Metabolic pathways, New York, 1967, Academic Press, Inc., vol. 2; Science **146**:504, 1964.
41. Wolf, D. E., et al.: J. Amer. Chem. Soc. **78**:4499, 1956.
42. Keys, A.: Science **112**:79, 1950.
43. Keys, A., et al.: J. Nutr. **59**:39, 1956.
44. Trulson, M. F., et al.: J. Amer. Diet. Ass. **45**:225, 1964.
45. Yudkin, J.: Lancet **2**:6, 1964.
46. Grande, F., et al.: J. Nutr. **86**:313, 1965.
46a. Fredrickson, D. S., et al.: New Eng. J. Med. **276**:34, 94, 148, 215, 273, 1967.
47. Volk, B. W., et al.: Amer. J. Med. **36**:481, 1964.
48. Okado, S., and O'Brien, J. S.: Science **160**:1002, 1968.
49. Steiner, G.: New Eng. J. Med. **279**:70, 1968.
50. Brady, R. O.: Med. Clin. N. Amer. **53**:827, 1969.

CHAPTER 13

METABOLISM OF AMINO ACIDS

s was discussed earlier (Chapter 5), some 18 or possibly 20 amino acids in varying amounts and sequences make up the proteins of plants and animals. The chemical structures and properties of these vital constituents of living matter have been considered, as have the structures, properties, and functions of proteins formed from them (Chapter 7). It is now appropriate to consider the metabolism of the amino acids themselves.

Amino acids perform many important functions in living matter. As the "building blocks" of proteins, they are essential constituents of the protoplasm of cells. They are incorporated into cellular structural proteins, e.g., collagen, elastin (p. 543); functional proteins, e.g., myosin of muscle, hemoglobin of blood; protective proteins, e.g., keratins of skin, hair, and nervous tissue; catalytic proteins for metabolic reactions in the form of enzymes; transport proteins, e.g., transferrin (p. 581); and regulatory proteins in the form of protein hormones. They are involved in the hereditary process as nucleoproteins of genes. As such, amino acids participate in the biosynthesis of many other essential cellular constituents—creatine, choline, purines, pyrimidines, porphyrins, epinephrine, thyroxin, niacin, melanin, bile acids, detoxication products, and even glucose and ketone bodies. Some of these substances have been discussed in the preceding pages. Others will be considered later. Amino acids also may be oxidized in the body, supplying about 4 kcal. of energy per gram and some 15% to 20% of the total energy requirement of the average human adult.

Most of the amino acids utilized by the animal organism are supplied in the form of macromolecular constituents of foods, the food proteins. Thus, as in the case of carbohydrates and lipids, before they can be utilized, the food proteins must be digested into their constituent amino acids and these must be absorbed through the intestinal mucosa into the blood plasma and transported to the various organs and tissues of the body.

DIGESTION OF PROTEINS

Unlike the carbohydrates and lipids, a significant amount of digestion of proteins occurs in the stomach. This was observed grossly by Beaumont in his classic studies on Alexis St. Martin in the 1820's. Beaumont actually observed pieces of meat and other proteins "liquify" in the stomach of this man. Most proteins are acted upon in the stomach by the proteolytic enzyme *pepsin* at the acid pH (approximately 1.0) of gastric juice and converted to smaller peptides. Pepsin is not a highly specific proteolytic enzyme and hydrolyzes a variety of peptide linkages. It preferentially hydrolyzes those linkages involving the amino group of the aromatic amino acids, tryptophan, phenylalanine, and tyrosine, at least in synthetic peptide substrates (p. 113). However, in natural protein substrates, pepsin splits other peptide bonds similar to those of aromatic amino acids at a relatively rapid rate, e.g., Leu-Glu, Glu-Asn, Leu-Val, Val-Cys. The peptide bonds attacked by pepsin need not be adjacent to a free carboxyl or an α-amino group. Therefore pepsin can act on the "interior" of peptide chains and is accordingly sometimes termed an *endopeptidase*.

Although pepsin digests proteins mainly into polypeptides of varying length, some short-chain peptides and free amino acids, notably tyrosine and phenylalanine, may be formed.

Pepsin is not secreted as such by the "chief" cells of the gastric mucosa; rather, it is secreted as a zymogen form, *pepsinogen* (p. 112). Pepsinogen is converted to the active enzyme by hydrogen ions at a pH of 4.65 or below and also autocatalytically by pepsin itself.

$$\text{Pepsinogen} \xrightarrow[\text{H}^+ + \text{Pepsin}]{\text{H}^+ \text{ or}} \text{Pepsin} + \text{Peptides}$$

The conversion of pepsinogen to pepsin involves the hydrolysis of several, probably five, peptides from the zymogen form, including an "inhibitor" peptide, which is responsible for the inactivity of pepsinogen.

Both pepsinogen and pepsin have been isolated in crystalline form and are proteins. Homogeneous crystalline porcine pepsinogen contains about 363 amino acid residues, whereas crystalline pepsin derived from it contains 321 residues. Thus in the activation process, some 42 amino acid residues are split off, including nine lysine, two histidine, and two arginine. The partial amino acid sequences of both porcine pepsinogen and pepsin are now known.[1] The final 27 amino acids of pepsin are characterized by the absence of positive charges, which probably contributes to the acid stability and alkali lability of the enzyme.

The optimum pH for pepsin activity varies from 1.5 to 2.2, depending on the substrate.

A small amount of pepsinogen apparently is secreted into gastric tissue fluid and is carried via the blood plasma to the kidney, where it is excreted as *uropepsin*.[2] This may be determined clinically and may be of some value in studies of gastric function.

There is some evidence that two forms of pepsin may exist, one secreted by the chief cells, the other by the pyloric cells.[3] The optimum pH values of these forms differ somewhat.

Another proteolytic enzyme, a weak proteinase active at a neutral pH, also has been described in gastric juice. It apparently contributes little to protein digestion in the stomach under ordinary circumstances.

Still another proteolytic enzyme, *rennin*, is secreted in the fourth stomach of the calf and probably other young ruminants. Its action is to clot milk. This is accomplished by the slight hydrolysis of the casein of milk to produce paracasein, which coagulates in the presence of calcium ions, resulting in an insoluble calcium paracaseinate curd:

$$\text{Casein} \xrightarrow{\text{Rennin}} \text{Paracasein} \xrightarrow{\text{Ca}^{++}} \begin{array}{c} \text{Ca-paracaseinate} \\ \text{(insoluble curd)} \end{array}$$

Certain desserts are made with commercially prepared rennin.

Apparently pepsin, or perhaps pepsin plus some other proteolytic enzyme, has a similar action in older animals since evidently no rennin is present in the gastric juice of the adult, at least in man.

The secretion of gastric juice is stimulated by the hormone *gastrin* (p. 457) from the pyloric mucosa. Apparently products of protein digestion, peptides, and other factors, in turn, cause an increase in gastrin formation.

The gastric digestion of proteins is thus incomplete, producing mainly larger peptides from only a limited number of proteins. The major digestion of proteins is accomplished, therefore, in the small intestine, where several powerful proteolytic enzymes are secreted.

Pancreatic juice contains a number of important proteinases, including *trypsin, chymotrypsin, elastase,* and two *carboxypeptidases.* Trypsin and chymotrypsin are secreted in zymogen forms, trypsinogen and chymotrypsinogen, respectively, and there are two chymotrypsinogens, A and B. Chymotrypsinogen-A has been crystallized and more intensively studied than chymotrypsinogen-B. Trypsinogen is changed to trypsin by *enterokinase* secreted by the intestinal mucosa. This agent, sometimes termed an "activator" of the enzyme, has been definitely shown by Kunitz to be an enzyme. Trypsinogen can also be converted to trypsin autocatalytically; i.e., as soon as some trypsin is formed, it acts on trypsinogen. The amino acid sequences of both trypsinogen and trypsin are now completely known.[4] Trypsinogen consists of a single, folded polypeptide chain of 229 amino acids. Trypsin has a similar conformation apparently, but with 223 amino acids, six less, in the chain. The conversion of trypsinogen to trypsin involves the splitting off of a hexapeptide (with the sequence Val-[Asp]$_4$-Lys). This is an example of the activation of a proenzyme by the removal of a "masking" peptide. Apparently, the active site of trypsin involves the histidine region of the molecule and the serine region. The conformation of these regions has been partially determined.[5] Similarly, chymotrypsinogens A and B are transformed into the active chymotrypsin by trypsin by the splitting off of smaller peptides, e.g., serylarginine, threonylasparagine (p. 113). These peptides, as well as the peptide bond at position 15-16, may be split in different sequences by trypsin or chymotrypsin, producing several intermediary forms, termed *neochymotrypsinogens* and π-, δ-, and α-chymotrypsins. Several of these forms have proteolytic activity, but apparently α-chymotrypsin is the final, more stable, active form of the enzyme. The parent chymotrypsinogen molecule is made up of 245 amino acids forming a single folded chain. Its amino acid sequence, as well as those of its derivatives, is now known.[5] The activation of chymotrypsinogen by trypsin involves the cleavage of the chain between the fifteenth and sixteenth amino acid residues (Asn-Cys). No peptide fragment is released by the cleavage because the residue is tied to the remainder of the molecule by a disulfide bond. However, hydrolysis of the molecule can go somewhat further because the chymotrypsin thus formed, π-chymotrypsin, is active and can act as a proteolytic enzyme on itself and cleave three additional peptide bonds. The two peptides just mentioned (Ser-Arg and Thr-Asn) are split off in this manner.

Remarkable is the fact that the active site of chymotrypsin is almost identical with that of trypsin[5] (p. 110). Also striking is the fact that there are many similarities in the amino acid sequences of chymotrypsin and trypsin. Indeed, about 40% of the positions in the two chains are occupied by the same amino acids. This is reminiscent of the similarities between the various chains of hemoglobin and is suggestive, likewise, of some functional and perhaps evolutionary relationship. The three-dimensional structures of chymotrypsin and trypsin have been reasonably well established.

The activation of the zymogen forms of both trypsin and chymotrypsin may involve a change in the conformation of the molecule to expose the *catalytic* site. A separate but adjacent "binding" site for the substrate is apparently exposed in the zymogen form, since the latter binds the active enzyme's substrate. Neurath[5] suggested that this relationship is analogous to a folding chair. The *back* of the chair is the exposed specific binding site, and the *seat* is the catalytic site. Only after the chair (zymogen) is unfolded does it become functional.

The optimum pH for both trypsin and chymotrypsin is in the neighborhood of 8 to 9. Each attacks proteins, splitting off peptide chains of varying length, and amino acids. Trypsin, however, is most effective on partially digested proteins. In fact, it digests collagen, ovalbumin, serum globulins, and hemoglobin very slowly, unless they have been denatured. However, trypsin attacks certain proteins (protamines, histones) that cannot be digested by pepsin. Each of the proteinases is quite specific with regard to the configuration of the peptide bonds it "unlocks." The peptide linkage specially attacked by trypsin is one containing the carboxyl group of either lysine or arginine (p. 114); i.e., there is a positive charge in the side group immediately adjacent to the point of attack. The net result of trypsin activity is to break down the products of peptic digestion still further and to digest those proteins that pepsin cannot attack. The products are amino acids and various polypeptides.

Several proteinlike substances that block the action of trypsin and related enzymes have been described. They are called *trypsin inhibitors*. One of these is present in the plasma and also has antithrombin activity (p. 628). It apparently is an α_1-globulin and is a glycoprotein. Another is present in pancreatic juice and is secreted in zymogen granules along with trypsinogen. It appears to be a peptide containing some 56 amino acid residues and has a molecular weight of about 6155. It is strongly acidic and has a relatively high content of glutamic and aspartic acids. It reacts rapidly with trypsin in a stoichiometric manner. Its function apparently is to protect pancreatic tissue from the proteolytic action of trypsin, which might be activated from trypsinogen. Pancreatic tissue (bovine) contains a similar basic polypeptide with analogous protective properties.

The occurrence of a hereditary deficiency of trypsinogen in an 8-week-old infant was reported recently.[6] The symptoms included severe growth failure, marked hypoproteinemia, edema, and diarrhea. Specific pancreatic proteolytic enzyme assays disclosed a complete absence of trypsinogen, with a secondary failure in the activation of chymotrypsinogen and procarboxypeptidase. These and other pancreatic enzymes appeared to be present in normal amounts. The disorder responded favorably to dietary management with the parenteral, then oral, administration of protein hydrolysates. Two brothers of the infant had previously died, one at birth, the other at about 1 month of age, with symptoms identical to those just described.

Chymotrypsin catalyzes the hydrolysis of the various protein breakdown products resulting from peptic and tryptic action. Again definite linkages are involved. Chymotrypsin preferentially splits peptide bonds involving the carboxyl group of the aromatic amino acids (Tyr, Phe, and Trp), but it also splits peptide linkages of leucine, methionine, asparagine, and histidine. The products are amino acids and simpler polypeptides.

There is an enzyme in pancreatic juice that specifically attacks collagen. It is capable of digesting collagenous fibers present in food. It would also account in part for the tissue necrosis associated with pancreatitis and for the digestion of other tissue that comes in contact with pancreatic juice from a pancreatic fistula.

Other proteolytic enzymes are present in pancreatic juice. Elastase attacks not only elastin but, in addition, a wide variety of proteins. It is secreted by the pancreas as the zymogen, which is converted to the active enzyme by trypsin and enterokinase. While elastase is capable of hydrolyzing many proteins, it has an unusual ability to digest elastin. The amino acid sequence of elastase has been partially determined, including that at the active site. Considerable homology exists between the amino acid sequences of elastase, trypsin, and chymotrypsin-B, suggestive of a common genetic origin of these proteases.

An elastomucoproteinase and a collagen mucoproteinase hydrolyze the proteins indicated by their names.

At least two peptidases are present in pancreatic juice, carboxypeptidases A and B. They attack an end-peptide linkage—that end having a free carboxyl group. Thus free amino acids are split off from dipeptides and higher peptides. These enzymes were formerly referred to as erepsin. Their optimum pH is about 7.4.

Carboxypeptidases A and B are apparently secreted in a zymogen form, *procarboxypeptidases* A and B, and are activated by trypsin. The activation of procarboxypeptidase-A, which exists as an aggregate of three large subunits, involves the conversion of one of these subunits by trypsin into carboxypeptidase-A. A second unit is apparently converted to a chymotrypsin-like substance. The role of the third unit is unknown. Carboxypeptidase-A contains in its active center a firmly bound atom of a metal, usually zinc, that is essential for its activity. Carboxypeptidase is composed of a single-chain polypeptide of some 300 amino acids. Its complete amino acid sequence and its conformation are still unknown. Carboxypeptidase-A acts preferentially on peptide bonds adjacent to C-terminal aromatic amino acids (Tyr, Phe, and Trp). It also splits the carboxyl terminal peptide bonds of a number of aliphatic side group–containing amino acids. Carboxypeptidase-B, however, apparently prefers peptide bonds adjacent to C-terminal amino acids whose side groups end in an amino group (Lys or Arg).

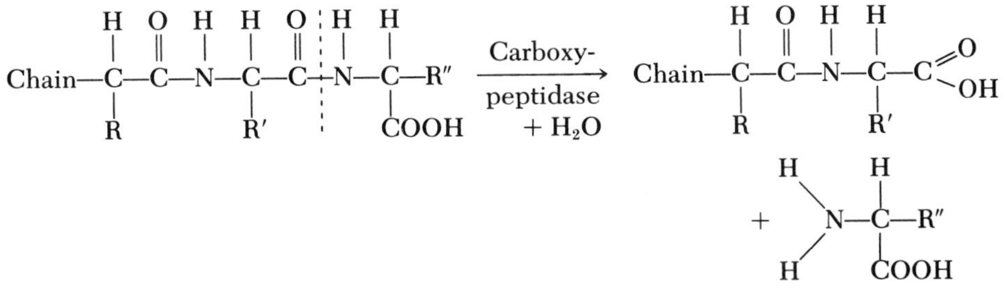

The secretion of pancreatic enzymes is controlled by the hormone *pancreozymin* (p. 457). It is found in the upper intestinal mucosa and is released into the bloodstream by the presence of a variety of substances, including proteins, peptides, and carbohydrates in the duodenum. The hormone *secretin* (p. 457), also found in the mucosa of the upper small intestine, likewise stimulates the secretion of pancreatic juice. However, the secretin-stimulated pancreatic juice is rich in bicarbonates rather than enzymes.

The digestion of proteins and the products of hydrolysis by pepsin, trypsin, chymotrypsin, and the carboxypeptidases is completed by the proteases secreted by the mucosa of the small intestine. These enzymes were formerly believed to be contained in an intestinal juice or *succus entericus*, analogous to gastric and pancreatic juices. However, they now appear to be primarily intracellular enzymes present in mucosal cells; some of these cells become detached and are released into the lumen of the small intestine.[7] Desquamation and replacement of intestinal mucosal cells are apparently a continuous and rather rapid process, the half-life of the cells being a period of only a few days. The enzyme content of the intestinal mucosal cells is increased by the hormone *enterocrinin* (p. 458), elaborated by the intestinal mucosa. A variety of digestive products stimulate the release of this hormone.

A number of peptidases are present in the intestinal mucosa cells and/or in the secretions of these cells. Included are a group of *aminopeptidases* and a group of *dipeptidases*. The aminopeptidases split a wide variety of N-terminal peptide linkages as shown below. Leucine aminopeptidase is an example of this type of enzyme. Aminopeptidases require magnesium or manganese ions for their activity. The dipeptidases are more specific in their action. For example, glycylglycine dipeptidase splits glycylglycine but not glycylglycylglycine. This dipeptidase requires the presence of cobalt or manganese ions for activity.

343

$$
\underset{\substack{\text{R}'-\text{C}-\text{C}- \\ | \\ \text{NH}_2}}{\overset{\substack{\text{H} \quad \text{O} \\ | \quad \| }}{}} \; \Big| \; \underset{\substack{-\text{N}-\text{C}-\text{C}-\text{N}-\text{C}-\text{Chain} \\ \quad | \quad \quad \quad | \\ \quad \text{R}'' \quad \quad \text{R}}}{\overset{\substack{\text{H} \quad \text{H} \quad \text{O} \quad \text{H} \quad \text{H} \\ | \quad | \quad \| \quad | \quad |}}{}} \quad \xrightarrow[\substack{\text{peptidase} \\ + \text{H}_2\text{O}}]{\text{Amino-}} \quad \underset{\substack{\text{R}'-\text{C}-\text{C} \\ | \quad \quad \diagdown \\ \text{NH}_2 \quad \text{OH}}}{\overset{\substack{\text{H} \quad \quad \text{O} \\ | \quad \quad \diagup\!\!\|}}{}}
$$

$$
+ \quad \underset{\substack{\diagup \quad \quad | \quad \quad \quad | \\ \text{H} \quad \text{R}'' \quad \quad \text{R}}}{\overset{\substack{\text{H} \quad \quad \text{H} \quad \text{O} \quad \text{H} \quad \text{H} \\ \diagdown \quad | \quad \| \quad | \quad | }}{\text{N}-\text{C}-\text{C}-\text{N}-\text{C}-\text{Chain}}}
$$

The hydrolysis of most proteins is thus completed to the constituent amino acids, which are then ready for absorption into the blood plasma. A few proteins, e.g., silk and several other albuminoids, are resistant to digestion. However, the digestion of the majority of proteins is about 95% complete in the normal human subject.

Some individuals apparently lack an enzyme necessary for the hydrolysis of N-glutamyl peptides in the small intestine. As a result, such persons are intolerant of proteins yielding these peptides on digestion. The chief offending proteins are the glutens from wheat, oats, barley, and rye. The undigested N-glutamyl peptides derived from the glutens exert a toxic effect on the mucosa of the small intestine, producing diarrhea, weight loss, malaise, and weakness. Anemia, edema, and bleeding tendencies may occur. These symptoms are apparently secondary to impaired intestinal absorption of all nutrients (especially fat, but also amino acids, glucose, vitamins, and calcium). This condition, termed *gluten-sensitive enteropathy,* is also called nontropical sprue or adult celiac disease.

ABSORPTION OF AMINO ACIDS

As described above, most food proteins are almost completely digested to amino acids in the gastrointestinal tract and are absorbed as such from the small intestine. There is mounting evidence that the absorption of amino acids involves an active transport mechanism (p. 14) and that specific transport proteins in the intestinal mucosal cells are required. Studies on the absorption of various individual amino acids and their mixtures from isolated ileal loops in dogs and in two human subjects[8] have demonstrated relations indicative of active transport. L-Amino acids are absorbed much more rapidly than the unnatural D-isomers. There are differences in the rates of absorption of individual amino acids and differences in preferential absorption or inhibition of absorption of some amino acids from mixtures of L-isomers.[8] The pattern of amino acid absorption from the small intestine depends on both the qualitative and the quantitative composition of the mixture of amino acids present. Several amino acids appear to share the same transport protein, e.g., one transport protein for the basic amino acids arginine and lysine and a different one for the acidic amino acids glutamic and aspartic. Evidence for this fact is that added lysine inhibits the absorption of arginine, indicating competition for the binding site on the transport protein.[8,9] A leucine-binding transport protein has been prepared from *E. coli.* Recent studies employing an immunologic procedure have demonstrated that this transport protein is present *only* in the cell envelope of *E. coli*, not in the cytoplasm. Transport proteins are characteristically located in the cell membrane (p. 15).

The absorption of amino acids is inhibited by antibiotics that block protein synthesis, e.g., puromycin,[11] actinomycin-D.[12] These antibiotics apparently prevent the synthesis of the transport protein in the intestinal mucosal cell.

After active absorption by the intestinal mucosal cell, the amino acids are taken up primarily by the blood capillaries of the mucosa and are transported in the plasma and erythrocytes to the liver and other organs and tissues of the body for metabolic utilization. A significant amount of the absorbed amino acids also appears in lymph.

Under some conditions small amounts of intact proteins apparently are absorbed through the intestinal mucosa. This leads to the formation of antibodies against the "foreign" protein, and anaphylactic reactions or other immunologic phenomena may occur following the subsequent absorption of the same intact protein. Thus we have the basis for the common allergies to food proteins. In some instances the reaction to the foreign protein may be severe enough to cause violent sneezing, cutaneous rashes, headache, vomiting, and even anaphylactic shock and death. It is interesting that intact proteins may also cross the pulmonary alveolar membrane and induce anaphylactic reactions.

GENERAL PATHS OF AMINO ACIDS IN THE BODY

Amino acids derived from the digestion of food proteins, i.e., *exogenous* sources, are absorbed and transported primarily by the blood as free amino acids to the liver and other organs and tissues of the body for utilization. In addition, however, amino acids derived from the hydrolysis of worn-out tissue proteins, *endogenous* amino acids, are added to form the labile amino acid metabolic pool of the body. The endogenous source of amino acids is by no means insignificant, current estimates being that *two thirds* of the amino acid pool is derived from the turnover of tissue proteins. Thus apparently only about one third of the amino acids utilized by the body are derived from food proteins. Isotopic studies of the turnover rates of different tissue proteins support these estimates. The half-life (T/2) of liver proteins, for example, is approximately 10 days. Plasma proteins also have a T/2 of about 10 days; muscle proteins, 180 days; and collagen, considerably longer. Some proteins, on the contrary, have much shorter T/2 values. The proteins of the intestinal mucosal cells turn over very rapidly, in a few days, and the T/2 of protein hormones and enzymes is also very short. The T/2 of insulin has been estimated as 6.5 to 9.0 minutes (p. 463). The average T/2 of the total body proteins of man is approximately 80 days. The overall significance of these facts is that, from a quantitative standpoint, the utilization of amino acids for the formation and replacement of tissue proteins is the *major* function of amino acids in the body.

The number of different tissue proteins in man is large but difficult to estimate. There are several hundred, perhaps more than 600, different enzymes alone. The total number of tissue proteins in man thus may well be several thousand. If this number is multiplied by the number of species of animals

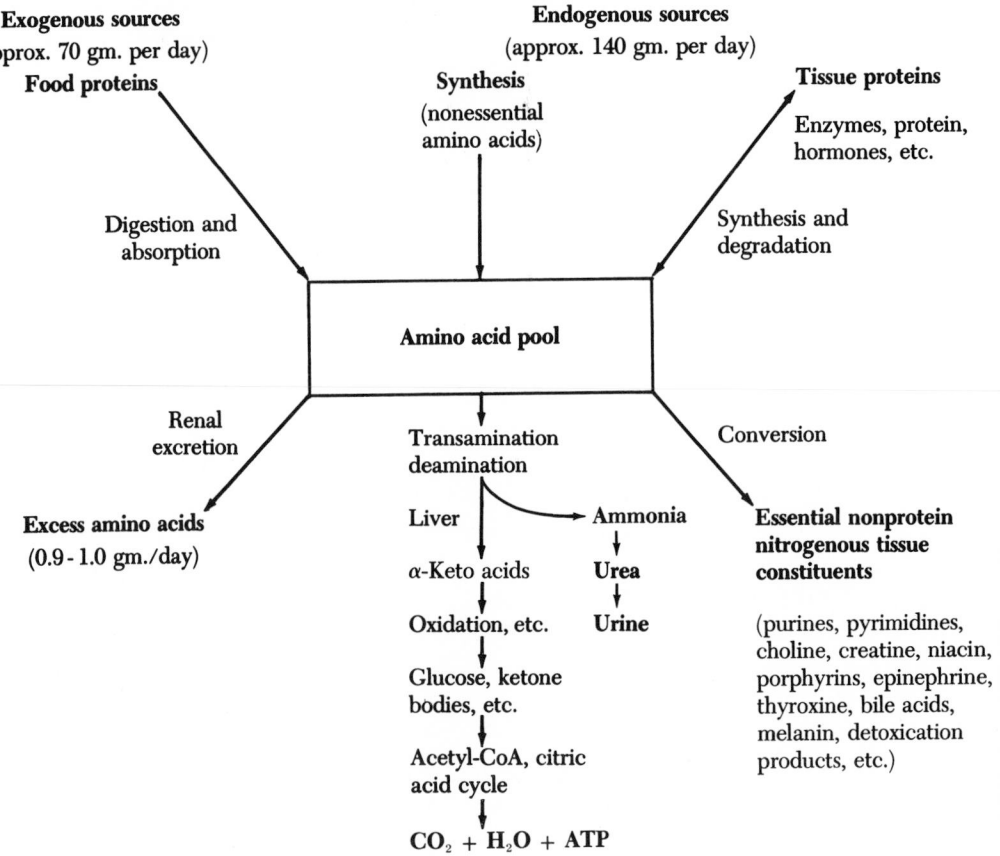

Fig. 13-1. Schematic representation of the general paths of amino acids in metabolism (average man).

and the number of other forms of life, including plant and microorganisms, the ascertainable total of proteins in living matter becomes enormous indeed. However, such variety is made possible because of the large size and multi-amino acid composition of proteins.

In addition to their primary role in the synthesis of tissue proteins, amino acids may be converted to other essential metabolites, as listed previously (p. 338), or may be oxidized to yield energy after the removal of the amino group (transamination, p. 350), deamination (p. 357). Small amounts of excess amino acids, some 0.9 to 1.0 gm. per day in the adult male, are excreted in the urine.

General paths for the metabolism of amino acids are shown schematically in Fig. 13-1.

NITROGEN BALANCE

One of the most interesting features of the metabolism of amino acids is the wide difference in the fate of amino acids during growth, on the one hand, and during adulthood, on the other. In a normal adult, under usual conditions, an amount of amino acids equal to the total taken in by the body undergoes degradation and the nitrogen is excreted each day. This means that the amount of nitrogen lost in a 24-hour period is approximately the same as that consumed, since the nitrogen ingested is chiefly protein nitrogen. In a growing child, in contrast, only part of the amino acids suffer degradation; the remainder enter into the net synthesis of protein that is characteristic of growth. The nitrogen that is lost from the body is nitrogen of the urine, feces, perspiration, and such functions as the desquamation of epidermis, the growth of hair and nails, and the secretion of nasal mucus, tears, etc. In striking a nitrogen balance, ordinarily only the outgo in the urine and feces is determined and is compared with the intake of food nitrogen. Usually the urinary nitrogen is estimated daily, whereas that of the feces, because of technical difficulties, is often collected over a 3- or 5-day period and the daily average computed.

In the normal average adult male, approximately 70 gm. of dietary protein per day (the "recommended dietary allowance" of the Food and Nutrition Board, National Research Council, 1968, p. 841) is adequate for the maintenance of nitrogen balance. A sufficient amount of *each* of the essential amino acids (p. 349) is also required for nitrogen balance. If any one of the eight amino acids essential for the adult (10 for the growing child, p. 349) is lacking, nitrogen balance becomes proportionally negative. Addition of the missing essential amino acid promptly restores nitrogen balance. Indeed, the balance may become positive for a period of time until the protein deficiency is made up. A sufficient quantity of the nonessential amino acids is likewise required for the maintenance of nitrogen balance. However, the amount of each individual nonessential amino acid is not critical since these acids are readily synthesized or interconverted in the body. For example, if the proteins ingested by the subject contain an inadequate amount of alanine but more than sufficient glutamic acid, the latter can be converted to alanine by transamination as follows:

$$\text{Glutamic acid + Pyruvate} \xrightarrow{\text{Transaminase}} \text{Alanine + Ketoglutarate}$$

A person is said to be in nitrogen equilibrium when the intake and output of nitrogen are equal to each other. A positive balance is that condition in which nitrogen is retained, and a negative balance is one in which more nitrogen is lost than is ingested. Positive balances occur during growth of children and convalescence of patients and during pregnancy. In all these cases protein is being reconstructed and therefore the amino acid nitrogen is retained. For growth to occur in young animals, growth hormone and insulin are required (p. 488). These hormones also exert an influence in other types of positive nitrogen balance. Other hormones concerned in the regulation of protein metabolism are the thyroid hormone, testosterone, adrenocortical hormones of the cortisone type, and ACTH. Negative balances are seen in starvation, malnutrition, fevers, after extensive burns or trauma, and postoperatively. Postoperative loss of nitrogen is a very common occurrence and is far greater than is usually appreciated. The severity depends on the extent of tissue damage and the degree of mobilization of amino acids for tissue repair. Under these conditions the body draws upon its tissue and plasma proteins, and hypoproteinemia may develop.

347

If an individual is in nitrogen equilibrium on a diet that is fairly constant in the amount of its protein and the level of protein intake is changed, he will, after a day or a few days, again become established in equilibrium at the new level. An interval of adjustment or "lag" is almost always seen (Table 13-1).

The organism does not store protein in the same way or to the same extent that it stores carbohydrate and fat. Nevertheless, during periods of high protein intake, considerable amounts of protein are stored in the liver and smaller quantities in the other tissues, probably built up into new tissue; i.e., when the liver hypertrophies after high protein feeding, the increase is due to an addition of functioning liver tissue rather than a deposition of inert storage material in the liver cells. As stated previously, if animals are kept on different levels of dietary protein, the various organs increase in weight and absorb protein at different rates, each organ responding optimally to a certain amount of protein in the diet. This indicates that the amount of new protoplasm in a tissue depends on the type of tissue and on the supply of amino acids. The amount probably also depends on the kinds of protein eaten, i.e., the assortment of amino acids available. Moreover, new protoplasm can increase and decrease only within certain limits. Organs that acquire protein rapidly, e.g., liver, intestine, kidney, are the first to lose the protein when fasting occurs. In other words, "labile" nitrogen is not distinguished primarily by a differ-

Table 13-1. Example of adjustment to changes in protein intake*

Day	Nitrogen in food (grams)	Nitrogen in feces (grams)	Nitrogen absorbed (grams)	Nitrogen in urine (grams)	Nitrogen balance (grams)
			Experiment 1		
Before	> 16.96				
1	16.96	0.94	16.02	18.2	−2.18
2	16.96	0.94	16.02	17.0	−0.98
3	16.96	0.94	16.02	15.8	+0.22
4	16.96	0.94	16.02	16.0	+0.02
5	16.96	0.94	16.02	15.7	+0.32
			Experiment 2		
1	14.40	0.70	13.70	13.60	+0.10
2	14.40	0.70	13.70	13.80	−0.10
3	14.40	0.70	13.70	13.60	+0.10
4	20.96	0.82	20.14	16.80	+3.34
5	20.96	0.82	20.14	18.20	+1.94
6	20.96	0.82	20.14	19.50	+0.64
7	20.96	0.82	20.14	20.00	+0.14

The subject was a young woman weighing 58 kg., at rest in bed. The first experiment is an example of adjustment to a lowered protein intake because it was known that the subject had previously been on a high-protein diet. Equilibrium occurred after the second day. The second experiment shows the effect of increasing the protein intake. In this case 3 days elapsed before the subject was in nitrogen equilibrium.

° After von Noorden, from Sherman, H. C.: Chemistry of food and nutrition, ed. 8, New York, 1952, The Macmillan Co.

ence in composition but by its location. Furthermore, it appears that nuclei of cells are spared longer than other parts of the cell.

ESSENTIAL AMINO ACIDS

In Chapter 5, a distinction between essential and nonessential amino acids was made. It is now advisable to clarify some phases of this subject and perhaps modify some rather arbitrary statements. Among the latter was the statement that the essential amino acids could not be synthesized by the body. However, it has been found (p. 353) that young animals can grow on a methionine-free diet if homocystine and either choline or betaine are present. The reason for this is plain, but it indicates that special conditions may arise whereby the body might be able to synthesize an essential amino acid if all the special "ingredients" were at hand and conditions were favorable.

Block, in 1956, suggested a classification of the amino acids into dispensable, semi-indispensable, and indispensable (Table 13-2). Arginine and histidine are called semi-indispensable because they are synthesized by man but not at an optimal rate. Glycine is not essential for the rat or the human being under usual conditions but is necessary for optimal growth of fowls. Another group of amino acids is semi-indispensable from another standpoint. These are nonessential only if a closely related amino acid is provided in the diet in quantities sufficient to cover the needs of both. Cystine, for example, has no effect on growth if methionine, from which it can be synthesized, is abundantly supplied; but cystine will stimulate growth if methionine is not present in the diet in sufficient amounts. Tyrosine bears a similar relation to phenylalanine. Methionine is not necessary in the diet if homocystine and choline are supplied. For the present, methionine should be considered an essential amino acid for man.

Table 13-2. Nutritive classification of the amino acids*

Essential (indispensable)	Semiessential (semi-indispensable)	Nonessential (dispensable)
Lysine	Arginine†	Glutamic acid
Tryptophan‡	Tyrosine‡	Aspartic acid
Phenylalanine	Cystine‡	Alanine
Methionine	Glycine†	Proline
Threonine	Serine†	Hydroxyproline
Leucine	Histidine	
Isoleucine		
Valine		

* Adapted from Block, R. J.: Borden Rev. Nutr. Res. **17**:75, 1956.
† Arginine and glycine are essential for chicks and turkeys. Serine spares or replaces glycine.
‡ Tyrosine spares but does not completely replace phenylalanine. Cystine spares but does not completely replace methionine. Nicotinic acid spares but does not completely replace tryptophan.

It should be noted that a mixture of amino acids deficient in one or more of the essential acids is of little nutritive value as regards its ability to build or replace body proteins. Such a mixture is deaminated to a considerable extent and used for the production of energy but does not contribute to a positive nitrogen balance. Even a subsequent administration of the missing essential amino acids is of no avail, because amino acids are not stored in the tissues for any considerable length of time. Only that portion of the essential amino acids present in the proper amount can be used to build body protein. In other words, no protein can be fabricated by the organism unless every amino acid of which it is composed is available at the site of synthesis. Furthermore, the quantity of protein that can be produced is limited by the essential amino acid available in relatively the smallest amount. This applies to either the oral or the parenteral administration of amino acids or protein hydrolysates and also to the feeding of incomplete proteins (like gelatin), when unaccompanied by other proteins to supplement them.

The nonessential amino acids must not be considered valueless. As mentioned earlier (Chapter 5), they may be considered so important that the body has "learned" to synthesize them. It would be better to designate them as "synthesizable." For the synthesis of the nonnitrogenous portion, both the carboxyl and the methyl carbons of acetate and, to a less extent, the carbon of bicarbonate are used. This was determined by using ^{14}C-labeled salts. The amino group is probably obtained from deamination reactions in the liver. These amino acids contribute to the makeup of body protein, as do the essential ones, but they are more interchangeable, more versatile, and more easily procurable. Glycine, one of the semiessentials, is used to make creatine and to detoxicate benzoic acid. Citrulline forms a part of the arginine-urea cycle; and other examples of specific usefulness could be memtioned. However, if any of these semiessential amino acids are lacking, the body can synthesize them from others. Indeed, it has been claimed[13] that "unessential" nitrogen is really an essential dietary factor under certain conditions. If a deficient diet is provided (decreased milk), the addition of glycine, or even urea, restores the ability to grow.

Biochemical transformations of amino acids In the laboratory, amino acids are relatively stable, but in the body they are highly reactive. They are synthesized into the form of proteins with extreme rapidity. Certain ones take part in the formation of urea in the ornithine-citrulline cycle, which will be discussed shortly (p. 359). Some are easily changed to hormones, e.g., epinephrine, insulin, thyroxine. The phenomena of transamination, transmethylation, and transpeptidation, which will be described, indicate how some of the amino acids take part in physiologic transformations.

Transamination. As the word indicates, transamination is the transfer of amino groups from one compound to another. L-Glutamic acid, under the influence of a transaminase, loses its amino group to a keto acid, the latter thereby becoming an amino acid; and the glutamic acid becomes a keto acid, namely, α-ketoglutaric. L-Aspartic acid may replace glutamic acid, but the reaction is slower. The phenomenon was first discovered in 1937. One such reaction is as shown on p. 351.

$$
\begin{array}{cccc}
\text{COOH} & & \text{COOH} & \\
| & & | & \\
\text{CH}_2 & \text{CH}_3 & \text{CH}_2 & \text{CH}_3 \\
| & | & | & | \\
\text{CH}_2 \quad + \quad \text{C}{=}\text{O} & \rightleftarrows & \text{CH}_2 \quad + \quad \text{CHNH}_2 \\
| & | & | & | \\
\text{CHNH}_2 & \text{COOH} & \text{C}{=}\text{O} & \text{COOH} \\
| & & | & \\
\text{COOH} & & \text{COOH} & \\
\end{array}
$$

Glutamic acid   Pyruvic acid   α-Ketoglutaric acid   Alanine

The transaminases occur in practically all animal tissues but in higher concentrations in heart muscle, brain, kidney, liver, and testes.

Most of the natural amino acids are now known to participate in transamination, the possible exceptions being glycine, threonine, and lysine. In isotope experiments using ^{15}N-labeled glycine, the ^{15}N appeared in the amino groups of all amino acids except threonine and lysine. Likewise, liver transaminases have been prepared which specifically transfer the amino group of glutamic acid to keto acid derivatives of each of the corresponding keto acids of the naturally occurring amino acids, with the exception of glycine, threonine, and lysine. A phosphate ester of pyridoxal or, as the case might be, pyridoxamine is the prosthetic group of transaminase acting as an amino group carrier (p. 352). The tissues of vitamin B$_6$–deficient animals exhibit a lowered level of transaminase activity. In the reaction shown, pyruvic acid, a product of carbohydrate metabolism, is transformed to an amino acid, thus showing how the body is able to synthesize some of its amino acids. In this case it is one of the simplest amino acids. The reverse reaction indicates how the more complex glutamic acid might be produced from alanine and another intermediate in carbohydrate metabolism, α-ketoglutaric acid. From another standpoint, transamination may be important. The nonnitrogenous compounds formed in these two-way reactions — pyruvic acid, α-ketoglutaric acid, oxaloacetic acid — are concerned in oxidation-reduction systems, some of which have been discussed. It thus appears that transamination may be a "shuttle" mechanism in which protein and carbohydrate metabolites are interconverted as needed. One of the most rapid transamination reactions is as follows:

Glutamic acid + Oxaloacetic acid $\rightleftarrows$ α-Ketoglutaric acid + Aspartic acid

The reaction toward the right is twice as fast as the one in the opposite direction.

The mechanism of transamination involves the formation of intermediate complexes, by the condensation of the amino acid with the coenzyme pyridoxine. The scheme[14] in Fig. 13-2 indicates how this may occur. In the upper reaction, note the coenzyme, in the form of pyridoxal phosphate, exchanging its O for the NH_2 of the R_1–amino acid, forming the R_1–keto acid and pyridoxamine. In the second line the R_2–keto acid exchanges its O for the NH_2 of pyridoxamine phosphate to finally yield the R_2–amino acid and pyridoxal. Note that in the first step in the first line, H_2O is lost; in the next step an intramolecular shift of H occurs; and in the third step H_2O is regained. These steps are reversed in the second set of reactions. The protein enzyme is, of course, associated with both substrate and coenzyme.

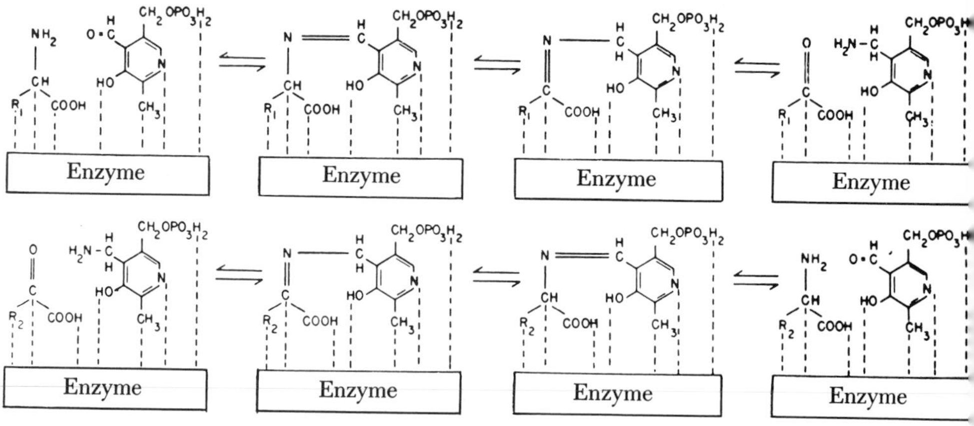

Fig. 13-2. Diagrammatic representation of transamination involving the amino acid R_1—CH with NH$_2$ and COOH, the keto acid R_2—C with O and COOH, pyridoxal phosphate, and pyridoxamine phosphate. (From Meister, A.: Advances Enzym. **16**:185, 1955.)

Thus in one cycle, one molecule of amino acid–R_1 forms one molecule of keto acid–R_1 and one molecule of keto acid–R_2 forms one molecule of amino acid–R_2. In this way transamination is complete and a different amino acid–R_2 is formed.

There is considerable evidence that the pyridoxal phosphate coenzyme is linked to a lysine ε-amino group as a Schiff base in the pyridoxal form of transaminase.

Transaminations are of great importance in the metabolism of many different amino acids and account for numerous transformations, as will be brought out from time to time. Transamination explains why the α-keto acids of analogous essential amino acids are, in certain instances, capable of substituting for these amino acids in the nutrition of rats and, perhaps, also of human beings. Since the transaminases are present in heart and liver tissues in relatively high concentrations, damage to these organs leads to transaminase leakage into the blood serum. As a result, determination of the concentration of different transaminases in blood serum is used to gain definite knowledge that transaminases are present and to assess the degree of cardiac and hepatic damage. This will be discussed in later sections.

Transmethylation. The methyl group of methionine, $CH_3SCH_2CH_2CH$-$(NH_2)COOH$, may likewise be transferred from that compound to a suitable receptor. This phenomenon, transmethylation, was discovered and has been studied by du Vigneaud.[15] One of the results of transmethylation is the formation of choline and creatine, both methylated compounds and both of utmost biologic significance.

The occurrence of methylated compounds has long been known, as has the recognition of their special importance in biochemistry. In fact, in 1894, Hofmeister proposed a hypothesis that has now been largely substantiated. He suggested that the body is unable to manufacture methyl groups and consequently must obtain them in the diet. As will be seen, this is not quite true, since methyl groups can be synthesized by the organism if conditions are favorable. Once absorbed, the methyl group may be transferred from one compound to another as a unit but only to and from certain compounds and not indiscriminately. This does not depend upon the methyl group, which has but one form, but upon the entire molecule. Certain compounds are methyl donors, the chief of which are choline, methionine, and betaine. The *labile* methyl is attached to either a nitrogen or a sulfur atom in the molecule. The fact that a methyl group is removable from a compound does not necessarily mean that it is "labile," i.e., transferable to another compound. Sarcosine, $CH_2NH(CH_3)COOH$, may lose its methyl group in the body, but the methyl group does not seem to be available for transmethylation reactions except to a very slight extent.

The starting point is the fact that, although methionine is an indispensable amino acid, young animals can grow on a methionine-free diet containing homocysteine, provided choline or betaine is also present. Choline and betaine both contain methyl groups, and the explanation is that the methyl groups are labile and are easily transferable to homocysteine, to change this amino acid to methionine. Since homocysteine alone would not permit growth, it was inferred that the animal organism is incapable of generating methyl groups for this methylation. By providing the suitable constituents, the body is able to synthesize the essential amino acid (methionine). This was later substantiated by isotope experiments. If choline, containing deuterium in the methyl group, was fed to animals along with homocysteine, the methionine isolated from the proteins of the animal's tissues was found to contain deuterium.

The reverse process also occurs. This was proved by feeding methionine containing deuterium in the methyl group to animals. On a diet free of choline and ordinary methionine, the administration of *deuteriomethionine* led to the discovery of choline containing deuterium in the tissues. The methyl group had been used to form new choline. Furthermore, some had also been used to form creatine. The demethylation of methionine is therefore a reversible reaction. A similar experiment has been performed on man, thus showing that transmethylation reactions also take place in the human organism.

Since the methyl group of methionine can be used to form creatine, the possibility was suggested that choline's methyl group might similarly be used. Isotope experiments proved that this could occur. *Deuteriocholine* given to animals on an otherwise choline-free, methionine-free diet was found to result in the presence in the urine of creatinine containing deuterium.

In transmethylations the substance yielding the methyl group is called the *methyl donor*, and the one receiving it the methyl acceptor. For the synthesis of choline, ethanolamine is considered the methyl acceptor. Feeding of this compound, labeled with ^{15}N, resulted in the formation of choline containing [15]N. In the synthesis of methionine, homocysteine is the methyl acceptor; and in creatine synthesis, glycocyamine (guanidoacetic acid) functions in the same way. Creatine does not become a source of methyl groups when it is present in the diet or when it is formed in the course of a transmethylation.

The labile methyl group can also be synthesized by the animal. This has been demonstrated by giving animals heavy water to drink and finding deuterium in some of the choline of their tissues. Since the animals were raised in the absence of bacteria, synthesis by microorganisms was ruled out. However, very young animals do not possess this capability, and the biologically labile methyl groups are placed in a position analogous to that which arginine holds among the essential amino acids. They can be synthesized but not at a rate rapid enough for the welfare of the young animal.

The labile methyl group may be produced by the body from a variety of compounds. Following the discovery by Sakami that ^{14}C-methyl–labeled acetone, after administration to rats, results in the ^{14}C being placed as a β-carbon of serine, the reverse reaction was attempted by Arnstein. He found that serine carrying a labeled β-carbon yields choline bearing labeled methyl groups. Other effective precursors are formaldehyde, formate, methanol, and the α-carbon of glycine. In other experiments it was discovered that acetone, sarcosine, histidine, and tryptophan, in their metabolic reactions, yield either methyl groups directly or one-carbon units that are easily converted to methyl groups. Methyl groups from these sources, or from choline or betaine, may be transferred to form methionine. It is likely that choline acts only indirectly as a methyl donor, in that it must first be oxidized to betaine. As betaine loses a methyl group, it becomes dimethylglycine, which, in turn, loses a methyl group to form sarcosine and formaldehyde. The latter reaction occurs with the aid of an oxidizing enzyme from liver. Then sarcosine may lose its N-methyl group through the action of another hepatic enzyme to yield glycine; the methyl group may be oxidized to formaldehyde and formate.

$$CH_3-\overset{\overset{\textstyle CH_3}{|}}{\underset{\underset{\textstyle CH_3}{|}}{N^+}}-CH_2-COO^- \rightarrow \boxed{CH_3} + (CH_3)_2\,N-CH_2-COOH$$

Betaine   **Dimethylglycine**

$$\boxed{CH_3} \rightarrow HCOOH \leftarrow HCHO$$

$$CH_3NH-CH_2COOH \rightarrow CH_3 + NH_2-CH_2COOH$$

Sarcosine   **Glycine**
(methylglycine)

The formaldehyde or formate resulting from the oxidation of the methyl groups of choline, as shown, is then added to the "one-carbon pool" for utilization as N^{10}-hydroxymethyltetrahydrofolic acid, as will be described later (p. 821). For such transfers not much energy is required and hence ATP is not involved. On the other hand, ATP participates in those transmethylations in which methionine is the donor. Here ATP first converts methionine into *active* methionine.

$$\text{Methionine} + \text{ATP} \xrightarrow[\text{Mg}^{++}]{\text{GSH}} \text{Active methionine} + \text{Orthophosphate} + \text{Pyrophosphate}$$

Active methionine is S-adenosylmethionine:

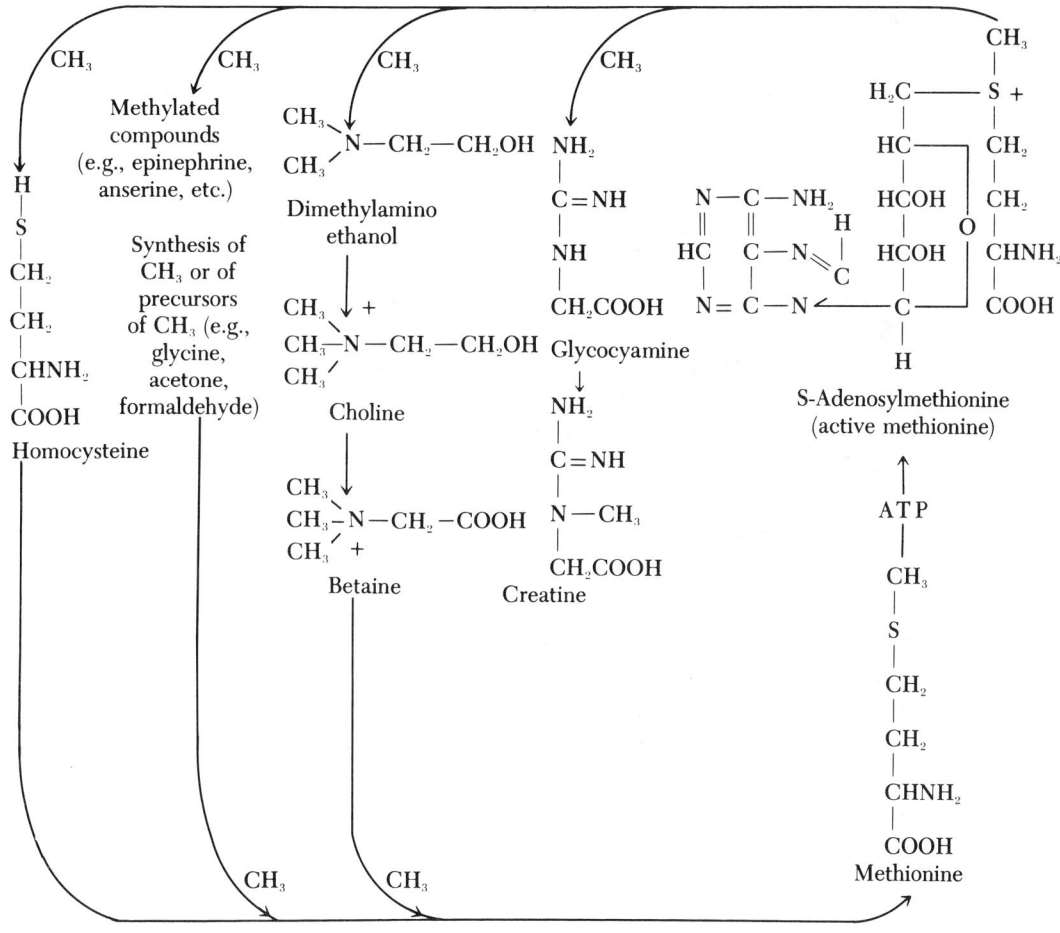

Once in this form, methionine can act as a methyl donor, even in the absence of ATP. Some of the transmethylation reactions discussed are shown schematically in Fig. 13-3.

Probably other methylated compounds derive their methyl groups from such reactions. These compounds include epinephrine and anserine as well as N'-methylnicotinamide, the form in which some of the nicotinamide is

Fig. 13-3. Transmethylation reactions.

excreted in the urine. Epinephrine not only is synthesized in part by methylation, but it and norepinephrine are inactivated by O-methylation to yield metanephrine and normetanephrine, respectively. These are then either conjugated with glucuronic acid or deaminated to 3-methoxy-4-hydroxymandelic acid. A specific enzyme, catechol-O-methyl transferase, catalyzes the reaction, S-adenosylmethionine serving as the methyl donor.

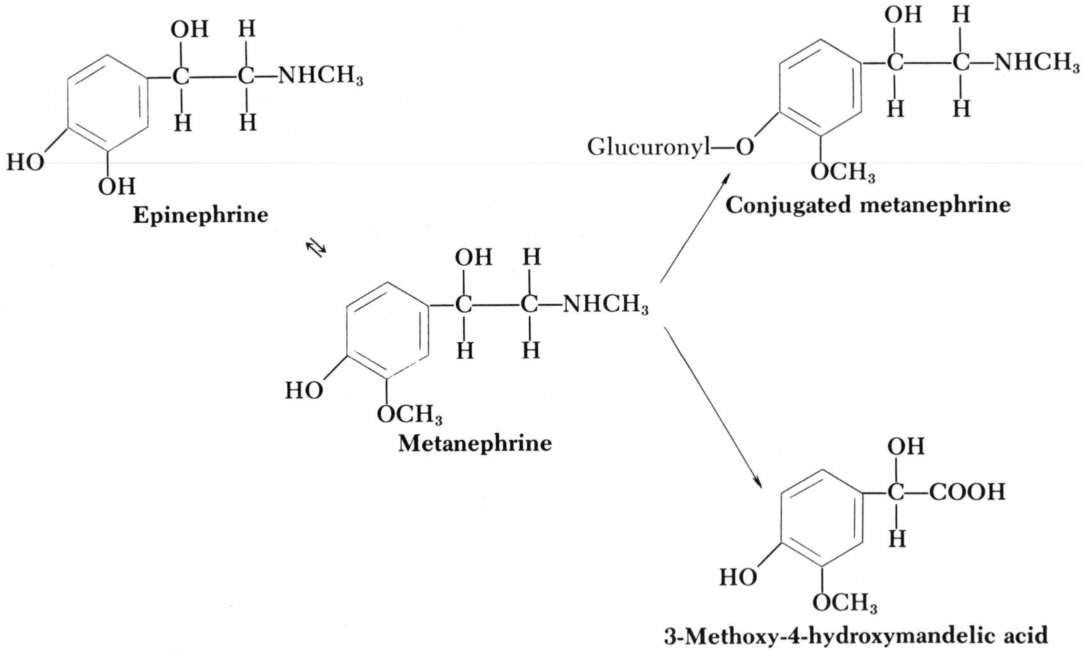

Epinephrine

Conjugated metanephrine

Metanephrine

3-Methoxy-4-hydroxymandelic acid

In addition to its role as promotor of growth in the presence of homocysteine and absence of methionine, the labile methyl group has other effects. It has a lipotropic action; i.e., it inhibits fatty liver formation under certain circumstances. It prevents perosis or slipped tendon disease in chicks and hemorrhagic degeneration of various organs. Thus labile methyl groups resemble choline in function (p. 352), and, of course, the reason is obvious — choline is an important source of labile methyl groups. The labile methyl group of methionine can be oxidized to carbon dioxide. Methionine containing ^{14}C in the methyl group was fed to a rat, with the result that some of the expired carbon dioxide contained ^{14}C. It is probable that excess labile methyl groups from methionine and other methyl donors are disposed of in this way.

Transpeptidation. Since the reaction peptide $\rightleftharpoons$ amino acids is reversible, theoretically the synthesis of peptides, and eventually proteins, is possible by means of the reverse reaction. However, the equilibrium lies far on the side of hydrolysis, i.e., toward the right. Synthesis is likely to occur therefore only if the peptide can be removed from the system rapidly enough, and, although this has been accomplished by using amino acids that yield insoluble peptides, it does not usually happen.

A different method of accomplishing syntheses of peptides, or of rearranging them, was discovered by Bergmann and Fraenkel-Conrat and others, namely, transpeptidation. This is the term applied to the transfer of amino acids or peptides to amines, to other amino acids, or to peptides. Transpeptidations require little energy because the energy of the broken peptide bond is utilized for the synthesis of the new peptide bond. An intermediate compound is assumed to be formed, and in the new peptide the carboxyl group of the transferred amino acid is attached to the initial amino group.

Among the enzymes that have been shown to take part in such transfers are cathepsin, trypsin, and chymotrypsin, and it is probable that all enzymes that catalyze hydrolytic reactions involving peptide bonds also catalyze transpeptidations.

Of particular importance is the γ-glutamyl radical, because of its incorporation in glutamine and glutathione. In mammalian kidney, liver, and brain there is a γ-glutamyl transpeptidase that transfers this group from glutathione to various amino acids. For example:

$$
\begin{array}{llll}
\text{COOH} & & \text{COOH} & \\
| & & | & \\
\text{CHNH}_2 & & \text{CHNH}_2 & \\
| & \text{C}_4\text{H}_9 & | & \\
\text{CH}_2 & \;+\; \text{HC—COOH} \;\rightarrow\; & \text{CH}_2 \quad \text{C}_4\text{H}_9 & +\text{ Cysteinylglycine} \\
| & | & | & \\
\text{CH}_2 & \text{NH}_2 & \text{CH}_2 \quad \text{HC—COOH} & \\
| & & | \qquad\qquad | & \\
\text{O=C—Cysteinylglycine} & & \text{O=C———NH} & \\
\textbf{Glutathione} & \textbf{L-Leucine} & \boldsymbol{\gamma}\textbf{-Glutamyl-L-leucine} &
\end{array}
$$

The reverse of this, namely, the synthesis of glutathione, has been accomplished in the presence of a suitable enzyme.

γ-Glutamylglycine + Cysteinylglycine $\rightarrow$ Glutamylcysteinylglycine + Glycine

If a new peptide bond is formed, a phosphate donor must be present. An example of this is the production of hippuric acid from benzoic acid and glycine (p. 751). ATP is required and is changed to ADP.

Deamination and deamidation It has been stated that after absorption from the alimentary tract, a large share of the amino acids are picked up by the liver and are soon freed of their amino groups. This undoubtedly holds true for the amino acids originating in the tissue proteins as well as for the excess derived from food proteins. The kidney and other organs share this function, but only to a minor degree. There are perhaps several types of reaction, but only the two major ones will be discussed here. The first type is a deamination. It may be brought about by the combined action of a transaminase and a dehydrogenase. The site of these reactions is also the liver and kidney.

With alanine as a typical L-amino acid, there is first a transamination with α-ketoglutaric acid, yielding an α-keto acid and glutamic acid.

$$
\begin{array}{llllll}
\text{COOH} & & \text{CH}_3 & \text{CH}_3 & & \text{COOH} \\
| & & | & | & & | \\
\text{CH}_2 & + & \text{HCNH}_2 & \rightleftarrows \quad \text{C=O} & + & \text{CH}_2 \\
| & & | & | & & | \\
\text{CH}_2 & & \text{COOH} & \text{COOH} & & \text{CH}_2 \\
| & & & & & | \\
\text{CO} & & & & & \text{CHNH}_2 \\
| & & & & & | \\
\text{COOH} & & & & & \text{COOH} \\
\boldsymbol{\alpha}\textbf{-Ketoglutaric acid} & & \textbf{Alanine} & \textbf{Pyruvic acid} & & \textbf{L-Glutamic acid}
\end{array}
$$

357

The glutamic acid is now oxidatively deaminated by a special dehydrogenase system that reversibly converts glutamic acid to α-ketoglutaric acid and ammonia.

$$
\begin{array}{ccc}
\text{COOH} & & \text{COOH} \\
| & & | \\
\text{CH}_2 & & \text{CH}_2 \\
| & & | \\
\text{CH}_2 & + \tfrac{1}{2}\,\text{O}_2 \rightleftarrows & \text{CH}_2 \quad + \text{NH}_3 \\
| & & | \\
\text{CHNH}_2 & & \text{CO} \\
| & & | \\
\text{COOH} & & \text{COOH}
\end{array}
$$

The glutamic dehydrogenase system represents a significant link between the metabolism of proteins and carbohydrates. It also provides a pathway for the conversion of α-amino groups to ammonia and other nitrogen-containing products.

The fact that a given amino acid can participate in transamination does not mean that transamination is obligatory for the metabolism. In fact, direct oxidative deamination by means of an L-amino acid oxidase is known to occur. This acts in the presence of atmospheric oxygen, with FAD serving as a cofactor. The reaction is as follows:

$$\text{R—CHNH}_2\text{—COOH} + \text{O}_2 + \text{H}_2\text{O} \rightarrow \text{R—CO—COOH} + \text{H}_2\text{O}_2 + \text{NH}_3$$

In the presence of catalase, hydrogen peroxide is decomposed to molecular oxygen and water, and the net reaction is therefore as follows:

$$\text{R—CHNH}_2\text{COOH} + \tfrac{1}{2}\,\text{O}_2 \rightarrow \text{R—CO—COOH} + \text{NH}_3$$

Thus, although the result is the same as in the case of glutamic acid, the enzymes and mechanism involved are different. The following L-amino acids have similarly been shown to be oxidized by these enzymes: leucine, phenylalanine, norleucine, isoleucine, valine, cystine, histidine, tyrosine, proline, methionine, alanine, and tryptophan.

Deamination of most amino acids may also result from dehydrogenation. Apparently glycine and the hydroxy amino acids are exceptions. This type of deamination is catalyzed by L-amino oxidases, perhaps more accurately termed dehydrogenases. The steps involved appear to be as follows:

$$
\underset{\text{Amino acid}}{\text{R—}\overset{\displaystyle \text{H}}{\underset{\displaystyle \underset{\displaystyle \text{H}_2}{\text{N}}}{\text{C}}}\text{—COOH}}
\xrightleftharpoons[\quad]{\text{FAD} \quad \text{FADH}_2}
\underset{\text{Imino acid}}{\text{R—}\overset{\displaystyle}{\underset{\displaystyle \underset{\displaystyle \text{H}}{\text{N}}}{\text{C}}}\text{—COOH}}
\xrightleftharpoons[\quad]{+\ \text{H}_2\text{O}}
\underset{\text{Keto acid}}{\text{R—}\overset{\displaystyle}{\underset{\displaystyle \text{O}}{\text{C}}}\text{—COOH} + \text{NH}_3}
$$

The L-amino oxidases are flavoproteins.

The second type of reaction is a simple hydrolysis of an amino acid amide, e.g., glutamine, asparagine, yielding the corresponding amino acid, glutamic or aspartic, respectively. This is a deamidation and the enzyme required is an amidase. These two amino acid amides are present in the proteins as such to a considerable extent.

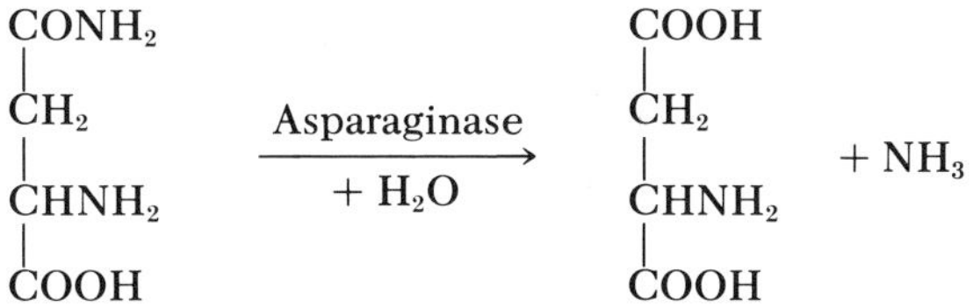

$$
\begin{array}{ccc}
\begin{array}{c}
\text{CONH}_2 \\
| \\
\text{CH}_2 \\
| \\
\text{CHNH}_2 \\
| \\
\text{COOH}
\end{array}
&
\xrightarrow[\text{+ H}_2\text{O}]{\text{Asparaginase}}
&
\begin{array}{c}
\text{COOH} \\
| \\
\text{CH}_2 \\
| \\
\text{CHNH}_2 \\
| \\
\text{COOH}
\end{array}
\quad + \text{NH}_3
\end{array}
$$

Asparagine   **Aspartic acid**

UREA FORMATION

The ammonia formed by deamination is converted to urea in the liver. This had been suspected for a long time, but Bollman, Mann, and Magath confirmed it in 1924 by showing that hepatectomized dogs are unable to form urea. After such an operation the amino acids and ammonia accumulated in the blood, but the urea of the blood and tissues decreased in concentration. If the kidneys were ligated in such animals, the blood urea remained at a constant level. It is therefore apparent that the liver, and only the liver, produces urea. Furthermore, we know that there is present in the liver an enzyme, arginase, that splits urea off from arginine, leaving ornithine, another amino acid, as a residue.

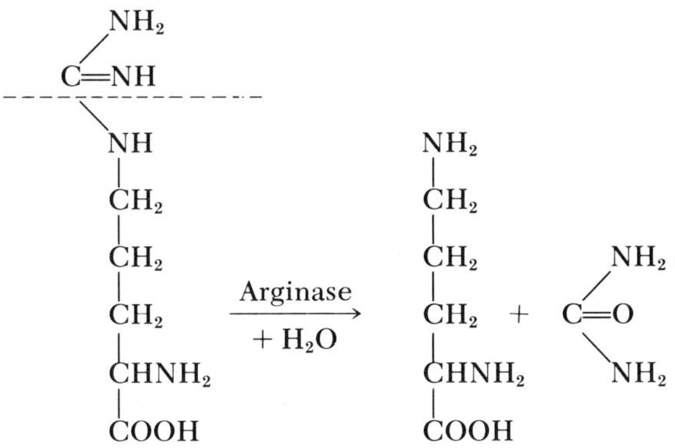

$$
\begin{array}{c}
\quad\quad\quad \text{NH}_2 \\
\quad\quad\quad / \\
\text{-----C=NH-----} \\
\quad\quad\quad \backslash \\
\quad\quad\quad \text{NH} \\
\quad\quad\quad | \\
\quad\quad\quad \text{CH}_2 \\
\quad\quad\quad | \\
\quad\quad\quad \text{CH}_2 \\
\quad\quad\quad | \\
\quad\quad\quad \text{CH}_2 \\
\quad\quad\quad | \\
\quad\quad\quad \text{CHNH}_2 \\
\quad\quad\quad | \\
\quad\quad\quad \text{COOH}
\end{array}
\quad
\xrightarrow[\text{+ H}_2\text{O}]{\text{Arginase}}
\quad
\begin{array}{c}
\text{NH}_2 \\
| \\
\text{CH}_2 \\
| \\
\text{CH}_2 \\
| \\
\text{CH}_2 \\
| \\
\text{CHNH}_2 \\
| \\
\text{COOH}
\end{array}
\quad + \quad
\begin{array}{c}
\quad\quad \text{NH}_2 \\
\quad\quad / \\
\text{C=O} \\
\quad\quad \backslash \\
\quad\quad \text{NH}_2
\end{array}
$$

Arginine   **Ornithine**   **Urea**

Krebs and Henseleit studied this reaction by the use of slices of liver tissue in an oxygenated nutrient medium containing ammonium salts. They were able to obtain urea formation only with liver tissue, thus confirming the fact that liver is the sole site of urea formation. The amino acids ornithine and citrulline catalyze the reaction to a marked degree. It was soon discovered that the formation of urea from arginine, as shown above, is really the last of a series of enzymic reactions. These include the synthesis of citrulline from ornithine and carbamyl phosphate, the synthesis of arginine from citrulline and aspartate, and the splitting off of urea from arginine.

1. The ammonia from deamination and deamidation of amino acids presumably combines with carbon dioxide or some carbon dioxide–yielding compound to form carbamic acid. It is thought that the compound utilized is an active carbon dioxide derivative of N-acetyl-L-glutamate

(AGA). ATP is required, and inorganic phosphate (P_i), as well as ADP, is formed. Thus:

$$(1) \quad ATP + HOCO_2^- + AGA \rightarrow ADP + P_i + AGA\text{-}CO_2^-$$

$$AGA\text{-}CO_2^- + ATP + NH_3 \rightleftharpoons \underset{\substack{\text{Carbamyl} \\ \text{phosphate}}}{NH_2\overset{\overset{\displaystyle O}{\|}}{C}OPO_3^=} + ADP + AGA$$

AGA–carbon dioxide may be as follows:

2. Carbamyl phosphate then reacts with ornithine to yield citrulline and P_i. Magnesium ions are required for Reaction 1 but not for Reaction 2. An enzyme, a transcarbamylase, is necessary for Reaction 2, and biotin also seems to be involved.

$$(2) \quad H_2N\text{—}\overset{\overset{\displaystyle O}{\|}}{C}\text{—}O\text{—}PO_3H_2 + \text{Ornithine} \rightleftharpoons \text{Citrulline} + H_3PO_4$$

Carbamyl phosphate   Ornithine   Citrulline

3. Citrulline, in its enol form, reacts with aspartic acid to form an intermediate addition compound, argininosuccinic acid, that yields arginine and fumaric acid. ATP is required in the first of these two steps, possibly to phosphorylate the hydroxyl group of the enol form of citrulline.

Citrulline   Enol form   Aspartic acid   Argininosuccinic acid

$$\rightleftarrows \quad \begin{array}{l} NH \\ \parallel \\ C-NH_2 \\ \mid \\ NH \\ \mid \\ (CH_2)_3 \\ \mid \\ CH-NH_2 \\ \mid \\ COOH \end{array} \quad + \quad \begin{array}{l} COOH \\ \mid \\ CH \\ \parallel \\ CH \\ \mid \\ COOH \end{array}$$

Arginine Fumaric acid

4. The arginine formed is decomposed by arginase, with the formation of urea and ornithine. The ornithine is again ready to take up carbon dioxide and ammonia via carbamyl phosphate. The ammonia, it should be remembered, is derived from amino acids, and the carbon dioxide from the metabolism of carbohydrates, fats, or the nonnitrogenous residue of amino acids.

Urea formation involves at least seven enzyme reactions — three in the formation of citrulline, three in the formation of arginine, and one in the formation of ornithine, with the concomitant splitting off of urea. A scheme of this cycle is shown in Fig. 13-4.

Amount of urea excreted. Urea is the chief nitrogenous end product of amino acid metabolism and thus of protein metabolism. Small amounts are also derived from the breakdown of other products, but these are negligible. On a normal or a high-protein diet the urea (about 25 to 30 gm.)

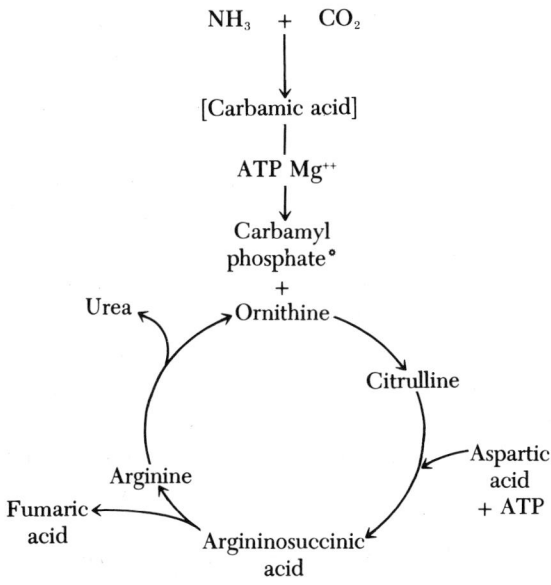

°N-acetyl-L-glutamate is very likely involved in the reactions leading to the formation of carbamyl phosphate.

Fig. 13-4. Scheme showing formation of urea.

361

comprises the greatest part of the urinary nitrogen; from 85% to 92% of the total nitrogen is urea nitrogen. On a low-protein diet the urinary urea nitrogen forms a smaller fraction. It may be as low as 60% of the total nitrogen. The reason for this is that certain nitrogenous constituents of the urine, e.g., uric acid, ammonia, and creatinine, are present in comparatively small amounts even on a high-nitrogen diet; and when the protein intake is lowered, they continue to be excreted in almost the same amount. They arise from other phases of metabolism not directly concerned with the breakdown of protein.

Urea itself has no very marked physiologic effects. It has some diuretic action. Consequently on a high-protein diet the volume of urine eliminated tends to be increased. This may be the reason for the feeling of thirst one often experiences after a very hearty meal.

Ammonia formation Ammonia, from a quantitative standpoint, is quite unimpressive when compared with urea. It amounts to about only 2.5% to 4.5% of the total urinary nitrogen under ordinary conditions. However, it is of considerable importance as a neutralizing agent for acids. As such it conserves fixed bases, such as sodium, potassium, and calcium. If an increased amount of fixed acid is present, more ammonia is formed to neutralize it and thus the loss of these elements is prevented. The same is true when an acidosis occurs and the reverse when there is an alkalosis (Chapter 20).

Nash and Benedict showed that ammonia formation occurs in the kidney. They ligated both kidneys and demonstrated that the ammonium salts of the blood did not accumulate as they would have done if ammonia were formed in some other organ. They also showed that the blood of the renal vein contains more ammonium salts than blood from other parts of the circulatory system. This indicated that the kidney manufactures ammonia, a small amount of which diffuses into the blood for neutralizing purposes. Most of it is eliminated by the kidney and forms the ammonia fraction of urine.

The source of ammonia has been the subject of much investigation as well as controversy. The use of isotopic compounds has helped to clarify the matter. The feeding of isotopic ammonia was followed by the excretion of isotopic urea, almost exclusively. Similarly the administration of isotopic urea was followed by the excretion of isotopic urea. Ammonium salts, which might arise in digestion to a slight extent, and urea are therefore both excluded as sources of urinary ammonia. However, when various amino acids containing isotopic nitrogen were fed, a large portion of the nitrogen was found in the urinary ammonia. Probably the urinary ammonia is formed by direct deamination of the amino acids, without urea as an intermediate. Van Slyke has designated glutamine, the amino acid amide, as the chief source of ammonia. Dogs were prepared with kidneys explanted, i.e., transferred to positions under the skin. In this way blood could be withdrawn from the renal vein by skin puncture. By special methods of analysis, he found that glutamine is the major source of ammonia, with α-amino acids a minor one. Glutamine makes up about one fourth to one fifth of the free amino acids present in plasma.

NH₂—CH—COOH
    |
CH₂   + HOH → (Glutaminase)
    |
CH₂—CONH₂

$$NH_2-CH-COOH \quad (CH_2) \quad (CH_2-CONH_2) + HOH \xrightarrow{Glutaminase} NH_2-CH-COOH \quad (CH_2) \quad (CH_2-COOH) + NH_3$$

Glutamine   **Glutamic acid**

The ammonia formed by other amino acids is probably via oxidative de-amination by L-amino oxidase (a flavoprotein containing FAD as the prosthetic group). D-Amino oxidase, also a flavoprotein, probably serves in a similar capacity for glycine, as glycine oxidase.

The various amino acids have been classified on the basis of their effect on ammonia excretion in the perfused kidney (dog) as follows:

A. Greatly enhance excretion of ammonia	B. Moderately increase excretion of ammonia	C. No effect on excretion of ammonia
L-Glutamine	L-Aspartic acid	L-Glutamic acid
L-Asparagine	L-Methionine	L-Lysine
L-Alanine	Glycine	L-Arginine
D-Alanine	L-Cysteine	
L-Histidine	L-Leucine	

Fate of nonnitrogenous residues The α-keto acids remaining after the deamination of amino acids are transformed to glucose, to acetoacetic acid and related compounds, and to other products. The structure of the amino acid determines the substance to which the amino acid is changed. This has been determined chiefly on dogs or other animals made diabetic either by pancreatectomy or by the injection of phlorizin. Such diabetic animals excrete glucose even when starved or on a diet containing only protein. It is evident that when all the fat and glycogen stores have been used up any glucose excreted in the urine must be derived from protein. Since the nitrogen content of proteins is known (approximately 16%), a determination of both urinary nitrogen and glucose should indicate the proportion of sugar that can be derived from protein. This has led to the formulation of the glucose:nitrogen (G:N) ratio, formerly called D:N or dextrose:nitrogen. Minkowski's figure for the G:N ratio in depancreatized dogs was 2.8. The G:N ratio in phlorizin diabetes (p. 222) was placed at 3.65 by Graham Lusk, and the latter value has been assumed the better one to use. Although a great deal of doubt has been cast upon the accuracy of this figure and, indeed, upon part of the theoretic basis for this figure,[13] its use may be continued until the subject is in a less confusing state. Now, if the G:N ratio is 3.65 on a protein diet, the indication is that the amount of glucose derived from 100 gm. of protein ingested is 58 gm.

$$\frac{G \text{ (Glucose of the protein)}}{N \text{ (Nitrogen of the protein)}}, \quad \text{or} \quad \frac{x}{16} = 3.65, \text{ and } 3.65 \times 16 = 58.4$$

The process of forming glucose from protein is called *gluconeogenesis*, and hence the gluconeogenic value of proteins in general is 58%. When diets are planned for diabetic patients, and the approximate amount of potential glucose in the food must be known with some degree of accuracy, this figure is of value. Fifty-eight percent of the protein ingested is added to the amount of carbohydrate (plus about 10% of the fat, representing the glycerol fraction)

363

for a total glucose value of the diet. This 58%, it must be understood, represents the glucose derivable from a *mixture* of proteins. Single purified proteins yield different amounts of glucose and nitrogen. Janney gave the following results: casein yields 48% glucose; ovalbumin, 54%; serum albumin, 55%; gelatin, 68%; fibrin, 53%; edestin, 65%; gliadin, 80%; and zein, 53%. These divergent figures are due to the differences in composition of the proteins. Feeding pure amino acids to diabetic animals results in the interesting observation that only certain ones give rise to glucose in this way, namely, glycine, alanine, valine, serine, threonine, cysteine (and cystine), methionine, aspartic acid, glutamic acid, arginine, histidine, proline, hydroxyproline, and tryptophan.

The mechanism of this conversion to glucose is complex. However, it has been seen that keto acids are the first step. The simplest keto acid, pyruvic, is a well-known intermediate in all carbohydrate transformations, but whether the longer keto acids must be cut down to pyruvic first or not is still uncertain. Possibly this is so because only three of the carbon atoms in each glucogenic amino acid go to form sugar. In the case of glycine, of course, only two are so converted. There is some evidence that the glucogenic amino acids may not in all cases be actually converted to glucose. The glucose formed may come from some other metabolite, which the amino acid spares. Gurin found that ^{14}C-alanine, when administered to phlorizinized dogs, results in a formation of glucose, to be sure, but the glucose is not labeled. Similar results have been obtained by other workers (Table 13-3).

Certain amino acids may be *glucogenic* under some conditions and *ketogenic* under others, i.e., form ketone bodies (p. 315). It should also be mentioned in this connection that, since many amino acids yield glucose, and since carbohydrates are convertible to fats (Chapter 12), the proteins indirectly may be fat formers. The opposite to glucose formation from proteins also occurs; i.e., glucose and many related compounds can be converted to the carbon chains of amino acids. For example, when sucrose containing ^{14}C was fed to mice, the labeled carbon was found in several of the nonessential amino acids of the tissues.

Table 13-3. Glucogenic and ketogenic amino acids

Glucogenic		Glucogenic and ketogenic	Ketogenic
Alanine	Hydroxyproline	Isoleucine	Leucine
Arginine	Methionine	Lysine	
Aspartic acid	Proline	Phenylalanine	
Cystine-cysteine	Serine	Tyrosine	
Glutamic acid	Threonine		
Glycine	Tryptophan		
Histidine	Valine		

Perhaps it should be added that the degradation of the carbon chain of amino acids may involve shortening by decarboxylation. This is accomplished by means of enzymes, the carboxylases. Several of these decarboxylations have been fairly well characterized. The carboxylases for histidine, lysine, and tyrosine contain pyridoxal phosphate as the coenzyme, whereas the carboxylase for pyruvic acid, cocarboxylase, and the keto acids derived from several other amino acids contain thiamine pyrophosphate and lipoic acid. Histidine, lysine, and tyrosine apparently may be decarboxylated before deamination occurs.

Decarboxylation of amino acids by decarboxylases gives rise to many amines with physiologic activity, e.g., histamine, tyramine, serotonin. Many microorganisms have decarboxylases that form products such as cadaverine, from lysine, and putrescine, from ornithine. These are responsible for much of the odor of putrified protein.

In the degradation of amino acids, oxidative decarboxylation is an important step usually following the transamination of alanine, valine, leucine, isoleucine, and glutamic acid. CoA-derivatives are formed, as will be discussed later.

METABOLISM OF SOME INDIVIDUAL AMINO ACIDS

Most of the discussion of amino acid metabolism up to this point has been concerned with amino acids as a class. It is now necessary to consider them individually. They will be taken up in about the same order as they were listed in Chapter 5. The problem to be studied is how the amino acids are utilized by the liver or other tissues, when they are not being built into protoplasm, and, further, what are their special functions and uses.

The question of the biosynthesis of individual amino acids should be mentioned but will not be treated in any detail in this chapter. Only schematic diagrams with the precursors and major intermediates involved will be shown. Enzymes and, in some cases, cofactors concerned will not be included since they are uncertain as yet in some instances. Formulas will usually not be given since many of these would be repetitions of those included in the degradative pathways. For further information, refer to the general and special references at the end of the chapter, particularly the articles by Greenberg and by Meister. In general, the biosynthesis of the nonessential amino acids may involve a reversal of the catabolic pathways to be described. Usually different enzyme systems are required, however. Transamination of the corresponding α-keto acid with glutamic acid is usually the final step in the biosynthesis of the nonessential acids. The carbon chain "backbone" of the molecule is usually an intermediate of the glycolytic pathway or the citric acid cycle. The same is true in a general way of the essential amino acids. These, of course, cannot be synthesized in the animal organism, but their biosynthetic pathways and the enzymes and cofactors involved, in most instances, are fairly well documented in microorganisms.

Disorders of amino acid metabolism Since a number of enzymatically catalyzed reactions are involved in the metabolism of typical amino acids, there are possibilities of inherited disorders of amino acid metabolism. These may be *direct*, due to a single hereditary enzyme deficiency affecting the metabolism or transport of an amino acid. As a result, an increase in the plasma level and urinary excretion (amino-aciduria) of the amino acid or of one of its metabolites, depending on the site of the deficiency, can occur. Disorders of amino acid metabolism also may be *secondary* (or "indirect"), due to some other disease process, e.g., in the liver or kidney, impairing metabolism. Secondary disorders are either hereditary or acquired. Usually they are characterized by a generalized rather than a specific aminoaciduria as is true of the primary type. Typical examples are the generalized aminoacidurias seen in galactosemia (p. 216), Wilson's disease (p. 425), and a number of conditions (burns, poisonings, etc.) in which there is extensive tissue damage, especially of the liver or kidney.

Nearly 100 different primary hereditary disorders of amino acid metabolism have been described in the literature.[16] Examples of those that are supported by confirmatory evidence will be cited as the metabolism of the individual amino acids is discussed. Table 13-4 lists some of these disorders.

Glycine. Glycine may be oxidatively deaminated by glycine oxidase, an enzyme present in liver and kidney tissue.

$$CH_2(NH_2)COOH + \tfrac{1}{2}\,O_2 \;\rightleftarrows\; CHO{-}COOH + NH_3$$

$$\text{Glycine} \qquad\qquad\qquad \text{Glyoxylic acid}$$

The enzyme is a flavoprotein and apparently is a D-amino oxidase. Glyoxylic acid may be decarboxylated to yield formaldehyde and carbon dioxide, both of which take part in many biochemical reactions. Glyoxylate may also be converted to malate and then metabolized via the citric acid cycle. By isotope experiments, glycine has also been shown to be converted to acetic acid.

A further interesting pathway involves the participation of glycine in the synthesis of serine, which is then converted to pyruvic acid (p. 203), a carbohydrate metabolite:

$$CH_2(NH_2)COOH + 5\text{-Formyl-THFA} \;\rightleftarrows\; CH_2OH\cdot CH(NH_2)COOH$$

$$\text{Glycine} \qquad\qquad\qquad\qquad\qquad \text{Serine}$$

In 1946, Shemin showed that ^{13}C- or ^{15}N-labeled serine administered to rats gives rise to labeled glycine, showing that the reaction is reversible in vivo. This reversible reaction occurs in the liver and requires as a coenzyme a pteroylglutamic acid derivative and pyridoxal phosphate. In fact, it is not as simple a reaction as indicated above. Pyridoxal forms an addition product, a Schiff's base, with glycine. The folic acid derivative is the 5-formyl derivative of 5,6,7,8-tetrahydrofolic acid, which donates its formyl group to the glycine fraction. Serine is finally split off from this complex (p. 371).

Glycine, as a nonessential amino acid, may be readily synthesized in the animal organism from serine, as indicated above. By way of serine, it may be formed from 3-phosphoglyceric acid or, of course, in turn, from any intermediate of the glycolytic pathway.

Although glycine is the simplest of the amino acids chemically and is nonessential, it performs, perhaps, the most biochemical functions of any amino acid. The following include some of its special functions, which are, of course, in addition to its role as a constituent of various body tissue proteins, protein hormones, and enzymes: It is a prime precursor, along with succinyl-CoA, of the porphyrins and heme (p. 608). It contributes to the biosynthesis of purines (p. 403) and is glucogenic (p. 364), thus contributing indirectly via glycolytic intermediates to lipid synthesis, carbohydrate formation, the syntheses of other amino acids, and the syntheses of many other compounds of biologic importance. By way of glyoxylate, it may form a one-carbon fragment, which by complexing with tetrahydrofolic acid may be incorporated into a wide variety of biologically active compounds (p. 821).

Glycine is one of the substances necessary for the formation of creatine, and creatine is essential in muscle physiology. Glycine is also a part of the bile acid glycocholic acid and the tripeptide glutathione, which has certain oxidation-reduction functions.

When benzoic acid or its salts are included in the diet, glycine conjugates with them to form hippuric acid. This is a detoxifying action. It occurs even when no glycine is present in the diet; hence glycine must be readily obtainable from other amino acids and is therefore one of the nonessential amino acids.

Several hereditary diseases of glycine metabolism have been described (p. 394). In *glycinemia* (characterized by increased blood levels of glycine) mental retardation, ketosis, hypogammaglobulinemia, and blood dyscrasias are found clinically. The cause is unknown. A second condition, *glycinuria*,

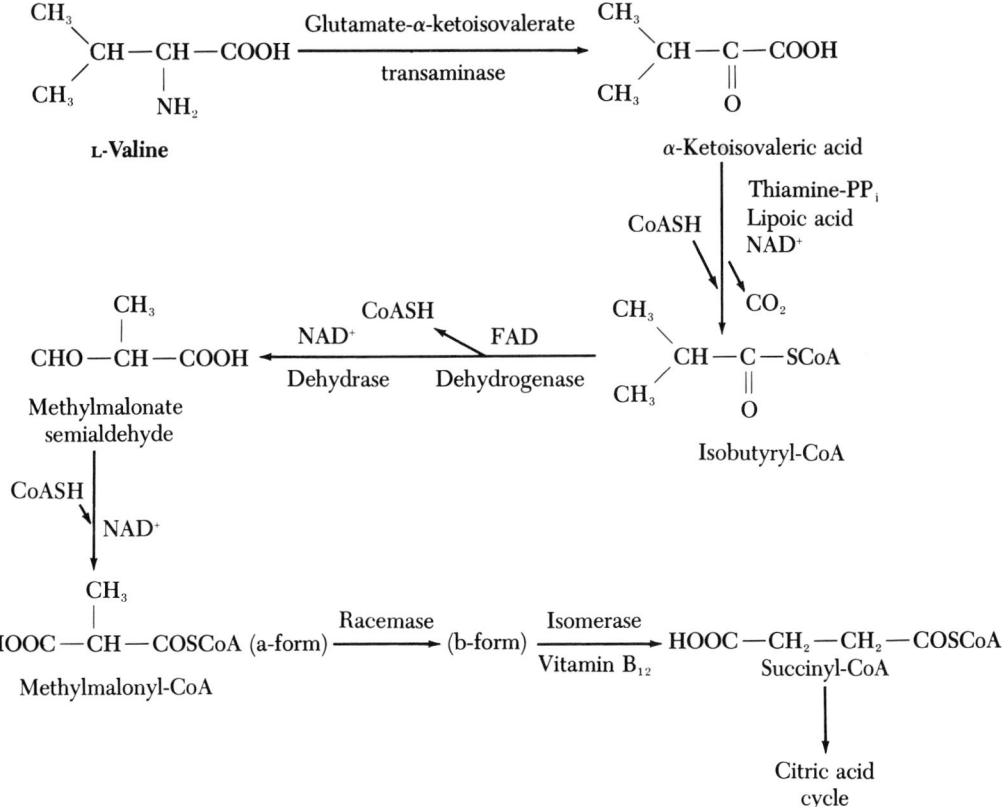

Fig. 13-5. Metabolic degradation of valine.

367

is apparently due to a defect in the renal transport system for glycine. An abnormally high renal excretion of glycine is found. The presence of calcium oxalate renal stones is the major clinical finding.

Alanine. It was shown previously (p. 351) that, by transamination, alanine can be converted to pyruvic acid. Pyruvic acid is an intermediate in the metabolism of carbohydrates. Here is a clear relation between the proteins and the carbohydrates. As has been seen, alanine fed to diabetic animals is converted to glucose. In normal animals it is similarly converted but is then utilized.

Alanine is a nonessential amino acid and is readily synthesized in the body by the transamination of pyruvate by glutamate or other amino acids. It is formed in plants and microorganisms apparently in this same manner.

Valine. The metabolic degradation of valine begins with a transamination yielding α-ketoisovaleric acid. The subsequent fate of this is pictured in Fig. 13-5, based on isotope experiments. Note that isobutyryl-CoA, rather than isobutyric acid, is formed in the decarboxylation of α-ketoisovaleric acid. This step is analogous to the conversion of pyruvate to acetyl-CoA (p. 203). Isobutyryl-CoA is converted in several steps to methylmalonyl-CoA and finally to succinyl-CoA by steps discussed on p. 828. Succinyl-CoA can be metabolized by way of the ctiric acid cycle and other pathways as described earlier (p. 263). The biosynthesis of valine, which is an essential amino acid, is limited to plants and microorganisms. The principal steps in its formation,[17] in *Salmonella*, for example, are shown in Fig. 13-6.

Leucine and isoleucine. Leucine and isoleucine undergo oxidative transamination to form the keto acid. It appears that the further degradation of leucine follows a break in the carbon chain between the β- and γ-carbons. Both fragments yield acetoacetate. This was determined by administering leucine containing ^{14}C in various positions in the molecule to animals, or incubating it with liver slices, and discovering the exact location of the tagged carbon of the acetoacetate formed in each case (Fig. 13-7). Obviously these reactions explain the origin of acetoacetic acid from L-leucine and reaffirm the fact that it is a *ketogenic* amino acid. The metabolic fate of acetoacetic acid was discussed earlier (p. 315).

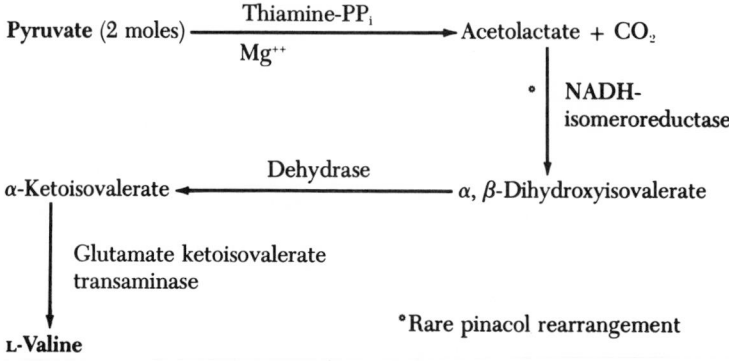

Fig. 13-6. Biosynthesis of L-valine.

HMG-CoA was discussed as an obligatory intermediate in the biosynthesis of cholesterol (p. 326) and in ketone body formation from acetyl-CoA (p. 315). This is another example of the interrelationship of protein, fat, and carbohydrate metabolisms.

Leucine is also an essential amino acid. It is synthesized in microorganisms and plants apparently by the pathway[17] shown in Fig. 13-8.

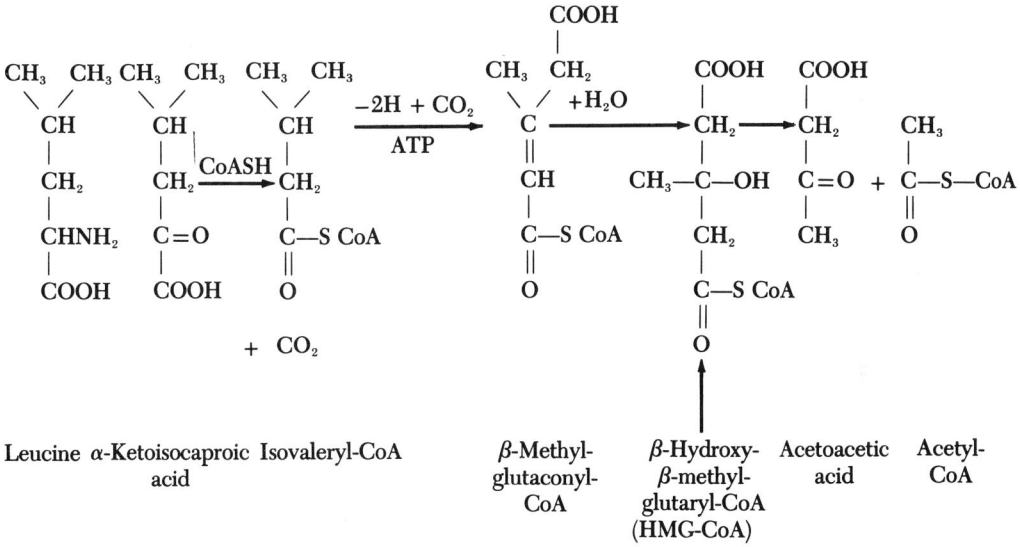

Fig. 13-7. Metabolic degradation of L-leucine.

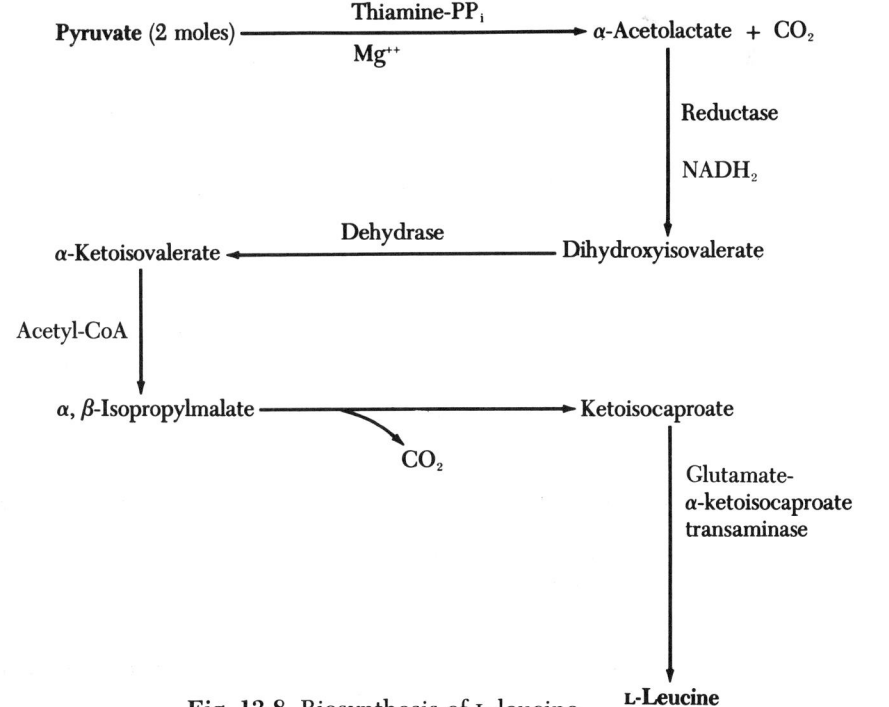

Fig. 13-8. Biosynthesis of L-leucine.

369

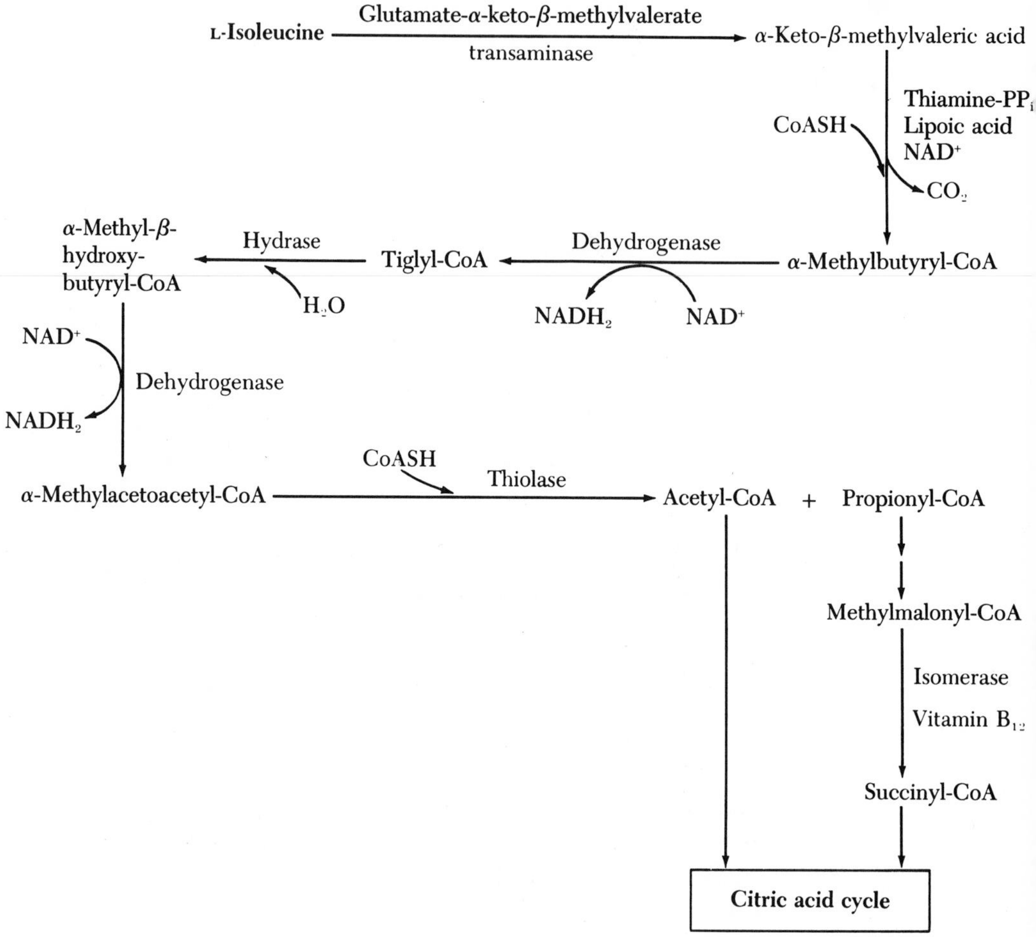

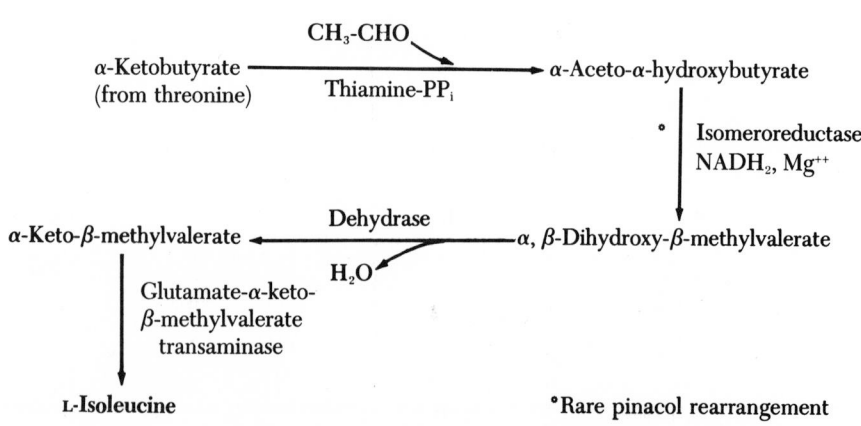

Fig. 13-9. Metabolic degradation of L-isoleucine.

Fig. 13-10. Biosynthesis of L-isoleucine.

There is now evidence from Coon's laboratory that clarifies the steps involved in the metabolism of isoleucine (Fig. 13-9). After transamination, the α-keto acid formed, α-keto-β-methylvaleric, is converted in several steps to propionyl-CoA and acetyl-CoA. These two products account for the weak ketogenic and glycogenic properties of isoleucine, mentioned previously. The propionyl-CoA is converted to methylmalonyl-CoA and then succinyl-CoA in several steps, as indicated previously (p. 368).

Isoleucine is an essential amino acid. It is synthesized in microorganisms as shown in Fig. 13-10.

A block in the metabolism of leucine, isoleucine, and valine results in an inborn error of metabolism in infants known as *maple syrup urine disease*, so called because the odor of the urine resembles that of maple sugar. The oxidative decarboxylation of the keto acids does not occur, and hence the branched-chain keto acid derivatives of leucine, isoleucine, and valine accumulate in the urine. A block in the metabolism of methylmalonic acid formed in the metabolism of valine and isoleucine, as shown in Fig. 13-10, has been described recently.[18] The hereditary condition is characterized by methylmalonic aciduria, long-chain ketonuria, intermittent hyperglycinemia, and profound metabolic acidosis. Methylmalonic acid can be derived, of course, from other metabolic sources, e.g., threonine, methionine (pp. 372, 383).

Serine. The anaerobic deamination of serine has been demonstrated. In this case, the reaction differs from the general one heretofore considered:

$$
\begin{array}{llll}
CH_2OH & CH_2 & CH_3 & \\
| & \parallel & | & \\
CHNH_2 \xrightarrow{-H_2O} & C-NH_2 \longrightarrow & C=NH & +H_2O \\
| & | & | & \\
COOH & COOH & COOH & \\
\text{Serine} & & & \\
\text{(as pyridoxal complex)} & & &
\end{array}
$$

$$
\begin{array}{l}
CH_3 \\
| \\
C=O + NH_3 \\
| \\
COOH \\
\textbf{Pyruvic acid}
\end{array}
$$

It is found to occur in liver extracts and in kidney and is catalyzed by the pyridoxal-dependent enzyme threonine aldolase. The possibility that β-hydroxypyruvic acid might be produced by an oxidative deamination is not excluded. Both pyruvic acid and β-hydroxypyruvic acid could easily enter into metabolism, and pyruvic acid would likewise be formed in the transamination of serine. Isotope experiments indicate that the carbon chain of serine can be converted to cystine (p. 380). Cystine is *dicysteine*, and cysteine has the same number of carbon atoms as serine.

Furthermore, serine and glycine have been found to be interconvertible. This was shown by isotope experiments on rats and guinea pigs.

$$
\begin{array}{lll}
CH_2{}^{13}COOH + H^{14}COOH & \rightleftarrows & {}^{14}CH_2CH^{13}COOH \\
| & & \quad\quad | \;\; | \\
NH_2 & & \quad\; OH\; NH_2 \\
\textbf{Glycine} \quad\quad \textbf{Formic acid} & & \textbf{Serine} \\
\quad\quad\quad\text{(as THFA derivative)} & &
\end{array}
$$

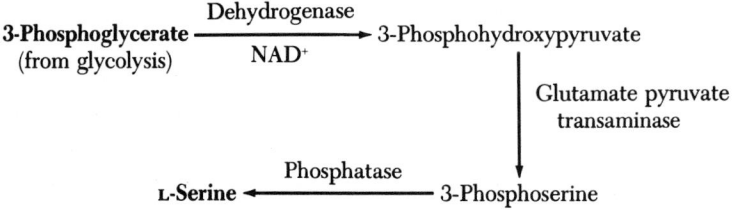

Fig. 13-11. Pathway for the formation of L-serine.

Serine may also be formed as indicated in Fig. 13-11. Other pathways for its synthesis from 3-phosphoglyceric acid also have been described.[19]

Serine is a constituent of one of the phosphatides found in brain. In addition, it can give rise to ethanolamine, which is one of the constituents of another phosphatide. Thus we see links between protein and lipid metabolism.

$$
\begin{array}{ccc}
CH_2OH & & CH_2OH \\
| & & | \\
CHNH_2 & \rightarrow & CH_2NH_2 \quad + CO_2 \\
| & & \\
COOH & & \\
\textbf{Serine} & & \textbf{Ethanolamine}
\end{array}
$$

Serine also takes part in the biologic synthesis of tryptophan in the mold *Neurospora*.

Threonine. Threonine is handled similarly to serine, since it also is a hydroxy amino acid.

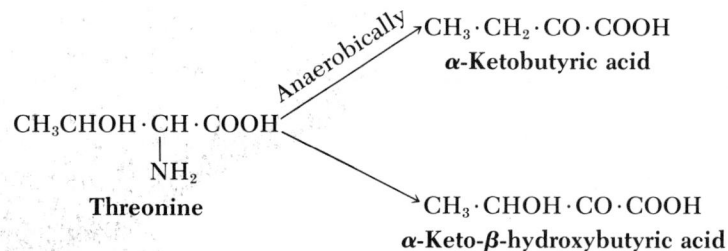

The α-ketobutyrate thus formed is converted to propionyl-CoA, which forms succinyl-CoA as previously shown (p. 370). Threonine is thus a glucogenic amino acid.

By an indirect method, another path for threonine has been indicated. It is an oxidation at the β-carbon, preliminary to a splitting of the four-carbon chain in half. The enzyme that catalyzes this reaction requires pyridoxal phosphate as coenzyme:

$$
\begin{array}{ccc}
CH_3 \cdot CH \cdot CH \cdot COOH & \rightarrow & CH_3 \cdot CHO + CH_2 \cdot COOH \\
\quad | \quad \ | & & | \\
\quad OH \ \ NH_2 & & NH_2 \\
\textbf{Threonine} & & \textbf{Acetaldehyde} \quad \textbf{Glycine}
\end{array}
$$

Thus threonine, like serine, participates in many of the reactions of glycine. Threonine was the last of the 10 essential amino acids to be discovered (p. 349). It is synthesized in microorganisms as shown in Fig. 13-12.

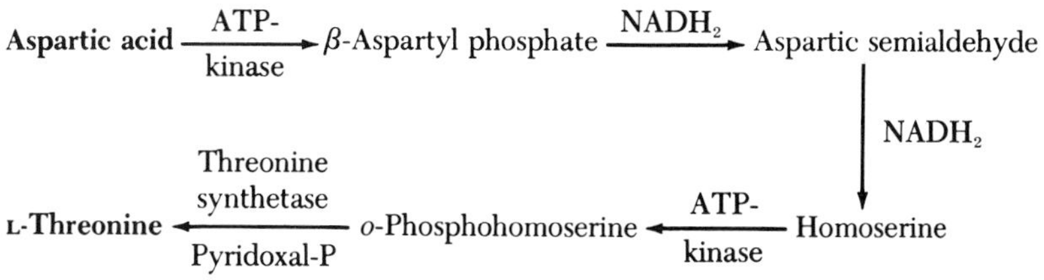

Aspartic acid $\xrightarrow[\text{kinase}]{\text{ATP-}}$ β-Aspartyl phosphate $\xrightarrow{\text{NADH}_2}$ Aspartic semialdehyde

$\Bigg\downarrow \text{NADH}_2$

L-Threonine $\xleftarrow[\text{Pyridoxal-P}]{\substack{\text{Threonine} \\ \text{synthetase}}}$ o-Phosphohomoserine $\xleftarrow[\text{kinase}]{\text{ATP-}}$ Homoserine

Fig. 13-12. Formation of L-threonine in microorganisms.

Phenylalanine and tyrosine. The animal body cannot synthesize the benzene ring, and phenylalanine and tyrosine are the chief source of it in food. Phenylalanine is converted to tyrosine in the body, which reaction appears to be the first step in its metabolism; the reverse reaction is not possible for the body. No doubt, this is the reason why phenylalanine is an indispensable amino acid and tyrosine is not; i.e., phenylalanine may be used by the organism, whenever either one is needed, whereas tyrosine cannot substitute for phenylalanine. Because of this relationship, these two compounds will be considered together (Fig. 13-13).

By transamination, tyrosine is converted to *p*-hydroxyphenylpyruvic acid, and phenylalanine to phenylpyruvic acid. The further transformations of these two have been deduced by the use of isotopically labeled intermediates and by studying two inborn errors of metabolism. In *alkaptonuria* and in *tyrosinosis* there is an inability to metabolize completely phenylalanine and tyrosine. The former is a hereditary disorder, occurring more frequently in men than in women. Homogentisic acid is formed, is excreted in the urine, and, on exposure to air, is oxidized to a blackish pigment that darkens the urine. This is a very rare condition, but still more uncommon is tyrosinosis. In this disease the aromatic amino acids are eliminated as tyrosine or as hydroxyphenylpyruvic acid.

If tyrosine is administered to patients with alkaptonuria, the excretion of homogentisic acid is increased. This probably indicates that homogentisic acid is intermediate in the normal metabolism of tyrosine but that in this curious condition the body cannot carry the breakdown further. In homogentisic acid there are two hydroxyls, neither of which is in the *para* position to the acetic acid radical. How this rearrangement takes place is not known.

In tyrosinosis, several cases of which have been reported, Medes found that there were excreted in the urine *p*-hydroxyphenylpyruvic acid and its reduction product, *p*-hydroxyphenyllactic acid, and tyrosine and its oxidation product, 3,4-dihydroxyphenylalanine. Apparently there was difficulty in the early steps of tyrosine breakdown. That this was so can be seen from the fact that feeding homogentisic acid resulted in the complete utilization of this compound. In other words, in tyrosinosis the introduction of a second hydroxyl group and the shift of the two hydroxyls cannot be accomplished; but if such 2,5-dihydroxyphenyl derivatives are available, they are catabolized. In alkaptonuria the early steps can be brought about but not the last ones.

Normally phenylalanine is partly converted to tyrosine. This has been demonstrated repeatedly. Moss and Schoenheimer replaced a hydrogen of the

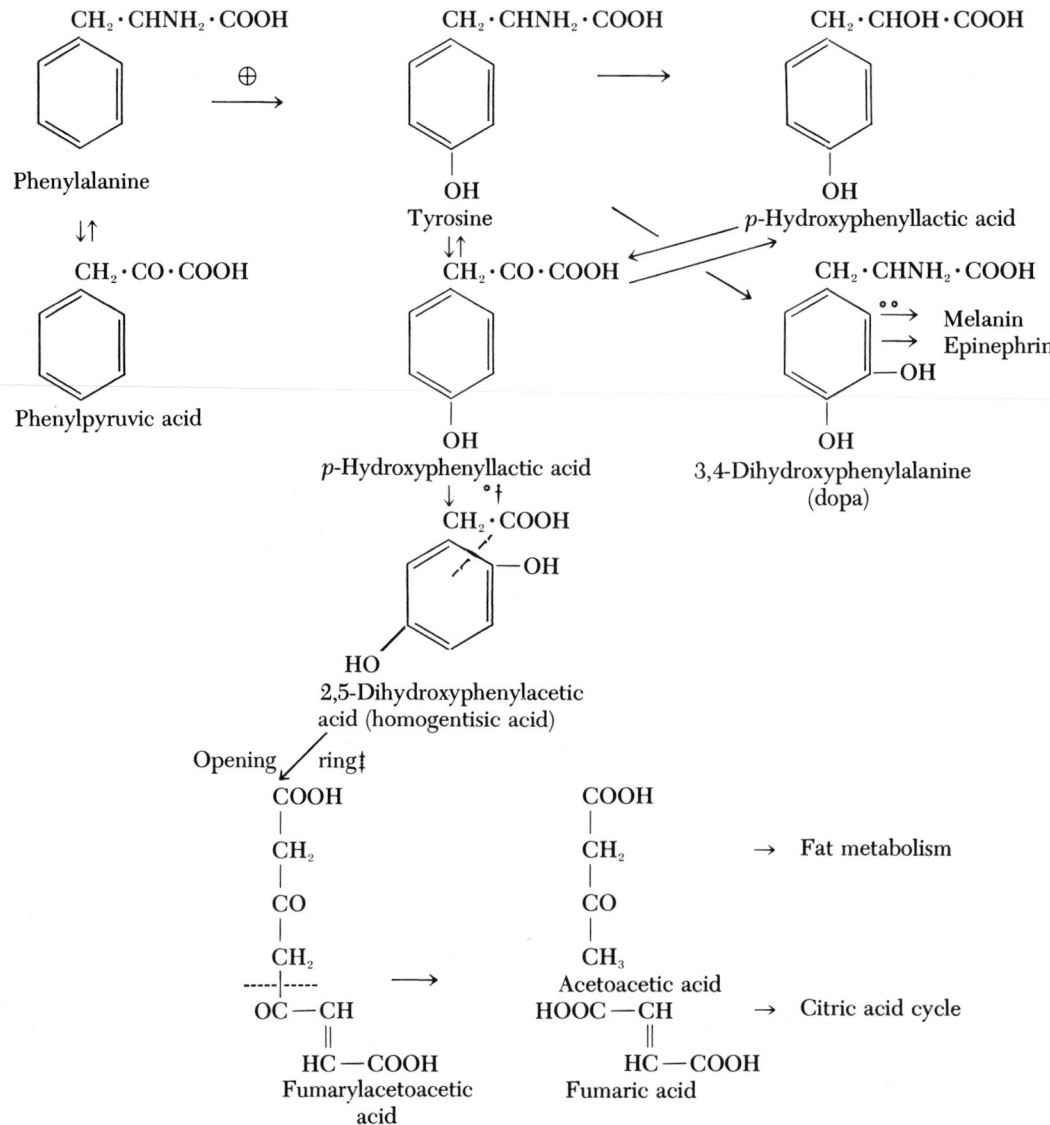

⊕ indicates point of blockage in phenylketonuria.
° indicates point of blockage in tyrosinosis.
† indicates point of blockage in vitamin C deficiency in human beings.
‡ indicates point of blockage in alkaptonuria and in vitamin C deficiency in guinea pigs.
°° indicates point of blockage in albinism.

Fig. 13-13. Metabolism of phenylalanine and tyrosine.

benzene ring with deuterium and fed the labeled phenylalanine to rats. Labeled tyrosine was recovered from the tissue proteins. This reaction occurs in the liver of man, the enzyme requiring oxygen as well as NAD$^+$ or NADP$^+$. Tyrosine is catabolized according to the middle vertical column of Fig. 13-13 by another enzyme system in the liver. Transamination is responsible for the loss of an amino group, α-ketoglutarate being the acceptor. Vitamin C is a necessary factor for further degradation. Phenylalanine is also partly oxidatively deaminated to phenylpyruvic acid.

Another intermediate appears to be 2,5-dihydroxyphenylpyruvic acid. Decarboxylation and oxidation yield 2,5-dihydroxyphenylacetic acid, known as homogentisic acid. The benzene ring is now opened, with the eventual formation of fumaric and acetoacetic acids. Both phenylalanine and tyrosine are completely utilized by the normal body.

Another interesting anomaly of metabolism is connected with phenylalanine. Fölling, in Norway, first observed that certain feebleminded children excrete a considerable amount of phenylpyruvic acid. This, as has been seen, is an intermediate in the breakdown of phenylalanine but not of tyrosine. The condition is called *phenylpyruvic oligophrenia* or simply *phenylketonuria* (PKU). Since these children are otherwise metabolically normal, they can apparently build phenylalanine into their body protein but cannot catabolize it in the normal manner, which is mostly via tyrosine. This biochemical error was shown to be a hereditary deficiency of the enzyme *phenylalanine hydroxylase*, resulting in an inability to introduce the hydroxyl group into the phenyl ring in the *para* position. Such patients can metabolize tyrosine, when they are fed it, just as well as normal persons can. As a consequence, phenylalanine accumulates in the blood and is excreted in the urine along with phenylpyruvic acid and its derivatives phenylacetic and phenyllactic acids. The latter two are probably responsible for the mental symptoms. This concept is supported by the fact that if the phenylalanine intake is restricted in infants with PKU the mental symptoms do not seem to develop. Special protein hydrolysate preparations of low phenylalanine content are available for therapeutic use in this condition. Woolley and associates[20] believe that a low serotonin content of the brain, due to an inhibition of the enzymatic synthesis of serotonin by phenyllactic and/or phenylpyruvic acid, is actually responsible for the mental aberrations of PKU. More recent studies, [20a]however, suggest that a chronic depletion of glutamine may be more directly involved in the damaging of the brain in PKU.

At the present time, tests for PKU are done routinely in most hospitals on all newborn infants before they are released. Some 30 states now require this early screening procedure before the brain-damaging process has begun. The older ferric chloride method of detection is now considered inadequate, due to insensitivity and nonspecificity. Blood levels of phenylalanine are usually determined by fluorometric or microbiologic methods.

Interesting recent work[21] demonstrated that phenylketonuria can be produced experimentally in infant monkeys by the feeding of a high-phenylalanine (5%) diet. The feeding of the diet is begun soon after birth. High blood levels of phenylalanine similar to those seen in human PKU patients are produced. Urinary levels of phenylpyruvic and phenyllactic acid are also high. The symptoms, grand mal convulsions and mental retardation, are also similar to those seen in human subjects.

Experimentally, phenylpyruvic acid appears in the urine when extra phenylalanine is fed to rats having a thiamine deficiency. Ascorbic acid also is involved in some of these transformations. If tyrosine is fed to guinea pigs deficient in this vitamin, homogentisic acid is excreted in the urine. Similarly, in prematurely born infants on vitamin C–deficient diets, tyrosine and phenylalanine are not metabolized in a normal manner, p-hydroxyphenyllactic acid and p-hydroxyphenylpyruvic acid being found in the urine. Since this condition is due to an absence of vitamin C, the administration of vitamin C restores metabolism to normal. ACTH (p. 494) has a similar effect, although it is not as effective as ascorbic acid; the adrenocortical hormones have inconsistent or no action.

Another interesting phase in which tyrosine takes part is the production of certain pigments. Tyrosine is oxidized to dihydroxyphenylalanine (dopa), then to a red indole compound, by an oxidizing enzyme, tyrosinase. This is subsequently converted to a melanin. The melanins are brown or black pigments of ill-defined composition. They are deposited in the skin and hair

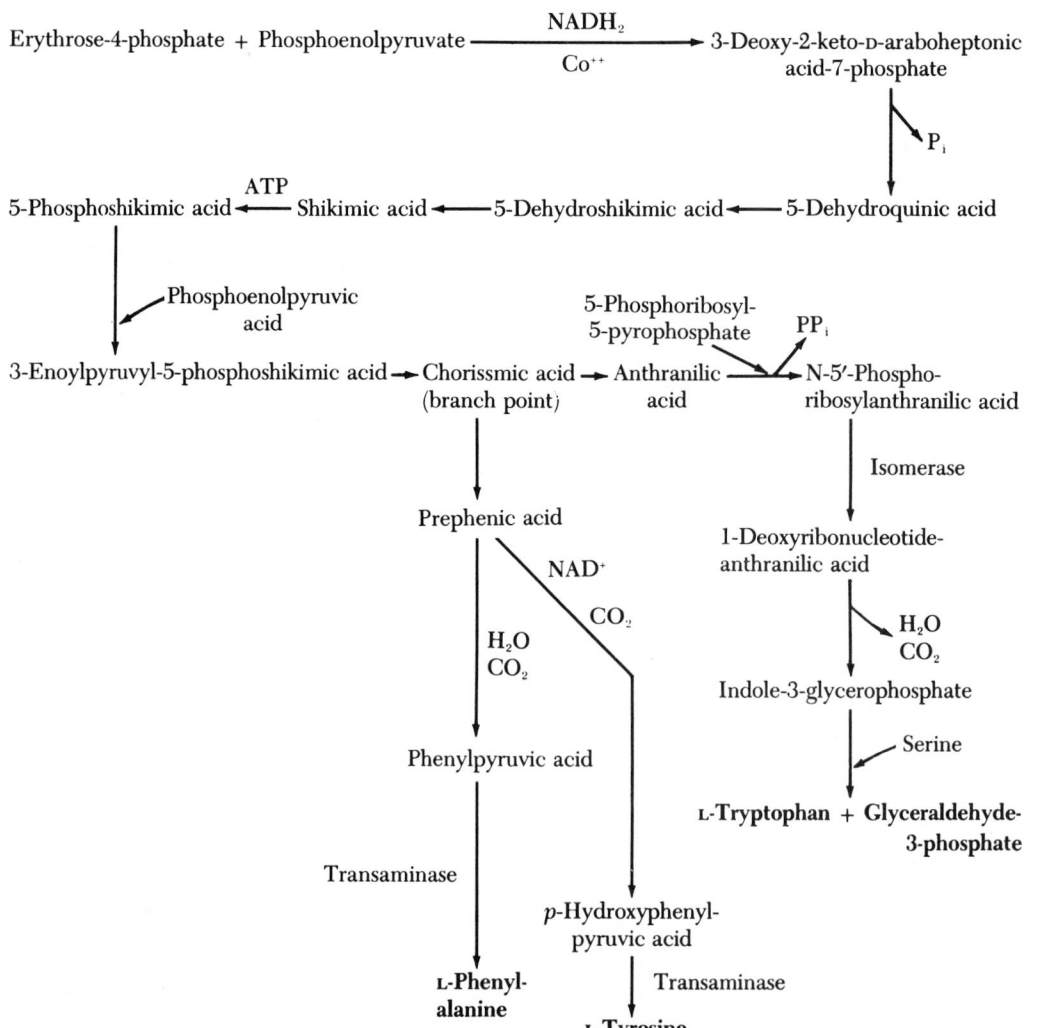

Fig. 13-14. Biosynthesis of phenylalanine, tyrosine, and tryptophan.

and in the choroid coat of the eye. Their formation is aided by light; the production of freckles and tanning of the skin are common examples. Melanins are also deposited in melanotic sarcomas. Still another congenital aberration in the metabolism of phenylalanine and tyrosine is found in *albinism*. The metabolic defect here is apparently a lack of the enzyme tyrosinase, required for the formation of melanin from dopa. As will be seen, tyrosine constitutes an integral part of thyroxine and epinephrine (Chapter 16) as well as of other compounds having biologic importance.

Another minor catabolic pathway of the metabolism of tyrosine is decarboxylation to form tyramine, which has the property of raising blood pressure. Tyramine is present in some varieties of cheese in significant amounts.

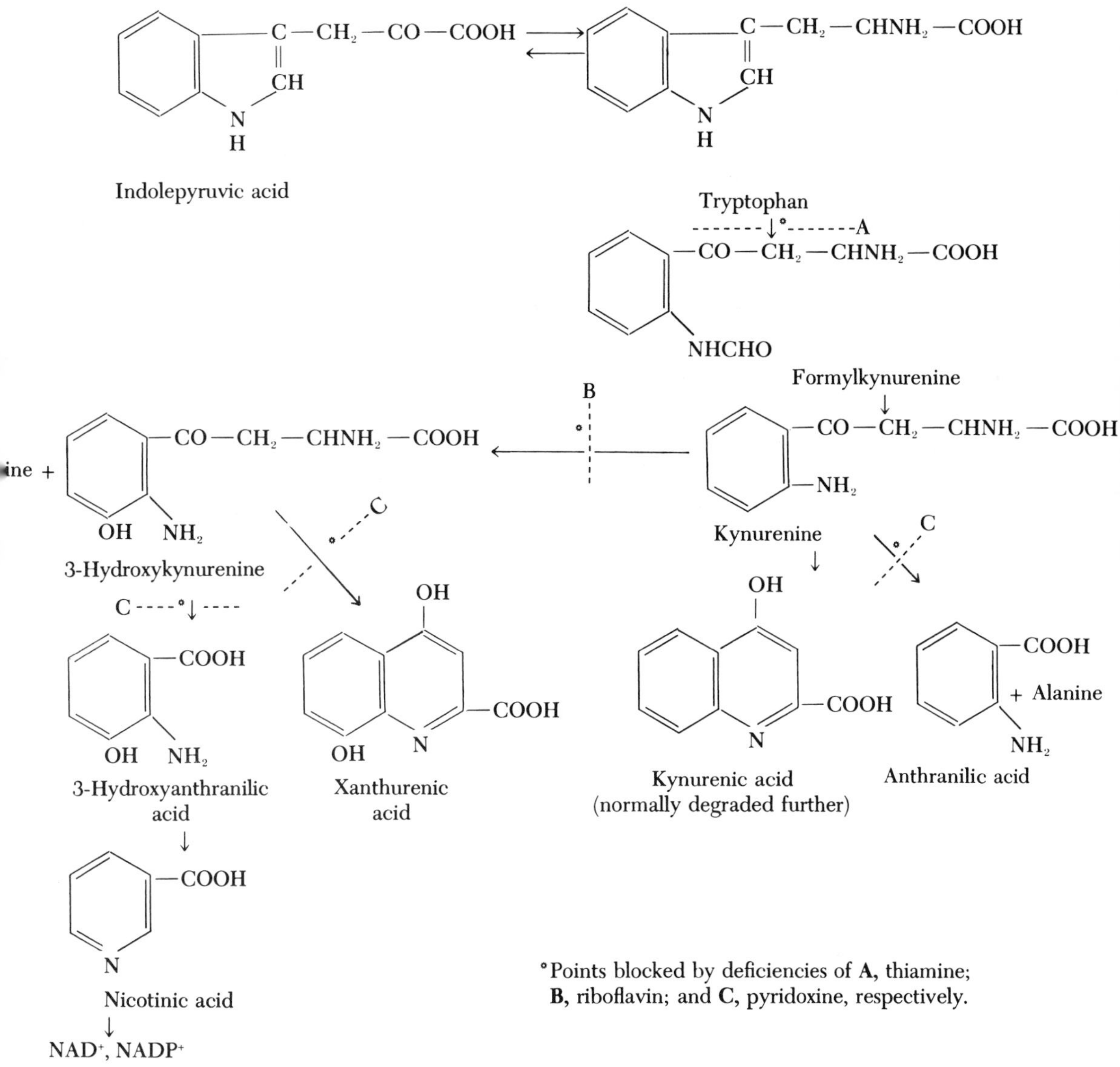

Fig. 13-15. Paths of tryptophan metabolism.

°Points blocked by deficiencies of **A**, thiamine; **B**, riboflavin; and **C**, pyridoxine, respectively.

377

This became important recently when patients who were being treated with monoamine oxidase inhibitors (MAOI), for the hypotensive action of these drugs in decreasing catecholamines, showed soaring blood pressures when they ingested cheese. The MAOI's prevented the oxidation of tyramine, which, in turn, increased the blood pressure.

Phenylalanine is an essential amino acid since the animal organism is unable to synthesize the benzene ring. Tyrosine is not essential since it can be formed by the hydroxylation of phenylalanine, although it "spares" phenylalanine and may reduce phenylalanine's requirement (p. 349). The biosynthetic pathway of these two aromatic amino acids, therefore, is especially interesting. As found in *E. coli,* the pathway may be summarized briefly in Fig. 13-14, along with the biosynthesis of tryptophan, which shares a portion of the same reactions.

Tryptophan. Tryptophan is an essential amino acid and is the only amino acid containing the indole ring. It undergoes reversible deamination in mammals, with the formation of the corresponding keto acid, β-3-indolepyruvic. This probably explains why either the D-form or the L-form of tryptophan or its keto acid can maintain nitrogen balance and growth in animals fed a low-tryptophan diet.

Many intermediate products of tryptophan degradation have been identified in the animal organism. Their formation from tryptophan is summarized in Fig. 13-15. One important metabolite of tryptophan is the B-vitamin nicotinic acid. The synthesis of this vitamin from tryptophan supplies about one half the total nicotinic acid requirement of man (p. 809). It has been estimated that 60 mg. of tryptophan in food proteins are converted to 1 mg. of nicotinic acid in man. Nicotinic acid (amide) forms the active group of NAD^+ and $NADP^+$ (p. 244).

The two major pathways for the degradation of tryptophan are (1) its oxidation to 5-hydroxytryptophan followed by decarboxylation to 5-hydroxytryptamine (serotonin), to be discussed later (p. 379), and (2) its oxidation

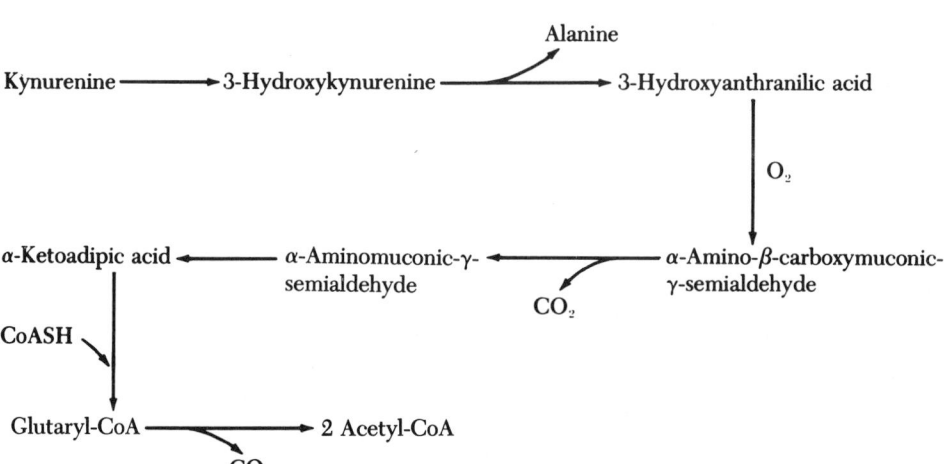

Fig. 13-16. Degradation of kynurenine (from tryptophan) to acetyl-CoA.

to kynurenine (Fig. 13-15), which is converted to a series of intermediates and by-products, some of which are excreted in the urine in relatively small amounts (kynurenic acid, quinaldic acid, xanthurenic acid, 8-hydroxyquinaldic acid, anthranilic acid, and 5-hydroxyanthranilic acid). These intermediates apparently have no known function in the body and are excreted in the urine, which fact emphasizes the inefficiency of the utilization of tryptophan in the body, despite its "essential" nature.

Kynurenine, however, may be metabolized further, as indicated in Fig. 13-16, to yield glutaryl-CoA and then two moles of acetyl-CoA. This accounts for glucogenesis from tryptophan (p. 364).

Still another pathway of the degradation of tryptophan, important because it occurs as a result of bacterial action in the large intestine, is the following:

$$\text{Tryptophan} \xrightarrow{\text{NH}_3} \text{Indolepyruvic acid} \xrightarrow{\text{CO}_2} \text{Indoleacetic acid}$$

$$\downarrow \text{CO}_2$$

$$\text{Indoxyl} \xleftarrow{\text{O}_2} \text{Indole} \xleftarrow[\text{CO}_2]{} \text{Skatoxyl} \xleftarrow{\text{O}_2} \text{Skatole}$$

Skatole and indole are partially responsible for the characteristic odor of feces. Some indoxyl may be reabsorbed from the large intestine, conjugated with sulfate in the liver, and excreted in the urine as indican (potassium salt).

Indican

If pyridoxine is lacking in the diet, nicotinic acid is not formed but xanthurenic acid results instead. Large amounts are excreted in the urine. Riboflavin also is needed for nicotinic acid formation (Fig. 13-16). It is interesting to note that pregnant women suffering from or threatened with eclampsia also have a deranged type of tryptophan metabolism. If given a test dose of tryptophan, they excrete in the urine much larger amounts of xanthurenic acid than do normally pregnant or nonpregnant women under the same conditions. Another derangement of tryptophan metabolism seems to occur in schizophrenia. It was found[22] that the output of urinary tryptamine (p. 696) in some patients is increased during periods of schizophrenic activity.

We have long known that after blood coagulates it possesses vasoconstrictor properties. In 1948, the active agent was isolated and crystallized by Page and others and was called *serotonin*. It was analyzed and found to be a complex of creatinine, sulfuric acid, and 5-hydroxytryptamine. Since the pharmacologic properties reside in the 5-hydroxytryptamine, which is separable from the complex, the name serotonin was assigned to this compound. It has been synthesized. Serotonin causes other types of tissue to contract, besides vascular tissue, and it may prove to be an important physiologic agent in other respects as well. Antimetabolites of serotonin have been produced. The derivation of serotonin from tryptophan is indicated below. Tryptophan is first oxidized to 5-hydroxytryptophan. This amino acid is then acted on by a specific decarboxylase to yield serotonin.

5-Hydroxytryptophan   5-Hydroxytryptamine
                                  (serotonin)

Tryptophan may be synthesized in certain microorganisms (*E. coli*) from erythrose-4-phosphate and phosphoenolpyruvate as precursors (refer again to Fig. 13-14).

Several hereditary disorders of tryptophan metabolism have been described. One of these is so-called *Hartnup disease*, named after the family in which it was discovered, due to the defective intestinal and renal transport of tryptophan and other monoamino-monocarboxylic acids. The neutral amino acids, including tryptophan, are excreted in the urine and feces in large amounts, at least five to 10 times the normal average. Fecal excretion of tryptophan is especially marked after a loading dose is given orally. There is also a high urinary excretion of indolylacetic acid and indican. A decreased conversion of tryptophan to kynurenine and nicotinamide occurs. The major clinical findings of a pellagra-like rash and mental aberrations and retardation appear to be due primarily to a lack of nicotinic acid formation from tryptophan. The biochemical defect in this disease is not known, although it would appear to be an impaired formation of the transport protein(s) for the neutral amino acids in the intestinal mucosa and renal tubule cells.

Another closely related hereditary disorder of tryptophan metabolism is the so-called *blue diaper syndrome* in infants (p. 394). It likewise appears to be due to impaired intestinal and renal absorption of tryptophan. The blue color of the diaper appears to be due to the oxidation of indole compounds excreted in the urine. The biochemical defect is not known, but an impaired biosynthesis of the intestinal and renal transport protein is suspected.

Cystine and cysteine. Since cystine and cysteine are readily interconvertible, it is probable that they undergo similar reactions in the body.

There is present in certain mammalian tissues an enzyme that rapidly converts cysteine to pyruvic acid, ammonia, and hydrogen sulfide. Possibly this reaction can occur to cysteine while it is in peptide linkage but only when it is at either end of the peptide chain. The formation of pyruvic acid accounts for the fact that cystine and cysteine are among the amino acids convertible to glucose. The sulfur may be oxidized and excreted as inorganic or organic sulfate or as part of the unoxidized sulfur of the urine.

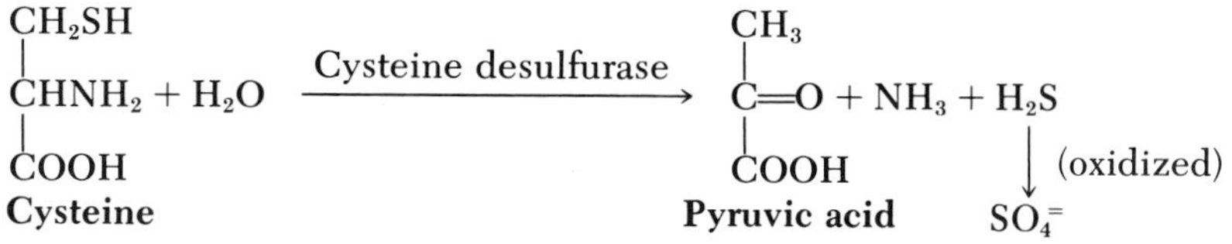

$$
\begin{array}{l}
\text{CH}_2\text{SH} \\
| \\
\text{CHNH}_2 + \text{H}_2\text{O} \xrightarrow{\text{Cysteine desulfurase}} \\
| \\
\text{COOH} \\
\textbf{Cysteine}
\end{array}
\qquad
\begin{array}{l}
\text{CH}_3 \\
| \\
\text{C=O} + \text{NH}_3 + \text{H}_2\text{S} \\
| \qquad\qquad\qquad | \;\;(\text{oxidized}) \\
\text{COOH} \qquad\quad \text{SO}_4^= \\
\textbf{Pyruvic acid}
\end{array}
$$

Cysteine may also be oxidized, in the rat, to cysteinesulfinic acid, which is then decarboxylated to form 2-aminoethanesulfinic acid, which has been named *hypotaurine*. Hypotaurine may be oxidized to taurine, or cysteine-

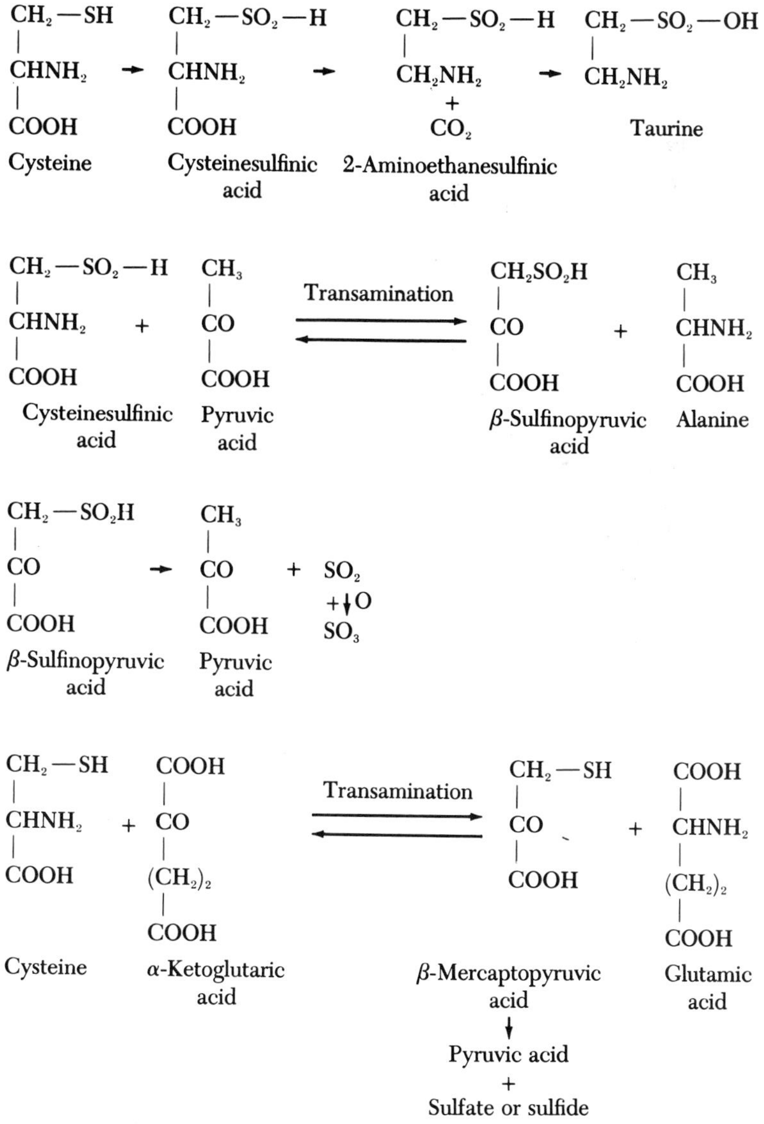

Fig. 13-17. Metabolic pathways of cysteine.

sulfinic acid may undergo transamination with pyruvic acid and eventually give rise to sulfur trioxide. Thus it is seen how sulfates are formed from cysteine.

A number of other reactions of cystine have been demonstrated. Some of them are shown in Fig. 13-17. Instead of pyruvic acid, α-ketoglutaric acid may enter into the transamination reaction, yielding glutamic acid. Cysteine itself may be transaminated with α-ketoglutaric acid, yielding β-mercapto-pyruvic acid, a compound rapidly converted to sulfate or sulfide, and pyruvic acid, by various tissues.[22] Besides taurine, other sulfur-containing compounds of physiologic importance are also derived from cysteine or cystine. Among these are insulin, coenzyme-A, glutathione, and vasopressin. Cysteine is also important in detoxication, as will be described later (p. 752).

Cysteine and cystine are formed in the animal organism from methionine, to be discussed on p. 383. Hence these amino acids are not classed as essential; they do, however, "spare" the requirement for methionine. Cystine occurs in the urine of certain individuals. *Cystinuria* is an inborn error of metabolism and is hereditary.[23] Persons suffering from cystinuria excrete this amino acid even on a protein-free diet. It has been shown that, in contrast to the normal subject, the individual with cystinuria excretes administered cystine rapidly with only a transient rise in the blood level. Indeed, the renal clearance of cystine in a patient with cystinuria was 30 times that in the normal subject, even though the blood level was somewhat lower. This observation is interpreted as evidence that the metabolic error is in the re-absorption of cystine in the renal tubule and that cystinuria is therefore renal in origin. Such an interpretation would also explain the presence of relatively large amounts of other amino acids in the urine of patients with cystinuria. The failure of cystine, when fed, to increase the urinary excretion of cystine in patients with cystinuria in earlier studies apparently is explainable on the basis of the insolubility and hence the poor intestinal absorption of cystine.

A second hereditary abnormality of cystine metabolism, *cystinosis* or cystine-storage disease, differing from cystinuria, has also been described. There is an excessive deposition of cystine, sometimes as distinct crystals, in various tissues, including the cornea and conjunctiva and the peripheral leukocytes.[24] The condition may appear in adults as well as in children. There is a generalized aminoaciduria, glycosuria, and in some cases rickets or osteomalacia. The cause of the condition is unknown but may be an impaired conversion of cystine to cysteine in the involved tissue due to a congenital deficiency of the enzyme cystine reductase.

L-Cysteine may be synthesized in the yeast and certain other microorganisms from L-serine as follows:

$$\text{L-Serine} + H_2S \xrightarrow[\text{sulfhydrase}]{\text{Serine}} \text{L-Cysteine}$$

Hydrogen sulfide is apparently formed in microorganisms from inorganic sulfate by the following route:

$$SO_4^= \xrightarrow[Mg^{++}]{ATP} \text{Adenosine-5'-phosphosulfate}$$

$$\begin{array}{cc} Mg^{++} & ATP \end{array}$$

$$H_2S \xleftarrow[\text{reductase}]{\text{Sulfite}} SO_3^= \xleftarrow{\text{Reductase}} \text{3'-Phosphoadenosine-5'-phosphosulfate}$$

Methionine. Methionine has two, perhaps three, principal metabolic pathways. The two primary routes involve transmethylation first, as will be discussed in some detail next. The remaining portion is then metabolized as indicated in Fig. 13-18. Transamination to the corresponding keto acid is thought to be a relatively minor pathway.

As is evident from Figs. 13-18 and 13-19, the principal routes of methionine involve the transfer of its methyl group by way of S-adenosylmethionine or N^5-methyltetrahydrofolic acid. These are discussed in more detail on pp. 355 and 821, respectively. The methyl group may be accepted by a variety of substances to form such important biochemical agents as creatine, epinephrine,

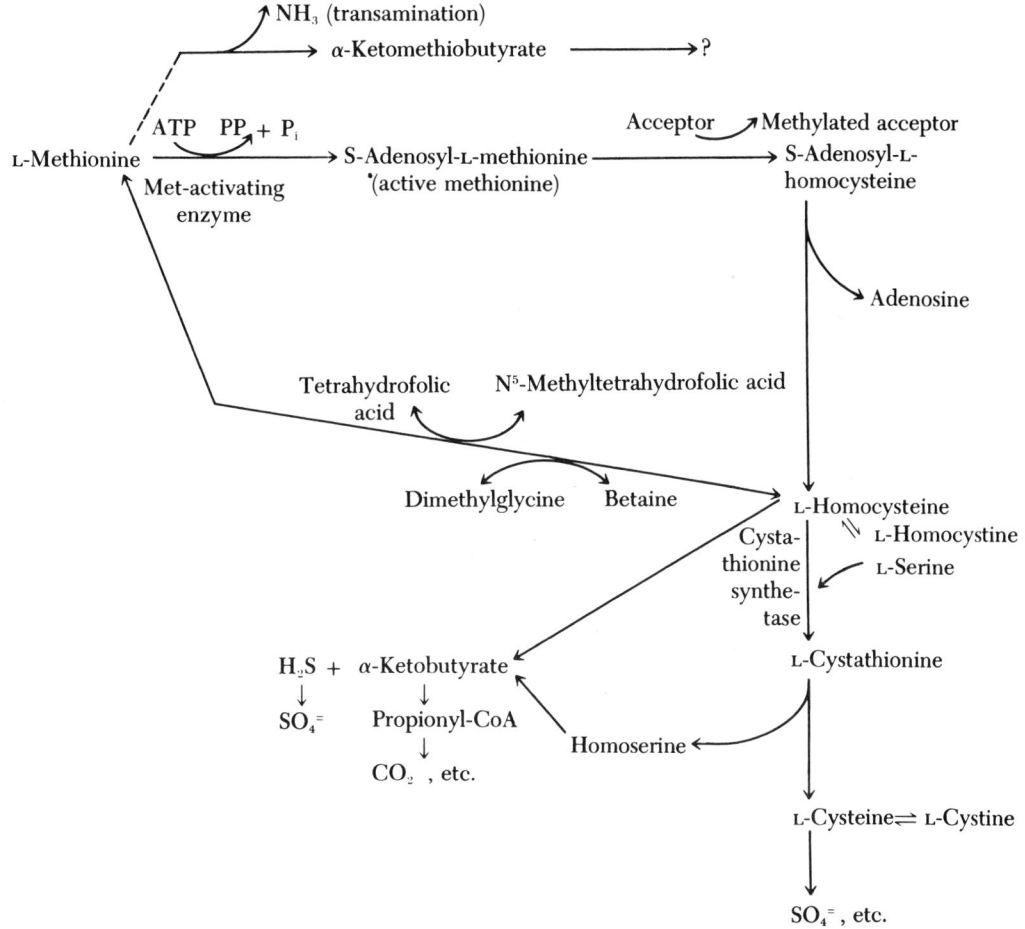

Fig. 13-18. Summary of major catabolic pathways for methionine.

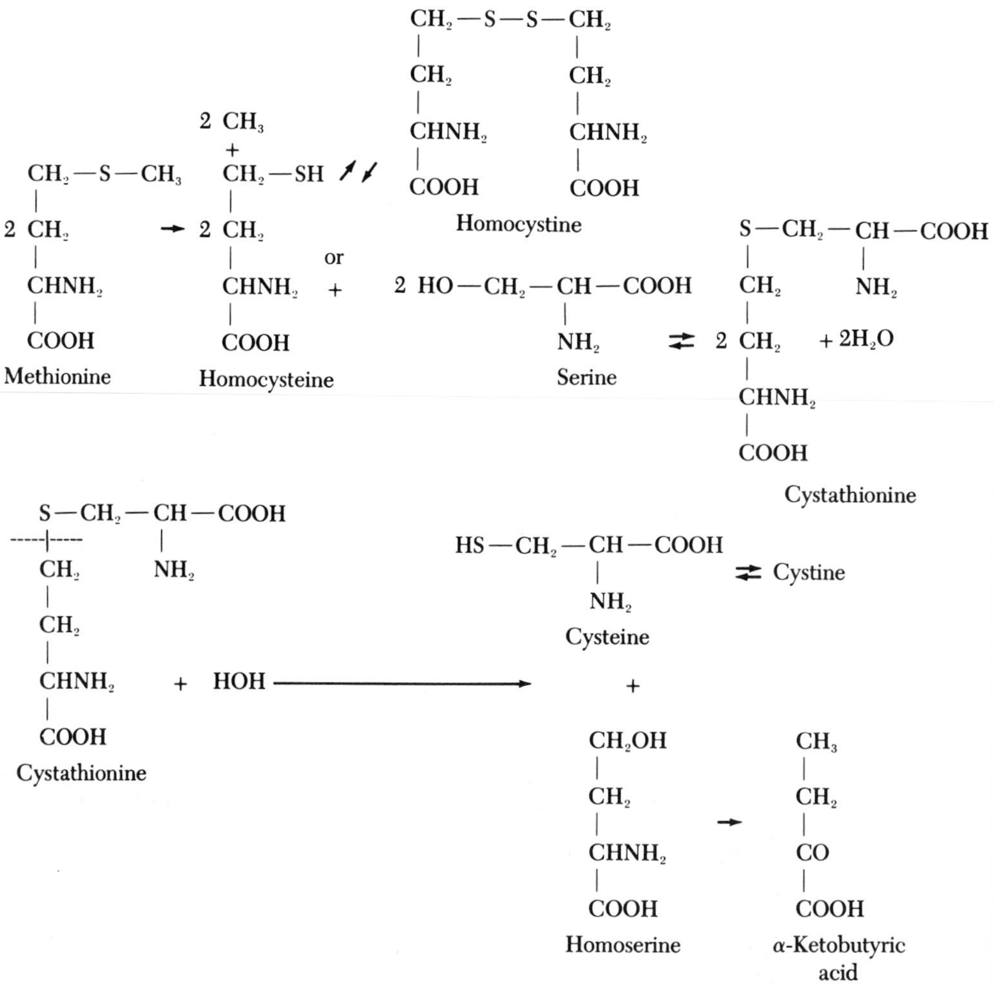

$$CH_2-S-S-CH_2$$

$$
\begin{array}{cc}
CH_2 & CH_2 \\
| & | \\
CHNH_2 & CHNH_2 \\
| & | \\
COOH & COOH
\end{array}
$$

Homocystine

$$
\begin{array}{ccc}
 & 2\ CH_3 & \\
 & + & \\
CH_2-S-CH_3 & CH_2-SH & \\
| & | & \\
2\ CH_2 & \longrightarrow\ 2\ CH_2 & \quad\text{or} \\
| & | & \\
CHNH_2 & CHNH_2 & +\quad 2\ HO-CH_2-CH-COOH \\
| & | & \\
COOH & COOH & NH_2 \\
\text{Methionine} & \text{Homocysteine} & \text{Serine}
\end{array}
$$

$$
\begin{array}{c}
S-CH_2-CH-COOH \\
| \qquad\qquad | \\
CH_2 \qquad\quad NH_2 \\
| \\
\rightleftarrows\ 2\ CH_2 \qquad +\ 2H_2O \\
| \\
CHNH_2 \\
| \\
COOH
\end{array}
$$

Cystathionine

$$
\begin{array}{c}
S-CH_2-CH-COOH \\
\text{-----|-----} \qquad | \\
CH_2 \qquad\quad NH_2 \\
| \\
CH_2 \\
| \\
CHNH_2 \qquad +\quad HOH \longrightarrow \\
| \\
COOH
\end{array}
$$

Cystathionine

$$HS-CH_2-CH-COOH$$
$$NH_2 \quad \rightleftarrows\ \text{Cystine}$$
Cysteine

$$+$$

$$
\begin{array}{cc}
CH_2OH & CH_3 \\
| & | \\
CH_2 & CH_2 \\
| & \longrightarrow \quad | \\
CHNH_2 & CO \\
| & | \\
COOH & COOH \\
\text{Homoserine} & \alpha\text{-Ketobutyric} \\
 & \text{acid}
\end{array}
$$

Fig. 13-19. Degradation of methionine.

choline, and trigonelline. Indeed, Meister lists some 54 compounds whose methyl groups are derived from methionine.

Methionine is an essential amino acid, whereas cystine is not; evidently the former can be changed to the latter, but cystine cannot be transformed to methionine. When methionine, containing isotopic sulfur, ^{35}S, was fed to animals, the isotopic sulfur was isolated from the tissue proteins. By similar experiments the pathway was indicated to be methionine $\rightarrow$ homocysteine, with the loss of a methyl group. The methyl group may be oxidized to carbon dioxide and water or may enter transmethylation reactions as described below. Homocysteine then may be oxidized to homocystine, or be converted to cysteine, after having been coupled with serine to yield cystathionine as an intermediate product. The cysteine then may be oxidized to cystine. The further catabolic pathway of cystine is the same as that described in the discussion of that amino acid. The remainder of the molecule may be converted to α-ketobutyric acid as indicated. The enzymes responsible for the formation of cystathionine and for its cleavage have been found to require pyridoxal phosphate as their coenzyme.

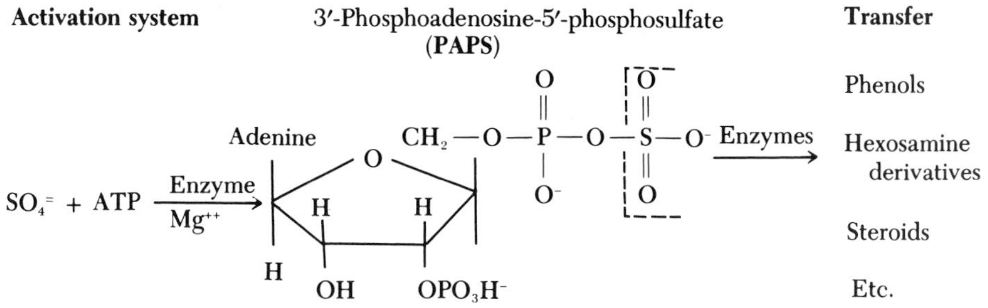

Fig. 13-20. Sulfate activation.

A hereditary defect of methionine metabolism, known as *cystathioninuria*, has been found in man. It appears to be caused by a failure of the cystathionine cleavage enzyme to bind pyridoxal phosphate to its apoenzyme.

A new inborn error of metabolism, *homocystinuria*, which involves the catabolism of methionine or more specifically its metabolic intermediates, homocysteine and homocystine, has been described.[25] Elevation of homocystine occurs in the plasma, resulting in an "overflow" into the urine amounting to as much as 50 to 100 mg. per day. It is associated usually with mental retardation in children or surviving adults. Skeletal deformities involving the spine, thorax, and vertebrae ("codfish vertebrae") may occur. Some affected individuals are extraordinarily tall with long extremities, frequently with flat feet, which "toe out." All have abnormal electroencephalographs and some experience seizures. There is a curious dislocation of the lens of the eye, which may be used as a clue to homocystinuria. The disease is apparently due to an autosomal recessive trait and occurs in approximately one in 20,000 live births. The basic biochemical lesion in the disease appears to be a deficiency in, or defect of, connective tissue, perhaps of the intercellular cement substance. It apparently is due to a genetic deficiency or absence of the enzyme cystathionine synthetase in the liver. As indicated previously, this enzyme converts homocysteine plus serine to cystathionine. Hence its deficiency results in an increase in the plasma level of homocystine and homocystinuria results.

Since sulfate is formed in the metabolism of sulfur-containing amino acids, the mechanism by which sulfate is metabolized should be considered next. Sulfate occurs, mostly in ester linkage, in a wide variety of physiologic compounds. The sulfate mucopolysaccharides, e.g., chondroitin sulfate and heparin, are important examples. The ethereal sulfates of the urine are conjugation products of phenols, indoxyl, and other compounds; these represent detoxication products. They are formed by sulfate transfer in which active sulfate is the mediator. Active sulfate is formed from inorganic sulfate and ATP, and then, with the aid of transfer enzymes, it transmits the sulfate to the compounds that are to be sulfated. The scheme shown in Fig. 13-20 illustrates these reactions.

Since methionine is an essential amino acid and cannot be formed in animal tissues, its synthesis in plants and microorganisms is of interest. Fig. 13-21

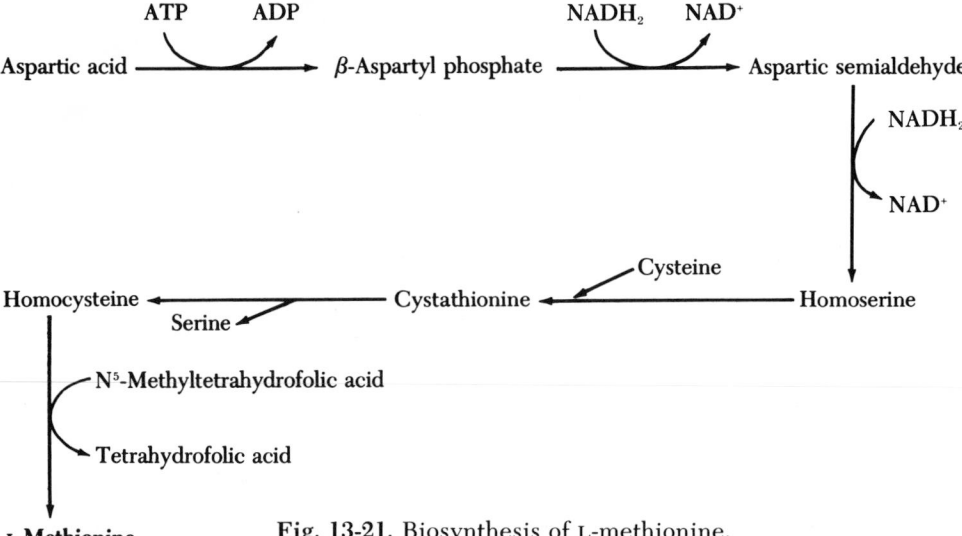

Fig. 13-21. Biosynthesis of L-methionine.

is a schematic diagram of the formation of methionine from aspartic acid in *E. coli*.

Aspartic acid, glutamic acid, asparagine, and glutamine. Under anaerobic conditions, succinic, fumaric, and malic acids have been found to arise from aspartic acid when it is added to minced muscle.

COOH	COOH	COOH	COOH
CH_2	CH_2	CH_2	CH
$CHNH_2$	CHOH	CH_2	CH
COOH	COOH	COOH	COOH
Aspartic acid	**Malic acid**	**Succinic acid**	**Fumaric acid**

Anaerobically, we would expect ketosuccinic acid (oxaloacetic acid) to be an intermediate in the catabolism of aspartic acid. Glutamic acid also gives rise to succinic acid anaerobically, but by oxidative deamination it is transformed to α-ketoglutaric acid.

COOH		COOH		COOH	
CH_2		CH_2		CH_2	
CH_2	$\xrightarrow{-H_2}$	CH_2	$\xrightarrow{+H_2O}$	CH_2	$+NH_3$
$CHNH_2$		C=NH		C=O	
COOH		COOH		COOH	
Glutamic acid		**α-Iminoglutaric acid**		**α-Ketoglutaric acid**	

Transamination also converts glutamic acid to α-ketoglutaric acid and aspartic acid to oxaloacetic acid. Both of these amino acids yield glucose in diabetic animals, and in each case three carbons are so utilized. Both bind ammonia, forming acid amides, and because of this are of importance in ammonia transport and also in ammonia formation.

$$
\begin{array}{ccc}
\begin{array}{c}
\text{COOH} \\
| \\
\text{CH}_2 \\
| \\
\text{CH}_2 \\
| \\
\text{CHNH}_2 \\
| \\
\text{COOH} \\
\textbf{Glutamic acid}
\end{array}
&
+ \text{NH}_3 \xrightarrow[\text{ATP, Mg}^{++}]{\text{Enzyme}}
&
\begin{array}{c}
\text{CONH}_2 \\
| \\
\text{CH}_2 \\
| \\
\text{CH}_2 \\
| \\
\text{CHNH}_2 \\
| \\
\text{COOH} \\
\textbf{Glutamine}
\end{array}
\quad + \text{H}_2\text{O}
\end{array}
$$

Glutamine synthetase, the enzyme that can effect this reaction, is present in kidney, brain, and retina. The mechanism for accomplishing this is as follows:

$$\text{Enzyme} + \text{ATP} \rightleftarrows \text{Enzyme-P} + \text{ADP}$$

$$\text{Enzyme-P} + \text{Glutamic acid} \rightleftarrows \text{Enzyme(glutamic acid)} + \text{P}$$

$$\text{Enzyme(glutamic acid)} + \text{NH}_3 \rightleftarrows \text{Enzyme} + \text{Glutamine}$$

On p. 560 it is mentioned that γ-aminobutyric acid is found in brain tissue. This arises from the decarboxylation of glutamic acid by a specific decarboxylase in brain tissue. It can then be transaminated with α-ketoglutaric to form glutamic acid again and succinic semialdehyde.

$$
\begin{array}{ccccccc}
\begin{array}{c}
\text{COOH} \\
| \\
\text{CHNH}_2 \\
| \\
\text{CH}_2 \\
| \\
\text{CH}_2 \\
| \\
\text{COOH} \\
\textbf{Glutamic acid}
\end{array}
& \rightleftarrows &
\begin{array}{c}
\text{NH}_2 \\
| \\
\text{CH}_2 \\
| \\
\text{CH}_2 \\
| \\
\text{CH}_2 \\
| \\
\text{COOH} \\
\textbf{γ-Aminobutyric} \\
\textbf{acid} + \textbf{CO}_2
\end{array}
& + &
\begin{array}{c}
\text{COOH} \\
| \\
\text{CH}_2 \\
| \\
\text{CH}_2 \\
| \\
\text{CO} \\
| \\
\text{COOH} \\
\textbf{α-Ketoglutaric} \\
\textbf{acid}
\end{array}
& \rightleftarrows &
\begin{array}{c}
\text{CHO} \\
| \\
\text{CH}_2 \\
| \\
\text{CH}_2 \\
| \\
\text{COOH} \\
\\
\textbf{Succinic} \\
\textbf{semialdehyde}
\end{array}
\; + \;
\begin{array}{c}
\text{COOH} \\
| \\
\text{CH}_2 \\
| \\
\text{CH}_2 \\
| \\
\text{CHNH}_2 \\
| \\
\text{COOH} \\
\textbf{Glutamic} \\
\textbf{acid}
\end{array}
\end{array}
$$

The hydrolysis of glutamine is catalyzed by glutaminases—there are two of them with different optimum pH's. Thus the enzyme that synthesizes glutamine is different from the one or ones that decompose it.

$$\text{Glutamine} + \text{H}_2\text{O} \xrightarrow[\text{Glutaminase}]{} \text{Glutamic acid} + \text{NH}_3$$

Another fact of interest in connection with glutamine is that it is capable of transamination with a variety of α-keto acids to yield α-ketoglutaramic acid. The latter is then hydrolyzed by a specific deamidase to produce α-ketoglutaric acid and ammonia. An example follows:

$$
\begin{array}{ccccc}
\begin{array}{c}
\diagup\text{NH}_2 \\
\text{C}{=}\text{O} \\
| \\
\text{CH}_2 \\
| \\
\text{CH}_2 \\
| \\
\text{CHNH}_2 \\
| \\
\text{COOH} \\
\textbf{Glutamine}
\end{array}
& + &
\begin{array}{c}
\text{CH}_3 \\
| \\
\text{C}{=}\text{O} \\
| \\
\text{COOH} \\
\textbf{Pyruvic acid}
\end{array}
& \rightleftarrows &
\begin{array}{c}
\diagup\text{NH}_2 \\
\text{C}{=}\text{O} \\
| \\
\text{CH}_2 \\
| \\
\text{CH}_2 \\
| \\
\text{C}{=}\text{O} \\
| \\
\text{COOH} \\
\textbf{α-Ketoglutaramic acid}
\end{array}
\; + \;
\begin{array}{c}
\text{CH}_3 \\
| \\
\text{HC}{-}\text{NH}_2 \\
| \\
\text{COOH} \\
\textbf{Alanine}
\end{array}
\end{array}
$$

$$\alpha\text{-Ketoglutaramic acid} \rightarrow \alpha\text{-Ketoglutaric acid} + \text{NH}_3$$

387

The corresponding acid amide of aspartic acid is asparagine. Asparagine apparently undergoes deamidation by asparaginase, and also transamination, in much the same manner as described above for glutamine. However, the enzymatic synthesis of asparagine has not yet been demonstrated from aspartic acid; but the formation of asparagine from α-ketosuccinamic acid has been demonstrated:

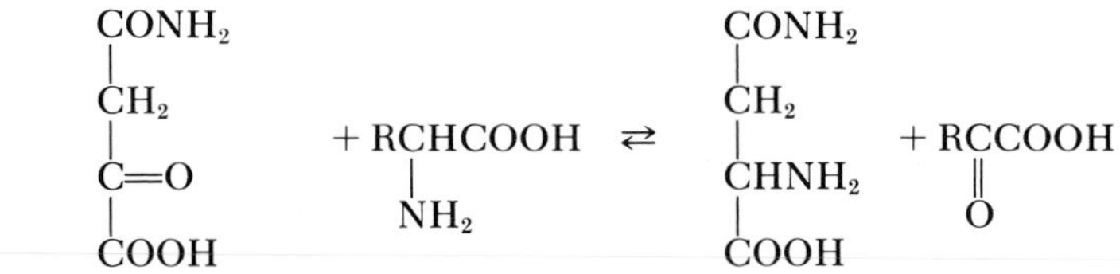

$$
\begin{array}{ccc}
\underset{\substack{| \\ \text{CH}_2 \\ | \\ \text{C}=\text{O} \\ | \\ \text{COOH}}}{\text{CONH}_2} + \underset{\substack{| \\ \text{NH}_2}}{\text{RCHCOOH}} \rightleftarrows & \underset{\substack{| \\ \text{CH}_2 \\ | \\ \text{CHNH}_2 \\ | \\ \text{COOH}}}{\text{CONH}_2} + \underset{\substack{\| \\ \text{O}}}{\text{RCCOOH}}
\end{array}
$$

α-Ketosuccinamic acid   Asparagine

Apparently glutamic and aspartic acids are formed in microorganisms and plants by the transamination of α-ketoglutaric and oxaloacetic acids, respectively, as they are in animals.

Lysine. Lysine, a diaminomonocarboxylic acid, is in a class by itself. It is the only amino acid that, once present in tissues, does not exchange its nitrogen by transamination with other amino acids circulating in the body fluids. When lysine is fed, however, it can give up its nitrogen to those amino acids

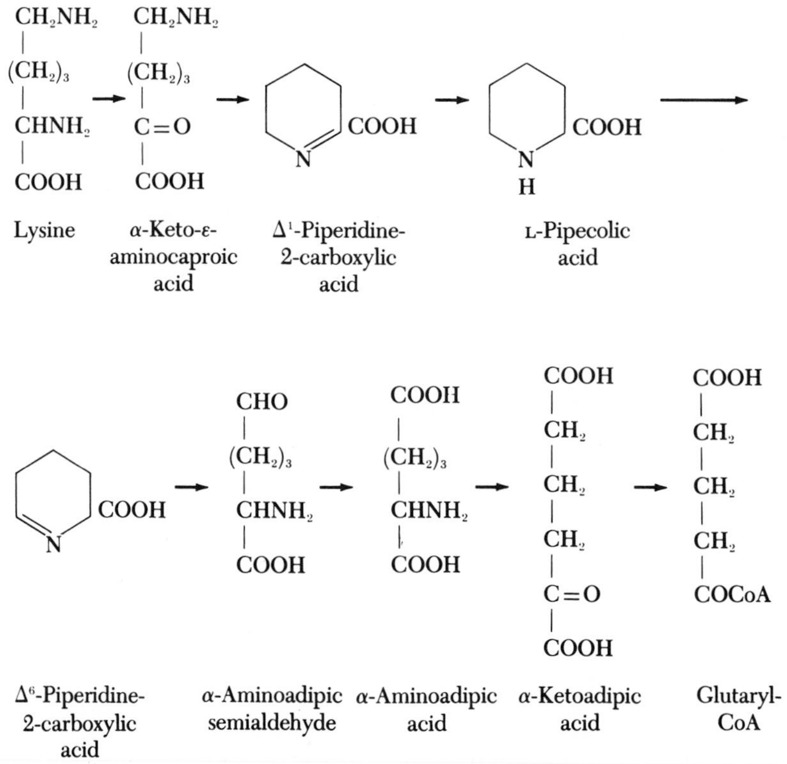

Fig. 13-22. Suggested pathway for the degradation of lysine.

present in the tissues just as the others do, but if it has lost its nitrogen, it cannot be reaminated. Since lysine can contribute its nitrogen in the direction just mentioned, it is deaminated. The nonnitrogenous residue does not yield either glucose or acetoacetic acid.

Using lysine containing an ϵ-labeled carbon, Borsook found that guinea pig liver converts lysine in vitro to α-aminoadipic acid. When the latter, similarly labeled, was the starting point, it was oxidatively deaminated to α-ketoadipic acid, which was then oxidatively decarboxylated to glutaric acid. (In the formulas below, labeled carbons are indicated by asterisks.)

$$
\begin{array}{cccc}
H_2C^*{-}NH_2 & C^*OOH & C^*OOH & C^*OOH \\
| & | & | & | \\
CH_2 & CH_2 & CH_2 & CH_2 \\
| & | & | & | \\
CH_2 \rightarrow & CH_2 \rightarrow & CH_2 \rightarrow & CH_2 \\
| & | & | & | \\
CH_2 & CH_2 & CH_2 & CH_2 \\
| & | & | & | \\
HC{-}NH_2 & HC{-}NH_2 & C{=}O & C^*OOH \\
| & | & | & \\
COOH & COOH & COOH & \\
\text{Lysine} & \text{α-Aminoadipic} & \text{α-Ketoadipic} & \text{Glutaric} \\
& \text{acid} & \text{acid} & \text{acid}
\end{array}
$$

Other studies have shown that L-pipecolic acid may be involved in this and perhaps other pathways of lysine metabolism (Fig. 13-22).

There is some doubt about the disposition of glutaric acid. Two pathways have been under consideration.

The above pathways (A and B) explain why lysine may be either glucogenic or ketogenic under different situations.

Several pathways for the biosynthesis of lysine appear to be available. That occurring in yeast is shown schematically in Fig. 13-23. Not all the reactions, especially the first, are completely understood at the present time.

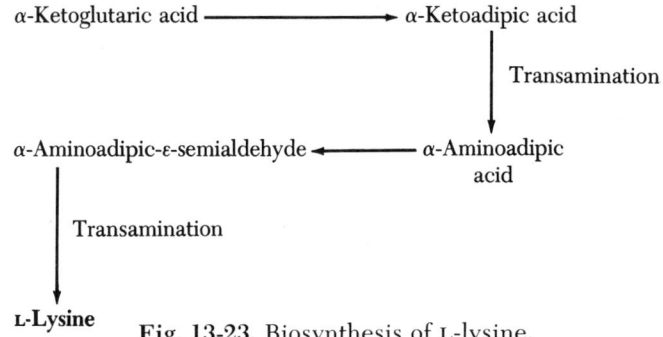

Fig. 13-23. Biosynthesis of L-lysine.

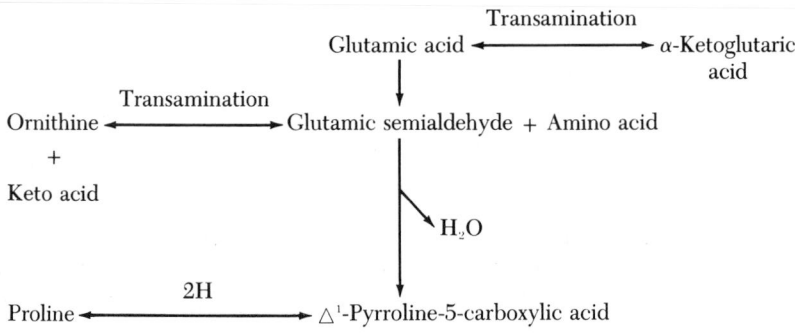

Fig. 13-24. Interconversions of ornithine, proline, and glutamic acid.

Arginine. Arginine takes part in the formation of urea (p. 359), yielding ornithine. All the ornithine thus formed does not continue in that cycle. Some may be converted to proline and glutamic acid. The conversion of ornithine to proline and glutamic acid is by way of glutamic semialdehyde (Fig. 13-24). Thus the ornithine from arginine may be converted to glutamic acid, then by transamination form α-ketoglutaric acid, and eventually via the citric acid cycle (p. 263) be metabolized or form glucose (p. 364).

Arginine, as will be seen, also contributes to the synthesis of creatine. It may be synthesized in the animal body from α-ketoglutaric acid or glutamic acid or proline by the reversal of the above process. The ornithine thus produced reacts with carbamyl phosphate, as in the formation of urea (p. 359), thus forming arginine.

Arginine is considered to be a semiessential amino acid. It can be synthesized in animal tissues at a rate sufficient for maintenance in the adult but not rapidly enough to support growth in the young animal. It is thus an essential amino acid for growth but not for maintenance.

Histidine. Histidine, like arginine, is a semiessential amino acid. A dietary protein source of histidine is needed for growth of the young animal (rat) because this amino acid is not synthesized in vivo at a sufficiently rapid rate. However, an amount adequate for the maintenance of nitrogen balance in the fully grown animal, including man, may be synthesized.

Histidine has several other important functions in addition to the general role of amino acids in tissue protein formation. Upon decarboxylation it forms histamine, which reduces blood pressure, is a vasodilator, and increases the

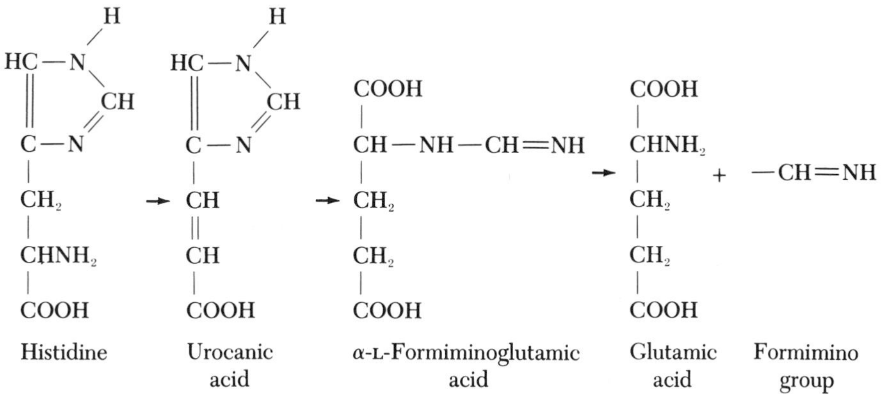

Fig. 13-25. Degradative pathway for histidine.

secretion of gastric juice. Allergic reactions appear to stimulate an excessive liberation of histamine. Histamine is converted to β-imidazoleacetic acid by the enzyme histaminase and is excreted in the urine. Histaminase is found in most tissues, a notable exception being the lungs. Consequently, large quantities of histamine may accumulate in lung tissue. Carnosine and anserine present in muscle extracts (p. 566) are β-alanyl dipeptides of histidine and 1-methylhistidine, respectively. Ergothionine, present in erythrocytes, liver, and brain, is the betaine of thiolhistidine. The functions of these dipeptides are not understood.

The degradation of histidine in animals occurs mainly in the liver. The major pathway and principal intermediates are shown in Fig. 13-25. Histidine is first converted to urocanic acid by the enzyme *histidase*, with the loss of ammonia from the amino group and adjacent hydrogen atom. The imidazole ring is then hydrolytically cleaved at the nitrogen-3, carbon-4 position by the enzyme *urocanase* to form an intermediate imidazolone propionic acid then formimino-L-glutamic acid. In the presence of tetrahydrofolic acid, the formimino group is removed as N^5-formiminotetrahydrofolic acid, or N^{10}-formyltetrahydrofolic acid plus ammonia, leaving L-glutamic acid, which is converted to α-ketoglutaric acid by transamination or metabolized otherwise, as described previously (p. 319). Histidine is thus a glucogenic amino acid (p. 364). N^5-Formiminoglutamic acid (FIGLU) and N^{10}-formyltetrahydrofolic acid may be used in one-carbon metabolism (p. 352). Interesting in this connection is the fact that FIGLU is excreted in the urine in folic acid deficiency (p. 821).

Another minor pathway for the degradation of histidine by transamination with pyruvate to form imidazolepyruvic acid, which is converted to imidazoleacetic acid and excreted in the urine, is known. During pregnancy, large amounts of histidine are excreted in the urine. This occurs from about the fifth week of pregnancy until a few days postpartum. The absence of histidase from the liver during this period accounts for the phenomenon, and the explanation given is that nature thus provides the fetus with a superabundance of this indispensable amino acid.

A hereditary disorder of histidine metabolism, histidinemia, has been described. Elevated levels of plasma and urinary histidine are found. The urine gives a greenish color when treated with ferric chloride, sometimes leading to the erroneous diagnosis of phenylketonuria. There is a deficiency of the enzyme histidase so that some histidine is diverted to alternate pathways. The metabolites imidazolepyruvic acid, imidazolelactic acid, and imidazoleacetic acid are also excreted in the urine. The disorder is rather benign, the principal symptom being speech defects, which may appear during childhood.

Histidine is synthesized in microorganisms by a rather complex series of reactions, similar to some of those involved in purine formation (p. 403). The pathway may be summarized schematically as in Fig. 13-26.

Proline and hydroxyproline. Malherbe and Krebs, after incubating kidney tissue with proline, found α-ketoglutaric acid, ammonia, and a substance believed to be glutamine. Other evidence in favor of this discovery is the fact that both proline and glutamic acid are glucogenic. The conversion of proline to glutamic acid and ornithine may be via the route shown below:

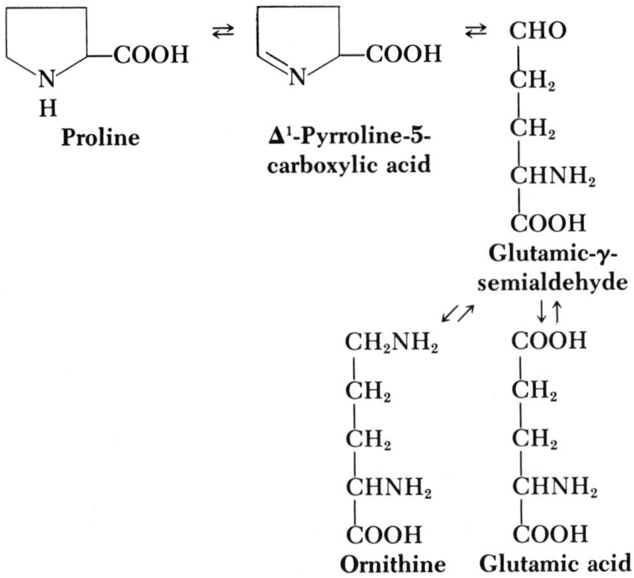

The first reaction is catalyzed by proline oxidase, and the second by a dehydrogenase. Both enzymes are found in liver mitochondria. The proline ring can also be opened by cleavage at a Δ^5–double bond by proline oxidase, as already mentioned. In this case, α-keto-δ-aminovaleric acid is produced.

Proline and ornithine are readily interconverted in the body (Fig. 13-24). Thus, another metabolic route is seen; i.e., proline may yield ornithine for urea synthesis, or ornithine may be broken down via proline. Proline is a nonessential amino acid and is readily formed in the organism from glutamic acid or ornithine by a reversal of the above reactions.

Hydroxyproline is metabolized by routes similar to those of proline. In fact, there is evidence from studies using purified enzyme systems from *Pseudomonas striata* that the L-hydroxyproline is converted to α-ketoglutaric semialdehyde. Hydroxyproline, like proline, is classed as a glycogenic amino acid. It is an important constituent of collagen (p. 545) and is formed from

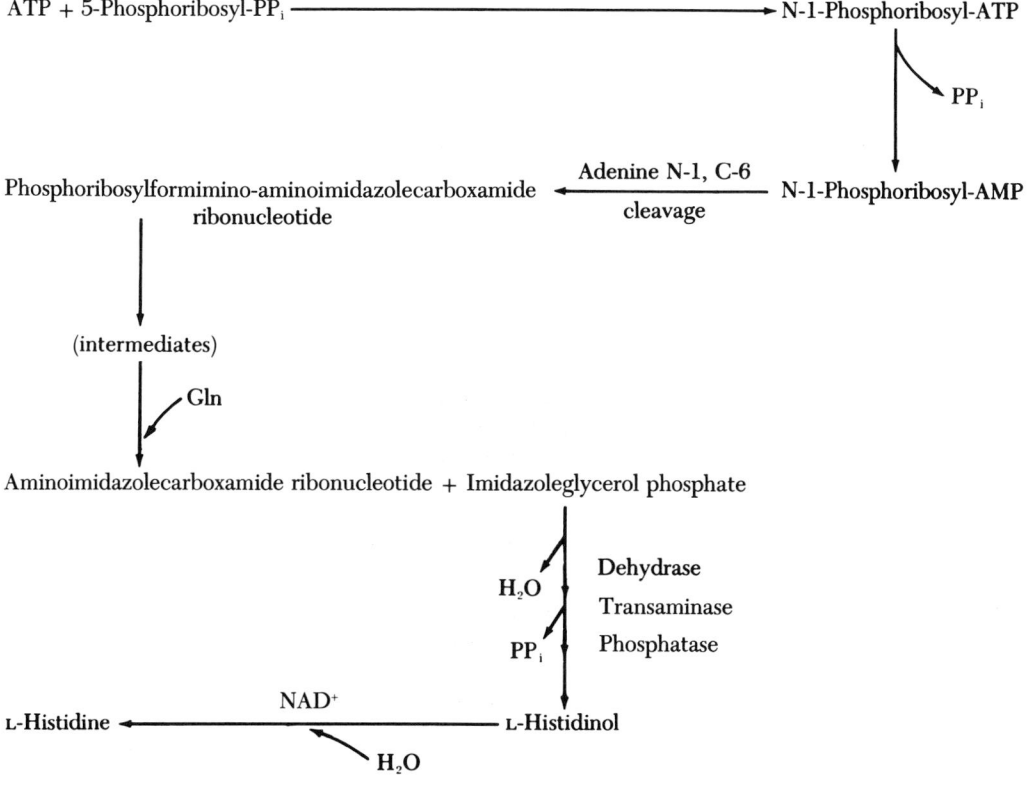

Fig. 13-26. Formation of L-histidine.

proline by the ascorbic acid–dependent, oxygen-utilizing hydroxylation of proline (p. 800), apparently after it has been incorporated into a polypeptide in collagen biosynthesis.

Hydroxyproline is metabolized in the liver by conversion into γ-hydroxyglutamic acid through Δ¹-pyrroline-3-hydroxy-5-carboxylic acid as an intermediate. Transamination then occurs with oxaloacetate to form α-hydroxy-γ-ketoglutaric acid and aspartic acid. The former is split by an aldolase-type reaction into glyoxylic acid and pyruvic acid, which are finally metabolized by now familiar routes.

The common form of hydroxyproline is 4-hydroxy and has been known for many years.

$$\begin{array}{c} \text{HO} \qquad\qquad \text{H}_2 \\ \text{H}_2 \qquad\quad\; \text{COOH} \\ \text{N} \\ \text{H} \end{array}$$
3-Hydroxyproline

3-Hydroxyproline also has been isolated recently from beef tendon collagen. Apparently the same enzymes act on it as on the 4-hydroxy form, resulting in similar reactions.

Table 13-4. Some primary hereditary disorders of amino acid metabolism

Disorder	Biochemical defect	Principal metabolite° increased in blood• and/or urine°
Albinism	Tyrosinase	Tyrosine metabolites°
Alkaptonuria	Homogentisic acid oxidase	Homogentisic acid•°
β-Aminoisobutyrate aciduria	BAIB-Glu transaminase	β-Aminoisobutyrate°
Ammonemia	Ornithine transcarboxylase	Ammonia•
Argininosuccinic aciduria	Argininosuccinidase	Argininosuccinic acid°
Blue diaper syndrome	Renal and intestinal transport of tryptophan	Indole derivatives,° tryptophan (feces)
Cerebromacular degeneration	Unknown (renal transport of histidine?)	Histidine and derivatives°
Citrullinuria	Argininosuccinate synthetase	Citrulline°
Cystathioninuria	Cystathionase	Cystathionine°
Cystinosis	Unknown (excess cystine deposit in tissue?)	Generalized aminoaciduria°
Cystinuria	Renal reabsorption	Cystine°
Glycinemia	Unknown	Glycine•
Glycinuria	Renal reabsorption	Glycine°
Hartnup disease	Intestinal and renal transport (TRP)	Tryptophan° and other neutral amino acids°
Histidinemia	Histidase	Histidine• and derivatives°
Homocystinuria	Cystathionine synthetase	Homocystine°°
Hyperlysinemia	Unknown	Lysine•
Hyperprolinemia—type I	Proline oxidase	Proline•° (also Gly, Hypro)
Hyperprolinemia—type II	Proline dehydrogenase	Proline•°
Hydroxyprolinemia	Hydroxyproline oxidase (?)	Hydroxyproline•° (also Pro, Gly)
Leucine intolerance	Unknown	Hypoglycemia
Lysine intolerance	Lysine transport	Lysine in feces
Maple syrup urine disease	Branched-chain keto acid decarboxylase	Keto acids of Leu, Ileu, Val, Met°
Mastocytosis	Histidine decarboxylase (excess)	Histidine and imidazole derivatives°
Methionine malabsorption	Intestinal transport	Methionine (in feces)
Methylmalonate aciduria	Methylmalonyl-CoA isomerase (vitamin B_{12})	Methylmalonate°
Phenylketonuria	Phenylalanine hydroxylase	Phenylalanine,•° phenylpyruvate, etc.°
Pheochromocytoma	Excess decarboxylase, Tyr → norepineprine, epinephrine	Norepinephrine,° epinephrine, etc.°
Tyrosinosis	p-Hydroxyphenylpyruvate oxidase (?)	Tyrosine,° p-hydroxyphenyl-pyruvate°
Valinemia	Valine transaminase (?)	Valine•°

° Solid circle (•) signifies increased in blood; open circle (°), increased in urine.

Several hereditary disorders of proline and hydroxyproline metabolism have been described (p. 394).

Two types of hyperprolinemia, resulting in increased blood and urine levels of proline, are known. The deficient enzymes are proline oxidase and Δ^1-pyrroline-5-carboxylic acid dehydrogenase, respectively. Both disorders are characterized clinically by mental retardation. Renal damage is also found in the first type. Hydroxyprolinemia possibly due to a lack of hydroxyproline oxidase has also been described. Increased urinary excretion of proline, hydroxyproline, and glycine is reported. Mental retardation and hematuria are prominent clinical features. Impaired renal reabsorption of proline and hydroxyproline, as well as of glycine, has been reported in *glycinuria*. Calcium oxalate kidney stones are a prominent clinical finding in this condition. (See Table 13-4.)

CREATINE AND CREATININE

Although creatine and creatinine are not α-amino acids and are not present as such in proteins, it is perhaps logical to consider them at this time since they are important biologic substances derived from the three amino acids glycine, arginine, and methionine.

Creatine is methylguanidineacetic acid and creatinine is its anhydride. Their close relation and the formula for phosphocreatine are shown below.

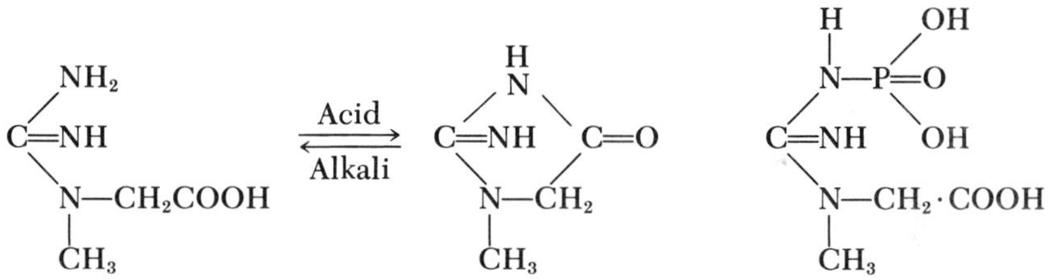

$$
\begin{array}{ccc}
\begin{array}{l}
\text{NH}_2 \\
| \\
\text{C}=\text{NH} \\
| \\
\text{N}-\text{CH}_2\text{COOH} \\
| \\
\text{CH}_3 \\
\textbf{Creatine}
\end{array}
&
\xrightarrow[\text{Alkali}]{\text{Acid}}
&
\begin{array}{l}
\text{H} \\
\text{N} \\
\text{C}=\text{NH} \quad \text{C}=\text{O} \\
| \\
\text{N}-\text{CH}_2 \\
| \\
\text{CH}_3 \\
\textbf{Creatinine}
\end{array}
\qquad
\begin{array}{l}
\text{H} \quad \text{OH} \\
\text{N}-\text{P}=\text{O} \\
\text{C}=\text{NH} \quad \text{OH} \\
| \\
\text{N}-\text{CH}_2\cdot\text{COOH} \\
| \\
\text{CH}_3 \\
\textbf{Phosphocreatine}
\end{array}
\end{array}
$$

The conversion of creatine to creatinine by acid is a quantitative reaction and is the method used when estimating this substance, since creatinine is easily determined. The reverse reaction is not quantitative. Phosphocreatine is a creatine derivative containing a labile high-energy phosphate bond (p. 254) and yields energy during muscle contraction. The physiologic relations between creatine and creatinine have puzzled biochemists for many years, and although many facts concerning these compounds are now known, there is still a great deal that is obscure. About 120 gm. of creatine and phosphocreatine are present in the human body, mostly in the muscles. Very little creatinine is found there. Neither creatine nor creatinine has been found among the hydrolysis products of any protein. Consequently, the origin of both creatine and creatinine presents a problem. A small part of this origin was considered in the discussion of transmethylation, i.e., of the methyl group. We should, however, inquire into the normal and pathologic occurrence of both compounds and their behavior, when administered, as well as any other available pertinent facts.

Since creatine is present in muscle tissue and is water soluble, it is found in meat, meat gravies, meat soups, and meat extracts. Phosphocreatine is so easily hydrolyzed to creatine and phosphoric acid that no phosphocreatine as such is present in our food.

Children regularly eliminate creatine in their urine in larger amounts than do adults. It was formerly believed that normal adult males excrete no creatine in their urine but that normal adult women excrete moderate amounts at irregular intervals. This has been the subject of controversy, but now creatine is recognized as a normal component of the urine of healthy men. It constitutes about 6% of the total creatine-creatinine output, i.e., about 60 to 150 mg. per day. Most women excrete about twice as much as men and do so much more irregularly. In about 20% of females, the excretion of creatine does not exceed that of the male. During pregnancy the output of creatine increases, and for 2 or 3 weeks postpartum it is found in even greater amounts than previously. The probable explanation for most of these facts is that the reaction creatine → creatinine takes place in the muscles and does so only when the muscles are functioning efficiently. The adult musculature is ordinarily more efficient than that of the child. In pregnancy, a large amount of uterine muscular tissue is formed and is not functioning, and postpartum the reduction of this tissue may release creatine stored up there. However, the same increased creatine output occurs after cesarean section and removal of the uterus. The output of creatine is also greater in starvation, carbohydrate deprivation, diabetes, hyperthyroidism, fevers, and malnutrition. In all these conditions there is an increased catabolism either of muscular tissue or of tissue proteins in general. Diseases peculiar to the musculature frequently are accompanied by creatinuria. In myasthenia gravis it is not always found, and in myotonia congenita it is seldom found; but in dystrophia myotonia (progressive muscular dystrophy) and in amyotonia congenita, creatine invariably appears in the urine. Creatine elimination is greatly increased in rheumatoid arthritis but not in osteoarthritis.

The relation of creatine to creatinine was investigated at an early date by feeding creatine to animals. The first trials seemed to indicate that creatine is not converted to creatinine in the body. Rose fed doses of 10 or 20 gm. of creatine to men and found increases in urinary creatinine of only about 0.2 to 0.5 gm., the bulk of the creatine being eliminated unchanged. Administration of creatinine, however, did not lead to a formation of creatine, and most of the creatinine was excreted. No urea was formed from either compound. It is evident, then, that creatine → creatinine in the body is not reversible. This was corroborated by Benedict and Osterberg, who fed a dog small amounts of creatine daily for 70 days. Appreciable amounts of creatine began to be excreted after 10 days, and "extra" creatinine appeared after a week of creatine feeding. The creatinuria occurred as long as the feeding continued, but the increased elimination of creatinine persisted much longer. Almost half the creatine fed could not be accounted for. The experiment therefore indicates that although creatine is converted to creatinine in the body this is not the only pathway for its catabolism. Isotope experiments have given more direct evidence of this relationship. Bloch and Schoenheimer[26] fed small amounts of creatine containing ^{15}N to adult rats. This ^{15}N was found to be present in the creatine of muscle and internal organs, as well as in urinary creatinine. In a second series the tissue creatine was labeled with isotopic nitrogen by feeding isotopic creatine during a preliminary period. Then, when creatine feeding was discontinued, the isotopic content of the urinary creatinine was identical with that of the body creatine. These facts indicate (1) that creatine in the diet can be absorbed and can replace the creatine of the tissues and (2) that on a creatine-free diet, the tissue creatine is the sole source of urinary creatinine. When isotopic creatinine was fed, however, no isotopic nitrogen was found in the tissue creatine, again emphasizing the fact that creatine $\rightarrow$ creatinine is biologically irreversible.

Creatinine is always present in the urine. It is an end product of creatine metabolism. The daily output on a creatine-creatinine–free diet is almost constant for a given individual, and the amount in milligrams excreted per day per kilogram of body weight is called the creatinine *coefficient*. The creatine present in the urine should be added to the creatinine. For most normal men the creatinine coefficient varies between 18 and 32, with an average of about 25, and for women the normal range is between 9 and 26, with an average of about 18. Children have lower values. In general, the better the muscular development, the higher is the creatinine coefficient. Consequently, obese individuals are likely to have low coefficients because much of their weight is not muscle. This indicates that every individual has a characteristic creatine-creatinine turnover dependent, in a general way, on the amount of functioning muscle *tissue* but independent of the degree of muscular *activity*. Lindquist found that when phosphocreatine is hydrolyzed in vitro at 38° C. about 10% is converted to creatinine. This led him to surmise that similarly, in the living organism, part of the phosphocreatine spontaneously goes to form creatinine; hence the fact that the daily output of creatinine varies with the *total amount of musculature* was deduced. The reaction of phosphocreatine, resulting in the transfer of phosphate to some acceptor, does not yield creatinine, which harmonizes with the fact that the creatinine output is not related to muscular activity.

The creatine content of the body is derived, in part, from creatine in the diet. Any creatinine in the diet, of course, cannot be utilized as such. However, as has been said, on a creatine-creatinine–free diet there is a constant output of creatinine. This indicates a synthesis of creatine by the body. How does such a synthesis arise? We cannot even touch on the many earlier experiments in this field. Suffice it that Bloch and Schoenheimer[26] by isotopic experiments very beautifully elucidated the mechanism, although it must be said that many investigators had previously brought evidence tending in the same direction. Feeding a number of possible precursors containing ^{15}N, they found that arginine and glycine are the only natural amino acids investigated so far that are precursors, to any considerable extent, of creatine. Each of these two supplies nitrogen to different parts of the creatine molecule, as the scheme below shows. The methyl group may be derived from methionine, choline, or betaine.

$$
\begin{array}{ccccccc}
\underset{\text{proteins}}{\overset{\text{From}}{\downarrow}} & \underset{\text{arginine}}{\overset{\text{From}}{\downarrow}} & & & \underset{\text{or choline}}{\overset{\text{From methionine}}{\downarrow}} & & \\
\underset{|}{NH_2} & \underset{|}{NH_2} & & NH_2 & \overset{+\,CH_3}{} & NH_2 & \\
CH_2COOH & +\ C{=}NH & \xrightarrow{\text{(in kidney)}} & C{=}NH & \xrightarrow{\text{(in liver)}} & C{=}NH & \\
& | & & NH & & N{-}CH_3 & \\
& & & CH_2COOH & & CH_2COOH &
\end{array}
$$

Glycine **Amidine group** **Guanidoacetic acid or glycocyamine** **Creatine**

Very small amounts of isotopic creatine were found to arise after feeding isotopic ammonia, leucine, tyrosine, and glutamic acid. Apparently these are indirect creatine precursors. When isotopically labeled glycine was fed to patients with severe progressive muscular dystrophy, differences in the distribution of the isotope in the creatine and creatinine excreted indicated that urinary creatine does not originate in muscle but represents freshly synthesized creatine that cannot be absorbed by muscle. It is presumably synthesized in liver in this disease, which may also be the case normally.

To summarize creatine and creatinine metabolism:

1. Creatine is an essential physiologic constituent of the body. Under conditions of maximum muscular efficiency, it is not excreted as such.
2. Creatine is converted to creatinine physiologically. The amount of creatinine excreted is fairly constant and bears some relation to total musculature.
3. Tissue creatine may be obtained from food creatine but is largely synthesized. Glycine and the guanidine group from arginine unite to form glycocyamine; then a methyl group from methionine is added to complete the synthesis.
4. Creatinine is a waste product and is not converted to creatine.

References

GENERAL

Beaumont, W.: Experiments and observations on the gastric juice and the physiology of digestion, 1833 (facsimile of original edition), New York, 1959, Dover Publications, Inc.

Bender, M. L., and Kézdy, F. J.: Mechanism of action of proteolytic enzymes, Ann. Rev. Biochem. 34:49, 1965.

Blondy, P. K., and Rosenberg, L. E., editors: Duncan's diseases of metabolism, ed. 6, Philadelphia, 1969, W. B. Saunders Co.

Effron, M. L.: Aminoacidurias, New Eng. J. Med. 272:1058, 1965.

Greenberg, D. M., editor: Metabolic pathways, ed. 3, New York, 1969, Academic Press, Inc., vols. 1, 3.

Greenstein, J. P., and Winitz, M.: Chemistry of the amino acids, New York, 1961, John Wiley & Sons, Inc.

Hsai, D. Y.: Inborn errors of metabolism, ed. 2, Chicago, 1966, Year Book Medical Publishers, Inc.

Meister, A.: Biochemistry of amino acids, New York, 1965, Academic Press, Inc.

Munro, H. N., and Allison, J. B., editors: Mammalian protein metabolism, New York, 1964, Academic Press, Inc.

Neurath, H., editor: The proteins: composition, structure, and function, ed. 2, New York, 1963-1966, Academic Press, Inc.

Schoenheimer, R.: The dynamic state of body constituents, Cambridge, Mass., 1942, Harvard University Press.

Stanbury, J. B., Wyngaarden, J. B., and Fredrickson, D. S., editors: The metabolic basis of inherited disease, ed. 2, New York, 1966, McGraw-Hill Book Co.

Umbarger, H. E.: Regulation of amino acid metabolism, Ann. Rev. Biochem. 38:323, 1969.

Wiseman, G.: Absorption from the intestine, New York, 1964, Academic Press, Inc.

SPECIAL

1. Dopheide, T. A. A., et al.: J. Biol. Chem. **242**:1833, 1967.
2. Janowitz, H. D., and Hollander, F.: Gastroenterology **17**:591, 1961.
3. Taylor, H. H.: Physiol. Rev. **42**:519, 1962.
4. Walsh, K. A., et al.: Proc. Nat. Acad. Sci. **51**:301, 1964.
5. Neurath, H.: Sci. Amer. **211**:68, 1964.
6. Townes, P. L.: J. Pediat. **66**:275, 1965.
7. Miller, D., and Crane, R. K.: Amer. J. Clin. Nutr. **12**:220, 1963.
8. Orten, A. U.: J. Mich. Med. Soc. **58**:767, 1959; Fed. Proc. Sympos. **22**:1103, 1963.
9. Christensen, H. N.: Science **158**:525, 1967.
10. Oxender, D. L., et al.: Science **161**:182, 1968.
11. Elsas, L. J., and Rosenberg, L. E.: Proc. Nat. Acad. Sci. **57**:377, 1967.
12. Swendseid, M. E., et al.: Science **158**:129, 1967.
13. Snyderman, S. E., et al.: J. Nutr. **78**:57, 1962.
14. Meister, A.: Advances Enzym. **16**:185, 1955.
15. Du Vigneaud, V.: Biol. Sympos. **5**:234, 1941.
16. Rosenberg, L. E.: New Eng. J. Med. **281**:145, 1969.
17. Calvo, R. A., and Calvo, J. M.: Science **151**:1107, 1967.
18. Lilljequist, A. C., and Hsai, Y. E.: New Eng. J. Med. **278**:1319, 1968.
19. Fallon, H. J., et al.: J. Nutr. **96**:220, 1969.
20. Woolley, D. W., et al.: Science **144**:883, 1964.
20a.Perry, T. L., et al.: New Eng. J. Med. **282**:761, 1970.
21. Waisman, H. A., and Harlow, H. F.: Science **147**:685, 1965.
22. Brune, C. G., and Himwich, H. E.: Recent Advances Biol. Psychiat. **5**:144, 1963.
23. Rosenberg, L. E.: Science **154**:1341, 1966.
24. Schneider, J. A., et al.: New Eng. J. Med. **279**:1253, 1968.
25. Gerritson, T., et al.: Arch. Dis. Child. **38**:425, 1963; Mudd, S. H., et al.: Science **143**:1443, 1964.
26. Bloch, K., and Schoenheimer, R.: J. Biol. Chem. **131**:111, 1939.

CHAPTER 14

METABOLISM OF NUCLEOTIDES AND PURINE AND PYRIMIDINE BASES

After nucleic acids are liberated in the intestinal tract from food nucleoproteins by the action of proteases, the polynucleotides are depolymerized and split into their constituent nucleotides by the *nucleases* found in the small intestine. The nucleotides are attacked by *nucleotidases*, yielding phosphoric acid and purine and pyrimidine nucleosides. These nucleosides are probably absorbed as such and are then further degraded by a phosphorolytic process to yield the individual purine and pyrimidine bases.

Despite the existence in the cell of mechanisms for utilizing preformed purines and pyrimidines, most of the bases actually used for synthetic purposes are synthesized from very simple metabolic precursors. The dietary purines are excreted as uric acid, while the pyrimidines are further degraded and metabolized via other metabolic pathways.

METABOLIC FATE OF NUCLEIC ACIDS

At the present time, it is presumed that the intestinal digestion of nucleic acids and their catabolism in tissues proceed by relatively similar pathways. In either situation the initial process is one of depolymerization by enzymes called *deoxyribonuclease* and *ribonuclease*, which are specific for DNA and RNA, respectively. The deoxyribonuclease found in the pancreas, essential for the digestion of dietary DNA, is an enzyme that splits the 3',5'-phosphodiester linkages to produce large pieces, or oligonucleotides, with 5'-phospho terminal ends. It does not produce a large amount of mononucleotides. Another phosphodiesterase or deoxyribonuclease is found in the spleen. This enzyme also produces large pieces but hydrolyzes the bond between the phosphate and the 5'-carbon of the nucleotide. Thus its products are 3'-phospho terminal nucleotides. Intestinal mucosa and various organs, e.g., the liver, contain a ribonuclease that is a phosphodiesterase acting on the phosphate bonds of RNA linked to the 5'-carbon, thus releasing 3'-phosphonucleotides. This enzyme requires a pyrimidine base to be part of the nucleoside contributing the 3'-phospho terminus (diagram below). An intermediate stage in the hydrolysis of RNA by ribonuclease is the formation of a 2',3'-phosphodiester linkage (p. 116). When this step is prohibited, as when the 2'-carbon is reduced (DNA), or blocked, as by methylation (p. 352), the activity of the enzyme is abolished.

Pancreatic RNase

In the intestine the oligonucleotides are further hydrolyzed to individual nucleotides, which, in turn, are attacked by phosphatases removing the terminal phosphoric acid. These enzymes are called *nucleotidases;* their products are nucleosides. Intestinal absorption of nucleic acid breakdown products appears to occur primarily at this stage. The nucleosides absorbed are then degraded in the liver and other tissues by *nucleosidases,* which release the purine and pyrimidine bases by a phosphorolytic process.

$$\text{Purine nucleoside} \xrightarrow[P_i]{} \text{Ribose-1-P} + \text{Purine}$$

A similar process yields pyrimidines.

The adenine from dietary nucleic acids may be used, in part at least, for the synthesis of nucleic acids in the tissues. This scavenging process is, however, not essential to nucleic acid production; most is derived from nucleotides newly synthesized in the cells.

CATABOLISM OF PURINES

Adenine is degraded further in mammals beginning at the nucleoside stage. Thus, adenosine is deaminated by means of a specific enzyme, *adenosine deaminase*. Guanine, on the other hand, is deaminated as the purine base by the enzyme *guanase*. The product, xanthine, is then oxidized to uric acid by the flavoprotein enzyme, *xanthine oxidase*. The reaction with xanthine is as follows:

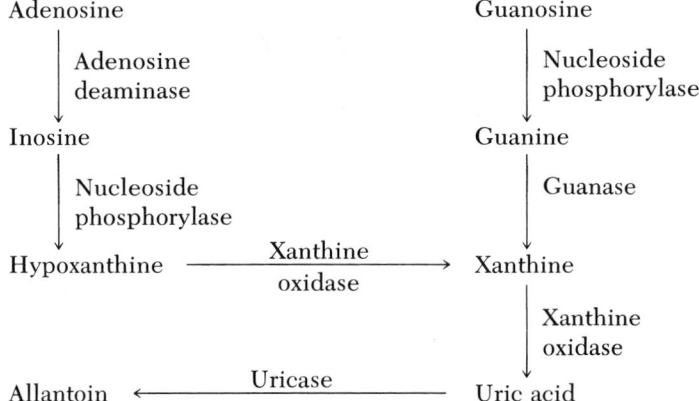

The same enzyme oxidizes hypoxanthine in an analogous manner. The overall pathway for the degradation of purines has been suggested to be as follows

Adenosine   Guanosine

    Adenosine   Nucleoside
    deaminase   phosphorylase

Inosine   Guanine

    Nucleoside   Guanase
    phosphorylase

Hypoxanthine   → Xanthine → Xanthine
         oxidase

                            Xanthine
                            oxidase

Allantoin   ← Uricase   Uric acid

Uric acid, the end product of purine metabolism in man, is excreted in the urine at a rate of 0.4 to 0.8 gm. per 24 hours. This level of excretion is somewhat dependent on the diet so that with diets rich in nucleoproteins or purines the uric acid content is much higher than ordinarily. The urinary excretion of uric acid by human subjects is partly regulated by the endocrine hormones. The administration of 11-hydroxysteroids of the adrenal cortex or of ACTH causes an increased excretion. It is not known whether this is due to an increased biosynthesis or to an increased elimination of uric acid.

In many mammals, with the exception of man and the anthropoid ape, uric acid is further degraded to allantoin by the enzyme uricase.

CATABOLISM OF PYRIMIDINE

The metabolic fate of the pyrimidines is still not completely known. However, cytosine appears to be deaminated to uracil and then oxidized through several steps to β-alanine and malonic semialdehyde. The ultimate product, succinyl-CoA, is utilized in the citric acid cycle. Thymine is oxidized via a similar sequence of steps to methylmalonyl semialdehyde and then to succinyl-CoA and the citric acid cycle. The steps involved in the degradation of pyrimidines by the liver are shown in the following scheme:

As has already been indicated, preformed dietary purines and pyrimidine bases do not represent essential precursors for the biosynthesis of nucleic acids.

BIOSYNTHESIS OF PURINES

Early experiments using isotopically labeled compounds showed that both purines and pyrimidines are synthesized from amino acids, carbon dioxide, and formate. For example, Barnes and Schoenheimer fed ammonium salts labeled with the heavy isotope of nitrogen (^{15}N) to pigeons and rats. Pigeons were first used because birds excrete a larger part of their waste nitrogen as uric acid rather than as urea. The ^{15}N was found in the uric acid of the excreta as well as in the purines and pyrimidines isolated from nucleic acids. In rats the same observations were made although the amount of purines and pyimidines synthesized was not as great because a large fraction of the isotopic nitrogen was lost as urea.

When ^{15}N-labeled glycine was fed to man, the end product of purine catabolism, uric acid (p. 402), was found to contain the isotope in the 7-position. In other words, nitrogen-7 of the purine ring is derived from the amino acid glycine. Other studies showed that nitrogen in position-1 (N-1) is from the amino group of aspartic acid (or glutamic acid) whereas the amide nitrogen of glutamine becomes N-9 and probably N-3. Glycine contributes its carboxyl carbon to the 4-position (C-4) and its α-carbon to C-5. This amino acid provides C-4 and C-5 as well as N-7 in a single intact unit. Formate, carried as the formyl derivative of tetrahydrofolic acid, contributes C-2 and C-8, while carbon dioxide becomes C-6. Thus it appears that the precursors of purines are glycine and other amino acids from proteins, carbon dioxide, formate, and a number of other intermediates that yield these compounds in metabolism.

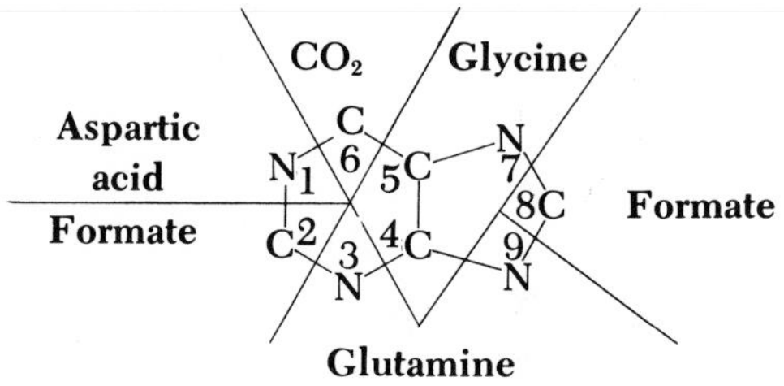

Sources of individual atoms in the purine complex

The biosynthesis of purines begins with ribose-5-phosphate, an intermediate in carbohydrate metabolism (p. 209). Ribose-5-phosphate is converted to 5-phosphoribosyl-1-pyrophosphate (PRPP) by the transfer of the pyrophosphate group from ATP to C-1 of the ribose.

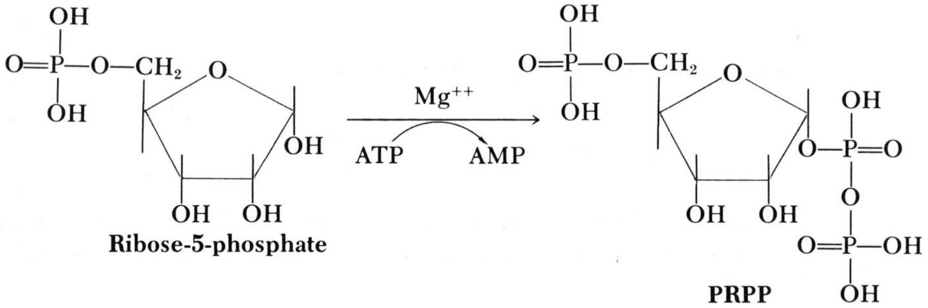

PRPP is subsequently aminated, by the addition of an amino group from glutamine, to form the amino sugar 5-phosphoribosyl-1-amine. The diagram below shows that C-1 now has the β-configuration:

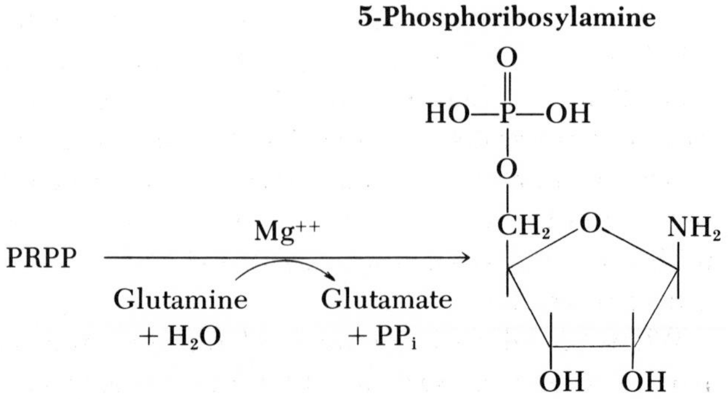

The amino sugar is combined next with the amino acid glycine to yield the amide, glycinamide ribonucleotide, which is often abbreviated GAR.

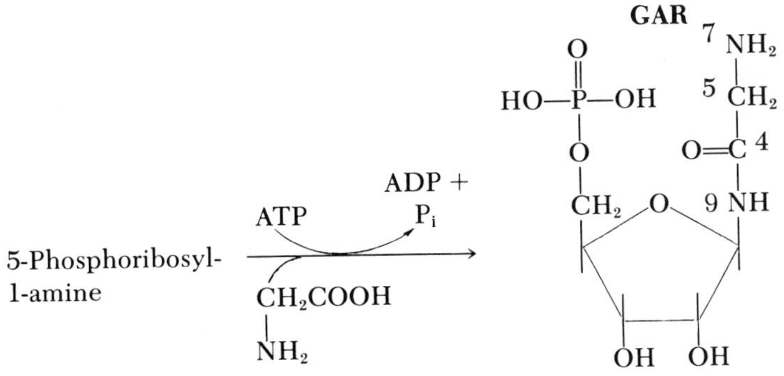

This compound serves as the source of C-4 and C-5 as well as N-7 and N-9 in the purine ring structure (the numbers in the diagram refer to the positions of C and N in the purine ring). The remaining atoms are then added as indicated in Fig. 14-1. A formyl group is transferred to the free amino group of GAR to form N-formylglycinamide ribonucleotide (FGAR). The vitamin tetrahydrofolic acid is important at this stage because its formylated derivative serves as a carrier of the C-1 entity. Glutamine and ATP are again involved in the amination of C-4 to yield the glycinamidine compound FGAM. When ring closure occurs, the product is 5-aminoimidazole ribonucleotide (AIR).

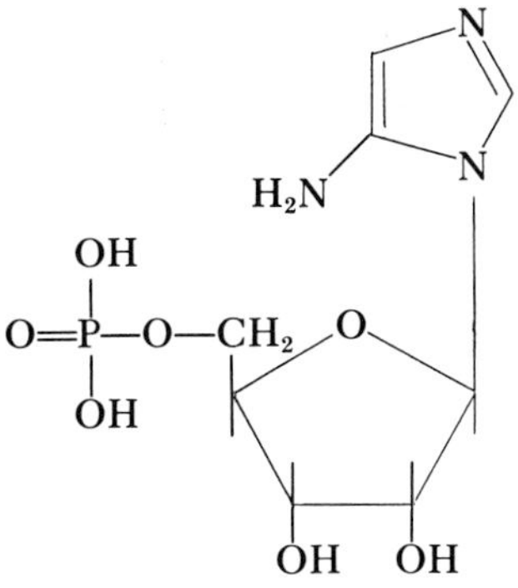

AIR

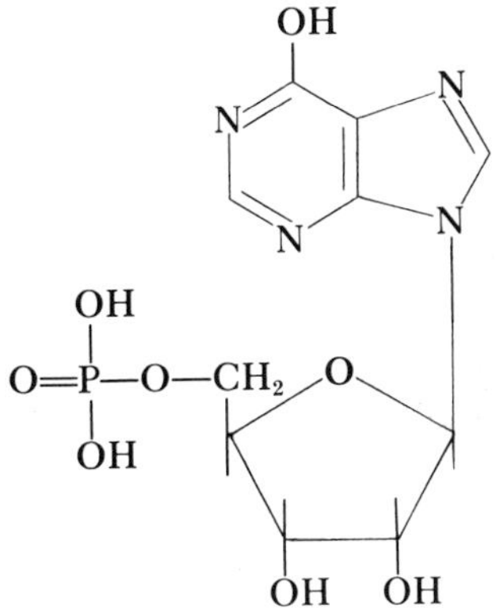

Inosinic acid

The remaining steps of the biosynthetic pathway are indicated diagrammatically in Fig. 14-1. The various enzymes[1] and cofactors, with the numbers corresponding to those on the diagram, are as follows: (1) amidotransferase; (2) ATP, Mg^{++}; (3) transformylase, THFA; (4) and (5) ATP, Mg^{++}; (6) kinosynthetase, biotin, ATP, Mg^{++}; (7) adenylosuccinase; (8) transformylase; (9) $NADPH_2$; (10) NAD^+; (11) ATP, Mg^{++}; (12) adenylosuccinate synthetase, GTP, Mg^{++}; (13) adenylosuccinase.

Inosinic acid is the first purine nucleotide formed.

Adenylic acid and guanylic acid are then formed by the amination of inosinic acid via the nitrogen of glutamine and aspartic acid. These nucleotides are incorporated into nucleic acids, or they may serve other metabolic purposes.

405

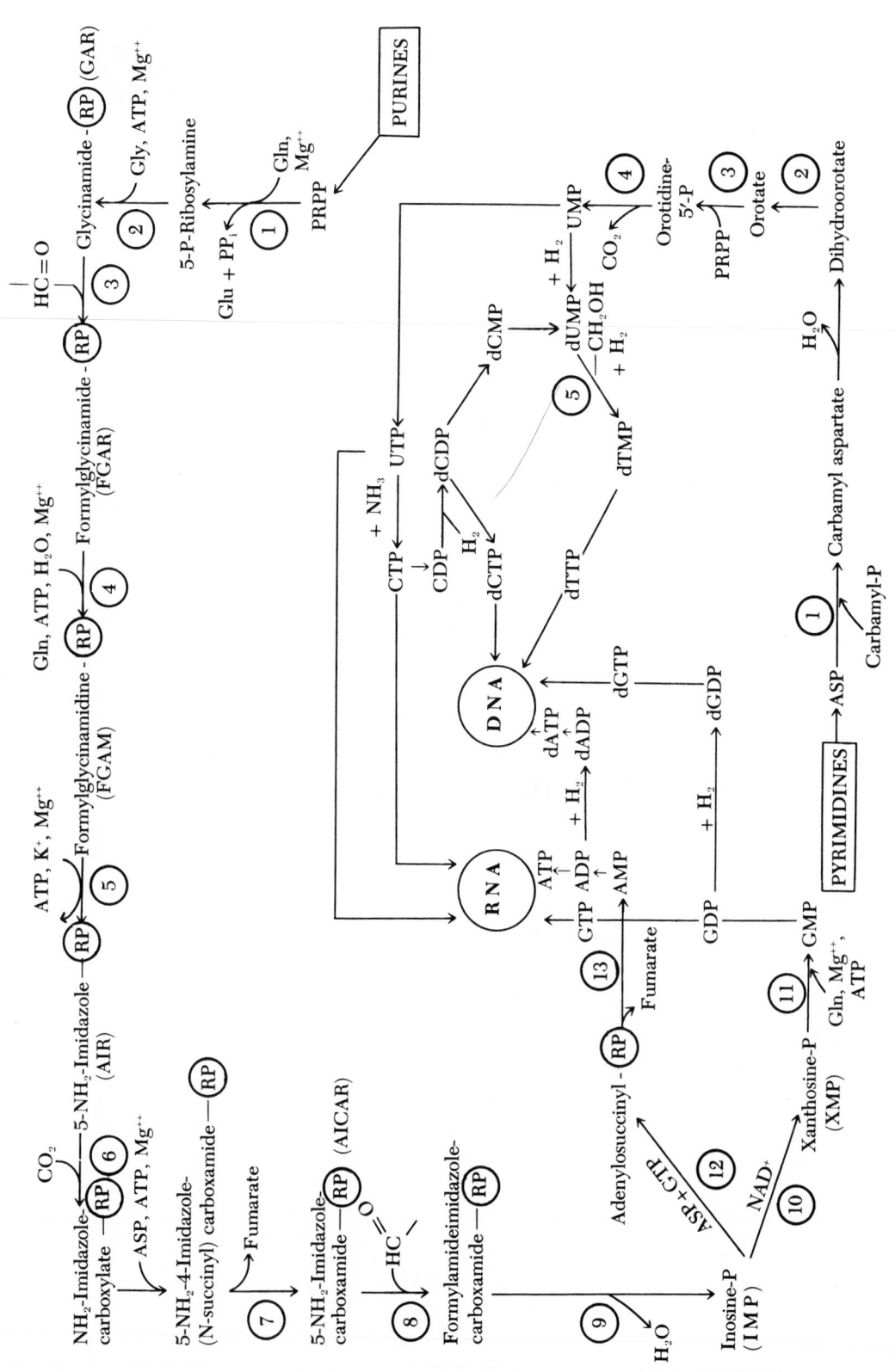

Fig. 14-1. Biosynthetic pathways of the purines and pyrimidines. Where known, the enzymes and cofactors required for the various steps are shown with corresponding numbers in the text.

BIOSYNTHESIS OF PYRIMIDINES

The pyrimidines also are formed from relatively simple precursors, namely, an amino acid, aspartic acid, carbamyl phosphate, and the carbohydrate derivative PRPP. In the first step, the carbamyl group of carbamyl phosphate is transferred to the nitrogen of aspartic acid to yield N-carbamylaspartic acid. The enzyme involved in this reaction is aspartyltranscarbamylase. Dehydration results in ring closure and the formation of *dihydroorotic acid.* Orotic acid, formed by the dehydrogenation of dihydroorotic acid, is an important intermediate in the biosynthetic scheme. (Studies of the mechanisms controlling RNA synthesis in living organisms often begin by administering

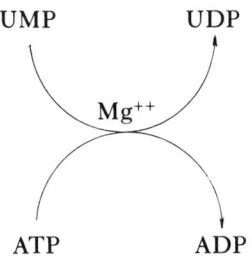

Orotic acid   **Dihydroorotic acid**

radioactive orotic acid.) Next, the orotic acid reacts with PRPP and then is decarboxylated to yield uridylic acid (UMP). (See p. 408.)

The stepwise formation of pyrimidines is also outlined in Fig. 14-1. The corresponding enzymes[2] and cofactors required are as follows: (1) aspartate transcarbamylase; (2) dihydroorotase, NAD^+; (3) orotidylic acid pyrophosphorylase; (4) orotidylic acid decarboxylase; (5) thymidylic acid synthetase.

NUCLEOSIDE TRIPHOSPHATES

As is apparent from the biosynthetic pathways outlined for purines and pyrimidines, the monophosphates are the products. These are further phosphorylated in the presence of ATP, a reaction catalyzed by a group of enzymes called *kinases:*

UMP   UDP

Mg^{++}

ATP   ADP

Orotic acid

PRPP → PPi

CO_2

Uridylic acid

The enzyme that catalyzes this phosphorylation reaction is called *nucleoside monophosphate kinase:*

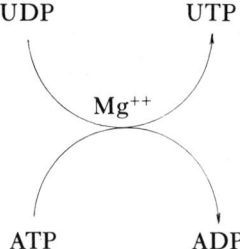

UDP → UTP

Mg^{++}

ATP → ADP

In this reaction the enzyme responsible is called a *nucleoside diphosphate kinase.*

The reduction of carbon-2 of ribose to deoxyribose occurs at the nucleoside diphosphate stage and depends on the enzyme *nucleoside diphosphate reductase.* The source of hydrogen atoms for this reductive step is a reduced protein cofactor, called *thioredoxin.* The overall reaction is:

$$CDP \xrightarrow[\text{Reduced thioredoxin}]{Mg^{++}} dCTP \qquad GDP \xrightarrow[\text{Reduced thioredoxin}]{Mg^{++}} dGTP$$

Another conversion required for the formation of various nucleosides is the transfer of an amino group from glutamine, in the presence of ATP, to UTP, to form CTP. The overall synthesis of thymidylic acid, beginning with cytidine diphosphate, is as follows:

$$CDP \rightarrow dCDP \rightarrow dCMP \rightarrow dUMP \rightarrow dTMP$$

The enzyme required is *thymidylate synthetase*, which uses methylene-tetrahydrofolic acid as a carrier of a single methylene carbon and the hydrogen atoms necessary to reduce this one-carbon unit to the methyl group.

In addition to their role in the biosynthesis of nucleic acids, the nucleoside triphosphates are needed in various areas of metabolism. For example, ATP is used wherever energy is required as well as in the formation of S-adenosylmethionine (p. 385) and amino acid activation (p. 94); UTP is used in carbohydrate metabolism (p. 189); GTP in protein synthesis (p. 100); CTP in phospholipid (p. 322) and mucopolysaccharide synthesis (p. 547).

An understanding of the biosynthetic pathways for the formation of purines and pyrimidines has had a number of practical consequences. The entire biosynthetic scheme depends on interrelations with other metabolic processes, namely, carbohydrate and protein metabolism.[3] By administering analogues of various intermediates, e.g., of the amino acid glutamine or the vitamin folic acid, a competition with the natural compounds results that inhibits purine synthesis.

In this way, the biosynthesis of DNA can be blocked, thereby slowing growth. *Azaserine*, which is an analogue of glutamine, retards the growth of tumors and, therefore, has therapeutic value.

Likewise, the analogues of folic acid *aminopterin* and *amethopterin* have been used to treat leukemia. Other substances used to control conditions are 6-mercaptopurine, 8-azaguanine, 5-fluorouracil, 5-iodouracil, and 5-fluoroorotate.

6-Mercaptopurine   8-Azaguanine   5-Fluorouracil

409

Understanding biosynthetic pathways for the formation of purines and pyrimidines has also clarified the nature of some diseases; e.g., gout, a disease for many years associated with "high living," is now known to be hereditary in some instances and caused by a defect in purine biosynthesis. Gout involves an accumulation in the joints of the end product of purine catabolism, uric acid. In 1954, Stetten administered ^{15}N-glycine to patients with this disease and observed that the amount of heavy nitrogen excreted as uric acid was three times normal. It now appears that hereditary gout is caused by an overproduction of inosinic acid, which is then converted to uric acid (p. 402).

Another hereditary condition involving nucleic acid precursors is *orotic aciduria*, characterized by a severe anemia that is refractory to the usual therapeutic measures. A deficiency of the enzymes orotidylate pyrophosphorylase and orotidylate decarboxylase is probably the biochemical defect.

References

GENERAL

Boyer, P. D., Lardy, H., and Myrbäck, K., editors: The enzymes, New York, 1961, Academic Press, Inc., vol. 5.

Colowick, S. P., and Kaplan, N. O., editors: Methods in enzymology, New York, 1967, Academic Press, Inc., vol. 14, parts A, B.

Davidson, J. N.: The biochemistry of the nucleic acids, ed. 5, New York, 1965, John Wiley & Sons, Inc.

Davidson, J. N., and Cohn, W. E.: Progress in nucleic acid research and molecular biology, New York, 1903–1967, Academic Press, Inc.

Glaser, L.: Biosynthesis of deoxysugars, Physiol. Rev. **43**:215, 1963.

Greenberg, D. M., editor: Metabolic pathways, New York, 1961, Academic Press., Inc., vol. 2.

Hutchinson, D. W.: Nucleotides and coenzymes, New York, 1964, John Wiley & Sons, Inc.

Schoenheimer, R.: The dynamic state of body constituents, Cambridge, Mass., 1942, Harvard University Press.

SPECIAL

1. Buchanan, J. M., and Hartman, S. C.: Advances Enzym. **21**:199, 1959.
2. Richard, P.: Advances Enzym. **21**:263, 1959.
3. Blakley, R. L., and Vitols, E.: Ann. Rev. Biochem. **37**:201, 1968.

CHAPTER 15

INORGANIC METABOLISM AND WATER BALANCE

Although the inorganic constituents of the body are only a small fraction of the total amount of body tissue, they must not be considered unimportant. They are, in fact, becoming recognized more and more as essential cogs in the human machine. They range in amount from calcium, which makes up about 2% of the average body weight, to cobalt, which is present to the extent of perhaps 0.00004%, and other "trace elements" that may occur in even smaller amounts. The inorganic compounds are required for several purposes: (1) They are needed to provide a suitable medium for protoplasmic activity. The irritability of muscle and nerve cells, the permeability of cell membranes, and the normal functioning of all cells depend on a proper balance of the diverse ions, particularly H^+, Na^+, K^+, Ca^{++}, Mg^{++}, OH^-, HCO_3^-, Cl^-, $HPO_4^=$, and $SO_4^=$. (2) They play a primary role in osmotic phenomena. These have much to do with the flow of tissue fluids, absorption, and secretion. (3) Several salts are also of utmost importance in acid-base equilibria. (4) Certain tissues, especially bones and teeth, have a high mineral content, which accounts for their hardness and rigidity. (5) Some mineral elements become parts of specialized physiologic compounds. Hemoglobin's iron and thyroxine's iodine are examples. (6) Other ions are essential to a number of enzyme systems. Manganese, magnesium, and potassium, as has been seen, are examples of ions needed by enzymes in metabolism. (7) Other trace elements, e.g., Co^{++}, Cu^{++}, Zn^{++}, and Mo, appear to be essential for reasons still not fully understood.

Studies in this field have been facilitated in the past few years by improvements in the techniques for determining small amounts of inorganic elements in biologic materials, including refinements in flame photometry and the development of other sensitive specific analytic procedures, e.g., atomic absorption spectrophotometry. Atomic absorption devices are particularly useful in determining trace elements as well as Na^+, K^+, Ca^{++}, and Mg^{++} in body fluids and tissues.

INORGANIC COMPOSITION OF THE BODY

Seven elements comprise from 60% to 80% of all inorganic matter in the body. They are calcium, magnesium, sodium, potassium, phosphorus, sulfur, and chlorine. They are the principal elements in nutrition—at least from a quantitative standpoint. With an increase in age, the total ash, or mineral matter of the body, increases; but a decrease in magnesium, sodium, potassium, chlorine, and sulfur occurs also. This is shown in Table 15-1.

Table 15-1. Inorganic composition of the body*

| Age | Body weight (kilograms) | Total ash (grams) | Percentage of total ash | | | | | | | |
			Ca	Mg	Na	K	P	Cl	S	Total
Fetus, 6 wk.	0.88	19	28	0.9	10	7	17	8	8	79
Fetus, 7 mo.	1.16	30	23	0.8	8	7	14	10	6	69
Newborn infant	2.9	100	24	0.7	5	5	14	5	6	60
Adult	70	3,000	39	0.7	2	5	22	3	4	76

* Calculated from values given by Shohl, from Macy, I. G.: J.A.M.A. **120**:35, 1942.

Under average conditions a healthy normal man excretes about 20 to 30 gm. of inorganic material daily. This consists chiefly of the chlorides, sulfates, and phosphates of sodium, potassium, calcium, magnesium, and ammonium. Normally the intake should equal the outgo, except in growth and pregnancy. In Table 15-2 is shown the amount of inorganic salts in 150 American diets.

Table 15-2. Inorganic elements in 150 American diets*

| Elements | Per man per day | | | Per 3000 kcal. | | |
	Minimum (grams)	Maximum (grams)	Average (grams)	Minimum (grams)	Maximum (grams)	Average (grams)
Calcium	0.24	1.87	0.73	0.35	1.47	0.73
Magnesium	0.14	0.67	0.34	0.17	0.53	0.34
Potassium	1.43	6.54	3.39	1.63	5.27	3.40
Sodium†	0.19	4.61	1.94	0.22	4.83	1.95
Phosphorus	0.60	2.79	1.58	0.72	2.30	1.59
Chlorine†	0.88	5.83	2.83	0.83	7.26	2.88
Sulfur	0.51	2.82	1.28	0.80	2.35	1.30
Iron	0.0080	0.0307	0.0173	0.0090	0.0234	0.0174

* From Sherman, H. C.: Chemistry of food and nutrition, ed. 8, New York, 1952, The Macmillan Co.
† Since these dietary records did not show the quantities of table salt used, the figures for sodium and chlorine cover only the amounts in the food as purchased and may be greatly below the actual intake of these elements.

Study of these figures reveals the great variation in every element determined. Since this might be due to a divergence in the amounts of food consumed, the figures were also calculated to a uniform basis of 3000 kcal. Even these figures show great differences between the minimum and maximum. The question naturally arises as to whether some of these amounts are too low and others too high for optimal physiologic activity or whether only a minimum of each is required and the remainder is an unnecessary excess, or a "factor of safety."

It is generally felt that some excess is desirable, especially in the case of calcium, iron, and phosphorus. A diminution of the inorganic salt intake to a very low level is quite deleterious to health. Osborne and Mendel found that young rats cease to grow on an otherwise suitable diet when the total amount of an adequate salt mixture is greatly restricted. A. H. Smith[1] extended these studies. He found that under the conditions mentioned the bones grow somewhat, in spite of the stunting of the animal as a whole, but the animal does not gain weight. There is also a hypertrophy of the kidney and a polycythemia (excessive formation of erythrocytes). Nevertheless the total hemoglobin of the blood is decreased because the erythrocytes, although containing a normal percentage of hemoglobin, are smaller in size. Feeding an adequate diet with a complete salt mixture to such stunted animals changes the picture completely. They increase in size, the total number of erythrocytes diminishes, and the total amount of hemoglobin returns to a normal value. Substitution of calcium for the complete salt mixture gives only partial return toward the normal.

Two factors that enter into inorganic salt metabolism, namely, ammonia formation and sulfur metabolism, have already been considered (Chapter 13). These will be taken up only incidentally in this chapter.

Calcium   *Functions of calcium.* Calcium is needed by all cells. It is one of the ions required for physiologic balance, as mentioned previously. It is present in blood serum, about half in the ionized form and the rest un-ionized, probably bound to protein for the most part and, to a minor degree, in a calcium-citrate complex. Normally the concentration is about 10 to 11 mg. per 100 ml. of serum. The calcium that is readily available for metabolic use, i.e., the freely moving calcium in soft tissues, extracellular fluid, and blood, is termed the *miscible calcium pool of the body.*

A particular and important effect of the calcium ion is on nervous tissue. If the ionic calcium of the blood falls, the nervous system becomes hyperirritable. This may lead to tetany. On the other hand, a high calcium content depresses nervous irritability. Hence the administration of calcium salts is indicated in the alleviation of tetany arising from low calcium. Calcium is involved in the contraction and relaxation of muscle, as will be described later (p. 563).

Calcium is, of course, required for bone and tooth formation. If the diet is deficient in this element, either or both may suffer. This is also true if the absorption of calcium is inefficient, even in the presence of an adequate amount in the diet. Growing children, particularly, require an abundance of calcium for teeth and bones as well as for other tissues. During pregnancy and lactation there is likewise a great demand for it in the diet to provide for the growing fetus and for the secretion of the calcium-rich milk. The requirement for calcium ions in blood clotting need only be mentioned at this point.

Absorption of calcium. The absorption of calcium is quite a variable factor. Calcium forms insoluble salts with a number of anions that occur in the intestinal tract. Thus we may find much of the calcium precipitated as the phosphate, carbonate, oxalate, or sulfate, or as calcium soaps, which are also insoluble and therefore unabsorbable. This depends on the amount of soluble calcium salts present, the negative ions, the pH, and the state of fat digestion and absorption. Calcium salts are more soluble in acid than in basic solutions. Furthermore, all food calcium does not behave in the same way. For example, the calcium of all vegetables is not uniformly absorbed, and in some cases the vegetables actually tend to depress the absorption of calcium from other foods. This may be due to the presence or formation of oxalates or phosphates or to an influence on the pH of the intestinal contents. Insoluble calcium soaps form if fatty acids are present in large amount, resulting, of course, in diminished calcium absorption. Phytic acid and its compounds also interfere with the absorption of calcium. These substances are abundant in unrefined cereals.

At this point it may be well to mention the importance of vitamin D in aiding the absorption of calcium and phosphorus. As will be discussed in more detail later, vitamin D appears to induce the biosynthesis of a transport protein for calcium in the intestinal mucosal cells (p. 785). This calcium-binding protein has been isolated and prepared in a purified form from the intestinal mucosa of several species of animals.

However, at best, normal adults absorb only small amounts of calcium, perhaps 100 to 200 mg. per day, this amounting to 10% to 20% of that in the foods eaten.

Lactose exerts a rather striking favorable effect on the absorption of calcium, at least experimentally in the rat. Investigations,[2] using the amount of ^{45}Ca (and ^{85}Sr) deposited in the femur of the rat as an index of absorption, demonstrated that lactose significantly increases calcium absorption when given orally but not when administered parenterally. The beneficial effect is proportional to the amount of lactose fed and may be due to chelation of calcium by lactose, resulting in the formation of a soluble complex of low molecular weight. L-Sorbose, cellobiose, D-xylose, raffinose, melibiose, D-glucosamine, D-mannitol, and D-sorbitol also favor calcium absorption to some extent. D-Glucose, D-galactose, D-fructose, and sucrose are without apparent effect. Of interest in this general connection is the fact that the amino acids lysine and glycine also increase the solubilities of certain calcium salts.

Excretion of calcium. The excretion of calcium is partly through the kidneys but mostly by way of the small intestine. Excretion into the feces continues even when the intake is low, and accordingly a negative balance is possible. The intestinal elimination of calcium may be increased by a lack of vitamin D and diminished by a suitable amount in the diet. Measurable amounts of calcium may also be lost in sweat. It is questionable whether an individual on a low-calcium diet ever attains calcium balance under heavy sweating conditions. Since calcium levels have a profound effect on nervous irritability, it can be appreciated that a negative calcium balance, if continued long enough, would cause hyperirritability and even tetany as well as decalcification of the skeleton. These are conditions to be guarded against in pregnancy and lactation. In these states the demand for calcium is so great that supplements of calcium and vitamin D should always be provided.

Calcium excretion in the urine is increased by the ingestion of carbohydrates, particularly glucose and sucrose.[3] This may favor calcium salt precipitation in patients who form calcium oxalate types of kidney stones.

Calcium requirement. The amount of calcium retained by the body depends not only on the amount in the diet but also on the efficiency of absorption and on excretion. Hence it is difficult to set an absolute standard for the calcium requirement. Moreover, it has been shown by investigations of many authorities[4,5] that the need for calcium is flexible. In certain parts of the world where the calcium content of the diet is low, the adult population gets along well with little of this element. Apparently, however, such diets must start in childhood and extend throughout life, and adaptation occurs early under such circumstances. This idea is in conflict with the concept that each individual has a definite daily need for calcium, which, if not met by the diet, leads to nutritive disaster in time. The adaptive process must be a gradual one. An abrupt change from a high- to a low-calcium ration may lead to a negative calcium balance.

The preceding facts should be kept in mind when considering the recommended dietary allowances (see p. 841 for the 1968 revised values of the Food and Nutrition Board), which are as follows: for children up to 9 years of age, 0.7 to 0.9 gm.; for teen-age girls, 1.2 to 1.3 gm.; for boys, 1.2 to 1.4 gm.; for adults, 0.8 gm. but increasing to 1.2 to 1.3 gm. during the second and third trimesters of pregnancy and during lactation. A quart of milk supplies about 1.2 gm. of calcium in a readily assimilable form. Consequently, a safe rule to follow is a pint of milk a day for every adult and a quart for every child. (For other sources of calcium in foods, see p. 436.) However, milk has another virtue in this connection, in addition to its high content of calcium. Milk sugar, lactose, also plays a role in calcium absorption, as mentioned above.

The recommended dietary allowance for calcium established by the Food and Nutrition Board of the National Research Council is based on the average daily loss of calcium adjusted for the average percent absorption of food calcium in the normal human subject. For example, if urinary excretion is 175 mg./day, endogenous fecal excretion is 125 mg./day, and losses in sweat are 20 mg./day, then a total excretion of 320 mg./day would occur. Assuming a 40% average absorption of food calcium (a figure actually obtained experimentally), a total intake of 800 mg. calcium/day would be necessary to replace the excretory loss. There is substantial evidence that an inadequate calcium intake over a period of years contributes to the relatively high prevalence of osteoporosis in older persons.

Regulation of blood calcium. About 99% of the calcium of the body is present in the bones and is in the form of hydroxyapatite (see p. 549). This is in equilibrium with the plasma calcium, which is kept at a fairly constant level. The bone salt and plasma calcium shift back and forth as necessary to maintain this constancy.[6] Thus the bones are continually being resorbed and rebuilt. The amount of calcium that can be absorbed from the intestine is, of course, very important in preventing a drain on stored bone calcium, which would result in a negative balance. Although only a small portion of the total body calcium is in solution in the blood plasma, this calcium is of great physiologic importance, and its regulation is not a simple matter.

According to McLean and Urist,[7] there are two main direct mechanisms for regulating plasma calcium levels: (1) the physical equilibrium between the plasma and the soluble bone salts; (2) the mobilization of calcium from the less soluble bone salts under the control of *parathormone.* Bone calcium is in two forms, the more soluble intercrystalline material and the less soluble crystalline hydroxyapatite (p. 549). The more soluble fraction is in equilibrium with the calcium salts of the blood plasma and tends to keep the calcium level up, for the most part, perhaps to 70% of the normal calcium content. The remainder is supplied by a feedback mechanism under the control of the parathyroid glands. When the level of calcium ions of the plasma falls below normal, the parathyroid glands increase their secretion of parathormone. This promotes the solution of the bone salt and adds calcium ions to the blood. The parathyroid glands thus exercise a regulatory effect on the level of calcium in the serum. Removal of these glands experimentally results in increased excretion of calcium in the urine and low serum calcium levels, leading to tetany and eventually to death. The symptoms may be relieved by injections of calcium salt solution, but as soon as this calcium is excreted the symptoms recur. Administration of parathormone raises the serum calcium to a normal level, and this also causes a temporary cessation of the tetany.

Another important hormonal regulatory mechanism for the plasma calcium level has been demonstrated in recent studies—the secretion of a calcium-lowering hormone by the parathyroid glands called *calcitonin* or *thyrocalcitonin.* This hormone, therefore, has the opposite action of parathormone on plasma calcium. It thus aids in balancing parathormone and in maintaining a constant plasma level. Calcitonin is discussed in some detail later (p. 481).

Parathormone also causes an inhibition of renal tubular reabsorption of phosphorus. This results in an increased excretion of phosphorus in the urine and a fall in the level of blood phosphorus, with an attendant rise in blood calcium. The constancy of the serum calcium level depends chiefly on these mechanisms along with the absorption of calcium from the intestine, which is influenced by vitamin D (p. 785).

The action of parathormone and of vitamin D, as well as the mechanism of calcification, may involve citrate.[7] The precipitate of calcium, phosphate, and citrate, which can be demonstrated in vitro, is a complex similar to that existing in bone. The solubility of this product is increased by the presence of additional citrate and magnesium ions in the solution. Citrate injections cause the serum calcium to become more ultrafiltrable so that a rapid excretion of calcium takes place. The rise in serum calcium, caused by parathormone, was found to be accompanied by a rise in serum citrate, and the microscopic picture of the bone was found to be similar following both of these procedures. High doses of vitamin D also raised both serum calcium and serum citrate.

Whenever the plasma calcium is lowered, tetany is likely to result. This occurs occasionally in the newborn infant and sometimes in rickets and in fatty diarrhea. In the last instance, a loss of fat-soluble vitamin D accounts for a diminished calcium absorption, resulting in a plasma calcium level too low to be compensated by the parathyroid glands.

Contrary to common opinion, the calcium of teeth is not regulated in the same way as the calcium of bone. The adult tooth, already fully formed and calcified, is not subject to decalcification readily when the body requires calcium. This is true in pregnancy and lactation as well, and the old saying "a tooth for every child" has no scientific justification. Disturbances of calcification are of importance only in the *growing* tooth. Therefore, children must have an abundance of calcium with vitamin D or sunshine to help them absorb the calcium for tooth as well as skeletal development.

Phosphorus   The vital part played by phosphorus compounds in many phases of metabolism and in acid-base regulation indicates how necessary this element, in sufficient amount, is.

Vitamin D aids in the absorption of phosphates from the gastrointestinal tract, just as it aids in calcium absorption. As a rule, in the absence of vitamin D, a low serum phosphorus results. In rickets there is usually a normal serum calcium with a low serum phosphorus. Other cases of rickets occur in which both calcium and phosphorus are low in the serum or calcium is low and phosphorus is normal. The typical and usual disease, however, is characterized by a low phosphorus and normal calcium. An empiric index for determining whether a child is rachitic is the product of the serum phosphorus and serum calcium (in milligrams per 100 ml.). If the index is below 30, rickets is present or will develop, but not if it is above 40.

The ratio of calcium to phosphorus in the food intake has an important influence on the metabolism of both elements. If either is inadequately present, the other is not utilized properly, even though it be present in normal quantity. In the infant and growing child the ratio (Ca:P) should be somewhere between 1:1 and 1:2; i.e., the phosphorus intake should be equal to or about twice as great as the calcium intake. In adult life the ratio should be about 1:1.5. However, as Sherman stated, "Obviously when intakes of both elements are right, the ratio cannot be wrong"; i.e., from a practical nutritional standpoint the calcium to phosphorus ratio is likely to be right if the recommended quantities are present in the diet. For phosphorus this amounts to about 1 gm. per day. Again, in pregnancy and lactation a greater amount must be provided.

Phosphorus is normally abundant in our food, and there is little likelihood of a deficiency in this element. The same cannot be said for calcium. Most American diets are below the minimum level of calcium for safety or are dangerously close to it. Sherman stated that about one half of the American diets studied by him were below the safe level and 16% were even below the minimum requirement. If the vitamin D intake should happen to be diminished in these cases, serious consequences would result.

Requirement of phosphorus. The recommended dietary allowance for phosphorus (p. 841) has been established on the basis of a 1:1 relationship with calcium, as just stated, at ages above 1 year. In the first 2 months of life, a calcium to phosphorus ratio of 2:1 is used (based on the Ca:P ratio in human milk). For older infants up to 1 year of age, the phosphorus allowance is increased to about 80% of the calcium allowance, based on the 1.2:1 ratio in cow's milk generally used at this age. The recommended daily allowance for both men and women is 0.8 gm. For infants and children the values range from 0.2 to 1.0 gm., depending on age (see p. 841). The amount during pregnancy and lactation should be increased 0.4 and 0.5 gm. per day, respectively. The recommended 1 pint or more of milk per day for the adult and 1 quart for the child and during pregnancy and lactation to satisfy the calcium requirement will also nearly supply the need for phosphorus.

Magnesium   Magnesium is an essential element. Magnesium-free diets can be prepared experimentally, and animals on such diets have circulatory disturbances, increased irritability, and finally convulsions and death. It is the essential metal in chlorophyl and therefore occurs in all green plants. The skeletons of some marine forms are rich in magnesium. This is undoubtedly related to the fact that seawater contains more magnesium than calcium.

Magnesium occurs in bones, muscles, and nervous tissue of man. Its distribution is uneven, probably because it can replace calcium to some extent, and this depends largely on the amount of calcium available. Human blood serum, however, has a constant magnesium content, 1 to 3.5 mg. per 100 ml. (0.8 to 2.9 mEq. per liter). The blood plasma level is about 2 mEq. per liter and that of the red blood cells is 5.3 mEq. per liter.

The Food and Nutrition Board of the National Research Council now places the requirement of the adult man at 350 mg. per day. As is true of other nutrients, more magnesium is required during pregnancy and lactation, 450 mg. per day. The recommended dietary allowance for the infant and child is less than that for the adult, depending on age.

Zeelig[8] maintains that the frequent claim that an adult cannot have a magnesium deficiency on an ordinary diet is simply untrue. For instance, there is a large loss of magnesium during diabetic acidosis[9] and in alcoholism.

The magnesium ion influences tissue irritability. Thus when introduced in large amounts parenterally, it is a central depressant, having anesthetic and anticonvulsant effects. These effects are completely antagonized by calcium, and this antagonism has not been explained. Curiously, however, low serum concentrations of either magnesium or calcium lead to the same pharmacologic effects, namely, hyperirritability and convulsions. Magnesium deficiency in rats produced by the feeding of a magnesium-deficient diet is likewise characterized by the development of hyperirritability and convulsions. A decrease in growth, a decrease in the efficiency of food utilization, and a striking vasodilatation also occur. The tissues most likely to be damaged by chronic magnesium depletion are cardiovascular, renal, and neuromuscular. Magnesium ions also function as cofactors in a number of enzyme reactions.

Magnesium is excreted by way of the intestine, for the most part. A fraction is eliminated by the kidneys. One of the characteristic crystal forms frequently seen in urinary sediments is the "coffin plate" crystal of ammonium magnesium phosphate ($NH_4MgPO_4 \cdot 6H_2O$).

Iron   The role of iron in the body is closely associated with that of hemoglobin. The great importance of iron is quite out of proportion to the amount present in the entire body, which is the insignificant value of 3 to 5 gm. This small amount is used over and over again in the body. Iron is not like the vitamins or most other organic or even inorganic substances, which are either inactivated or excreted in the course of their physiologic functions. Very little iron is lost from the body normally; and, since it is a small part of the hemoglobin molecule (about 0.3%), comparatively little is needed. Iron is also a constituent of many tissues besides blood (e.g., the myoglobin of muscle) and is essential for the composition of such catalysts as the cytochromes, peroxidases, and catalases.

Iron is also a constituent of the nonheme iron-containing protein *ferredoxin*. This protein is widely distributed in plant and animal tissues and plays an important role in photosynthesis (p. 219); it is also involved in methemoglobin reduction, $NADP^+$ reduction, pyruvate metabolism, and nitrogen fixation. It has been crystallized from certain bacteria and from spinach leaf, and its amino acid composition and sequence have been determined.[10] Similarities of the amino acid sequence of spinach ferredoxin to that of bacterial ferredoxin suggest a common evolutionary origin. The ferredoxins have relatively low oxidation-reduction potentials and serve as electron carriers in certain anaerobic bacteria and in photosynthetic organisms. The extremely electronegative character of the ferredoxins suggests that they may have existed as a biologic catalyst during the era of the earth's reducing atmosphere before green plants emerged.

Iron has been called a "one-way substance." It may be absorbed in small amounts. Any excess over and above the amount absorbed is eliminated in the feces. This cannot be considered a true excretion but rather an oversupply, which is thus wasted. However, there is some actual excretion, as determined by following isotopic iron administered intravenously. This is of the order of 0.5 to 1 mg. per day and occurs mainly through the small intestine. Almost none is found in the urine,[11] and careful studies of the intake and output have never revealed any appreciable negative balances except in early infancy.

Hypochromic anemias usually do not result from negative iron balances but from losses of blood, which may be very difficult to detect. Hypochromic anemias are those conditions in which there is a greater diminution in the concentration of hemoglobin than in the number of red cells and, accordingly, the red cells are paler than normal. Positive iron balances occur in growing children and in pregnant women. In both instances more iron is absorbed than is excreted, which corresponds with the need to synthesize hemoglobin for the expanding blood volume.

Absorption of iron. The absorption of iron takes place chiefly in the upper part of the small intestine. Although normally very little is absorbed, under certain conditions larger quantities may pass into the body. After a severe hemorrhage, the absorption of iron may be increased 10 to 20 times, but there is usually a delay before this occurs. In hypochromic anemia, iron is absorbed more than normally, and in hemochromatosis an astonishing amount may be found in the tissues. This is a disorder of iron metabolism that is characterized by large deposits in the liver and other organs of two pigments, *hemosiderin* and *hemofuscin,* the first of which contains iron. Hemosiderin is probably derived from hemoglobin and other sources of iron. Its iron content may vary between 9% and 55% and is in the form of ferric hydroxide stabilized by protein. It is also present normally to some extent. Defective absorption of iron may result from gastrointestinal disturbances, e.g., achlorhydria or diarrhea, leading to anemias that readily yield to large doses of iron.

The absorption of iron appears to involve the release of food iron by gastric hydrochloric acid (as Fe^{++}), which then forms a chelate with ascorbic acid and certain sugars and amino acids.[12] These chelates remain soluble in the more alkaline fluids of the duodenum and jejunum, and hence iron absorption is enhanced. It is possible that mucosal receptors in the upper small intestine (apoferritin?) control the absorption of iron. Thus when there is iron need in the body, usually as a result of blood loss and resulting increased compensatory erythropoiesis, iron is removed from the intestinal mucosal cell receptor and increased absorption of food iron occurs to replace it. This continues until the body's stores of iron, particularly that of the intestinal mucosal cells, are replenished. The iron-saturated mucosal receptor then once again refuses to absorb available iron. There is also recent evidence[13] that copper is involved in the intestinal transport of iron. ^{59}Fe fed to copper-deficient swine was absorbed by the intestinal mucosal cell, but its transfer to the plasma was impaired. Likewise, injected ^{59}Fe was taken up by cells of the hepatic parenchyma and reticuloendothelial system. The investigators therefore concluded that copper is required for the release of ferrous iron into the plasma for subsequent utilization. This may entail its oxidation to ferric. The copper-containing protein ceruloplasmin may promote the incorporation of ferric iron into transferrin, and hence its utilization, by serving as a ferroxidase.[14]

The iron in foods is not all equally available. Iron in the heme combination, it has been claimed, is not as assimilable as salts of the metal. In administering iron therapeutically, inorganic iron is probably as useful as organic, and, although ferrous iron is preferable, ferric is usually converted to ferrous in the body and is absorbed as such. It should be emphasized, however, that only small amounts are absorbed. By giving massive doses, slightly larger quantities can be forced, but there is a regulatory mechanism that hinders unlimited absorption no matter how much is available. Several investigators[15] consider this regulatory mechanism to depend on the interesting substance ferritin.

Ferritin. Ferritin is a protein that may contain as much as 23% iron by weight. The iron is present as micelles or colloidal particles, composed of a ferric hydroxide–ferric phosphate complex, bound rather firmly to the protein. It can be freed of iron without denaturing the protein, and this protein, *apoferritin*, is homogeneous, with a molecular weight of 460,000. Both ferritin and apoferritin can be crystallized with cadmium sulfate. Ferritin has been isolated from bone marrow, spleen, and liver of a number of different animals and has also been found in the gastrointestinal mucosa. Experiments indicate that apoferritin may not always be present in appreciable amounts in the intestinal mucosa but is formed in response to iron feeding; i.e., the feeding of iron in some way brings about the formation of the particular protein that combines with it.

As the iron of the food passes down the gastrointestinal tract, it is reduced to the ferrous state, if it is not already in that state, by gastric acidity, sulfhydryl groups, ascorbic acid, or other reducing agents in the food and secretions. This ferrous iron is absorbed into the mucosal cells of the duodenum and jejunum. The cells of the mucosa regulate iron absorption by maintaining within the other tissue cells of the body a level of ferrous iron, governed in part by the oxidation-reduction potential of these other cells. The body cells possess a special mechanism for the one-way transfer of ferrous iron into them. Radioiron studies have shown that this mechanism or "bloc" adjusts the uptake of iron in accordance with body needs for iron and previous iron feedings. The ferrous iron is oxidized, combined with phosphate, and united with apoferritin to form ferritin. This is stored in the mucosal cell. Thus the ferrous iron of the body cells is in equilibrium with the ferritin (Fe^{+++}) of the mucosal cells and the plasma iron (Fe^{+++}) of the bloodstream. The amount of ferrous iron moving into the cell thus depends upon the level of ferrous iron in the cell and indirectly upon the ferritin concentration. From the mucosa the ferrous iron passes into the bloodstream, the amount being dependent on the relative redox level of the body cells, and this is related to the oxygen tension in the blood. Only ferrous iron can pass into the blood. It has been suggested that the reductant responsible for this action is ascorbic acid. The ferrous iron is then autoxidized and becomes attached to one of the β_1-globulins, called *transferrin*.

$$2\ Fe^{++} + O_2 + \text{Transferrin} \quad \rightarrow \quad Fe_2^{+++} \cdot \text{Transferrin}$$

This complex is also in equilibrium with the ferrous iron and ferritin in the liver (the chief storage site for iron) and the spleen and bone marrow. Each transferrin molecule binds two atoms of ferric iron and two molecules of carbonate. In the bone marrow the ferrous iron is converted to heme by combining with protoporphyrin, and thus the store of ferritin there has an immediate use. However, the ferritin in the other tissues is, of course, convertible to the ferrous form for transport to the bone marrow for the same purpose.

If there is need for iron by the body, e.g., following hemorrhage or debilitating disease, the bone marrow, liver, and spleen are called upon first to give up their ferritin, for these are the organs with the largest amounts of this protein. Hemosiderin, another form of iron storage, is less soluble than ferritin and probably is not used until ferritin has reached a low level. Only when these major sources have been depleted and the plasma iron concentration diminished, is the mucosa called upon for its iron. When this occurs and the physiologic saturation of the mucosal cells with respect to ferrous ions is no longer maintained, iron can be absorbed. Thus the ferritin content of the mucosa acts as a valve, permitting the absorption of only enough iron to preserve equilibrium. This is a fortunate provision of nature, for ferric ions are rather toxic.

Fig. 15-1 indicates these relationships in a general way. It also shows how this hypothesis accounts for the saving of iron in the catabolism of hemoglobin. When the erythrocytes have finished their life cycle, the iron is reutilized. Recent investigations using radioactive iron showed that this iron from the "old" erythrocytes is used in preference to storage iron. Thus we see that low absorption of iron is compensated for by the efficient reutilization of iron and by the intricate mechanism of storage.

Requirement. The recommended dietary allowance for iron has been recently revised (p. 841) by the Food and Nutrition Board of the National Research Council. The intake for adult men should be 10 mg. per day, and for adult women 18 mg. per day. The recommended dietary allowance for girls from the age of 10 years and for premenopausal women also has been increased to 18 mg. per day. Iron needs for women are higher than for men because of menstrual losses and the demands of pregnancy and lactation. This increase is based on recent findings that iron stores are reduced or absent in about two thirds of menstruating women and in the majority of pregnant women. The increased recommended dietary allowance cannot easily be met by customary diets so, for certain age categories of women and also for infants, increased iron fortification of foods may be desirable. These iron-intake values are considerably higher than the actual amounts of iron required. Allowance is thus made for the fact that only about 10% of food iron is absorbed by the normal adult.

As stated previously, pregnancy demands additional iron for the growing fetus. When the infant is born, he has a considerable store of iron for future

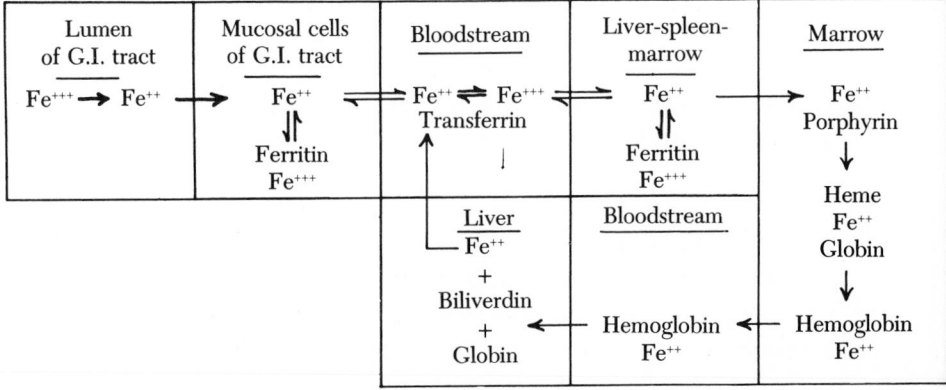

Fig. 15-1. Scheme showing the role of ferritin in the absorption and storage of Fe.

use. This is fortunate because milk is extremely low in its content of this element. There is a supply of iron in the infant's spleen and liver, but neither is as great as was formerly believed. The amount of liver iron ranges from a negligible quantity to 60 mg. The chief location of the infant's iron is the hemoglobin of the blood. With a concentration of 22 to 23 gm. of hemoglobin per 100 ml., this is higher than at any later period in the individual's life. During the first few weeks with a constant loss of iron, and almost no iron in the milk ingested, there is an appreciable negative balance of iron; but after the second month this balance tends to approach zero. The iron comes, for the most part, from the physiologic destruction of hemoglobin. Premature babies or twins may be deficient in iron for obvious reasons, and anemia may result unless iron medication is given. Hypochromic anemia of infants is the most common nutritional deficiency in North America.[16]

Iron deficiency is not at all uncommon in the United States, nor, indeed, is it uncommon in most of the world in infants and in pregnant women.[17] The deficiency is readily detectable if sensitive measurements such as plasma iron and iron-binding capacity of the plasma (transferrin) are employed. Prophylactic iron administration daily is justified, therefore, in such infants and during the latter half of pregnancy.

Metabolism of iron. As indicated in Fig. 15-2, the major amount of iron is

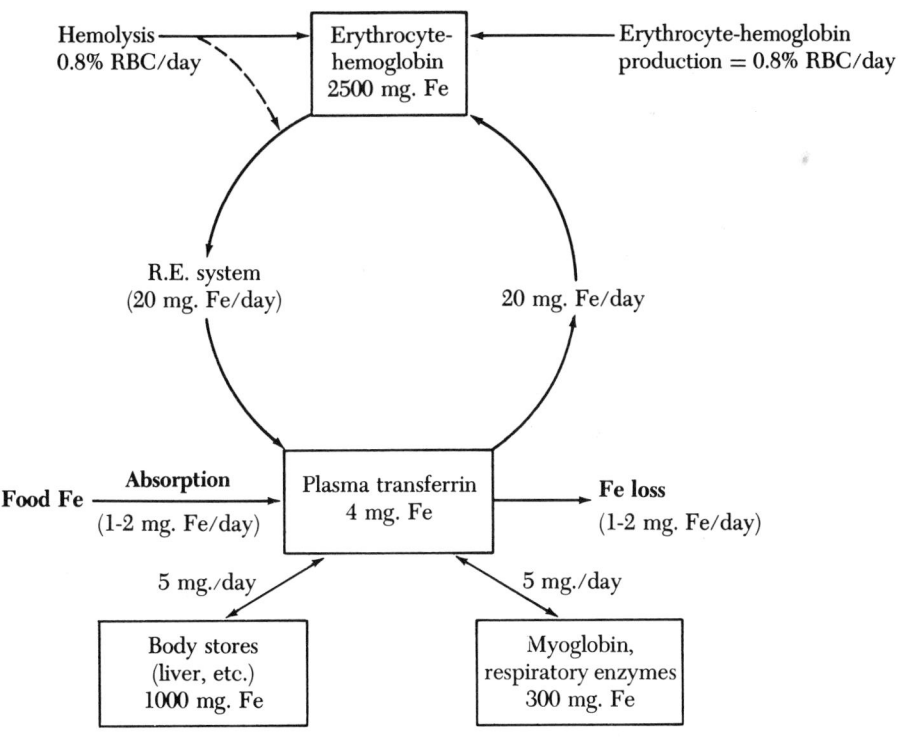

Fig. 15-2. Metabolism of Fe in the human adult. (Adapted from Conrad, M. E.: Borden Rev. Nutr. Res. **28:**49, 1967.)

present in the hemoglobin of erythrocytes. About 0.8% of the circulating erythrocytes "wear out" daily, having reached their normal life-span in man of about 120 days (p. 596), and are hemolyzed. The hemoglobin iron is carefully conserved and reutilized in the biosynthesis of new hemoglobin and erythrocytes in the bone marrow. Body stores of iron in the liver and other tissues may be called upon to replenish plasma iron if needed. Iron present in muscle as myoglobin or in all tissues as cytochromes and other respiratory enzymes appears to be relatively nonavailable for blood hemoglobin formation. The small iron loss daily, 1 to 2 mg., usually in the form of intestinal secretions, desquamated, epithelial cells, etc., is compensated for by the absorption of an equal amount of food iron as described. In the adult woman, approximately 30 mg. of iron are lost during the menstrual period. In pregnancy, some 600 mg. are transferred to the fetus. These amounts must be replaced by either increased absorption of food iron or therapeutic doses of iron salts. The principal cause of an iron deficiency in man is *blood loss*.

Copper and other trace elements

Copper. For the formation of hemoglobin, minute amounts of copper are believed to be needed. This is certainly true in the regeneration of hemoglobin after dietary anemias in experimental animals and possibly also after nutritional anemias in children. Apparently copper is used over and over again as iron is, and the loss is limited to the amount excreted in the urine and in the feces. The average daily loss of copper in young women is 0.04 mg., half being attributable to menstruation. However, 2 to 2.5 mg. of copper per day are recommended as a daily allowance in the diet. In men the average daily loss is probably less than 0.02 mg. Copper occurs in certain oxidases and possibly in other enzymes. Copper is also present to the extent of about 0.34% in one of the plasma α_2-globulins, *ceruloplasmin*. The latter apparently serves to transport copper to the tissues. Copper occurs in many foods, and the estimated daily requirement of from 2 to 2.5 mg. is usually ingested.

Investigations in experimental animals during the past few years demonstrated that a deficiency of copper produces a variety of striking pathologic changes. In sheep, the wool becomes straight instead of curly and black wool loses its pigmentation, becoming a grayish white. By adding molybdenum salts, which interfere with copper metabolism, to the diet periodically, a black and white striped wool results. Everson and co-workers[18] showed that copper deficiency in lambs and pigs results in ataxia, gross brain abnormalities, swayback, and aneurysms of the aortic arch or abdominal aorta. Anemia may also occur. These investigators attributed such diffuse pathologic changes in tissues to a basic defect from copper deficiency in cytochrome oxidase activity, producing an impairment, particularly in phospholipid synthesis, which, in turn, results in structural defects of and pathologic lesions in the vascular system, brain, and nervous tissue.

Similar results were reported recently[19] in weanling rats maintained on a copper-deficient diet. Neural lesions characterized by hyperirritability, catatonic posture, and convulsive seizures developed. The gross and histologic appearance of the brain and nervous tissue was analogous to that produced by severe tissue anoxia.

O'Dell's group[20] observed similar dissecting aneurysms of the aorta in copper-deficient chicks, which they attributed to defective elastin formation. There was a decreased monoamine oxidase activity (p. 750) in the aorta, cartilage, tendons, and skin. These workers, therefore, concluded that copper is essential as a catalyst for the cross-linking of collagen (p. 546).

It will be recalled that copper plays a role in the absorption and utilization of iron, possibly by acting as ferroxidase (p. 420). Thus, copper, in the form of ceruloplasmin and possibly other oxidases, appears to be vitally and fundamentally involved in cellular oxidation-reduction reactions, as yet only incompletely understood.

In hemochromatosis, the condition in which iron is retained in large amounts in the form of hemosiderin, there is also an increased amount of copper in the liver and other organs. Copper has been found in amounts greater than normal in the brain and liver of persons dying of hepatolenticular degeneration (Wilson's disease). This is an uncommon disease of the nervous system in which there is an associated hepatic disorder; it is generally regarded as incurable. High urinary copper figures have been reported in such cases. In view of this fact, several patients with Wilson's disease were treated with 2,3-dimercaptopropanol (BAL, or British anti-Lewisite), which is known to promote excretion of copper, as well as with various other heavy metals and arsenic. A greatly increased excretion of copper resulted. The condition of these patients was favorably affected, sometimes to a remarkable degree.

Zinc. Zinc is an essential element for rats, mice, and young lambs, and it is necessary for the human being also. In young men, deficiency causes stunted growth, anemia (due to concomitant iron deficiency), enlarged liver and spleen, and underdevelopment of genitals and secondary sex characteristics.[21] Deficiency of zinc may be due to the nature of the diet (high in phytic acid), to the excretion of zinc in perspiration, or to blood loss if there is parasitic infection. In animals, zinc deficiency causes hyperirritability, anorexia, retardation of growth, loss of hair, and changes in the skin and sometimes in the cornea. Probably the reason for these changes is the fact that zinc is a constituent of several vitally important enzymes. Among these are carbonic anhydrase, carboxypeptidase, alkaline phosphatase, lactic acid, and alcohol dehydrogenases. The last-named enzymes occur in the eye, and, indeed, the eye contains a considerable amount of this metal, as do the testes and the teeth.[22] The blood also has a small amount. Zinc seems to be present in the pancreas, and it accompanies insulin when this hormone is crystallized. Diabetic pancreatic tissue contains only half as much zinc as does normal tissue. Zinc is present in the insulin molecule but is not essential to the activity of insulin (p. 460). Other investigators have claimed that zinc is localized in the α-cells of the pancreas and have suggested that it is related more to glucagon content than to insulin.

There is increasing evidence that zinc plays an important role in protein biosynthesis and utilization. The addition of small amounts of zinc to a diet containing suboptimal amounts of a vegetable protein, as indicated by the growth of young rats, causes a marked increase in protein utilization and growth. Prasad and his co-workers considered this to result from a failure in adequate RNA synthesis. Zinc apparently inhibits the enzyme ribonuclease.

Thus, in zinc deficiency, excessive destruction of RNA could occur, which might result in the defects of protein synthesis seen in zinc deficiency as well as the other sequelae observed.

The adult human being ingests from 12 to 20 mg. of zinc per day. This element is widely distributed, and to find a diet deficient in it would be a difficult task, indeed. An intake of 0.3 mg. per kilogram of body weight is believed to be adequate for children.

Manganese. It is now generally agreed that manganese is an essential element. It occurs rather widely in plant and animal tissues. The richest sources are liver, kidney, muscle, lettuce, spinach, and whole-grain cereals. Male rats fed diets deficient in manganese become sterile and have testicular degeneration. Young rats that are born of females on similar diets do not survive long, and the mothers are unable to suckle normal young animals. These symptoms in the female may be cured or prevented by the addition of manganese to the diet. Manganese is also needed by rats for growth. In the chick the presence of manganese in the diet prevents the development of a condition known as perosis; this is an osteodystrophy. The tibial-metatarsal joint becomes enlarged, the distal end of the tibia and the proximal end of the tarsometatarsus are twisted and bent, and the gastrocnemius tendon slips from its condyles. As a result the chicks have shortened leg bones and vertebral columns. Whether a deficiency in man would have results resembling those observed in the rat or chick cannot be said, since no case of manganese deficiency in man has been observed.

Recent interesting studies by Everson and co-workers[24] demonstrated that manganese deficiency during the pre- and postnatal period in young guinea pigs is associated with a reduction in the size of the pancreas. In some animals the pancreas was entirely absent. These animals died at birth or shortly thereafter. The manganese-deficient guinea pigs showed a diabetic-like tolerance curve to glucose administered either orally or intravenously. The administration of manganese resulted in the gradual development of a normal tolerance to glucose.

Manganese is an activator of several different enzymes, phosphatases in particular. Other enzymes are more active in the presence of manganese, e.g. phosphoglucomutase, intestinal peptidases, cholinesterase, isocitric dehydrogenase, the carboxylases, arginase, and adenosine triphosphatase. For most of these, although manganese is considered the physiologic activator, other ions (e.g., magnesium, cobalt) may replace them. However, several important enzymes demand manganese exclusively. These include the peptidases, prolidase, which splits the dipeptide glycylproline, and succinic dehydrogenase. The first is an intestinal digestive enzyme, the latter one of the enzymes involved in the citric acid cycle.

The exact human requirement for manganese is not known. Possibly from 0.2 to 0.3 mg. per kilogram of body weight should be ingested by children daily, but probably that amount or more is regularly available. After oral or parenteral administration, manganese is excreted almost entirely in the feces with extremely small quantities in the urine.

Cobalt. Cobalt is an essential element for some animal species but possibly not for others. For example, cattle and sheep in certain regions develop a peculiar disease characterized by emaciation and anemia. This has been traced to a deficiency of cobalt, and the administration of cobalt is effective in the treatment of the condition. Horses grazing on the same lands remain healthy. A slight excess of cobalt in either metallic or ionic form produces polycythemia in rats and in a number of other species. Rats fed a copper-deficient diet fail to develop this cobalt polycythemia.[25] The administration of cobalt to experimental animals significantly increases the level of the hormone erythropoietin (p. 507) in the blood and produces a polycythemia.

Since cobalt is a constituent of the vitamin B_{12} molecule, it is evidently necessary for hemoglobin formation and must be regarded as essential. As mentioned above, cobalt may substitute for manganese as an activator of certain enzymes. It is a specific activator for glycylglycine dipeptidase and perhaps for others. Human foods containing over 0.2 p.p.m. include buckwheat, figs, cabbage, lettuce, spinach, beet greens, and watercress, and there are smaller quantities in other vegetable and animal products. It is also a contaminant of many medicinal preparations of iron.

Molybdenum. During the past several years, molybdenum has been found to be a constituent of certain enzymes, including xanthine oxidase and aldehyde oxidase. For this reason molybdenum perhaps should now be classed as an essential mineral element.

Iodide. Normally the total iodide content of the body approximates 20 to 50 mg., distributed as follows: muscles, 50%; skin, 10%; skeletal structure, 7%; thyroid, 20%; other endocrine organs plus the central nervous system, 13%. The concentration of iodine in the thyroid gland is more than a thousand times that in muscle and 10,000 times that in blood. Thyroxine and triiodothyronine, the physiologically active substances that are manufactured by the thyroid, are iodine compounds, but only one fourth or one fifth of the total iodine in the gland is present in those forms (p. 477). Probably most of the remainder is in the form of organic precursors of thyroxine, and 1% or less is iodide ion. Little is known of the function of iodide except in the thyroid. The blood plasma normally contains from 4 to 8 μg. of protein-bound iodine (PBI) per 100 ml.

A lack of iodide in the food and drinking water is related to the occurrence of simple goiter. McClendon showed that the drinking water in different localities in the United States varies in its iodide content from 0.01 to 73.3 parts per billion. Goiter occurs more frequently in persons living in those regions where the drinking water has a low iodide content. It was also shown that, in general, simple goiter is more prevalent far from the ocean or in sections where ocean winds cannot carry their moisture. The reason is that seawater contains iodide, and, when the sea spray is deposited on coastal regions, it enriches the soil and drinking water with this element. Vegetables grown in these regions take up iodide from the soil, and thus the inhabitants of coastal areas get iodide from drinking water and vegetables, as well as from sea food.

Until recently, goiter was common in Switzerland. Although not far from the sea, Switzerland is surrounded by high mountains that cause the ocean breezes to deposit their moisture on the outer sides. As a result, Swiss soil and drinking water are low in iodide. Marine and Kimball[26] demonstrated that simple goiter can be prevented by an intake of sufficient iodide. This may be accomplished by adding inorganic iodides to the source of water supply or more simply by the addition of iodides to table salt (1:5000 to 1:200,000)

Recent surveys[27] showed that endemic goiter is still prevalent in many parts of the world, especially in mountainous areas remote from the oceans. Frank endemic goiter and cretinism, for example, are present in as much as 54% of the population of rural villages in the Andes regions of Ecuador. The iodine content of the drinking water there is low. Laboratory thyroid function tests (^{131}I uptake, PBI, basal metabolic rate, etc.) showed values typical of endemic goiter. Apparently *coto*, the Indian term for "goiter," was noted by the Spanish explorers of this area in the early 1500's. The art and sculpture of that era in Ecuador also clearly show the presence of goiter. Iodine prophylaxis in the form of iodized salt is being instituted in this region.

It is well known that not all goiters are due to a lack of iodide. There is, for example, a goiter due to infection. Exophthalmic goiter is a hyperthyroid condition that is not a result of low iodine intake. Experimentally the feeding of agents that block formation of the thyroid hormone (p. 477) causes a hyperplasia of the thyroid gland, resembling goiters. Thiourea, thiouracil, and large amounts of certain vegetables, notably cabbage and cauliflower, have this effect.

Iodine or iodides may be absorbed from mucous surfaces or from the skin. They are excreted chiefly in the urine and, to a minor degree, in the sweat and feces. If given in large amounts, they are also found in tears, saliva, and bile.

In the 1968 revision of *Recommended Dietary Allowances*, of the Food and Nutrition Board, National Academy of Sciences, iodine is included for the first time. The recommended intake for the adult is 90 to 150 μg. per day. Smaller amounts are recommended for infants and children, depending on size. During pregnancy and lactation, 125 to 150 μg. daily are recommended. In order to ensure adequate dietary iodine, it is desirable to use *iodized salt*. The Food and Nutrition Board has currently recommended federal legislation requiring such iodization.

Fluoride. Fluoride is rather widely distributed in nature and is found in varying amounts in drinking water and in foods. In those localities where the fluoride concentration is relatively high, it usually has deleterious effects on the teeth. If it is ingested in toxic quantities during childhood while the teeth are undergoing calcification, characteristic signs appear. Instead of the normal glistening translucent appearance, the teeth acquire dull white patches, or even the entire surface may look chalky. Pitting, due to the breaking off of the ends of the enamel prisms, is a common occurrence. The teeth also may have a brown stain, "mottling" (Fig. 15-3). McCollum demonstrated that the inclusion of fluoride in the diets of experimental animals produces fragility of the teeth and bones; and there is much other evidence that it affects calcium and phosphorus metabolism. It is an inhibitor of various enzymes, notably enolase. Fluoride is sometimes added to blood that is to be analyzed for glucose, because it inhibits glycolysis.

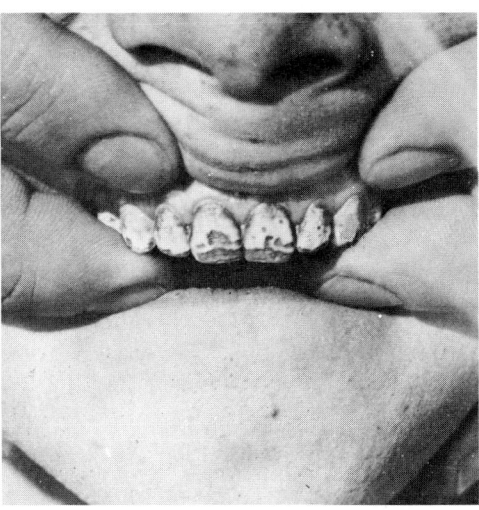

Fig. 15-3. Mottled enamel (endemic dental fluorosis) of severe degree. Teeth calcified using water containing 14 p.p.m. of fluoride. (From Dean, H. T., McKay, F. S., and Elvove, E.: Pub. Health Rep. **53**:1736, 1938; courtesy F. A. Arnold, Jr.)

The effect of the fluoride ion is not always unfavorable physiologically. Smaller amounts, i.e., traces, check the occurrence of dental caries. Armstrong and Brekhus[28] found that the enamel of sound teeth contains more fluoride than that of carious teeth. This is the only element known to vary in such a manner, and it was suggested that the increased fluoride may be the effective factor in the prevention of caries. Many other observations point in the same direction. Either the fluoride actually imparts to the tooth structure caries-resistant properties, or it inhibits bacterial action on food particles and on dental tissue. Perhaps both occur. The optimum concentration of fluoride in drinking water that provides a balance between the power to resist caries and the tendency to cause mottling has been calculated to be 0.75 p.p.m. The presently accepted level is 1 to 2 p.p.m. A large-scale test began in 1945 in two cities in the state of New York. The drinking water of Newburgh had traces of sodium fluoride (F, 1 p.p.m.) added, whereas Kingston, a nearby city of about the same population, served as a control with nothing added to its water supply. The school children in each community had their teeth examined at the beginning of the test and once a year thereafter. At the end of 10 years, the Newburgh children, who had been drinking fluoridated water all their lives, had 58% less caries in their permanent teeth than did the Kingston children of the same age group. The 10-to-12-, 13-to-14-, and 16-year-old Newburgh children, who had partaken of fluoridated water for the last 10 years of their lives, had 52%, 48%, and 41% less caries, respectively, than did their Kingston controls. There was no mottled enamel noted in the teeth of the Newburgh children and very little dental fluorosis.[29] Similar results have been obtained in carefully controlled studies in Michigan and in other parts of the United States and Canada.

On the basis of the favorable results obtained in the above pioneer studies, some 3200 communities in the United States now adjust the fluoride conten of their public water supplies to the optimal level of about 1 p.p.m. It is es timated that at the present time approximately 72 million people in the Unite States drink fluoridated water. Another 10 million live in areas where th drinking water supply contains enough natural fluorides to inhibit tooth de cay.

Controlled fluoridation of public water supplies has been included by som authorities in the four great mass preventive health measures of all time the others being pasteurization of milk, purification of water, and immuniza tion against disease. In each case bitter opposition initially was followed b controversy centered around a set of difficult scientific and political prob lems. The ultimate fate of fluoridation, however, has been decided largely b public referendum, whereas the fates of the others were decided, more prop erly, by administrative and legislative means. The fluoridation question ha been characterized as the most extensively studied public health problem i the history of mankind.

It has been shown[30] that intake of sodium fluoride by patients suffering fron osteoporosis (which seems to be more prevalent in low-fluoride vicinities leads to a diminution of urinary loss of calcium, symptomatic relief, and im provement in bone formation.

Bromide. Small amounts of bromide sometimes are found in table salt an also in certain vegetables. Normal human serum contains about 1 mg. pe 100 ml. Bromides are absorbed, distributed, and eliminated by the body i almost exactly the same manner as the chlorides; i.e., they are absorbed fron the gastrointestinal tract, pass into the various body fluids, penetrate the re cell but not other cell membranes, and are eliminated by the kidney, just a chlorides are. If present in sufficient amounts, bromide tends to replace chlo ride in the body, doing so in a quantitative manner. It has a sedative effect o nerve tissue, which may be a result of the decrease in concentration of chlo ride displaced by bromide in the extracellular fluid. Bromide poisoning known as bromism, is fairly common because bromides may be obtained with out a physician's prescription. The advanced stages are characterized b mental and neurologic disturbances.

Selenium. For a number of years selenium has been known to occur i significant amounts in the soil and vegetation in certain parts of the wester United States. Animals grazing in these regions have developed alkali dis ease. Recent studies,[31] however, indicate that traces of selenium may be a essential factor in tissue respiration, as a component of the electron-transfe system in cells. This observation resulted from a study by Schwarz and co workers on the identity of "factor 3," a dietary substance that protects agains hepatic necrosis produced in the rat by the feeding of a diet low in cystin and vitamin E. Factor 3 was found to be an organic compound containin selenium. Inorganic selenium salts, e.g., selenite, were likewise active i amounts as small as 2 to 4 μg. per 100 gm. of diet (2 parts in 100,000,000 part of diet!). Selenium salts were 500 times more effective than vitamin E and 250,000 times more active than L-cystine. This element seems to be essentia for a number of animal species, including chickens, lambs, and calves. The muscular system is particularly dependent on it, and vision may also be involved.

A recent study[32] demonstrated that lambs fed a hay–raw cull kidney bean ration develop muscular dystrophy. Selenium plus vitamin E administration prevented the condition. Apparently the raw beans contain a heat labile anti-selenium or antivitamin E factor or both. Autoclaving the beans destroys the factor.

Chromium. In studies of hepatic necrosis produced by dietary means in the rat, Schwarz and co-workers reported, in 1955, that a low tolerance to intravenously administered glucose is also characteristic of this condition. Selenium salts prevented or cured the degenerative changes in the liver but had no effect on the low tolerance to glucose. In further extensive studies, trivalent chromium compounds were found to be extremely effective in correcting the impaired tolerance to glucose. The diet employed in producing the hepatic necrosis syndrome proved to be deficient in chromium as well as selenium and the other factors involved. Furthermore, minute quantities of chromium, a few micrograms, were found to be essential along with insulin in promoting the utilization of glucose by epididymal tissue for fat synthesis in vitro. Neither chromium nor insulin alone was effective.

Subsequent studies[33] supported the hypothesis that chromium (III) acts as a cofactor for insulin in increasing not only glucose utilization but also the transport of amino acids into cells (heart, liver, and diaphragm). Chromium may also be related to maturity-onset diabetes.[34] Other recent studies[35] indicated that very small amounts of chromium (0.02 p.p.m. in drinking water) lower the serum cholesterol level, as well as serum glucose level, in rats fed refined sugar.

Vanadium. There is some evidence that vanadium may be involved in the mineralization of bones and teeth. This element also appears to increase the resistance of rats to experimentally produced dental caries.

Lead. Lead is found in some foods, especially in drinking water. It is stored in the bones and, to a lesser extent, in the liver. In large amounts it is toxic. Its deposition in bones may be explained by postulating that lead, phosphorus, and vitamin D form a system of lead deposition analogous to the deposition of calcium in bones. Lead is a potent inhibitor of certain enzymes dependent on sulfhydryl groups for their activity. δ-Aminolevulinic acid dehydratase, involved in the biosynthesis of heme (p. 608), is an example. For this reason, the determination of δ-aminolevulinic acid in urine is a sensitive procedure for the early detection of lead poisoning in man.

Nickel. There is some evidence that nickel plays a role as an enzyme activator and in maintaining the conformation of protein molecules. It is consistently found associated with RNA.

Lithium. Lithium salts inhibit the release of norepinephrine and serotonin from brain slices stimulated by an electric current. Lithium salts were found effective in the treatment of mania and related mental disorders in which there is a disturbance of amine metabolism.[36]

Cadmium. According to some current work, cadmium may be involved in essential hypertension.

Tin. Tin also occurs in the body; the largest quantities are found in the tongue and skin. In the concentrations usually occurring in foods, as a result of their having been preserved in tin containers, this metal has no deleterious effects.

Silicon. Silicon, as silicates, enters the body chiefly in vegetable foods. Soluble silicates are easily absorbed. Human blood serum ordinarily carries about 1 mg. per 100 ml. After the ingestion of silicates, this level does not rise because the excess is rapidly excreted by the kidneys. Varying quantities are found in the different organs and tissues. The lungs are highest in silicon because of the inhalation of insoluble particles that lodge there. In industries in which silica dust is produced in large amounts, e.g., stonecutting, the workmen inhaling this dust develop silicosis. In this condition the lung tissue is replaced by nodular connective tissue overgrowths. Naturally the silicon content of such lung tissue is comparatively high. Similar pathologic states result from breathing dusts of other types—coal, steel, etc.

Other elements. Many other elements are present in traces in foods and in body tissues, e.g., boron, rubidium, arsenic, titanium, aluminum, and silver, to list only a few. As far as is now known these are "incidental" constituents of tissues and have no physiologic function or significance.

Sodium, potassium, and chloride Sodium chloride is added to food in cooking and at the table in an amount greater than is usually present in the uncooked food. It is the only salt that is commonly added to the diet and is needed for both its positive and its negative ions. This requirement for salt is shared with herbivorous animals. They do not obtain sufficient sodium from plants, which are rich in potassium; consequently they seek out deposits of sodium chloride, the so-called "salt licks."

The effects of severe deficiencies of both sodium and potassium have been studied in rats. A lack of sodium results in retarded growth, both somatic and skeletal, atrophy of muscles and testes, and diffuse degenerative changes in

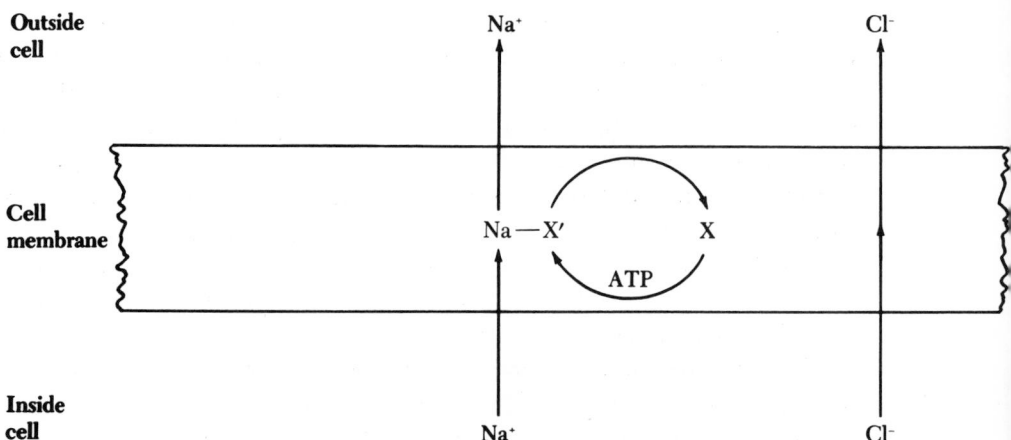

Fig. 15-4. "Sodium pump." X, Carrier or transport protein for active transport of Na^+; Cl^- follows Na^+ to maintain electroneutrality. ATP may cause a change in the conformation of the transport protein, X to X', and thus effect active transport (see Fig. 2-3).

many other tissues. A deficiency of potassium likewise produces poor somatic growth, fragility of the bones, sterility in both males and females, renal hypertrophy, paralysis, and a slow heart rate. Chloride deficiency in rats also results in poor growth but apparently few other significant gross changes.

In the body, sodium ions predominate in the plasma and other body fluids, whereas potassium occurs to a greater extent within the cells, both of the blood and of the tissues in general. The sodium content of cells is kept at low levels by a postulated "sodium pump" mechanism, shown diagrammatically in Fig. 15-4.

However, current evidence also indicates that the energy required for the maintenance of such a sodium pump mechanism is exorbitant, being some three times the total energy generated by the cell. This contradiction may be avoided if cellular water is regarded as being in a semicrystalline state, an assumption supported by current research. These studies indicate that most of the water in brain and muscle tissue is not in its familiar liquid state but instead exists as a highly organized semicrystalline or icelike structure. If these findings of two independent research laboratories, based on nuclear magnetic resonance studies, are confirmed, established theories of such basic phenomena as membrane transport of ions and the transmission of electric impulses along nerve fibers will need to be completely revised.

There is recent evidence that most of the sodium ions in tissues are not free but are bound to macromolecules. Apparently as much as 60% of the sodium ions in muscle, kidney, and brain are associated with protein and other molecules. Similar complexing of potassium ions to cellular macromolecules also occurs.

Sodium and potassium usually have a reciprocal influence on each other, i.e., as one increases in a certain fluid or tissue, the other decreases. Thus a sudden increase of potassium salts in the diet experimentally causes a fall in the sodium content because of a concurrent increase in sodium and chloride elimination in the urine. Since many foods are higher in potassium than sodium, this might easily occur and result in a subnormal sodium content of the body were it not for the addition of sodium to our food. However, if the high potassium intake is continued for several days, the chloride output is diminished even to a point below the amount ingested. Conversely, the toxic symptoms seen when there is a deficiency of potassium are related to the presence of large amounts of sodium as much as they are to a lack of potassium.

Sodium chloride and other salts aid in keeping the serum globulin in solution, and they function in the various other ways mentioned earlier. For example, an excised heart continues to beat for hours if, under suitable conditions, it is perfused with an oxygenated solution of salts. The optimum concentrations of these salts vary with the type of animal, but in all cases sodium, potassium, and calcium must be present. Calcium and potassium seem to be antagonistic to each other in such a nutrient solution. The required osmotic state is produced chiefly by the predominance of chloride, but the sodium ion itself is essential and, of course, the pH must be suitable. An example of such a solution is Locke's (containing 0.92% $NaCl$, 0.024% $CaCl_2$, 0.042% KCl, 0.018% $NaHCO_3$, and 0.1% glucose).

More sodium than potassium is needed by the body. The usual daily intake of sodium chloride is about 10 to 15 gm., or 170 to 256 mEq. This is far greater than is required, but the amount is used chiefly because of its flavor. About 98% is eliminated by way of the urine, and 2% via the feces. The usual amount of potassium in the diet, on the other hand, is only 2 to 4 gm., or 50 to 100 mEq., per day.

Although loss of fluid and loss of salt generally accompany each other, deficit of sodium chloride alone may be encountered. The symptoms are weakness, fatigue, lack of appetite, nausea, and a diminution of mental acuity. Impairment of renal function with delayed diuresis follows. A thirst that cannot be allayed by drinking develops. Salt, however, does alleviate it.

Chloride is an essential anion. It is closely connected with sodium in food and in body tissues and fluids and excretions. It is needed in the chloride shift and the formation of gastric hydrochloric acid. Chloride is excreted mostly as sodium chloride and chiefly by way of the kidney. About 2% is eliminated in the feces and perhaps 4% or 5% in perspiration.

Ordinary diets contain sufficient sodium, potassium, and chloride, but when there is excessive excretion of any of them, more must be provided. Adrenal insufficiency and acidosis are examples; diarrhea and excessive perspiration are others. Men working in industries in which they encounter intense heat and perspire freely must have salt supplied with their drinking water to make up for this loss of electrolytes.

No other cation can entirely replace potassium for the performance of a great number of cellular functions. Therefore, potassium is an essential element. It can move in and out of most cells more easily than sodium according to the demands of shifting membrane equilibria. Probably changes in acid-base balance influence these shifts considerably. Under normal conditions the respective concentrations of sodium and potassium ions are held within a fairly narrow range, although, as shown by tracer studies with radioactive isotopes, these ions move freely across cell membranes.

In the building of cells, the potassium ions are taken up; this appears to be essential for growth. In infancy and childhood and during pregnancy and lactation, there is a comparatively high potassium retention. During muscular contraction there is a loss of potassium from the muscle cells to the extracellular fluid. Subsequently, this lost fraction returns to the muscle tissue. The significance of the movement of potassium during muscle contraction is unknown, but the movement seems to be related to the contractile process rather than to the neuromuscular transmission of the stimulus. In the steady state the loss due to contraction is probably just equal to the gain due to recovery. Undoubtedly this is the condition in cardiac contraction, for potassium ions are essential to heart rhythm.

Potassium also is necessary for nerve activity, and the same type of movement of the ion occurs here. Nerve fibers are exceptionally rich in potassium. When the nerve is stimulated, potassium diffuses into the surrounding fluid very rapidly; during rest, it diffuses back. This diffusion seems to be associated with a change in potential that occurs during the conduction of the nerve impulse, but its exact physiologic role is not known.

We are now certain that potassium is related to carbohydrate metabolism. The potassium level of the plasma rises and falls with the lactic acid level and with the concentration of blood sugar. It falls after insulin administration and rises after epinephrine is given. Glycogen formation from either glucose or pyruvate requires potassium ions. The exact manner by which these ions influence glycogenesis in liver has not been ascertained, but the maintenance of a normal intracellular ionic environment is believed to be essential. Other ions probably needed are magnesium, calcium, bicarbonate, and chloride. Since glycogen deposition in the liver is accompanied by the deposition of potassium, the administration of insulin may, under certain conditions, tend to shift potassium from the extracellular fluid into the cells.

In diabetic acidosis, apparently the failure to metabolize glucose properly is associated with loss of potassium from the cells. There follows an increased excretion of potassium in the urine if the kidneys are functioning efficiently. Often there is vomiting, with further loss of potassium. However, the plasma level of potassium is usually not below normal, because the urinary excretion cannot keep pace with the influx of potassium from the cells. When insulin is administered, the extracellular fluid potassium is shifted into the cells, and a hypopotassemia occurs. This may lead to several alarming symptoms, including paralysis of the respiratory muscles. Hence, under such circumstances, the replacement infusion fluid should contain potassium (Table 15-5).

In certain types of hypertension, rigid restriction of sodium in the diet has been found by some investigators to be beneficial (p. 870). This is a controversial subject. In hypertensive rats the sodium content of the entire body is elevated, whereas potassium remains unchanged. The data indicate a penetration of the intracellular compartment by sodium. If this occurs, it must be because sodium displaces some other intracellular cation or is in an osmotically inactive state. Other interrelationships of sodium, potassium, and chloride will be taken up in connection with water balance.

There is some evidence in the literature[37] that a relation between excessive salt consumption and the pathogenesis of essential hypertension exists. Data from an interesting recent comparison[38] between the sodium intake and blood pressure levels of two Polynesian populations are pertinent in this connection. The subjects male and female, numbering 51 in one group and 60 in the other, were inhabitants of two Polynesian islands, Rarotonga and Puka Puka. They were similar ethnically but observed different dietary, social, and economic habits. The mean blood pressure of the Rarotonga group was significantly higher than that of the Puka Puka group and increased with age, especially in females. Only a slight rise with age was seen in the latter group. The blood pressure differences between the two populations showed no correlation with height or weight but correlated significantly with the sodium intake. The sodium intake, as determined by dietary surveys and urinalyses, averaged 50 mEq. per day higher in the Rarotonga group than in the Puka Puka group.

A brief summary of the metabolism of inorganic elements is presented in Table 15-3.

Table 15-3. Summary of metabolism of inorganic elements

Element[°] and total amount in human body	Best food sources	RDA[†] 1968	Absorption and metabolism	Principal metabolic functions	Clinical manifestations of deficiency
Sodium (Na^+) 1.8 gm./kg.	Table salt, salty foods, animal foods, milk, baking soda, baking powder, some vegetables	About 3–5 gm.[‡]	Readily absorbed, extracellular, excreted in urine and sweat; aldosterone increases reabsorption in renal tubules	Buffer constituent, acid-base balance, water balance, osmotic pressure, CO_2 transport, cell membrane permeability, muscle irritability	Dehydration; acidosis; tissue atrophy; excess leads to edema, hypertension
Potassium (K^+) 2.6 gm./kg.	Vegetables, fruits, whole grains, meat, milk, legumes	About 1.5–4.5 gm.[‡]	Readily absorbed, intracellular; secreted by kidney	Buffer constituent, acid-base balance, water balance, CO_2 transport, membrane transport, neuromuscular irritability	Acidosis; renal damage
Calcium (Ca^{++}) 22 gm./kg.	Milk, milk products, fish bones (cooked)	0.8 gm.	Poorly absorbed (20%–40%) according to body need; absorption aided by vitamin D, lactose, acidity; hindered by excess fat, phytate, oxalate; excreted in feces; parathormone mobilizes bone Ca^{++}	Formation of apatite in bones, teeth; blood clotting; cell membrane permeability; neuromuscular irritability	Rickets (child), poor growth; osteoporosis (adult), hyperexcitability

[°] The inorganic elements included are those for which evidence exists that they are *essential* for man. Other elements not included but present in the human body in trace amounts, for which there is fragmenting evidence for some biochemical function, include cadmium, lithium, nickel, vanadium. Other elements present in human tissues in trace amounts as incidental constituents of no known significance include Ag, Au, Al, As, Br, Pb, Rb, Si, Ti, B. The amounts of the element present in the entire human body are averages from the literature (Dairy Council Digest 39:26, 1968). They are expressed as grams or milligrams per kilogram of body weight (*fat-free basis*) or as milligrams in entire body.

[†] Recommended dietary allowance per day, established by the Food and Nutrition Board, National Research Council, 1968. The values given are for a normal adult male, 22 years of age. (See Table 25-1, for values for females and other age groups.)

[‡] An estimated value is given if no RDA value has been established. The estimated value is the average daily dietary intake of a normal adult.

Table 15-3. Summary of metabolism of inorganic elements—cont'd

Element° and total amount in human body	Best food sources	RDA† 1968	Absorption and metabolism	Principal metabolic functions	Clinical manifestations of deficiency
Phosphorous ($PO_4^{\equiv}$) 12 gm./kg.	Milk, milk products, egg yolk, meat, whole grains, legumes, nuts	0.8 gm.	Readily absorbed; excreted by kidney	Constituent of bones, teeth; constituent of buffers; constituent of ATP, NAD, FAD, etc.; constituent of metabolic intermediates, nucleoproteins, phospholipids, phosphoproteins	Osteomalacia (rare); renal rickets; cardiac arrythmia
Magnesium (Mg^{++}) 0.5 gm./kg.	Chlorophyll, nuts, legumes, whole grains	350 mg.	Absorbed; competes with Ca^{++} for transport	Cofactor for PO_4-transferring enzymes; constituent of bones, teeth; decreases neuromuscular irritability	Magnesium-conditioned deficiency, muscular tremor, choreiform movements, confusion; vasodilatation, hyper-irritability
Iron (Fe^{++} or Fe^{+++}) 75 mg./kg.	Liver, meats, egg yolk, green leafy vegetables, whole grains, enriched bread and cereals	10 mg. male; 18 mg. female	Absorbed according to body need; aided by HCl, ascorbic acid	Constituent of hemoglobin, myoglobin, catalase, ferredoxin, cytochromes; electron transport, enzyme cofactor	Anemia, hypochromic; pregnancy demands; excess → hemochromatosis
Iodine (I^-)	Seafoods, iodized salt	140 μg. male; 100 μg. female	Concentrates in thyroid; transported as PBI	Constituent of thyroxin, triiodothyronine; regulator of cellular oxidations	Endemic (simple) goiter (hypothyroidism); cretinism
Zinc (Zn^{++}) 28 mg./kg.	Liver, pancreas, shellfish; widely distributed in animal and plant tissue	10–15 mg.‡	1–2 mg. absorbed; phytate decreases absorption	Constituent of insulin, carbonic anhydrase, carboxypeptidase, lactic dehydrogenase, alcohol dehydrogenase, alkaline phosphatase	Anemia; stunted growth; hypogonadism in male
Copper (Cu^{++}) 2 mg./kg.	Liver, kidney, egg yolk, whole grains	2–3 mg.‡	Limited absorption; transport by ceruloplasmin; stored in liver; excretion via bile	Formation of hemoglobin (increases iron utilization); constituent of oxidase enzymes (tyrosinase, cytochrome oxidase, ascorbic acid oxidase)	Hypochromic anemia; excessive hepatic storage in Wilson's disease

continued.

437

Table 15-3. Summary of metabolism of inorganic elements—cont'd

Element° and total amount in human body	Best food sources	RDA† 1968	Absorption and metabolism	Principal metabolic functions	Clinical manifestations of deficiency
Cobalt (Co^{++}) 3 mg.	Liver, pancreas, mushrooms	1–2 mg.‡	Limited absorption; stored in liver; excretion via bile	Constituent of vitamin B_{12}	Anemia in animals; deficiency as vitamin B_{12} → pernicious anemia; excess → polycythemia
Manganese (Mn^{++}) 20 mg.	Liver, kidney, wheat germ, legumes, nuts	3–9 mg.‡	Stored in liver mitochondria and bone; excreted via bile	Cofactor for number of enzymes—arginase, carboxylase, kinases, etc.	Unknown in man; in animals → decreased glucose tolerance, perosis, congenital ataxia
Molybdenum (Mo) 5 mg.	Liver, kidney, whole grains, legumes, leafy vegetables	Trace ‡	Readily absorbed; excreted in urine and bile	Constituent of xanthine oxidase, aldehyde oxidase	Unknown
Chromium (Cr^{+++})	Liver, animal and plant tissue	Trace ‡		Involved in carbohydrate utilization	Unknown; deficiency in diabetes claimed; decreased glucose tolerance in rats; possible relation to cardiovascular disease
Selenium (Se)	Liver, kidney, heart	Trace ‡	Excreted in urine	Constituent of factor 3; acts with vitamin E to prevent liver necrosis and muscular dystrophy in animals; inhibits lipid peroxidation	Unknown; excess → alkali disease in cattle, sheep
Chloride (Cl^{-}) 50 mEq./kg.	Animal foods, table salt	Intake 5–10 gm. as NaCl‡	Rapid absorption; excreted in urine; high renal threshold; not stored	Electrolyte, osmotic balance; gastric HCl; acid-base balance	Hypochloremic alkalosis (pernicious vomiting)

Table 15-3. Summary of metabolism of inorganic elements—cont'd

Element° and total amount in human body	Best food sources	RDA† 1968	Absorption and metabolism	Principal metabolic functions	Clinical manifestations of deficiency
Fluoride (F⁻)	Seafoods, some drinking water	1 mg.‡ (1 p.p.m. in drinking water)	Easily absorbed; excreted in urine; deposited in bones and teeth	Constituent of fluoroapatite—tooth enamel	Dental caries; osteoporosis; excess (5–8 p.p.m. in water) → mottled enamel.
Sulfur (SO₄⁼)	Plant and animal proteins as Cys and Met	2–3 gm.‡	Derived from metabolism of Cys and Met; excreted in urine	Constituent of proteins, mucopolysaccharides, heparin, thiamine, biotin, lipoic acid; detoxication	Cystinuria; cystine renal calculi

WATER BALANCE

The study of water regulation in the body has made great strides in recent years. As might be expected, water balance is clearly bound up with sodium and potassium distribution, although other factors also are concerned. Among these are acid-base equilibrium; the intermediary metabolism of proteins, carbohydrates, and fats; some of the hormones; and certain physical factors, particularly external temperatures.

Pathways of salts and water The necessity for the various salts has been discussed in the first part of this chapter. Salts must, of course, be in solution in order to be absorbed. The water is derived from water and other beverages ingested, from the water content of solid foods, and from metabolic water. Most of the absorption is through the mucosa of the upper intestine. Besides the water actually present in food and drink, a small amount is produced in metabolism by the oxidation

Table 15-4. Typical daily water balance

Water intake	Grams	Water output	Grams	
Drinking water	400	Skin	500	
Water in other beverages	580	Expired air	350	
Preformed water in solid foods	720	Urine	1,100	
Metabolic water	320	Feces	150	
Total	2,020	Total	2,100	Balance = −80 gm.

of the hydrogen of metabolites. The amount of this varies but is generally thought to be from 300 to 350 gm. According to Magnus-Levy, 100 gm. of fat yield 107 gm. of water; 100 gm. of starch, 55 gm. of water; and 100 gm. of protein, 41 gm. of water. The water absorbed goes first into the interstitial fluid, i.e., lymph, tissue juices. From here it passes into cells or blood plasma and wanders back and forth, depending on conditions. Eventually it is excreted by four channels — skin, lungs, kidneys, intestines. Salts accompany the water into the sweat, urine, and intestinal secretions.

In children the daily water intake varies from about 700 ml. in the newborn infant to about 1300 ml. for 10-year-olds.[39] A typical daily water balance for an average-sized man is given in Table 15-4.

General distribution of body fluids The total amount of fluid in the body is about 70% of the body weight. About 5% of the body weight is blood plasma, roughly 3.5 liters in a person weighing 70 kg. (It will be remembered that the blood makes up about one twelfth of the body weight, or 8.33%, and about 60% of this is plasma, i.e., 5% of the body weight.) The lymph and other extracellular fluids or juices comprise the interstitial fluid and total about 15% of the body weight, or 10.5 liters. The intracellular fluid is estimated at 50%, in this case, about 35 liters. (Fig. 15-5). The figure for intracellular fluid is an estimate based on determinations on animals. The other values have been obtained by experimental methods.

The estimation of total body water presented an interesting problem. Most of the procedures aimed at injecting intravenously a substance that would distribute itself uniformly in the total body water and then determining its concentration. It had to be a harmless substance that was not destroyed quickly. Most of the substances tested were unsuitable because of their uneven distribution among the different tissues. However, heavy water, deuterium oxide, and tritiated water were successfully employed. The last contains a small fraction of tritium, the radioactive isotope of hydrogen of mass 3. These heavy waters are ideal for this purpose because, although they differ enough from ordinary water to permit their determination when mixed with it, they are handled by the body exactly in the same way as ordinary water. A few milliliters of tritiated water were injected after the water's radioactivity was determined. At different intervals samples of blood were removed and the radioactivity of the plasma measured. By taking the average after 1, 2, and 3 hours, the figure of 60% of body weight was obtained for the total body water in the human subject.[40] The half-life of body water in man was found to be about 9.3 days.

The interstitial fluid is the "middleman" of body fluids. It is the medium through which nutrient materials pass from the blood to the cells and sometimes in the reverse direction. Through it also travel waste products from the cells to the blood. The hydrogen ion concentration and osmotic pressure of the interstitial fluid must be in equilibrium with both the plasma and the intracellular fluids. The interstitial fluid shrinks or expands in volume easily as the various physiologic functions add to or subtract from the body water. In rapidly occurring pathologic disturbances of fluid balance, the total interstitial fluid may fluctuate tremendously, and thus it protects both the blood

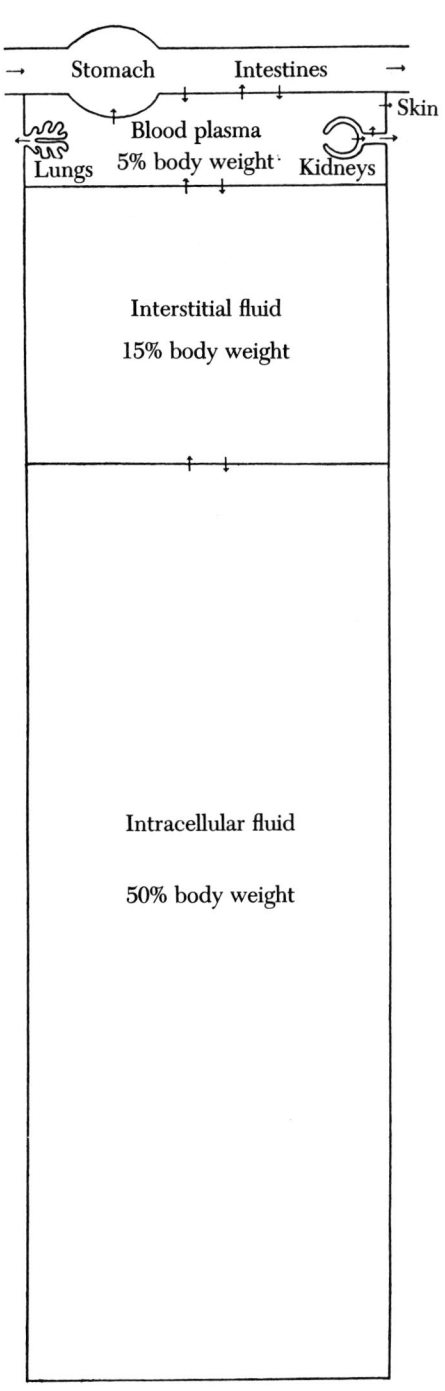

Fig. 15-5. Distribution of body fluids. (Modified from Gamble, J. L.: Chemical anatomy, physiology and pathology of extracellular fluid, Cambridge, Mass., 1958, Harvard University Press.)

volume and the cellular fluid from sudden change. In this manner the interstitial fluid is instrumental in preserving a normal constant equilibrium, a homeostasis. When extreme fluid loss occurs, plasma fluid is the second to be depleted, the interstitial fluid being first. The intracellular fluid, the most vital, is preserved to the end. However, when fluid loss is gradual, as in water deprivation, all three compartments suffer equally.

Electrolyte content of body fluids The concentrations of electrolytes in the three "compartments" of fluid, as they are called, are maintained within narrow ranges during health. The cells are the last to suffer any changes in electrolyte concentration; the interstitial fluid and blood plasma bear the brunt of any fluctuations.

The electrolyte composition of blood plasma is shown in Fig 15-6.

The values are expressed in milliequivalents per liter. A milliequivalent weight is one thousandth of an equivalent weight. Milliequivalents per liter may be calculated from the number of milligrams per liter by the following formula:

$$\text{Milliequivalents per liter} = \frac{\text{Milligrams per liter} \times \text{Valence}}{\text{Atomic weight}}$$

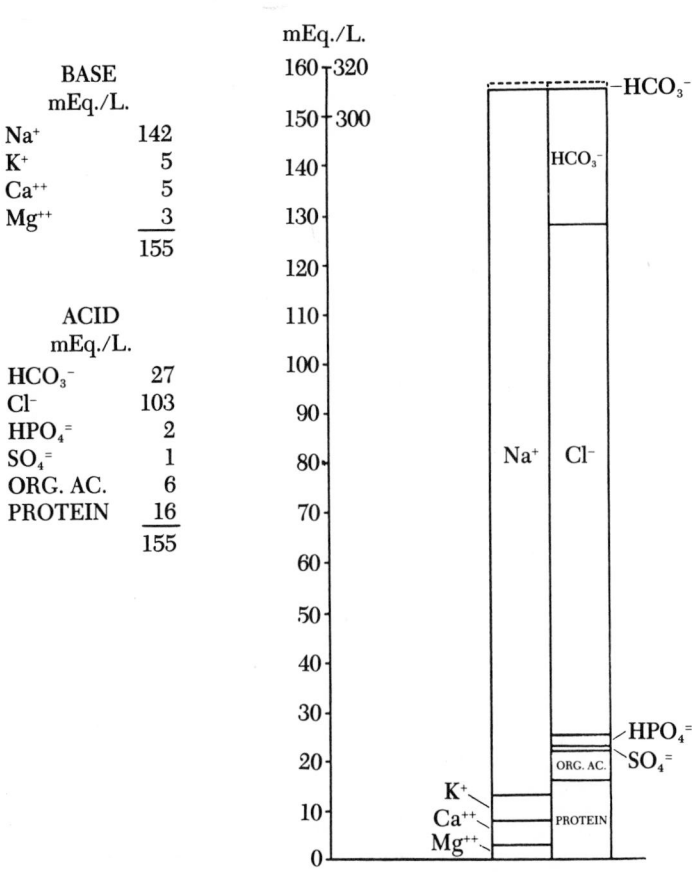

Fig. 15-6. Acid-base composition of blood plasma. (From Gamble, J. L.: Chemical anatomy, physiology and pathology of extracellular fluid, Cambridge, Mass., 1958, Harvard University Press.)

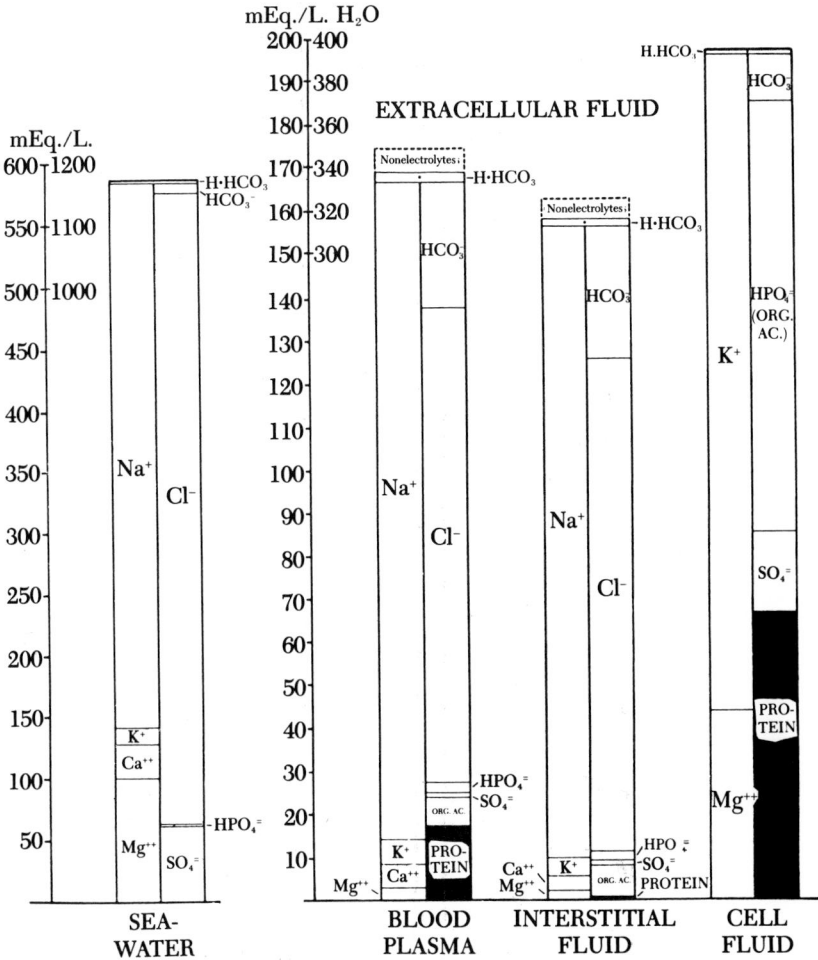

Fig. 15-7. Chemical composition of extracellular fluids and of seawater and cell fluid. Note that the values are given as milliequivalents per liter of H_2O contained in the fluid instead of per liter of plasma, as in Fig. 15-6. Note also that the patterns of blood plasma and interstitial fluid are almost identical; the greatest single item of difference is in the amounts of protein. This makes necessary adjustment of the concentrations of the diffusible ions, which will preserve the total cation-anion equivalence (Donnan equilibrium). The nonelectrolyte concentration (glucose, urea, etc.) is seen to be very small in comparison with that of the electrolytes although the total quantity carried to the tissue cells and into the urine over a unit of time is several times larger. The history of extracellular fluid is clearly indicated by the resemblance of its chemical pattern to that of seawater, which is roughly three times more concentrated than plasma. Note the predominance of K^+ and the high protein content of cell fluid. (From Gamble, J. L.: Chemical anatomy, physiology and pathology of extracellular fluid, Cambridge, Mass., 1958, Harvard University Press.)

Thus a milliequivalent of any one element or ion is equivalent to a milliequivalent of any other. The fact that there are 5 mEq. of potassium per liter and 5 of calcium in plasma conveys the idea instantly that these two are of the same relative value as bases; whereas the figures 200 mg. of potassium per liter and 100 mg. of calcium per liter would not.

Venous plasma has approximately the same electrolyte composition as has arterial, except for the bicarbonate, which is higher. Interstitial fluid probably has very nearly the same inorganic composition as plasma; however, because of a lower concentration of protein than in plasma, the distribution of the diffusible ions is somewhat different, as a result of a Gibbs-Donnan equilibrium effect. Partly for the same reason the distribution of the diffusible ions in the cells is also different, since the nondiffusible protein in the cells is much higher than in the interstitial fluid (Fig. 15-7). Sodium and chloride are the predominant ions in the extracellular fluids, but potassium and phosphate are the major intracellular ions. Protein contributes its important colloidal osmotic pressure effect (p. 582). Bicarbonate, which occurs in all three compartments, fluctuates considerably since it is formed and excreted constantly, and both bicarbonate and phosphate contribute to the regulation of acid-base balance.

Intake of water The total amount of water absorbed by the body depends on a number of factors. In health, an important influence on the amount of water ingested is the external temperature since water is concerned in the regulation of body temperature. Ordinarily a person satisfies his water requirements by ingesting food and drink in moderate amounts and does not experience the sensation of thirst. Thirst appears in health when there is an inadequate amount of water in the body. Although the exact cause of thirst is not known, it appears to depend on decreased water content and possibly increased osmotic pressure of the cells. Usually the sensation is alleviated by drinking water. However, thirst associated with dehydration probably is a sign of a lack of salt as well. Man cannot discriminate between salt hunger and water hunger as animals can. It is therefore important under some conditions to provide salt with the drinking water to replenish the electrolytes of extracellular fluid.

Output of water and salts The loss of water and salts by way of the skin, lungs, and intestinal tract is governed by physiologic needs. The excretion of water through the skin and lungs is chiefly a matter of heat regulation and bears little relation to the intake of fluid. The water secreted by the intestine is the solvent for excretory products and is needed to ensure suitable consistency of the feces. Renal secretion normally is highly flexible. If a large amount of water has been ingested or produced, the kidney excretes the excess. If the water intake is low, this organ can and does produce a concentrated urine so that little water is lost from the body. Similarly, the kidney can conserve or eliminate salt, depending on dietary intake.

The inspired air at ordinary temperatures contains very small amounts of water. Expired air, on the contrary, is almost saturated. The familiar condensation of moisture after breathing on a cold glass object is evidence of this. Consequently, any increase in pulmonary ventilation increases the water loss by this pathway. The evaporation of water from the lungs is one of the body's methods of losing excess heat.

Perspiration. Sweating is an important means of getting rid of body heat, since heat is used in evaporation. At moderate temperatures this evaporation keeps pace with secretion and no actual drops of sweat form. This is called insensible perspiration Some carbon dioxide is lost with insensible perspiration. With higher temperatures the sweat glands become more active and secrete more freely. Evaporation is faster, unless the humidity of the air is high. Sweating is accelerated also, for the purpose of dissipating heat, when there is considerable muscular activity. Therefore the amount of perspiration normally secreted depends on the temperature and relative humidity of the atmosphere and on the muscular activity of the individual. The insensible perspiration range is from 300 to 700 ml. per day; sensible perspiration is any additional quantity.

It is, of course, difficult to obtain sweat for analysis, but by the employment of microchemical and microbiologic methods our knowledge of sweat composition is becoming more complete. Sweat has a specific gravity of about 1.002 to 1.003, with a pH reputed to be anywhere from 5.2 to 7.3. Urea is present in a concentration four or five times that of blood. Glucose is present in minute amounts, much less than in blood. Ten free amino acids have been found by microbiologic methods. Most of these acids are in about the same concentrations as in blood, but a few are much higher in sweat—arginine and histidine are about six times higher in sweat. Sweat is said to have about one fifth to one half as high a concentration of sodium chloride as found in blood plasma. It is therefore evident that many of the constituents of sweat are not merely a result of filtration from the blood plasma. Usually less than 0.1 gm. of nitrogen is secreted in the perspiration each day, but if sweating is profuse, as much as 0.2 gm. may be eliminated in a single hour. In addition to sodium chloride, some potassium salts, appreciable amounts of calcium, magnesium, and phosphorus, and traces of copper and manganese are found in sweat.

Gastrointestinal secretion of water. The water that leaves the body by way of the intestinal canal is small in amount under ordinary circumstances because the water of the digestive fluids is largely reabsorbed along with the water of food and drink. Some materials are actively secreted and must be held in solution; thus the feces should not be permitted to become too hard and dry. When diarrhea or vomiting occurs, large amounts of water and electrolytes may be lost, especially Na^+, K^+, H^+, Cl^-, and HCO_3^-. The gastrointestinal secretions contain potassium in concentrations higher than those of extracellular fluid, although lower than those present within the cells. Consequently the loss of potassium by this route is of great importance, since it may lead to grave potassium deficits.

Secretion of urine The water-excreting function of the kidneys is by no means their only function. The kidneys excrete waste products, aid in acid-base regulation both by excreting acids or bases and by producing ammonia, and, in addition, produce physiologically active substances. At the moment we are concerned with their activities in excreting water and salts. As stated earlier, the renal excretion of water and salts is highly flexible and is rapidly adjustable to the needs of the body. If excessive amounts of water or salts are ingested, the kidney promptly eliminates the excess under normal conditions. If the water or salt intake is low, renal conservation occurs. The antidiuretic hormone of the posterior pituitary controls renal water loss (p. 486), and aldosterone (p. 470) regulates sodium loss by increasing the tubular reabsorption of sodium. The mechanisms involved will be considered in more detail in Chapter 23.

Dehydration. Dehydration may result from an inadequate intake or excessive loss of water, or both, and is of two types: (1) that due to deprivation of water alone and (2) that resulting from pathologic loss of water and electrolytes (Fig. 15-8). The output of water may be due to diuresis, to a loss of water from the gastrointestinal tract as a result of diarrhea, or, more frequently, to persistent vomiting. There are all degrees of dehydration, from a mild state to an

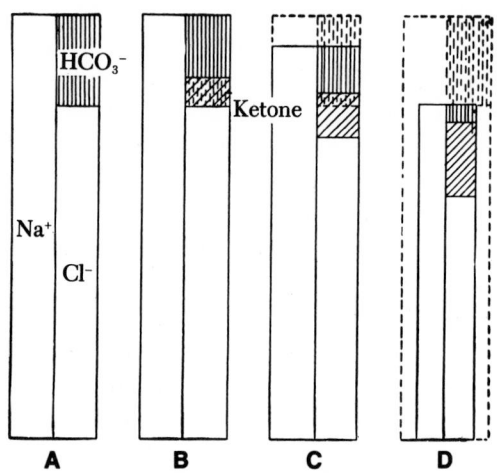

Fig. 15-8. Schematic representation of the effect of diabetic acidosis on the volume and composition of extracellular fluid. The vertical dimension represents osmolar concentration, and the horizontal, volume of fluid. For purposes of simplification, only Na^+, Cl^-, and HCO_3^- are depicted. The broken lines in each case indicate the pattern of normal interstitial fluid for comparison. The β-hydroxybutyric and acetoacetic acids in excess displace the HCO_3^- as shown in **B.** This results in the excretion of some Na^+ as salts of these acids and the elimination of CO_2 by the lungs. For some unknown reason NaCl is also excreted in large amounts. These salts take H_2O along with them and dehydration is accelerated. The Cl^- continues to be excreted even after its concentration in the blood serum is greatly diminished, **C.** The patient experiences extreme thirst but is unable to retain H_2O by mouth because of nausea and vomiting. In fact, these add to the salt depletion and dehydration. In the attempt to excrete CO_2 through the lungs, overventilation occurs, which takes away more H_2O. The final stage is suggested by **D.** Here the dehydration is caused in part by the high glucose in the blood, which is diuretic. The acetoacetic acid and β-hydroxybutyric acid are buffered by blood HCO_3^-, thus lowering the HCO_3^-. They also must be excreted. Despite an increased formation of NH_3 by the kidney to help neutralize these acids so that they can be excreted, the acids take away some Na^+ into the urine. Consequently there is a loss of fixed base from the blood along with a lowered bicarbonate. (From Peters, J. P.: In Duncan, G. G., editor: Diseases of metabolism; detailed methods of diagnosis and treatment, ed. 3, Philadelphia, 1952, W. B. Saunders Co.)

exceedingly severe one, which may establish itself more rapidly than one would believe possible. At first the interstitial fluid suffers a shrinkage and not much harm is done; in this situation, if water is taken by mouth, there is a restoration of normal conditions. Losses of the second type require calculated replacement of electrolytes and water.

Pathologic dehydration and related conditions   At this point it may be well to repeat the statement that normally the total osmotic effects of the plasma, the interstitial fluids, and the intracellular fluid are all the same. This does not hold for secretions, e.g., sweat, saliva, which are secreted onto relatively impermeable stratified epithelium, but it does hold for all truly internal fluids. The osmotic effect is due to nonelectrolytes, glucose, urea in some measure, and to proteins in a very minute degree; but most of the osmotic effect is attributable to the inorganic ions. Consequently, gains or losses of electrolytes, especially sodium or potassium ions, or changes in their concentrations, are usually followed by shifts of fluid to restore osmotic equilibrium.

The volume of blood in an adult's body is roughly 5 liters, of which about 3 liters are plasma. From this blood plasma, of course, all secretions, as well as the interstitial fluid, are derived. As an example of the effect of loss of secreted fluid on water and salt balance, the following illustration may be given: Assume that 500 ml. of mixed jejunal and ileal fluids have been secreted and lost from the body. A mixture of equal parts of these two secretions resembles blood plasma in composition except that it contains less protein. Consequently, removing a mixture such as this is like removing 500 ml. of protein-free plasma. The results to be expected are as follows:

1. Reduction in plasma volume from 3000 to 2500 ml.
2. Reduction in total blood volume of 500 ml., i.e., from 5000 to 4500 ml.
3. Rise in erythrocyte count because of blood concentration
4. Increase in the concentration of plasma proteins by 20% with a rise in colloidal osmotic pressure
5. No change in *concentration* of the plasma electrolytes and hence little change in the total osmotic pressure

This would result in no change in the size of the body cells because of the constancy of osmotic pressure. However, additional losses of other body fluids would have other effects. Such losses are caused by longer periods of dehydration, pyloric stenosis, intestinal obstruction, sweating, trauma, and severe burns.

If dehydration and loss of extracellular electrolytes are continued, the volume of the blood plasma decreases, and the plasma is found to have become concentrated. Serum proteins increase in concentration. Blood urea rises, and a negative balance of nitrogen and potassium occurs, which indicates that a generalized tissue disintegration has set in. Since the cells contain potassium, this element thus gets into the interstitial fluid and thence into the plasma and is excreted in the urine. However, prolonged dehydration from any cause has been shown to result in a greater loss of intracellular potassium than can be accounted for by protein catabolism. A continued dehydration, with concentration of blood and loss of cations, eventually leads to death.

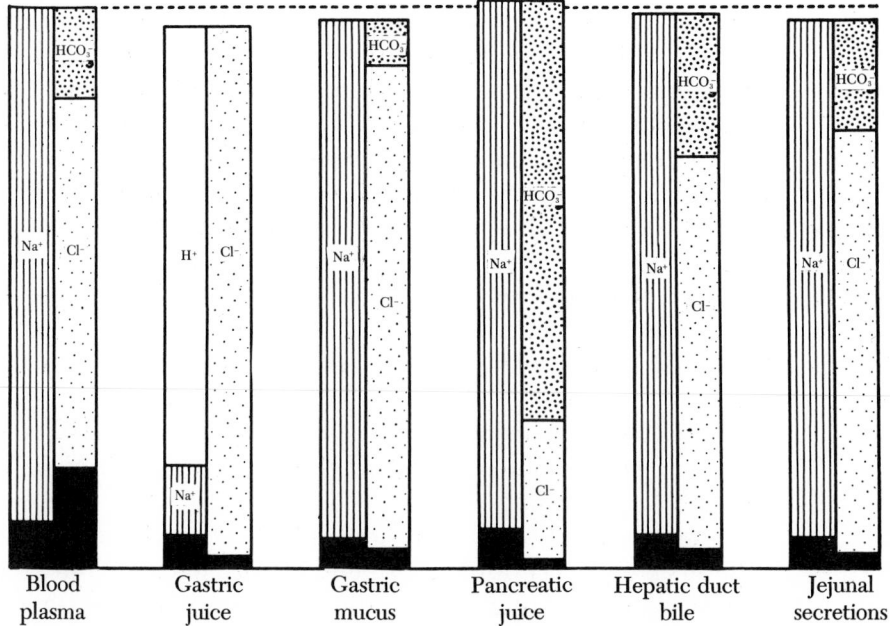

Fig. 15-9. Electrolyte composition of gastrointestinal secretions. The K^+ present in these secretions (included in the black block beneath the Na^+) is usually two to five times that of plasma K^+. Gastric vomitus usually is a mixture of gastric juice and gastric mucus, and the Na^+ may be less than, equal to, or greater than the Cl^-. (From Gamble, J. L.: Chemical anatomy, physiology and pathology of extracellular fluid, Cambridge, Mass., 1958, Harvard University Press.)

Pyloric stenosis or obstruction results in excessive loss of fluid by vomiting. The fluid lost is gastric secretion, which is a varying mixture of sodium chloride, potassium chloride and hydrochloric acid. Therefore a drop in the chloride ion concentration of the plasma occurs. There is a compensatory rise in bicarbonate ion (derived from carbon dioxide) to preserve electric neutrality. Plasma potassium may also be reduced if this ion is not included in the replacement solution.

Darrow and Hellerstein[41] showed that diarrhea in infants is accompanied by a decrease in extracellular water due to a loss of sodium, chloride, and bicarbonate in the watery stools. These ions are derived from the alkaline intestinal secretions, particularly pancreatic juice and bile (Fig. 15-9). As sodium leaves the plasma and interstitial fluid, potassium salts move out of the cells. As a result, intracellular potassium is lost in tremendous quantities. For this reason potassium salts are added to therapeutic solutions containing sodium salts (Table 15-5). Since heart block is produced when potassium rises to a certain level in the plasma, care must be exercised in the intravenous administration of such fluids; hence oral administration is recommended.

Similarly, in any condition involving an excessive loss of sodium chloride and water from the body, e.g., hemorrhage, intestinal obstruction, potassium tends to leave the cells and go into the blood plasma. The potassium salts are

Table 15-5. Comparison of plasma with replacement solutions (all concentrations in milliequivalents per liter)*

Solution	Na^+	Cl^-	HCO_3^-	K^+	Ca^{++}	Mg^{++}
Plasma	140	103	27	5	5	3
Balanced electrolyte solution (Fox)	140	103	55†	10	5	3
0.9% Sodium chloride	154	154	0	0	0	0
M/6 Sodium lactate	167	0	167‡	0	0	0
Ringer's solution, USP	147	155.5	0	4	4.5	0
Lactate Ringer's solution, USP	130	109	28‡	4	3	0
Darrow's solution	122	104	53‡	35	0	0

*From Fox, C. L., Jr., et al.: J.A.M.A. **148**:827, 1952.
†Obtained by metabolism of acetate and citrate.
‡Obtained by the theoretic 100% metabolism of D,L-lactate.

excreted in the urine if renal function is satisfactory; but if this function stops, potassium accumulates in the plasma and toxicity is manifested. Potassium also leaves the muscles and other organs in certain disease states and after surgical trauma. Under these circumstances sodium frequently accumulates in excess of the potassium lost.

In untreated diabetes there is a loss of water, together with sodium and potassium; these ions are excreted in the urine as salts of the keto acids. When acidosis occurs, such losses are increased. Plasma bicarbonate is diminished. Since vomiting frequently occurs, marked dehydration results from losses of electrolytes and water, with effects pictured in Fig. 15-8. However, the administration of insulin and replacement solutions halts ketosis and further loss of water and electrolytes. The acidoses of childhood and of starvation are also accompanied by similar losses of water and salts.

The adrenal cortex has a profound influence on electrolyte metabolism. More specifically, it controls the level of sodium ions. In adrenalectomized animals there is a decreased concentration of sodium in the plasma and an increase in the potassium. Attention at first was centered on this rise in the potassium, but the sodium now appears to be the more important factor. In Addison's disease, which is a condition involving adrenal insufficiency, the same relationships are seen. The low plasma sodium is a result of increased excretion of sodium by the kidneys. Sodium is lost not merely from the plasma but also from the interstitial fluid, especially in the muscles, which at the same time gain water, in a manner analogous to the swelling of erythrocytes when placed in hypotonic saline solutions. Treatment with sodium chloride alleviates the symptoms of patients suffering from this disease. Administration of one of the adrenocortical hormones, deoxycorticosterone, cortisone, or aldosterone, in large amounts to animals with acute adrenal insufficiency results in an increased sodium concentration in the blood serum. This probably is due to a shift of interstitial fluid (tissue fluid) to the blood, resulting in a dilution of the blood with this fluid, which contains sodium salts. A more rapid excretion of water then occurs and a diminished excretion of sodium salts, with a consequent improvement of the condition. In edematous states, e.g., nephroses, cortisone frequently causes a diuresis of sodium and water. The drugs acetazolamide (a carbonic anhydrase inhibitor) and chlorothiazide (a diuretic) are sometimes used for this purpose.

The high potassium content of the blood in adrenal insufficiency seems to be due to a diminished ability of the kidney to excrete potassium. Along with an increase in the potassium content of the serum, there is also an augmentation in the potassium of the muscle cells. The large doses of adrenocortical extract, which raise serum sodium in adrenal insufficiency, decrease serum potassium by enabling the kidney to excrete it.

In shock due to trauma or burns, there is no overall loss of salt from the body, but there is internal loss and a marked change of the electrolyte pattern. The injured or burned tissues lose potassium, apparently by extrusion from the cells. Sodium passes into the cells in exchange for the potassium. These changes are proportional to the mass of damaged tissue. There is also a considerable gain of extracellular fluid (water, sodium), which is probably the source of the increment of intracellular sodium. The sodium present in the injured cells is really lost from the plasma and interstitial fluid and other uninjured functioning tissue. Tissues remote from the site of injury or burn do not show much change in water content but do show a loss of sodium and a gain of potassium, pointing to extracellular dehydration with intracellular swelling.

The loss of salts and water by sweating may be considerable. When strenuous work is done, especially at high temperatures, as by miners or blast furnace workers, as much as 10 to 15 liters may be lost in 8 hours of work. If each liter contains 3 gm. of sodium chloride, this represents a tremendous depletion of the salts of the interstitial fluid. When these stores are gone, first the plasma and then the cells suffer. Violent cramps (stoker's or miner's cramps) and prostration may result from the combined loss of salt and fluid. Replacement of the water alone may make matters worse by diluting the plasma. To guard against this, the drinking water for such workers should contain 0.1% to 0.15% sodium chloride. This does not have an unpleasant flavor and allays thirst quite as well as unsalted water. In fevers, patients may lose large amounts of moisture and electrolytes in perspiration. These should be replaced if ill effects are to be prevented. A moderately increased salt intake during hot weather has also been recommended for most people because of this loss of salt in the perspiration. In cases of renal insufficiency or edema more cautious replacement is necessary.

The simplest way to restore fluid in dehydration is to administer saline parenterally, usually 0.9% sodium chloride. If there is acidosis, some alkaline salt may be used. Sodium lactate and sodium acetate, both of which are metabolically converted to bicarbonate, are generally preferred to sodium bicarbonate (Table 15-5). Glucose should not be administered unless there is ketosis because it tends to cause or increase diuresis, thereby accentuating the dehydration. Excellent results have been obtained by the oral administration of isotonic sodium lactate solution to restore fluid and salt balance in severe extensive third-degree burns. In infantile diarrhea the addition of potassium to a mixture of sodium chloride and sodium lactate was found to improve the clinical results. When large volumes of fluid are administered in a variety of clinical conditions, the inclusion of potassium and other mineral supplementation is advisable to assist in obtaining normal extracellular fluid composition. The readily available solutions for intravenous therapy are compared in Table 15-5. The frequent occurrence of multiple ionic alterations and the critical interrelationships among the various cations suggest the desirability of some type of balanced electrolyte solution.

References

GENERAL

Aikawa, T. K.: The role of magnesium in biological processes, Springfield, Ill., 1963, Charles C Thomas, Publisher.

Bothwell, T. H., and Finch, C. A.: Iron metabolism, Boston, 1962, Little, Brown & Co.

Bowen, H. J. A.: Trace elements in biochemistry, New York, 1966, Academic Press, Inc.

Comar, C. L., and Bronner, F., editors: Mineral metabolism, New York, 1960–1964, Academic Press, Inc.

Early, L. E., and Daugharty, T. M.: Sodium metabolism, New Eng. J. Med. 281:72, 1969.

Elkinton, J. R., and Danowski, T. S.: The body fluids, Baltimore, 1955, The Williams & Wilkins Co.

Frieden, E.: The biochemistry of copper, Sci. Amer. 219:102, 1968.

Gamble, J. L.: Chemical anatomy, physiology, and pathology of extracellular fluid, ed. 6, Cambridge, Mass., 1958, Harvard University Press.

Morgane, P. J., editor: Neural regulation of food and water intake, Ann. N.Y. Acad. Sci. 157:531, 1969.

Muntwyler, E.: Water and electrolyte metabolism and acid-base balance, St. Louis, 1968, The C. V. Mosby Co.

Peisach, J., Aisen, P., and Blumberg, W., editors: The biochemistry of copper, New York, 1966, Academic Press, Inc.

Pitts, R. F.: Physiology of the kidney and body fluids, Chicago, 1963, Year Book Medical Publishers, Inc.

Rosenfeld, I., and Beath, O. A.: Selenium, New York, 1964, Academic Press, Inc.

Underwood, E. J.: Trace elements in human and animal nutrition, New York, 1962, Academic Press, Inc.

Wasserman, R. H.: The transfer of calcium and strontium across biological membranes, New York, 1963, Academic Press, Inc.

Wolf, A. V.: Body water, Sci. Amer. 199:125, 1958.

SPECIAL

1. Swanson, P. P., and Smith, A. H.: J. Biol. Chem. 98:479, 499, 1932; Brooke, R. O., and Smith, A. H.: J. Biol. Chem. 104:141, 1934; Smith, P. K., and Smith, A. H.: J. Biol. Chem. 105:lxxxi, 1934.
2. Wasserman, R. H., and Lengemann, F. W.: J. Nutr. 70:377, 1960.
3. Lemann, J., Jr., et al.: New Eng. J. Med. 280:232, 1969.
4. Mitchell, H. H.: Mod. Med. 23:85, 1955.
5. Gershoff, S. N., et al.: J. Nutr. 64:303, 1958.
6. Harris, W. J., and Heaney, R. P.: New Eng. J. Med. 280:193, 253, 1969.
7. McLean, F. C., and Urist, M. R.: Bone: an introduction to the physiology of skeletal tissue, Chicago, 1955, University of Chicago Press.
8. Zeelig, M. S.: Amer. J. Clin. Nutr. 14:342, 1964.
9. Wacker, W. E. C., and Parisi, A. F.: New Eng. J. Med. 278:712, 1968.
10. Matsubara, H., et al.: Proc. Nat. Acad. Sci. 57:439, 1967.
11. Dubach, R., et al.: J. Lab. Clin. Med. 45:599, 1955.
12. Crosby, W. H.: J.A.M.A. 208:347, 1969.
13. Lee, G. B., et al.: J. Clin Invest. 47:2058, 1968.
14. Osaki, S.: J. Biol. Chem. 241:2746, 5053, 1966.
15. Granick, S.: Physiol. Rev. 31:489, 1951.
16. Goldsmith, G. A.: Nutr. Rev. 23:1, 1965.
17. Review: J.A.M.A. 203:407, 1968.
18. Everson, G. J., et al.: J. Nutr. 93:533, 1967.
19. Carlton, W. W., and Kelly, W. A.: J. Nutr. 97:42, 52, 1969.
20. Chou, W. S., et al.: Proc. Soc. Exp. Biol. Med. 128:948, 1968.
21. Prasad, A. S., editor: Zinc metabolism, Springfield, Ill., 1966, Charles C Thomas, Publisher.

22. Brudevold, F., et al.: Arch. Oral Biol. 8:155, 1963.
23. Prasad, A. S.: Fed. Proc. Sympos. 26:172, 1967.
24. Everson, G. J., and Shrader, R. E.: J. Nutr. 94:89, 1968.
25. Orten, J. M.: Amer. J. Physiol. 114:414, 1936.
26. Marine, D., and Kimball, O. P.: J.A.M.A. 77:1068, 1921.
27. Fierro-Benitez, R., et al.: New Eng. J. Med. 280:296, 1969.
28. Armstrong, W. D., and Brekhus, P. J.: J. Dent. Res. 17:393, 1938.
29. Ast, D. B., et al.: J. Amer. Dent. Ass. 52:290, 1956.
30. Stare, F., and Bernstein, D.: Med. World News, April 23, 1965.
31. Schwarz, K., and Foltz, C. M.: J. Biol. Chem. 233:245, 1958.
32. Gardner, R. W., and Hogue, D. E.: J. Nutr. 93:418, 1967.
33. Roginski, E. E., and Mertz, W.: J. Nutr. 97:525, 1969.
34. Mertz, W.: Fed. Proc. Sympos. 26:186, 1967.
35. Schroeder, H. A.: J. Nutr. 97:237, 1969.
36. Katz, R. I., et al.: Science 162:466, 1968. Editorial: New Eng. J. Med. 280:560, 1969.
37. Dahl, L. K.: Amer. J. Cardiol. 8:571, 1961.
38. Prior, I. A. M., et al.: New Eng. J. Med. 279:515, 1968.
39. Walker, J. S., et al.: Science 140:890, 1963.
40. Gaebler, O. H., and Choitz, H. C.: Clin. Chem. 10:13, 1964.
41. Darrow, D. C., and Hellerstein, S.: Physiol. Rev. 38:114, 1958.

CHAPTER 16

HORMONES

ormones are substances manufactured by cells in minute amounts; they produce characteristic biochemical and physiologic effects on other cells, usually in some *target* organ or tissue remote from the source of the hormone. They are secreted directly into the bloodstream and are transported in the plasma to the target or *effector* cell where they exert their characteristic effect. In many instances they are relatively ineffective when administered by mouth and, therefore, if given for medical purposes, are usually injected parenterally.

Hormones are, strictly speaking, stimulating substances (Greek, *hormān*, "to excite"). However, some endocrine secretions inhibit functional activity, and these have been designated chalones.

The need for extracellular neural and hormonal mechanisms for the control of physiologic processes apparently arose with the evolutionary development of multicellular organisms. These, of course, are supplementary to enzymatic and genetic control mechanisms, which, in general, operate intracellularly. Indeed, recent evidence has apparently established an involvement of the central nervous system, primarily the hypothalamus, in the control of the secretion of certain hormones, as will be described later. This area of biochemistry is sometimes called *neuroendocrinology*. Likewise, certain hormones appear to regulate genetic mechanisms (RNA formation), which, in turn, control enzyme and protein synthesis in their target tissues. Thus, there appears to be a delicately balanced interrelationship between the hormones, the central nervous system, and genetic-enzymic mechanisms in the regulation of cellular metabolic processes.

The major hormone-secreting glands include the intestinal mucosa, pancreas, adrenals, thyroid, parathyroids, pituitary, ovaries, and testes. Several other glandular tissues are alleged to secrete hormones. For example, the juxtaglomerular cells of the kidney may produce the hormone erythropoietin, which regulates erythrocyte maturation (p. 507). Also, the thymus may regulate immunologic mechanisms in the body by means of a hormonal secretion.[1] The pineal gland may likewise secrete one or more hormones, at least in certain species.

The hormones can be classified chemically into three major groups: (1) *steroids*, e.g., androgens, estrogens, and adrenocorticoids; (2) *amino acid derivatives*, epinephrine and thyroxine; and (3) *peptide-proteins*, insulin, glucagon, parathormone, oxytocin, vasopressin, probably most of the hormones secreted by the intestinal mucosa, and the seven or eight so-called tropic hormones of the anterior pituitary. Each of these is apparently synthesized in its respective glandular tissue from simple precursors. Presumably, after the molecule has served its biologic function, it is converted to an inactive form, usually in the liver, and excreted or destroyed. The major steps in the biosynthesis and degradation of most hormones are fairly completely known and will be discussed later. A delicately controlled balance between these two processes is maintained in the normal organism so that an optimal level of the hormone is present in body fluids at all times.

Although the physiologic, apparently secondary, effects of most hormones have been rather completely known for a number of years, the primary biochemical mechanisms of action of hormones at a cellular-molecular level are just beginning to be understood. Indeed, one of the more exciting newer developments in biochemistry is the current indication that certain hormones serve as inducers or repressors in the genetically controlled synthesis of certain key cellular enzymes. In this indirect way, hormones exert their control over the metabolic processes of the cell. Thus, one important general type of action of hormones (e.g., insulin, the adrenocorticoids, and possibly the androgens, estrogens, and erythropoietin) is the modulation of gene activity in controlling enzyme induction and repression.

A second, primary, type of action of several hormones (e.g., epinephrine, glucagon) is the regulation of enzyme activity by way of cyclic-AMP (p. 455). A third type of action (e.g., of parathormone, aldosterone, growth hormone, and possibly thyroxine and insulin) is the serving as agents for the control of membrane transport.

These three basic biochemical mechanisms of action are manifested in the whole organism as the more gross physiologic effects of the hormones, e.g., the raising or lowering of the blood sugar level, increasing or decreasing basal metabolism, or changing protein synthesis in the target tissue of the hormone in question. This extremely active area of biochemical research will be considered in some detail as each hormone is discussed.

IMMUNOASSAY OF HORMONES

The rapid advances made in the past few years in knowledge of the chemical nature and mode of action of the hormones have been a result of the application of newer, more sophisticated techniques to these problems. One in particular should be mentioned at this point, the technique of immunoassay.[2] By this procedure, applicable only to protein hormones, it is possible to quantitatively assay the extremely small amounts of protein hormones present in the blood plasma and other body fluids and tissues. Needless to say, the availability of such an ultrasensitive and specific quantitative method of assay has made feasible studies of hormone action heretofore not possible. Hormones now determined by this technique include insulin, growth hormone, the gonadotropins, parathormone, and gastrin. It should be applicable to any protein hormone that has significant antigenic properties.

The principle of the immunoassay technique, briefly, is as follows: antibodies to the protein hormone are produced in an animal, usually a rabbit, and antisera are thus prepared; the antiserum reacts specifically with and precipitates the hormone, which may be labeled with a radioactive isotope, e.g., ^{131}I or ^{125}I, or with a fluorescent dye, making possible its immunoassay; typically this is accomplished in a radioimmunoassay by determining the isotope dilution effect of an unlabeled unknown hormone sample (e.g., plasma insulin) on a standard ^{131}I- or ^{125}I-labeled hormone preparation; an additional step, the use of a second antibody (e.g., goat-antirabbit γ-globulin), to increase the sensitivity of the procedure, is sometimes employed.

ROLE OF CYCLIC-AMP IN HORMONE ACTIONS

One of the interesting developments in the hormone field in the past decade is the mounting evidence that cyclic adenosine-3′,5′-monophosphate, cyclic-AMP (p. 36), is involved as a "second messenger," mediating the cellular response to the hormone or "first messenger." The effect of cyclic-AMP on the action of a hormone was first described, in 1960, by Sutherland and Rall[3]. It was observed then that the effect of epinephrine on hepatic glycogenolysis is a result of the conversion of inactive phosphorylase-b into an active form by cyclic-AMP. Epinephrine was found to activate the enzyme adenyl cyclase, which in turn, converts ATP to cyclic-AMP (p. 194). Since these pioneer observations, cyclic-AMP has been found to mediate the effect of a number of hormones, including epinephrine, glucagon, parathyroid hormone (PTH), vasopressin, ACTH, TSH, interstitial cell–stimulating hormone (ICSH) or luteinizing hormone (LH), and α-melanocyte–stimulating hormone (α-MSH). Several hormones are also known to *decrease* cyclic-AMP levels and produce an opposite effect to the stimulation by cyclic-AMP. These include[4] insulin, the prostaglandins, the α-adrenergics, and melatonin. From the size of this list, it would appear that hormone action *not* mediated by cyclic-AMP may prove to be the exception rather than the rule. The specific effects of cyclic-AMP on individual hormone action will be discussed later in this chapter. A schematic diagram showing the effect of cyclic-AMP on hormone action is shown in Fig. 16-1. The hormone apparently activates the target cell membrane enzyme, called adenyl cyclase, which, in turn, catalyzes the transformation of ATP to cyclic-AMP. The increased cyclic-AMP, acting within the target cell, then carries out the specific work of the hormone by affecting the activity of enzymes, the permeability or transport processes, the release of other hormones (third messengers), etc.

Cyclic-AMP is apparently inactivated rapidly by a cellular enzyme, a phosphodiesterase, which, like adenyl cyclase, is present in practically all tissues. Phosphodiesterase is inhibited by pyrophosphate, methylxanthines, citrate, and several nucleotides.

Questions may arise in regard to harmonizing the variety of functions performed by cyclic-AMP (e.g., increasing lypolysis in adipose tissue, decreasing gluconeogenesis in the liver) with the high degree of specificity of the hor-

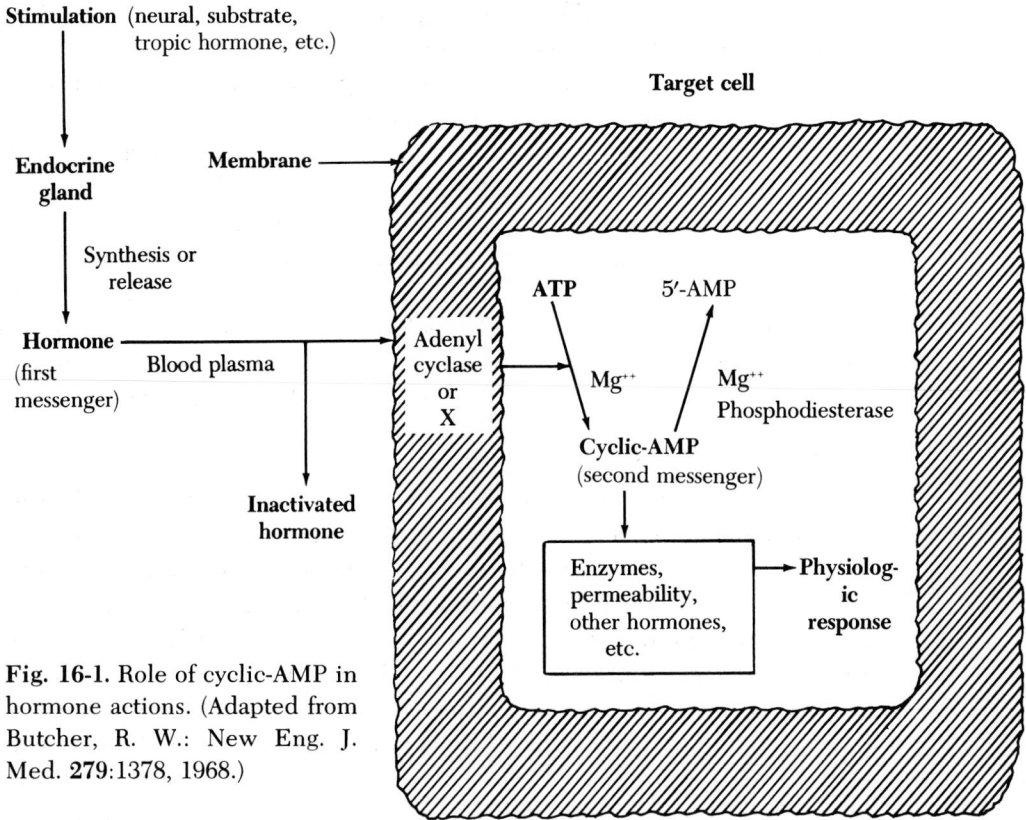

Fig. 16-1. Role of cyclic-AMP in hormone actions. (Adapted from Butcher, R. W.: New Eng. J. Med. **279**:1378, 1968.)

mones whose actions they mediate. Undoubtedly the answers lie in the enzyme profile of the individual target cell itself. In other words, what cyclic-AMP does in a particular effector cell is determined by the cell itself rather than by cyclic-AMP.

HORMONES OF THE GASTROINTESTINAL TRACT

During the past few years, substantial progress has been made in the isolation and purification of various hormones of the gastrointestinal tract. All are proteins, and the amino acid sequences of at least four (gastrin, secretin, pancreozymin, cholecystokinin) have been determined. The structural overlap among the various gastrointestinal hormones is indeed remarkable. The structural similarities account for the overlapping of functional activity of several gastrointestinal hormones and have led to questions of the hormones' existence for many years. For example, pancreozymin and cholecystokinin are remarkably similar, almost like "twins." Jorpes[5] believes they are identical. Also, secretin and glucagon (from the pancreas) each are composed of 27 amino acids, and at least 14 of these acids are in the same positions in the two hormones. Other characteristics of the gastrointestinal hormones will be considered as they are discussed individually.

Undoubtedly one of the reasons for recent rapid progress in knowledge of this group of hormones is the fact that the hormones are proteins and thus can be quantitatively determined in small amounts by radioimmunoassay procedures just mentioned. As well stated by one investigator, "Grinding up of gastric and duodenal mucosa of pigs and other animals will after some 50 years redound to the benefit of the patient."

Gastrin   Gastrin is produced by the pyloric mucosa, which is apparently stimulated by proteins or polypeptides present in or derived from food, or possibly by hydrochloric acid. Mechanical stimulation caused by distention of the stomach also results in the production of gastrin. The hormone is absorbed into the bloodstream and is carried to the fundic cells, causing them to secrete hydrochloric acid actively. The possibility that a hormone (perhaps gastrin), also involved in gastric secretion, is secreted by the antrum is discussed on p. 672. The chemical nature of gastrin was determined recently. Gastrin is apparently a heptapeptide, and its amino acid sequence has been determined. The active portion of the molecule according to Gregory[6] is a tetrapeptide with a C-terminal end sequence of Trp-Met-Phe-Asn. The Trp-Met-Phe sequence seems to serve as the binding site(s). There may be a second form of gastrin differing slightly in its amino acid composition.

Secretin and cholecystokinin   Secretin is formed by the upper intestinal mucosa and is liberated by the hydrochloric acid present in the acid chyme. Secretin is carried by the bloodstream to the pancreas, which it stimulates, thus causing a flow of pancreatic juice rich in bicarbonate. This occurs even if the nerves supplying the pancreas are cut and is therefore a true hormonal action. Further evidence in favor of this theory is the fact that if the blood from an animal, in the process of forming pancreatic juice due to the presence of hydrochloric acid in the duodenum, is injected into the veins of a starving animal the pancreas of the latter is also stimulated to secrete. Secretin has been obtained in crystalline form and appears to be a polypeptide (p. 72). It is very effective by the intravenous route. Mellanby was of the opinion that secretin controls the volume and bicarbonate content of pancreatic juice while the enzyme content is under the control of the vagus nerve. In 1943, however, another hormone, cholecystokinin, was separated from the mucosal extract of the small intestine. Cholecystokinin stimulates the secretion of a juice that is rich in enzymes, and thus pancreatic secretion is under both hormonal and nervous control. Cholecystokinin also stimulates the contraction of the gallbladder (p. 680).

Secretin stimulates the production of fluid low in enzymes but containing bicarbonate. It produces the same effects in man as it does in animals and is being employed in tests for pancreatic function. Secretin probably also stimulates the flow of intestinal juice and is one of the factors that increase the secretion of bile by the liver.

Pancreozymin   Another hormone, called pancreozymin, is present in the mucosa of the upper small intestine. It is thermostable and is not destroyed by acid, but it is destroyed by alkali. It may be separated from secretin in alcoholic solution by the precipitation of secretin by bile salts and the precipitation of pancreozymin by saturation with sodium chloride.

Pancreozymin is a protein and has been prepared in pure form. Its amino acid sequence has been determined; there are 33 amino acids in its molecule.

The five terminal amino acids are the same as those of gastrin. Pancreozymin is similar in amino acid composition to cholecystokinin; in fact, Jorpes[5] believes they are identical. The release of pancreozymin is said to be brought about by the presence of any one of a variety of substances, including peptone, casein, dextrin, maltose, lactose, saline, and even distilled water.

The pancreatic juice stimulated by pancreozymin is rich in enzymes, or their zymogens, as well as in bicarbonate. The enzymes (or zymogens) include trypsinogen, chymotrypsinogen, lipase, nuclease, and carboxypeptidase (p. 678). Possibly similar stimulants are also effective in causing the release of secretin.

Entero-gastrone
Enterogastrone is a hormone that has been shown to be present in duodenal mucosa. It has not been crystallized or identified but apparently is a polypeptide. Its formation is associated with the presence of fat, and other substances derived from food, in the duodenum, and its function is to inhibit gastric secretion and gastric motility. When fat reaches the duodenum, it causes the secretion of enterogastrone, which then slows up gastric digestion and motility, including hunger contractions. There is a diminution in the volume of juice secreted, with a lower concentration of hydrochloric acid and a smaller amount of pepsin. The effect is to permit digestion to be more completely accomplished. From human urine a substance having similar effects has been isolated. It has been called *urogastrone* and may be an excretory product of enterogastrone. It seems also to inhibit pancreatic secretion.

Parotin
Although salivary secretion does not appear to be under hormonal control, extracts of gastrointestinal mucosa may produce changes in the salivary glands demonstrable by histologic procedures. It has been claimed[7] that the salivary glands elaborate parotin, a protein hormone with several effects. Parotin is said to stimulate calcification of the teeth, decrease the calcium content of the serum, and increase the phosphorus level of the serum.

Other alleged hormones
The flow of intestinal juice is also controlled by a hormone of the intestinal mucosa, called *enterocrinin*, which is apparently protein in nature and is distinct from secretin in that it stimulates the secretion of both fluid and enzymes by the intestinal mucosa. Various digestive products effect its release from the mucosa. Furthermore, extracts of intestinal mucosa contain cholecystokinin, which stimulates contraction of the gallbladder. This hormone can be separated from secretin and is set free through the agency of many different substances. The most effective are fats, fatty acids, dilute hydrochloric acid, and peptone. Another alleged related hormone, called *hepatocrinin*, is believed to stimulate the secretion of a dilute, low-salt type of bile.

Although there is good evidence for all the humoral agents mentioned, some authorities believe that gastrin, secretin, and cholecystokinin are the only gastrointestinal hormones that have been fully established as such, according to strict physiologic and biochemical standards.

INSULIN

Insulin is the hormone elaborated by the β-cells of the islets of Langerhans. It is essential in carbohydrate metabolism. Its discovery, properties, physiologic effects, and the theories of its mode of action have been described in Chapter 9. However, current work indicates that the biochemical function of insulin at the cellular level apparently is to act also as an inducer or suppressor (p. 230) of key enzymes of the glycolytic or gluconeogenic pathways of carbohydrate metabolism,[8] at least in the liver. Apparently insulin serves as an inducer for the hepatic synthesis of the glycolytic enzymes pyruvate kinase, glucokinase, and phosphofructokinase but as a suppressor for the key gluconeogenic enzymes glucose-6-phosphatase, fructose-1,6-diphosphatase, phosphoenolpyruvate carboxykinase, and pyruvate carboxylase. The adrenoglucocorticoid hormones (p. 466), on the other hand, act as inducers for the latter four gluconeogenic enzymes. These two sets of enzymes appear to be produced on two functional genome units.[8] However, if, indeed, insulin does prove to act primarily as an inducer or suppressor of the hepatic formation of key enzymes involved in carbohydrate metabolism, the long-standing enigma of the biochemical mechanism of insulin action may at last have been elucidated. There is also evidence that insulin may serve as an inducer for acetyl carboxylase, which is involved in fatty acid synthesis.

Although its chief use is in the control of diabetes, insulin has been recommended in other conditions as well, including certain liver diseases. Possibly glucose alone would be just as useful in some of these conditions, but more likely the hepatic dysfunctions are affected by insulin in some specific way. It is also known that insulin hypoglycemia is accompanied by increased tonus and motility of the stomach, resulting in hunger and sometimes increased appetite. Overdoses of insulin to produce a state of insulin shock are sometimes used in the treatment of certain mental disorders, often with beneficial effect.

Insulin is a protein with a molecular weight of 5734. Its isoelectric point is pH 5.3 to 5.36. It is inactivated by alkali, which liberates ammonia, and by proteolytic enzymes, which digest it. Its structure and amino acid sequence were described on p. 76. It contains sulfur as disulfide linkages. Attempts are being made to ascertain whether the disulfide or other characteristic groups are responsible for the activity of the hormone.

Proinsulin. During the past 2 years, evidence has been presented that insulin is not initially secreted as such by the β-cells of the pancreas but rather as a larger single-chain precursor protein, called proinsulin. Steiner and his co-workers[9] found that slices of β-cell tumors from a human pancreas incubated with ^{14}C-labeled amino acids incorporate the radioactivity first into a larger protein (separated by gel filtration) and then into insulin. Subsequent work by these and other investigators established the fact that proinsulin is a single-chain protein composed of 84 amino acids, in contrast to the 51 of insulin, and a molecular weight of approximately 9100. Proinsulin is apparently converted to insulin by proteolytic enzyme (trypsinlike) cleavage of a 33 amino acid–connecting peptide chain, shown diagrammatically at the top of p. 460.

Proinsulin appears to have a half-life of about an hour and comprises only 5% of the total insulinlike protein of islet tissue. It is therefore not a storage form of insulin but rather appears to be necessary in the formation of the

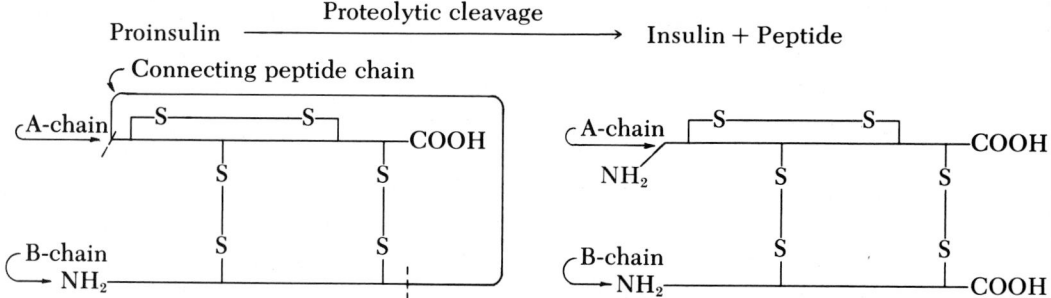

Proteolytic cleavage

Proinsulin ────────────────────────→ Insulin + Peptide

disulfide bonds essential for the biologic activity of insulin. Proinsulin formation has been demonstrated in bovine, porcine, and rat pancreatic tissue as well as in human pancreas.

Structure of insulin It has been known for quite some time that there are slight differences between the insulins of different species, even though the biologic activities of different insulins (p. 27) are identical. Sanger and Smith[10] determined the amino acid sequence of insulins from five different species and found the sequences to be identical, with the exception of the identity and sequence of only three amino acids in the 8- to 10-positions in the A-chain. The species and differences are shown in Table 16-1. This is indeed a most significant observation with respect not only to insulin but to other animal proteins as well because of possible implications in the problem of the species specificity of proteins in general.

Abel[11] succeeded in crystallizing insulin; and now, by a more simplified procedure, crystalline insulin is produced commercially (Fig. 16-2). This is sometimes termed zinc insulin. Zinc is present in the insulin molecule in loosely bound form. The addition of zinc (or cobalt, cadmium, or nickel) also aids in the crystallizing process.

An extremely significant advance in the elucidation of three-dimensional architecture of insulin was reported at recent meetings of two international congresses by D. M. Hodgkin and co-workers, of Oxford University. Porcine insulin and presumably also bovine insulin (the types used for injection in man) were shown to be hexameric molecules composed of three subunits,

Table 16-1. Differences in amino acid sequences in insulin of various species

Species	Position		
	8	9	10
Cattle	Ala	Ser	Val
Pig	Thr	Ser	Ileu
Sheep	Ala	Gly	Val
Horse	Thr	Gly	Ileu
Whale	Thr	Ser	Ileu

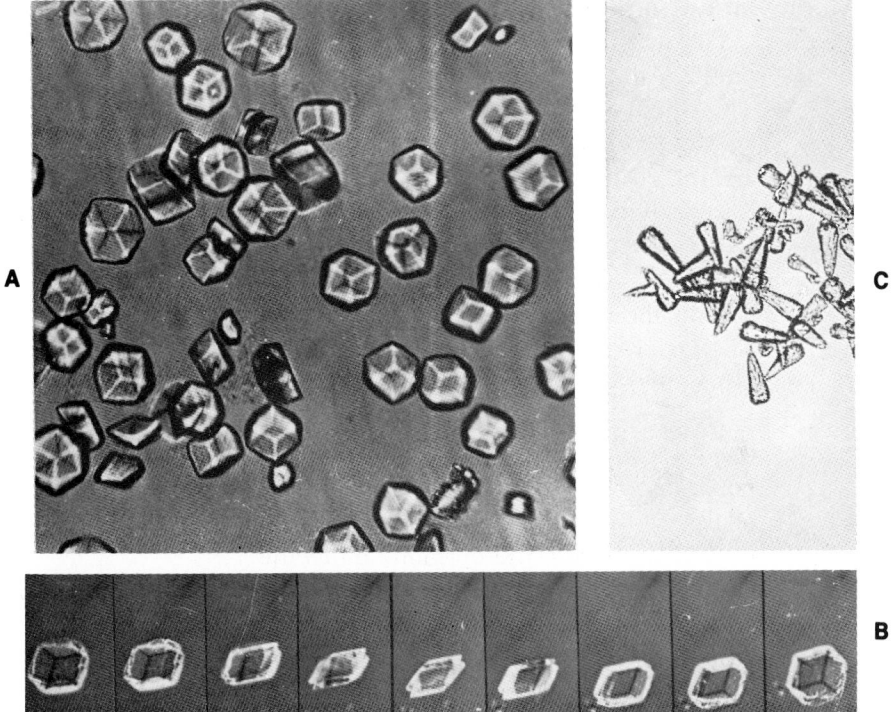

Fig. 16-2. Crystalline zinc insulin. **A,** Zn-insulin crystals formed at about pH 6. **B,** One of the same crystals, taken on motion picture film, as it rolls across the field. **C,** Zn-insulin crystals formed at about pH 5. (From Scott, D. A.: Endocrinology **25:**437, 1939.)

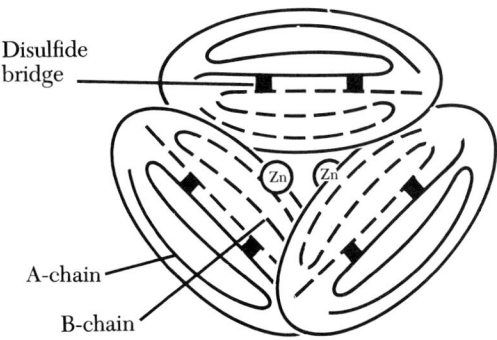

Fig. 16-3. Schematic representation of the three-dimensional structure of insulin, a hexamer consisting of three dimers, each composed of an A- and a B-polypeptide chain. Two Zn atoms are apparently involved in the formation of the quaternary structure.

each of which, in turn, is a dimer composed of the two polypeptide chains, A and B. The multicomponent molecule of insulin thus formed is a triangular ringlike structure consisting of three tilted, football-like dimers around two central zinc atoms in the core. The present concept of the structure is shown schematically in Fig. 16-3.

The hexamer is held together by a variety of forces. The ends of the overlapping dimers are apparently joined by interlocking phenylalanine groups. The dimers are also secured by hydrogen bonding between dual glutamic acid groups midway in each dimer. The A- and B-chains of the monomers are linked by hydrogen and hydrophobic interactions and by two disulfide bridges between the chains. The role of the two zinc atoms in the quaternary structure is as yet uncertain.

The present definition of the structure of insulin resulted from a study of tens of thousands of x-ray reflections of insulin crystals at 2.8 Å resolution. The Oxford group now plans to further refine the elucidation of the structure of insulin through even higher resolution measurements.

The present remarkable investigation represents the first resolution of the three-dimensional structure of a protein hormone. This work is an important step forward in ultimately understanding the mechanism of action of this vital hormone, which is undoubtedly dependent on the spatial arrangement within the hormone molecule.

The potency of an insulin preparation is expressed in *units*. A unit is that amount of insulin required to reduce the blood sugar level of a normal 2 kg. rabbit, which has been fasted for 24 hours, from 120 to 45 mg. per 100 ml. in 5 hours. A more exact definition refers to a standard preparation of zinc insulin crystals kept by the National Institute for Medical Research in London. A unit corresponds to $\frac{1}{22}$ mg. of this preparation. As sold for clinical purposes, insulin comes in concentrations designated *U-40*, *U-80*, *U-100*, and *U-500*, which indicate the number of units per milliliter. Protamine insulin and other types of slowly absorbed insulin are discussed on p. 229.

Functions of insulin The role of insulin in carbohydrate metabolism was discussed in some detail in Chapter 9. You will recall that hyperglycemia and glycosuria result from a deficient supply of insulin, due, in turn, to impaired glucose utilization by tissues. This results from an impaired transport of glucose into the cell and also from decreased activity of hepatic microsomal glucokinase and probably also from decreased activity of two other key glycolytic enzymes, pyruvate kinase and phosphofructokinase. There is also reduced activity of glycogen synthetase, at least in muscle.

Insulin affects protein and nucleic acid metabolism, apparently independent of its role in glucose utilization. It facilitates the entry of amino acids into cells. It increases the incorporation of amino acids into proteins, liver, and most other tissues, and it augments the synthesis of ribosomal proteins. Insulin apparently affects the translation of messenger RNA for the above enzymes.

Insulin, likewise, has a profound effect on lipid metabolism. It markedly increases lipogenesis from glucose in liver and adipose tissue. Syntheses of fatty acids, triglycerides, and phospholipids from glucose are all augmented in adipose tissue in vitro. Fatty acid release from the tissue is inhibited in the presence of insulin.

Plasma levels of insulin   As pointed out earlier (p. 454), the development of a specific, sensitive radioimmunoassay method for the quantitative estimation of insulin in blood plasma is proving extremely valuable in further understanding the normal and abnormal metabolism of carbohydrate. For example, in normal subjects, the plasma insulin level increases rapidly after administration of glucose. It then decreases to a normal value as the blood glucose level recedes. Low plasma insulin levels occur in only about 20% of diabetics.[12] Plasma insulin is uniformly low in juvenile-type diabetes. However, in the maturity-onset type of diabetes, it varies widely. Indeed, it may even be high for reasons as yet incompletely understood. The pancreatic reserve of insulin, however, is characteristically decreased. Certain substances that have a diabetogenic effect (e.g., overdoses of diphenylhydantoin) produce a low plasma insulin level. Interesting is the fact that arginine and other amino acids augment the secretion of insulin produced by carbohydrate administration.

Insulin appears to be rapidly metabolized or destroyed in the liver and other tissues by an enzyme, *insulinase*. The half-life of insulin in the normal human adult is determined as 6.5 to 9.0 minutes. No evidence for significant change in its decay rate has been found in certain types of diabetes.

GLUCAGON

Glucagon is produced by the islets of Langerhans, specifically by the α-cells. It has an effect just opposite that of insulin, since, on parenteral administration, it causes hyperglycemia.

You will recall that glucagon increases the blood glucose level by increasing hepatic glycogenolysis (p. 194). Glucagon activates the enzyme adenyl cyclase, which converts ATP to cyclic-AMP, which, in turn, activates phosphorylase kinase, which activates phosphorylase-b. The latter then splits glucose-1-phosphate from liver glycogen, ultimately yielding free blood glucose (p. 194).

Glucagon is a protein and has been isolated and crystallized. The crystals are rather insoluble in water at pH 7 but dissolve at a pH of 10 or higher or at a pH of about 4. It appears to be a straight-chain polypeptide containing 29 amino acids and has a molecular weight of about 3482.

The sequence of amino acids in the glucagon molecule, determined by the Sanger technique (p. 74), appears to be as follows[13]:

His Ser Gln Gly Thr Phe Thr Ser Asp Tyr Ser Lys Tyr Leu Asp Ser Arg

Arg Ala Gln Asp Phe Val Gln Try Leu Met Asn Thr

It will be noted that the only sulfur-containing amino acid is methionine and the amount of this is rather low. The complete synthesis of glucagon has been reported and significant yields of the hormone are feasible.

Recent studies[14] indicated that glucagon depresses the appetite and reduces feelings of hunger and food intake in man. It is suggested that glucagon may exert this effect by maintaining the blood glucose level or that it may act on some central neural structures in depressing appetite and food intake.

EPINEPHRINE AND NOREPINEPHRINE

Epinephrine, adrenaline, or adrenine is produced by the medulla of the adrenal glands. It was first isolated by Abel. Its structure has been determined, and it has been produced synthetically by Stoltz. Examination of its formula reveals that it is closely related to tyrosine and phenylalanine. Experiments have been performed in which isotopically labeled phenylalanine was fed to animals and was shown to be converted to epinephrine. The radioactive carbon was located in the carboxyl and α-carbon positions of the amino acid, and the epinephrine recovered was found to bear a ^{14}C at the position corresponding to the α-carbon.

Apparently phenylalanine is first converted to tyrosine by the action of phenylalanine hydroxylase (p. 373), which, in turn, is converted to dihydroxytyrosine by tyrosine hydroxylase, a rate-limiting step. The details of the conversion of tyrosine to epinephrine and norepinephrine have not yet been established.

| Tyrosine | Epinephrine | Norepinephrine |

Since epinephrine possesses an asymmetric carbon, two stereoisomers are possible. The natural (L) form is levorotatory and is 15 times more potent than the dextrorotatory (D) form. It is isolated from adrenal tissue by extraction with dilute acid, precipitation of the protein with alcohol, and treatment of the filtrate with ammonium hydroxide. This precipitates the free base, a white substance that on exposure to air is easily decomposed and becomes pink, red, and finally brown.

Norepinephrine has been isolated and characterized physiologically as well as chemically. Norepinephrine, also called noradrenaline and L-arterenol, differs from epinephrine structurally in having a hydrogen in place of the methyl group. The commonly available epinephrine or "adrenaline," therefore, is a mixture of these two hormones (usually about 10% to 20% norepinephrine), and its effects are a resultant of the actions of the two hormones, which differ somewhat from each other. These effects include constriction of the arterioles of the skin, the mucous membranes, and the splanchnic viscera. The vessels of the muscles and the coronaries dilate under the influence of epinephrine. The constricting effect has a greater influence than the dilating effect on blood pressure, and therefore epinephrine generally produces a rise in blood pressure.

The mixture has an inhibitory effect on muscular tone of the stomach, intestine, bronchioles, and wall of the urinary bladder and on movements of the gastrointestinal tract. On the other hand, the sphincter muscles of the bladder and the intestine contract. The effect on the uterus varies with the species and the state of the uterus, i.e., whether it is gravid or not. In the human being, epinephrine causes the pregnant uterus to contract. The nonpregnant uterus is inhibited. The pupil dilates as a result of contraction of the radiating fibers of the iris. Epinephrine also increases the rate and force of contractions of the heart.

The actions of the two hormones may be summarized as follows: Epinephrine increases cardiac output and thus raises blood pressure. It causes vasodilatation of skeletal and cardiac muscle blood vessels but vasoconstriction of skin and splanchnic vessels. It has no effect on cerebral blood flow but decreases the blood flow through the kidneys. Whereas epinephrine causes an increase in pulse rate, norepinephrine acts in an opposite manner in this respect.

Norepinephrine, having little effect on the heart, is a peripheral vasoconstrictor and thus also raises blood pressure; yet, on the other hand, it increases the size of the splanchnic bed. Norepinephrine apparently is the physiologic neurotransmitter in the adrenergic nervous system.

The injection of epinephrine and, to a lesser degree, norepinephrine causes hyperglycemia and glycosuria. This is because epinephrine increases liver glycogenolysis by increasing cyclic-AMP formation (p. 194). In this way it can relieve the hypoglycemia produced by insulin. Its effect here is, of course, greatest if there is a goodly store of glycogen in the liver. A similar effect on muscle glycogen can also be brought about by epinephrine, resulting in increased lactic acid. The lactic acid may be transported to the liver, where it is resynthesized to glycogen at the expense of muscle glycogen.

Solutions of epinephrine have wide application in medicine. The constriction of blood vessels and shrinking of mucous membranes make it useful in hemostasis. Also, in conjunction with local anesthetic solutions, it tends to localize, intensify, and prolong the anesthetic effects. It is used to relax the bronchioles in asthmatic attacks and frequently combats allergic manifestations in a dramatic manner.

Despite the varied and definite physiologic effects of its characteristic hormone, the adrenal medulla does not appear to be essential to life. Animals may be deprived of the adrenal medulla and get along quite well. No clinical syndrome attributable to a deficiency or disease of the adrenal medulla is known. Consequently, the exact importance of the adrenal medulla is really undetermined. Cannon's theory that epinephrine is secreted in emergencies in order to raise the blood sugar to provide ready fuel for the necessary activity ("for fight or flight") and, at the same time, to cause a shift of blood from the skin and gastrointestinal tract to the muscles warrants consideration. If this is the true function of the adrenal medulla, we may have the reason why this gland is not absolutely essential to life although probably useful for optimum physiologic performance.

The metabolism of epinephrine and norepinephrine involves the O-methylation of these substances to yield metanephrine and normetanephrine, respectively. These are physiologically inactive and are then conjugated (with sulfate or glucuronic acid) or deaminated to 3-methoxy-4-hydroxy-mandelic acid. The O-methylation is accomplished by the enzyme catechol-O-methyl transferase.

Epinephrine ⇌ **Metanephrine**

Deamination / Conjugation

3-Methoxy-4-hydroxymandelic acid   **Conjugated metanephrine**

ADRENOCORTICOIDS

Although epinephrine and the adrenal medulla are dispensable, the same is not true of the adrenal cortex. An animal with both adrenal glands completely removed survives only 1 or 2 weeks. This is almost certainly due to the absence of adrenocortical tissue.

The chief symptoms that occur in such animals are as follows:

1. A disturbance of the electrolyte and water balance occurs. There is increased excretion of sodium, chloride, and water and retention of potassium. As a result, the sodium and chloride content of the blood decreases, potassium increases, and there is hemoconcentration. Although an excess of potassium is generally considered deleterious, we are not certain that death results from potassium toxicity in adrenal deficiency.

2. The urea content of the blood rises. This may be due, in part, to a decrease in renal blood flow; in part, to decreased kidney function.

3. There is great muscular weakness. This is probably secondary to the effects on carbohydrate metabolism and on the salt and water balance.

4. There is a decrease in liver glycogen, with hypoglycemia and a greater sensitivity toward insulin. These disturbances in carbohydrate metabolism are generally believed to result from a diminished utilization of carbohydrate and a decreased formation of sugar from proteins (gluconeogenesis). The "Long animal" strikingly illustrates this general effect. It is an animal with both the pancreas and the adrenals removed. The pancreatic diabetes is not as severe when the adrenal cortex is absent as when the adrenal cortex is present, thus demonstrating the opposing effects of insulin and the cortical carbohydrate hormone. Moreover, the average length of life after operation is about three times as great for those animals that have been both adrenalectomized and depancreat-

ized as it is for those that have been only depancreatized. The administration of extracts of adrenal cortex to normal animals results in an increase in blood sugar, liver glycogen, and muscle glycogen.

Along with a decreased formation of sugar from proteins in adrenalectomized animals, there occurs a *decrease* in the quantity of protein catabolized. As would be expected, the injection of cortical hormones into normal fasting animals *increases* the rate of protein breakdown. The adrenocortical hormone must accelerate protein catabolism and simultaneously diminish protein anabolism. Consequently, the administration of adrenocortical hormones to a normal young animal retards its growth because they specifically stimulate the breakdown of protein tissues.

5. There is a reduced ability to withstand stress, e.g., cold, or mechanical or chemical shock. This is also probably referable to the primary effects on carbohydrate and electrolyte metabolism.

6. Retardation of growth occurs if adrenalectomy is performed on a young animal. This undoubtedly results from the inhibition of protein anabolism mentioned above, whereas the more specific symptoms previously mentioned indicate the most prominent effects on individual organs.

Administration of cortical extracts remedies all these symptoms, returns the chemical picture practically to normal, and extends the life of the adrenalectomized animals for months. The production of potent extracts suitable for use in human beings has resulted from these experiments. We owe our knowledge, and many patients their lives, to the fundamental work of Rogoff, Hartman, Swingle, and Grollman.

From an organic chemical standpoint, Kendall, Reichstein, and Wintersteiner have been particularly active and successful. They isolated 28 crystalline steroids from the adrenal cortex. The structure and configuration of these steroids are known in detail, and some have been synthesized. Six or seven have been found to be active physiologically in prolonging the life of adrenalectomized animals or in preventing or curing single symptoms present in such animals. They are often grouped into two classes from a functional standpoint: the *mineralocorticoids*, with a predominant action on electrolyte metabolism, and the *glucocorticoids*, with a pronounced effect on carbohydrate metabolism.

The most important of the latter group is compound-F, 17-hydroxycorticosterone, which is of great value in carbohydrate and protein metabolism. Another glucocorticoid is corticosterone, but this is not secreted in large amounts in man. Another of the natural steroids, possessing one less oxygen than corticosterone, is deoxycorticosterone. It is a mineralocorticoid and has been prepared synthetically; it is much more powerful than corticosterone in its effect on electrolyte balance, although it does not have a favorable effect on carbohydrate metabolism. The most powerful mineralocorticoid, however, is aldosterone, which has been isolated from the amorphous fraction. It was crystallized, its structure established, and its real nature as a hormone indicated by its isolation from adrenal and systemic venous blood and from urine. Aldosterone is 30 times more active than deoxycorticosterone. It is probably the chief regulator of sodium, potassium, and chloride metabolism. However, its primary effect appears to be to increase the reabsorption of sodium ions in the distal convoluted tubules of the kidney. In addition to its electrolyte-regulating powers, it also has some slight effects similar to those of compound-F.

Aldosterone is relatively insensitive to ACTH stimulation. An increase in its secretion may be triggered by a decrease in blood volume (or blood pressure) via the renal juxtaglomerular cells and the secretion of renin and angiotension, the latter actually increasing aldosterone secretion. This mechanism would thus increase sodium retention, and concomitantly fluid retention, raising blood pressure and volume to normal values.

A pathologic condition, known as *primary aldosteronism*, was described by Conn.[15] A patient suffering from this condition, which is caused by an aldosterone-secreting tumor of the adrenal cortex, secretes in his urine large amounts of this hormone and retains too much sodium at the expense of potassium. The blood serum has low potassium and high sodium levels. Muscular weakness, hypertension, and a polyuria, which does not yield to posterior pituitary hormone therapy, occur. Alkalosis is present, with increased carbon dioxide combining power and tetany. The symptoms of Cushing's syndrome or of the adrenogenital syndrome are absent. There is evidence that aldosterone exists in solution in equilibrium with its hemiacetal, as illustrated on p. 470.

Compound-E, 11-dehydro-17-hydroxycorticosterone (cortisone), has had a dramatic impact on medicine. It was first found[16] to have a remarkably beneficial action on the severe symptoms of rheumatoid arthritis and later on other pathologic conditions, and it has proved to be a widely useful therapeutic agent. Cortisone is present in comparatively small amount in the venous blood leaving the adrenal gland.

The structural formulas of various adrenocortical hormones are shown below:

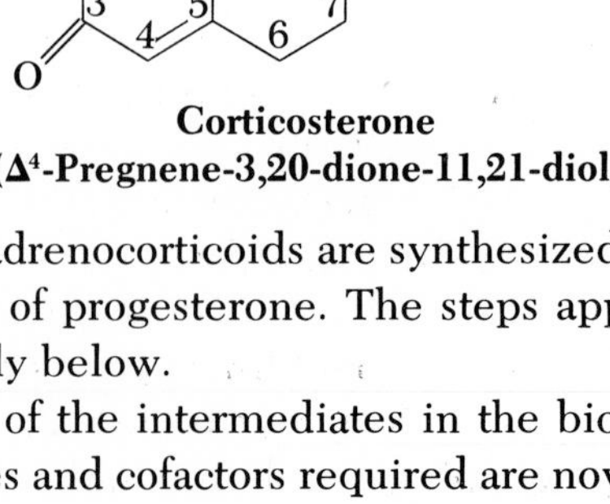

Corticosterone
(Δ⁴-Pregnene-3,20-dione-11,21-diol)

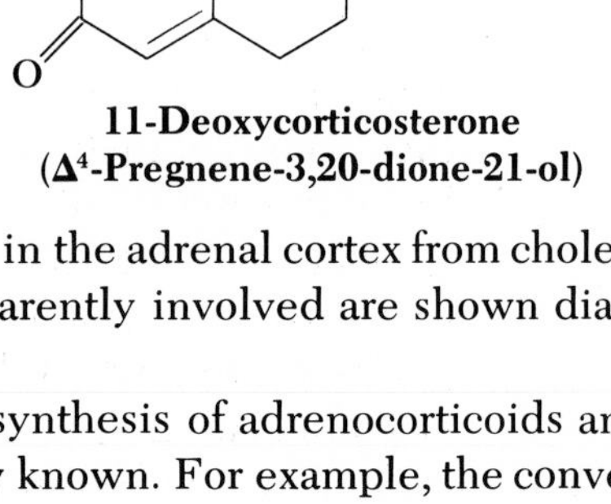

11-Deoxycorticosterone
(Δ⁴-Pregnene-3,20-dione-21-ol)

The adrenocorticoids are synthesized in the adrenal cortex from cholesterol by way of progesterone. The steps apparently involved are shown diagrammatically below.

Most of the intermediates in the biosynthesis of adrenocorticoids and the enzymes and cofactors required are now known. For example, the conversion of progesterone (p. 500) to 11-deoxycorticosterone and corticosterone involves the enzymes 21-hydroxylase and 11-β-hydroxylase, respectively. The conversion of corticosterone to aldosterone is catalyzed by an 18-hydroxylase. The conversion of 17-α-hydroxyprogesterone to hydrocortisone and then to cortisone is catalyzed by 21-hydroxylase and 11-β-hydroxylase, respectively. $NADP^+$ is required as a cofactor in each case. These hydroxylases are so-called mixed-function oxidases, as stated earlier (p. 242). ACTH stimulates adrenocorticoid synthesis (except aldosterone) at the point of the conversion of cholesterol (sulfate) to pregnenolone. A desmolase is the enzyme catalyzing this step.

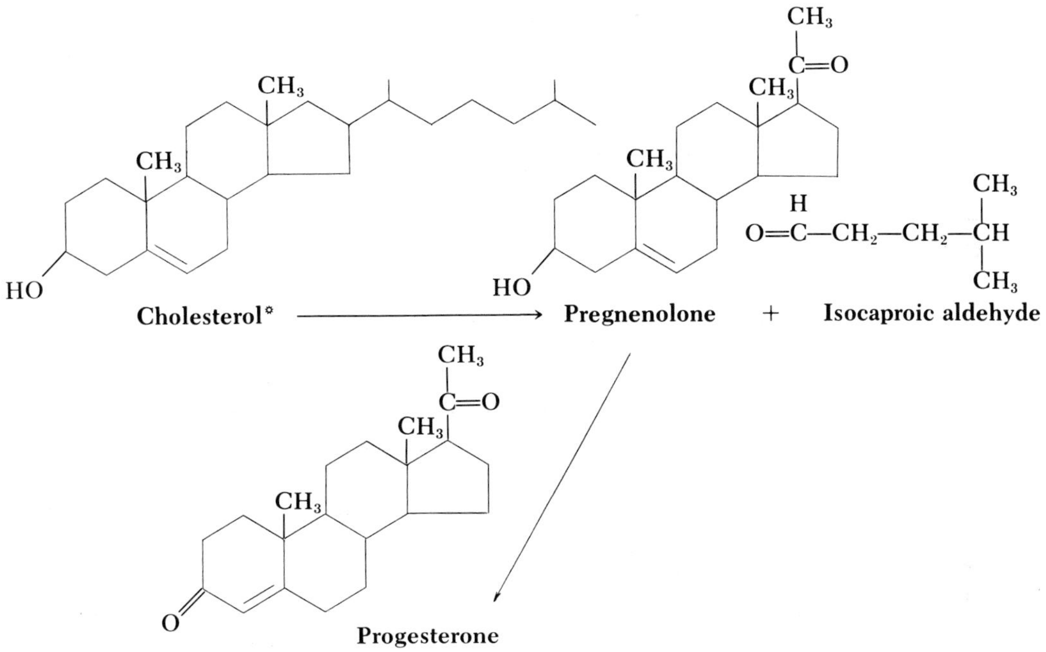

Cholesterol°   ⟶   Pregnenolone + Isocaproic aldehyde

Progesterone

Deoxycorticosterone   17-α-Hydroxyprogesterone
↓   ↓
Corticosterone   Hydrocortisone
↓   ↓
Aldosterone   Cortisone

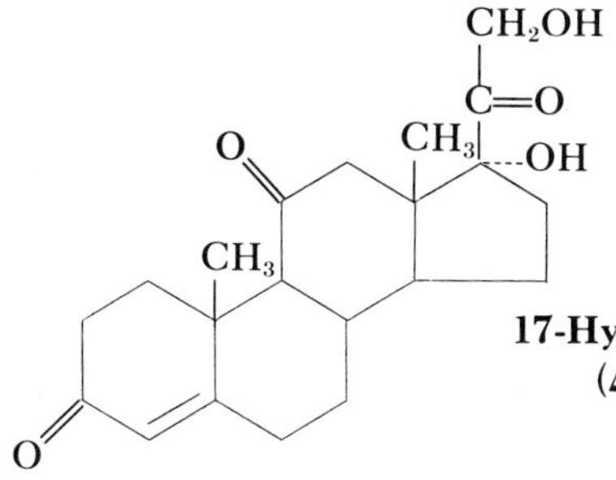

Cortisone
17-Hydroxy-11-dehydrocorticosterone
(Δ⁴-pregnene-3,11,20-trione-
17[α],21-diol)

° Hydroxylation occurs at carbon-20 and carbon-22 of the side chain of cholesterol, with the resultant splitting off of isocaproic aldehyde. $NADP^+$ is required as a cofactor.

Hydrocortisone (compound-F)
17-Hydroxycorticosterone
(Δ^4-pregnene-3,20-dione-
11,17[α],21-triol)

Aldosterone
(Δ^4-pregnene-11[β],21-diol-3,20-dione-18-al)

It has been estimated that in the normal adult man approximately 10 to 20 mg. of hydrocortisone, 3 mg. of corticosterone, and 0.3 mg. of aldosterone are synthesized daily.

The adrenocortical hormones are transported in the plasma to the respective target tissues bound loosely to plasma proteins, mainly α_1-globulins. One of these, *transcortin*, is involved in the transport of cortisol. A syndrome that appears to result from low cortisol-binding capacity of the plasma has been described recently. The adrenocorticoids are inactivated in the liver. This occurs apparently at a rate equivalent to that of formation, so a balance with a constant level of the hormones in body fluids is maintained. The primary mechanism of inactivation appears to be reduction of the ketone group on carbon-3 of ring-A. The saturated derivatives are then conjugated with glucuronic acid primarily and excreted in the urine as glucuronides. The side chain may also be split further to form 17-ketosteroids (androstenone, etio-cholanone, etc.) and may be excreted in the urine as glucuronides or, to a lesser extent, as sulfate derivatives. Normally about 10 to 20 mg. of keto-steroids are excreted in the urine daily.

While the many physiologic effects of the adrenocorticoids on carbohydrate and mineral metabolism have been recognized for a number of years, only recently has the fundamental biochemical role of these steroids begun to be understood. As mentioned earlier (p. 231), the adrenoglucocorticoids (cortisone, 17-hydroxycorticosterone, etc.) apparently serve as inducers of the synthesis of key gluconeogenic enzymes, glucose-6-phosphatase, fructose-1,6-diphosphatase, phosphoenolpyruvate carboxykinase, and pyruvate carbox-ylase. Insulin apparently acts as a suppressor of the synthesis of these same enzymes but as an inducer of the formation of key glycolytic enzymes. The precise role of aldosterone in regulating the renal reabsorption of sodium ions is still not known other than its increasing the reabsorption of sodium ions in the distal convoluted tubules of the kidney.

In man the syndrome of Addison's disease represents a hypofunction of

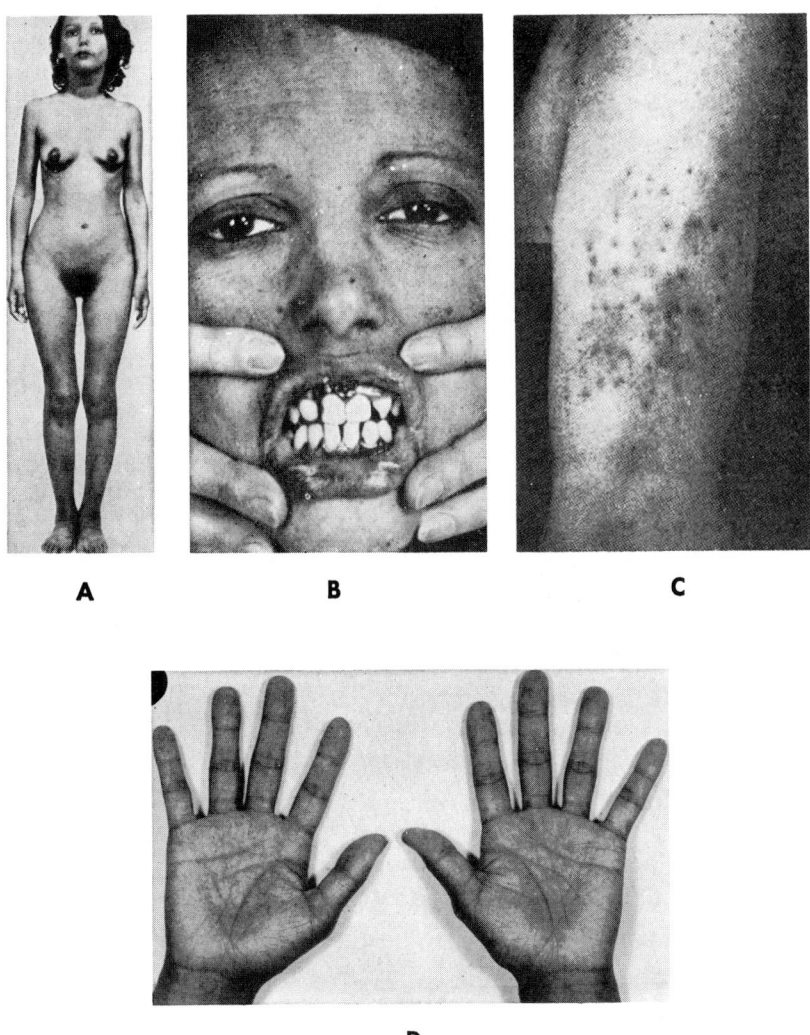

Fig. 16-4. Addison's disease. Note the generalized pigmentation, **A**, especially dark and pronounced about the face, nipples, and ankles. Characteristic pigmented spots are evident on the gums and buccal mucosa of the lower lip, **B**, elbow, with extensive jet black freckles of the arm, **C**, and folds and creases of the palms and fingers, **D**. (**A** and **B** from Goldzieher, M. A.: The adrenal glands in health and disease, Philadelphia, 1944, F. A. Davis Co.; **C** from Rowntree, L. G., and Snell, A. M.: A clinical study of Addison's disease, Philadelphia, 1931, W. B. Saunders Co.; **D** from Lisser, H., and Escamilla, R. F.: Atlas of clinical endocrinology, St. Louis, 1962, The C. V. Mosby Co.; Pediatric clinic, University of California School of Medicine, San Francisco.)

the adrenal cortex. Many of the symptoms resemble those of adrenalecto-mized animals. These were described in 1855 by the discoverer of this syndrome, Thomas Addison, in the following words: "The leading and characteristic features of the morbid state to which I would direct attention are anemia, general languor and debility, remarkable feebleness of the heart's action, irritability of the stomach, and a peculiar change of color in the skin, occurring in connection with a diseased condition of the 'supra-renal' capsules." To these symptoms today would be added low blood pressure, lowered basal metabolic rate, subnormal temperature, and a disturbance in the water and electrolyte balance. This includes loss of sodium and chloride ions, retention of potassium ions, and a loss of body water. There is also a hypoglycemia, which indicates that a profound effect on carbohydrate metabolism is occurring. The kidneys are affected, resulting in urea retention. Skin pigmentation occurs in those locations where the normal pigmentation is greatest. Frequently the face and neck and backs of the hands are so deeply bronzed as to cause the afflicted individual to look like a mulatto (Fig. 16-4).

Treatment of Addison's disease with extracts of the adrenal cortex has been very successful since its beginning in about 1929. Because this is substitution therapy, as most endocrine therapy is, the constant administration of potent extracts is essential. The administration of the natural cortical extracts to patients suffering from this disease resulted in marked improvement in many cases. Today modifications of cortisone are used to control the symptoms of Addison's disease and as replacement therapy for adrenalectomized patients, and they are just as efficient as glandular extracts. Δ^1-Hydrocortisone (prednisolone) and Δ^1-cortisone (prednisone) are examples of such modifications. Cortisone is now made by partial synthesis from naturally occurring steroidal starting materials. Total synthesis of cortisone has also been accomplished.

Loeb showed that the administration of sodium chloride alone is of immense value to suffers from Addison's disease. It corrects the electrolyte and water imbalance and leads to decided improvement of the clinical symptoms. Before deoxycorticosterone or cortisone was available, many patients were brought out of severe crises of this disease by the parenteral administration of physiologic solutions of sodium chloride.

The administration of deoxycorticosterone, usually as the acetate, or aldosterone affects almost exclusively electrolyte and water metabolism. Both cause retention of sodium and restore the blood sodium level to normal. A retention of water is brought about, thus increasing the volume of the blood plasma and the interstitial fluid. They increase the elimination of potassium, resulting in a reduction of serum potassium to normal and even subnormal levels. Renal function is restored, so urea and other nonprotein nitrogenous (NPN) constituents are excreted, leading to a diminution in the blood NPN. There is also a decrease in the total protein, calcium, and cholesterol of the blood serum, probably as a result of the retention of water and dilution of these constituents (Fig. 16-5).

The adrenal cortex has a high concentration of both cholesterol and ascorbic acid. In fact, vitamin C was first isolated from adrenocortical tissue, by Szent-Györgyi. However, since the glands are extremely small, the actual amounts

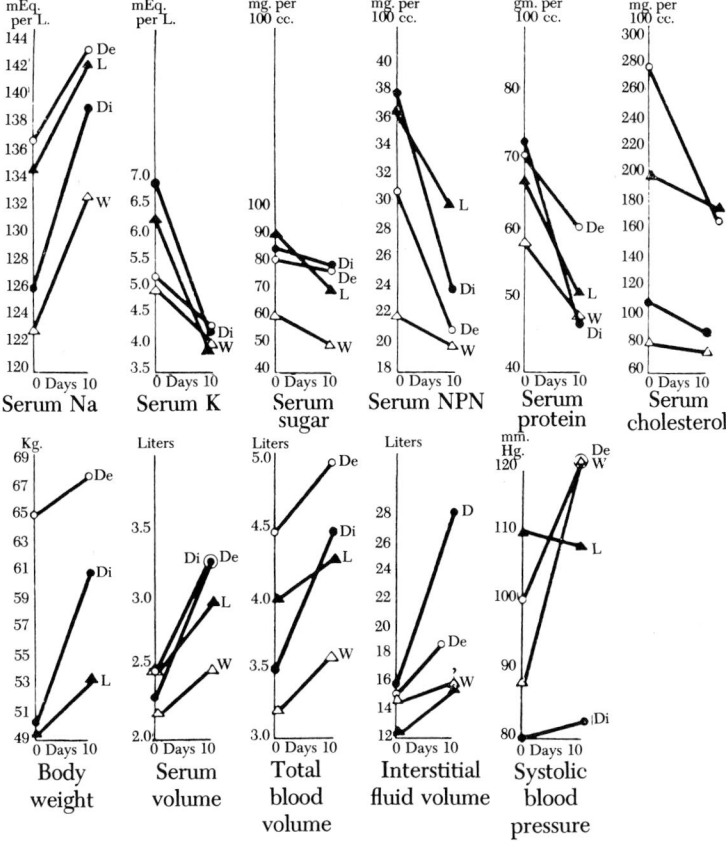

Fig. 16-5. Summary of the effects of deoxycorticosterone propionate observed after 10 days' treatment of a group of patients with Addison's disease maintained on a standard regimen. The serum Na rose and the serum K fell. The serum NPN fell as a result of increased excretion of urea. The serum protein concentration fell because of an increased retention of all body fluids, which also accounts for the rise in body weight and the improvement in blood pressure. Serum sugar did not rise but, if anything, fell, perhaps because of dilution. (From Ferrebee, J. W., Ragan, C., Atchley, D. W., and Loeb, R. F.: J.A.M.A. **113**:1725, 1939.)

of cholesterol and ascorbic acid are not large in comparison with those present in other tissues. Apparently the cholesterol is a precursor of the steroid hormones elaborated by the cortex. The injection of adrenocorticotropic hormones, which will be described later, stimulates the adrenal cortex to secrete these hormones. When this occurs, both the cholesterol and the ascorbic acid contents of the adrenal cortex decrease in concentration.

The function of ascorbic acid in the adrenal glands is unknown. It may be related to cellular respiration and metabolic rate. In stress there is a greater requirement and utilization of adrenocortical hormones and therefore of ascorbic acid, which seems to be related to the increase in adrenocortical function. In scurvy, vitamin C avitaminosis and symptoms involving the joints are seen. Cortisone prevents these from occurring in the guinea pig, whereas deoxycorticosterone aggravates such symptoms. Hence, ascorbic acid may be a necessary component of the oxidation-reduction system that produces the oxy type of adrenal hormones, e.g., cortisone.

Pantothenic acid and biotin are also related to adrenocorticosteroids. Both vitamins increase the survival time of adrenalectomized animals. Animals on a diet deficient in pantothenate develop lesions of the adrenal cortex and fail to have satisfactory adrenocortical function. Pantothenate affects both the structure and the function of the adrenal cortex. It seems to be involved with adrenal cholesterol concentration and may act as a catalyst in the production of these hormones through their precursor, cholesterol. Moreover, since pantothenic acid is a part of coenzyme-A, it has a critical role in the intermediary metabolism of all cells, particularly those of the adrenal cortex.

Adrenogenital syndrome. The adrenal cortex seems to be the origin of many instances of abnormal sexual changes. Sometimes tumors of the cortical tissue have been found to account for these changes; but in other cases, tumors of the same types of cells have not been followed by these symptoms, and most of these sexually abnormal patients have shown at autopsy glands that were either grossly normal or more or less hyperplastic (i.e., increased in amount of tissue). The sexual changes are mostly toward the masculine side. If they occur early in life, they may produce, in the female, *pseudohermaphrodism;* i.e., the external genitals become masculinized to such an extent that they resemble male organs. There are also changes in the secondary sexual characteristics. In very young girls, occasionally the sex organs and the breasts may assume adult size and appearance, and menstruation may occur. In adult women, masculinization occurs — the voice deepens, the breasts atrophy, menstruation ceases, the pubic hair changes to the male pattern, and a beard may grow on the face. Boys likewise show precocious sexual development, and sometimes both boys and girls acquire unusual musculature. In the adult male this condition is rather rare, but when it occurs, there is sometimes an exaggerated male sexual development and desire, sometimes a feminization, but frequently no sexual changes whatever.

The cause of the adrenogenital syndrome is unknown. The prevailing view is that the syndrome is due to a congenital lack of the 11-β-hydroxylating enzyme; i.e., the normal hydroxylation of progesterone to hydrocortisone is defective. This results in a lowered production of glucocorticoids. Thus, instead of the normal production of hydrocortisone, some of the precursors of this hormone, e.g., 17-hydroxyprogesterone, are liberated. Some metabolites of these are androgens; hence a virilizing action on the body results.

Substances that in themselves are androgenic have been obtained from the adrenal glands. Reichstein and Shoppee isolated from beef adrenals adrenosterone, which has about one fifth the androgenic potency of androsterone, a "male" sex hormone to be discussed later. Its relation to one of the typical cortical steroids, 11-dehydro-17-hydroxycorticosterone, is shown below. The latter is one of the hormones capable of supporting life in an adrenalectomized animal. The urine of patients suffering from this syndrome frequently, but not always, contains increased amounts of androgenic substances, the neutral 17-ketosteroids (p. 503). Cortisone frequently has a beneficial effect in these patients.

11-Dehydro-17-hydroxycorticosterone
(Δ⁴-pregnene-3,11,20-trione-17[α],21-diol)

Adrenosterone
(Δ⁴-androstene-3,11,17-trione)

CORTISONE AND ACTH IN RHEUMATOID ARTHRITIS

Rheumatoid arthritis is a chronic disease affecting the joints. It is characterized by pain, deformity, limitation of motion, and sometimes bony ankylosis, and it results in debility and weakness. In the past the most useful therapeutic agents have been salicylates combined with improved hygienic conditions. Evaluation of new drugs has been difficult, because remissions frequently occur spontaneously for varying lengths of time. However, the discovery by the Mayo group, in 1949, of the effect of cortisone and ACTH was dramatic.

Twenty years previously, Hench had made the observation that if patients suffering from rheumatoid arthritis become pregnant or jaundiced there is a prompt relief of the arthritic symptoms. On this basis he tested many bile and hormonal derivatives for their value in this condition without avail, until finally Kendall's compound-E (p. 468) became available. This is 11-dehydro-17-hydroxycorticosterone, or cortisone. It effects a decrease in the stiffness, tenderness, and pain in the joints in a few hours or days. Diminution of the joint swellings, disappearance of soft tissue deformities, and general improvement in health occur more slowly. ACTH (p. 494), which, of course, stimulates the production of cortisone, has an effect resembling that of cortisone in every particular. Cortisone has been used not only for rheumatoid arthritis but also for a number of other ailments, including acute rheumatic fever, acute asthma, and Addison's disease. However, recently the use of cortisone has declined as newer, more potent, compounds that are less likely to cause sodium retention have been developed.

The explanation offered for the temporary suppression of arthritis during pregnancy and jaundice is that in these conditions the anterior pituitary is stimulated to increase its output of ACTH, which, in turn, causes the adrenal cortex to produce more cortisone; the cortisone produces the beneficial effect against arthritis.

As might be expected, cortisone sometimes has unpleasant side effects. Some of these remind one of the adrenogenital syndrome. Others are hypertension, headaches, skin eruptions, confused mental states, and even diabetes, which may disappear when the cortisone treatment is discontinued. As a result, there are quite a number of contraindications to its use.

Cushing's syndrome. Cushing's syndrome is a rather rare condition. It is associated with an oversecretion of all types of adrenocortical hormones as a

475

result of hyperplasia or tumor of the adrenal cortex. Changes in the basophil cells of the anterior pituitary are so commonly present that Harvey Cushing regarded them as the causal factor; but they may actually be a result rather than a cause. The syndrome is characterized by profound disturbances of protein, fat, carbohydrate, and calcium metabolism. There is a rapidly developing, often painful, adiposity of the face, neck, and trunk; rarefaction of the bones, with resulting curvature of the spine, and pain and general body weakness; and often hypertension and polycythemia. In men there is impotence, and in women, amenorrhea and masculinization. Thus Cushing's syndrome resembles somewhat the adrenogenital syndrome. The 17-ketosteroid excretion is usually moderately increased. Diabetes mellitus is often present and is usually insulin resistant. Evidently there is an increased secretion of glucocorticoids.

THYROID GLAND

Early work on the thyroid gland was complicated by the fact that investigators did not appreciate the importance of the parathyroid glands. The thyroid consists of two lobes, one on each side of the trachea just below and anterior to the larynx, with a connecting isthmus. It weighs about 30 gm. There are usually four parathyroids, two at or near the dorsal surface of each lobe of the thyroid, but there may be fewer than four or as many as eight and their location is similarly variable. The parathyroids are very small and are closely connected with, or embedded in, the thyroid tissue. Consequently, when the thyroid was removed for experimental purposes, the parathyroids were sometimes extirpated at the same time. This resulted in a loss of both the thyroid and the parathyroid secretions. In 1891, the importance of the parathyroids was recognized and the confusion was dispelled.

The thyroid gland is composed of a large number of tiny closed vesicles lined with epithelial cells and filled with a colloidal material commonly called *colloid*. It is richly supplied with blood vessels. The colloid material, which probably contains the hormone secreted by the cells, is believed to be reabsorbed by these cells and to be secreted into the bloodstream.

Any enlargement of the thyroid gland, except of an inflammatory or malignant character, is termed a *goiter*. Simple goiters are not accompanied by constitutional symptoms. They are said to occur more frequently in certain regions of the earth—those far from the ocean or shielded from sea breezes by high mountains. Seawater contains relatively high concentrations of iodide; and in general, a lack of iodide in the drinking water and foods of regions remote from the sea is associated with the prevalence of endemic goiter (p. 427). Other types of goiters are seen in both hypothyroidism (cretinism, myxedema) and hyperthyroidism (exophthalmic goiter, toxic adenoma).

The hormone secreted by the thyroid gland contains iodine. In fact, more than half of all the iodine in the body is concentrated in the thyroid gland. The secretion of the thyroid hormone is influenced by the supply of iodine available. If an iodine deficiency occurs, the rate of hormone secretion remains constant at first, but the iodine stores present in the gland become depleted. Under these conditions the thyroid removes the iodide from the blood more efficiently, and the secretion of the hormone may continue until the iodine deficit becomes acute. Then the pituitary responds with a secretion containing a greater amount of thyrotropic hormone (TSH) (p. 493), and the activity of the thyroid gland is again stimulated. These measures are usually adequate to prevent hypothyroidism, which may have been produced by artificially restricting dietary iodine.

Apparently the thyroid gland is a sort of trap for excess iodine. A gradient of iodide ion concentration is established so that the concentration of iodide in the thyroid is many times that in the circulating blood. Normally the blood contains about 0.5 μg. per 100 ml., and the thyroid tissue can hold about 10 μg. per 100 gm. This gradient of 20:1 is increased to several hundred to one by activation of the thyroid by TSH, by iodine deficiency, or in Graves' disease. This concentrated iodine is probably within the cells. The relation of iodine to the thyroid has long been known, and iodine has been used in the treatment of simple goiter for over a century. It is more effective in *preventing* simple goiter than in *curing* it. There is present in the gland an iodized protein called thyroglobulin or iodothyroglobulin. This has marked physiologic properties. In 1919, Kendall obtained a crystalline substance from thyroid that was highly active. He called it *thyroxine*, and Harington and Barger established its chemical formula as:

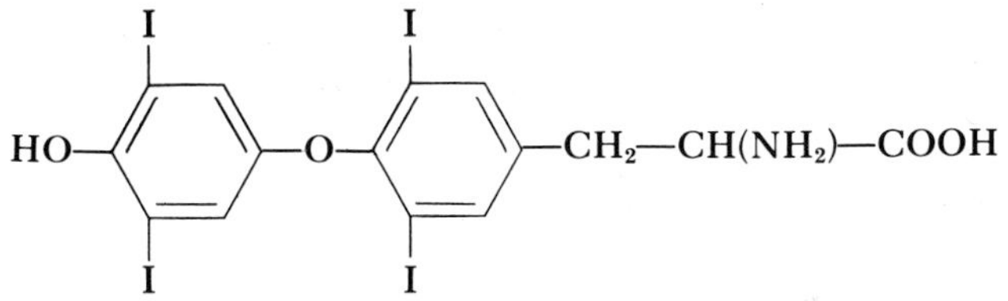

Thyroxine

It will be noted that thyroxine is closely related to tyrosine. In fact, much of the iodine present in the gland (about 70%) is present as an even closer relative to tyrosine, namely, diiodotyrosine, which has little physiologic activity, and some monoiodotyrosine.

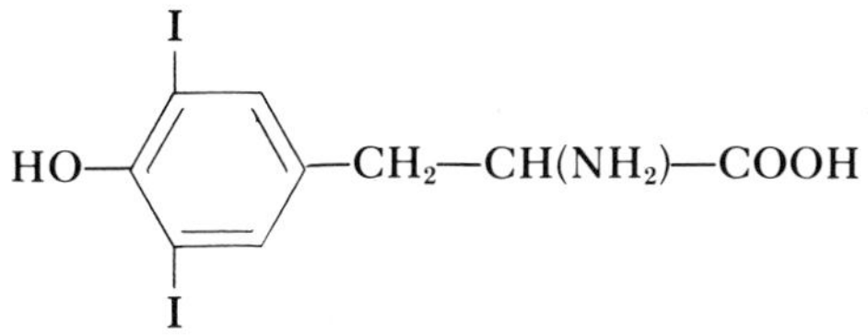

Diiodotyrosine

It is believed that diiodotyrosine is the precursor of thyroxine. This assumption is based on experiments in which radioactive iodine was used in both injection and tissue slice experiments. Evidence indicated that the tagged iodine goes through the diiodotyrosine stage before being incorporated into thyroxine.

Still another related compound is 3,5,3'-triiodothyronine. (Thyronine is the iodine-free skeleton of thyroxine.) This has five times the physiologic activity of thyroxine and is present in relatively small amounts. Apparently

477

the iodination of tyrosine, with the formation of diiodotyrosine, occurs after iodine in the form of iodide is taken up, concentrated from 30 to several hundred times by the thyroid gland, and incorporated in the thyroglobulin molecule of diiodotyrosine. The gland then converts diiodotyrosine to thyroxine, which, in turn, is changed to triiodothyronine, perhaps in the peripheral tissues. The circulating blood contains thyroxine and small amounts of triiodothyronine.

$$HO-\underset{I}{\bigcirc}-O-\underset{I}{\overset{I}{\bigcirc}}-CH_2-CH(NH_2)-COOH$$

3,5,3′-Triiodothyronine

There is present in blood plasma, bound to an α_1-globulin, a plasma protein known as thyroxine-binding globulin. This compound, with a molecular weight of 40,000 to 50,000, is critical in the estimation of protein-bound iodine (PBI) of blood plasma, which is considered a valuable measure of thyroid function. Measurement of the uptake of radioactive iodine (^{131}I) is also useful in the laboratory evaluation of thyroid function. Since a familial (genetic) deficiency of thyroxine-binding globulin is known to occur (e.g., in Turner's syndrome and possibly in other diseases involving thyroid hormone transport), the iodine-binding capacity of plasma is also sometimes determined.

It is possible that neither thyroxine nor triiodothyronine is the true thyroid hormone. Some authorities maintain that the true thyroid hormone is a much larger molecule, e.g., thyroglobulin or a peptide complex built around one or more of the iodine-containing compounds. Thyroglobulin has a greater activity than thyroxine in proportion to its iodine content.

As is stated later (p. 670), there is recent evidence that the salivary glands play a role in regulating the thyroxine level of the blood by deiodinating thyroxine. The iodine released is excreted in the saliva and reabsorbed in the small intestine, completing an iodine cycle.

Two functions are attributed to the thyroid gland: it has a profound effect on growth and development of the body; and it has a stimulating effect on total metabolism. Current studies[31] report that thyroxine causes an increased synthesis of all forms of RNA, nuclear, ribosomal, and transfer. This may well prove to be the fundamental biochemical effect of the thyroid hormone in affecting growth and development of the body and in stimulating total metabolism.

In young animals, removal of the thyroid glands without disturbance of the parathyroids results in an arrest of growth. In the human being a similar effect is seen when the thyroid is atrophied at birth. Apparently the human fetus can obtain little thyroid hormone in utero and must make its own, using available iodine. If there is not sufficient iodide or if the mother is under the influence of some goitrogenic factor, the fetus fails to develop normally. The resulting condition is termed cretinism. Cretins are abnormal dwarfs. They frequently have bowed legs, thick skin, and coarse hair. Although they may grow to adulthood, they do not develop mentally. The sex organs remain small and the abdomen becomes distended.

In the adult the clinical condition of hypothyroidism is known as myxedema. The symptoms include changes in appearance of the patient—the skin becomes thick and puffy, and there tend to be swellings under the eyes. This is said to be due to the deposition in the skin of additional protein material.

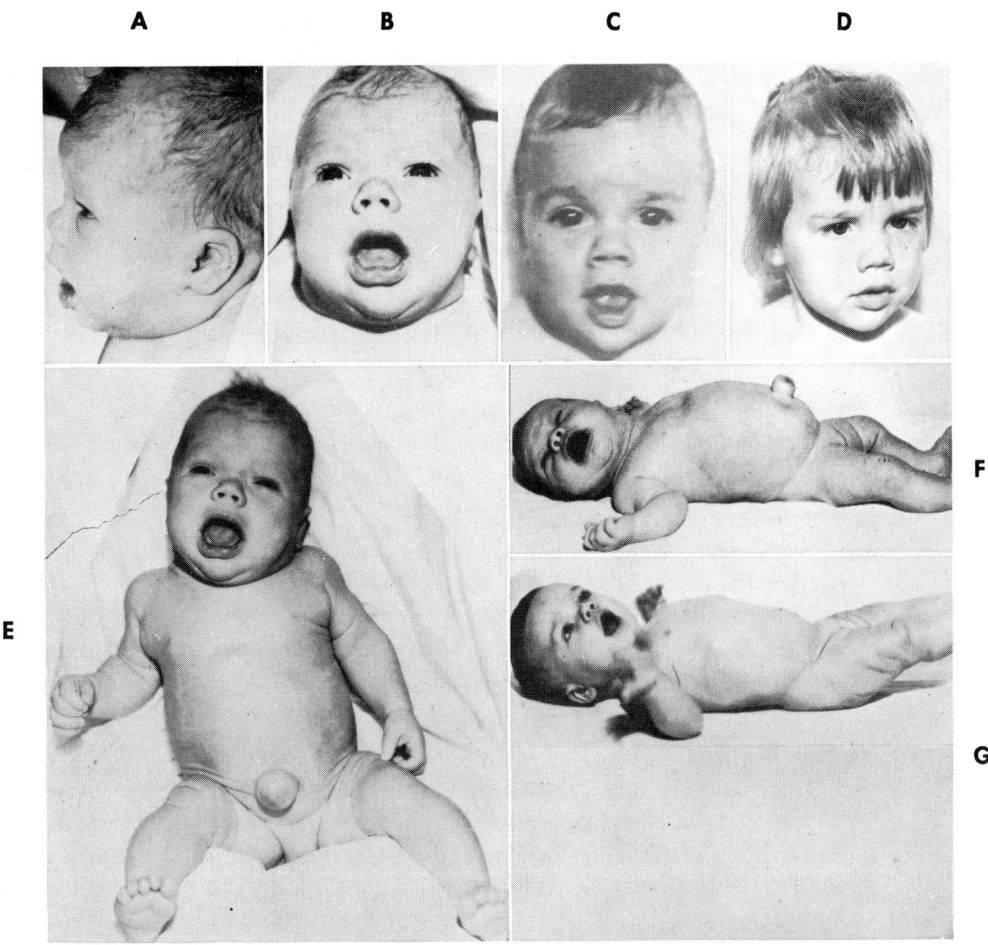

Fig. 16-6. Cretinism (or more accurately childhood myxedema for this type of severe hypothyroidism of childhood). **A** and **B**, Myxedematous infant, 9½ months of age. Note saddle nose, open mouth, thick, beefy, protruding tongue, puffy lips, and stupid expression. **C**, Appearance after 5½ months' treatment with thyroid. Note brighter, more intelligent appearance, loss of puffiness, and increased prominence of bridge of nose. **D**, Appearance after 21 months' treatment. Note further improvement. **E**, Same as **A**, infant lying down. Note protuberant abdomen and umbilical hernia. Skin dry, coarse, and cold. **F**, Same as **E**. **G**, Same as **C**. Note flattening of abdomen and disappearance of umbilical hernia. (From Lisser, H., and Escamilla, R. F.: Atlas of clinical endocrinology, St. Louis, 1962, The C. V. Mosby Co.; Pediatric clinic, University of California School of Medicine, San Francisco, F. H. Smyth, W. Deamer, and W. A. Reilly.)

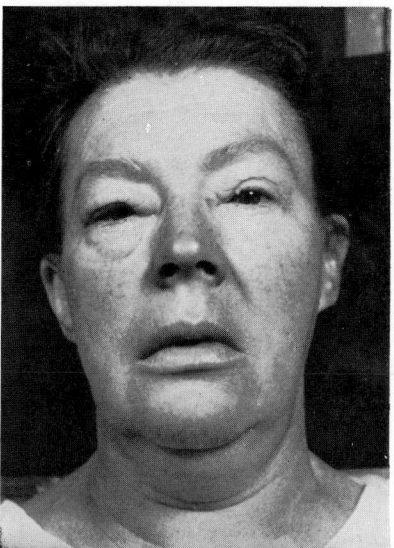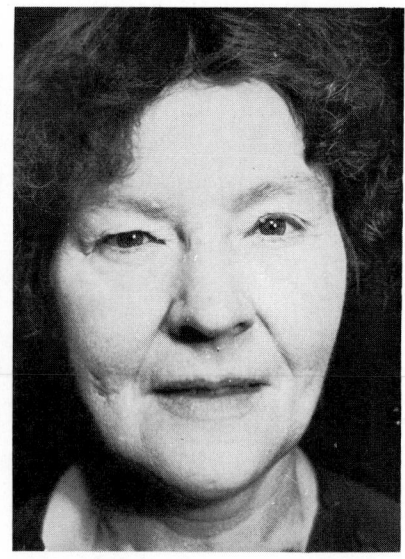

Fig. 16-7. Spontaneous myxedema before and after treatment with thyroid. (Courtesy E. Shorr; case of D. P. Barr.)

Although general intelligence is not impaired, the patient is slower in thinking as well as in movements. There is a low B.M.R., increased deposition of fat, and high blood cholesterol. The sexual functions are usually diminished.

In cretinism, treatment with thyroid preparations must be started early, to have any beneficial effect (Fig. 16-6), and must be continued as long as the thyroid gland fails to function. Mental retardation is usually, but not always, irreversible and permanent. Myxedema yields to treatment quite dramatically. Whether thyroid gland or thyroxine is given, the patient is usually brought back to a normal state (Figs. 16-6 and 16-7).

The influence of the thyroid on metabolism is more evident in cases of hyperthyroidism. In exophthalmic goiter the B.M.R. increases considerably above the normal figures—80% above normal is not unusual. Consequently, more food is consumed, in spite of which a loss of weight usually occurs. The high metabolic rate demands a more rapid glycogenolysis, resulting in a mild hyperglycemia and sometimes a small amount of glucose in the urine. The patient often feels hot because of the increased heat production. Other symptoms include protrusion of the eyeball and dilated pupil, mental excitement, and irritability. There is also an accelerated pulse, cardiac dilatation, and other cardiac effects. The hormone appears to act directly on heart muscle to produce this more rapid rate. Tissues from an animal that has had its thyroid removed have a decreased metabolism; addition of thyroglobulin increases the metabolism, but thyroxine does not. If the tissues derived from an animal that has been fed thyroid are tested, they also are found to have an increased metabolic rate.

Recent evidence indicates that the serum of patients with Graves' disease (diffuse goiter) contains a thyroid-stimulating factor, apparently a protein, that is different immunologically from TSH, of the anterior pituitary (p. 493).

When injected intravenously, this factor exerts its maximal thyroid-stimulating effect more slowly than TSH and it disappears more slowly from the plasma than does TSH. It has therefore been called long-acting thyroid-stimulating factor or LATS. Since the amounts of this substance in the plasma of patients with Graves' disease are increased, LATS is believed to be involved in the etiology of Graves' disease.

Hyperthyroidism may be combated by surgical removal of some of the overactive thyroid tissue. A chemical method of accomplishing the same effect is the administration of thiourea or thiouracil (or large doses of sulfonamides).

$$\begin{array}{cc} & O \\ & \| \\ H_2N & HN \\ | & \diagdown \\ S=C & S \\ | & \diagup \diagdown \\ H_2N & N \\ & | \\ & H \\ \textbf{Thiourea} & \textbf{Thiouracil} \end{array}$$

These antithyroid drugs cause inhibition of LATS synthesis by the gland, probably by preventing the coupling of two diiodotyrosine molecules to form thyroxine. They do not interfere with the action of the hormone if the hormone is administered simultaneously. The 6-propyl derivative of thiouracil is five times as potent as thiouracil itself and is much less toxic. Antabuse, which is used in treating alcoholism, has some antithyroid activity. It is tetraethylthiuram disulfide and contains —N—C—. Thus it resembles other anti-
$$\overset{\|}{S}$$
thyroid drugs. It has been shown to react with iodine to form a complex, which might render the iodine unavailable. Antithyroid substances are said to be present in certain foods excessive ingestion of which causes simple goiter, although this has been disputed. Since antithyroid substances inhibit the formation of the thyroid hormone, the pituitary gland secretes greater quantities of the thyrotropic factor, and a compensatory hypertrophy of the thyroid results (p. 493). Among the goitrogenic foods are cabbage and related vegetables, turnips, soybeans, peanuts, and the seeds of mustard. An antithyroid factor has been isolated from turnips and other goitrogenic vegetables. Evidence points to its identity as L-5-vinyl-2-thiooxazolidone.

Thyroid preparations are often used to increase the B.M.R. This may be necessary in certain types of obesity, especially if hypothyroidism is present. Because of the effects of such preparations on the circulation, this must necessarily be done with caution, for thyroid administration is quite dangerous in many cases. Not only thyroglobulin and thyroxine possess this calorigenic action, but also other closely related substances. These must have as a minimum requirement two atoms of iodine attached to a tyrosine nucleus. Simple iodination of a protein gives the protein thyroidlike properties.

Calcitonin   Recent studies[17] indicated that a hypocalcemic-hypophosphatemic substance exists in the thyroid glands of a number of mammalian species. The substance has been called calcitonin or thyrocalcitonin. Its effects, at least on the serum calcium level, are opposite those of parathormone, to be discussed next. It may thus be a balancing factor to parathormone. Calcitonin has been purified about five hundredfold from extracts of hog thyroids and appears to be a polypeptide. It is distinct from thyroxine and triiodothyronine.

In subsequent more current work,[18] calcitonin was isolated in pure form. It is a single-chain polypeptide, containing 32 amino acids, with a molecular weight of about 3600. It is rather unique in that it contains no isoleucine or lysine. Its amino acid sequence has been determined.[19] Its synthesis has been accomplished in two different laboratories.

Calcitonin, or thyrocalcitonin, is secreted by the parafollicular C-cells of the thyroid. Its secretion is stimulated by an increase in the blood calcium level; hence it counterbalances parathormone and aids in the maintenance of calcium homeostasis. Its mechanism of action is uncertain, but it rapidly inhibits calcium withdrawal from bones. This characteristic property gives calcitonin considerable promise as a therapeutic agent for the treatment of certain types of bone diseases. A radioimmunoassay procedure for its determination in blood has been described.[20]

PARATHYROID GLANDS

The close anatomic relation between the parathyroid and the thyroid glands has been mentioned. When both are removed experimentally, the animal develops severe tetany and often dies. This particular symptom is due to the loss of the parathyroids. Since tetany may also be produced by other methods, this type is called *tetania parathyreopriva* or *parathyroid tetany*. If the parathyroids are removed in a human being, either accidentally when the surgeon is excising thyroid tissue or in the case of a malignancy, tetany may occur. This is a danger even if a considerable proportion of parathyroid tissue remains, since the remaining tissue may not immediately produce a sufficient amount of the hormone. MacCallum and Voegtlin showed, in 1908, that parathyroidectomy is followed by a diminution in the calcium content of the blood serum, and Greenwald demonstrated a rise in the phosphorus. The calcium and phosphorus excretion in the urine is diminished. The tetanic symptoms seem to be due to a low calcium ion content of the serum, since the intravenous injection of calcium salts relieves these symptoms very quickly. It is now well established that the parathyroid hormone's role is to regulate the levels of calcium and phosphorus. Administration of this hormone, obtained by Collip from beef parathyroids, is also effective in parathyroid deficiency. It not only relieves the tetany within a few hours but also brings the calcium and phosphorus blood values back to normal.

The parathyroid hormone, parathormone (PTH), is a protein and can be digested by proteolytic enzymes. Rasmussen and Craig[21] purified it, making use of the countercurrent distribution method. It has a molecular weight of about 7000 and is a chain of 83 separate amino acid residues of 17 different amino acids. The amino acid composition appears to be as follows:

$$\text{Lys}_9 \text{ His}_4 \text{ Arg}_5 \text{ Asp}_9 \text{ Thr Ser}_6 \text{ Glu}_{11} \text{ Pro}_2 \text{ Gly}_4 \text{ Ala}_7 \text{ Val}_8$$

$$\text{Met}_2 \text{ Ileu}_3 \text{ Leu}_8 \text{ Tyr Phe}_2 \text{ Trp}$$

The exact sequence will undoubtedly be known soon.

A radioimmunoassay procedure for the determination of PTH has been developed.[22] The plasma level of the hormone is extremely high in patients with parathyroid adenomas, as might be expected.

Administration of PTH (1) raises the blood calcium and lowers blood phosphorus, (2) increases the elimination of both in the urine, (3) causes the migration of calcium from the bones if this element is not available in sufficient amounts in the food, and (4) increases the phosphatase activity of the serum. These actions are brought about by effects on both bone and kidney. In bone, parathormone increases the activity of the osteoclasts, those cells that break down bone tissue and release calcium.

It has been observed recently[23] that PTH increases bone resorption in tissue cultures of embryonic rat bone as evidenced by ^{45}Ca release. PTH apparently stimulates osteoclastic proliferation while inhibiting osteoblasts. Actinomycin-D inhibits the calcium-mobilizing effect of the hormone, which suggests that PTH exerts its calcemic effect by increasing osteoclast proliferation (RNA synthesis).

Other recent studies[24] in the rat suggest that PTH may activate renal adenyl cyclase to form cyclic-AMP, which, in turn, increases the transfer of calcium and phosphate in the proximal portion of the nephron. This would account for the increased urinary excretion of calcium and phosphates following PTH administration, as mentioned previously.

The secretory activity of the parathyroid glands is controlled by the level of calcium ions in the blood; i.e., as blood calcium falls, the parathyroid secretion increases, whereas a rise in the blood calcium automatically shuts off parathyroid activity (p. 553). As stated previously, vitamin D plays a role in calcium regulation, supplementing that of the parathyroid. PTH also influences the rate of exchange of calcium in the lactating mammary gland.

The normal level of calcium in blood serum is about 9.5 to 11 mg. per 100 ml.; in a completely parathyroidectomized person, it falls to 5 to 7 mg. All the symptoms of parathyroid deprivation may be referred to this low serum calcium. The object of therapy, therefore, is to bring the calcium level up to normal but not much higher, since hypercalcemia is as dangerous to life as is hypocalcemia. At a level of about 7.5 to 9 mg., the renal threshold occurs; above this, calcium is excreted in the urine. Consequently, if the calcium value can be raised until calcium appears in the urine, a safe level will probably be attained. Such a procedure would obviate the necessity of frequent blood examinations. The purified PTH is not yet available for clinical use. Therefore, clinicians recommend raising the blood calcium level by administering vitamin D until calcium appears in the urine. The amount of calcium in the urine can be quickly ascertained by using the Sulkowitch reagent, a buffered solution of oxalates that, when added to urine, produces an immediate precipitate of calcium oxalate, varying in density with the amount of calcium present. Of course, the patient must be on a diet containing sufficient calcium for his needs.

Hyperparathyroidism may occur in man. It is known as *osteitis fibrosa cystica* or von Recklinghausen's disease. High blood calcium, low phosphorus, and high plasma alkaline phosphatase levels are found. Decalcification of the bones leads to pains in them, deformities and fractures, and, frequently, urinary calculi. Cysts in the bones are another characteristic of this disease. Hyperparathyroidism is due to a tumor of a parathyroid gland, and the treatment consists of surgically removing the gland. This should be done as early as possible—before the bone changes have become irreversible.

PTH is sometimes given as treatment in lead poisoning. In chronic lead poisoning the metal is deposited in the bones, displacing calcium from the bone salt. The hormone tends to release the lead just as it does the osseous calcium, sending it into the blood and permitting its elimination by the kidneys. However, if this occurs too rapidly, the presence of large amounts of lead in the circulation may have serious ill effects.

PITUITARY GLAND

The pituitary or hypophysis is a small ovoid gland located at the base of the brain. It is attached to the infundibulum, the tubular stalk of the tuber cinereum, a diverticulum of the third ventricle, immediately behind the optic chiasma, and it occupies a depression of the sella turcica in the floor of the cranium. From our standpoint the gland may be considered to consist of (1) the anterior lobe, the largest part and the dominant endocrine structure; (2) the posterior lobe, which also possesses endocrine activities; and (3) the very small intermediate lobe, which lies between the other two and also has hormonal functions. Methods of study of the functions of the gland began with its removal from animals. Because of the gland's peculiar anatomic position, this is quite difficult procedure, and injury to the nearby nervous structures is likely to occur. However, in recent years the technique has been improved so that this operation is now frequently performed, even on human beings for therapeutic purposes, and much information has been gained. Birds such as pigeons and ducks have been used successfully in research activities connected with this gland, as have the common laboratory mammals, particularly the rat.

In the young mammal, hypophysectomy results in a cessation of growth and retardation in development both physically and mentally. The animals generally remain immature, their sexual glands do not develop, the epiphyses do not unite, and the first teeth are retained. If the operation is performed on an adult animal, there is an almost immediate effect on all the other glands of internal secretion. The testes, ovaries, and secondary sexual organs atrophy. The thyroid, parathyroids, and adrenal cortex become smaller in size and their activity diminishes. In addition, the animal is apathetic, loses its appetite, and becomes emaciated. Metabolism of protein, carbohydrate, and fat becomes deranged. One evidence is the hypersensitivity of the hypophysectomized animal to insulin and the animal's resistance to the hyperglycemic effect of epinephrine.

It is obvious that the pituitary must exert powerful influences on many other glands of internal secretion and, either directly or indirectly, on all physiologic activities (Fig. 16-8). In fact, the pituitary has been called the master gland, since its secretions seem to control those of most of the other important endocrine structures. However, it is now believed that the secre-

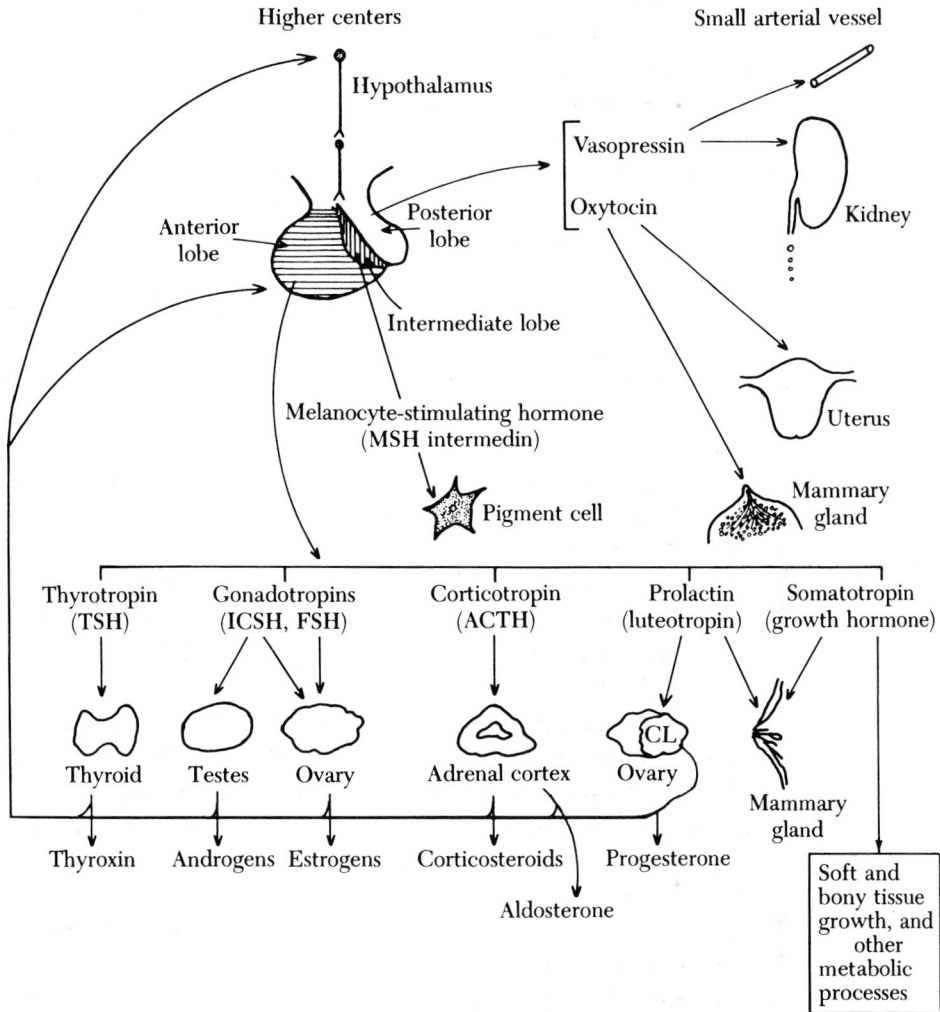

Fig. 16-8. Scheme illustrating the relationships among the anterior and posterior pituitary glands and their target structures. (Courtesy C. H. Li; presented at International Union of Pure and Applied Chemistry, Paris, July 25-29, 1957.)

tions of the posterior pituitary may be elaborated by the hypothalamus and then may be sent to the posterior pituitary gland cells for storage. The hypothalamus also controls the anterior pituitary but in a different way, as will be seen.

Posterior pituitary lobe The anterior lobe of the pituitary, or adenohypophysis, controls most vital activities. The posterior lobe, the neurohypophysis, should not, however, be disregarded, and for convenience it will be considered first.

It has been practically impossible thus far to remove the posterior lobe of the pituitary without injuring the anterior lobe or other structures. The most nearly successful experiments have resulted in an increased urinary output coupled with an increased water intake. This resembles the clinical condition known as diabetes insipidus, which undoubtedly is due to a lack of the hormone now thought to be antidiuretic hormone (ADH). This hormone is believed to be the same as vasopressin (p. 487).

In diabetes insipidus, tremendous quantities of water are taken in, as much as 30 liters a day, with an excretion of almost as much urine. Most cases yield to subcutaneous administration of posterior pituitary extract. Another effective and convenient method of administration is absorption of the extract through the nasal mucosa. Small wads of cotton soaked with the solution are inserted in the nostril, or the dry powdered extract is blown up the nostril with an insufflator.

The primary action of the hormone is to increase the reabsorption of water by the distal renal tubules, where about 10% of the glomerular filtrate is *actively* reabsorbed (p. 719). Fluctuations in the concentration of the blood plasma, of course, affect the blood's osmotic properties, and these changes influence the osmoreceptors in or near the brain. Increase in concentration stimulates the secretion of ADH by the posterior pituitary gland, preventing the loss of more water, whereas decrease in concentration lessens the secretion of hormone and permits more water to be lost in the urine. It has been reported that stimulation of the osmoregulatory center in the hypothalamus causes a release of ADH, which travels down the hypophyseal stalk as little "packets" to the posterior lobe of the pituitary, where the packets are stored and released into the blood plasma.

ADH (vasopressin) appears to exert its effect on the renal reabsorption of water via the formation of cyclic-3′,5′-AMP (p. 455) from ATP. The exact manner in which cyclic-3′,5′-AMP alters membrane permeability, "aqueous channels," in responsive membranes is still unknown. Some substances, e.g., ethyl alcohol, produce diuresis, apparently by suppressing the action of vasopressin.

Two other effects of posterior pituitary extracts were discovered as a result of studies of the pharmacologic effects of these extracts on animals and isolated tissues. The first is a marked rise in blood pressure, and the second a contraction of smooth muscle, particularly uterine muscle. Kamm separated the extract into two fractions: one, having preponderantly pressor and antidiuretic action, termed *vasopressin;* the other, having mainly an effect on smooth muscle, called *oxytocin.* Vasopressin and perhaps another substance elaborated by the hypothalamus stimulate the anterior pituitary to secrete corticotropin (p. 494). Therapeutic doses of these preparations have little effect on blood pressure in the human being, but oxytocin finds application in obstetrics when uterine contractions must be stimulated. Another function of oxytocin is to facilitate the expression of milk by the lactating mammary gland. In the gland there is a large amount of modified smooth muscle tissue, called myoepithelium. Contraction of this tissue is brought about by minute amounts of oxytocin. The response is known as milk "let-down." This effect is probably necessary in normal lactation.

Du Vigneaud and associates[25] purified both the oxytocic and the vasopressor fractions to a very high degree. Pure oxytocin, on hydrolysis, yields one equivalent each of leucine, isoleucine, tyrosine, proline, glutamic acid, aspartic acid, glycine, and cystine and three equivalents of ammonia. It is

$$
\begin{array}{c}
\text{C}_6\text{H}_4\text{OH} \qquad \text{C}_2\text{H}_5 \\
| \qquad\qquad\quad | \\
\text{NH}_2 \;\; \text{O} \qquad \text{CH}_2 \;\; \text{O} \qquad \text{CH---CH}_3 \\
| \qquad \| \qquad\quad | \qquad \| \qquad\quad | \\
\text{CH}_2\text{---CH---C---NH---CH---C---NH---CH} \\
| \qquad\qquad\qquad\qquad\qquad\qquad | \\
\text{S} \qquad\qquad\qquad\qquad\qquad\; \text{C}{=}\text{O} \\
| \\
\text{S} \qquad\qquad\qquad \text{O} \qquad\qquad \text{O} \;\; \text{NH} \\
| \qquad\qquad\qquad \| \qquad\qquad \| \;\; | \\
\text{CH}_2\text{---CH---NH---C---CH---NH---C---CH---(CH}_2)_2\text{---CONH}_2 \\
| \qquad\qquad\qquad\qquad | \\
\text{C}{=}\text{O} \qquad\qquad\quad \text{CH}_2 \\
| \qquad\qquad\qquad\qquad | \\
\qquad\qquad\qquad\qquad \text{CONH}_2 \\
\text{CH}_2\text{---N} \qquad\; \text{O} \qquad\qquad \text{O} \\
| \quad\;\; \backslash \qquad \| \qquad\qquad \| \\
| \qquad\; \text{CH---C---NH---CH---C---NH---CH}_2\text{---CONH}_2 \\
\text{CH}_2\text{---CH}_2 \qquad\qquad\quad | \\
\qquad\qquad\qquad\qquad \text{CH}_2 \\
\qquad\qquad\qquad\qquad | \\
\qquad\qquad\qquad\quad \text{CH(CH}_3)_2
\end{array}
$$

Oxytocin

a polypeptide, having a molecular weight of about 1000, with a cyclic disulfide structure. Substitution of some of these groups can cause a diminution of the oxytocic activity and can even enhance the pressor action. The preceding configuration has been assigned to it, and a substance has been synthesized on this basis, by the same investigators. The synthetic compound is identical with natural oxytocin physically, chemically, and physiologically.

Vasopressin also appears to be an octapeptide, containing the following amino acid sequence:

Cys Tyr Phe Asn Gln Pro Arg (or) Lys Gly

Du Vigneaud and co-workers suggested a structural formula for the compound. Six amino acids are common to both oxytocin and vasopressin. The two differ in the presence of leucine and isoleucine, in oxytocin, and phenylalanine and arginine (or lysine), in vasopressin.

Another group of hormones elaborated by this gland is the *intermedins*. Long thought to be limited to lower vertebrates, in which the pituitary has a definite intermediate lobe, they were recently isolated from the posterior pituitary of a mammal, the pig. In lower vertebrates they stimulate the expansion of melanocytes, but their function in higher vertebrates is unknown, although it may be related to pigmentation in human skin. They are two peptides, identical except for the terminal groups. The α-type has its terminal groups blocked, whereas the β-type end groups are free. The structure consists of a peptide of 18 amino acids with a molecular weight of 2177 and the sequence of amino acids (in beef β-MSH, melanocyte-stimulating hormone) as follows:

Asp Glu Gly Pro Tyr Lys Met Glu His Phe Arg

Try Gly Ser Pro Pro Lys Asp

Anterior pituitary lobe The anterior lobe or adenohypophysis secretes a number of important hormones. All of them are believed to be proteins, and several have been isolated in pure form. Those that cause other glands to function or increase their activity are termed tropic hormones, from the Greek *trepein*, "to turn," and this term is used as a suffix. Thus there are thyrotropic, adrenocorticotropic, gonadotropic, etc. hormones. Thyrotropic hormone (TSH) has the specific effect of increasing the amount of hormone released by the thyroid gland; adrenocorticotropic hormone (ACTH) affects the adrenal cortex similarly, etc. There is good evidence that the rate of secretion of a tropic hormone is inversely proportional to the concentration in the blood of the hormone with which it is related. For instance, a high blood level of thyroid hormone tends to inhibit the anterior pituitary secretion of TSH, and a low level causes an increased production of it. The regulatory effect of this mechanism is evident.

Hypothalamus and neurohormones The adenohypophysis also appears to be under the control of the hypothalamus. The exact mechanisms have not been worked out in every case, but a brief description of one mechanism, which may be the pattern of others, is that for ACTH (p. 494). Ordinarily, small amounts of this tropic hormone are secreted continuously by the adenohypophysis. When stress occurs, this secretion may be greatly increased and very quickly. Probably nervous stimuli, caused by stress, are first sent to the hypothalamus, which then secretes a product, called the *corticotropin-releasing factor* (CRF). CRF is sent via the hypophyseal portal system to the adenohypophysis, where it excites the glandular cells to secrete ACTH. Thyrotropin secretion (p. 493) likewise is mediated by an analogous *thyrotropin-releasing factor*, TRF; and the gonadotropins (p. 496) and somatotropin (below) are also under hypothalamic control, perhaps by similar mechanisms. CRF and TRF are neurohormones, i.e., produced by nerve cells.

Recent studies have demonstrated that TRF, also called thyrotropin-releasing hormone (TRH), is a tripeptide of glutamic acid, histidine, and proline. Its structure is pyro (Glu-His-Pro)-NH_2. It has been synthesized by Folkers and his co-workers. The elucidation of the structure and the synthesis of this neurohormone (TRH) is an extremely important current development in the endocrine field. It opens significant new possibilities in the treatment of diseases of the thyroid gland.

Growth (somatotropic) hormone. The presence of an anterior pituitary hormone that influences growth is indicated, on the one hand, by the fact that hypophysectomy inhibits growth and, on the other, by the occurrence of gigantism as a result of pituitary hyperfunction. Gigantism is not infrequent in man; the "tall man" in the circus is a person whose pituitary was overactive during childhood, before the closure of the epiphyses limited the further growth of his long bones.

An excellent example is an individual who claims to be the tallest man in the world. He is about 25 years of age, is 9 feet, 7 inches, tall, weighs 470 lb., and wears size 36 shoes (custom made). His birth weight was 16 lb., 3 oz. He has been in several movies and has appeared on television, in circuses, etc. His younger brother is 14 years old and is 7 feet, 4 inches, tall. His

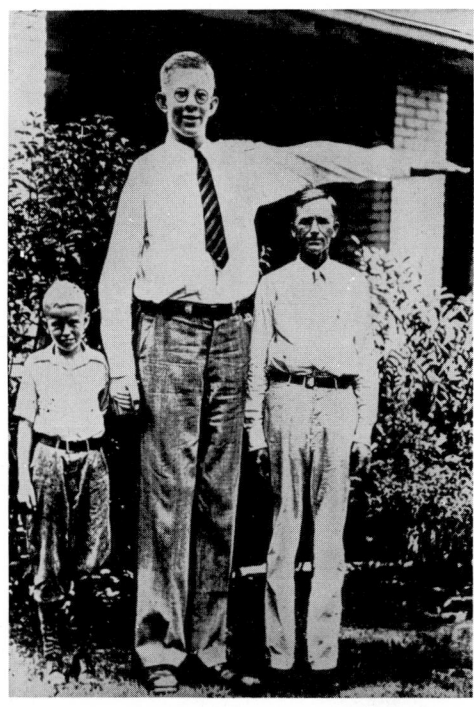

Fig. 16-9. Gigantism. The Alton giant at age 14 years, with his father and brother. Height, 7 feet, 6½ inches; weight, 360 lb. At the age of 18 years he reached a height of 8 feet, 3¼ inches, weighed 395 lb., wore a size 34 shoe, and consumed 6000 to 8000 calories daily. Note the disproportionate length of limbs. (From Lisser, H., and Escamilla, R. F.: Atlas of clinical endocrinology, St. Louis, 1962, The C. V. Mosby Co.)

father is 6 feet, 9 inches, tall, and his mother, 4 feet 11½ inches.* Such individuals may be quite normal mentally and, except for their size, physically (Fig. 16-9). It is considered dangerous to attempt to stop the growth of these individuals by irradiating their pituitary glands because of the possible harmful effects to the other important functions of the gland.

If the overactivity of the gland occurs in an adult, i.e., after the closure of the epiphyses, a condition known as acromegaly occurs. Here the bones become misshapen, particularly the bones of the face (Fig. 16-10). There is also an excessive growth of fibrous tissue, resulting in thickened nose, lips, eyelids, and broadened fingertips. Acromegaly is sometimes caused by a tumor of the anterior pituitary, and in such a case surgery may be attempted.

The opposite effect is seen in pituitary dwarfism. It is said that if no other adequate cause for retarded growth can be found, e.g., hypothyroidism, the trouble is likely to be hypopituitarism (Fig. 16-11). Children so affected are usually only half as tall as they should be for their age. Even though they may be well fed at mealtimes, they eat almost constantly from any source available – even garbage cans. They eventually attain a height of about 4 feet. In such dwarfs the bodily proportions are relatively normal, but the sex

---

*The Detroit News, October 13, 1967. The man's name is Ed Carmel.

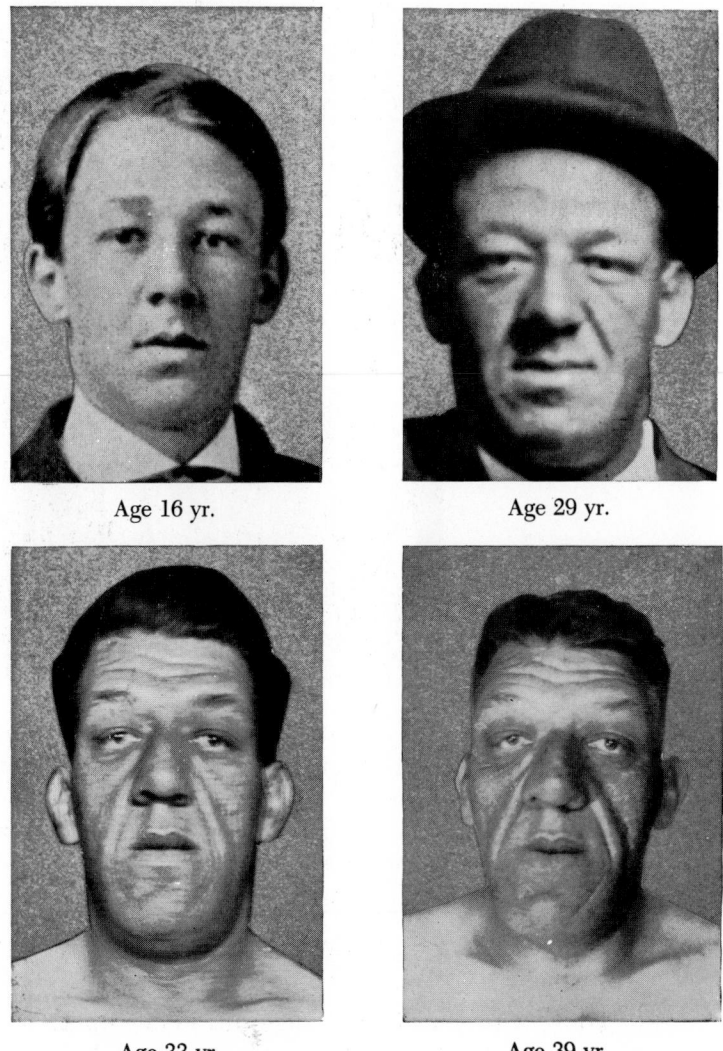

| Age 16 yr. | Age 29 yr. |

| Age 33 yr. | Age 39 yr. |

Fig. 16-10. Acromegaly of 25 years' duration. Note the changes in facial appearance with age. Note also the increase in size of the head, coarsening of the features, bulbous thickening of the end of the nose, and protrusion of the forehead and mandible. (From Goldberg, M. B., and Lisser, H.: J. Clin. Endocr. 2:477, 1942; University of California School of Medicine, San Francisco.)

organs are underdeveloped. The administration of anterior pituitary extracts or of thyroid and oral methyltestosterone (Fig. 16-11) sometimes results in considerable growth of such dwarfs, but this is not usual. However, it has been found that the growth hormone is species specific (see below), and, consequently, human pituitary dwarfs are more favorably affected by preparations from human glands.

Li and Evans[26] succeeded in isolating from the anterior lobes of ox pituitaries the pituitary growth hormone. It is a protein that can be destroyed by heat, inactivated by proteases, and precipitated by ordinary protein precipi-

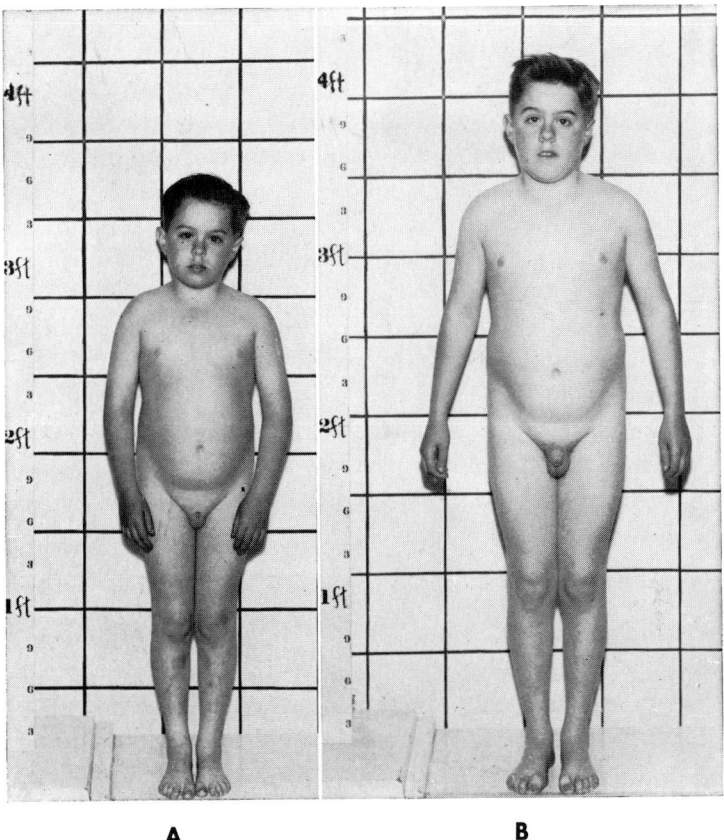

A **B**

Fig. 16-11. Male pituitary dwarf. **A,** Age, 9 years, 4 months; height, 3 feet, 6¼ inches; weight, 44½ lb.; bone age, 6 to 7 years. **B,** Two years, 1 month, later after treatment with thyroid and oral methyltestosterone. Height now, 4 feet, 1⅜ inches; weight, 70¼ lb. (From Lisser, H., and Escamilla, R. F.: Atlas of clinical endocrinology, St. Louis, 1962, The C. V. Mosby Co.; University of California School of Medicine, San Francisco.)

tants. It has a molecular weight of about 45,750 and behaves as a single substance in electrophoresis. This protein seems to consist of a branched polypeptide chain having two N-terminal residues and one C-terminal residue. The molecule appears to contain about 396 amino acid residues of 18 different amino acids. However, it has been shown that there is considerable variation among the growth hormone preparations from different species (human, monkey, whale, fish, bovine). They differ in their amino acid content and are somewhat species specific in their physiologic activities. For example, fish growth hormone acts on fish but not on rats; the hormone derived from the monkey acts on monkeys, whereas beef growth hormone does not. Human growth hormone has a molecular weight of about 26,000 with only one N-terminal residue. According to Li's current work, it contains 188 amino acid residues. Its complete amino acid sequence has been determined. The growth hormone may possibly have a much simpler active core.

Stimulation of the hypothalamus (ventromedial nucleus) in rats causes a prompt secretion of growth hormone.[27] In 5 minutes there is an increase in the plasma level of the growth hormone, as determined by radioimmuno-assay. Stimulation of the cerebral cortex in a similar manner produces no effect.

The pituitary growth hormone causes growth in hypophysectomized rats and is responsible for the effects on carbohydrate metabolism and ketogenesis, which will be discussed later. Indeed, the growth-promoting effect may be due to a depression of the oxidation of both proteins and carbohydrates, thus making these substances available for physiologic needs, including growth. Since the utilization of carbohydrates and of protein is dependent, to a considerable degree, on insulin, the increase in tissue protein anabolism or growth occurs as a result of the synergistic effect of these two hormones. Insulin alone cannot cause such action in normal animals, and growth hormone alone cannot do so in depancreatized animals. Thus the growth-promoting action of the anterior pituitary hormone depends on the availability of extra insulin, secreted *under its influence*. Li is of the opinion that growth hormone is a powerful protein anabolic agent. Indeed, it induces mammary gland development and milk secretion and enhances the action of the sex hormones. It also increases antibody formation and resistance to infection.

Recent investigations[31] have emphasized the fundamental role of growth hormone in regulating nucleic acid metabolism. Growth hormone has been shown to stimulate RNA synthesis in rat liver and other tissues. All forms of RNA, ribosomal, messenger, and transfer, are increased. It also stimulates the formation of RNA polymerase in rat liver nuclei. Thus the fundamental biochemical action of growth hormone on the growth and development of the organism now appears to be the stimulatory effect of this hormone on nucleic acid metabolism, as manifested by an increased formation of RNA polymerase and of all types of RNA.

The interrelations of several glands of internal secretion to pancreatic diabetes was discussed in Chapter 9. The particular influence of the pituitary may, however, be emphasized at this time.

You will remember that removal of the pancreas produces hyperglycemia and extirpation of the hypophysis results in hypoglycemia. The two glands seem to have opposing effects. This was shown strikingly by Houssay, in 1930. He found that removal of the pituitary gland lessens the severity of the diabetes produced by pancreatectomy. The animal is not cured of diabetes by any means. The hyperglycemia, however, is not as severe as in the animal deprived of only its pancreas. Moreover, survival of the Houssay animal is much longer than of the simple diabetic animal, if neither receives hormone therapy. The Houssay animal is more sensitive to the injection of insulin or anterior pituitary extract; i.e., insulin produces more profound hypoglycemia and pituitary extract more readily causes hyperglycemia in such animals, apparently because the antagonizing factor is absent in each case. This demonstrates beautifully the interplay of hormones. Seldom does one hormone have an isolated or unmodified effect.

In man the relation between the two glands is observed in acromegaly. In this condition of hyperactivity of the pituitary gland, hyperglycemia and glycosuria are frequently seen. These effects of the anterior pituitary are probably explained on the basis of the action of ACTH, since this hormone causes the adrenal cortex to secrete glucocorticoids.

Injection of anterior pituitary extracts has variable effects on the normal animal. In some cases a fall in blood sugar is seen, and in some, a rise. The rise or fall seems to depend on whether the animal is fasted or well fed, on the species of animal employed, on the number and amount of doses given, and on other factors. Therefore it is not surprising that the existence of a number of different principles was formerly postulated. These are called the pancreatotropic, glycostatic, and diabetogenic hormones. All of these effects can now definitely be ascribed to the growth hormone.

Thus, in addition to the influence of ACTH, which stimulates the production of the adrenocortical steroids and thus indirectly affects carbohydrate metabolism, the anterior pituitary has a direct effect. It has a marked anti-insulin action by inhibiting the peripheral utilization of sugar. On the other hand, a single injection administered to fasting rats produces a moderate hypoglycemia. These contradictory effects may be related to the fact that, whereas growth hormone stimulates the secretion of extra insulin, it also stimulates the secretion of glucagon and diminishes the sensitivity of tissues to insulin. Apparently the type of effect produced by the growth hormone depends on the balance of these two activities and on other factors. Usually in young animals the growth effect prevails, whereas in adult animals, especially carnivores, the diabetogenic action may be seen. The somatotropic hormone is also known to cause adrenal enlargement. Bois and Selye showed that this corticotropic effect can be greatly augmented by simultaneous treatment with small doses of thyroxine, thus indicating that the pituitary produces this action via the thyroid gland.

The injection of anterior pituitary extracts also causes an increase in the formation of ketone bodies. For a time this was believed to be a distinct hormone, a ketogenic factor, but it is now believed to be still another action of the growth hormone. This type of effect is best shown by injection of growth hormone into starving animals or those on a high-fat diet, i.e., animals having some degree of ketosis already. This action is, of course, an intensification of the normal production of ketone bodies from fatty acids by the liver, but there is as yet no definite proof of the exact mechanism of this ketosis.

Thyrotropic factor. Removal of the hypophysis results in a decrease in the size of the thyroid gland. This can be prevented by the injection of certain extracts of the anterior pituitary, and if such extracts are injected into normal animals, the thyroid hypertrophies. The active principle involved is called the thyrotropic factor or thyroid-stimulating hormone (TSH). This hormone has been obtained in a high degree of activity but not in a pure state. It is a protein with a molecular weight of about 26,000 to 30,000.

The action of TSH is on the thyroid gland, stimulating the gland to secrete thyroid hormone. Thus, TSH has an indirect action on general metabolism. Removal of the anterior pituitary, or inhibition of its secretory activity, has a result equivalent to hypothyroidism. Injection of the hormone, on the other hand, is similar to the administration of thyroid or the production of hyperthyroidism, with the following effects: (1) enlargement of the thyroid gland,

(2) rise in the B.M.R., (3) reduction in the iodine content of the thyroid gland, (4) increase in the iodine content of the blood, (5) greater rapidity of the heart rate, and (6) exophthalmos. There are other effects in addition to these, but they are probably due to the presence of other factors.

Current evidence[28] indicates that TSH regulates thyroid metabolism via the stimulation of adenyl cyclase and the generation of cyclic-AMP (p. 455).

The disorders of the thyroid gland, observed clinically, may thus be due to either a primary thyroid disease or some disorder of the anterior pituitary with a secondary effect on the thyroid. These two glands seem to have a reciprocal relationship; i.e., after thyroidectomy the pituitary glands become enlarged.

Another factor (p. 488) may again be mentioned. The hypothalamus secretes a hormone that stimulates the secretion of thyrotropin by the anterior pituitary. Thus, the hypothalamus seems to control the pituitary-thyroid system. The hypothalamic hormone is designated thyrotropin-releasing factor (TRF).

Adrenocorticotropic factor. One of the most important principles elaborated by the anterior pituitary is ACTH. This tropic substance causes the adrenal cortex to secrete its steroids more actively. The anterior pituitary is sensitive to the requirements of the body for adrenocortical hormones and secretes ACTH or adrenocorticotropin in increased quantities during stress. The ACTH then acts on the adrenal cortex, leading to an increased output of the adrenocortical hormones and causing hyperplasia to ensue. There is considerable evidence that this action is due to an acceleration of the *synthesis* of the corticosteroids rather than merely an acceleration of their rate of release from the adrenal cortex.

More specifically, ACTH appears to stimulate the formation of the enzyme *desmolase,* which is required for the biosynthesis of the adrenocorticosteroids (p. 466). This factor, in a manner analogous to that of TSH, can prevent regression of the adrenal cortex, which occurs when the hypophysis is removed. Evidence of the close relationship between these two glands is seen in the fact that in acromegaly, in which the pituitary is overactive, the adrenal cortex also shows an increase in size.

ACTH is a protein with a molecular weight of approximately 3500. It has been prepared in pure form from the pituitary glands of several species, including sheep, pigs, and cattle. The data now available[29] indicate that bovine corticotropin contains 39 amino acid residues and that the amino acid sequence is as shown in Fig. 16-12. Bovine, ovine, and porcine corticotropins are identical except in the region between amino acids 25 and 33, a portion rich in acidic amino acids. Recent investigations indicate that the activity may reside in a smaller peptide "core" with a sequence of over 16 amino acid residues. Li's group prepared synthetically a peptide corresponding to the sequence of the first 19 N-terminal amino acids, having considerable activity. Hofmann and his co-workers[30] synthesized one comprising amino acid residues from the same end of the ACTH sequence, which has physiologic activity equal to that of the entire 39 amino acid peptides.

If we compare the sequence of the amino acids in ACTH shown in Fig. 16-12 with that for the intermedins on p. 487, we can see that a part of each

Ser Tyr Ser Met Glu His Phe Arg Try Gly Lys Pro Val
1   2   3   4   5   6   7   8   9   10   11   12   13

Gly Lys Lys Arg Arg Pro Val Lys Val Tyr Pro Asp Gly
14   15   16   17   18   19   20   21   22   23   24   25   26

Glu Ala Glu Asp Ser Ala Gln Ala Phe Pro Leu Glu Phe
27   28   29   30   31   32   33   34   35   36   37   38   39

Fig. 16-12. Amino acid sequence of bovine corticotropin.

chain is identical with the other; namely, in intermedin, 7 (Met) through 13 (Gly) and, in ACTH, 4 (Met) through 10 (Gly). This is, indeed, a striking similarity. When injected into animals, ACTH, of course, produces all the varied effects that are caused by the adrenocortical hormones themselves. Furthermore, ACTH can evoke these effects in hypophysectomized animals.

The influence of ACTH, or indeed of any factor, on the adrenal cortex can be followed by determining either the cholesterol or the ascorbic acid content of the cortex. From such studies it has been shown that prior treatment with ACTH prevents the usual fall in ascorbic acid when the animal is exposed to cold, trauma, etc.; i.e., the blood level of ACTH seems to influence the rate of secretion of this hormone. Other factors also seem to be concerned in the regulation of the secretion of ACTH by the anterior pituitary. The hypothalamus may have some action, either by a nervous mechanism or by some secretion. Finally, there is evidence that epinephrine or, to a lesser degree, norepinephrine may stimulate the release of ACTH, especially during acute stress, which activates the sympathetic nervous system.

Prolactin. The demonstration of a factor of the anterior pituitary stimulating the secretion of milk was accomplished by Riddle, who called the hormone prolactin. This hormone can initiate lactation not only in the mature female breast but also in the breast of an immature female or of a male if the latter have been properly prepared by a preliminary treatment with gonadal hormones.

Prolactin was the first anterior pituitary hormone to be obtained in pure form. It is a protein and has been crystallized by White and associates (Fig. 16-13). It appears to be a single peptide chain, with a molecular weight of about 24,200. In this pure form it has no growth-promoting, thyrotropic, diabetogenic, adrenotropic, or gonadotropic activities. It is thermolabile and is destroyed by tryptic digestion.

Although prolactin alone has little or no influence on the growth or development of undeveloped mammary glands, it may have some effect on the growth of these glands in association with the hypertrophy coincident with induced lactation. The lactogenic hormone initiates lactation in mammary glands suitably prepared by gonadal hormones. The estrogenic hormones

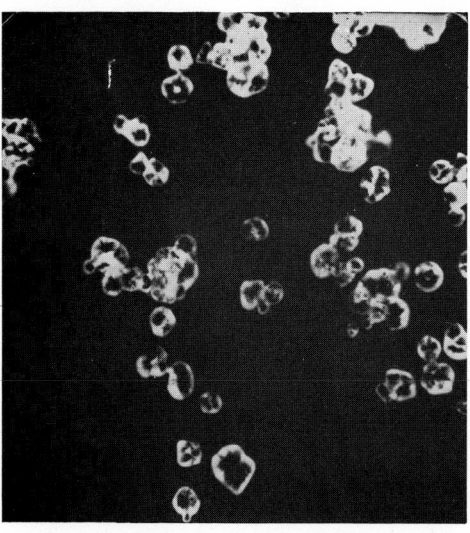

Fig. 16-13. Crystalline prolactin (×900). (From White, A., Bonsnes, R. W., and Long, C. N. H.: J. Biol. Chem. **143**:447, 1942.)

do not induce mammary growth in hypophysectomized animals. Growth does occur, however, in such animals if they receive lactogenic hormone in addition to estrogens. Prolactin also has gonadotropic properties, in the rat at least, in that it maintains functional corpora lutea in hypophysectomized animals.

Gonadotropic factors. Hypophysectomy results in atrophy of the primary and secondary sexual glands. These glands may be restored to normal function by the administration of extracts of the anterior lobe or by the implantation of living anterior lobe tissue. Since it makes no difference whether the pituitary glands are derived from males or females, the pituitary hormones involved are identical and the type of effect produced is determined by the sex of the animal affected.

Three anterior pituitary hormones are now recognized as gonadotropins, i.e., hormones that simulate the sex glands. All are active in the female, and only two in the male. They are follicle-stimulating hormone (FSH), luteinizing hormone or interstitial cell–stimulating hormone (LH or ICSH), and prolactin, also called luteotropic hormone (LTH) or luteotropin. The interrelationships of the gonadotropic and the sex hormones are exceedingly complicated. The simplified account that follows, although based on present knowledge, will no doubt require modification in the future as new facts are discovered.

In the female, FSH induces growth of a graafian follicle in the ovary preparatory to release of the ovum. During this phase of the menstrual cycle, the follicle itself secretes a female sex hormone, an estrogen called *estradiol*. This hormone induces a proliferation and thickening of the endometrium and an increase in the vascularity of the endometrium, thus preparing the uterine wall for the reception of the fertilized ovum. LH controls the development of the corpus luteum, which, in turn, secretes another sex hormone, *progesterone,* while the secretion of estrogen is gradually diminishing. Prolactin now maintains the corpus luteum in an active state for the continued production of progesterone, which, itself, is one of the hormones necessary for maintaining pregnancy.

In the male, FSH induces growth of the testes by causing proliferation of the sperm-forming tissue. Thus, mature spermatozoa are produced. The secretion of *testosterone,* the male sex hormone, is stimulated by ICSH. Testosterone sustains spermatogenesis and develops the secondary or accessory sex organs, the vas deferens, prostate gland, and the vesicles.

The specific biochemical action of the gonadotropins appears to be to stimulate the formation of the enzyme *desmolase,* required in the biosynthesis of androgens and estrogens (p. 503).

Both FSH and ICSH have been isolated after much difficulty. They are glycoproteins, which are soluble in water, and they are destroyed by tryptic digestion, by dilute acids and bases, and by heating above 50° C. FSH has a molecular weight of 67,000 and an isoelectric point of pH 4.5. In contrast to tryptic digestion, peptic digestion at pH 4.0 results in a product that retains the activity of the native protein. Prolactin differs from FSH and LH in that it contains no carbohydrate.

The secretion of FSH by the anterior pituitary gland is under feedback control by the estrogens. Feedback inhibition is apparently by way of the hypothalamic region of the brain. Similarly, the secretion of LH appears to be controlled by progesterone via a feedback mechanism involving the hypothalamus.

Only the most important aspects of the interrelations among the anterior pituitary hormones and the glands that they influence and that influence them have been discussed. Some of these, as well as the posterior pituitary hormones, are diagrammatically shown in Fig. 16-8.

Chorionic gonadotropin. Chorionic gonadotropin was discovered by Aschheim and Zondek in the urine of pregnant women and became the basis for a pregnancy test, bearing their name, as well as modifications of it. This hormone is produced by the placenta and appears in the urine shortly after pregnancy begins. It also is formed whenever there is abnormal chorionic proliferation, such as hydatidiform mole or chorionepithelioma. Such cases must be ruled out when making the test. The injection of urine containing this gonadotropin into immature female white mice under standard conditions causes hemorrhage of an ovarian follicle in about 96 hours. The Friedman modification uses a mature unmated female rabbit. In such an animal the injection of the hormone results in follicular rupture and corpus luteum formation within 24 to 48 hours. The results in both species can be observed macroscopically. This gonadotropin is now considered to possess more luteinizing than follicle-stimulating power.

Chorionic gonadotropin is a glycoprotein with a molecular weight of about 47,000 and has been purified to a high degree. The carbohydrate moiety contains some six components, including D-galactose, D-mannose, N-acetylglucosamine, N-acetylgalactosamine, L-fucose, and N-acetylneuraminic acid. The sequence and nature of the carbohydrate moiety are now partially known.

497

N-Acetylneuraminic acid is essential to the biologic activity of the hormone. Apparently all 18 common amino acids are present in the protein moiety, proline being especially high (about 20%). Chorionic gonadotropin is usually called the "anterior pituitary–like" hormone or APL, but this is not an accurate term because the hormone is not effective in hypophysectomized rats, whereas pituitary hormones are.

OVARIAN HORMONES

During growth of the follicle under the influence of FSH, estrogen is secreted. *Estrogen* is a generic term for a substance that induces estrus, which is a cyclic phenomenon of the female reproductive system. The stages and timing differ in various species, but, in general, first a proestrus period occurs, during which the follicle ripens and the organs of reproduction develop. This is followed by estrus, the period of heat, in which the female will receive the male. Ovulation takes place toward the end of estrus, either spontaneously or, as in the rabbit, after mating. Then follow a period of retrogression of the accessory reproductive organs and a period of sexual inactivity. In some animals, e.g., mice, rats, the estrus cycle is accompanied by characteristic changes in the vaginal epithelium. Vaginal smears, when viewed microscopically, reveal whether or not estrus is occurring, and this technique is used to determine qualitatively and quantitatively the estrogenic activity of synthetic substitutes for hormones.

In the human being the reproductive phenomena also show a periodicity, but this is not the same as estrus. The follicle matures and the ovum is discharged not during menstruation but at the midinterval of the cycle; during estrus in other animals, the vaginal bleeding occurs at a time near ovulation. However, the estrogen in the human subject has a definite effect on the female organs, inducing growth of the vagina, uterus, and mammary glands and accentuating secondary sex characteristics.

Crude extracts of ovary or follicular fluid produce estrus experimentally in immature rats. This was shown by Allen and Doisy and led to the isolation, crystallization, and identification of *theelin,* the name originally given to the first estrogenic substance obtained by Doisy. Now the term *estrone* is commonly used. There are known to be several naturally occurring estrogenic compounds. The most important ones are (1) estrone, (2) estriol, and (3) estradiol. These and several other natural estrogens are steroids. Their formulas are as follows:

Estrone
($\Delta^{1,3,5:10}$-estratriene-3-ol-17-one)

Estriol
($\Delta^{1,3,5:10}$-estratriene-3,16[α],17[β]-triol)

β-Estradiol
(Δ$^{1,3,5:10}$-estratriene-3,17[β]-diol)

Although estrone was the first of these to be isolated and for a long time was called the "female sex hormone," it is not as powerful as estradiol. In fact, there is a tendency to regard β-estradiol as the true follicular or ovarian hormone. The relative potencies of β-estradiol:α-estradiol:estrone:estriol are approximately 1000:10:100:30.

The ovarian hormones are synthesized from cholesterol by way of progesterone and, surprisingly, testosterone. The intermediates in their biosynthesis are shown schematically on p. 503. As β-estradiol circulates, it is converted by some organ to estrone, and this to estriol. The sequence of reactions is probably estrone → 16-ketoestrone → 16-keto-α-estriol → estriol. Estriol is then united with glucuronic acid, forming estriol glucuronide, which has little or no physiologic action. Just how much of the hormone is metabolized and excreted in this way is not known. Estrone itself may also be conjugated in part in the liver. Of interest is the fact that estrone is conjugated not only with glucuronic acid but also equally or perhaps to a greater extent with sulfate and to a lesser extent with phosphate. The conjugated forms, of course, may be excreted in the urine. When estradiol is administered to laboratory animals, less than 20% is excreted, partly in this conjugated form; the remaining 80% is destroyed in the body. The conjugation may be a step preliminary to the utilization of estradiol by tissues or to its ultimate destruction. The liver is the site of destruction of the estrogens in some experimental animals and also probably in the human being. The ability of the liver to metabolize these hormones is dependent on nutritional factors, among which is the intake of protein.

The amount of estrogens in the blood of women shows cyclic alteration, with peaks at approximately the fourteenth and twentieth days of the monthly cycle. As stated earlier, the amount of estrogen secreted by the ovarian follicle cells is increased by FSH, of the anterior pituitary gland. In turn, estrogens control the secretion of FSH by feedback inhibition.

The biochemical mechanism by which the estrogens exert their physiologic effects has received considerable attention. There is some evidence that estrogens serve as *transhydrogenases* in the shift of hydrogen atoms (and electrons) from reduced NADP$^+$ (NADPH$_2$) to NAD$^+$ to form NADH$_2$. Such a function would in this way serve to connect the NADP$^+$ system to NAD$^+$ and, in turn, to the main electron-transport system of biologic oxidation. However, the alleged role of the estrogens as transhydrogenases appears to be very uncertain at the present time. Estradiol, as the conjugate with sulfate, apparently is highly active in increasing RNA and protein synthesis in the target organ (rat uterus), which may well constitute the primary biochemical function of β-estradiol.

Indeed, recent studies[31] indicate that estrogens act on the mammalian uterus at the level of transcription within the cell nucleus to effect new RNA formation and thus protein biosynthesis. The estrogens, and probably other steroid hormones, may activate, or derepress (p. 105), certain functionally linked genes and allow transcription of the messenger RNA, which then would code for the synthesis of specific proteins (e.g., ovalbumin). An increase in the nuclear transcription of transfer RNA has also been observed.

Corpus luteum hormone. The corpus luteum produces progesterone, which seems to be responsible for continuing the development of the uterus, initiated by estradiol, and for converting the endometrium to a secretory stage. Indeed, it has very little effect unless uterine development has been started by the estrogenic hormone. Progesterone has a number of other effects, all of which bear somewhat upon the reproductive cycle. It inhibits ovulation and influences growth of the mammary glands, producing development of the acinar structures. The absence of this hormone, brought about by removal of the corpus luteum, results in interference with implantation of the ovum in human beings. In other animals the ovum or embryo may become implanted, but it is later expelled.

Although there may be several progestational hormones, the most active is progesterone, which has been isolated and has the following formula:

Progesterone
(Δ^4-pregnene-3,20-dione)

Pregnanediol

Note the close resemblance to the structure of 11-deoxycorticosterone (p. 468). It is not surprising, therefore, to find progesterone with certain adrenocortical properties — namely, those influencing salt and water. Indeed, as is shown in the schematic diagram of the biosynthesis of the adrenocorticoids (p. 469), progesterone serves as a precursor of these steroid hormones. It also serves as a precursor of the androgens and estrogens (p. 503). The chief metabolic product of progesterone found in urine is *pregnanediol*, which is excreted as the glucuronide. Progesterone is soluble in most organic solvents and in vegetable oils but is insoluble in water. It is used clinically to some extent, particularly in the treatment of amenorrhea (absence of menstruation in young women). Some oral contraceptives in use at the present time are derivatives similar to progesterone. The two major types are the 19-nor derivatives, which lack the methyl group on the nineteenth carbon, and the 17-hydroxyprogesterone diacetate or caproate derivatives.

Progesterone, like other steroid hormones, is biologically active in cell protein synthesis at the level of increasing new RNA transcription in the cell nucleus. Apparently progesterone specifically induces synthesis of the protein *avidin* in the oviduct. Avidin combines with the vitamin biotin (p. 817). Its role in the cytoplasm of the ovum is as yet unclear.

Menstrual cycle   At this point we should reconsider the effects of the various hormones on the menstrual cycle. True menstruation occurs only in human beings and in members of a closely related group of primates. Under the influence of the pituitary gonadotropic hormone, the follicle matures and an increasing amount of estradiol is formed. This occurs during the first 2 weeks of the cycle. Under the influence of estradiol, the endometrium increases in thickness and vascularity up to the time of ovulation. The follicle then ruptures and liberates a mature ovum, after which LH causes the ruptured follicle to change to a corpus luteum, which forms progesterone. Progesterone, in turn, causes the endometrium to assume a turgid secretory condition and to be ready to receive and maintain a fertilized ovum. If the ovum is not fertilized, the corpus luteum regresses, progesterone diminishes in amount, and the endometrium breaks down, with the occurrence of menstrual bleeding. If the ovum is fertilized, the secretion of progesterone continues, for this hormone is necessary in the maintenance of pregnancy. Prolactin aids in continuing the secretion of progesterone.

Other effects of estradiol. In addition to its action on the endometrium, estradiol seems to maintain the normal size and function of the various parts of the female reproductive organs. It promotes growth of the duct tissue in the breasts. It appears to have a controlling action on the secretion of the anterior pituitary so that the ovary and pituitary seem to have reciprocal effects. Thus, indirectly, the ovarian hormone may have an influence on the other endocrine glands through its action on the pituitary. A number of other effects have been shown to be due to estradiol, including stimulation of the growth of certain epithelial tissues, especially the mucosa of the vagina and the nose.

Therapeutic uses of estradiol. In common with the other sex hormones, and, indeed, with most of the hormones of whatever origin, estradiol has been recommended for many therapeutic purposes, often with no justification. It is a very potent substance and may have harmful effects if used indiscriminately. Fortunately, on cessation of administration, the unpleasant symptoms tend to disappear. If employed on the basis of its known physiologic effects, it becomes a useful agent to the physician.

Estradiol is said to be effective in developing the female sex organs in sexual infantilism. In juvenile vaginitis due to gonorrheal infection and in other forms of vaginitis, it is administered to stimulate proliferation of the mucosa. It promotes growth of the breasts under certain conditions but also is said to inhibit the pituitary in the control of excessive milk secretion.

This inhibiting effect on the pituitary gland is the basis for one hypothesis put forward to explain the use of estrogens in controlling abnormal symptoms of the menopause. The menopause is that period in which menstruation ceases and the woman is no longer capable of becoming pregnant. In most cases menopause occurs without particular disturbance; but in about 15%, a number of distressing symptoms ensue. These are chiefly cardiovascular, vasomotor, and nervous in nature. To some extent, they may be controlled by estrogenic substances. Since there is no marked decrease in the estrogenic content of the blood in these cases, the beneficial action of the estrogens is attributed to their presumed inhibitory action on the pituitary.

Stilbestrol. Stilbestrol is a synthetic product with marked estrogenic properties. As can be seen from its formula, it does not resemble the steroids from a chemical standpoint. However, it produces practically all the physiologic effects that estradiol does. It is administered by mouth, and in some cases unpleasant side effects are seen; but usually, if the dosage is carefully regulated, these do not occur. The formula of the more potent diethyl derivative is as follows:

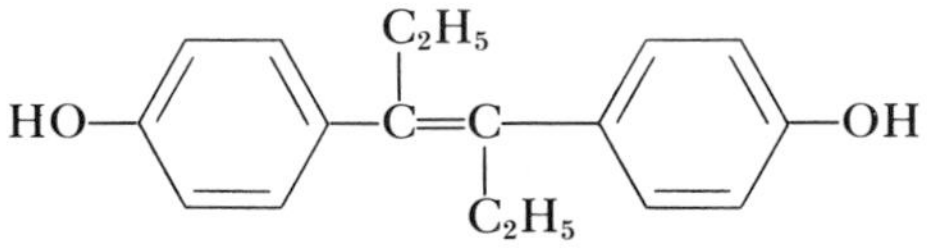

Diethylstilbestrol

Relaxin. Relaxin is a hormone (or group of hormones) produced and active during pregnancy. A preliminary priming with estrogen appears necessary. It was discovered by Hisaw, in 1926. It is a protein or polypeptide but has not yet been obtained in pure form, and, consequently, its structure has not been determined. It greatly hastens pubic relaxation, which is caused by estrogen alone, in the guinea pig and certain other species, and has other effects, e.g., promoting development of the mammary glands. Relaxin has been obtained from the blood, placenta, and reproductive tract of various mammals, including human placenta. However, its role in human physiology is problematic.

TESTICULAR HORMONES

One of the first attempts to demonstrate the presence of a male sex hormone was that of Brown-Séquard. In 1889, at the age of 72, he gave testicular extracts to himself and felt that he experienced increased vigor and strength. These and similar experiments have not been convincing, and there is no evidence that the testicular secretion has any relation to the phenomenon of aging. The testes, however, do secrete a definite hormone. The actual production of this secretion is regulated by the anterior pituitary and can be demonstrated in several test animals. For example, injection of testicular extracts into capons causes growth of the comb, wattles, and earlobes. It has a similar growth-promoting effect on the combs of male chicks. It also inhibits ovulation in hens and has the curious effect of causing the ovipositor of the female bitterling, a small fish, to increase in length, a phenomenon that occurs during the natural sexual cycle. The effective substance or substances can be isolated not only from testicular tissue but also from urine.

The *androgens*, as they are generically called, also have some slight estrogenic properties. Thus the term *male hormones* is not strictly applicable. Furthermore, the occurrence of estrogenic and androgenic substances is seen in the urine of both sexes, although androgens usually predominate in the urine of males and estrogens in the urine of females.

The structure and chemistry of the androgens have been worked out, largely by Butenandt and by Ruzicka and their colleagues. These compounds also are steroids. Testosterone is probably the characteristic hormone, and androsterone seems to be a transformation product of it. Intermediate products are Δ^4-androstene-3,17-dione and epitestosterone (Δ^4-androstene-3-one-17[β]-ol). The 3-keto group of testosterone is important to the biologic activity of this hormone, probably for steric reasons since it induces a flattening effect on the A-ring. The liver is most likely the site of the inactivation of androgens as well as of estrogens.

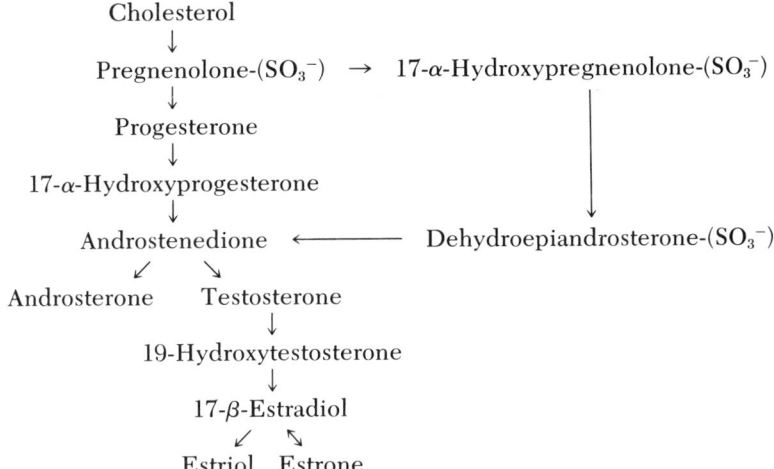

Testosterone
(Δ^4-androstene-3-one-17[α]-ol)

Androsterone
(androstane-3[α]-ol-17-one)

The probable biosynthetic pathway of the androgens, as well as that of the estrogens, is shown schematically below.

Cholesterol
↓
Pregnenolone-(SO_3^-) → 17-α-Hydroxypregnenolone-(SO_3^-)
↓
Progesterone
↓
17-α-Hydroxyprogesterone
↓
Androstenedione ←——— Dehydroepiandrosterone-(SO_3^-)
↙   ↘
Androsterone   Testosterone
↓
19-Hydroxytestosterone
↓
17-β-Estradiol
↙   ↘
Estriol   Estrone

The enzymes and cofactors involved in each of the above steps have been fairly well characterized. The enzymes required for the conversion of cholesterol to progesterone have already been discussed. From progesterone to testosterone, the enzymes required in sequence are: 17-α-hydroxylase, side chain–splitting enzyme, and 17-β-hydroxysteroid dehydrogenase. The conversion of testosterone to estradiol is catalyzed by an aromatizing enzyme system, not yet completely characterized. The interconversion of estradiol and estrone requires 17-β-hydroxysteroid dehydrogenase. In steps where hydrogenation is involved, $NADPH_2$ apparently serves as the cofactor.

By the perfusing of respective glands with solutions containing labeled acetate, it has been shown that the complex steroid hormones are synthesized from the simple two-carbon chain. Thus, adrenal hormones are produced by the adrenal gland; testosterone and Δ^4-androstene-3,17-dione by the testis; and estrone, β-estradiol, and cholesterol by the ovary. However, it is probable that the steroid hormones are produced to a greater extent from cholesterol. Deuterium-labeled cholesterol administered to a pregnant woman found its way into the urine as labeled pregnanediol. The synthesis of corticosterone in the adrenal gland can be traced from cholesterol through pregnenolone to progesterone. A 3-β-hydroxysteroid dehydrogenase system results in the removal of two hydrogens from the carboxyl group of pregnenolone at position-3, leaving a carbonyl group at that point. At the same time the double bond Δ^5 is shifted to Δ^4.

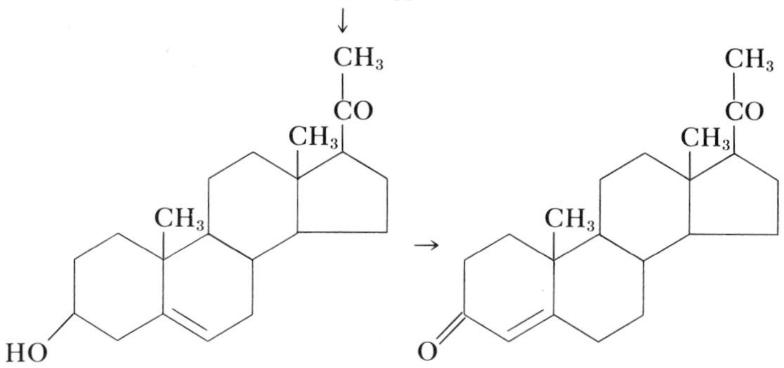

Cholesterol
↓

Pregnenolone   Progesterone

Progesterone can be converted to corticosterone by the introduction of a hydroxyl in position-11 and another in position-21.

Cholesterol also leads to the formation of the androgens by the testis. The steps are the same as those just described. Carbons 20 and 21 are oxidized off to form Δ^4-androstene-3,17-dione, which is reduced to testosterone.

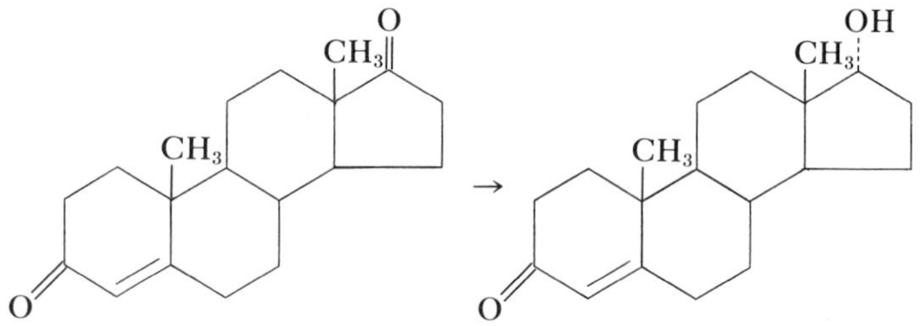

Δ^4-Androstene-3,17-dione   Testosterone

It has been found that placental tissue can cause the reverse of the above reaction to take place and that the resulting androstene compound can be converted to estrone.

The chief functions of testosterone are to produce normal development of the male reproductive organs and to maintain the secondary male characteristics. Under its influence the descent of the testes occurs. Testosterone is also effective in sustaining spermatogenesis. The secondary male characteristics that develop in its presence are the deep voice, the growth and pattern of facial and body hair, and the male type of skeletal muscular development. It inhibits mammary development and function and stimulates libido in both the male and the female. The male hormones constitute one factor in the production of baldness. Age and inheritance are other factors involved in bringing about this condition, but baldness does not ensue without androgenic stimulation.

At a molecular level, the primary action of testosterone is to increase protein synthesis in various target tissues. This apparently results from a stimulation by testosterone of RNA production within the nucleus of cells of affected tissues. Recent work[31] supports the concept that the increase in protein synthesis following the administration of androgens is mediated by the increased synthesis of RNA in the cell nucleus. The latter can be demonstrated within 20 minutes after androgen administration. The formation of all classes of RNA, messenger, ribosomal, and transfer (p. 42), is increased. Large transitory elevations of *DNA polymerase* are also seen. Thus the androgens appear to rapidly stimulate synthesis of DNA polymerase and DNA, as well as RNA polymerase and nucleolar RNA, in target tissues.

Clinically, testosterone is used if the testes are absent or are unable to function. Such males may have an effeminate appearance and build, with broad hips and prominent breasts, feminine pattern of pubic hair, slight growth of facial hair, and a high-pitched voice. They usually are easily fatigued and have a low basal metabolic rate. These symptoms vary greatly with the age of onset of the disorder. The administration of suitable doses of testosterone may relieve many of these symptoms. It often brings about enlargement of the sexual organs, prostatic secretion, growth of pubic and axillary hair as well as a beard, and deepening of the voice. Such individuals acquire sexual desire and may become parents if there is potentially functional testicular tissue present. The use of the gonadotropic hormones is theoretically more sound if there is testicular tissue that can be stimulated. The administration of large doses of testosterone to women may have masculinizing effects.

In cryptorchidism, i.e., failure of the testes to descend in the normal manner, testosterone seems to be of considerable value. If testosterone is administered in high therapeutic dosage for long periods of time (e.g., 25 mg. daily for 4 to 6 weeks), atrophy of the sperm is likely to result. However, such an effect may be reversed if treatment is discontinued for a similar length of time.

Steroid interrelationships. All the sex hormones are closely related chemically. Only slight changes in certain parts of the molecule are needed to transform a female to a male hormone. The adrenocortical hormones are also steroids, and abnormalities in sexual development are often traced to the adrenal cortex. Furthermore, the adrenal cortex can manufacture both androgens and estrogens, and, conversely, the sex hormones also have some adrenocortical functions; e.g., progesterone has some effect in ameliorating the symptoms resulting from adrenalectomy.

The interaction of the glands of internal secretion has been noted in several connections. Undoubtedly many other relationships obtain. Selye showed some of these in his hypothesis of the general adaptation syndrome, which states that the prolonged exposure of an individual to stress leads to (1) the alarm reaction, (2) the stage of resistance, and (3) exhaustion. Stress is defined as the rate of all wear and tear caused by life. It is the normal response of the body to any damaging agent, ranging from a burn or a severe infection to an intense emotional episode, which might even be a happy one. The effects of these factors are nonspecific, and all produce similar results, as contrasted with specific actions that may differ among themselves. In the current discussion we are concerned with nonspecific or stressor effects. Many nervous impulses come into play and are related to hormonal releases, especially those of the pituitary-adrenal system. However, from the purely biochemical standpoint, there is believed to be, during the first stage, a breakdown of body proteins with an increase in the content of protein catabolites and proteolytic enzymes in the blood. This seems to be due to a generalized disintegration of body cells. At the same time these stresses result in an enlargement of the adrenal cortex.

The stage of resistance, or the hormonal defense mechanism, is characterized by a *decreased* secretion of most of the anterior pituitary hormones but an *increased* output of ACTH. This causes the adrenal cortex to secrete its hormones, especially the glucocorticoids, in increased amounts. The effect of these hormones is manifold. There is involution of the thymus gland and other lymphatic organs. The blood count is greatly changed. Gluconeogenesis is stimulated, and a rise in blood sugar ensues. There are many other effects, and Selye considers it possible that a number of diseases may be listed as "diseases of adaptation." These, in general, are the results of breakdown in the normal response to stress. Among them are hypertensive diseases, nephrosclerosis, nephritis, periarteritis nodosa, rheumatic diseases, gastrointestinal ulcers, gout, diabetes mellitus, and Cushing's syndrome. The results of the mechanisms put into play may be a resistance, which results in a restoration of the normal state. However, it may lead to the third stage, namely, exhaustion, when the glands give up the struggle and death eventually ensues.

17-Ketosteroids The determination of the metabolic products of some steroids in the urine has become of considerable clinical importance. The 17-ketosteroids, in particular, are of interest. These are steroids possessing a ketone group at position-17. An example is androsterone, the formula of which is given on p. 503. Other important 17-ketosteroids are dehydroisoandrosterone, etiocholanolone, 11-hydroxyandrosterone, 11-ketoetiocholanolone, and estrone. The determination involves hydrolysis to free the steroids from their ester combinations, extraction with organic solvents, and removal of phenolic substances, including estrone. After further purification, typically by chromatography, including thin-layer chromatography, the steroids are determined quantitatively by color reactions. Since estrone has been removed, the figure obtained, i.e., the neutral 17-ketosteroid value, is an index of the steroid secretory activity of the adrenal glands in the female and of the adrenal glands and testes in the male.

In normal adults between the ages of 20 and 40 years, the 24-hour excretion of the neutral 17-ketosteroids ordinarily ranges from 7 to 12 mg. in women and from 12 to 17 mg. in men. The greater output by men is ascribed to the fraction produced by the testes. The values are expressed in terms of milligrams of androsterone. In childhood the amounts rise from 1 to 2 mg., for children at 3 or 4 years of age, to about 8 to 9 mg., at 11 years. Above 12 years, boys excrete 8 to 13 mg., and adult values are reached at the age of 18 years or even younger.

Pathologically, derangements of the adrenal cortex, testis, and anterior pituitary are accompanied by changes in the 17-ketosteroid output. Decreased amounts are excreted in hypopituitarism and also in acromegaly. In Addison's disease there is also a low elimination. In hypogonadism in both sexes a low output is sometimes but not always seen. High values are found in adrenocortical hyperfunction or in testicular hyperfunction, as in certain tumors of these glands. However, the adrenogenital syndrome does not always result in an increase in these steroids — if it does not, the increase may be the result of hyperplasia rather than a tumor.

It has been suggested that the determination of 17-hydroxycorticoid excretion in the urine affords a more sensitive measure of adrenal activity than does the alteration of 17-ketosteroid excretion. The 17-hydroxycorticoids that have been isolated from human urine include 11-dehydro-17-hydroxycorticosterone (cortisone), its dihydro and tetrahydro metabolic reduction products, 17-hydroxycorticosterone, estradiol, and estriol.

The relations of the steroids to cancer are assuming great importance. There is some experimental evidence that continued overdosage with estradiol produces tumors but discontinuous treatments are without this effect. Progesterone and testosterone have an antitumorigenic action on the tumors produced by estradiol. Some clinical improvement is seen in certain cases of metastatic carcinoma of the prostate when estrogens are administered. Castration, i.e., deprivation of androgens, has a similar effect. It is also noteworthy that two carcinogenic compounds, which are not steroids, are also estrogenic.

Other alleged hormones In addition to the hormones discussed in the preceding pages, a number of others have been postulated from time to time. Some of these were discarded because of lack of confirmation. Three other hormones, however, have been described in the past few years and have apparently become established by confirmatory evidence. These will be considered next.

Erythropoietin. Erythropoietin is one of the newer additions to the hormone field. Mounting evidence has established its endocrine nature beyond question. Erythropoietin, or the erythrocyte-stimulating factor (ESF), is secreted by the kidney. Its secretion is stimulated primarily by tissue anoxia, presumably in the renal cells.[32] Androgenic hormones and cobalt also stimulate its secretion or release. Apparently ESF is secreted as an inactive protein,[32] possibly an enzymelike substance, termed by Gordon and his group the renal erythropoietic factor (REF), that converts a plasma globulin to active erythropoietin:

$$\text{Plasma globulin} \xrightarrow[\text{(enzyme?)}]{\text{REF}} \text{Active erythropoietin}$$

Evidence for the renal origin of erythropoietin is threefold: (1) polycythemia is characteristically associated with renal neoplasms and cysts; (2)

anemia is commonly found in renal disease; (3) plasma levels of erythropoietin decrease in nephrectomized animals or animals with bilateral uretal ligation.

Erythropoietin has been prepared in highly active form from the plasma of anemic sheep and from the urine of human subjects with certain types of anemia. It is an α_1-globulin, a glycoprotein containing 8% to 12% total hexose. Its molecular weight by gel filtration is about 60,000. All the common amino acids are present in its molecule, with the possible exception of methionine. Its activity is destroyed by proteolytic enzymes and by hyaluronidase and neuraminidase.

Apparently there are species differences in the amino acid composition of erythropoietin, samples from mammals differing slightly from those of birds and amphibia in activity. Erythropoietin is immunogenic, sheep plasma preparations producing antibodies in rabbits.

The exact mechanism of action of erythropoietin is uncertain at this time. The target cell is the stem cell (hemohistioblast) of bone marrow and other erythroid tissue. Erythropoietin stimulates the differentiation of the stem cell into the erythroid series, increasing the numbers of proerythroblasts in the bone marrow. This is followed by increases in other nucleated erythrocytes and, finally, by increases in reticulocytes and mature erythrocytes in the peripheral circulation. Current studies[33] indicate that the earliest effect of erythropoietin is stimulation of the synthesis of a very large RNA (150 S) by bone marrow cells, which occurs within a few minutes after the addition of erythropoietin in vitro. Increases in smaller RNA molecules then rapidly occur, probably in ribosomal, transfer, and messenger RNA (p. 42). Erythropoietin increases the incorporation of ^{59}Fe into the hemoglobin of peripheral blood, which is the basis of the present method of erythropoietin assay. The action of erythropoietin is inhibited by the antibiotic actinomycin-D.

Prostaglandins. Another possible new addition to the hormone group is prostaglandin or more accurately the prostaglandins.[34] This group of hormone-like substances was originally found in seminal fluid of man and other species, hence the name. Since then, prostaglandins have been found in lung, brain, pancreas, and a number of other tissues. These substances are lipid soluble and have been isolated by counter-current extraction and by chromatography (p. 901). They are 20-carbon, unsaturated, cyclic, hydroxy fatty acids. There appear to be at least six primary prostaglandins, designated PGE_1, PGE_2, PGE_3, $PGF_{1\alpha}$, $PGF_{2\alpha}$, and $PGF_{3\alpha}$. There may be some 10 or 15 intermediate forms.

PGE_1 has been shown to have the formula:

The other prostaglandins are derivatives of PGE_1, varying in structural details, including the number of double bonds and hydroxyl groups and the stereoconfiguration of the hydroxyl groups.

The prostaglandins are synthesized in the various tissues cited, from arachidonic acid (p. 279), which forms PGE_2, or from bis-homo-γ-linolenic acid, plus a two-carbon fragment, which forms PGE_1 and $PGF_{1\alpha}$. The total chemical synthesis of five of the prostaglandins has been reported recently.

The primary physiologic effect of the prostaglandins seems to be to stimulate the smooth muscle of the uterus, particularly at the time of ovulation. This effect may be due to a chelation of calcium ions. Other metabolic effects of the prostaglandins include inhibition of lipolysis in adipose tissue, possibly by inhibiting the conversion of ATP to cyclic-AMP, and inhibition of platelet aggregation. The prostaglandins thus have the opposite effect of epinephrine, norepinephrine, glucagon, and ACTH on the release of fatty acids from adipose tissue. The prostaglandins also appear to control the secretion of gastric hydrochloric acid and to have some beneficial effect in the control of acid-induced experimental gastric ulcers.

The fact that prostaglandins are so widely distributed in tissues and appear to produce rather varied metabolic effects has led some to question the propriety of their being called hormones. Further studies are required to resolve this question.

Pineal gland. There is evidence that the pineal gland secretes one or more hormones that participate in the control of several reproductive processes.[35] This gland appears to be the only structure in the mammalian body that synthesizes melatonin (5-methoxy-N-acetyltryptamine), which inhibits the secretion of the luteinizing hormone (LH) of the pituitary. LH, it will be recalled, is involved in inducing ovulation in mammals. The pineal gland contains a high level of the enzyme hydroxyindole-O-methyl transferase (HIOMT), which catalyzes the formation of melatonin from serotonin (p. 380). Apparently, light inhibits HIOMT activity, and hence melatonin synthesis, whereas darkness increases melatonin formation. The sympathetic nervous system may also affect melatonin synthesis. Thus, such "biologic clock" phenomena as light-induced estrus in animals and dark-induced atrophy of the gonads may be related to the pineal gland and variations in its secretion of melatonin.

Antihormones and hormone antagonists. Antihormones are substances antagonistic to their respective hormones and may be produced when the hormone is administered in large amounts and over a very long period. Collip and Anderson found that an experimental animal can be made resistant to the thyrotropic hormone (TH) of the pituitary in this way. Only relatively few hormones have this action, and all are protein in nature. They are apparently analogous to antibodies and may be important in producing resistance to the action of the hormones involved. For example, *antierythropoietin* antibodies may be responsible for a certain type of refractory anemia found in man.

Another type of antagonist may arise from the synthesis of substances having structures that differ slightly from the effective natural product. Woolley produced compounds that antagonize thyroxine in its effect on the tadpole.

Several ethers of N-acetyldiiodotyrosine were found to protect these animals against the lethal action of thyroxine.

References

GENERAL

Cori, C. F., et al., editors: Perspectives in biology, New York, 1963, American Elsevier Publishing Co., Inc.

Davidson, E. H.: Hormones and genes, Sci. Amer. 213:36, 1965.

Danowski, T. S., editor: Diabetes mellitus and obesity, Ann. N.Y. Acad. Sci. 148:573 1968.

Dorfman, R. I., editor: Methods in hormone research, New York, 1968, Academic Press, Inc., vol. 1.

Foa, P.: Glucagon, Springfield, Ill., 1962, Charles C Thomas, Publisher.

Gray, C. H., and Bacharach, A. L., editors: Hormones in blood, New York, 1967, Academic Press, Inc.

Grossman, M. I.: Gastrin, Berkeley, 1964, University of California Press.

Karlson, P., editor: Mechanisms of hormone action, New York, 1965, Academic Press, Inc.

Kendall, E. C.: Hormones of adrenal cortex, Bull. N.Y. Acad. Med. 29:91, 1953.

Krahl, M. E.: The action of insulin on cells, New York, 1961, Academic Press, Inc.

McGavack, T. H.: The thyroid, St. Louis, 1951, The C. V. Mosby Co.

McKerns, K. W., editor: Biochemical endocrinology (A series), New York, 1968, Appleton-Century-Crofts.

Netter, F. H.: Ciba collection of medical illustrations, vol. 4, The endocrine system, Summit, N.J., 1965, The Ciba Pharmaceutical Co.

Pecile, A., and Müller, E. F., editors: Growth hormone, proceedings of an international symposium, Amsterdam, 1967, Excerpta Medica Foundation.

Pincus, G.: Recent progress in hormone research, New York, 1964, Academic Press, Inc., vol. 20.

Pincus, G., Thimann, K. V., and Astwood, E. B.: The hormones: physiology, chemistry and applications, New York, 1948–1965, Academic Press, Inc.

Pitt-Rivers, R., and Trotter, W. R., editors: The thyroid gland, Washington, D. C., 1964, Butterworth, Inc.

Polvani, F., and Crosignani, P., editors: Immunological properties of protein hormones, New York, 1966, Academic Press, Inc.

Weber, G., editor: Advances in Enzyme Regulation, vols. 1–6, 1963–1968.

Williams, R. H., editor: Textbook of endocrinology, ed. 3, Philadelphia, 1962, W. B. Saunders Co.

SPECIAL

1. Miller, J. F. A. P.: Science 144:1544, 1964; Levey, R. H.: Sci. Amer. 211:66, 1964.

2. Yalow, R. S., and Berson, S. A.: Science 154:907, 1966; Trans. N.Y. Acad. Sci. 28:1033, 1966; Harvey Lect. 62:107, 1967.

3. Sutherland, E. W., and Rall, T. W.: Pharmacol. Rev. 12:265, 1968.

4. Butcher, R. W.: New Eng. J. Med. 279:1378, 1968.

5. Jorpes, J. E.: Gastroenterology 55:157, 1968.

6. Gregory, R. A.: Gastroenterology 51:953, 1966.

7. Ito, Y.: J. Jap. Biochem. 25:143, 1953; Ann. N.Y. Acad. Sci. 85:228, 1960; Fleming, H. S.: Ann. N.Y. Acad. Sci. 85:313, 1960.

8. Weber, G., et al.: Fed. Proc. 24:745, 1965; Proc. Nat. Acad. Sci. 53:96, 1965; Science 149:65, 1965; Weinhouse, S., et al.: Advances Enzym. Regulat. 1:363, 1963; 2:189, 1964; Samuels, L. D.: New Eng. J. Med. 271:1252, 1964.

9. Steiner, D. F., et al.: Proc. Nat. Acad. Sci. 57:473, 1967; Science 157:697, 1967.

10. Sanger, F., and Smith, L. F.: Endeavour 16:48, 1957.

11. Abel, J. J.: Proc. Nat. Acad. Sci. 12:132, 1926.

12. Butterfield, W. J. H., and Van Westerling, W., editors: Tolbutamide after ten years, Amsterdam, 1967, Excerpta Medica Foundation.

13. Bromer, W. W., et al.: J. Amer. Chem. Soc. 78:3858, 1956.

14. Penick, S. B., and Smith, G. P.: J. Obesity 1:1, 1964.

15. Conn, J. W.: Harvey Lect. 62:257, 1967.

16. Hench, P. S.: Proc. Staff Meet. Mayo Clin. 25:474, 1950.

17. Copp, D. H., et al.: J. Lab Clin. Med. 61:1029, 1963; Hirsch, P. F., et al.: Science 146:412, 1964.

18. Brewer, H. B., et al.: J. Biol. Chem. 243:5739, 1968.

19. Foster, G. V.: New Eng. J. Med. 279:349, 1968.

20. Potts, J. T., et al.: Proc. Nat. Acad. Sci. 59:1321, 1968; 60:293, 1968.

21. Rasmussen, H.: J. Biol. Chem. 235:3442, 1960; Rasmussen, H., and Craig,

L. C.: J. Biol. Chem. **236**:759, 1083, 1961.

22. Berson, S. A., and Yalow, R. S.: Science **154**:907, 1966.

23. Raisz, L. G.: J. Clin. Invest. **44**:103, 1965; Proc. Soc. Exp. Biol. Med. **119**:614, 1965.

24. Chase, L. R., and Aurbach, G. D.: Science **159**:545, 1968.

25. Du Vigneaud, V., et al.: J. Amer. Chem. Soc. **75**:4879, 4880, 1953.

26. Li, C. H., and Evans, H. M.: Science **99**: 183, 1944; Li, C. H., and Chung, D.: J. Biol. Chem. **218**:33, 1956; Li, C. H., and Papkoff, H.: Science **124**:1293, 1956.

27. Frohman, L. A., et al.: Science **162**:580, 1968.

28. Kaneko, T., et al.: Science **163**:1062, 1969.

29. Cole, R. D., et al.: J. Biol. Chem. **219**: 903, 1956; Li, C. H., et al.: J. Amer. Chem. Soc. **82**:5760, 1960.

30. Hofmann, K., et al.: J. Amer. Chem. Soc. **83**:487, 1961.

31. O'Malley, B. W.: Trans. N.Y. Acad. Sci. **31**:478, 1969; Hamilton, T. H.: Science **161**:649, 1968.

32. Stohlman, F., Jr.: New Eng. J. Med. **279**: 1437, 1968; Jacobson, L. D., and Doyle, M., editors: Erythropoiesis, New York, 1962, Grune & Stratton, Inc.; Fisher, J. W., editor.: Ann. N.Y. Acad. Sci. **149**:1, 1968.

33. Gross, M., and Goldwasser, E.: Biochemistry **8**:1795, 1969.

34. Bergström, S.: Science **157**:382, 1967; Bergström, S., and Samuelsson, B.: Endeavour **27**:109, 1968; Nobel symposium no. 2, New York, 1968, John Wiley & Sons, Inc.

35. Martin, L., and Ganong, W. F., editors: Neuroendocrinology, New York, 1967, Academic Press, Inc., vol. 2.

CHAPTER 17

ENERGY METABOLISM

The demonstration of the laws of conservation of matter and energy has been made again and again for animate as well as inanimate matter. Matter is transformed chemically and physically, but none is lost and none gained; energy is changed from one form to another, but, here too, there is neither loss nor gain. When the products derived from foods are oxidized, there is an evolution of heat, in much the same way as when a substance is burned outside the body. The combustion is not as intense and is accomplished with the aid of complicated enzyme reactions; but in the end, it is an oxidation and there is an evolution of heat or other forms of energy. It was the great French scientist Lavoisier (1743–1794) who first demonstrated that animal heat is derived from oxidations of essentially the same sort as any other oxidation. He also showed that the amount of heat produced by the oxidation of a certain amount of carbon in an animal is equivalent to that produced by the combustion of the same amount of nonliving carbon.

In earlier chapters the material phases of metabolism, the building up and breaking down of tissues, were studied. Now the energy transformations involved in those processes will be discussed. Both phases make up *total metabolism.*

HEAT REGULATION OF THE BODY

The transformation of the potential energy of food into muscular contractions and other forms of kinetic energy by the animal body is, from a mechanical standpoint, more efficient than in most man-made machines. About 18% to 22% of our food may be converted to mechanical energy, the energy of work, etc., as compared with from 9% to 19% for the steam engine and 20% for the gasoline motor. The Diesel engine, however, is more efficient since it transforms from 29% to 35% of its fuel into kinetic energy. The rest of the energy transformed from food, about 80%, is liberated as heat. Usually the body is warmer than the surrounding atmosphere and loses heat to it. Sometimes, however, the reverse is the case, the atmospheric temperature being higher than that of the body, and the organism has the burden of losing heat, which is constantly being produced, against this gradient. When the environment is above body temperature, all of the excess heat must be eliminated by the evaporation of water.

Nevertheless the body temperature of the human being is remarkably constant. There are, to be sure, slight normal variations. In the early morning, between 2 and 5 A.M., the temperature is lowest, rising gradually to its highest point between 5 and 8 P.M. During sleep the temperature always goes down slightly. These variations do not exceed 1.8° F.; i.e., throughout the day, under ordinary conditions of work and rest, in a normal adult, the rectal temperature may range from 97.3° to 99.1° F. The temperatures of different parts of the body vary—that of the rectum is higher than that of the mouth, and that of the mouth higher than that of the axilla. In the normal woman there is a rather regular temperature rhythm dependent on the menstrual cycle. During the period between menstruation and ovulation there is a slow fall in body temperature, with occasionally a steeper drop just before ovulation. Immediately thereafter a sharp rise, to a flat or slowly ascending plateau, occurs. Shortly before the onset of menstruation, the temperature rapidly falls again. At the menopause this ovarian temperature cycle ceases. Muscular work causes an increased heat production, of course, but this usually changes the temperature of the body little because of the effectiveness of the heat-regulating mechanism. The temperature of the atmosphere usually does not affect body temperature, but prolonged hot or cold baths can raise or lower body temperature, respectively.

Heat is produced in both oxidative and nonoxidative reactions in all tissues of the body but chiefly in the muscles. There is, of course, some heat produced during digestion and in the various chemical reactions occurring in the liver and other organs. The contractions of nonstriated muscle, as in peristalsis, must give rise to some heat, and the heartbeat also accounts for a considerable amount. By far, the largest factor, however, is the heat produced by the skeletal muscles. Even during rest, between periods of activity, muscles have a large energy requirement, and during work this requirement may be increased enormously. When the external temperature is lowered, the muscles are called upon to produce more heat by shivering. Glands of internal secretion, particularly the thyroid, play a role in heat production by altering the rate of metabolism. In all these ways, heat production is affected, and each is thus a part of the heat-regulating mechanism.

On the other hand, there are several factors that regulate heat control by modifying the loss of heat from the body. There are three main paths by which heat is lost: the skin, the lungs, and the excretions. At least 85% of the heat loss is from the skin. This occurs by conduction, radiation, convection, and evaporation. The relative amounts lost by these different pathways vary with the conditions of the body and its environment. The amount of body fat, the clothing, the temperature of the air and walls of the room, the humidity, and the movement of air are all important factors. Heat loss by way of the lungs is partly by vaporization and partly by convection. The amount of heat transferred or lost from the body in feces and urine is relatively small.

The regulation of heat loss is partly voluntary and partly involuntary. The former is seen in the various devices adopted for warming the body: clothing, heating our buildings, warming our food and drink. The involuntary regulatory machinery includes the vasomotor mechanism and the secretion of sweat. When the external temperature is high, the cutaneous blood vessels dilate and the abdominal vessels constrict, thereby exposing more blood to the cooling influence of the external environment, which, although warm, is almost invariably cooler than body temperature. The cooled blood is brought to the interior of the body, where it is again warmed, and is returned again and again to the surface for cooling. The sweat glands are stimulated to increase their secretion when heat loss from the skin by physical means is insufficient. Then the evaporation of sweat becomes a cooling factor. If the secretion is extremely rapid or the external temperature and humidity are high, evaporation does not keep pace with secretion and beads of perspiration form.

The control of heat production and heat loss is vested in the central nervous system. The central mechanism for regulating heat production is located in the posterior hypothalamus, whereas that for heat loss is in the anterior hypothalamus.

Measurement of heat   In physiologic studies, heat is measured in *large calories* (Cal. or kcal.). A kilocalorie is equal to 1000 small calories and is therefore the amount of heat needed to raise 1000 gm. (1 kg.) of water 1° C., e.g., from 15° to 16° C. A bomb calorimeter is used to determine the caloric value of a given substance, e.g., a food. The calorimeter is a metal vessel in which the weighed food is ignited in an atmosphere of oxygen by means of an electric spark. The vessel is surrounded by a measured volume of water. The increase in temperature of the water multiplied by the weight of the water gives the number of calories liberated by the combustion of the food. By such measurements it has been found that, on the average:

1 gm. carbohydrate yields	4.1 kcal.
1 gm. fat yields	9.4 kcal.
1 gm. protein yields	5.6 kcal.

These figures are typical of the caloric equivalents of foods ordinarily present in the diet of man. However, specific members of each class may have values somewhat at variance with these typical or average values. For example, the 4.1 figure is applicable to starch $(C_6H_{10}O_5)_n$, but glucose, $C_6H_{12}O_6$, produces only 3.8 kcal. per gram. Individual fats also vary in their heat equivalents; olive oil yields 9.384 kcal., and butterfat 9.179 kcal., per gram. When the same substances are utilized by the body, it can be shown that carbohydrates and fats have the above caloric values, but proteins give rise to only 4.1 kcal. instead of 5.6. The reason for this is that the proteins are not completely oxidized in the body since urea, to which they give rise, could be oxidized still further in the bomb calorimeter. For practical purposes the following approximate figures are usually employed when dealing with animal calorimetry and nutrition:

1 gm. carbohydrate yields	4 kcal.
1 gm. fat yields	9 kcal.
1 gm. protein yields	4 kcal.

The heat produced by the animal body can similarly be directly measured by placing the animal in a calorimeter. Animal heat can also be estimated indirectly by measuring the amount of oxygen retained by the body and the amount of carbon dioxide excreted and calculating the heat represented by these values. The direct method is far more accurate but entails the construction of complicated and costly apparatus. Therefore it is used in relatively few institutions.

Atwater-Rosa-Benedict calorimeter. Fig. 17-1 is a diagram of the Atwater-Rosa-Benedict calorimeter. In such an apparatus not only is the heat measured, but the oxygen absorption and carbon dioxide output can also be determined. Thus the direct and indirect methods may be employed simultaneously and may be compared with each other. The animal, or man, occupies a chamber that has a double copper wall enclosed in an insulated wall. The heat lost from the body is removed by water flowing through coils of pipe. This is shown in the figure as a single tube with a thermometer, T, at the inlet and another at the outlet. The number of calories lost from the body is calculated from the difference in temperature and the volume of water flowing through the coils. In addition, the heat removed as latent heat of evaporation must be

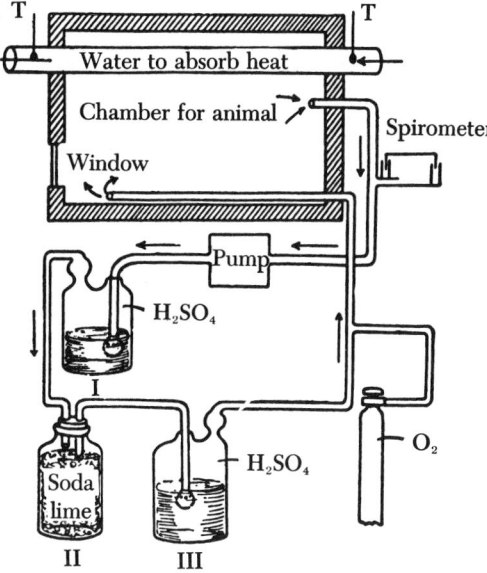

Fig. 17-1. Diagram of Atwater-Rosa-Benedict respiration calorimeter. Heat produced by the body is absorbed by a coil of pipe through which water flows (here shown as a single tube). T and T are thermometers registering the temperature of the inflowing and outflowing H_2O, the volume of which can be measured. This permits the calculation of "sensible heat." The pump blows the air in the direction of the arrows. The spirometer shows contraction of total air volume as the animal uses O_2. A corresponding amount of O_2 is delivered from the weighed O_2 cylinder. The increase in weight of bottle *I* gives the water lost by evaporation, and from this the latent heat of evaporation may be computed. The increase in weight of bottles *II* and *III* gives the CO_2 evolved. (From Bard, P., editor: Medical physiology, St. Louis, 1961, The C. V. Mosby Co.)

computed. This is done by absorbing the moisture from the air leaving the calorimeter and weighing it. Each gram of water vaporized requires 0.580 kcal. at 30° C., the temperature of the skin. Other losses of heat from the calorimeter are prevented by an elaborate system for keeping the inner and outer copper walls at the same temperature so that heat cannot flow in either direction. The air is circulated by a pump in the direction indicated by the arrows in Fig. 17-1. As the subject uses up oxygen from the air, the spirometer indicates the decrease in volume. Oxygen is then added from a weighed cylinder and the difference in weight gives the amount of oxygen used. Bottles of sulfuric acid and soda lime are also weighed at the beginning and end of the experiment. Bottle I absorbs the water vapor, which permits the estimation of the latent heat of evaporation. Bottle II absorbs carbon dioxide but liberates water in the reaction:

$$2\ NaOH + CO_2 \rightarrow Na_2CO_3 + H_2O$$

For that reason, bottle III is used to catch any water that may be lost from bottle II. Therefore the increase in weight of bottles II and III gives the amount of carbon dioxide liberated by the body. The air entering the chamber is freed of carbon dioxide and moisture and its oxygen content is restored. The chamber may have facilities for the subject or animal to do work, such as a bicycle ergometer, for a man, or a treadmill, for an animal, with suitable devices for measuring the work done. Thermometric measurements of the air and body temperature are likewise arranged for, and samples of air can also be obtained for analysis.

Using such an apparatus, Rubner, in about 1894, showed that for a dog the caloric equivalent of the food taken in is equal to the heat output plus the heat equivalent of the urine and feces. The error was within 1%. He also showed that the direct method checks with the indirect method, i.e., the heat production calculated from the gas exchange. Later, Atwater and Benedict brought out the same facts, using men as subjects. For example, the average results obtained for three men tested for 40 days each were as follows:

	Average kilocalories per day
Direct calorimetry	2,723
Indirect calorimetry	2,717
Difference	6 (or 0.2%)

RESPIRATORY QUOTIENT

The respiratory quotient (R.Q.) has an important bearing on many phases of energy metabolism, whether we are dealing with the intact animal or with tissue preparations. It is the ratio of the volume of carbon dioxide produced to the volume of oxygen used.

$$R.Q. = \frac{Vol.\ CO_2}{Vol.\ O_2}$$

For complete combustion of carbohydrates, the R.Q. is 1.0, as seen from the following equation in which glucose is oxidized:

$$C_6H_{12}O_6 + 6\ O_2 \quad \rightarrow \quad 6\ CO_2 + 6\ H_2O$$

From Avogadro's law, we know that a given volume, at constant temperature and pressure, contains the same number of molecules of *any* gas. Therefore, since six molecules of carbon dioxide occupy the same volume as six molecules of oxygen:

$$\text{R.Q. of } C_6H_{12}O_6 = \frac{6\ CO_2}{6\ O_2} = 1.0$$

The equation for the oxidation of a typical fat (triolein) is as follows:

$$C_{57}H_{104}O_6 + 80\ O_2 = 57\ CO_2 + 52\ H_2O$$

$$\text{R.Q. triolein} = \frac{57\ CO_2}{80\ O_2} = 0.71$$

The other fats have slightly different R.Q.'s, but all are about 0.7.

The respiratory quotient of protein is more difficult to determine since the protein molecule is not completely oxidized. Loewy estimated it in the following manner. One hundred grams of meat protein contain:

> 52.38 gm. C
> 7.27 gm. H
> 22.68 gm. O
> 16.65 gm. N
> 1.02 gm. S

After ingestion, all the nitrogen and sulfur and part of the hydrogen, oxygen, and carbon are excreted in the urine and feces. The amounts of carbon, hydrogen, and oxygen not excreted in the urine and feces are as follows:

> 41.50 gm. C
> 4.40 gm. H
> 7.69 gm. O

These, then, are available for oxidative processes. The 7.69 gm. of oxygen are sufficient to oxidize 0.96 gm. of hydrogen, leaving for further oxidation and, thus, for computation of the R.Q.:

> 41.50 gm. C
> 3.44 gm. H

The oxygen necessary for these oxidations would be 138.18 gm. or 96.59 liters (138.18 gm. $\times$ 0.699 liter, since 1 gm. O_2 occupies 0.699 liter of space). The carbon dioxide produced would be 152.17 gm. or 77.41 liters (152.17 gm. $\times$ 0.5087 liter, because each gram of CO_2 occupies 0.5087 liter). The R.Q. of the proteins is, accordingly:

$$\frac{77.41 \text{ liters } CO_2}{96.59 \text{ liters } O_2} = 0.801$$

In general, 0.8 is used for the respiratory quotient of proteins.

If an animal could oxidize exclusively one food at a time, when using carbohydrate, its R.Q. would be 1.0; when burning fat, it would be 0.7; and during protein utilization, it would be about 0.8. Since this is not the case and all three types of food are metabolized simultaneously, the R.Q. is always a resultant of all types of metabolism. On an ordinary mixed diet, the R.Q. is usually found to be about 0.85 for a normal individual. In the postabsorptive state, i.e., some 12 hours after the last meal, the R.Q. is usually slightly lower, about 0.82. However, foods high in any one of the three chief foodstuffs can be found to have a definite influence on the R.Q. Thus, in the normal individual, the feeding of carbohydrate tends to raise the R.Q. above 0.85, and the feeding of fat to lower it.

Since the three types of foodstuffs, with different caloric values, each have different R.Q.'s, the caloric value of 1 liter of oxygen absorbed depends on the particular foodstuff being oxidized. The same is true of the carbon dioxide produced. For example:

$$C_6H_{12}O_6 \quad + \quad 6\ O_2 \quad = \quad 6\ CO_2 \quad + \quad 6\ H_2O$$

180 gm.	192 gm.	264 gm.
	134 liters	134 liters

In other words, 134 liters of oxygen are required to oxidize 180 gm. of glucose or to produce 180×3.8 kcal., since each gram of glucose produces 3.8 kcal. of heat. Therefore, with a R.Q. of 1, a liter of oxygen is equivalent to $\dfrac{180 \times 3.8}{134}$ kcal., or about 5.1 kcal. Similarly, for a fat:

$$C_{57}H_{104}O_6 \quad + \quad 80\ O_2 \quad = \quad 57\ CO_2 \quad + \quad 52\ H_2O$$

884 gm.   1792 liters

In other words, 1792 liters of oxygen are required for 884 gm. of triolein or to produce 884×9 kcal. Therefore, with a R.Q. of 0.7, a liter of oxygen is equivalent to $\dfrac{884 \times 9}{1792} = 4.4$ kcal. If a person has a respiratory quotient of 1.0, not only can we assume that carbohydrate alone is burning, but, if the volume of oxygen consumed in a definite period of time can be ascertained, the amount of carbohydrate burned in that time can also be calculated. If the respiratory quotient is 0.7, the R.Q. of fat, the amount of fat being consumed, can similarly be ascertained. Since the R.Q. for protein is between these two figures, i.e., about 0.8, exclusive protein combustion cannot be assumed, since the simultaneous combustion of carbohydrate and fat and protein would result in an R.Q. of about this value.

As stated before, however, all three foodstuffs usually are consumed at the same time. Nevertheless, calculations that give us the amounts of protein, carbohydrate, and fat being consumed at the same time are possible. The protein catabolized during the experimental period can easily be found by obtaining the urine excreted during this time. The total nitrogen present is, of course, about 16% of the protein catabolized:

$$\frac{\text{Total N}}{0.16} \text{ or Total N} \times 6.25 = \text{Protein}$$

The volumes of carbon dioxide and oxygen represented can be calculated and subtracted from the total carbon dioxide and oxygen. The remainder is

Table 17-1. Analysis of the oxidation of mixtures of carbohydrate and fat*

R.Q.	Percentage of total oxygen consumed by		Percentage of heat produced by		Kilocalories per liter O_2
	Carbohydrate	Fat	Carbohydrate	Fat	
0.707	0	100.0	0	100.0	4.686
0.75	14.7	85.3	15.6	84.4	4.739
0.80	31.7	68.3	33.4	66.6	4.801
0.82	38.6	61.4	40.3	59.7	4.825
0.85	48.8	51.2	50.7	49.3	4.862
0.90	65.9	34.1	67.5	32.5	4.924
0.95	82.9	17.1	84.0	16.0	4.985
1.00	100.0	0	100.0	0	5.047

*From Lusk, G.: J. Biol. Chem. **59**:41, 1924. (Abbreviated.)

the nonprotein carbon dioxide and oxygen, from which the nonprotein R.Q. can be calculated. A nonprotein R.Q. must vary between 0.7 (the R.Q. for 100% fat and no carbohydrate consumption) and 1.0 (the R.Q. for 100% carbohydrate and no fat catabolism). All R.Q. figures between 0.7 and 1.0 indicate that a mixture of the two is being burned. Tables that give the amounts of each of these two constituents being burned (per liter of oxygen) are available for R.Q.'s between 0.7 and 1.0, and they also show the number of calories that 1 liter of oxygen represents in this combustion. Thus, knowing the total nitrogen output, the oxygen consumption, and the carbon dioxide output in a given period, we can estimate the number of grams of protein, carbohydrate, and fat catabolized.

In metabolism experiments it is desirable to calculate the heat production from the oxygen consumption. As has been seen, this would be easy to do rather accurately if only carbohydrate and fat were being utilized. The protein makes it more difficult. However, extreme accuracy is not necessary in the indirect methods of calorimetry employing this calculation. At a respiratory quotient of 0.71, the number of kilocalories produced per liter of oxygen is only about 6% less than that produced at a respiratory quotient of 1.0. These values are shown in Table 17-1. Boyd[1] demonstrated that the error arising from the assumption that the subject is metabolizing only fat and carbohydrates is only a little over 0.5%. For these reasons the caloric value for oxygen consumption is usually based on the R.Q. observed, or, if it is not determined, a standard R.Q. is assumed.

It should be mentioned that the respiratory quotient cannot be considered as the index of a single process. If carbohydrate is being converted to fat, this reaction by itself would result in a respiratory quotient greater than 1.0, because carbon dioxide is produced and no oxygen is used.

$$13\ C_6H_{12}O_6 \rightarrow C_{57}H_{104}O_6 + 21\ CO_2 + 26\ H_2O$$
$$\text{Glucose} \qquad\qquad \text{Triolein}$$

519

On the other hand, if fat were being transformed to carbohydrate, the R.Q. would be very low. For example, from the reaction

$$C_{57}H_{104}O_6 + 32\ O_2 \quad \rightarrow \quad 8\ C_6H_{12}O_6 + 9\ CO_2 + 4\ H_2O$$

Triolein   **Glucose**

we would have an R.Q. of about 0.28. The first of these reactions is accepted by all, and the second is claimed to occur by many authorities. The theoretic R.Q. for the conversion of protein to carbohydrate has been calculated as 0.6 to 0.7. There may be still other reactions that influence this value, including the fixation of carbon dioxide and physiologic and pathologic factors that modify it. Therefore, we can see that the total R.Q. is a figure representing a composite of the respiratory exchanges involved in all metabolic reactions. Nevertheless, since the oxidative processes predominate in the body over the synthetic ones just mentioned, the use of the R.Q. in studying heat production is justified.

It was observed[2] that athletic training results in a slight lowering of the R.Q. The reason for this lowering is not known, but the suggestion has been made that an increased amount of fat is being metabolized as the exercise progresses.

Metabolism of ethyl alcohol. Alcohol in moderate amounts is 90% to 95% utilized. The rate of utilization varies somewhat with the individual but not with the quantity ingested; i.e., the rate of oxidation is fairly constant. From 3.5 to 15 ml. of pure alcohol may be oxidized by the organism per hour. The R.Q. of ethyl alcohol is 0.67 and the caloric value is 7 kcal. per gram. Assuming an average utilization of 10 ml. or 8 gm. per hour, this would amount to 56 kcal. per hour. Thus, an individual could obtain an appreciable proportion of his caloric needs from alcohol alone. Minute amounts of both ethanol and methanol have been found[3] in human tissues and blood.

The oxidation of alcohol occurs mainly in the liver (p. 206). The products of alcohol catabolism are carbon dioxide and water. Since alcohol cannot be stored in the body but can be converted to the energy of heat and work, it spares carbohydrate and fat and thus may increase glycogen and fat deposition. It may even become a protein sparer if the diet is deficient in carbohydrate. It also enters into the formation of cholesterol and, to a lesser degree, fatty acids.[4] The small amount of alcohol that escapes utilization is eliminated mainly through the lungs and kidneys.

BASAL METABOLISM

There are several factors that contribute to the total heat production of the body. The principal ones are derived from the metabolism of the body at rest, the heat produced by work or exercise, and the heat due to specific effects of food. In addition, a low atmospheric temperature stimulates heat production, and sleep depresses it. Emotions, noises, and discomforts usually increase heat production also. The metabolism of the body at rest is called basal metabolism. More exactly, basal metabolism is defined as the heat production of the body when in a state of complete mental and physical rest and in the postabsorptive state.

The basal metabolic rate (B.M.R.) is frequently determined clinically. Since food, exercise, sleep, and external temperature all modify heat production, these factors must be excluded. Therefore, the subject is required to take the test after a 12 hour fast, i.e., in the postabsorptive state. He is made warm and comfortable in a room that is quiet and has subdued lighting. He must be informed about what is to be done so that he will not be alarmed, and in every possible way he must be put in a resting condition. Under such conditions the subject's metabolism is considered basal.

Heat production in the basal state may be determined directly by an Atwater-Rosa-Benedict calorimeter, which is the most accurate procedure. Since ordinarily this is not feasible, indirect methods based on the principles discussed have been devised. By the indirect methods, either the oxygen consumption and carbon dioxide output or only the oxygen consumption are determined. In the former instance the R.Q. can be determined, and this, as has been seen, permits us to get a more exact idea of the calorific value of the oxygen being consumed. If only the oxygen consumption is determined, the R.Q. must be assumed to be the average value usually found. In general, then, the B.M.R. for a given period is obtained by multiplying the volume of oxygen consumed during that period by the calorific value for oxygen corresponding to the observed (or assumed) respiratory quotient.

There are, in general, two systems available for the indirect determination of the B.M.R. These are the open-circuit system, in which both the oxygen consumption and the carbon dioxide output are measured, and the closed-circuit system, in which only the oxygen consumption is determined. Both can be used clinically, but the former requires a high degree of technical skill and more cumbersome apparatus and is less rapid. Since it is the more accurate, we will describe it first.

Open-circuit systems. The Tissot method and the Douglas method are both open-circuit systems. The subject breathes through a valve system, which is so arranged that he inspires pure atmospheric air and his expired air is collected in either a Tissot spirometer or a Douglas bag. The latter is a rubber pouch of 60 to 100 liters capacity. It has the advantage of being portable and thus is also useful in energy experiments involving exercise. The spirometer, on the other hand, is easily calibrated so that the volume of expired air can be accurately observed on the instrument itself. The passage of the air may be accomplished by having the subject breathe through a mouthpiece connected with the apparatus. In this case a clip prevents nose breathing. A more comfortable arrangement is the use of a mask of special design that can be made airtight. The valves used to ensure the passage of air in the right direction must have low resistance so that little extra work is done by the subject in overcoming this resistance. Fig. 17-2 is a diagram showing a Tissot or gasometer apparatus in use. The subject inspires fresh air and expires into the spirometer or gasometer. After a given period of time, the volume of expired air is measured and a sample is analyzed. The composition of inspired air is also determined by analysis. However, the *volume* of inspired air is not measured. It can be calculated from the percentages of nitrogen in both the inspired and the expired air, since nitrogen is an inert gas and the

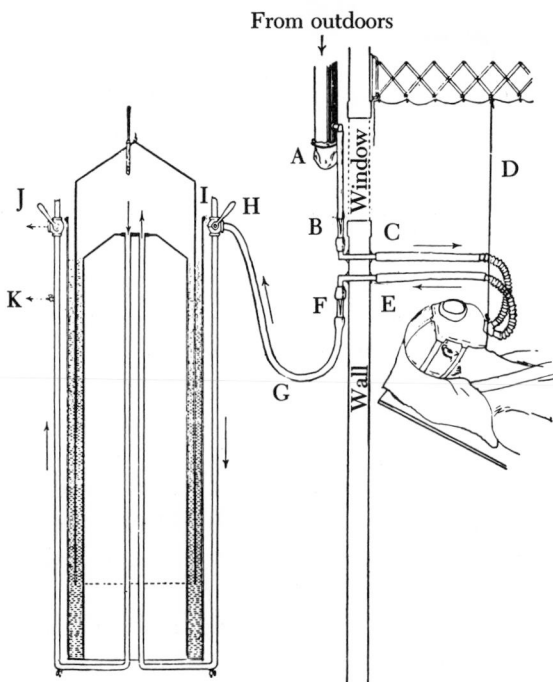

Fig. 17-2. Apparatus for the determination of the basal metabolism by the open circuit method. The subject, lying at rest on a cot and wearing a face mask, is separated by a wall and a window from the spirometer. *C* and *E* are pipes leading from the mask to outside air and spirometer, respectively; *B* and *F* are flutter valves that direct inspiratory air to the mask from outside and expiratory air to the spirometer from the mask. The spirometer consists of a bell arranged to rise freely as the expired air is collected under it. The entire dead space of the apparatus can be flushed out with expired air by allowing it to escape through the valve, *J*. On closing this valve, the expired air is caught in the spirometer bell. *H* is a valve that permits expired air to escape through *I*, a vent. (From Bailey, C. V.: J. Lab. Clin. Med. **6**:657, 1921.)

total volumes of nitrogen inspired and expired must be equal. Thus we can determine the volumes of oxygen utilized and carbon dioxide produced (having given the percentages of these gases in both inspired and expired air), as well as the volume of expired air. Consequently, the R.Q. is readily found. Since each liter of oxygen retained corresponds to a certain number of calories of heat for the respiratory quotient in question, it is a simple matter to calculate the number of calories produced during the experimental period.

Closed-circuit system. In closed-circuit systems, which are the more commonly used clinical procedures, the passage of air may be controlled by either a mouthpiece or a mask, as in the open-circuit systems. However, fresh air is not continually inspired. The system is filled with oxygen, and any diminution in the total volume is due to oxygen consumption because carbon dioxide and water from the lungs are absorbed by soda lime as fast as they are formed. In the closed system, the respired gas is breathed over and over again. The Benedict-Roth apparatus is shown in diagrammatic form in Fig. 17-3.

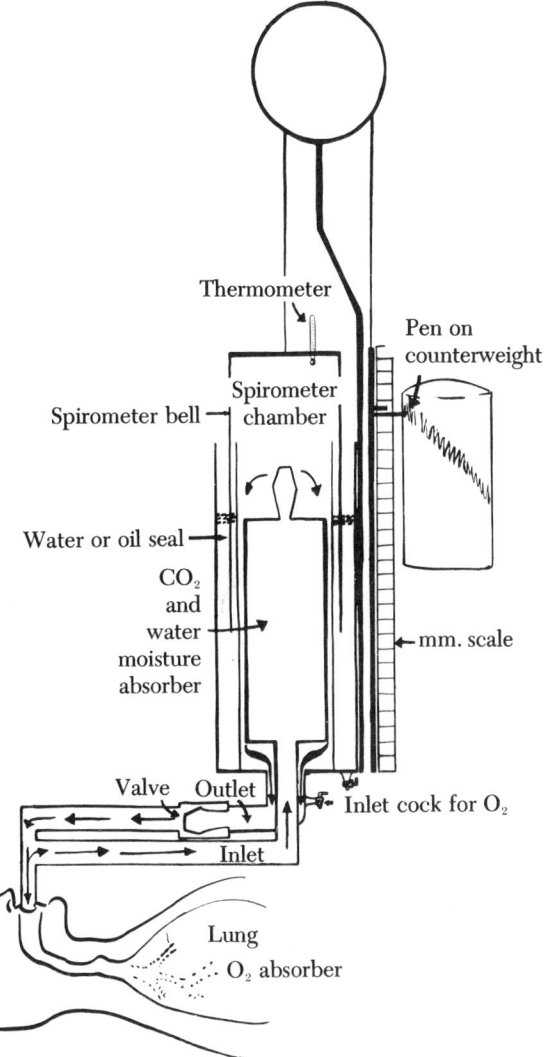

Fig. 17-3. Diagram of Benedict-Roth apparatus for the determination of basal metabolism. The patient breathes through a mouthpiece that fits between the gums and the lips; the nose is clamped. Two tubes connect the mouthpiece with the spirometer, and appropriate valves permit the air to flow only in the direction indicated. The expired air passes through soda lime, which absorbs CO_2 and H_2O. The calibrated spirometer bell is balanced by a counterweight carrying a pen that writes the record on a millimeter scale. The spirometer chamber is filled with O_2 when the test starts. As O_2 is absorbed by the subject, the volume of the gas in the chamber decreases and this decrease in volume is used as a basis for calculations. (Modified from Roth, P.: Boston Med. Surg. J. **186**:491, 1922.)

There is one respiration valve in the inspiration tube and a second one at the outlet of the carbon dioxide and water absorbed. These direct the air in the right path. There is a spirometer bell suspended by a cord that passes over a pulley and is balanced by a counterweight. With each respiration, the spirometer rises and falls and a pointer on the counterweight writes on a kymograph a record of this movement. Before the test is started, the spirometer is emptied of gas and is filled with oxygen. As the subject breathes, he retains some of this oxygen and expires a mixture of carbon dioxide, water, oxygen, and nitrogen. The carbon dioxide and water are absorbed by the soda lime, and the spirometer gradually falls as the oxygen is used up. The slope of the curve is used to measure the oxygen consumption in a 6-minute period.

Since the carbon dioxide is not measured in this method, a R.Q. of 0.82 is assumed. This gives a heat value for each liter of oxygen consumed as 4.825 kcal. (see Table 17-1). The spirometer bell is designed to have a volume of 20.73 ml. for every millimeter of height. Therefore each millimeter that the spirometer falls in 6 minutes is equivalent to $\frac{20.73}{1000}$ liter $\times$ 4.825 kcal., or 0.1 kcal. in 6 minutes, or 1 kcal. per hour. The kymograph paper is ruled in millimeters so that the heat production can be directly obtained by observation. Furthermore, timing is rendered unnecessary by having vertical lines spaced at intervals, each equivalent to 1 minute. Fig. 17-4 shows an oxygen line drawn in relation to the *calorie* and *time* lines. Corrections for temperature and barometric pressure must, of course, be made, but these and all calculations are explained on the back of the tracing paper.

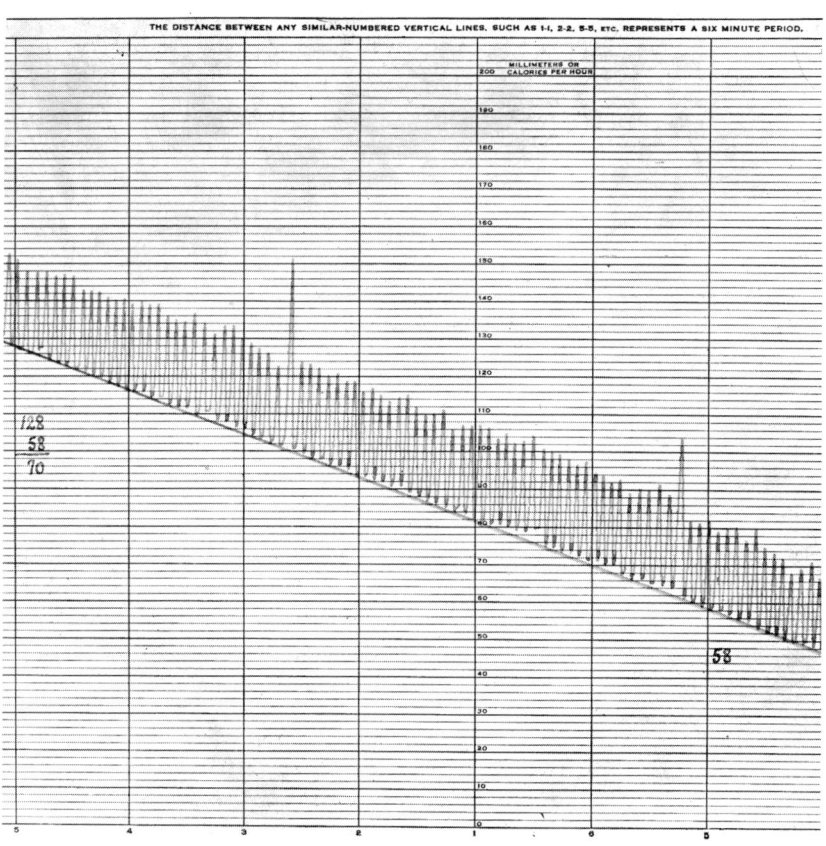

Fig. 17-4. Typical O_2 line in a basal metabolism test using a Benedict-Roth apparatus. (Courtesy Warren E. Collins, Inc., Boston, Mass.)

Calculating basal metabolic rate. Let it be assumed that the oxygen line, a straight line drawn through a majority of the lower peaks of the curves, intersects a vertical *minute* line at 58 mm. Another intersection six spaces from the first one is, perhaps, at 128 mm. (see Fig. 17-4). The oxygen consumption, then, in 6 minutes is represented by:

$$\begin{array}{r} 128 \\ -\ 58 \\ \hline 70 \ \text{mm.} \end{array}$$

Since each millimeter for 6 minutes is equivalent to 1 kcal. per hour, the heat output is 70 kcal. per hour. This must now be corrected for temperature and pressure. Assuming 20° C. and 750 mm., we find from a table (on the back of the tracing paper) the corresponding factor 0.902.

$$70 \times 0.902 = 63.1 \ \text{kcal. per hour}$$

The corrected figure is 63.1 kcal. per hour.

This must now be related to the normal values. If the subject is a woman, 50 years of age, 5 feet 4 inches tall, and weighing 108 lb., it may be found from Table 17-3 that her output should be 33.9 kcal. per square meter surface area per hour. From the nomogram (Fig. 17-5), a line

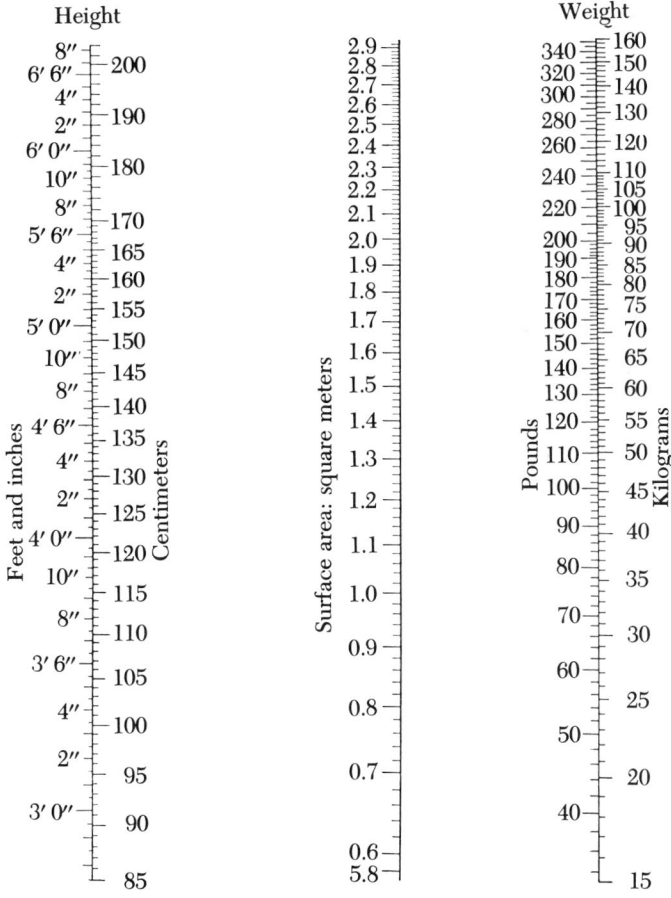

Fig. 17-5. Nomogram for estimating surface area from weight and height, according to DuBois' formula. A straight line drawn from a point corresponding to the height of the individual, on the left-hand scale, to that of his weight, on the right-hand scale, crosses the middle line at a point indicating his surface area. (Courtesy W. M. Boothby.)

drawn between the points indicating her height and weight crosses the middle line at 1.50 square meters of surface area. Therefore, the normal B.M.R. would be

$$33.9 \text{ kcal. per square meter} \times 1.5 \text{ square meters} = 50.9 \text{ kcal.}$$

This is now subtracted from the (corrected) figure found:

$$63.1 - 50.9 = 12.2 \text{ kcal. per hour above normal}$$

This excess is divided by the normal; i.e., $12.2/51.0 = +24\%$. In other words, in this instance the B.M.R. is 24% above the normal for a woman of the age, height, and weight given.

Normal influences From the data obtained by any of the methods outlined, the basal metabolic rate, i.e., the caloric output at rest, is determined. There are several factors that normally influence this. Consequently, in order to ascertain whether the B.M.R determined is normal or not, we must compare the reading in question with normal standards. (All these factors have been taken into consideration in the calculations of the hypothetic test described.)

Influence of size. It is of course true that the greater the size of an animal the greater will be the total heat production. However, the amount of heat produced is not proportional to the body *weight*. In 1901, Voit showed that heat production bears a much closer relationship to *surface area* than to weight; and, shortly after, Rubner proposed the law that the total metabolism is proportional to the superficial area of an animal. This is clearly evident from Table 17-2. Rubner's law holds true not only for different species but also for individuals of the same species of different sizes. Thus a small man has a greater heat output than a large man per pound, but when calculated to their surface areas, the heat output is about the same. For this reason either the B.M.R. is expressed as kilocalories per square meter of surface area or the total number of kilocalories produced is compared with the total calories that would be produced by a normal individual having the same surface area.

The surface area of a man is difficult to estimate accurately. Many measurements have been made, and a fairly constant relationship between body weight and height has been established. This is expressed by the formula of DuBois:

Surface area (in sq. cm.) = Weight (in kg.)$^{0.425}$ × Height (in cm.)$^{0.725}$ × 71.84

A graphic method of obtaining the same result is by the use of a nomogram, shown in Fig. 17-5.

It is now believed that, although there is a considerable correlation, the metabolic rate and the body surface are not quite as closely related as is indicated by Rubner's law. The figures found today for total daily heat production per square meter of body surface do not quite agree with those found by Rubner (Table 17-2), and authorities in this field suggest a power function of body weight as a standard instead of the surface area. Thus Brody adopts $W^{0.7}$ as the reference base, W representing body weight in kilograms. Kleiber[5] maintains that $W^{3/4}$ is more accurate. Because surface area for all animals is approximately equivalent to $W^{2/3}$, which is a value not far from those just given, the clinical measurements based on the DuBois formula or nomogram have been found to be sufficiently accurate for clinical purposes.

Table 17-2. Relation of heat production to body weight and surface area*

| | Weight in kilograms | Kilocalories in 24 hours | |
		Per kilogram of body weight	Per square meter of body surface
Pig	128	19	1,078
Man	64	32	1,042
Dog	15	52	1,039
Mouse	0.018	212	1,188

*From Rubner, M.: Die Gesetze des Energieverbrauchs bei der Ernährung, Leipzig, 1902, F. Deuticke, p. 282.

Influence of age and sex. At birth the basal metabolic rate is said to be very low, but after the infant begins to gain weight the B.M.R. increases rapidly, and it is very high for the first 3 to 6 years. Thereafter, heat production diminishes with increasing age, and the decrease is very gradual indeed during adult life. These facts have been obtained by thousands of measurements by the indirect method. As a result, we have data that show approximately the normal B.M.R. for any age and for either sex. Females have from 2% to 12% lower rates than males; adults from 10% to 12% lower than children. The relationships of sex and age are shown in Table 17-3. These normal standards are occasionally revised as more determinations under carefully controlled conditions are obtained.

Table 17-3. Newer standards of basal metabolism — kilocalories per square meter per hour*

Age (Years)	Males	Females	Age (Years)	Males	Females
1	53.0	53.0	17	40.8	36.3
2	52.4	52.4	18	40.0	35.9
3	51.3	51.2	19	39.2	35.5
4	50.3	49.8	20	38.6	35.3
5	49.3	48.4	25	37.5	35.2
6	48.3	47.0	30	36.8	35.1
7	47.3	45.4	35	36.5	35.0
8	46.3	43.8	40	36.3	34.9
9	45.2	42.8	45	36.2	34.5
10	44.0	42.5	50	35.8	33.9
11	43.0	42.0	55	35.4	33.3
12	42.5	41.3	60	34.9	32.7
13	42.3	40.3	65	34.4	32.2
14	42.1	39.2	70	33.8	31.7
15	41.8	37.9	75	33.2	31.3
16	41.4	36.9	80	33.0	30.9

*From Fleisch, A.: Helvet. Med. Acta **18**:23, 1951.

Other physiologic factors. The data mentioned were obtained in the United States on individuals of the various races that make up our population. However, there may be some variation in different parts of the world. Natives of Yucatan were found to have generally higher metabolic rates than Americans, whereas some Chinese women living in America had lower rates. White individuals usually show a decreased metabolism when they live in tropical countries. However, probably these racial and climatic difference are explained on other grounds. For example, Eskimos have been found to show significantly higher B.M.R. values than whites; but Rodahl[6] showed that this was due partly to apprehension of the subjects and partly to the Eskimo diet, which is a high-protein–high-fat diet with high specific dynamic action. When these two factors were eliminated, the metabolism was almost exactly the same as that of white controls.

The metabolism of women fluctuates much more than that of men. Before menstruation the rate usually rises and after menstruation it falls. These facts must be taken into consideration when studying the results of tests. It has also been shown that, although ordinarily the B.M.R. of women is from 2% to 12% below that of men, in a very warm environment it may be from 15% to 20% below that of men and in a cold climate it may be the same.

Normal pregnancy has little influence on the basal metabolic rate, although, of course, the total amount of heat produced is the sum of that produced by the mother and the fetus. Athletes and laborers usually have a somewhat higher rate than other people because of a greater degree of muscular development.

The determination of the basal metabolic rate in persons who are ill is best made in the same building where they spend the night. The excitement and disturbance of even a short ride is sufficient to increase the B.M.R. by as much as 50%. On the other hand, an ambulant patient may travel for an hour or more, rest for half an hour, and be in a basal condition. The novelty of the experience may, however, be a disturbing factor. Unless the operator understands how to reassure the patient, a first B.M.R. test is likely to be from 5% to 10% too high.

Pathologic influences The most important practical use for basal metabolic rate determinations is in the diagnosis and treatment of thyroid conditions. The hormone elaborated and secreted by the thyroid has the property of stimulating the metabolic activities of the cells. A hypersecretion, therefore, causes an increased B.M.R. A hyposecretion, on the other hand, results in a lowered B.M.R. Determinations of the B.M.R. prove extremely valuable before thyroid operations for hyperthyroidism, before administration of the hormone for hypothyroidism, and in following the effects of operations or treatment. Too much emphasis cannot be laid upon the necessity for careful technical work in performing these tests.

Fevers raise the B.M.R., increasing it by about 5% for each degree Fahrenheit above the normal body temperature. The reason for this is evident, since an increased body temperature is primarily due to increased cellular activity. It is therefore imperative when doing "basals" to take the temperature of the patient. If he has a subnormal temperature, he should be given additional covers, hot pads, etc. to bring his temperature to normal.

Because the adrenal gland secretes a hormone, epinephrine, that also increases cellular activity, affections of this gland may also change the B.M.R. Epinephrine's action, however, is ordinarily fleeting; nonetheless, it may account for the temporarily high rates that sometimes are encountered in nervous patients. This effect of epinephrine is also one of the reasons for requiring mental as well as physical repose when determining the B.M.R.: the emotional excitement causes increased secretion of epinephrine. In Addison's disease, a condition in which the adrenal cortex is damaged, the B.M.R. is low. This is probably not due to a lack of epinephrine, which is produced in the adrenal medulla, but to a deficiency of ACTH.

In the vast majority of cases, the B.M.R. is within normal limits, which are generally assumed to be from 10% above to 10% below the normal standard for the age, sex, and surface area of the individual studied. The pathologic variations mentioned may be from 40% below to 130% above the average normal. In addition to thyroid disorders, fevers, and Addison's disease, there are a few other pathologic conditions in which the basal metabolic rate may be altered. A more complete list is as follows, but it must be remembered that the effect on the B.M.R., except in the instances previously noted, is not invariable.

Basal metabolic rate below normal
Hypothyroidism
Addison's disease and other types of hypoadrenalism
Starvation and malnutrition
Hypopituitarism
Lipoid nephrosis
Shock
Vitamin D deficiency

Basal metabolic rate above normal
Hyperthyroidism
Cushing's syndrome (basophilic adenoma of pituitary)
Tumors of adrenal gland
Fever
Leukemia
Polycythemia
Anemia
Essential hypertension
Myocardial insufficiency
Diabetes insipidus

Effect of thiouracil on basal metabolic rate. The specific action of thiouracil and related compounds on the thyroid gland has been discussed in Chapter 16. It may be pointed out here, however, that this action results in a reduction of the B.M.R. Hence, any pathologic effect with a high B.M.R. may be treated by using this drug, provided the underlying cause is a hyperthyroidism. The opposite effect, i.e., an increase in the B.M.R., is produced by the administration of thyroxine or related substances (p. 477). An increase may also be accomplished by other drugs, notably dinitrophenol.

Instead of determining the basal metabolic rate, many clinicians now use the level of protein-bound iodine (PBI) in blood serum as an index of thyroid activity; or they use the determination of radioactive protein-bound iodine after the administration of tracer doses of [131]I (p. 428). However, such tests measure only thyroid secretion. Nevertheless, since fluctuations in the B.M.R. are usually due to thyroid derangement, this is ordinarily satisfactory. Normally the values for PBI are not altered appreciably by sex, and only in men by age.

Obesity. The deposition of excess fat in the body has led to many fallacious ideas on the subject. We frequently hear that a certain stout person eats very little, that it is his "nature" to be fat, that he has an endocrine condition, etc. There is no way of avoiding the fact that the law of conservation of matter and energy holds for the fat person as well as for the thin person discussed earlier (p. 526). If intake of food exceeds output of the equivalent amount of heat and energy, then the excess must be stored.[7] The storage forms are fat, glycogen, and, to a minor degree, protein. The only exceptions are those conditions in which food is not digested or absorbed properly. Such a state of affairs may account for the lack of adiposity that some heavy eaters exhibit. If food is normally digested and absorbed, however, and the calories ingested equal the total calories expended, there will be no appreciable change in weight. Why, then, is there a tendency to "put on weight" with increasing age? The answer is that the B.M.R. decreases as one gets older. Less food is needed, but the food habit or appetite remains. There is also the tendency to exercise less. Hence, less of the food intake is utilized and it is therefore stored chiefly as fat.

Another puzzling fact is the inability to lose weight frequently experienced by obese individuals when they go on a reducing diet. This was explained by Newburgh,[9] in careful water-balance experiments. Obese patients on a reducing diet frequently do not lose weight for as long as 2 weeks. Sometimes they even gain weight. This is due to a retention of water by the tissues. After a time, however, the water is eliminated and the weight drops. Fig. 17-6 is a typical graph.

Several endocrine conditions, other than those already mentioned, are commonly believed to be associated with a pathologic state of obesity. This may mean that the appetite is increased or water retention is enhanced, since there are very few cases of abnormally low B.M.R. among them. Indeed an abnormally low metabolism is as common among thin as among fat people. However, abnormalities of the endocrine system do affect the *distribution* of adipose tissue, and the conformation of the figure can thus aid in diagnosing the type of endocrine dysfunction.[10]

Obesity sometimes results when injury to the hypothalamus is suffered. Here, again, there is no specific mechanism involved that stimulates the laying down of adipose tissue. The hypothalamus has important regulatory functions, e.g., temperature control, water balance, appetite, gastrointestinal function, sleep. Thus damage to the paraventricular hypothalamic nuclei has resulted in voracious appetite, which began abruptly after the injury; therefore the obesity that followed was due simply to overeating.

Some authorities maintain that there may be genetic factors involved in some cases of obesity. A recent report[11] is interesting in this connection. The

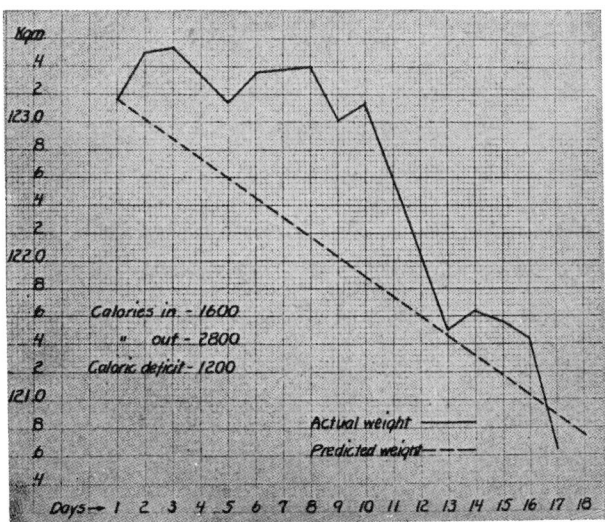

Fig. 17-6. Weight chart of an obese patient on a reducing diet. The increases in weight and failure to follow the predicted weight line are ascribed to addition and retention of water by the tissues. (From Newburgh, L. H.: Physiol. Rev. **24**:18, 1944.)

citrate-cleavage enzyme activities (p. 266) in livers of nonobese and obese litter-mate mice were compared. The specific activity of the enzyme was 3.3 *times* greater in the livers of the obese mice than in those of the nonobese. The investigators believed that an excessive amount of citrate from an intra-mitochondrial source is transferred across the mitochondrial membrane into the cell cytoplasm, where it is broken down at an increased rate by the citrate-cleavage enzyme to acetyl-CoA, which is then synthesized into fatty acids (p. 310) at an increased rate. Further studies of this type should aid in clarifying the importance of any genetic (enzymatic) factors in the etiology of obesity.

Specific If a person's basal metabolic rate is known, we would expect that the in-
dynamic gestion of an amount of food corresponding to this value would result in the
action of production of this same quantity of heat, provided the subject remained at
foods rest. The fact is that a greater amount of heat is produced than is represented by the calories ingested. For example, if the basal metabolic output is 1800 kcal. in 24 hours, or 900 kcal. in 12 hours, the ingestion of food equivalent to 900 kcal. will result in an output during the next 12 to 18 hours of perhaps 950 kcal. To furnish this extra energy, food stores of the body must be drawn upon. This is called the specific dynamic action (S.D.A.) of foods.

Protein has the greatest specific dynamic action, amounting to about 30% above its caloric value; carbohydrate causes an increase of about 5% or 6%; and fat, about 4%. Ordinarily the S.D.A. of all together amounts to about 6% of the B.M.R. The experiments of Forbes and associates[12] emphasized the fact that the S.D.A. of any combination of foodstuffs is not the sum of the individual values of the foodstuffs but is invariably less. Furthermore, when such mixtures are fed, protein does not dominate the S.D.A. as was formerly believed. Fat seems to be more potent than either of the other two nutrients

531

and apparently confers economy of utilization upon the food mixtures in which it occurs; i.e., it lowers the S.D.A. to a greater extent than does either of the others.

The explanation for specific dynamic action is not clear. It cannot be due to a production of heat as a result of digestion, because the feeding of the products of digestion is just as effective as the undigested substances. In fact, the intravenous injection of the amino acids gives rise to a S.D.A. of the same order as results from feeding. Several studies indicate that the S.D.A. of the various amino acids is best correlated with the metabolizable energy of the individual amino acid; i.e., it is not related to the nitrogen but rather to the nonnitrogenous fraction. This fraction undergoes oxidative and synthetic changes that liberate heat. In other words, heat is evolved during the intermediary metabolism of the carbon chains. The S.D.A. of glucose is increased if thiamine is administered at the same time. Since thiamine stimulates the formation of fat from glucose, the S.D.A. of glucose has been suggested as being due to the energy required to prepare it for deposition of fat. Possibly this is the explanation for the S.D.A. of all foodstuffs, i.e., the energy required to prepare the nonnitrogenous parts of the molecule for storage.

Isodynamic law. Rubner formulated a law to the effect that the different foodstuffs may replace each other in the diet for energy as well as for heat production in proportion to their calorific value; i.e., a certain number of calories in a given food are equivalent to the same number of calories in any other food, regardless of the proportion of protein, carbohydrate, and fat. Although this is true in a general way, it must not be forgotten that proteins are in a class by themselves and must be provided in every diet in a suitable amount and of the proper quality. We cannot therefore substitute carbohydrate and fat for protein, even though the total caloric value of the substitutes is the amount needed; nor would it be wise to make up a diet of protein and either carbohydrate or fat. Unusually large amounts of carbohydrate might lead to alimentary glycosuria, whereas an overabundance of fat in the diet might cause ketosis. A mixture of the three is more physiologic. Carbohydrate is a better protein sparer[13,14] than fat and is usually the least expensive of the foodstuffs. It has been found that when the percentage of fat in a diet is varied, while maintaining equal quantities of energy and protein, the animal exhibits certain differences in nutritional behavior. For instance, with a higher fat diet there is better economy of food utilization and increased activity.[15] However, the concept of isodynamic equivalent is a useful one from a dietetic standpoint. *One hundred–calorie portions* are commonly given in food tables or demonstrations and aid materially in computing diets.

INFLUENCE OF MUSCULAR WORK ON TOTAL METABOLISM

Muscular work is accomplished by the body at the expense of increased metabolism. The potential energy of the foodstuff is transformed to the free energy of work and the energy of heat. The latter, as has been seen, is greater than the former; and although the body is a good machine, as machines go, it is still not perfect. Therefore, in order to be able to do work or exercise, the organism must have potential energy for the work and for the excess heat that is simultaneously liberated. A man sitting quietly has a total metabolism, on the average, of about 100 kcal. per hour. When he stands up, his metabolism increases by about 10% because of the greater tonus of the muscles, and if he engages in active work, it may increase to 300 kcal. or more per hour. The type of work or exercise influences the total amount of energy output, heavy work requiring more energy than light. From Tables 17-4 and 17-5, you can see how various types of activity affect the total energy expenditure. Table 17-6 shows similar figures but in a different way; here the extra Calories, i.e., the amount *above* the basal rate, are shown, whereas in Tables 17-4 and 17-5 the figures are for the total caloric output. It is thus easy to understand

Table 17-4. Energy expenditure per hour under different conditions of muscular activity*

	Kilocalories per hour		
Form of activity	Per 70 kg.	Per kilogram	Per pound
Sleeping	65	0.93	0.43
Awake lying still	77	1.10	0.50
Sitting at rest	100	1.43	0.65
Reading aloud	105	1.50	0.69
Standing relaxed	105	1.50	0.69
Hand sewing	111	1.59	0.72
Standing at attention	115	1.63	0.74
Knitting (23 stitches per minute on sweater)	116	1.66	0.75
Dressing and undressing	118	1.69	0.77
Singing	122	1.74	0.79
Tailoring	135	1.93	0.88
Typewriting rapidly	140	2.00	0.91
Ironing (with five-pound iron)	144	2.06	0.93
Dishwashing (plates, bowls, cups, and saucers)	144	2.06	0.93
Sweeping bare floor (38 strokes per minute)	169	2.41	1.09
Bookbinding	170	2.43	1.10
"Light exercise"	170	2.43	1.10
Shoemaking	180	2.57	1.17
Walking slowly (2.6 miles per hour)	200	2.86	1.30
Carpentry, metalworking, industrial painting	240	3.43	1.56
"Active exercise"	290	4.14	1.88
Walking moderately fast (3.75 miles per hour)	300	4.28	1.95
Walking down stairs	364	5.20	2.36
Stoneworking	400	5.71	2.60
"Severe exercise"	450	6.43	2.92
Sawing wood	480	6.86	3.12
Swimming	500	7.14	3.25
Running (5.3 miles per hour)	570	8.14	3.70
"Very severe exercise"	600	8.57	3.90
Walking very fast (5.3 miles per hour)	650	9.28	4.22
Walking up stairs	1100	15.8	7.18

*Compiled by Rose, M. S.; from Sherman, H. C.: Chemistry of food and nutrition, ed. 6, New York, 1941, The Macmillan Co.

Table 17-5. Total caloric requirements for 24 hours*

Men	Kilocalories	Women	Kilocalories
Shoemaker	2,000–2,400	Seamstress (needle)	1,800
Carpenter or mason	2,700–3,200	Seamstress (machine)	1,900–2,100
Farmer	3,200–4,000	Household servant	2,300–2,900
Lumberman	5,000 or more	Laundress	2,600–3,400

* Data from Tigerstedt and from Lusk.

Table 17-6. Extra calories of metabolism attributable to occupation*

Occupations	Extra kilocalories per hour
Men	
Tailor	44
Bookbinder	81
Shoemaker	90
Metalworker, filing and hammering	141
Carpenter, making table	164
Stonemason, chiseling stone	300
Man, sawing wood	378
Women	
Seamstress, needlework	6
Typist, 50 words per minute	24
Seamstress, using sewing machine	57
Housemaid, moderate work	81
Laundress, moderate work	124
Housemaid, hard work	157
Laundress, hard work	214

* After Harrop.

why different types of workers liberate varying amounts of energy and therefore require different amounts of calories in their diets.

INFLUENCE OF MENTAL WORK ON TOTAL METABOLISM

Mental work results in very little increase in total metabolism. Benedict found, for instance, that the effort involved in solving mathematic problems increases metabolism by only 3% or 4%. This does not mean that the metabolism of the brain is low. In fact, just the opposite is the case. Brain tissue has a high *basal* metabolism, amounting to about one tenth of that for the entire body, but the additional work it performs in thinking does not result in much of an increase over this high basal figure.

INFLUENCE OF SLEEP

During normal sleep the muscles are relaxed and the total metabolism is correspondingly low. It is usually 10% below the B.M.R. In fact, if the metabolic rate could be determined routinely during sleep, this would be the true B.M.R. since it is the minimal physiologic rate. Since this is usually not possible, the conditions previously outlined are always advised.

TOTAL HEAT PRODUCTION

All the factors that go to make up the total heat production of an individual may now be listed. From such calculations, figures like those in Table 17-5 have been obtained. Take, for instance, the figures for a carpenter. From a determination of the B.M.R., we get, perhaps, 1500 kcal. Then, from Table 17-6, it may be seen that he expends 164 kcal. per hour while working 8 hours, and it may be assumed that he expends 74 kcal. per hour (20% above basal) during the remaining 8 hours. During sleep there is a diminished heat production, and the specific dynamic action adds about 6% of the B.M.R.

Basal metabolism – 24 hours	1,500 kcal.
8 hours' sleep	−50 kcal. for sleep (10% of basal for eight hours)
8 hours' work (extra calories)	1,312 kcal. (8 × 164)
8 hours' sedentary or light exercise	592 kcal. (8 × 74)
Specific dynamic factor	90 kcal. (1,500 × 0.06)
Total	3,444 kcal.

Using the data in Table 17-4, also for a man engaged in carpentry, we get:

8 hours' sleep at 65 kcal.	520 kcal.
2 hours' light exercise at 170 kcal.	340 kcal.
8 hours' carpenter work at 240 kcal.	1,920 kcal.
6 hours' sitting at rest at 100 kcal.	600 kcal.
Specific dynamic action	90 kcal.
Total	3,470 kcal.

The two hypothetic carpenters, therefore, have about the same total caloric output. In the first case, we began with a basal output and added and subtracted the additional energy factors. In the second, the total caloric output per hour was tabulated plus the specific dynamic action.

METABOLISM OF CHILDREN

The total metabolism in childhood is relatively much greater than in adult life. There is, in the first place, the high B.M.R. of childhood. In addition, the physical activity of children is usually greater, despite the fact that their period of sleep is longer than that of the adult. Their games and play involve a tremendous amount of muscular exercise. The food intake, therefore, must cover these caloric needs in addition to the extra food required for growth. A child of 12 years consequently needs about the same amount of food as an adult, whereas an active boy of 16 years requires 3800 kcal. or more per day.

PRACTICAL CONSIDERATIONS

Having in mind the various factors mentioned, we should be able to calculate roughly the number of calories required by a given individual. The B.M.R. for normal persons can be estimated from Table 17-3 if the subject's

Table 17-7. Total caloric requirements

	Male		Female	
Age in years	Weight (pounds)	Kilocalories per day	Weight (pounds)	Kilocalories per day
Adults				
18–35	154	2,800	128	2,000†
35–55	154	2,600	128	1,850†
55–75	154	2,400	128	1,700
Children				
0– 1	18	kg. × 120–100	–	kg. × 120–100
1– 3	27	1,100–1,250	–	1,100–1,250
3– 6	40	1,400–1,600	–	1,400–1,600
6– 9	53	2,000–2,200	–	2,000–2,200
9–12	72	2,200–2,500	72	2,200–2,250
12–15	98	2,500–2,800	103	2,250–2,300
15–18	134	2,800–3,000	117	2,300–2,400

*Calorie allowances for infants are gradually reduced from 120 kcal./kg. at birth to 100 kcal./kg. by the end of the first year.
†Plus 200 during pregnancy (second and third trimesters); plus 1000 during lactation.

height and weight are known. Although the normal person's B.M.R. may be up to 10% above or below this standard normal value and although the B.M.R. for a given individual is not constant from day to day, we can get a rough idea of that factor. According to DuBois and Chambers,[16] 10% may be added to the B.M.R. to estimate the caloric requirement of a person quiet in bed, 30% for a moderately active patient, and 50% for a patient out of bed but indoors and moderately quiet. For activities of normal subjects, Tables 17-4, 17-5, and 17-6 may be used as mentioned previously.

The Food and Nutrition Board of the National Research Council has made revisions in its 1968 recommendations, which are summarized in Table 17-7. The values given for adults are for individuals in good health and moderately active physically. In the 1968 revision cited, it is stated that although physical activity is a major variable affecting energy requirements no simple procedure is available for estimating the extent of the adjustment required. The best rule of thumb appears to be, "The proper calorie allowance for an individual is that on which he maintains body weight and health at a level most conducive to his well-being." Some authorities regard an individual's weight at 25 years of age as being his ideal lifelong body weight.

In normal people, appetite generally regulates the intake of food so as to provide enough for caloric needs, replacement, growth, etc. However, in disease and obesity the appetite is a poor guide indeed, and the physician and nutritionist must have in mind the basic principles indicated in this chapter so as to approximate the requirements of the individual.

References

GENERAL

Brody, S.: Bioenergetics and growth, New York, 1945, Reinhold Publishing Corp.

Kleiber, M.: Energy metabolism, Ann. Rev. Physiol. **18**:35, 1956.

Lusk, G.: The elements of the science of nutrition, ed. 4, Philadelphia, 1928, W. B. Saunders Co.

Swift, R. W., and French, C. E.: Energy metabolism and nutrition, Washington, D.C., 1953, The Scarecrow Press.

SPECIAL

1. Boyd, W. C.: J. Appl. Physiol. **6**:711, 1954.
2. Nutr. Rev. **21**:127, 1963.
3. Nutr. Rev. **21**:326, 1963.
4. Nutr. Rev. **22**:15, 1964.
5. Kleiber, M.: Physiol. Rev. **27**:511, 1947.
6. Rodahl, K.: J. Nutr. **48**:359, 1952.
7. Schachter, S.: Science **161**:751, 1968.
8. Review: Dairy Council Dig. **39**:1, 1966.
9. Newburgh, L. H.: Physiol. Rev. **24**:18, 1944.
10. Conn, J. W.: Physiol. Rev. **24**:31, 1944.
11. Kornacker, M. S., and Lowenstein, J. M.: Science **144**:1027, 1964.
12. Forbes, E. B., et al.: J. Nutr. **31**:203, 1946.
13. Braucher, P. F.: University of Maryland Agricultural Experiment Station, Bull. A, 120, 1962.
14. Munro, H. N., and Wikramanayake, T. W.: J. Nutr. **52**:99, 1954.
15. Forbes, E. B., and Swift, R. W.: J. Nutr. **27**:453, 1944; Black, A., et al.: J. Nutr. **37**:275, 1949.
16. DuBois, E. F., and Chambers, W. H.: J.A.M.A. **119**:1183, 1942.

BIOCHEMISTRY OF SPECIALIZED TISSUES AND BODY FLUIDS

CHAPTER 18

BIOCHEMISTRY OF SPECIALIZED TISSUES

By definition, tissues are an aggregation of similarly specialized cells united in the performance of a particular function. Thus the cells of nervous tissue are specialized for the transmission of the electric nerve impulse, muscle cells for contraction and the performance of mechanical work, etc. The cells of tissues have the general properties of typical cells as discussed in Chapter 2. However, modified or additional properties adapt them chemically for the performance of their particular tasks. In this chapter we will consider the biochemical adaptations of tissue cells that enable them to carry out their specialized function.

Epidermal tissues The epidermis consists of several layers. The lowest layer is the most active physiologically and contains the most water; it is the *stratum germinativum*. As the cells lose water and are displaced by new ones, they are moved toward the surface. They are pushed into the next layer, the *stratum granulosum*, which is made up of cells containing granules that are deeply stainable by basic dyes. These granules are composed of an albuminoid called keratohyaline, which is believed to be the precursor of eleidin, a semifluid substance occurring in the next highest layer, the *stratum lucidum*. The cells composing the stratum lucidum are shiny and refractile and do not stain with basic dyes. Evidently some marked chemical change occurs in the transition of keratohyaline to eleidin. Another change occurs when eleidin is transformed into keratin, the characteristic constituent of the uppermost layer, the *stratum corneum*. This layer is not as refractile as the lower one; the cells are tightly packed, and the nuclei are gone.

Keratin, from the Greek word for "horn," is a specialized protein first evolved in lower vertebrates to form a tough, insoluble outer coat that served to prevent the loss of body fluids. It retains this function in higher animals; and in modified forms, e.g., in hair, feathers, horns, claws, nails, quills, hoofs, beaks, scale, and the outer layer of skin, the keratins have added functions including protection and defense.

Mammalian (α) keratin is an albuminoid of great insolubility in all neutral solvents, making it an ideal protective covering for the body. The keratins are soluble in strong acids on the application of heat and in strong alkali.

They are also dissolved by alkali sulfides and alkali earths. Undoubtedly solubility in such strong reagents is due to the breaking of disulfide bonds, which form intermolecular bridges cross-linking the polypeptide chains that make up the keratins. As long as these disulfide bridges are intact, the keratins are insoluble and resistant to enzyme cleavage.

Treatment of α-keratins with oxidizing or reducing agents also renders them soluble and cleaves them into two different types of proteins. The major fraction is a low-sulfur, fibrous type of protein. The high-sulfur fraction is a globular protein. The low-sulfur protein can be split by the enzyme *pronase*, a proteolytic enzyme from *Streptomyces griseus*, into helical "cores" and nonhelical "tails." α-Keratin of mammals thus appears to have a microfibrillar structure consisting of linear aggregates of low-sulfur proteins. The helical sections of the molecule are twisted to form intermittent two-strand and three-strand "ropes." The microfibrils of the α-keratins, thus formed, are embedded in a matrix containing the sulfur-rich proteins. Other keratins, e.g., the β-type in feathers, appear to consist of similar microfibrils embedded in a sulfur-rich matrix.

Mammalian keratins are characterized by a relatively high content of lysine and arginine as well as of cystine. Interesting is the fact that the feeding of cystine to animals on a low-protein diet promotes the growth of hair. The turnover time of the epidermis, and presumably of its major constituent, α-keratin, has been estimated to be about 30 days. The constant replacement of keratin thus represents an important metabolic function of epidermal tissue and drain of amino acids from the metabolic pool (p. 345).

Skin also contains a small amount of lipid. In the subcutaneous tissues there is a considerable quantity of lipid, and about one fifth of this consists of sterols. One of these sterols, on irradiation by ultraviolet light, is changed to vitamin D (p. 778). Fat, fatty acids, phospholipids, and carotene are also present, and there is a sex difference[2] in the lipid content of the epidermis of human extremities, women having a higher percentage of triglycerides and men having a higher percentage of cholesterol and phospholipids. Lanolin or wool fat, which finds some use in medicine, consists of esters of palmitic, stearic, and oleic acids with cholesterol and other sterols. Human sebum contains a considerable amount of hydrocarbons, about one third of which is squalene. Cholesterol and other lipids are also present, but there is little protein. Cerumen, or earwax, is composed of over 40% proteins and about 13% neutral fats, with smaller amounts of phospholipids, cholesterol, and other lipids. Carbohydrates in the skin include pentoses, glucose, and glycogen. It has been claimed that the skin may act as a temporary storage depot for glucose when glucose is present in the blood in large amounts. In psoriasis and certain other scaling skin diseases, there is an increased content of free reducing substances, particularly pentoses. Inorganic radicals present in all human tissues are found in epidermal tissue. Toxic heavy metals, however absorbed, seem to find their way, in part, to the skin and are deposited there. In silver poisoning, argyrism, the skin may become bluish in color and remain so for years. Significant amounts of lead are deposited in the skin and hair in lead poisoning.

The chief pigment of skin is *melanin*. Melanin formation is under both hormonal and neurogenic control. It is produced by the melanocytes in the basal layer of the epidermis and occurs in variable amounts as fine granules in the cells and between the cells of the stratum germinativum. The activity of the melanocytes of dark-skinned races is greater than that of the white race, and brunettes more than of blondes. Albinos form no melanin, probably because of the absence of an enzyme that produces melanin from tyrosine through 3,4-dihydroxyphenylalanine, or dopa (p. 374). *Tyrosinase*, an enzyme in the skin, converts dopa to melanin, as described in Chapter 13. This conversion is aided by the tanning action of sunlight, but the mechanism of action, as well as the structure of melanin itself, is unknown. Melanin is a very complex substance of high molecular weight. It may be combined with protein in the tissues. It is a dark brown substance, quite insoluble in all ordinary reagents except alkalies, although some melanins do not dissolve readily even in alkaline reagents. The relationship of the melanins to tyrosine and epinephrine is discussed in Chapter 13.

Connective tissue Connective tissue is a system of insoluble protein fibers embedded in a continuous matrix called the *ground substance*. Connective tissues are widely distributed in the body, e.g., in the dermis (stratum corneum), tendons, ligaments, cartilage, and matrix of bone. Its chief function is supportive and is performed by the fibrils of the insoluble proteins *collagen* and *elastin*. The characteristics of connective tissues depend on the proportions of collagen and elastin as well as on the amount of ground substance. Achilles tendon, for instance, a tissue of great strength, is 32% collagen and 2.6% elastin. Ligamentum nuchae, an elastic tissue, contains 32% elastin and only 7% collagen. While cartilage is rich in ground substance, the areolar connective tissue contains little of the liquid matrix.

The protein collagen, which represents almost 30% of the total body protein, is formed by fibroblasts embedded in the connective tissues.[3] Electron micrographs of collagen reveal a characteristic banding of 640 Å (Fig. 18-1). Since electron micrographs are prepared by treating the sample with an electron-dense material, e.g., phosphotungstic acid, the anions of this material are bound at regularly spaced regions of polar amino acids.

The formation of insoluble fibers such as collagen by individual cells is difficult to visualize. It is necessary to propose the prior formation of small soluble subunits that can be produced by the cell in accord with the usual processes of protein synthesis (Chapter 6). These subunits presumably leave the cell and aggregate in a regular manner in the extracellular fluid or ground substance. The existence of such subunits was shown by the extraction of connective tissues with cold neutral salt solutions.[4] This removes a readily soluble collagen protein. Warming such solutions results in the re-formation of a fibrillar mass showing, by electron microscopy, the characteristically regular spacing of 640 Å. The solubilized collagen is now called *tropocollagen* and is considered to be the subunit of the mature fibers.

Tropocollagen is a highly asymmetric molecule, a relatively rigid rod, with a molecular weight of approximately 300,000 and dimensions of 50 by 2900 Å. It is composed of three polypeptide chains, each in a left-handed helical

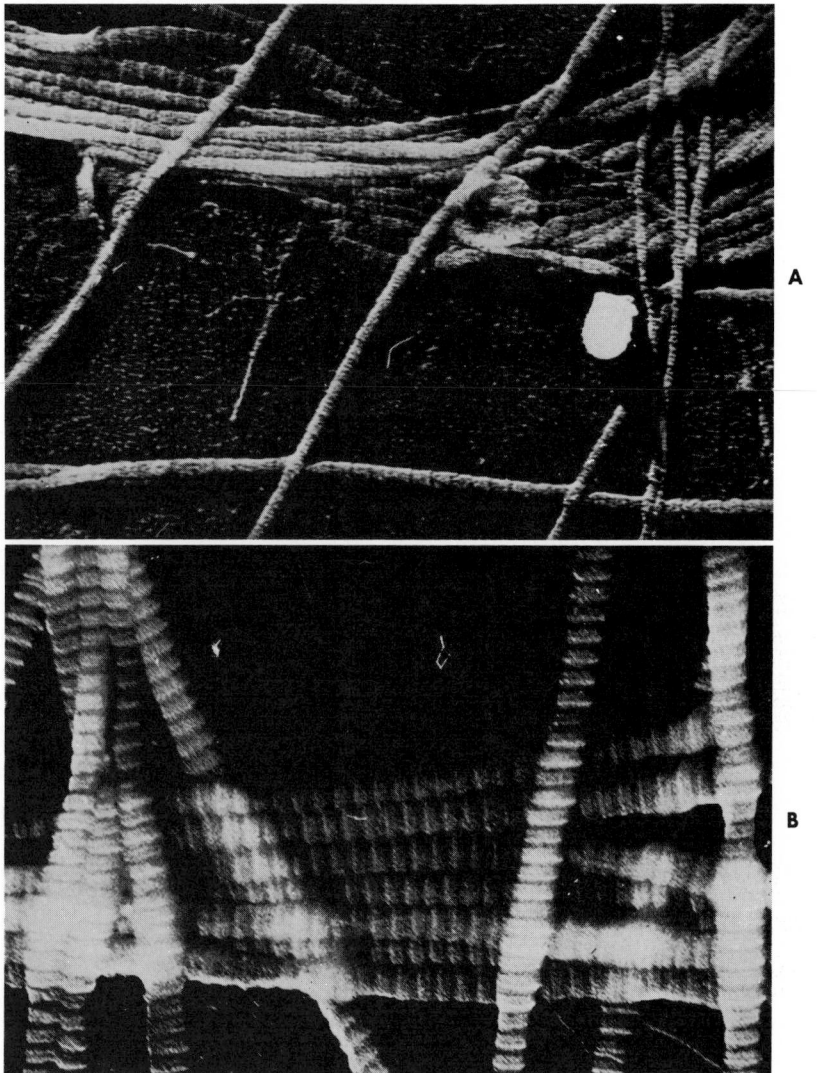

Fig. 18-1. Electron micrographs of connective tissues, showing reticular fibers, **A**, and collagen, **B**. Both fibers show a characteristic periodicity of 640 Å. (Courtesy J. Gross; from Bevelander, G.: Essentials of histology, ed. 6, St. Louis, 1970, The C. V. Mosby Co.)

conformation. The three helices together then wind in a right-handed coil (super helix). Hydrogen bonds between the three chains appear to be the primary linkage holding the structure together (Fig. 18-2). Although helical in conformation, tropocollagen does not exhibit the typical α-helix described for other proteins (p. 81). The high concentrations of prolines and glycine (Table 5-1) prevent this conformation, which requires the presence of 3.6 amino acid residues per turn. Instead, there are three residues per turn. Each of the constituent polypeptides has a molecular weight of approximately 100,000. Apparently a further subunit is present since each of the three

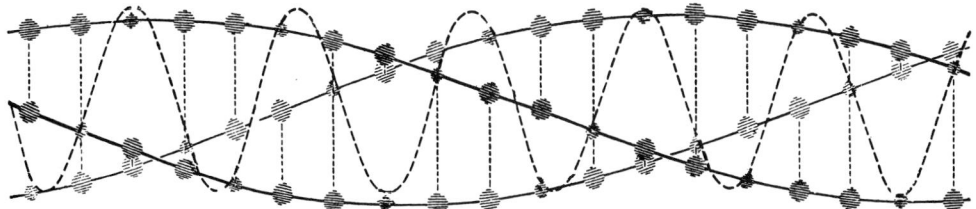

Fig. 18-2. Diagram of tropocollagen molecule. This is a triple helix. The wavy broken line indicates the H bonds between glycine units. The straight broken lines indicate the H bonds that link hydroxyproline units and give greater stability to collagens in which they are found. (From Doty, P.: Sci. Amer. **197**:173, 1957.)

polypeptides may consist, in turn, of four smaller chains held together by covalent bonds.

The three polypeptide chains represent two α_1-chains of the same amino acid composition and one α_2-chain of different composition. The primary structure of these polypeptides consists of regions of highly polar amino acids separated by regions rich in glycine, proline, and hydroxyproline. The following is a suggested arrangement of amino acids to show (in tropocollagen) the asymmetric pattern of polar and nonpolar residues:

(Polar region-Pro-X)–([Gly-Pro-X]$_7$-[Gly-Pro-(polar region)-Pro-X]-

[Gly-Pro-X]$_7$-[Gly-Pro-(polar region)-Pro-X])$_4$–(Gly-Pro-[polar region])

(The polar regions $= $ Gly$_4$-Glu$_2$-Asp-Lys-Ala$_2$-Ser-X)

Tropocollagen subunits are synthesized in a manner similar to that described previously for other proteins (p. 98). It appears, however, that hydroxyproline is not incorporated into the peptide chain by way of hypro-tRNA but rather by a subsequent hydroxylation of proline already present in the growing polypeptide. Hydroxylation requires a *proline hydroxylase*, ascorbic acid, ferrous iron, α-ketoglutarate, and oxygen. It becomes apparent why scurvy, vitamin C deficiency, has a profound affect on connective tissue formation.

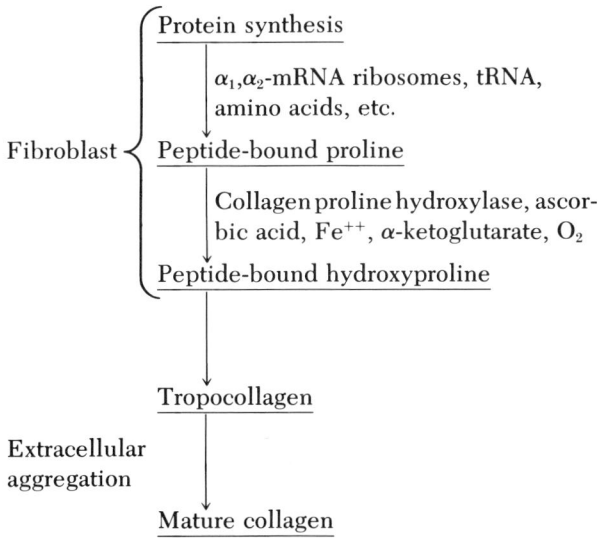

Protein synthesis

α_1,α_2-mRNA ribosomes, tRNA, amino acids, etc.

Fibroblast — Peptide-bound proline

Collagen proline hydroxylase, ascorbic acid, Fe^{++}, α-ketoglutarate, O$_2$

Peptide-bound hydroxyproline

Tropocollagen

Extracellular aggregation

Mature collagen

The helical groups of three chains that form the tropocollagen molecule aggregate in the extracellular environment in a quarter-staggered array of molecules.

Fig. 18-3 illustrates how individual tropocollagen molecules are thought to align themselves in a parallel manner to create a quarter-staggered effect. These are arranged so that one end of a tropocollagen molecule, represented by a knob, is one fourth the length of a single unit (2800 Å) from the knob of its neighbor in a parallel row. In this way a series of knobs separated by 700 Å results. In Fig. 18-3, every fifth knob is seen to be a repeat of the first knob. To emphasize this point, the repeats are connected by black lines. If these knobs are rich in basic amino acids (polar regions), then phosphotungstic acid binds at them. Electron microscopy reveals the polar regions as electron-dense zones separated by regular intervals of approximately 700 Å, creating a banded effect.

In tissue the newly formed tropocollagen is readily extractable with neutral salt solutions because little or no cross-linking has occurred. Upon aging, the collagen becomes increasingly cross-linked and no longer readily extractable. At one point this collagen is still soluble in a dilute acidic medium, e.g., a solution of citric acid. More extensive cross-linking results in fibers that remain insoluble in dilute alkaline and acidic media.

Collagen is unique in its transformation into gelatin upon heating. This is usually accomplished by boiling in water for a long time or in acid solution for a shorter time. The formation of gelatin appears to result from the untwisting of the triple-strand helix accompanied by a breaking of hydrogen bonds. Although collagen is only slowly digested by pepsin and trypsin, gelatin is readily hydrolyzed. Because of its digestibility, gelatin is a common article of food.

Elastin is a protein having distinctly elastic properties as well as high mechanical strength. Compared with that of collagen, our knowledge of elastin is extremely meager. Electron micrographs show elastin to be amorphous in structure; i.e., it consists of fibers without the obvious structural detail seen in collagen. Elastin has a low content of polar side chains, especially of the basic and acidic amino acids. The only way in which the amino acid content of the two proteins is similar is in the high content of glycine (27%), alanine (23%), and proline (13.5%) and the low concentration of tyrosine.

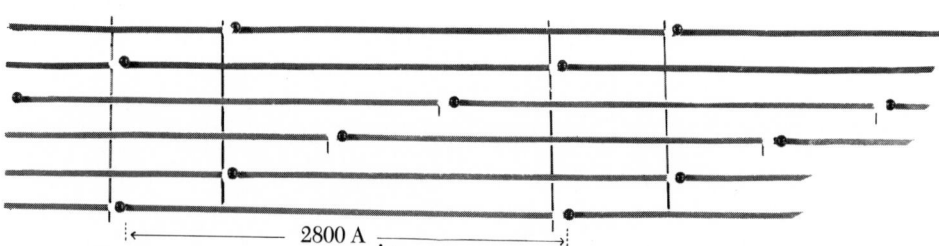

2800 A

Fig. 18-3. Quarter-staggered arrangement of parallel rows of tropocollagen to produce repeated regions of like composition separated by 700 Å.

Elastin is also insoluble in all solvents that do not change its chemical nature. It is not, however, converted to gelatin, as is collagen.

A third fibrous protein found in connective tissues is known as *reticulin*. This albuminoid resembles collagen in terms of its amino acid composition as well as its 640 Å axial repeating period, characteristic of the electron micrographs. It appears to be distinctive, however, because of its association with lipids and carbohydrates.

Ground substance may be viewed as a modified dialysate of plasma. It contains some proteins derived from plasma by a certain degree of capillary permeability. The fluid matrix, however, is unique in terms of its content of mucopolysaccharides (p. 174). The mucopolysaccharides present are hyaluronic acid and chondroitins A, B, and C. These polysaccharides are also synthesized by the fibroblasts.

Hyaluronic acid is an unbranched polymer of high molecular weight (1 to 1.5×10^6) of a repeating disaccharide consisting of glucuronic acid and N-acetylglucosamine (p. 174). The chondroitin sulfates are sulfated polysaccharides. Chondroitin sulfate–A is a polysaccharide of glucuronic acid and N-acetylgalactosamine bearing a sulfate ester group on carbon-4 of the amino sugar. Chondroitin sulfate–C differs from –A only in being sulfated on carbon-6 of the amino sugar. Chondroitin sulfate–B is similar to –A except that the uronic acid is of the sugar L-idose rather than D-glucose.

Mucopolysaccharides are thought to be complexed with protein found in the ground substance. Hyaluronic acid combines with proteins possibly in a somewhat similar manner to the way in which nucleic acid combines with proteins; however, the nature of the uniting forces is currently unclear. The chondroitin sulfates, on the other hand, are not as large as the hyaluronic acid, each polysaccharide having a molecular weight of approximately 50,000. Numerous such polysaccharide units are combined with a single protein core to produce a total unit of large molecular weight (4×10^6). The binding forces here are thought to be covalent in nature.

The mucopolysaccharide-protein complexes play numerous roles. They have a particular ability to bind water, forming a gel. This is important in structural terms, e.g., maintaining the turgidity of the skin and other tissues. Hyaluronic acid is an important constituent of vitreous humor and the umbilical cord. It imparts the lubricative quality to the synovial fluid of the joints. Mucopolysaccharides help prevent the invasion of the body through the skin by disease-producing microorganisms. Many bacteria, however, produce an enzyme, *hyaluronidase*, that catalyzes the depolymerization of mucopolysaccharides, thereby increasing the invasiveness of the bacteria. Hyaluronidase is a β-glucosaminidase, therefore hydrolyzing the β-1,4-glycosidic bond between N-acetylhexosamine and the neighboring uronic acid (p. 174). This enzyme is also found in spermatozoa and may be functional in facilitating the penetration and thus the fertilization of the ovum. Highly purified hyaluronidase is used clinically for the intradermal administration of large volumes of fluid when intravenous injections are contraindicated. The enzyme is given prior to, or simultaneously with, the fluid and hastens the flow and absorption of the fluid. Hyaluronidase may also be used to enable edematous patients to excrete accumulated tissue fluid more rapidly. It can facilitate the penetration of drugs, e.g., penicillin, into mucous membranes, and it can help spread the effect of local anesthetics over a wider area. Hyaluronidase has been found useful as an adjuvant in infiltration and nerve block anesthesia, increasing the area and depth but decreasing the duration of anesthesia. Another interesting application of the enzyme is to facilitate the separation of closely adherent structures and thus aid in surgical dissection. A few minutes after the application of a sponge moistened with the warm enzyme solution, adherent tissues are more easily separated. Of course, the use of hyaluronidase in infected areas and in malignancy is not advised since the enzyme might tend to spread the offending material.

The composition of ground substance changes with aging. In children, chondroitin sulfate–A predominates, while in the adult chondroitin sulfate–C is the major component.

Cartilage is also a connective tissue and contains collagen, some noncollagenous protein, and ground substance. The acid mucopolysaccharide chondroitin sulfates A and C are attached to the noncollagenous protein. The collagen appears to be the same as that in other connective tissues although the cartilage is devoid of large collagen fibers exhibiting the characteristic 640 Å periodicity. Fibers of elastin are present in elastic cartilage, tending to give added flexibility to this tissue. Articular cartilage is exceedingly elastic; it recovers quickly and completely from intermittent pressures. This property, which enables cartilage to absorb the shocks to which the body is subjected, is lost on drying but regained when water is restored. Vitamin D is quite possibly related to the development and health of cartilage, in addition to being involved in the normal conversion of cartilage to bone.

Chronic rheumatoid arthritis in man is characterized by disruption of collagenous structures. Recent investigations have indicated that this may result from an excessive production of the enzyme *collagenase* by cells of the proliferating synovium. Several investigators reported high collagenase activity in synovial specimens from patients with rheumatoid arthritis whereas none was demonstrable in specimens from control subjects. The amount of collagenase activity was directly proportional to the degree of local and systemic disease activity. This could account for the destruction of collagen in and about the joints, tendons, capsules, ligaments, cartilage, and bone in patients with this type of arthritis.

Bone The organic matrix of bone is the supporting lattice in which the bone salts are deposited to form a rigid structure. The organic matrix is flexible and extremely strong.

Table 18-1 shows that collagen is the principal organic substance present in the bone. It is apparently identical with the collagen of connective tissues[5] (p. 543) and is formed by the osteoblasts. The collagen is embedded in the ground substance containing mucopolysaccharides. The ground substance varies in consistency, from interstitial fluid to thick gel, thus forming the interconnection with the tissue fluid that permits an exchange of ions and other substances with the blood.

Analysis of bone and ash reveals a preponderance of calcium, a small

Table 18-1. Composition of bone*

	Percent of bovine compact bone
Ash	71.0
Water	8.2
Collagen	18.6
Protein-polysaccharide complex	0.2
Other proteins	1.0
Fat	0.0
Sugars, other than mucopolysaccharides	0.0
Total	99.0

* From Eastoe, J. M., and Eastoe, J. M., Jr.: Biochem. J. **57**:453, 1954.

amount of sodium, and less magnesium and other cations. The anions are chiefly phosphate with some carbonate and citrate and small amounts of chloride and fluoride. In general the mineral of bone is in the form of a *hydroxyapatite*, having the following formula:

$$3Ca_3(PO_4)_2 \cdot Ca(OH)_2$$

This formula accounts for the calcium and phosphate but not for the carbonate, citrate, and small amounts of chloride, fluoride, and other ions that are occasionally found. It was formerly held that bone salt was an apatite of changing composition and that these other elements or ions were introduced and withdrawn as they fluctuated in concentration in the blood plasma. Now there is evidence that these other salts are present in the intercrystalline material, perhaps in suspension in a semiliquid medium, which transports materials from the blood to the bone and vice versa. These two phases of the mineral structure of bone have quite different physical, chemical, and probably physiologic properties. The hydroxyapatite crystals (Fig. 18-4) are relatively stable in structure and are not easily soluble in aqueous fluids but are subject to rapid ion exchange reactions at their surfaces. They are extremely small and hence have an enormous surface area. The intercrystalline fraction is far smaller in amount than the crystalline fraction, about 4% as great. However, it is much more soluble and its calcium and other metallic elements go back to the blood by the simple process of solution. The importance of these facts will appear in a subsequent discussion (p. 552).

The hardness and rigidity of bone are chiefly due to the inorganic salts, whereas the elasticity and toughness are attributable to the organic matter. This can be illustrated by two simple experiments. If a small piece of bone is incinerated, a white ash with the form of the original fragment of bone results. When this is ground in a mortar, it is brittle and can be ground to a fine powder the hardness of which is apparent. On the other hand, if a bone is subjected to the action of dilute hydrochloric acid for a number of days, the inorganic salts are removed and the material left is again seen to have the

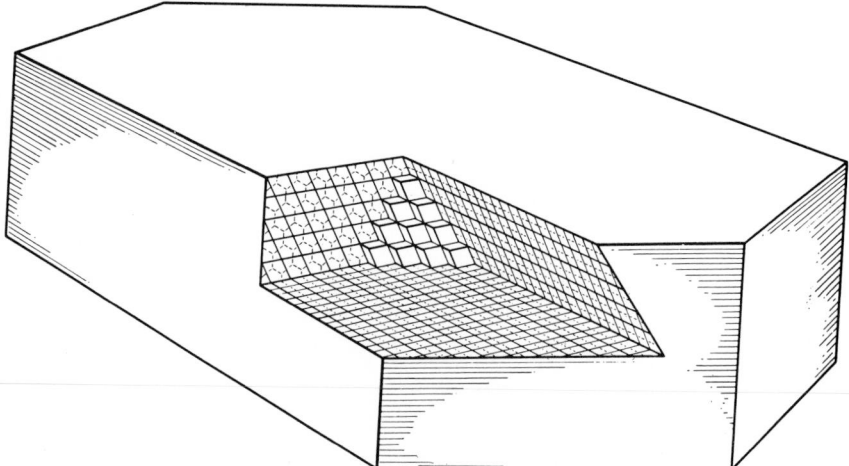

Fig. 18-4. Diagrammatic representation of a crystal of hydroxyapatite. This model of a single crystal is cut to show the unit cells of its molecular structure. The model enlarges the crystal about 5 million times. (From McLean, F. C.: Sci. Amer. **192**:84, 1955.)

exact form of the original bone. However, it no longer is hard and rigid but tough and flexible. The combination of these inorganic and organic fractions results in a very strong tissue with high tensile strength. A feature of bones adding greatly to their strength is the fact that bones are hollow tubes. It is a well-known physical principle that a given weight of rigid material is much stronger when fashioned in the form of a tube than when fashioned as a solid rod. The space within the tube is not empty but is filled with bone marrow, which will be discussed later.

Since bone is laid down first as cartilage or membrane that becomes impregnated more and more with inorganic salts, we can easily see why children's bones are less easily broken than adults'.

Citrate has been discovered as a constituent of human bone, to the extent of about 1% of the dry weight of bone, which may be as much as 70% of the citrate of the whole body. Nevertheless, when means are employed to increase the output of citrate by the kidneys, this "extra" citrate does not come from the stores in bone. Although the citrate content of bone is not constant, the stores there are apparently for another function, as yet unknown. Bone citrate may be a source of energy in the metabolism of bone or other tissue, but it probably has a special role in the metabolism of calcium by virtue of its power to bind calcium. The calcium-citrate complex is soluble and diffusible but is un-ionized.

In the formation of the complex bone salt, the concentration of the various ions involved must exceed the saturation point at the site of deposition. Since calcium and phosphate make up the greater part of this salt, evidently these are the ions chiefly involved.

In the process of bone formation, two enzymes appear to be involved: phosphorylase and phosphatase. The epiphyses of the bones of growing mammals have been shown to contain a phosphorylase. This enzyme catalyzes the conversion of glycogen to glucose-1-phosphate. The phosphatase hydrolyzes this substrate, in addition to any other phosphoric acid esters that may be available. Thus the hexose phosphates, glycerophosphates, and nucleotides are potential sources of phosphate ions. The phosphatase that is found in high concentration wherever bone is being formed is probably produced by the osteoblasts; the concentration of phosphate ions is raised locally near these cells as a result of enzyme action. Calcium is present in blood in both ionized and un-ionized form. The un-ionized calcium is partly diffusible and partly not. The nondiffusible calcium is largely that fraction combined with protein, whereas the calcium-citrate complex forms most of the un-ionized diffusible part. Probably the chondroitin sulfate of growing bone unites with calcium to provide a local surplus of available calcium. Normally the concentrations are such that the product of ionic calcium and phosphate is about 36 to 40 mg. per 100 ml. of plasma. Products above 40 are found when bone growth or healing is taking place, whereas products below 40 generally are seen in active rickets and in other conditions in which bone formation is not occurring properly. When the concentration of both calcium ions and phosphate ions is increased beyond the saturation point, the formation of colloidal calcium phosphate occurs. How this is changed to bone salt is undetermined. One view is that it occurs in a series of steps until finally the apatite molecule is produced and additions or substitutions occur until a more stable and insoluble salt is achieved. This has been demonstrated by following the course of radioactive phosphorus, ^{32}P. After administration, ^{32}P is rapidly taken up by bone and built into the apatite structure. Enzyme conditions are favorable for the production of citric acid in calcifying areas of bone, and probably citric acid is coprecipitated during deposition of bone salt. Citric acid is thus available for the re-solution of calcium when that is brought about, and a high citric acid concentration may even reverse calcification and solubilize bone salt that has already been laid down.

The phosphatase is present in large amounts in the layer of osteoblasts on the surface of growing bone and in smaller amounts in adult bone, but it is absent from cartilage that is not undergoing ossification. The optimum pH at which phosphatase acts is an important factor. This is about pH 9. Just prior to ossification, chondroitin usually disappears from those areas in which osteoblastic activity is exerted, thus changing the pH in an alkaline direction. However, phosphatase is present in certain tissues that do not ossify, e.g., the intestine, and is absent sometimes when pathologic calcification is taking place, as in the arteries. Therefore the phosphatase theory of bone formation (Robison's) evidently does not tell the whole story. Significant also is the fact that an accumulation of glycogen occurs in the cells of epiphyseal cartilage prior to calcification. This is undoubtedly due to the presence of a phosphorylase, which thus provides not only organic phosphate but also, perhaps, a supply of energy that may be required in some enzymatic phase of calcification.

Another enzyme, carbonic anhydrase, may be involved in the deposition of calcium salts in bones and teeth.[6] In vitro experiments showed that carbonate hydroxyapatite is deposited on glass plummets immersed intermit-

Cross-banding of collagen fibril

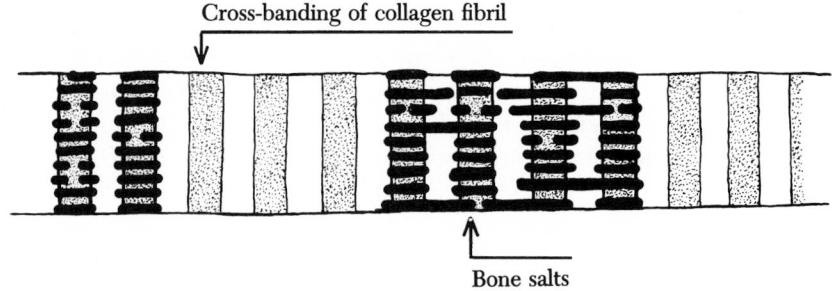

Bone salts

Fig. 18-5. Collagen fibril of bone, showing the relation of inorganic crystals to cross-banding. (Adapted from Robinson, R. A., and Watson, M. L.: Ann. N. Y. Acad. Sci. **60:**620, 1955.)

tently in either saliva or a synthetic solution containing sodium phosphate and calcium chloride and buffer, provided carbonic anhydrase is present. This enzyme apparently makes available the carbonate ion for the formation of the bone salt, carbonate hydroxyapatite.

The antibiotic tetracycline has been found to influence bone formation as well as to be distributed in detectable amounts in bones and teeth. A concentration of 1 μg. per milliliter prevents mineralization of embryonic bone in vitro with tissue culture.[7] The inhibition may be reversible by transferring the treated bone to a normal medium. However, a maldeveloped bone results. The tetracycline effect on bone may be related to the alleged chelating activity of tetracycline with certain inorganic ions.

Examination of the ultrastructure of bone by means of the electron microscope reveals an interesting relation between the bone salts and the supporting collagen fibers. The long axes of the bone salt crystals are invariably oriented with the long axes of the collagen fibrils and are arranged around the cross-banding of the fibrils, forming a type of sheath. This is depicted diagrammatically in Fig. 18-5.

It should be noted that the bone calcium is in equilibrium with the calcium of the blood. Consequently, the blood calcium can be kept at a fairly steady concentration by a slight shift of calcium from the bones to the blood or vice versa. The mechanism whereby this constancy is maintained is dual in character and apparently depends on the two phases of the mineral structure described previously[8] (p. 549). The total calcium of the blood amounts to about 10 mg. per 100 ml. Most of this is derived from the intercrystalline material by simple solution, which depends only on physical and chemical factors; i.e., as the level of blood calcium ions diminishes, more calcium is dissolved into the surrounding fluid and thus into the blood. This process usually keeps the level at about 7 mg. per 100 ml. The remaining 3 mg., more or less, are supplied in just the amount needed by means of a feedback mechanism under the control of the parathyroid glands (Fig. 18-6). PTH (p. 482) acts on the organic matrix, causing the dissolution of the mineral constituents, both the intercrystalline substance and the stable apatite crystals themselves. This process of decalcification and recalcification is under the control of various other factors besides the PTH. Some of these other factors are cal-

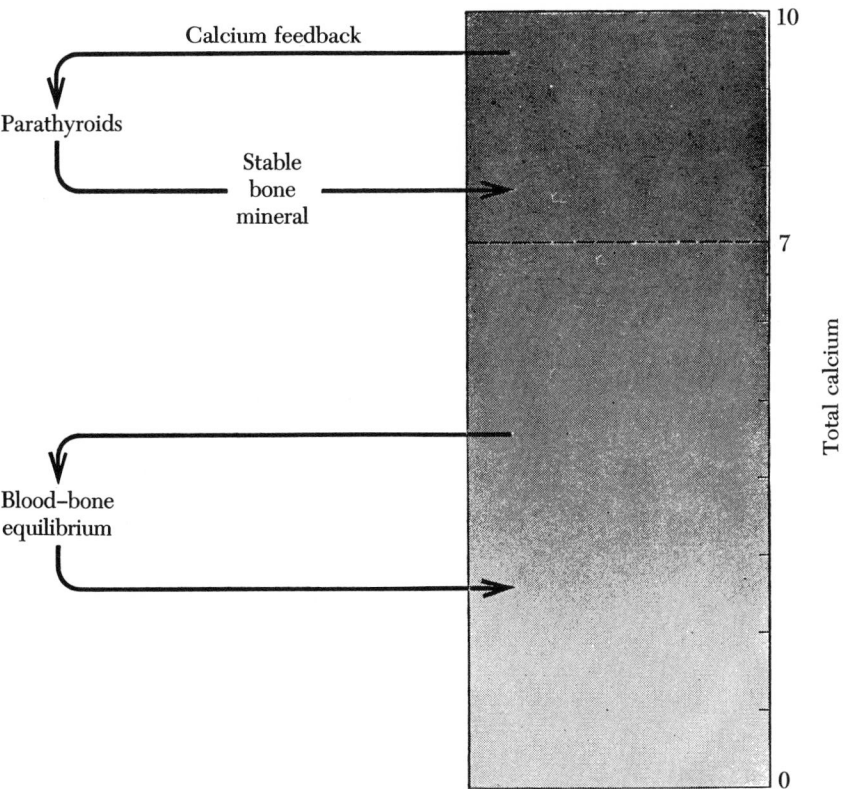

Fig. 18-6. Diagram of feedback mechanism regulating the level of Ca in the blood. The normal Ca concentration in the blood plasma is about 10 mg. per 100 ml. Seven milligrams of this are supplied by the more soluble fractions of bone mineral between the hydroxyapatite crystals. The parathormone promotes the release of Ca from the hydroxyapatite crystals, the stable crystalline reserve, and also from the intercrystalline substance when the Ca level falls below 7 mg. (From McLean, F. C.: Sci. Amer. **192:**84, 1955.)

citonin (p. 481), vitamins D, C, and A, and the anterior pituitary gland secretions. It is self-evident that the amounts of calcium and phosphorus in the diet are important as are various factors controlling the absorption and metabolism of calcium and phosphorus, e.g., the amounts and proportions of dietary protein and fat, the acid-base balance, and the vitamins and hormones present.

In rickets the amount of calcium phosphate in the bones is much below normal. This deficiency is usually the result of inadequate vitamin D, which has an inhibiting effect on the absorption and utilization of calcium and phosphorus. Since the concentration of minerals in the bones is low, the bones become less rigid and consequently bend, resulting in bowlegs or other deformities (Chapter 23). Vitamin A deficiency retards the growth of bone, particularly endochondral bone formation in rats. If the deficiency is established very early in life, skeletal growth is inhibited considerably before the effect on total increase in weight can be observed.

Vitamin C also is essential to bone development. In scurvy there are lesions of the epiphyseal junctions of growing bones. Subperiosteal hemorrhages are likely to occur in both growing and adult bone. Rarefaction of the alveolar bone leads to loosening of the teeth; dentine is resorbed; and the gums become spongy.

The effect of parathyroid secretion on blood calcium by removing calcium salts from the bones, thus tending to raise the calcium level of the blood, may be carried to excess and the bones may be weakened. The anterior pituitary gland has a marked effect on bone growth. In general, a hyperactivity causes increased rate of growth as seen in overgrowth of the skull in acromegaly and in huge bones in gigantism; a deficient activity is seen in the small bones of pituitary dwarfs. Thus hormones, diet, and vitamins share in the complex metabolism of bones.

Bone marrow. Bone marrow is of two kinds: yellow and red. The yellow marrow is composed of connective tissue and large amounts of fat. It has nothing to do with the function of forming red cells. That function belongs to the red marrow; but the yellow marrow may, under some circumstances, be converted to red marrow, which produces the red cells, some of the white cells, and perhaps the platelets (Chapter 19). Red marrow is higher in protein but much lower in fat. Both types contain albumins, globulins, nucleoproteins, fibrinogen, polypeptides, phospholipids, cholesterol, and extractives.

Teeth The teeth resemble bone chemically to a certain extent. Fig. 18-7 is a diagram of a typical tooth. Over the upper surface of the tooth is the enamel. This is the hardest substance in the body, a property of great value for the masticating and grinding action of the teeth. Only about 5% of enamel is water. The remaining 95% consists of inorganic material chiefly embedded in an organic matrix. This organic matrix of enamel is composed of a protein, resembling keratin but containing no cystine, and a mucopolysaccharide. The inorganic material is hydroxyapatite, a calcium phosphate with the formula $Ca_{10}(PO_4)_6 \cdot (OH)_2$. The greater part of the tooth is dentin, which is identical with bone from a chemical standpoint although differing from it histologically. Dentin protein is largely collagen,[9] and there is chondroitin sulfate present. The inorganic basis is again an apatite, similar to the bone salt.

Administration of labeled phosphorus is followed by rapid uptake of the tracer by developing teeth. Once the teeth are completely formed and calcified, this continuing metabolism is reduced to a minimum. Thus the teeth are not drawn upon for calcium in time of need, as are the bones.

Vitamins A, C, and D are all necessary for proper tooth development and calcification. Lack of vitamins A and C affects the functional activities of the formative cells. Deficiency of vitamin A results in hypoplastic enamel, imperfectly calcified. Lack of ascorbic acid affects the calcification of dentin. Vitamin D not only aids in the absorption of calcium but also promotes the deposition of calcium and phosphorus in teeth.

Dental caries When the enamel breaks and the underlying dentin is exposed, dental caries develop. The cause of this formation of tooth cavities has been a matter of dispute for years and is still unsettled.

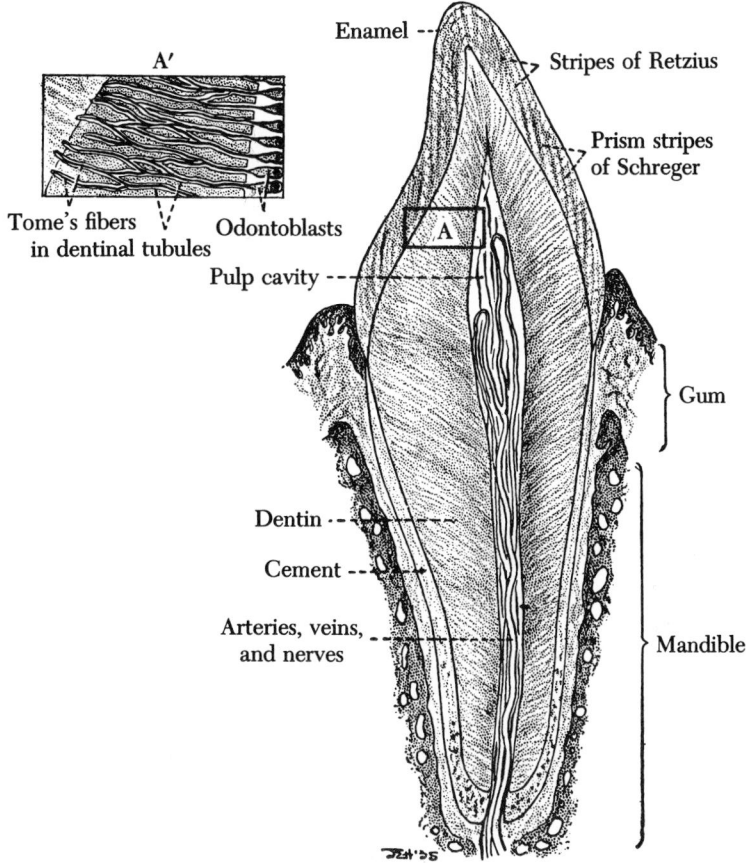

Fig. 18-7. Longitudinal section of an incisor tooth. The part *A* is shown at high magnification in *A'*. (From McClendon, J. F., and Pettibone, C. J. V.: Physiological chemistry, St. Louis, 1936, The C. V. Mosby Co.)

Dental caries are one of the most widespread of human diseases, and a tremendous amount of investigation has been instituted to determine the cause and effect a cure. The results up to the present time have been rather conflicting. In caries the enamel and other hard structures are dissolved by chemical action and washed away, thus producing a cavity. The formation of cavities in the teeth is not only a source of pain and discomfort, necessitating dental attention, but is also likely to lead to interference with mastication and hence with proper nutrition. Furthermore, infectious processes occurring in cavities may result in the absorption of toxins or lead to secondary infections in other parts of the body.

In general, there are two schools of thought regarding the initiation of caries; both allow for the possibility that genetic factors, which determine many dental characteristics, are involved also. Advocates of one point of view believe that local factors are entirely or, at any rate, chiefly responsible. Food particles lodging between the teeth or in recesses in the surface of teeth become breeding spots for bacteria. If they are not removed promptly, enough

555

acid is produced to dissolve the mineral constituents of the enamel and dentin. Foods particularly rich in carbohydrates, e.g., soft cereals, candies, pastries, are most easily fermented and, consequently, are most likely to lead to the formation of caries. Although saliva has no bactericidal power, the character of the saliva is believed to play a role: the more mucin saliva contains, the less effective it is in cleaning the teeth. The adherents of this chemicoparasitic theory advocate oral hygiene and prophylaxis as a deterrent to caries. The possibility of a proteolytic factor has attracted considerable attention. According to this view, caries are a proteolytic process, or perhaps the proteolytic and glycolytic processes go on side by side. It is assumed that bacteria, possessing proteolytic enzymes, multiply at the surface of the teeth and cause disintegration of the lamellae (the flattened bands of organic protein-containing matter extending through the enamel). This permits the easy entrance of fermenting organisms with their production of acid and consequent solution of the inorganic portion of the enamel. The possible formation of amino acid–calcium chelates as a factor in caries development has been mentioned previously (p. 70).

Advocates of the other view believe that, although caries are a local action and always begin at the exterior of the tooth, the structure of the tooth determines whether or not decay will occur. An excellent nutritive condition of the individual is responsible for perfection of the structure, and since the formation of teeth begins in fetal life, the food of the mother is just as important as that of the child. Vitamins A, C, and D and the elements calcium and phosphorus, with traces of fluorine, are all considered essential for the building of healthy teeth.

The influence of fluoride, which was discussed on p. 428, must be emphasized. If the amount of fluoride in drinking water is adequate (1.0 to 1.2 p.p.m.), the enamel seems to be *more resistant* to the development of dental caries. It should be noted that fluoride is probably most effective if it is present during the period of tooth development. There are several explanations for the possible inhibiting action of fluoride on caries. One is that fluoride is an essential or, at any rate, highly desirable component of enamel; i.e., fluoride reacts with the tooth substance to form a less soluble complex, a compound less susceptible to the solvent action of acids. Support of this hypothesis has recently been offered. Using isotope-exchange and ion-competition techniques, it was found that fluoride can replace hydroxyl or bicarbonate ions on the surface of bone, forming an insoluble and resistant fluoroapatite. Perhaps the same phenomenon occurs in the mouth. The fluoride content of the surface layers of enamel is normally approximately 10 times higher than that of the layers near the dentin-enamel junction. Another hypothesis is that fluoride acts as an enzyme inhibitor, thus interrupting the chain of fermentative reactions and preventing the formation of organic acids in proximity to the enamel. The use of fluoride in the water supplies of communities (p. 429) is being advocated as a method of preventing dental caries. In this connection it is interesting to note that the hardness of drinking water may also play a part. Mills stated that there is a lower incidence of carious lesions in regions where the drinking water is hard than in those in which it is soft. This opinion has been substantiated. Whether a nutritional effect of the additional calcium or magnesium present exists or a local effect is not apparent.

Another halogen, namely, iodine, may be involved in dental caries. Muhler recently showed that the feeding of desiccated thyroid has a marked anti-cariogenic effect in rats. It is just as effective as the administration of sodium fluoride. Following this, Ryan accumulated evidence that explains the fact. There is hyperfunction of the salivary glands in hyperthyroidism and hypo-function of the salivary glands in hypothyroidism. The anticariogenic action of desiccated thyroid may well come from an increased flow of saliva, together with an increased concentration of salivary iodide.

Several investigations[10] indicate that a cariostatic agent or agents may be present in certain foods. Both inorganic and organic phosphates in the diet of rats were shown to have a cariostatic effect. The effective organic phos-phates included phytin, sodium phytate, β-glycerophosphate, and fructose-1,6-diphosphate. No explanation was found for the mechanism of this effect. Another observation was that people who habitually chew sugar cane but do not eat refined sugar also have a low caries rate. These observations suggest that some natural constituent of cereal grains, or seed bulbs, and unrefined sugar may be an effective cariostatic agent.

Adipose tissue   Two types of tissue fat are to be distinguished: protoplasmic fat (*élément constant*) and depot fat (*élément variable*). The former is an essential con-stituent of protoplasm and includes other lipids besides neutral fat. It is not reduced in amount during starvation. The depot fat, on the other hand, is true adipose tissue and is largely a reserve food supply. A cell of adipose tissue is literally a droplet of fat contained within a thin membranous living cell. In order for the droplet of fat to be removed from such tissue, the tissue must be heated, the cell membranes and supporting tissues ruptured, and the fat poured and strained off. When fat is "tried out" or rendered in this way, little protein matter is left behind. Although the distribution of adipose tissue varies in different individuals, a large part of it is in the subcutaneous tissue. Other locations are near the kidneys, in the omentum, and in most other tissues except the brain. A "brown fat" is deposited in the interscapular glands of the embryo and sometimes of the adult and between the kidneys of hibernating animals. The latter is sometimes called hibernation fat (see p. 302).

According to recent isotopic investigations, fat must be deposited in tissues before it can be utilized. Depot triglyceride is thus very active metabolically. Its "half-life" has been estimated by isotopic techniques as some 5 days. Even when given in small amounts to a starving animal, fat apparently is not burned directly as so much fuel but is used only after it has been incorporated into adipose tissue or cellular fat. The mechanisms involved in the deposition and mobilization of storage fat were discussed earlier (p. 301).

In obesity there is an abnormal amount of fat laid down as adipose tissue. This is a result of a surplus of food calories over the amount expended. How-ever, there are a number of other factors that enter into the problem (Chapters 12 and 17). Excess obese tissue can be removed surgically—and this is frequently done—for cosmetic reasons.

Nervous tissue   Nervous tissue makes up only about one fortieth of the total weight of the body, yet the brain and nervous system dominate most of the functions of the body. This domination is either directly, by nerve impulses sent to the tissue or organ, or indirectly, by nervous control of the blood supply to the organs. We would expect, therefore, such a remarkable type of tissue to have a chemical makeup quite different from other tissues.

Nervous tissue is characterized by the presence of a large proportion of lipids.[11] Fat, however, is not among the lipids of nervous tissue. Like all other active tissues, there is a large amount of water present—more in embryonic and young nervous tissue and increasingly less with age. Nearly half the dry matter of the human brain consists of proteins (Table 18-2). The gray matter is much richer in proteins than the white matter, as can be seen from the table. *Corpus callosum*, which is composed entirely of white matter, contains 27% proteins, and whole brain, 37%. The proteins of nervous tissue include an albumin, several globulins, a nucleoprotein, and neurokeratin. Neurokeratin is the material remaining after nervous tissue is subjected to digestion by gastric and pancreatic juices and is then extracted with organic solvents, dilute acid, and alkali. This protein has the physical properties of keratins, to be sure, but contains the amino acids in different proportions from those present in keratins obtained from true epidermal tissue. The amino acid content of neurokeratin and of the combined brain proteins was determined by Block. The relative amounts of cystine, tryptophan, histidine, tyrosine, lysine, arginine are about the same in a number of different animals. There is a remarkable constancy in the ratio of lysine to arginine in all species except man and monkey. In the other species the ratio lysine:arginine is 100:103-105. In man and monkey it is 100:95-96. The percentage of nitrogen in human brain proteins is rather low, namely, 13.4%. The nitrogen content of nucleoprotein is low, but nucleoprotein seems to contain a typical deoxyribonucleic acid. Glycogen also is low in nervous tissue; in other words, the brain has little reserve supply of carbohydrate. For its proper functioning the brain requires a normal concentration of glucose in the blood in addition to a

Table 18-2. Solids of the human brain*

	Whole brain (child) (percent)	Whole brain (adult) (percent)	Corpus callosum (percent)
Proteins	46.6	37.1	27.1
Extractives	12.0	6.7	3.9
Ash	8.3	4.2	2.4
Phospholipids	24.2	27.3	31.0
Cerebrosides	6.9	13.6	18.0
Lipid sulfur	0.1	0.3	0.5
Cholesterol	1.8	10.9	17.1

*From Koch, W.: Z. Physiol. Chem. **63**:432, 1909.

small amount of hexose phosphate, which apparently comes into the tissue by diffusion. When the blood sugar becomes too low, e.g., after an overdose of insulin, the brain is affected and symptoms of dizziness, mental confusion, weakness, delirium, and even convulsions may ensue. The insulin shock therapy for schizophrenia utilizes this mechanism with some degree of success.

Abnormal metabolism of carbohydrate may also be related to certain neuroses. It was shown recently[12] that patients with anxiety neuroses have an excessively high blood lactate level. This may be related to a chronic overproduction of epinephrine, resulting in excessive lactate production. Small amounts of phosphocreatine, ATP, inositol, and other extractives* are also present, as well as various inorganic salts, particularly alkaline phosphates.

As can be seen from Table 18-2, large amounts of lipids are present in brain tissue. In the adult brain they make up more than half the total solids. The phospholipids are present most abundantly, with the glycolipids next, then cholesterol, and the sulfolipids last. White matter contains more lipids than does gray matter, in general. However, no true fat is present in nervous tissue, and experimental work has shown that the metabolic turnover of fatty acids present is very slow in nervous tissue as compared with that in other organs.

Another marked chemical difference between gray and white matter is in the mineral content. The ash of the *corpus callosum* makes up 2.4% of the solids, whereas it is 4.2% of whole brain solids; i.e., ash is higher in the gray matter than in the white.

Chemical transmitters of nerve impulse — acetylcholine. The only specific chemical transmitter of the nerve impulse definitely identified in the mammalian central nervous system is acetylcholine,[13] as shown originally by Loewy and confirmed and extended later by others. Agents like norepinephrine and serotonin (5-hydroxytryptamine) may be involved also. During the transmission of the nerve impulse, the chemical transmitter (acetylcholine, etc.) is ejected by some unknown mechanism from a special knoblike extension of one nerve cell into the synaptic cleft and thence into the next nerve cell. Although the mechanism of action of acetylcholine has not been established with certainty, a summary of a current concept is as follows: Acetylcholine, formed as shown in Fig. 18-8 and stored in synaptic vesicles of the nerve cell bound to its membrane, is released upon stimulation of the nerve cell and in the presence of calcium ions (Mg^{++} ions inhibit). The released acetylcholine apparently then attaches to the synaptic membrane, changing its conformation, with the resultant development of pores, through which sodium ions flow. This shift of sodium ions results in the development of an action potential, with a resultant electric transmission of the nerve impulse. Some authorities believe that the foregoing process occurs also in the axons of nerve cells as well as at the synapse and is thus involved in the propagation of the nerve impulse along the entire nerve cell. Meanwhile, the liberated acetylcholine is destroyed by cholinesterase, as indicated in Fig. 18-8. The

---

*The term "extractives" is rather loosely applied to substances that may be extracted from tissues by boiling water. It usually excludes proteins and inorganic salts.

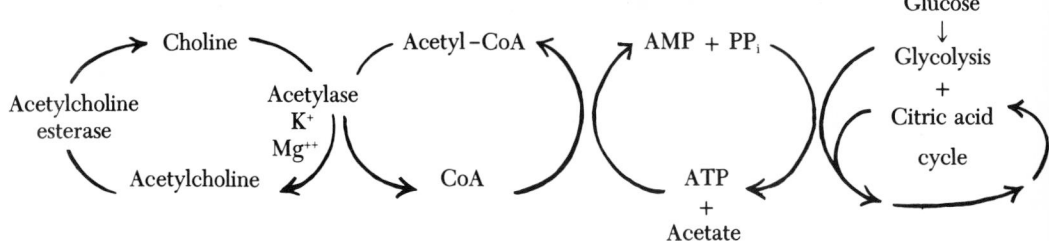

Fig. 18-8. Diagram of the mechanism of formation of acetylcholine in the nerve cell. (Adapted from Nachmansohn, D.: Science **134**:1962, 1961.)

process is ready then for repetition. The entire process occurs extremely rapidly, the turnover time being estimated at 30 to 50 μsec. Thus a nerve can conduct hundreds or perhaps a thousand or more impulses per second.

Cannon presented evidence in favor of the existence of sympathin, an analogous substance liberated at sympathetic postganglionic endings; but sympathin is now recognized as identical with norepinephrine (p. 464).

Acetylcholine has marked pharmacologic properties when introduced intravenously into an animal. It slows the heart rate, dilates the arterioles, constricts the bronchi, and has many other effects. There is present in the bloodstream, in the tissues, and especially in the axon and just beneath the cell surface of the ganglion cell an enzyme capable of hydrolyzing acetylcholine into choline and acetic acid, compounds that are much less active than the parent substance. This enzyme has been named *cholinesterase* (or acetylcholine esterase).

$$\underset{\text{Acetylcholine}}{CH_3-\overset{+}{\underset{CH_3}{\overset{CH_3}{N}}}-CH_2-CH_2-O-\overset{O}{\overset{\|}{C}}-CH_3} \xrightarrow{\text{Cholinesterase}} \underset{\text{Choline}}{CH_3-\overset{+}{\underset{CH_3}{\overset{CH_3}{N}}}-CH_2-CH_2-OH} + \underset{\text{Acetic acid}}{CH_3COOH}$$

Cholinesterase may be irreversibly inhibited by a number of substances, including diisopropylfluorophosphate (DFP). This fact has been made use of in the development of certain alkyl phosphate insecticides and the nerve gases. Here the effects are due to the resulting accumulation of acetylcholine. Cholinesterase inhibitors are also used in ophthalmology as miotics, i.e., substances that cause the pupil to contract.

The mechanism of formation of acetylcholine in the nerve cell may be depicted diagrammatically as shown in Fig. 18-8. This illustration also emphasizes the many biochemical requirements for the normal functioning of nervous tissue, i.e., complete pathways for the anaerobic and aerobic oxidation of glucose, adequate supply of ATP, acetate, coenzyme-A, as well as other cofactors and certain specific enzymes.

There is current evidence that γ-aminobutyric acid, derived from glutamic acid by decarboxylation, is involved in retarding or inhibiting the transmission of nerve impulses.

Biochemistry of memory. Biochemical processes involved in the storage of information, "memory," and its retrieval in the brain have been the center of intensive study in the past few years. Controversial claims of the transfer of knowledge from trained animals into naive animals using extracts of brain have also stimulated research in this area. RNA has been suggested as the active constituent of such extracts. Brain RNA has also been suggested as being involved in short-term memory.

More recent investigations by Agranoff and his co-workers, Flexner, and others (see "General References" at end of chapter), however, indicate that protein synthesis in the brain is involved in both short-term and long-term memory. The blocking of protein synthesis by puromycin and certain other substances when injected directly into the brain during or very soon after the learning situation does not affect the animal's ability to learn or its short-term memory but interferes dramatically with the formation of long-term memory. If the blocking agent is injected a short time after learning, there is no interference with long-term memory. Protein synthesis in the brain may also be necessary for converting short-term memory to long-term memory. Other recent work indicates that three key glycoproteins may be involved—two in short-term memory and one in long-term memory.

Further studies along these lines as well as investigations employing memory drugs give promise of elucidating the specific biochemical changes within the nerve cells of the brain that are responsible for the heretofore baffling phenomena of "learning" and remembering.

Muscle tissue Muscle forms a large proportion of the active tissue of the body. In normal adults it is fully two fifths of the body weight; but about half the metabolic, or chemical and physical, activity of the body takes place in our muscles even during rest. When the muscles are contracting, while doing work, fully three fourths of the total metabolism can be assigned to them. The three types of muscle, voluntary, involuntary, and cardiac, differ somewhat in their chemistry, but they have the same general characteristics. In muscle we find the following:

Water
Proteins
  Albumins, globulins, nucleoproteins, myoglobin
  Albuminoids
Lipids
  Cholesterol
  Phospholipids
  Triglycerides
Extractives
  Nonnitrogenous: glycogen, glucose, inositol, hexose phosphates, lactates
  Nitrogenous: creatine, creatine phosphate, creatinine, inosinic acid, adenylic acid, adenosine triphosphate, glutathione, purines, pyrimidines, carnosine, anserine, choline, acetylcholine
Enzymes, hormones, vitamins
Inorganic salts

In adult muscle there is from 72% to 78% water. As in the case of nervous tissue, the water content of the muscle of the young and of the fetus is even higher. Here the similarity ends, however. The solids of muscular tissue are largely protein in nature, whereas those of nervous tissue are largely lipid. The total lipid of muscle amounts to only about 3% and the glycogen less than 1%, but the protein content is about 19% or 20%.

Muscle proteins. Striated muscle is composed of fibers made up of innumerable fibrils arranged parallel to each other and parallel to the axis of the fiber. These fibrils are about 1μ in diameter and are separated from each other by about half that distance. The fibrils consist of two proteins, actin and myosin, that form a complex called *actomyosin.* Other proteins and protein complexes have been described. One is called *tropomyosin,* which is found to a greater degree in smooth muscle. The sarcoplasm that surrounds the fibrils is a mixture of globulin-like and albumin-like proteins. Around and among the muscle cells are found connective tissue fibers that ultimately become attached to the tendon. These consist of collagen, elastin, and some vascular substance and comprise the extracellular proteins, whereas the proteins of the fibrils and sarcoplasm are intracellular.

If fresh muscle is hashed and extracted with dilute potassium chloride at pH 7 to 8, a viscous fluid containing most of the intracellular proteins is obtained. From this the actomyosin can be precipitated by dilution with water or by the addition of certain salts. This protein is present in larger amounts than any of the others. The other intracellular proteins, i.e., proteins of the sarcoplasm, include another globulin, *globulin-X,* which is second largest in amount, an albumin, *myogen,* and small amounts of a second albumin, *myoalbumin.* In addition, *muscle hemoglobin* is present (1 to 3 gm. per 100 gm. of dry weight in human muscle),[14] and this gives a pink hue to some of the extracts. Muscle hemoglobin or myoglobin has been isolated in crystalline form. Its molecular weight, isoelectric point, and absorption bands differ from those of blood hemoglobin. Its affinity for oxygen is greater than that of the hemoglobin of blood, but its function is storage of oxygen within the cell rather than transport.

There appear to be three or possibly four different types of human myoglobin separable by electrophoresis.[15] A remarkable decrease in one type, the Mb_1 *fraction,* has been reported in patients with progressive muscular dystrophy.

Szent-Györgyi[16] presented evidence indicating that actomyosin is a complex of two proteins, *myosin* and *actin.* When these are mixed, they combine and an increase in viscosity is seen. Actin has two forms, a globular and a fibrous form, whereas myosin occurs only in the fibrous form. Together they form threads of actomyosin. Globular actin, or *G-actin,* is a globular shaped protein with a molecular weight of about 60,000. It is a monomer. In a 0.1 M solution and in the presence of ADP and magnesium ions, it polymerizes to form *F-actin,* the fibrous form. F-Actin exists as a fibrous double-strand helix with a molecular weight of over 1,000,000. F-Actin depolymerizes in the presence of ATP to again form G-actin, as a reversible reaction. F-Actin reacts with myosin to form actomyosin. These relationships are shown diagrammatically at the top of the following page.

$$\text{G-Actin} \xrightleftharpoons[\text{ATP}]{\substack{\text{0.1M KCl} \\ \text{ADP, Ca}^{++}}} \text{F-actin;} \quad \text{F-actin + Myosin} \rightleftharpoons \text{Actomyosin}$$

Under the influence of potassium and magnesium ions, ATP (p. 35) is adsorbed upon the actomyosin. When this occurs, the viscosity decreases. An enzyme that decomposes ATP, adenosine triphosphatase (ATPase), seems to be closely associated with actomyosin, or it may even be a part of this unique protein. The effect of the enzyme is to cause a small amount of energy to be released upon the protein, initiating the contraction of the actin fibers. ATP apparently performs a dual role in muscle. When dephosphorylation cannot take place, the presence of this compound keeps the muscle plastic and extensible; but when dephosphorylation can take place, the presence of ATP causes contraction.[17] Subsequently, more energy is released to induce relaxation. This energy is stored until the deposition of the first small amount of energy acts as a trigger to set off the next contraction. In contraction the fibrous actin changes to the globular form, and this causes the actomyosin to curl and become shorter. However, there is no visible folding or wrinkling during contraction, except for connective tissue; the contracting muscle becomes stiffer and resists extension, but no coiling of the fibers can actually be observed. Thus, when a muscle contracts, the following major events *appear* to take place: The detailed steps are somewhat more complex, however, as described in a recent review.[17]

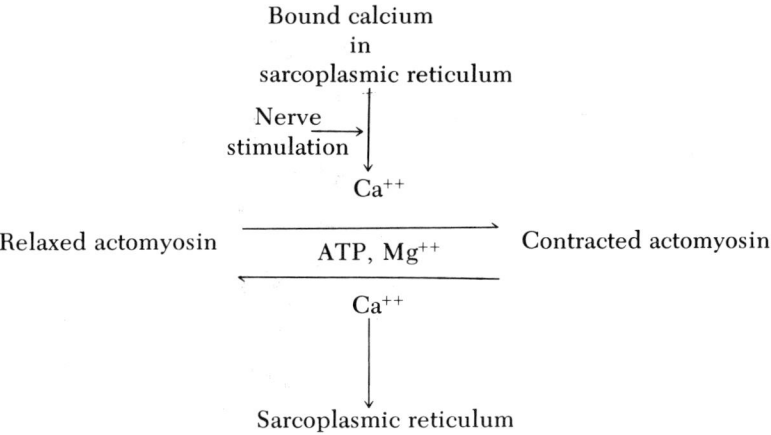

The reverse of this process takes place when relaxation of the contracted actomyosin occurs. Calcium ions return into the sarcoplasmic reticulum. Thus the contraction-relaxation cycle in muscle appears to be regulated by the shuttling of calcium ions out of and into the sarcoplasmic reticulum.

Actin and myosin or actomyosin-like complexes are generally considered the basis for all forms of contractility and motility. There is some evidence for the existence, however, of another protein concerned with maintaining tonus whereas actomyosin is responsible for the twitch and tetanic contractions. This may be tropomyosin.

There is also recent evidence that tropomyosin and/or another protein, troponin, which are associated with actomyosin, control the sensitivity of

563

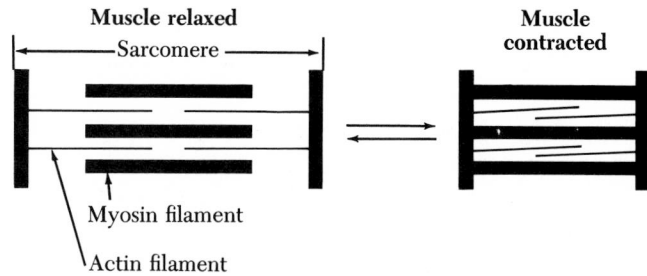

Fig. 18-9. Schematic representation of the "sliding filament" theory of muscle contraction. (Adapted from Huxley, H. E.: Endeavour **15**:177, 1956.)

actomyosin-ATPase to calcium ions. Troponin is believed to interact with calcium ions to modify the active ATPase site of actomyosin.

An important contribution to the understanding of muscle contraction came in 1955 with the postulation of the sliding-filament concept of Hanson and Huxley.[18] In essence, this theory states that during the contraction process, the secondary filaments (actin) are pulled in between the primary filaments (myosin), resulting in a narrowing of the I-band, as shown schematically in Fig. 18-9. This theory appears to be supported by ample experimental evidence and to be well established at the present time[19].

Most recently, Huxley[18] postulated that the actin filaments are pulled by cross-bridges projecting out from the myosin filaments. These projecting cross-bridges have a globular head carrying ATPase and actin binding sites. A slight rotation of the globular head apparently shortens the cross-bridge and pulls the interdigitating actin filaments, thus shortening the sarcomer units of the muscle fibrils. The rotation of the globular head of the myosin molecule is also associated with the splitting of ATP.

The foregoing process requires energy from the breakdown of ATP, with myosin or actomyosin apparently serving as the ATPase. The mechanism of the liberation of this energy as a result of neurogenic stimulation and of its relation to the sliding of the filaments remains to be determined.

Somewhat more chemical concepts of the mechanism of muscle contraction have been proposed. These involve, for example, the loss of hydrogen atoms between hydroxyl and/or sulfhydryl groups and adjacent phosphorus groups, ATP serving to mediate the change. A "looping" and hence shortening of the actomyosin molecule would result. However, there appears to be a lack of evidence to support such theories.

The mechanism of relaxation of the contracted muscle fibril has likewise received considerable attention recently. It is essentially the reverse of the process of contraction. An as yet unidentified relaxing factor[20] as well as ATP appear to be required. The relaxing factor serves to bind calcium, which is released during the process of relaxation. The relaxing factor is derived from the process of relaxation. The relaxing factor is derived from the sarcoplasmic reticulum and serves as type of "calcium pump"[21] to reduce calcium ion levels and reverse the steps just described in actomyosin formation and contraction. This may be shown schematically as follows:

$$\text{Actomyosin-Ca + Relaxing factor} \xrightleftharpoons[\text{ATP}]{\text{ATP}} \text{Actomyosin + Relaxing}$$

complex   (relaxed)   factor–Ca

(contracted)   complex

Muscle lipids. Besides variable amounts of fat, muscle is found to contain small amounts of cholesterol and larger quantities of phospholipid. Here there are definite differences among the three types of muscle. Smooth muscle has the greatest amount of cholesterol, cardiac muscle next, and striated muscle the least. The ratio of phospholipid to cholesterol is high for skeletal and cardiac muscle and low for smooth muscle. These findings indicate that cholesterol has some relation to the spontaneous muscular activity of cardiac and smooth muscle, and phospholipids are involved in some way with the greater energy production of cardiac and striated muscle.

Extractives. If muscle tissue is ground and repeatedly extracted with hot water, a light tan fluid with droplets of fat floating on its surface and particles of coagulated protein suspended is obtained. When this is filtered and concentrated, a dark brown sticky material, commonly known as beef extract, is left. This is composed of all the soluble inorganic salts and all the extractives mentioned on p. 561. The glycogen and some of the other compounds, of course, have been hydrolyzed in the process. Aside from the small amounts of carbohydrate, amino acids, and peptides present, there is little food value in beef extract. As a basis for soups and flavoring for other foods, it adds savor and may reflexly stimulate the flow of digestive juices. Some of the constituents, e.g., inositol, may have specific virtues, but the clear bouillon has little nutritive value.

Some of the individual extractives deserve mention at this point. One of them is inositol, $C_6H_{12}O_6$, or better, $C_6H_6(OH)_6$. There are a number of isomers of inositol in nature. The most important one was renamed *myoinositol* by Lardy, instead of "mesoinositol":

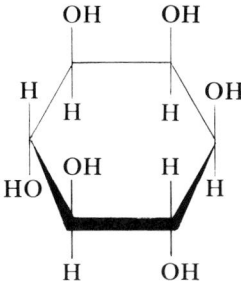

The other isomers differ from this in the arrangement of the hydroxyl groups and hydrogens in space. Although not a sugar, it has a sweet taste. This is a property common to many polyatomic alcohols, including glycerol. It is widely distributed in the plant and animal kingdoms and is sometimes considered part of the vitamin B complex. Inositol is possibly an intermediate between carbohydrates and aromatic substances. This transformation has been accomplished biologically as well as chemically. Isotopic myoinositol also was converted to glucose by phlorizinized rats, although by no means efficiently. In sharks and certain other fish, inositol is stored instead of glycogen. This substance thus may play a role in carbohydrate metabolism, either as a substitute for glycogen or as an intermediate in the transformation of one monosaccharide to another.

Salts of lactic acid are present because they result from carbohydrate breakdown in muscle metabolism. Creatine and creatine phosphate (p. 395) are also involved in muscle metabolism. Their formulas as well as the structurally related creatinine are as follows:

Creatine   Creatine phosphate   Creatinine

Creatine is methylguanidineacetic acid, and creatinine is its anhydride. Creatin phosphate is a very unstable compound. In muscle contraction, creatine phosphate plays an important role, its great instability being partly responsible for the release of energy in a series of reactions (p. 254). In human striated muscle, there are about 350 to 400 mg. of creatine per 100 gm. but only about one-fifth as much in nonstriated muscle. Extremely little creatinine is present — only about 5 to 10 mg. in striated and even less in nonstriated muscle.

Another constituent that is an important cog in the machinery of muscle contraction is ATP. When this compound loses two of its phosphoric acid groups, with the release of energy, adenylic acid results. Inosinic acid is another nucleotide present. The purines and pyrimidines found in extractives are probably decomposition products of nucleotides.

At least three peptides have been isolated from muscle extracts. *Carnosine* is β-alanylhistidine, and *anserine* is β-alanylmethylhistidine. The presence of a β-amino acid is rather extraordinary since the usual amino acids resulting from protein breakdown have the amino group in the α-position. Carnosine has a stimulating action on both the motor and the secretory activities of the intestines, and thus its presence in beef extract may be of some value. The third peptide present in muscle extractives is *glutathione*, a tripeptide, with the composition glutamylcysteinylglycine (p. 70). This compound is a hydrogen acceptor and as such must play a role in tissue reactions. Just what that role is cannot be said with certainty as yet. It is found in many tissues other than muscle, especially liver, red blood cells, brain, and kidney. It is also present in the lens of the eye and is reduced in amount when cataract occurs. *Carnitine*, a betaine, is also a muscle extractive and is also found in most tissues. Its formula is as follows:

Although its function in muscle is unknown, carnitine is an essential food factor for the yellow mealworm. A recent study suggested that carnitine may play a role in the oxidation of fatty acids in muscle tissue, possibly by facilitating their transfer to fatty acid oxidation sites (p. 305).

Other constituents. Other constituents include glycogen (0.5% to 1%), important as a source of energy for the formation of ATP, traces of free amino acids, a number of enzymes, and inorganic ions, including potassium, magnesium, and sodium as the principal cations in descending amount, and phosphate, sulfate, and bicarbonate as the main anions similarly.

BIOCHEMISTRY OF MALIGNANT NEOPLASMS (CANCER)

Cancer may be defined as a neoplastic growth that has the ability to invade surrounding tissues and be disseminated via the bloodstream and lymphatics. Numerous biochemical studies[22] have been undertaken in an attempt to define biochemical alterations associated with the development of cancerous changes (carcinogenesis), biochemical characterization or differentiation of cancerous from normal tissues, and systematic changes in the tumor host.

Carcinogenesis. In 1775, Pott drew attention to the fact that chimney sweeps frequently had cancer of the scrotum, a result of contact of the abraded skin with chimney soot. This was later correlated with coal tar, which was definitely established as a substance capable of causing cancer in man. In the early part of the twentieth century it was shown that frequent application of gasworks tar to the rabbit's ear produces cancer. Following this, Cook investigated the effects of many organic compounds, some of which are present in tar but many of which are not found in nature or in industrial products. Soon other laboratories joined in the search; today many definite chemical compounds with carcinogenic properties are known. At present no definite relation can be shown between chemical constitution and cancer-producing properties. The only active compound that has been isolated from coal tar is benzpyrene. One of the most powerful carcinogens thus far discovered is methylcholanthrene. It is particularly interesting from a biochemical standpoint, because it was synthesized by Fieser, using cholic acid as a starting point. Cholic acid (p. 686) is a bile acid, as well as a part of the molecule of the other bile acids. The relation of this to cholesterol and to one of the sex hormones is shown in the following series of formulas.

Cholesterol

567

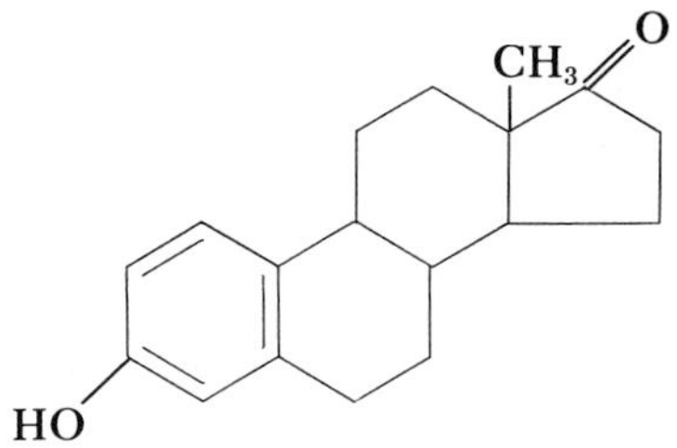

Estrone

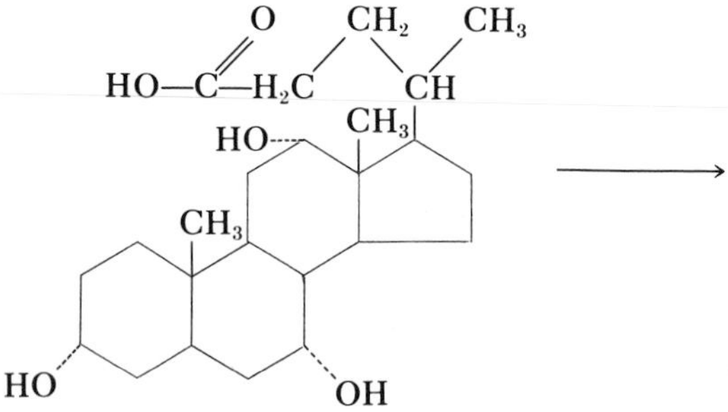

Cholic acid

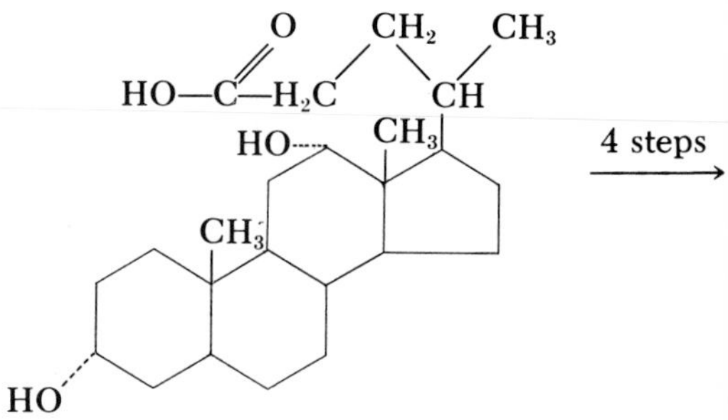

Deoxycholic acid

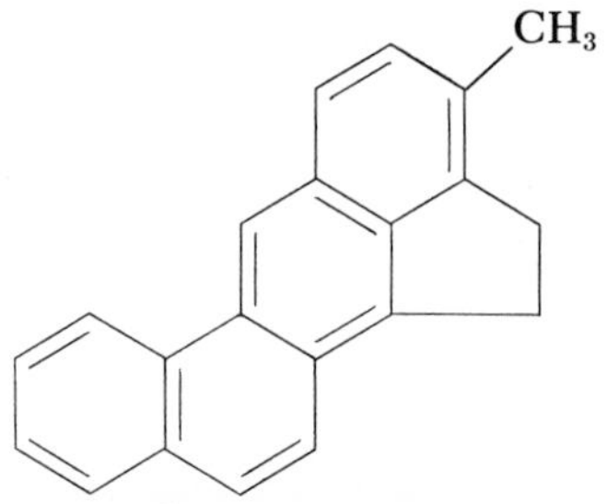

4 steps

Methylcholanthrene
(extremely potent)

Methylcholanthrene, cholanthrene, and 3,4-benzpyrene are powerful carcinogenic agents when administered to experimental animals.

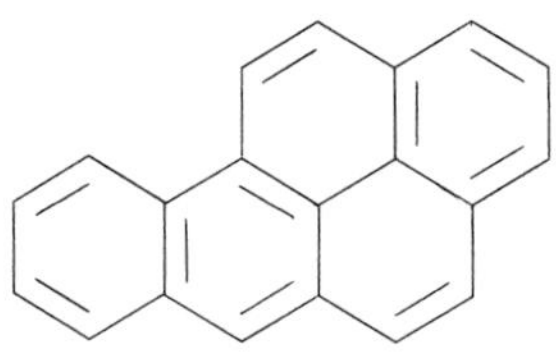

3,4-Benzpyrene 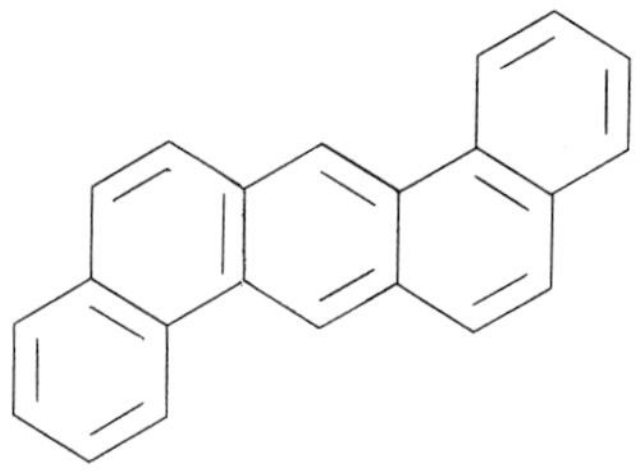   **1,2,5,6-Dibenzanthracene**

Some instructive studies have been carried out with 1,2,5,6-dibenzanthracene, which is also carcinogenic for certain experimental animals. Definite amounts of this, incorporated in cholesterol pellets, were inserted under the skin. After tumors had appeared, the pellets were removed, and, upon analysis, minute amounts of the causative agent were found in the tumors; but after repeated transplanting, the tumors were found to be still cancerous in the fifth or sixth generation, at which point the tissue contained none of the originally used substance. In other words, although these toxic substances *initiate* tumor growth, the cells themselves are cancerous and continue their unrestrained capacity for growth independently.

It was also found that some of the carcinogenic compounds are estrogenic (p. 498) when suitably tested. On the other hand, in mice and guinea pigs the estrogenic hormones may produce cancer. The latter effect does not hold true for all species. It apparently does not occur in human beings, since thousands of parenteral injections of estrogens are made daily and no increase in cancer incidence has been reported. However, one interesting development in the study of prostatic tumors relates to another sex hormone. The normal development of the prostate gland apparently depends on hormones elaborated by the testes. The prostate regresses and atrophy of the epithelium occurs when castration is performed. In animals under such circumstances, administration of the male hormone causes regeneration of the prostate. These facts led to the idea of treating prostatic tumors by deprivation of male hormones. This was tested by two methods: (1) surgical removal of the testes or (2) administration of estrogens, since, in a general way, estrogens and androgens are antagonistic. The results were favorable in a number of instances, so again we have evidence of the biochemical nature of the factors involved in tumor causation and possible tumor control.

Species differences also hold for some of the carcinogenic compounds already discussed. None of the *synthetic* compounds seems to affect primates, and rabbits are almost immune. It is possible that some mechanism for detoxicating the compounds is operative. In the rabbit, dibenzanthracene is hydroxylated and excreted in the urine. When this dihydroxy compound is administered to a mouse, which is susceptible to dibenzanthracene, no tumor results. If mice could hydroxylate the compound, they also, presumably, would be immune to its effects.

That vitamins and enzymes may be concerned in protection against carcinogenic compounds came out of the studies of Rhoads, du Vigneaud, and others. A dye, *p*-dimethylaminoazobenzene or "butter yellow," produces cancer of the liver in rats on a deficient diet. Supplements of yeast and casein to such diets have a pronounced protective action. This led to a search for one of the B-complex vitamins as an effective anticarcinogenic agent, another being presumably a peptide. Riboflavin was found to be quite potent, especially in combination with casein. Biotin was another possibility, but it was found to have just the opposite action; i.e., when biotin is added to a highly protective diet, butter yellow is more potent than without it.

Industrial factors in human carcinogenesis. There has been a considerable rise in the number and variety of occupational cancers, paralleling the enormous modern industrial expansion. Many of the agents and physical factors causing them are known, but it is safe to assume that many more are still unknown, particularly those carcinogens of low potency. A partial list of *environmental carcinogens* and their sites of action in man follows: anthracene (crude), arsenic, burns (thermic), mineral oil (crude), paraffin oil (crude), pitch, radioactive substances, roentgen rays, soot, spindle oil, tar, and ultraviolet light, all acting on the skin and appendages; chromates and radioactive substances, affecting the respiratory system; β-naphthylamine and schistosomiasis, affecting the urinary system; benzol, acting on the reticuloendothelial system; radioactive substances and roentgen rays, also acting on the reticuloendothelial system and on mesenchymal tissue; and arsenic, mineral oil (crude), pitch, and ultraviolet light, affecting the eye and surrounding tissues. Currently, there is considerable interest in the alleged relationship between excessive cigarette smoking and the incidence of lung cancer in man.

Chemistry of tumor tissue Greenstein made the following generalizations regarding the chemical pattern of normal tissues and of transplanted tumor tissues:

(a) Each normal tissue is characterized by the possession of an individual pattern of enzymic activity which may serve to distinguish it from all other tissues.

(b) Tumors have qualitatively the same enzymes as normal tissues.

(c) The enzymatic pattern of a tumor is largely independent of its age, of its growth rate, and of the strain of animal in which it is grown.

(d) The range of activity of each enzyme and of concentration of such components as the vitamins is much narrower among tumors than among normal tissues; *i.e.*, tumors possess a more uniform and less diverse chemical pattern than normal tissues.

(e) When a normal tissue becomes neoplastic many of the specific functional activities markedly decrease or are lost altogether.

(f) The range of values for the tumors is usually between the extremes of the corresponding values for normal tissues. . . . It cannot be said, therefore, that "tumors are lower (or higher) in activity than normal tissues," but only that their activity is lower (or higher) in respect to certain specified normal tissues. Tumors do not stand outside the metabolic range of normal tissues.°

Thus, mouse and rat tumors have a relatively elevated content of dehydropeptidase-I, benzoylarginine amidase, and xanthine dehydrogenase and a diminished activity of catalase, cytochrome oxidase, alkaline phosphatase, esterase, cystine desulfurase, and dehydropeptidase-II. In adenosarcoma of the colon, the following enzyme activities are higher than in the adjacent uninvolved tissues: lactic dehydrogenase, malic dehydrogenase, and enolase.[23]

It should be emphasized, however, that, as yet, no biochemical representation of the essential nature of cancer tissue has been defined. In addition, there is evidence of considerable biochemical and biologic variation between individual cancer tissues of the same sites of origin. Nevertheless, attention has been directed to nucleoprotein alterations, since these compounds apparently play a dominant role in metabolism. Therapeutic benefit might accrue if we could interfere in a selective manner with some of the steps in nucleoprotein synthesis in tumor cells. To some extent, this is true. Urethane, mustards, anifols (antimetabolites of folic acid), and 6-mercaptopurine interfere with nucleoprotein synthesis; and the tumor destruction caused by these agents seems to parallel this biochemical activity. However, these therapeutic effects might be secondary to the interference with anabolic synthesis, the primary action being something quite different.

Moreover, in studying the biochemistry of tumors, we must consider the nucleoproteins from another standpoint, i.e., in reference to tumor viruses. Viruses are known to be nucleoprotein in nature, and the implication of viruses as specific carcinogens is now firmly established, thanks to the work

---

° From Greenstein, J. P.: Biochemistry of cancer, New York, 1947, Academic Press, Inc.

of Rous, Bittner, Stanley, and others. Among the tumors known to have such a causative factor are rabbit papilloma, chicken sarcoma, mouse mammary carcinoma, and, most recently, a type of bone cancer in mice. Indeed, many investigators in the field accept the theory that most, if not all, cancers are caused by viruses.

The cell appears to defend itself ordinarily against viruses by means of a protein called *interferon*.[24] Indeed, this protein protects the cell against all foreign acids and is a second defense against viruses, the first being the well-known immune reaction.

Systemic changes in the cancer host. A wide variety of systemic alterations occur in the host coincidentally with malignant neoplasms. Some of these

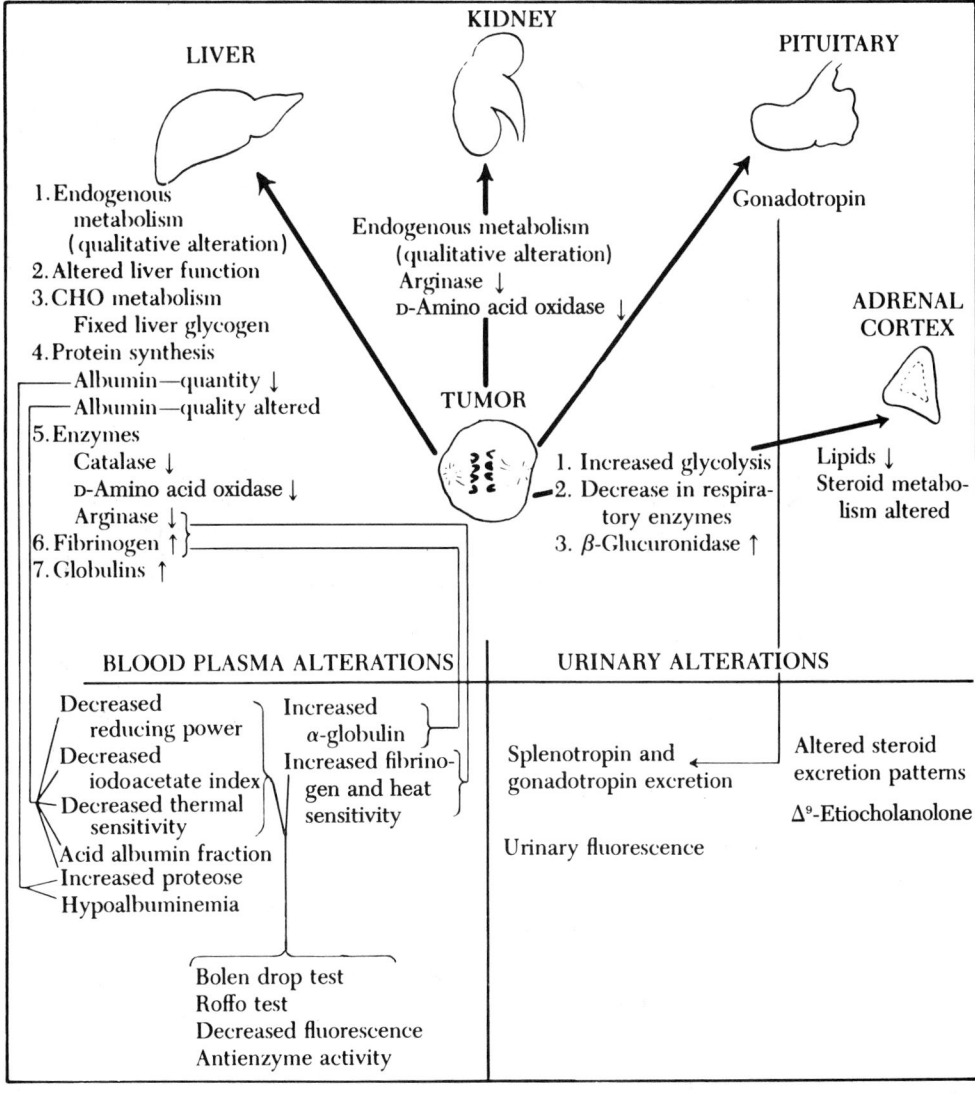

Fig. 18-10. Systemic effects of malignant tumors. (From Black, M. M., and Speer, F. D.: Amer. J. Clin. Path. **20**:446, 1950.)

changes are depicted in Fig. 18-10. Although the changes are not specific for cancer, they do provide evidence of the complexity of the systemic alterations involved and indicate the need for a more adequate study of cancer as a systemic disease.

References

GENERAL

Bartley, W.: The biochemistry of tissues, New York, 1968, John Wiley & Sons, Inc.

Bibby, B. G.: Nutrition and dental health, Nutr. News 30:1, 1967.

Bjorksten, J.: The cross-linkage theory of aging, J. Amer. Geriat. Soc. 16:408, 1968.

Bogoch, S.: The biochemistry of memory, New York, 1968, Oxford University Press, Inc.

Bourne, G. H.: The structure and function of muscle, New York, 1960, Academic Press, Inc.

Bourne, G. H.: The structure and function of nervous tissue, New York, 1968, Academic Press, Inc., vol. 1.

Brimacombe, J. S., and Webber, J. M.: Mucopolysaccharides, Amsterdam, 1964, Elsevier Publishing Co., vol. 6.

Busch, H, editor: Methods in cancer research, New York, 1967-1968, Academic Press, Inc.

Elliott, K. A. C., Page, I. H., and Quastel, J. H.: Neurochemistry, ed. 2, Springfield, Ill., 1962, Charles C Thomas, Publisher.

Flexner, L. B.: Dissection of memory in mice with antibiotics, Amer. Sci. 56:52, 1968.

Glassman, E.: Biochemistry of learning, Ann. Rev. Biochem. 38:605, 1969.

Harris, W. H., and Heaney, R. P.: Skeletal renewal and metabolic bone disease, New Eng. J. Med. 280:193, 1969.

Lajtha, A., editor: Handbook of neurochemistry, New York, 1969, Plenum Publishing Corp.

McLean, F. C., and Urist, M. R.: Bone—fundamentals of the physiology of skeletal tissue, ed. 3, Chicago, 1968, University of Chicago Press.

Meyer, K.: Chemistry of the mesodermal ground substance, Harvey Lect. 51:88, 1955.

Rodahl, K., Nicholson, J. T., and Brown, E., editors: Bone as a tissue, New York, 1961, McGraw-Hill Book Co.

Rothman, S.: Physiology and biochemistry of the skin, Chicago, 1954, University of Chicago Press.

Savara, B. S.: Nutrition and dental health, Nutr. News 31:1, 1968.

Seifer, S., and Gallup, P. M.: The structure of proteins. In Neurath, H., editor:

The proteins — composition, structure and function, New York, 1966, Academic Press, Inc., vol. 4.

Westenholme, G. E. W., and O'Connor, M., editors: Chemistry and biology of the mucopolysaccharides, Boston, 1958, Little, Brown & Co.

SPECIAL

1. Fraser, R. D. B.: Sci. Amer. 221:87, 1969.
2. Caruthers, C.: Proc. Soc. Exp. Biol. Med. 115:214, 1964.
3. Gross, J.: Sci. Amer. 204:120, 1961.
4. Gustavson, K. H.: Fed. Proc. 23:613, 1964.
5. Miller, E. J., and Martin, G. R.: Clin. Orthop. 59:195, 1968.
6. McConnell, D., et al.: Science 133:281, 1961.
7. Saxen, L.: Science 149:870, 1965.
8. McLean, R. C., and Urist, M. R.: Bone, an introduction to the physiology of skeletal tissue, Chicago, 1955, University of Chicago Press.
9. Lavine, L. S., et al.: Bull. N. Y. Acad. Med. 39:269, 1963.
10. McClure, F. J.: Science 144:1336, 1964; J. Dent. Res. 42:693, 1963.
11. Roberts, E., and Baxter, C. F.: Ann. Rev. Biochem. 32:513, 1963.
12. Pitts, F. N.: Sci. Amer. 220:69, 1969.
13. Eccles, J.: Sci. Amer. 212:56, 1965.
14. Akeson, A., et al.: Acta Med. Scand. 183:307, 1968.
15. Miyoshi, K., et al.: Science 159:736, 1968.
16. Szent-Györgyi, A.: Chemistry of muscle contraction, New York, 1947, Academic Press, Inc.; Science 128:699, 1958.
17. Davies, R. E.: Essays in Biochemistry 1:29, 1965.
18. Huxley, H. E.: Endeavour 15:177, 1956; Sci. Amer. 213:18, 1965; Science 164:1356, 1969.
19. Young, M.: Ann. Rev. Biochem. 38:913, 1969.
20. Parker, C. J., Jr., and Gergely, J.: J. Biol. Chem. 236:411, 1961.
21. Gergely, J.: Fed. Proc. 23:885, 1964.
22. Busch, H., and Starbuck, W. C.: Ann. Rev. Biochem. 33:519, 1964.
23. Ames, I. H., et al.: Proc. Soc. Exp. Biol. Med. 116:1013, 1964.
24. Isaacs, A.: Sci. Amer. 209:46, 1963.

CHAPTER 19

BLOOD

The cells of the tissues of the body are in contact with body fluids, which, in turn, are in equilibrium with the fluid portion of the blood. In the course of the development of the higher animals, this relation of the organism to its environment was even more direct. Early unicellular organisms were surrounded by seawater, and probably their mineral content was quite similar to it, qualitatively and quantitatively. Lakes that are of Pre-Cambrian origin have a far different distribution of ions from what is found in ocean water today, and this, together with other data, indicates that seawater in early geologic ages differed from modern seawater considerably. Thus potassium was probably present in greater concentration than sodium, whereas the reverse is true in present-day seawater.

As time went on, the electrolyte content of ocean water gradually changed because of the weathering of rocks, solution of minerals, precipitation of salts, and consequent shifting of equilibria. Such changes in the environment would make stabilization of conditions within the cell difficult. Apparently evolution provided a mechanism for maintaining internal equilibrium, despite a constantly changing external medium. This change was evidenced by an increase in sodium ions and a decrease in potassium ions. Although both sodium and potassium salts were deposited on land by rainfall, wind, and inundations, the sodium salts were washed back in larger proportion than the potassium salts because the latter formed insoluble compounds with silicon and aluminum and living organisms retained more potassium than sodium. Thus seawater gradually changed until, in early Cambrian times, when many multicellular organisms had evolved and the vascular tube had been sealed, the seawater, and hence the circulating tissue fluids, contained more sodium than potassium, less calcium, and still less magnesium. This early Cambrian seawater closely resembled modern mammalian blood serum in electrolyte content.[1]

Functions   Blood has a multitude of functions, all of which are highly necessary to health and to life itself. This is so apparent to the layman that he often becomes unduly alarmed at the loss of even a small quantity of it. Since blood makes up one eleventh to one twelfth of the body weight, evidently a person weighing only 120 lb. has about 10 lb. of blood and the loss of a pint (approximately a pound) would not be very serious. Indeed, thousands of persons have donated considerable amounts of blood for whole-blood transfusions and for the production of plasma. However, although single donations do not ordinarily cause more than slight discomfort, they should not be repeated too frequently, and evidence of complete blood regeneration should be required.

Among the chief functions of blood are the following:

1. Transportation of foods, or the products resulting from their digestion, from the intestines and chyle ducts to the tissues, from the liver to the tissues and back to the liver, and from one tissue to another
2. Exchange of the respiratory gases between the lungs and the tissues
3. Transporation of waste products arising in metabolism, such as urea and uric acid, to the kidneys, skin, intestines, liver for excretion
4. Distribution of hormones, enzymes, vitamins, and other substances, by which the effective agent is brought almost instantaneously to the organ or tissue to be stimulated or inhibited
5. Protection against microorganisms (leukocytes, antitoxins, other factors aid in combating these foreign invaders)
6. Aid in acid-base balance, electrolyte balance, and water balance
7. Heat regulation of the body, largely by shifting to or from the surface of the body
8. Prevention of excessive hemorrhage by coagulation

Some of these functions have been discussed in other chapters and one (5) belongs properly in the province of microbiology.

General composition Circulating blood consists of a fluid portion (plasma) and the formed elements. The plasma constitutes 55% to 60% by volume of whole blood. The formed elements are the red blood cells, or erythrocytes; the white blood cells, or leukocytes; and the blood platelets. The average number of erythrocytes is normally 5,400,000 per cubic millimeter for men and 4,900,000 for women, but higher figures are not uncommon. There is a slight fluctuation in the number of erythrocytes during the day: it is lowest during sleep, rises on awakening, and continues to rise during the rest of the day. Persons living at high altitudes usually have a higher erythrocyte count than do those living at sea level. High erythrocyte counts also follow muscular exercise, emotional excitement, and increased atmospheric temperature. These are temporary changes, resulting from a flow of concentrated blood from the spleen. Any condition that tends to lower the oxygen content of the blood causes an increase in the number of erythrocytes. On the other hand, any condition that increases the oxygen of the blood causes a decrease in erythrocyte count. High barometric pressure is an example. Pathologically, increases and decreases in the number of erythrocytes frequently occur. A condition in which there is an increased erythrocyte count is called a *polycythemia;* an *anemia* is a condition in which there is either a lowered count or a subnormal concentration of hemoglobin.

If blood is removed from an artery or vein, it clots or coagulates in a few minutes. The whole mass becomes gelatinous. If it is left undisturbed, a clear straw-colored fluid is gradually squeezed out; this is *serum*. In this case, the formed elements have become enmeshed in the clot. Blood *plasma* may be separated from the formed elements if, immediately after the blood is obtained, it is placed in paraffin-lined vessels and centrifuged in a cold atmosphere. A fluid that is also clear and straw colored is obtained; this fluid clots in a short time, gradually squeezing out serum from the clot in the process.

Whole blood − Formed elements = Plasma

Whole blood − (formed elements + clotting factors) = Serum

Plasma − Clotting factors = Serum

Clotting, of course, is a process that protects the individual from excessive loss of blood.

For purposes of chemical analysis or other studies, it is often inconvenient to have the blood clot; therefore methods to prevent clotting are used. Whipping or defibrinating blood accomplishes this. Blood is beaten with feathers, or twigs, or is shaken in a bottle with glass beads. The blood fibrin, which forms the clot, clings to the foreign object and the fluid blood remains. However, this is not really preventing clotting but causing clotting and removing the fibrin conveniently. Defibrinated blood is whole blood minus the clotting factors. Addition of anticoagulants, e.g., soluble oxalates, citrates, or fluorides, to blood as it flows from a blood vessel prevents it from clotting in vitro by precipitating calcium or changing it to an un-ionized form, since calcium ions are necessary for clotting. Hirudin, a substance derived from the salivary gland of the medicinal leech, and heparin, from liver and other tissues, prevent blood from clotting even if injected into the animal. The injection of toxic doses of protein digests (proteoses and peptones) likewise prevents the blood from clotting, but these digests do not act on blood in vitro. As indicated above, both paraffin-lined containers and cold inhibit, but do not prevent, clotting.

Physical characteristics   Arterial blood is a bright crimson in color; venous blood is a darker red but is not purple or blue. Blood is more viscid than water, the viscosity being due to the many corpuscles present and to the high protein content. The pH is approximately 7.4, with a normal range from 7.3 to 7.5. The mechanisms for maintaining this constancy of reaction are varied and will be taken up in Chapter 20. The specific gravity of blood ranges from 1.035 to 1.075. This may be determined clinically by Hammerschlag's method, which consists simply of letting drops of blood fall into mixtures of varying proportions of chloroform and benzene, or xylene and bromobenzene, or methyl salicylate and mineral oil. If the drop does not rise or sink in one mixture, it evidently has the same specific gravity as that mixture, which can easily be determined by a hydrometer.

A convenient, practical modification of the falling-drop method for determining the specific gravity of whole blood or plasma, using solutions of copper sulfate of increasing concentrations, has been described.[2] The method also permits estimation of the hemoglobin content of whole blood and the protein concentration in the plasma (p. 579).

Table 19-1. Composition of normal human blood (postabsorptive state)*

Whole blood	Grams percent
Total solids	19–23
Water	77–81
Hemoglobin	
Adult males	15.8
Adult females	13.8
Children	12.0
Total nitrogen	3.5

	Volumes percent
Carbon dioxide content (venous)	50–60
Carbon dioxide content (arterial)	45–55
Oxygen capacity	16–24
Oxygen content (venous)	10–18
Oxygen content (arterial)	15–23

	Milligrams per 100 ml.
Uric acid (serum)	3–6
Creatinine	1–2
Creatine	3–7
Glucose	70–120 (depending on method used)
Total combined fatty acids	300–400
Cholesterol	150–190
Total ketone bodies (as acetone)	1–5
Iron	52
Nonprotein nitrogen	25–35
Urea	22–33
Urea nitrogen	10–15
Amino acid nitrogen	5–8
Ammonia nitrogen	0.1–0.2
Undetermined nitrogen	4–10
Lecithin (as lipid phosphorus)	5–12
Lecithin (as lecithin)	125–300
Chloride (as NaCl)	450–500
Lactic acid	5–20

Plasma	Milligrams per 100 ml.	Milliequivalents per liter
Fibrinogen	200–400	
Total lipids	500–600	
Neutral fat	80–200	
Inorganic phosphorus		
Adults	3–4.5	1.7–2.5
Children	4–6	2.2–3.3
Chloride (as NaCl)	580–630	
(as Na)	226–248	99–108
(as Cl)	352–382	99–108
Carbon dioxide capacity	55–75 vol.%	20–33

Serum	Percent
Total protein	6.5–8.5
Albumin	3.6–5.4
Globulin	1.5–3.4

*Revised from Kleiner, I. S., and Dotti, L. B.: Laboratory instructions in biochemistry, ed. 7, St. Louis, 1966, The C. V. Mosby Co.

Table 19-1. Composition of normal human blood (postabsorptive state)*—cont'd

	Milligrams per 100 ml.	Milliequivalents per liter
Bilirubin, indirect	0.2–0.8	
Calcium	9–11	4.5–5.5
Cholesterol, total	150–300	
Cholesterol, ester	105–210	
Ester:total (ratio)	0.7	
Creatinine	1.0–1.8	
Iron	0.028–0.210	
Sulfate, inorganic (as S)	0.9–1.1	0.6–1.1
Phosphate	3–4.5	1–2
Magnesium	1.0–3.0	0.9–2.5
Potassium	16–22	4.1–5.6
Sodium	310–333	135–145
Uric acid	3.0–5.0	

Erythrocytes	Percent
Hemoglobin	35

	Milligrams per 100 ml.
Potassium	420
Sodium	25
Magnesium	6.6
Calcium	Small amount

Enzymes	Units per 100 ml. serum
Amylase, Somogyi	80 to 160
Acid phosphatase, Gutman	0.5–2.0
Acid phosphatase, King	1.4–4.5
Alkaline phosphatase (Bodansky units)	
Adult	2.0–3.5
Child	5.0–14.0
Alkaline phosphatase (King units)	
Adult	5.0–10.0
Child	15.0–20.0
Cholinesterase	39–51
Glutamate oxaloacetate transaminase	
Adult	4–40 per ml.
Infants	13–120 per ml.
Glutamate pyruvate transaminase	
Adults	5–30 per ml.
Infants	12–90 per ml.
Lactic dehydrogenase	200–690 per ml.
Phosphoglucomutase	19–84
Phosphohexoisomerase	14–28

Hormones	
ACTH	15 μg. per 100 ml. blood
Androgen	2.8 mg. per 100 ml. plasma
Corticosteroids	0.25 mg. per 100 ml. plasma
17-Hydroxycorticosteroids	6–44 μg. per 100 ml. plasma
Estrogen (as estradiol) during pregnancy	0.2–0.5 μg. per 100 ml. blood
Progesterone during pregnancy	530 μg. per 100 ml. plasma
Thyroxine	6–12 μg. per 100 ml. serum

Continued.

Table 19-1. Composition of normal human blood (postabsorptive state)* — cont'd

Vitamins	
A (as carotene)	120 μg. per 100 ml. blood
B₁₂	350–750 μg. per 100 ml. serum
Biotin	1.2 μg. per 100 ml. blood
Ascorbic acid	0.6 mg. per 100 ml. blood
	0.1–1.7 mg. per 100 ml. plasma
D (as D₂)	2.8 μg. per 100 ml. plasma
E	0.9–1.9 mg. per 100 ml. plasma
Niacin	0.6 mg. per 100 ml. blood
Pantothenic acid	30 μg. per 100 ml. blood
Folic acid	3.4 μg. per 100 ml. blood
Riboflavin	2.6–3.7 μg. per 100 ml. plasma
Thiamine	7.6–8.9 μg. per 100 ml. blood
Thiamine + Cocarboxylase	10 μg. per 100 ml. blood

Miscellaneous constituents†	*Milligrams per 100 ml.*
Bromide (serum)	0.252
Copper (plasma or serum)	0.086–0.161
Fluorine (whole blood)	0.28
Iodine (protein bound) (plasma or serum)	0.006–0.008
Lead (whole blood)	0.009–0.05
Manganese (whole blood)	0.005–0.02
Sialic acid (serum)	60.0‡ (adults)
	40.0‡ (infants)
Silica (soluble) (whole blood)	1.5 (as SiO₃)
Silica (total) (whole blood)	9.0 (as SiO₃)
Zinc (plasma or serum)	0.12–0.48

†Krebs, H. A.: Ann. Rev. Biochem. 19:409, 1950.
‡Higher values found in rickets, severe burns, rheumatic disease, tuberculosis.

When blood is removed from the circulation, the erythrocytes slowly settle out if clotting is prevented. The rate of settling, or *sedimentation rate*, is frequently determined for clinical purposes. Erythrocytes from men generally sediment more slowly than do those from women. Newborn infant red cells sediment very slowly. The sedimentation rate is markedly increased in menstruation and in normal pregnancy. Increased rates are found pathologically in septicemia and pulmonary tuberculosis. The probable explanation for the increased sedimentation rate is a clumping or agglutination of erythrocytes due to an increased globulin and fibrinogen content of the plasma. An increase in the ratio of cholesterol to phospholipid in the plasma also increases the sedimentation rate.

Quantitative composition. Average values or usual range of the principal constituents of blood of the normal human adult in the postabsorptive state are given in Table 19-1. The values are given for whole blood, for plasma, and for serum and in the units commonly used by clinical laboratories. Since many of these values vary after meals, it is desirable that the subject studied be in a postabsorptive state, usually 8 to 12 hours after the last meal. This is the procedure commonly followed in clinical laboratories for diagnostic purposes.

The quantitative composition of the blood of a normal human subject varies with respect to not only the types and amounts of food ingested but also the age, sex, and activity of the subject and other factors. The range may deviate markedly from normal in a number of diseases. It has been said that the blood "mirrors" metabolic and pathologic events in the cells and tissues of the body. This fact is of great practical importance today in modern medical diagnosis and therapy. Examples of the relationship appear repeatedly throughout this text.

BLOOD PLASMA

Blood plasma is a light straw-colored fluid with a specific gravity from 1.015 to 1.035. The higher specific gravity of whole blood must be ascribed to the erythrocytes, whose specific gravity is about 1.090. As previously stated, the specific gravity of plasma is related to the protein content, and an approximation of the total protein of plasma may be obtained by determining the specific gravity and applying the following formula[2]:

Percentage of total protein = 373 (specific gravity, 1.007)

Human plasma contains from 90% to 92% water. Blood owes much of its physiologic importance to high water content, for not only is water the medium in which the water-soluble and water-dispersible substances are carried; it also is needed for maintaining blood pressure, osmotic conditions, and heat regulation. As regards heat regulation, water has (1) high specific heat, (2) high heat conductivity, and (3) high latent heat of evaporation. Thus, water has great heat-storage properties; i.e., more calories of heat are required to raise the temperature of water a given number of degrees than for most fluids. Its high conductivity results in the rapid removal of heat from the interior of the body by conduction through the water in all the soft tissues and body fluids, as well as in the blood. Finally, a great deal of heat is lost through evaporation from skin and lungs, the water coming largely from the blood plasma.

Proteins Proteins form most of the solid matter of plasma. They total between 6% and 8% of the plasma. They include fibrinogen, albumin, and globulin. The globulin fraction consists of more than one individual protein. The approximate concentrations of these in human plasma, as determined by electrophoretic and chemical analyses, are shown in Table 19-2.

The globulin fraction of the plasma proteins contains a number of components that are of great and varied physiologic importance (Table 19-3). Interesting is the fact that the majority of the plasma proteins appear to be conjugated, e.g., glycoproteins, lipoproteins.

Fibrinogen Fibrinogen is the protein that, when blood is shed, is converted to fibrin, the basis of the blood clot. It resembles the globulins in most of the properties but has a few different precipitation reactions. Like globulins, it is precipitated by half saturation with ammonium sulfate; but globulins require full saturation with sodium chloride, whereas fibrinogen requires only half satura-

579

Table 19-2. Distribution of human plasma protein components in normal adults as determined by electrophoretic and sodium sulfate fractionation[*]

	Electrophoretic fractionation[†]			*Sodium sulfate fractionation*	
Component	*Percentage of total protein*[‡]	*Concentration (grams/100 ml.)*	*Component*	*Percentage of total protein*[†]	*Concentration (grams/100 ml.)*
Total protein		6.03–6.72	Total protein		6.0 –8.0
Albumin	55	3.32–4.04	Albumin	67	4.3 –5.0
Globulin					
Alpha-1	5	0.31–0.32	Pseudoglobulin-II	7	0.2 –0.8
Alpha-2	9	0.48–0.52			
Beta	13	0.78–0.81	Pseudoglobulin-I	19	0.8 –1.9
Gamma	11	0.66–0.74	Euglobulin	4	0.1 –0.4
Fibrinogen	7	0.34–0.43	Fibrinogen	3	0.17–0.25
Total	45	2.71–2.72	Total globulin	33	1.9 –3.3

[*] From Metcoff, J., and Stare, F. J.: New Eng. J. Med. **236**:26, 1947.
[†] The distribution of components in normal pooled human plasma as derived from electrophoretic analysis is based on the total refractive increment contributed by each component. The quantitative amount of each fraction is based on nitrogen analyis, assuming the conventional conversion factor of 6.25. A further assumption tentatively assigns a similar refractive increment per gram of nitrogen to all components. Data derived from several studies. Fractionation in diethylbarbiturate buffer at pH 8.6.
[‡] Percentage of total protein represents an approximation.

tion. It is formed in the liver. Animals deprived of their liver by surgical operation (hepatectomy) rapidly lose the fibrinogen of their blood. The fibrinogen content of plasma increases when inflammatory or infectious processes exist, and during menstruation and pregnancy.

The liver is also the site of formation of the albumin, prothrombin, and probably more than 80% of the globulins. Normally the plasma proteins are broken down or catabolized continuously, but rather slowly, and the rebuilding process or anabolism keeps pace with this, so the level of these proteins remains constant. Similarly, the fetal plasma proteins, except γ-globulin, are all synthesized in the fetal liver. The γ-globulin is probably derived from the mother.[3]

Recent studies[4] have shown that fetal serum proteins, like fetal hemoglobin (as will be discussed later), differ immunochemically from those of the adult. An α_1-fetoglobulin or fetuin, discovered first in calf serum, is an example. Fetuin comprises nearly half the total plasma protein of calf serum. It is a glycoprotein with a molecular weight of about 48,000. It is present in bovine fetal serum until the third trimester of pregnancy, when it gradually decreases and is almost absent at birth. Its function is unknown, but it promotes growth of the mammalian cells in tissue culture and may increase the adhesion of tissue culture cells to a glass surface.

Albumin and globulins Albumin and globulins comprise most of the proteins of blood plasma. The relative concentrations of these two proteins, along with the total protein content, are of great importance because under normal conditions the colloidal

Table 19-3. Properties and functions of some purified plasma globulins

Fraction	Component	Approximate amount (grams/100 ml.)	Molecular weight	Iso-electric point	Carbo-hydrate (percent)	Function
α_1	Lipoprotein	0.3–0.8	200,000	5.2	1.5	Transport of fat, steroids, phospholipids, carotenoids
	Orosomucoid	0.05–0.15	44,100	3.0	41.4	? ?
	Thyroxine-binding protein	0.0001	50,000	—	—	Transport of thyroxine
	Transcortin	0.0007	—	—	14.1	Transport of cortisol
α_2	Glycoproteins	0.8	300,000	4.9	16.0	? ?
	Mucoproteins	0.5	—	4.9	13.0	? ?
	Haptoglobin	0.1–0.22	85,000	4.1	19.3	Transport of free hemoglobin from destroyed red blood cells
	Lipoprotein	0.2	5,000,000 to 20,000,000	—	1.7	Transport of lipids and triglycerides
	Ceruloplasmin	0.02–0.5	150,000	4.4	8.0	Contains (transports?) copper
	Prothrombin (bovine)	0.01	68,900	4.2	11.0	Proenzyme of thrombin
	Angiotensinogen	—	—	—		Precursor of angiotensin
	Erythropoietin	<0.006	60,000	3.3		Erythropoietic hormone
β_1	Lipoprotein	0.4–1.0	Up to 3,000,000	5.5	1.8	Transport of various lipids
	Hemopexin	0.1	80,000	—	22.6	Heme-binding globulin
	Plasminogen	0.03	143,000	5.6	—	Profibrinolysin
	Fibrinogen	0.3	341,000	5.8	2.5	Coagulation factor I
$\beta_1\beta_2$	Complement components	0.01–0.15	—	—	—	Complement fixation reactions
	Metal-binding protein (transferrin)	0.2–0.4	90,000	5.8	5.8	Transport of iron (transferrin), copper, zinc
β_2	Unknown	0.2	—	6.3		? ? ?
	Glycoproteins	0.03	40,000	—	5.7–18.8	Unknown
γ	Blood group globulins	0.8	150,000 to 1,000,000	6.3–7.3		Contains antibodies, blood group globulins, complement c_1, c_2, etc.
	Immunoglobulin G, A, M	0.01–2.0	150,000 to 1,000,000	6.3–7.3	3.0–12.0	Antibodies to variety of antigens (bacterial, viral, toxinic, etc.)
	Cryoglobulins	0.01	—	—		? ? (insoluble in cold)

osmotic pressure of the blood, due almost entirely to the proteins of the plasma, is the force that opposes the hydrostatic pressure in the capillaries. The term "osmotic pressure" is not quite correct from the physicochemical standpoint since (1) there is no perfect semipermeable membrane and (2) a solution does not exert an osmotic pressure unless it is separated from another solution by such a membrane. In this discussion, the term "potential osmotic pressure" or osmotic tendency or quality might be better. With that in mind, we may proceed.

The *total* osmotic pressure is the osmotic pressure due to the electrolytes and organic crystalloids present plus that due to the colloids. The electrolytes and organic crystalloids are quite diffusible and pass through the capillary walls into the tissue fluids rather freely. Hence the osmotic pressure exerted by them is the same on both sides of the capillary. The plasma proteins, however, are not as freely diffusible and are greater in amount within the capillaries than without. Therefore the osmotic pressure exerted by them, small though it is, is greater inside than outside the capillaries. This is a pressure exerted inward, and normally it just balances the hydrostatic pressure (due to the heartbeat, elasticity of the arteries, etc.) exerted outward. The total osmotic pressure of plasma is about 6.5 atmospheres or 4940 mm. of mercury. This is *almost* balanced by a similar osmotic pressure of the tissue fluids bathing the capillaries. The slight difference is due to the difference in protein concentration between the plasma and the tissue fluids.

Osmotic pressure of plasma proteins = about 28 mm. Hg

Osmotic pressure of tissue fluid proteins = about 10 mm. Hg

Difference (oncotic pressure)   18 mm. Hg

Therefore the *effective* potential osmotic pressure of the plasma proteins, sometimes called the *oncotic pressure*, is 18 mm. Hg. The hydrostatic pressure inside and outside the capillaries varies in different locations and under different conditions; but assuming that the effective hydrostatic pressure is 32 mm. Hg on the arterial side of a given capillary and falls to 12 mm. on the venous side, we can see that the following state of affairs would then exist.

Arterial side	→	Capillary	→	Venous side
32 mm.	18 mm.	12 mm.	18 mm.	

As a result, on the arterial side the hydrostatic pressure exceeds the colloidal osmotic pressure ($32 - 18 = 14$ mm.) and fluid tends to be forced out. On the venous side the reverse is true ($12 - 18 = -6$ mm.) and fluid is drawn back. Thus filtration is favored on the arterial side, and absorption on the venous side. If the protein content of the plasma were to fall, the effective colloidal osmotic pressure would drop, more water would be forced out, and less would be absorbed. The water of the blood would pass into the tissues and *edema* would result. More than 80% of this colloidal osmotic effect is attributable to the albumin fraction, because there is more albumin, with a comparatively low molecular weight (about 70,000), than globulin, most of which have molecular weights over 100,000.

Pathologically, damaged kidneys eliminate proteins in about the same relative proportions as proteins are present in normal plasma. This means a greater loss of albumin than globulin, a particularly unfavorable occurrence if the plasma is already low in albumin. Experimentally, such an edema may be produced by plasmapheresis. This procedure consists of repeatedly bleeding an animal and injecting blood cells after they have been washed and suspended in a protein-free saline solution. When the protein content of the plasma falls below a critical level, edema occurs. There are a number of mechanisms that might lead to a low plasma protein content, e.g., loss of protein via the kidney (as in nephrosis), inadequate or improper protein intake, inhibition of plasma protein synthesis, loss of protein as a result of increased permeability of the capillaries.

Edema may result from a number of other causes besides the one described. The principal causes are related to general or local changes in capillary blood pressure; i.e., if the arterial pressure is relatively lower than the venous pressure, there is a back pressure and a slowing up of capillary flow, with a distention of the capillaries and a consequent forcing out of fluid by this increased capillary pressure. Such a condition frequently results from heart failure or mechanical obstruction of the large veins. Increased permeability of the capillaries may also produce edema; but in this case, edema is usually secondary to the changes in capillary pressure, or it may be brought about by avitaminosis (e.g., in beriberi and scurvy), by bacterial or other toxins, or by extreme heat.

As stated previously, two or possibly three albumin fractions are present in adult human plasma. The major fraction is present in amounts varying from 3.5 to 5.5 gm. per 100 ml. of plasma. This fraction has a molecular weight of 69,000 and contains approximately 0.8% carbohydrate. A small electrophoretically distinguishable fraction, termed *prealbumin,* is present in an amount of about 0.025%. This fraction has a molecular weight of approximately 61,000 and contains about 0.08% carbohydrate. A third *postalbumin* fraction, actually an α_1-globulin, contains approximately 10% carbohydrate. Specific functions of these minor fractions are unknown.

In addition to their primary function of retaining fluid within the vascular compartment, as described above, plasma albumins are important in the transport of fatty acids, bilirubin, and certain drugs, e.g., the sulfonamides. They are also important for their buffering capacity and for their nutritive effects. The plasma globulins also share in these functions as well as in the transport of certain specific substances, as summarized in Table 19-3.

Most of the substances concerned in immunologic reactions are of protein nature. At any rate, the *antibodies* that are present in blood, or are produced there, are modified plasma γ-globulins. When a foreign protein, an *antigen,* is injected parenterally into an animal, an antibody that is present in the serum of the animal is formed; this may be demonstrated by tests in vitro. The reactions in such tests are termed *precipitin* reactions if the antigen used is of molecular size. They are called *agglutinin* reactions if the antigen is of cellular size, and *lytic* reactions if the cellular antigen is lysed. Interferons are naturally occurring substances produced by vertebrates in response to viral infections. They are of protein or polypeptide nature.[5]

The γ-globulins represent some 10% to 18% of the total plasma proteins. Most of the antibodies found in plasma are associated with the γ-globulin fraction, although a minor portion is found in the β-globulin fractions. The γ-globulins are formed extrahepatically, apparently in the plasma cells of lymph tissue.

The γ-globulins were originally so-named because they move more slowly than any plasma protein fraction on electrophoresis at an alkaline pH. They are heterogeneous, being comprised of a number of distinctly different proteins. At least 25 or 30 different immunoglobulins have been prepared from human γ-globulins. The γ-globulins may be separated into subfractions by ultracentrifugation and by column chromatography on ion-exchange resins, agar gel, and other adsorbents. These subfractions vary widely in molecular weight (from 150,000 to over 1,000,000) and in isoelectric point (from 6.3 to 7.3) as well as in other physicochemical properties. The γ-globulins are glycoproteins, containing 2% to 12% carbohydrate, including mannose, galactose, fucose, glucosamine, and a sialic acid. They apparently differ only in minor ways with respect to amino acid composition. Their differing physical and immunologic properties appear to be due mainly to variations in amino acid sequences and conformational differences particularly at the active site of the molecule. The fact that the γ-globulins may be partially digested with certain proteolytic enzymes without a loss of immunologic properties is significant.

Upon ultracentrifugation the γ-globulins separate into at least *three* major fractions and several minor fractions. Several different systems of nomenclature are used for these fractions, making for some confusion. The current preferred biochemical nomenclature[6,7] for the three major fractions, together with synonyms indicated in parentheses, is as follows: γM (IgM, 19 S, macroglobulins); γG (IgG, 7 S); and γA (IgA, β_2A, 6.6 to 13 S). The S in each case refers to the number of Svedbergs (p. 904) characteristic of the γ-globulin (1 Svedberg = 1×10^{-13} second and represents the time required for the particle to move a specified distance in an ultracentrifugal field under specific conditions[8]). Most of the antibodies are in the γG (7 S)-fraction, which represents some 70% of the total γ-globulins. This fraction has a molecular weight of about 150,000 and contains 2% to 3% carbohydrate. The γA-fraction also has a molecular weight of 180,000 to 390,000. The γM-, or macroglobulin, fraction has a molecular weight of approximately 1,000,000 and a carbohydrate content of about 10%. A study[9] of a human macroglobulin, purified by agar gel chromatography, showed the molecular weight of the macroglobulin to be 890,000. Upon treatment with thiol reagents, the molecule splits into five subunits, each having a molecular weight of about 185,000.

The different types of γ-globulins are made up of subunit peptide chains

Table 19-4. Some characteristics of the major types of immunoglobulins*

Type	Subunit composition	Molecular weight	Carbohydrate content (percent)	Serum level (milligrams/ milliliter)	Synthetic rate (grams/day— 70 kg. man)	Half-life (days)
IgG (γG)						
Type I	$\gamma_2\kappa_2$	150,000	2.5	12	2.3	25
Type II	$\gamma_2\lambda_2$					
IgA (γA)						
Type I	$\alpha_2\kappa_2$	180,000 to	5.0 to	1.8	2.7	6
Type II	$\alpha_2\lambda_2$	390,000	10.0			
IgM (γM)						
Type I	$(\mu_2\kappa_2)_n$	900,000	5.0 to	1.0	0.4	5
Type II	$(\mu_2\lambda_2)_n$		10			
	(n = 5,					
	6, etc.)					

° Adapted from Tomasi, T. B.: New Eng. J. Med. **279**:1327, 1968.

apparently in much the same manner as hemoglobin (p. 596). Two general sizes of chains are found, a heavy chain, sometimes called A, and a light chain, or B. The former has a molecular weight of about 40,000; the latter, about 20,000. Three types of heavy chains have been described and termed μ (*mu*), γ (*gamma*), and α (*alpha*), after the major fractions of γ-globulin from which they are derived. Two types of light chains have been characterized, κ (*kappa*) and λ (*lambda*).

Some of the characteristic properties of the major types of human immunoglobulins,[10] together with their subunit compositions, are summarized in Table 19-4. The relatively rapid turnover and synthesis rates of the various immunoglobulins are evident from the data given. Also interesting is the fact that adult blood levels of the immunoglobulins are not attained until 2, 4 to 8, and 1 years of age for G-, A-, and M-types, respectively. The structures and amino acid sequences of the light and heavy chains comprising the immunoglobulins and their evolutionary relationships are the subject of current intensive study.[11] The complete amino acid sequences of several human subunits, including (light) λ-chains (164 amino acids) and κ-chains (213 to 221 amino acids) have been determined. The heavy chains, μ-, γ-, and α-, also contain a *variable* portion, having a variable amino acid sequence. The variable portion appears to be related to the specific antibody response of the immunoglobulin, which feature would account for the enormous number of chemically similar but biologically distinct molecules of immunoglobulins that are possible.[12] The light chains, κ- or λ-, are common to most types of γ-globulins. Their amino acid sequences and antibody sites have been partially determined. They, as well as the heavy chains, appear to be linked together in the whole γ-globulin molecule by means of disulfide linkages.

A schematic representation of the gross structure of a typical immunoglobulin-G (IgG) is shown in Fig. 19-1. The molecular weight is about 150,000.

585

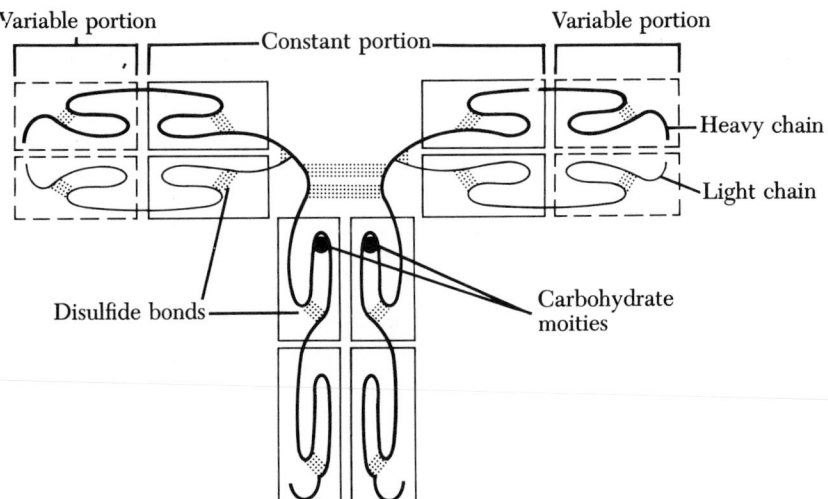

Fig. 19-1. Schematic representation of the gross structure of an immunoglobulin (IgG). (Adapted from Gottlieb, P. D., et al.: Proc. Nat. Acad. Sci. **61**:168, 1968; Rutishauser, U., et al.: Proc. Nat. Acad. Sci. **61**:1414, 1968.)

The immunoglobulin is composed of four subunits, two light and two heavy chains, having molecular weights of about 24,000 and 50,000, respectively. The conformation of the molecule is maintained, in part at least, by the 16 disulfide bonds shown. The carbohydrate moieties of the molecule may be attached to the heavy chains.

As indicated by the rectangular boxes in the diagram, the two polypeptide chains comprising the immunoglobulin molecule may be divided into 12 segments, each containing approximately 110 amino acids. Eight of these contain the two heavy chains, each of which is made up of about 440 amino acids. The other four contain two light chains, each made up of about 220 amino acids.

The eight solid rectangles enclose the so-called *constant* portion of the molecule, which is apparently the same for all immunoglobulins. The broken lines enclose the variable portion, whose amino acid sequence and composition vary for each different immunoglobulin. This feature is responsible for the specificity of a given antibody against the antigen that stimulated its formation.

There are two identical variable portions of the molecule, each made up of one half light chain (about 108 amino acids) and one fourth heavy chain (about 110 amino acids). These thus form two specific *active* sites for each molecule, which means that each molecule of this immunoglobulin can bind two molecules of antigen. The variations in the amino acid composition and sequence in this portion of the molecule are also responsible for the enormous number of possible antibodies—optimally one for each invading bacterial, viral, or other toxic antigen. Apparently the plasma cell, which forms antibodies, is "instructed" in some specific manner to synthesize a type of meshing conformation in the variable portions of the two light and heavy chains that will be complementary to the conformation of a portion of the antigen, and this instruction serves as a "lock" for the antigen. The antibody thus combines with the antigen to form an insoluble complex that is taken up by phagocytes and destroyed—a truly remarkable example of the biochemical adaptation of a molecule for the performance of a specific function.

The amino acid composition and sequence for the light-chain component of certain myeloma γ-globulins have been determined on preparations of Bence Jones protein (p. 588) made from the plasma and/or urine of patients with Bence Jones albumosuria. Apparently such proteins are constant in a given patient but vary from one patient to another.

The amino acid sequence of the constant portion of immunoglobulins has not yet been completely determined. When it is, the information should aid in clarifying the function of this portion of the molecule. The constant portion is now believed to be involved in attacking the cell wall of invading bacteria, e.g., lysing the wall and thus aiding in the destruction of the bacteria.

Although the amino acid sequences of certain γ-globulins and the locations of the disulfide bonds appear to be established, full reconstruction of the molecule's three-dimensional conformation must await x-ray analysis of the immunoglobulin crystal. Attempts to crystallize immunoglobulins are now being made at several laboratories as the next step in this direction.

Two other immunoglobulins, *IgD* (D) and *IgE* (E), apparently occur in human plasma in very small amounts, 1 to 40 mg. per 100 ml. IgD has a molecular weight of about 150,000. The functions of these two immunoglobulins are unknown.

Another alleged type of γ-globulin is the 3 S or microglobulin. This type is also heterogeneous, with molecular weights varying from 10,000 to 40,000. It contains no carbohydrate. It may be found in small amounts in plasma, in spinal fluid, and in urine. It may consist mainly of free light chains, but its biochemical function is unknown.

A deficiency of dietary protein is now generally believed to result in decreased antibody response. Recent studies[14] demonstrated that a deficiency of either tryptophan or phenylalanine, but not of methionine, in rats particularly decreases antibody response.

Quantitative changes in the amounts of γ-globulins in the plasma and/or urine are known in several pathologic conditions in man. A deficiency of γ-globulins is found in a rare hereditary disease, *agammaglobulinemia*. Individuals with this disorder lack the ability to synthesize the γ-globulin type of plasma protein, apparently for genetic reasons. As might be expected, such people are particularly susceptible to infectious diseases. Therapy consists of the parenteral administration of γ-globulin preparations.

Abnormally large amounts of certain γ-globulins may be found in the plasma in several diseases of man. An increase in γM, macroglobulins, termed a *macroglobulinemia*, may occur in neoplastic diseases, collagen disorders, chronic infections, amyloidosis, and hepatic cirrhosis. The major component found is the 19 S fraction, but heavier (24 to 40 S) and lighter (14 to 16 S) components may also appear. An explanation of this condition at a biochemical level is not now possible.

Increased amounts of a remarkable type of γ-globulin are found in the plasma (also the urine, p. 587) of patients with *multiple myeloma*. This is the so-called Bence Jones protein, named after its discoverer. The sedimentation rate of this globulin is 3.5 S, and its molecular weight is about 45,000. It usually appears in the γ-globulin fraction in electrophoresis, although it may be in the β- or even α-fractions. The Bence Jones proteins appear to be either monomers or possibly dimers of the light chains, probably κ_2- or λ_2-. They have the remarkable characteristic of precipitating on heating to 50° to 60° C., then redissolving with more heating.

Another unusual type of plasma protein, most commonly associated with the γ-globulins, but occasionally with the β- or α-fractions, is the so-called cryoglobulin. This protein precipitates or even gels when plasma or serum in which it is present is cooled, a phenomenon that can be demonstrated in vitro. Traces of cryoglobulin are found in normal serum. Increased amounts, up to 10 gm. per 100 ml., may be found in a variety of disorders, e.g., rheumatoid arthritis, chronic lymphocytic leukemia, multiple myeloma, hepatic cirrhosis, coronary artery disease, lymphosarcoma. Massive precipitation of the protein may occur at levels of about 1 gm.%. The molecular weight of the cryoglobulins appears to vary widely from about 165,000 to 600,000. The biochemical etiology of *cryoglobulinemia* is unknown.

Included in the various plasma protein fractions are also small amounts of a number of enzymes, e.g., several transaminases, dehydrogenases, peptidases, acid and alkaline phosphatases, aldolase, amylase, an invertase, lipase, catalase, cholinesterase, and β-glucuronidase. These appear to be derived from the tissues in which they are secreted, perhaps representing a leakage at least in some cases. The quantitative determination of certain of these enzymes in plasma is assuming considerable clinical significance.

Regeneration of plasma proteins. Fibrinogen is produced by the body with remarkable speed. If rabbits are bled until most of the fibrinogen is removed and the defibrinated blood is reinjected, the fibrinogen is almost completely regenerated in 5 or 6 hours. This does not occur if the animals have been hepatectomized. The other plasma proteins are not replaced as quickly, however.

Whipple and associates[15] studied this problem extensively, using plasmapheresis to deplete the organism of plasma proteins. First, they found that if the proteins are reduced to a concentration of between 1% to 2% in the plasma death usually occurs; second, if the proteins are reduced to about half the normal value regeneration is fairly rapid for the first 24 hours, during which about one third of the deficit is restored; thereafter, regeneration proceeds more slowly until the full quota of protein is restored, in from 7 to 14 days. The diet of the animal plays an important role in plasma protein formation; proteins containing a suitable assortment of amino acids are necessary for rapid regeneration. These studies showed that the liver is the chief site of formation of these proteins although the intestine may have some part in this function. Normally there is a considerable reserve of plasma protein–forming material in the body. This reserve may be reduced by a low-protein diet, by fasting, or by plasma depletion (plasmapheresis or hemorrhage). When such depletion occurs, the animal is much less resistant to infection or stress. However, such states can be remedied readily by feeding adequate protein together with other suitable nutritive factors.

More recent studies employing better techniques, e.g., in vitro liver perfusion, immunoelectrophoresis, fluorescent antibody procedures, confirmed the fact that the liver is the chief site of formation of most of the plasma proteins,[16] including not only fibrinogen but also plasma albumin(s) and α_1-, α_2-, β_1-, and β_2-globulins. The γ-globulins and probably certain generically related β-globulins appear to be formed extrahepatically, for the most part, probably in the plasma cells of the reticuloendothelial system. Prothrombin synthesis has been found to occur exclusively in the parenchymal cells of the liver,[17] possibly in the ribosomal particulate fraction of these cells.

Degradation of plasma proteins. The question of the site of degradation of the plasma proteins is still unsettled. There is some evidence, however, that the lumen of the intestine may be involved. Serum albumin labeled with ^{131}I was found to pass into isolated loops of duodenum (rabbits). If this transfer occurs in a considerable portion of the intestinal tract, the intestinal enzymatic digestion of plasma albumin so transferred could account for most of the in vivo degradation of this plasma protein. Whether the same site of degradation is also that for the plasma globulins remains to be determined.

Electrophoretic analysis. Electrophoretic studies of blood plasma and serum have increased in number and interest. The chief difficulty until now was the size and cost of the apparatus required, but technical improvements have remedied this problem considerably, as has the development of relatively simple, inexpensive electrophoretic methods employing filter paper, starch, or thin-layer silica gel plates. A brief discussion of electrophoresis is found on p. 903.

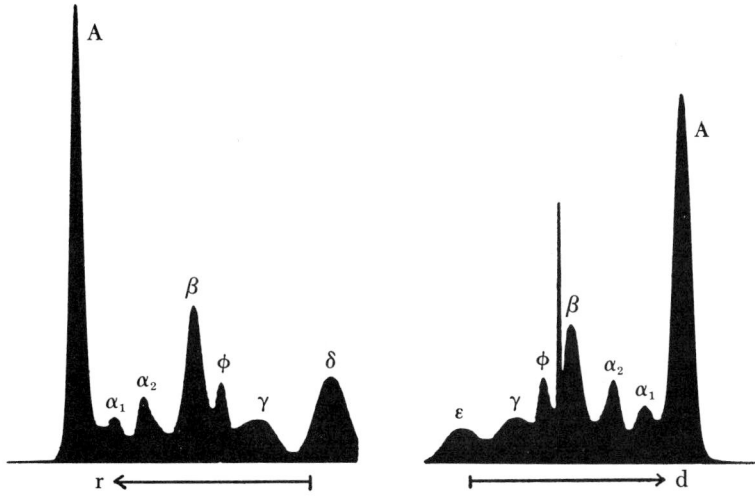

Fig. 19-2. Electrophoretic pattern of normal human plasma at pH 8.6. The peaks shown are, from the extreme ends inward, albumin, α_1-, α_2-, and β-globulin, fibrinogen, γ-globulin, and the anomalous peak. (From Longsworth, L. G.: Chem. Rev. **30**:323, 1942.)

Proteins move in an electric field because of the electric charges they carry. In the Tiselius[18] apparatus the diluted and dialyzed serum or plasma is overlaid with a buffer solution. During electrophoresis the various proteins at the boundary between the buffer solution and the plasma become separated and move at different rates of speed. As they move, the relative positions and widths of the protein boundaries may be either visibly projected on a ground-glass screen or recorded on a photographic plate. The albumin fraction moves faster than the globulins or fibrinogen, and a study of the patterns obtained reveals six distinct proteins (Fig. 19-2). The area of each hump measures the concentration of the protein moving with that particular mobility. Careful study has shown that fractions formerly designated *pseudoglobulin, euglobulin*, etc., which were obtained by salting-out methods, are really mixtures of several globulins. The older terminology has therefore been abandoned and the nomenclature of Tiselius[18] is now generally adopted. The proteins shown to be present are albumin, α_1-, α_2-, β_1-, β_2-, and γ-globulins, and fibrinogen. It should be mentioned that the patterns differ with different species and also, even in the case of the same sample, with the buffer used and with the period of electrophoresis. As seen in Fig. 19-2, the albumin peak is the tallest and best defined, whereas the globulin and fibrinogen peaks are lower and often spread over a greater distance. The ascending and descending boundaries are not identical.

Studies of pathologic plasma and body fluids have been made, and a few generalizations are permissible. In pneumonia, for example, and probably in all febrile conditions, the α-globulin fraction is increased. In most conditions in which an antigen-antibody system is involved, the γ-globulin fraction is found to be definitely elevated. The blood serum in cirrhosis of the liver is extremely abnormal. The same is true of nephrosis; and the protein-contain-

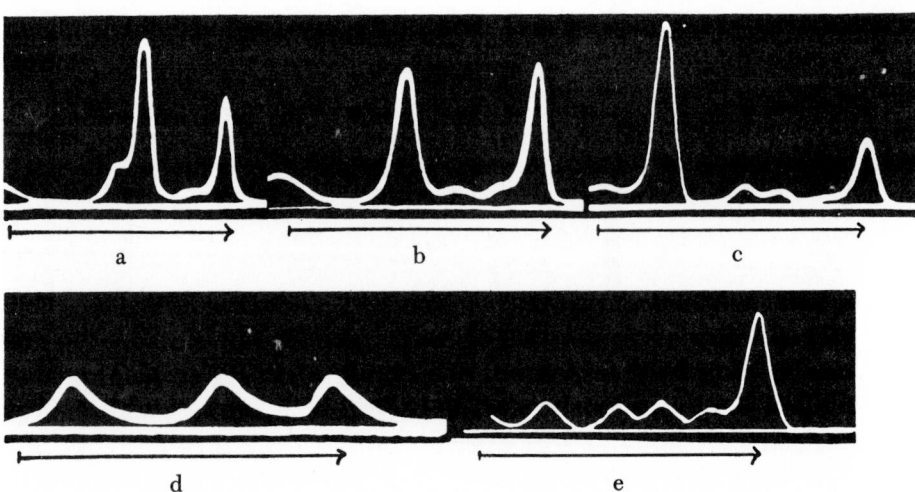

Fig. 19-3. Representative electrophoresis diagrams of sera of patients with multiple myeloma. *a*, α-Type; *b*, β-type; *c*, γ-type; *d*, multiple peaks; *e*, minor anomalies. Ascending boundaries. (From Reiner, M., and Stern, K. G.: Acta Haemat. 9:19, 1953.)

ing urine of nephrotic subjects produces an electrophoretic pattern closely resembling normal serum, which indicates that in nephrosis the urinary protein is not entirely albumin as was formerly believed. In multiple myelomatosis, a malignant disease of the bone marrow, a variety of electrophoretic patterns are encountered (Fig. 19-3).

Electrophoresis does not separate the protein components into *chemically pure* substances. According to Tiselius, the albumin component contains bilirubin and the β-globulin cholesterol. All the protein fractions contain carbohydrate and some lipid material. During *chemical* separation most of these combinations are broken; consequently, it is highly probable that the "purified" products ordinarily isolated are really derivatives of the protein complexes as they circulate in the blood and as they are prepared by electrophoresis.

During World War II, Cohn and his co-workers[19] developed chemical procedures for the separation of protein fractions from plasma in which there was little modification of the proteins. They precipitated the proteins at low temperatures with different concentrations of ethanol. The pH and ionic strength were also controlled meticulously, and large-scale methods were employed in order to obtain enough material for comprehensive studies of the functions of the various fractions (see also p. 581). All fractions take part in the osmotic phenomena previously described, but the albumins, having a smaller size, lower molecular weight, and higher concentration than the others, contribute most to these phenomena. The albumins and probably other plasma proteins are involved in nutritive functions, although albumins themselves are actually rather poor proteins nutritionally (since they contain little isoleucine and tryptophan). Plasma proteins, upon intravenous injection, are metabolized, and, it is presumed, those proteins normally circulating in the blood are similarly utilized. Antibodies, for the most part, associate with the γ-globulin fraction, as stated previously (p. 583). Among these antibodies are ones reacting with diphtheria toxin and with the viruses of mumps, influenza, and poliomyelitis. The function of fibrinogen in blood clotting will be discussed in a subsequent section of this chapter. One protein, *transferrin* or siderophilin, in the β-globulin fraction, carries iron.

Immunoelectrophoresis. Valuable as the various modifications of electrophorests have been, e.g., the foregoing Tiselius "moving-boundary" procedure and the several types of "zone" electrophoresis on filter paper or agar plates, these methods do not give a clear separation of closely related mixed proteins such as are present in human plasma. The newer technique of immunoelectrophoresis appears to be more satisfactory in this respect. Essentially, this procedure combines the electrophoretic separation of mixed proteins with the antigen-antibody reaction. The proteins are separated as a series of spots on an agar-covered glass plate by the usual electrophoretic procedure. The current is turned off and the proteins diffuse outward. Meanwhile, an antihuman immune serum from rabbit, horse, etc., which contains antibodies for the human serum protein under investigation, is placed in a trough at the side of the agar plate, parallel to the electrophoretic migration. The antibody diffuses inward, and, when it meets the antigen, the familiar

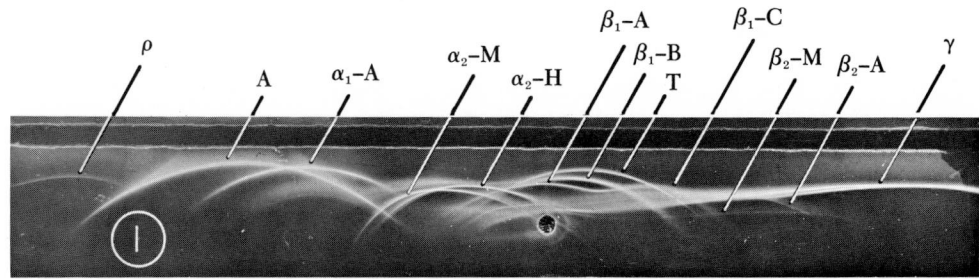

Fig. 19-4. Immunoelectrophoretic pattern for normal human serum. A sample was introduced into a small round starting well. After electrophoresis in the buffered agar layer, an antiserum was pipetted into the trough (above). The specific antibodies diffusing from the trough are precipitated by their corresponding serum protein antigens previously distributed in the gel, according to their electrophoretic mobilities. From left to right (anode to cathode) known constitutents are labeled in order of decreasing mobility. ρ, Rh_0, a minor component moving in advance of albumin; another ρ-component has been identified as a lipoprotein; A, albumin; α_1-A, α-1-glycoprotein; α_2-M, α-2-macroglobulin, molecular weight 900,000; α_2-H, haptoglobin, hemoglobulin-binding protein; β_1-A, conversion product of β_1-C associated with complement activity; β_1-B, β-1-mucoprotein; T, transferrin, β-1 Fe-binding protein; β_1-C, active component of the complement system; inactivation involves conversion to β_1-A; β_2-M, macroglobulin (molecular weight about 1,000,000) with antibody activity, aberrant in some types of multiple myeloma; β_2-A, globulin with some antigenic similarity to α-globulin that is aberrant in some types of multiple myeloma; γ, α-globulin. (Courtesy C. A. Williams, Jr.)

precipitation occurs, forming an opaque arc. It has been possible thus far to identify more than 25 distinct human serum proteins by this technique, using an antibody-rich horse serum. The possible applications appear to be extensive. For example, the technique should prove useful in studies of the serum proteins in various diseases, in studies of the embryologic development of tissues, and in investigations of bacterial proteins. The pattern obtained by immunoelectrophoresis of samples of human serum proteins is shown in Fig. 19-4.

Plasma proteins in liver disease. Since the liver is the chief site for the synthesis of plasma albumin and fibrinogen, it is not surprising to find that the quantitative relations of these proteins are disturbed in liver diseases. The liver also plays some part in the synthesis of the globulins. Serum albumin concentrations are lowered in cirrhosis, in viral hepatitis, in nutritional liver diseases, and in hepatic malignancies. The causes are (1) impaired synthesis because of decreased amount of functioning tissue, (2) losses by transudation into ascitic and edematous fluid, (3) hemorrhage, (4) increase in plasma volume, and (5) diminished ingestion of protein.

It would, therefore, seem logical to study blood proteins in abnormal liver conditions. Paper electrophoresis has been used with some success, and the quantitative measurement of γ-globulin has been employed. However, largely for technical reasons, the various semiempiric flocculation and turbidity tests have been more popular. More than a dozen of these tests have been described. The most widely used are the cephalin-cholesterol flocculation test, the zinc turbidity test, and the thymol test.

In 1939, Hanger showed that emulsions of mixtures of cephalin and cholesterol are distinctly flocculated by sera from patients having active disturbances of the hepatic parenchyma whereas sera from normal persons or from patients with obstructive jaundice are rendered diffusely turbid. This test is therefore looked upon as an index of parenchymatous function only. The test is said to depend on the capacity of γ-globulin in serum to unite with the colloidal constituents of the emulsion, to produce flocculation.

The zinc turbidity test depends on the low solubility of zinc compounds of γ-globulin in solutions of low ionic strength. Maclagan's thymol turbidity test is based on the fact that a saturated solution of thymol in barbital buffer produces a dense turbidity when added to serum from patients suffering from extensive liver disease. These and other flocculation or turbidity tests are valuable in aiding the differential diagnosis of various liver diseases.

Other constituents of plasma Included in the remaining fraction of plasma solids are amino acids and lower peptides, glucose, lipids, lactic acid, citric and other organic acids, the ketone bodies, nitrogenous waste products, pigments, inorganic salts, and small amounts of various enzymes, vitamins, and hormones. *Glucose* is present in a concentration of approximately 0.1%. It is most probably α,β-D-glucose. Both the *amino acids* and glucose vary in amount with the state of digestion and nutrition. This is also true of the *lipids*. In general, all three of these components increase after meals, reach a high point, level off, and then fall. Abnormally, all vary to a greater or lesser degree. These fluctuations were considered in earlier chapters. The lipids of plasma are fats, fatty acids, phospholipids, cholesterol, and cholesterol esters. The phospholipids include lecithin, a smaller amount of sphingomyelin, and a little cephalin. Most of the lipid is bound as the β-lipoprotein, which represents about 5% of the normal plasma proteins. *Lactic acid* is present normally in small amounts and increases with exercise and also under pathologic conditions. It is a product of carbohydrate metabolism. Traces of the *ketone bodies,* namely, acetone, acetoacetic acid, and β-hydroxybutyric acid, also are normally present. They are derived from fatty acids and are increased when there is increased fat metabolism. The *nitrogenous waste products* result from the breakdown of proteins, purines, and other organic nitrogen-containing substances present in food and tissues. Included are urea, uric acid, creatinine, hippuric acid, and others. Their presence in blood is an indication of the transportation of waste products by the bloodstream to the kidneys and other organs of elimination. Creatine is also present in minute amounts. The pigments of normal plasma probably include the urinary pigments, bile pigments, and carotene, all in traces, but abnormally these may be increased and others added.

The positive *inorganic* ions present in blood in appreciable amounts are Na^+, K^+, Ca^{++}, and Mg^{++}. The negative are Cl^-, HCO_3^-, $SO_4^=$, and $HPO_4^=$ (see Fig. 15-6). In addition, lactic, citric, and other organic acids and proteins contribute somewhat to the ionic picture. In plasma and, in fact, in all body fluids, the concentration of sodium ions exceeds that of potassium; in the blood cells and other cells, the reverse is true. The bicarbonates and the phosphates are quite important as buffers, and the shifting of the chloride ion in and out of the erythrocytes has a definite role in acid-base balance. Changes in the concentrations of many of these ions occur under pathologic conditions; e.g., Na^+ and Cl^- fall, K^+ rises in Addison's disease, Ca^{++} is diminished when parathyroid function fails. Similarly there are fluctuations of some of the elements and ions present in traces, e.g., iodine and iodides, sulfocyanates, copper, iron.

ERYTHROCYTES

The erythrocytes, or red blood cells, are formed in bone marrow. This long-established fact was reaffirmed[20] in human subjects. Injected ^{59}Fe was followed by visualization of various body areas after some 16 hours by means of a scintillation counter. In the normal adult, the major uptake of the labeled iron, and hence, under the conditions employed, the major erythropoietic tissue, was found to be in the bone marrow of the pelvis, spine, ribs, scapula, and proximal ends of the bones of the extremities. The liver and spleen did not accumulate sufficient iron to be visualized. In disease processes in which erythropoiesis is markedly increased (e.g., cyanotic congenital heart disease), there was an extension of the erythrocyte-forming marrow into the entire femur, the proximal portion of the tibia, and even the tarsal bones, the middle of the forearm, and the wrist. The control of the production of erythrocytes depends on a hematopoietic hormone, *erythropoietin* (p. 507), and a "maturation factor," now known to be vitamin B_{12}, as well as vitamin E. The mechanism of the action of vitamin B_{12} will be described in greater detail later (p. 823). In addition to these factors, there are required for normal erythropoiesis suitable and adequate dietary protein,[21] folic acid and perhaps pyridoxine, niacin, and ascorbic acid (Chapter 11), available iron salts, and traces of copper and cobalt.

The erythrocytes contain less water than do the cells of most tissues, namely, about 60%. Most of the solid matter is hemoglobin, the conjugated protein that is the red coloring matter of blood. The stroma or meshwork is composed of other proteins and lipids, to which the hemoglobin is probably bound intimately. The lipids are chiefly cholesterol, lecithin, and cephalin, and the proteins include an albuminoid, stromatin, and a lipoprotein, elinin. Another protein of the stroma is hemocuprein, a bluish copper-containing substance whose function is unknown. The erythrocyte has a membrane, an extremely delicate covering, composed of lipoprotein. The ratio of lipid to protein is from 1:1.6 to 1:1.8. The protein portion is a fibrous protein, and the lipid consists of cephalins and cholesterol, with smaller amounts of lecithin and sphingomyelin.

Various enzymes are present, including carbonic anhydrase, catalase, peptidases, cholinesterase, and the enzymes of the glycolytic system (p. 196). All the glutathione of blood is located in the erythrocytes. Adenosine di- and triphosphates (p. 252) and di- and triphosphopyridine nucleotides (p. 244) are also important constituents of the erythrocytes. Soluble organic crystalloids present include urea, amino acids, creatinine, and glucose. The concentration of glucose in the erythrocyte is about the same as in plasma.

The electrolyte composition of the erythrocytes is qualitatively similar to that of the plasma. It differs quantitatively, however. There is more potassium than sodium—just the reverse of the relation of these two elements in plasma. The osmotic pressure of the interior of the erythrocyte is equal to that of the plasma (i.e., normally equivalent to the osmotic pressure of 0.9% NaCl solution, which is termed *normal* or, better, *physiologic* saline, since it is not the same as a chemically "normal" solution). Changes in osmotic pressure of the medium surrounding red blood cells influence the size of the cells. If the medium is hypotonic, water passes into the cell and the size of the cell increases. Not a very great increase occurs before the cell bursts and the hemoglobin is released. This process is called hemolysis or laking, and such blood, which is a clear transparent crimson fluid, is laked or hemolyzed blood. When erythrocytes are put in a hypertonic solution, i.e., one with a higher osmotic pressure than 0.9% NaCl, they shrink and take on a shriveled appearance. These are described as crenated cells.

Hemolysis may be produced by other means besides the one mentioned. Substances that dissolve or change the physical state of lipids, e.g., ether, chloroform, bile salts, soaps, accomplish this also. Certain biologic toxins, especially those produced by venomous snakes and hemolytic bacteria, also cause the laking of erythrocytes. Some toxins contain enzymes that hydrolyze lecithin, and others act by solution of, or combination with, lipids. Physical forces, e.g., irradiation with ultraviolet rays, alternate freezing and thawing, may so alter the structure of the cell as to cause the release of hemoglobin. Aging also has a similar effect, and this is why whole citrated blood, kept in blood banks, cannot be used after 5 to 7 days. The erythrocytes become more and more fragile. The addition of glucose prolongs their serviceable period to 16 to 30 days, under proper conditions. Hemolysis may occur in the human body under pathologic conditions, but it never occurs in the body as a result of lowering osmotic pressure. When it does occur, as a result of the action of bacteria, venoms, or other agents, the hemoglobin released into circulation is excreted by the kidney, resulting in hemoglobinuria.

Erythrocytes, like other living cells, require energy to maintain their vital processes. Glucose appears to be the major substance oxidized to supply this requirement. Nucleated erythrocytes derive their energy mainly by the oxidation of glucose through the citric acid cycle[22] (p. 263). Nonnucleated erythrocytes, on the other hand, including those of man, appear to metabolize glucose primarily by way of anaerobic glycolysis (p. 196) and by the phosphogluconate shunt (p. 208). The latter requires $NADP^+$ with the appropriate dehydrogenase and is linked to cytochrome-c and oxygen by a hemoprotein enzyme, $NADPH_2$ oxidase. In this connection, an interesting congenital hemolytic anemia, called *hereditary spherocytosis*, appears to be due to a disturbance of glucose oxidation in the patient's erythrocytes. The condition is apparently caused by a congenital defect in intracellular glycolysis, probably due to a deficiency of enolase, the enzyme that converts 2-phosphoglycerate to phosphoenolpyruvate (p. 201). A decrease occurs in available energy-rich phosphate bonds (ATP), which seem to be required for the maintenance of the biconcave shape of the normal erythrocyte. Spherocytosis results and the erythrocytes are more susceptible to lysis and destruction. The characteristic anemia follows. Hereditary spherocytosis occurs once in about 20,000 live births. Similarly, a hereditary deficiency of *glucose-6-phosphate dehydrogenase*, which supplies $NADPH_2$ to the erythrocyte by way of the pentose pathway (p. 208), may result in increased hemolysis and a severe hemolytic anemia. The anemia may not become evident in some cases unless a drug (e.g., the antimalarial agent primaquine) or substances (fava beans) that have a hemolytic effect are ingested. The incidence of this enzyme deficiency has been estimated to be about 1% in Caucasian races and 13% in the American Negro male. A congenital deficiency of the enzyme *pyruvate kinase* may likewise be responsible for hereditary hemolytic anemia. This enzyme is required for a glycolysis, specifically for ATP formation from phosphoenolpyruvate (p. 202). As many as 80% of the erythrocytes in such cases may appear as bizarre, spiculated forms that are extremely fragile and readily hemolyzed. The three foregoing hereditary diseases thus emphasize the importance of energy-producing mechanisms in the erythrocyte for maintaining cellular structure and integrity.

Tracer nitrogen (^{15}N) was used to study the life-span of red cells. After the feeding of labeled glycine was stopped, the concentration of labeled heme did not level off and decrease as would be expected if the red cells were rapidly being catabolized. It continued to increase for nearly 25 days and then leveled off until about the seventieth day. At this time the ^{15}N content began to diminish. The life-span of the average red cell was found to be about 120 days for man and for the dog and 100 days for the rat.

HEMOGLOBIN

Hemoglobin is a conjugated protein in which a prosthetic group, heme, is attached to each of four subunits, two α- and two β-polypeptide chains, in the case of adult hemoglobin-A. The α- and β-chains of hemoglobin-A are characterized by a relatively high content of histidine and lysine and a small amount of isoleucine. By means of isotope tracer technique, the α- and β-chains were shown to be formed from amino acids derived, of course, from dietary protein. The peptide chain part of hemoglobin is responsible for the species specificity of the hemoglobin of the species. The pigmentary property and chief respiratory functions are associated with heme, the iron-containing pigment, but the globin fraction plays a role in carrying carbon dioxide (p. 649) as well as oxygen. Hemoglobin is a crystallizable protein, and, according to Reichert, each species has its own peculiar crystalline form. It has the power of uniting in loose combination with atmospheric oxygen, forming oxyhemoglobin. This occurs in the capillaries surrounding the alveoli of the lungs; the oxygen is thus transported in the arterial blood to the tissues, where part of it is released, and the venous blood, somewhat depleted of its oxygen supply, returns to the lungs for oxygenation.

Structure of hemoglobin. The structure of the hemoglobin molecule has been extensively studied—probably more than that of any other protein.

Most if not all mammalian hemoglobins are composed of four subunits (tetramers), consisting of four peptide chains to each of which is attached one heme group. The amino acid composition and sequence of the peptide chains have been determined in a number of species, as will be discussed later. The composite mammalian hemoglobin molecule is nearly spheric due to the remarkable fit of the subunit peptide chains. In the case of horse hemoglobin,[23] the molecule is a spheroid measuring $64 \times 55 \times 50$ Å. Most mammalian hemoglobins have a molecular weight of approximately 67,000. Of interest, however, is the fact that the copper-containing respiratory pigment, hemocyanin, of the octopus is a decamer with a molecular weight of about 2,800,000.

Normal human hemoglobin is of several types, containing four subunits made up of various combinations of four or possibly five different yet related peptide chains. They are designated α, β-, γ-, and δ-, with the alleged fifth type being tentatively represented as ϵ-. Most human hemoglobins contain two α-chains plus two other chains, usually either β-, γ-, or δ-. Thus, normal adult hemoglobin, commonly called Hb-A, consists of two α- and two β-chains and is designated therefore $\alpha_2^A \beta_2^A$, or, more simply, $\alpha_2 \beta_2$. Approximately 90% of the hemoglobin of the normal adult is of this type (Hb-A). Human fetal hemoglobin is designated Hb-F and is $\alpha_2 \gamma_2$. A minor component of normal adult hemoglobin, present usually to the extent of about 2.5% of the total erythrocyte hemoglobin, is called Hb-A_2 and is designated $\alpha_2 \delta_2$. Another alleged form, embryonic hemoglobin, is apparently $\alpha_2 \epsilon_2$. The four peptide chains of normal human hemoglobins appear to be held together by noncovalent forces (p. 598).

Apparently multiple forms of adult hemoglobin, as well as fetal and embryonic forms, occur in many species of animals and in man. These have been demonstrated in various mammals, including monkeys and chimpanzees, cattle, pigs, sheep, deer, goats, cats, dogs, rats, and mice. Multiple forms of hemoglobin, monomeric in some cases, are also found in lower species of animals, including fish and insects. The value of multiple forms of hemoglobin to the animal organism is unknown at the present time. These forms may represent fine molecular adaptations to a changing environment with the development and aging of the organism.

In a brilliant series of investigations using x-ray diffraction analysis, Nobel Laureate M. F. Perutz[23] and his colleagues of the University of Cambridge, aided by knowledge of the amino acid sequence of various hemoglobins obtained in other laboratories, succeeded recently in elucidating the complete tertiary structure of horse hemoglobin. As shown in Fig. 5-10, a photograph of a model constructed in Dr. Perutz' laboratory, the molecule is nearly spheric as a result of the remarkable fit of the two α- and β-chains. The helical nature of the four chains and their folding into the final convoluted subunits are evident.

The conformation of the α- and β-chains is shown more clearly in Fig. 5-12, in separate models of the two chains with superimposed lines showing the course of the central chain. It may be noted that both the α- and β-chains partially enfold and protect the heme groups located in "crevices" near their surface. Also striking is the fact that the folding of the two chains is quite similar. Even more remarkable is the resemblance of the conformation, particularly that of the β-chain, to the tertiary structure of myoglobin (Fig. 5-9), prepared from the sperm whale by Kendrew and his group. The significance of this structural similarity will be mentioned again in a discussion of the evolution of hemoglobin.

More recently the Perutz group[24] extended their studies on the conformation of horse oxyhemoglobin by much more precise x-ray diffraction analysis and three-dimensional Fourier synthesis at 2.8 Å resolution, rather than at 5.5 Å resolution, used in the earlier work[23] just described. Fifteen months were required to measure the intensities of some 100,000 reflections in the diffractometer. The phase angles of 8000 reflections were determined. The resulting electron density maps showed the positions of nearly all the amino acid residues of the hemoglobin molecule, the orientations of the side chains, and some details of the heme groups. On the basis of the results, combined with the known stereochemistry and sequence of the amino acids involved, a new atomic model of oxyhemoglobin (horse) was constructed.[24] In construction of this model, the x-ray analysis data of the hemoglobin crystals were subjected to a mathematic model building and refinement procedure programmed in Fortran for a digital computer. The general conformation of hemoglobin in the new model confirms that given in the earlier model (Figs. 5-10 and 5-12). However, much more detail is visible. Each polypeptide chain is made up of helical and nonhelical segments, similar to those described earlier (p. 81) in sperm whale myoglobin. The heme groups have similar surroundings. The center of the molecule is a cavity filled with water. The contacts between unlike subunits are chiefly nonpolar, while those between like subunits, if present, are polar. Thus, when the tetramer $(\alpha\beta)_2$ dissociates into two dimers, it probably breaks at the contacts between $\alpha_1\beta_2$ and $\alpha_2\beta_1$. Dissociation is favored by high concentrations of neutral electrolytes. The structure of the contacts between unlike subunits (α and β) suggests that the *tetramer,* rather than the $\alpha\beta$ dimer, as some have proposed, is the *functional unit of hemoglobin.*

The general features of horse oxyhemoglobin revealed in the new model are that polar residues are excluded from the interior of the molecule except for an occasional serine or threonine. Glycine and alanine occur anywhere in the molecule. The larger nonpolar side chains of amino acids are located in the interior or in surface crevices of the subunits or at the boundaries of unlike subunits. The heme groups lie in nonpolar "pockets" of the α- and β-chains. There are about 60 interactions between the atoms of the heme groups and those of the surrounding α- and β-chains. All but three are nonpolar.

Two kinds of contacts between the α- and β-chains are present. The great majority are nonpolar interactions. Only five probable hydrogen bonds are apparent. The exact locations of the various contacts between the four subunits of hemoglobin and other detailed features are described in this monumental work.[24]

Thus the tertiary and quaternary structures of hemoglobin derive their coherence from weak secondary forces—a few hydrogen bonds and a large number of nonpolar interactions. The ability of the ferrous iron of hemoglobin to combine reversibly with molecular oxygen is apparently dependent on these nonpolar surroundings.

The complete amino acid sequences of the α-, β-, γ-, and δ-chains of normal human hemoglobins have been determined in the past few years by the composite work of Konigsberg, Braunitzer, and Schroeder[25] and their colleagues. The procedure used was similar to that developed by Sanger (p. 74) for de-

Table 19-5. Amino acid sequences of the α-, β-, and γ-chains of human hemoglobin*

	1	2	3	4	5					10					15				
α	Val-		-Leu-Ser-Pro-Ala-Asp-Lys-Thr-Asn-Val-Lys-Ala-Ala-Try-Gly-Lys-Val-Gly-Ala-
β	Val-His-Leu-Thr-Pro-Glu-Glu-Lys-Ser-Ala-Val-Thr-Ala-Leu-Try-Gly-Lys-Val-Asn-
γ	Gly-His-Phe-Thr-Glu-Glu-Asp-Lys-Ala-Thr-Ile-Thr-Ser-Leu-Try-Gly-Lys-Val-Asn-
	1	2	3	4	5					10					15				

	20				25					30					35				
α	His-Ala-Gly-Glu-Tyr-Gly-Ala-Glu-Ala-Leu-Glu-Arg-Met-Phe-Leu-Ser-Phe-Pro-Thr-
β	-Val-Asp-Glu-Val-Gly-Gly-Glu-Ala-Leu-Gly-Arg-Leu-Leu-Val-Val-Tyr-Pro-Try
γ	-Val-Glu-Asp-Ala-Gly-Gly-Glu-Thr-Leu-Gly-Arg-Leu-Leu-Val-Val-Tyr-Pro-Try
	20				25				29	30					35				

	40				45					50									
α	Thr-Lys-Thr-Tyr-Phe-Pro-His-Phe-		-Asp-Leu-Ser-His-Gly-Ser-Ala-	-	-	-
β	Thr-Gln-Arg-Phe-Phe-Glu-Ser-Phe-Gly-Asp-Leu-Ser-Thr-Pro-Asp-Ala-Val-Met-Gly
γ	Thr-Gln-Arg-Phe-Phe-Asp-Ser-Phe-Gly-Asn-Leu-Ser-Ser-Ala-Ser-Ala-Ile-Met-Gly
	40				45					50					55				

	55				60					65					70				
α	-		-Gln-Val-Lys-Gly-His-Gly-Lys-Lys-Val-Ala-Asp-Ala-Leu-Thr-Asn-Ala-Val-Ala
β	Asn-Pro-Lys-Val-Lys-Ala-His-Gly-Lys-Lys-Val-Leu-Gly-Ala-Phe-Ser-Asp-Gly-Leu-Ala
γ	Asn-Pro-Lys-Val-Lys-Ala-His-Gly-Lys-Lys-Val-Leu-Thr-Ser-Leu-Gly-Asp-Ala-Ile-Lys
	60				65					70					75				

	75				80					85					90				
α	His-Val-Asp-Asp-Met-Pro-Asn-Ala-Leu-Ser-Ala-Leu-Ser-Asp-Leu-His-Ala-His-Lys
β	His-Leu-Asp-Asn-Leu-Lys-Gly-Thr-Phe-Ala-Thr-Leu-Ser-Glu-Leu-His-Cys-Asp-Lys
γ	His-Leu-Asp-Asp-Leu-Lys-Gly-Thr-Phe-Ala-Gln-Leu-Ser-Glu-Leu-His-Cys-Asp-Lys
	80				85					90					95				

	95				100					105									
α	Leu-Arg-Val-Asp-Pro-Val-Asp-Phe-Lys-Leu-Leu-Ser-His-Cys-Leu-Leu-Val-Thr-Leu
β	Leu-His-Val-Asp-Pro-Glu-Asn-Phe-Arg-Leu-Leu-Gly-Asn-Val-Leu-Val-Cys-Val-Leu
γ	Leu-His-Val-Asp-Pro-Glu-Asn-Phe-Lys-Leu-Leu-Gly-Asn-Val-Leu-Val-Thr-Val-Leu
	100				105					110									

	110				115					120					125				
α	Ala-Ala-His-Leu-Pro-Ala-Glu-Phe-Thr-Pro-Ala-Val-His-Ala-Ser-Leu-Asp-Lys-Phe-Leu
β	Ala-His-His-Phe-Gly-Lys-Glu-Phe-Thr-Pro-Pro-Val-Gln-Ala-Ala-Tyr-Gln-Lys-Val-Val
γ	Ala-Ile-His-Phe-Gly-Lys-Glu-Phe-Thr-Pro-Glu-Val-Gln-Ala-Ser-Try-Gln-Lys-Met-Val
	115				120					125					130				

	130				135					140	141								
α	Ala-Ser-Val-Ser-Thr-Val-Leu-Thr-Ser-Lys- Tyr- Arg
β	Ala-Gly-Val-Ala-Asp-Ala-Leu-Ala-His-Lys-Tyr-His
γ	Thr-Gly-Val-Ala-Ser-Ala-Leu-Ser-Ser-Arg-Tyr-His
	135				140	141	142	143	144	145	146								

* Gaps have been introduced into the sequences of the peptide chains in order to show the similarities in the sequences of the chains. These gaps do not actually exist in the hemoglobin molecule.

termining the amino acid sequence in insulin. As shown in Table 19-5, the α-chain is made up of 141 amino acids, and the β- and γ-chains are composed of 146 amino acids. The δ-chain, not shown, also is made up of 146 amino acids.

It may be noted that there are differences in the amino acid sequences of the three chains. However, more remarkable is the fact that there are many striking *similarities*, e.g., 24 consecutive identical amino acids (positions 88 to 111) in the β- and γ-chains, also 65 identical amino acid placements in the α- and β-chains, 108 in the β- and γ-chains, 55 the same in all three chains. Subsequent work showed that the β- and δ-chains are even more similar, with 138 identical amino acid positions out of a total of 146. Likewise, there is a surprising similarity between the β-chain of human hemoglobin and the amino acid sequence of myoglobin from sperm whale muscle. There are actually 22 identical amino acid positions in these two chains — obtained from such widely different species. The significance of these similarities in amino acid sequence, like those of the tertiary conformations just mentioned, will be discussed later in connection with the evolution of hemoglobins.

Evolutionary changes in hemoglobin. As mentioned previously, these striking similarities led Ingram[26] and others to propose that a genetic, evolutionary relationship existed. He suggested that the α-chain is probably the oldest form, from an evolutionary standpoint, because of its similarity in amino acid sequence to that of lamprey hemoglobin, a monomeric primitive form of hemoglobin. He further postulated that by gene duplication the γ-, β-, and δ-chains evolved in succession in that order. Calculations from the numbers of variant amino acid residues between chains have indicated that the time (in millions of years) of divergence from a proposed common ancestral chain is: α- and γ-, 600; α- and β-, 565; β- and γ-, 260; β- and δ-, 44. The divergence of myoglobin and the α-chain from the primitive ancestral chain presumably occurred over 600 million years ago.

Subsequent determinations of amino acid sequences of the α- and β-chains of various primates by Hill and Buettner-Janusch,[27] and of other species,[28,29] supported and extended Ingram's proposal. The following generalizations were made from the data: (1) Amino acid sequence differences vary directly with evolutionary relationships. The closer the species to man, the more similar is the amino acid sequence to that of human hemoglobin. (2) The β-chain varies more than the α-chain. (3) Sequences *essential* to the function of the molecule *do not vary*. This has been found true in all the mammals studied thus far. The functional portions of the molecule conserved include the basic and hydrophobic clusters, the binding groups to heme, and the C-terminus. (4) Amino acids with desirable but not essential properties show a lesser degree of evolutionary restraint. (5) Other amino acids simply take up space and vary widely.

Another interesting point found in these studies is the striking resemblance between the β-chain of lemurs and shrews and the γ-chain of human fetal hemoglobin.

The foregoing studies have also shown that there is a surprising correlation between the evolutionary times calculated from variant amino acid residues in hemoglobins of various species and paleontologic records. For example, the latter show that man and the horse separated from a common ancestor about 100 to 150 million years ago. The amino acids of the α-chains of these two species differ in 18 positions. Assuming that there were nine mutations in each species, evidently each mutation occurred at an interval of approximately 12 to 15 million years. Using this figure, application to the number of substitutions in the β-chains of primates gives values agreeing well with paleontologic data for these species. Likewise, application of the calculation to the numbers of variant amino acid residues in cytochrome-c (a heme-protein related to hemoglobin), as obtained in the work of Margoliash and Smith[30] in various species, gives values agreeing well with paleontologic records. Thus, the times in millions of years for the divergence of the following species compared with man calculate to be approximately as follows: pig, 83; horse, 130; chicken, 160; tuna, 230; and yeast, 500. As was pointed out earlier (p. 6), the cytochrome molecule is believed to have existed some 2 billion years. In view of some similarities between the hemoglobin, myoglobin, and cytochrome molecules, many authorities believe that the three are derived from a common primordial ancestor that existed some 1 to 2 billion years ago!

Biosynthesis of hemoglobin. The biosynthetic pathway of the heme portion of the hemoglobin molecule will be considered later (p. 608). The globin moiety is formed from amino acids from the body pool in amounts of about 8 gm. per day in the normal adult. Thus, about 14% of the amino acids from the average daily protein intake are used for globin formation. Apparently, globin biosynthesis has a "high priority" call on the labile amino acid pool of the body.[21] A number of studies using ^{14}C-labeled amino acids (leucine, lysine, glycine, etc.) demonstrated that the process occurs primarily in the nucleated erythrocyte (normoblast) of the bone marrow and also in the reticulocyte. The mechanism involved in the biosynthesis of globin has probably been studied more extensively than that for any other protein because of the relative ease of obtaining the necessary synthetic system, even in cell-free form, from reticulocytes. Apparently globin synthesis occurs on ribosomes[31] in much the same manner as that of other proteins. This process has been described in some detail (p. 98). Ultracentrifugal data and electron micrographic studies[32] indicated that hemoglobin synthesis in the reticulocyte occurs on a multiple ribosomal structure containing five ribosomes. These ribosomes appear to be strung on an RNA strand, possibly messenger RNA. An interesting study[33] reported, however, that hemoglobin synthesis occurs in the nucleus of nucleated avian erythrocytes. The nucleus of human nucleated erythrocytes (bone marrow), in contrast, does not appear to synthesize significant amounts of hemoglobin.[34] The formation of the α- and β-chains of globin does not appear to involve any special mechanisms or genetic factors. The two types of chains are apparently formed independently under the control of different genes although normally at the same rate. Bruns and London[35] found that hemin increases the rate of globin synthesis in rabbit reticulocytes while decreasing that of heme synthesis. Thus heme may serve as part of a control mechanism to maintain the synthesis of globin and presumably its constituent α- and β-chains at a near 1:1 molecular ratio. Protoporphyrin-IX has also been reported to increase globin synthesis.[36] In a rare genetic defect in man, there is apparently a suppression of the biosynthesis of α-chains so that an abnormal hemoglobin, Hb-H, with four β-chains (β_4) results. The four β-chains appear to form a tetramer much as do two α- and two β-chains. A similar genetic defect also seems to occur in Bart's hemoglobin, which is γ_4. Other genetic defects occur in the biosynthesis of globin, resulting in the production of the so-called abnormal hemoglobins or hemoglobin variants. These will be considered next.

Abnormal hemoglobins. The abnormal hemoglobins result from some genetic defect or alteration in the mechanism, presumably in the respective DNA molecule itself (p. 101), for globin synthesis or, more accurately, for the synthesis of its constituent α-, β-, γ-, or δ-chains. It represents one of the most completely studied effects of gene mutations on the structure of protein molecules and hence is of added general biochemical significance. Pauling and his associates[37] aptly called these conditions "molecular diseases."

Since Pauling's classic pioneer studies on hemoglobin-S and sickle-cell anemia, there has been widespread application of peptide mapping and amino acid analysis to hemoglobin isolated from patients with diverse abnormalities of red cell function. As a result, nearly 150 different mutant human types have been described in the literature at the present time. A few selected examples will be considered. For details on other abnormal hemoglobins, the reviews of Perutz[38] and others[39] and the general references at the end of this chapter should be consulted.

The abnormal hemoglobins may be grouped into two general types: (1) hemoglobins in which there are altered combinations of the normal α-, β-, γ-, or δ-chains; examples are Hb-H,β_4, and Hb-Bart's, γ_4, previously discussed; (2) hemoglobins in which there is an altered sequence of amino acids in usually one of the constituent chains; the α- or β-chain is affected and normally there is a *single* amino acid substitution, as originally shown in the classic work of Ingram[40] on sickle cell hemoglobin. Such substitutions may alter the net charge on the hemoglobin molecule, thus changing the isoelectric point and electrophoretic mobility of the molecule. Thus the substitution of valine for glutamic acid in sickle-cell hemoglobin changes the net charge +2 from Hb-A. This fact is, of course, the basis for the separation of various abnormal hemoglobins by electrophoresis. Amino acid substitutions also may change the solubility of the abnormal form. In the case of sickle-cell hemoglobin, for example, the deoxygenated form is much less soluble than that of Hb-A and hence tends to form insoluble tactoids, increasing the rate of destruction of the transporting erythrocyte and leading to the hemolytic anemia characteristic of this disease.

Most of the known substitutions in amino acid sequence in the abnormal hemoglobins do not significantly impair the oxygen-transport ability of the hemoglobin affected. An interesting exception, however, is hemoglobin-M types, in which the histidine residue in position-58 of the α-chain or in position-63 of the β-chain is replaced by tyrosine. Since this histidine is the one that apparently alternates with oxygen in attaching to the iron of heme, impairment of oxygen transport occurs. The ferrous iron of this type of hemoglobin becomes converted to ferric and thus to methemoglobin (p. 615) and is then useless for subsequent oxygen transport. This apparently explains the striking cyanosis seen in individuals with hereditary methemoglobinemia, resulting from the presence of hemoglobin-M. Hemoglobin-H (β_4) likewise has an altered capacity for oxygen transport as a result of its increased affinity for oxygen.

The description of the new more precise model of three-dimensional conformation of horse oxyhemoglobin (p. 598) has made possible the logical categorization of the new mutants of human hemoglobin and the prediction of their possible functional defects in oxygen transport and the clinical sequelae.[38] The three structural features of the hemoglobin molecule, apparent from studies of the new three-dimensional model, that are of primary functional importance in oxygen transport are (1) the points of contact binding the two symmetric α,β-dimers of hemoglobin; (2) the heme-binding contacts with α- and β-chains; and (3) the invariant sequence of the nonpolar amino acids in the helical portions of the α- and β-chains. Amino acid substitutions affecting these three vital structural features may seriously affect oxygen transport by the mutant hemoglobin and lead to gross clinical manifestations. Substitutions in other parts of the molecule, especially on the surface, should have little or no effect on oxygen transport and therefore produce no clinical symptoms. This prediction has been supported by studies of abnormal human hemoglobin, to be discussed next.

Substitutions altering the points of contact between the α,β-dimers (1) thus might be expected to produce an increased affinity of the molecule for oxygen (p. 646), leading to tissue hypoxia and, in turn, clinically to cyanosis and/or a compensatory polycythemia. Substitutions (or deletions) affecting the binding of the heme groups by the α- and β-chains (2) should result in an unstable hemoglobin that could precipitate in the erythrocyte as inclusion or Heinz bodies and lead to structural weakness of the cell and hemolytic anemia clinically. Substitutions affecting the invariant, nonpolar amino acids in the helical portions of the α- or β-chains (3) might allow internal bonding with ferrous heme, forming ferric heme and methemoglobin, which cannot carry oxygen. This would be manifested clinically by a methemoglobinemia and possibly weakness and other symptoms.

Substitutions involving predominantly polar amino acids on the external surface of the molecule may be placed in a fourth category. These form the largest group of abnormal hemoglobins at the present time. For the most part, there is no impairment in the oxygen transport of these mutant hemoglobins, hence no clinical symptoms. In the few exceptions, e.g., hemoglobins S and C, hemolytic anemia may occur in *homozygotes only* due apparently to mechanical damage to the erythrocyte transporting the mutant hemoglobin. Heterozygotes usually remain symptom free.

Selected examples of these four different types of abnormal hemoglobins[38] are given in Table 19-6, together with the amino acid substitutions involved and the clinical manifestations resulting.

Since the atypical hemoglobins are usually found in population surveys using electrophoretic methods at pH 8.6 or by examination of patients show-

Table 19-6. Some selected abnormal human hemoglobins with position of amino acid substitution

Designation	Substitution From	To	Position	Clinical symptoms
1. Substitution of amino acids in contact with heme groups				
α-Chain				
Torino	Phe	Val	43	Inclusion body anemia
M-Boston	His	Tyr	58	Cyanosis, methemoglinemia
β-Chain				
Hammersmith	Phe	Ser	42	Inclusion body anemia, cyanosis
Zurich	His	Arg	63	Inclusion body anemia (on treatment with sulfonamides)
M–Hyde Park	His	Tyr	62	Cyanosis, methemoglobinemia
Sabine	Leu	Pro	91	Methemoglobinemia; inclusion body anemia
2. Substitution of amino acids at contacts between α- and β- chains				
α-Chain				
Chesapeake	Arg	Leu	92	Polycythemia (high O_2 affinity; decreased heme-heme interaction)
J-Capetown	Arg	Gln	92	Mild polycythemia
β-Chain				
E	Glu	Lys	26	Mild hemolytic anemia (homozygotes only)
Yakima	Asp	His	96	Polycythemia (increased O_2 affinity)
New York	Val	Gly	113	None reported
3. Substitution of amino acids in general positions				
α-Chain				
Etobioke	Ser	Arg	84	None reported
Manitoba	Ser	Arg	102	None reported
β-Chain				
Freiburg	Val	?	23	Cyanosis (high O_2 affinity)
Gun Hill	(deletion of 5-amino between 91 and 97)			Hemolytic anemia
Rainier	Tyr	His	145	Polycythemia
4. External substitutions of amino acids				
α-Chain				
J-Oxford	Gly	Asp	15	No clinical symptoms in heterozygotes
Mexico	Gln	Glu	54	No clinical symptoms in heterozygotes
O-Indonesia	Glu	Lys	116	No clinical symptoms in heterozygotes
β-Chain				
S	Glu	Val	6	No clinical symptoms in heterozygotes (severe sickle-cell anemia in homozygotes)
C	Glu	Lys	6	No clinical symptoms in heterozygotes (mild anemia in homozygotes)
N-Seattle	Lys	Glu	61	No clinical symptoms in heterozygotes

Table 19-6. Some selected abnormal human hemoglobins with position of amino acid substitution—cont'd

Designation	Substitution From	To	Position	Clinical symptoms
4. External substitutions of amino acids—cont'd				
			δ-Chain	
F-Texas (I)	Glu	Lys	5	Apparently no clinical effects
F-Alexandra	Thr	Lys	12	Apparently no clinical effects
F-Hull	Glu	Lys	121	Apparently no clinical effects
			δ-Chain	
A₂	Gly	Arg	16	Apparently no clinical effects
A₂-Flatbush	Ala	Glu	22	Apparently no clinical effects
A₂-Bahinga	Gly	Asp	136	Apparently no clinical effects

ing clinical symptoms, it is probable that many mutations involving neutral amino acids are missed. As many as one in every 600 persons may carry a mutant hemoglobin.

The mechanical injury to the erythrocyte produced by certain abnormal hemoglobins was shown clearly in the case of hemoglobin Sabine. The "half-life" of erythrocytes from one patient was found by the ^{51}Cr method to be only 4 days, in contrast to about 28 days for normal subjects. One explanation for the mechanical damage to the erythrocyte is that the amino acid substitution in the vicinity of heme attachment lessens the avidity of the α- and β-chains for heme, liberating free heme, which is metabolized to dipyrroles and excreted in the urine. The remaining free globin moiety is unstable and precipitates in the erythrocyte, forming the inclusion bodies or Heinz bodies frequently seen clinically in certain blood dyscrasias. The inclusion bodies attach to the erythrocyte membrane and alter its permeability, resulting in osmotic damage to the cell, early destruction, and the characteristic hemolytic anemia. One patient showed severe hemolytic anemia even though only 8% of her total hemoglobin was Hb-Sabine,[41] which suggests that clinical symptoms can occur in heterozygotes as well as in homozygotes having this mutant hemoglobin.

Abnormal hemoglobins are known to occur in animals also. Sickling of erythrocytes and a type of hemoglobin-S has been described in deer.

Apparently, several of the abnormal hemoglobins (F, I, Lepore, A₂) bind to human haptoglobin an α_2-globulin that transports free hemoglobin from destroyed erythrocytes to the reticuloendothelial system for catabolism (p. 681), to the same degree as does Hb-A. However, Hb-H and Hb-Bart's fail to bind to human haptoglobin.

The foregoing monumental expansion of knowledge of the conformation and biosynthesis of normal and abnormal hemoglobins is of far-reaching significance not only in itself but also insofar as it is prophetic of future similar developments for other proteins of equal biologic importance (of which there may be an estimated 10^5 to 10^6 in man alone).

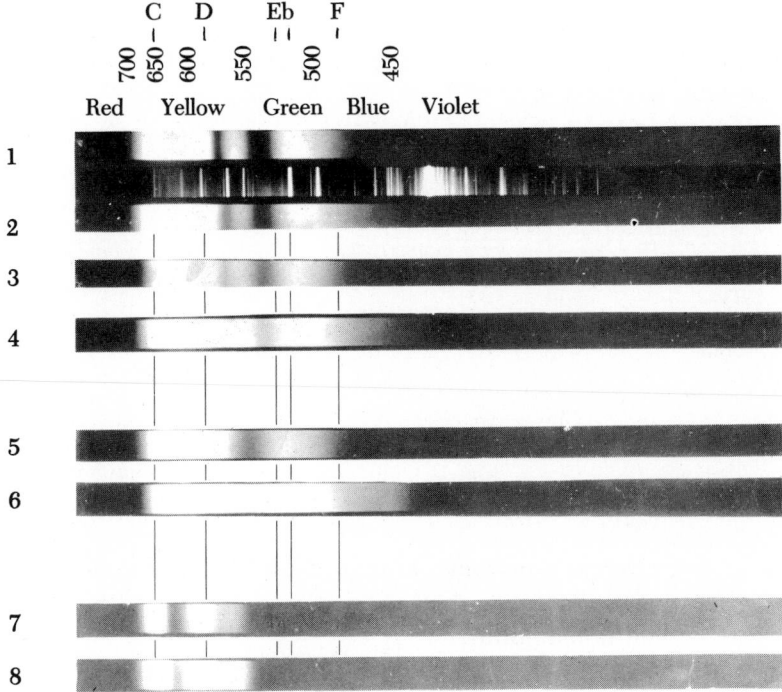

Fig. 19-5. Absorption spectra. At the top are shown the positions of the reference lines; next is a millimicron scale, below which are indicated the positions of the colors of the solar spectrum. The spectra below must be pictured as having these same spectral colors wherever light appears, the dark portions appearing black because of absorption of the light rays. *1*, Oxyhemoglobin; *2, 3,* and *4,* carbon monoxide hemoglobin of different concentrations (compare with *1* and note the slight but definite difference in the position of the two bands and also the disappearance of one absorption band in the most dilute solution, *4*); *5* and *6,* reduced hemoglobin of different concentrations; *7* and *8,* methemoglobin of different concentrations.

Absorption spectra of hemoglobin and its derivatives. Hemoglobin, its derivatives, and other related compounds have characteristic absorption spectra; i.e., if such a solution is interposed between a source of white light and the prism of a spectroscope, the light of certain wavelengths is absorbed and dark bands or shadows appear in the spectrum wherever the light has been taken out. Thus hemoglobin, in the deoxygenated state (reduced hemoglobin), has one broad band in the yellow-green section, its center being at 559 mμ.* Oxyhemoglobin has two narrow bands. One, the narrower of the two, is in the yellow, with its center at 579 mμ; the other, the wider, is nearer the green, with its center at 542 mμ. On great dilution, the wider one disappears first. Dilute solutions of hemoglobin may be detected spectroscopically.

The absorption spectrum of carbon monoxide hemoglobin is similar to that of oxyhemoglobin, having two main absorption bands. However, the absorp-

---

*Millimicrons (mμ) are now frequently expressed as "nanometers" or "nM." 1 nM $= 1 \times 10^{-9}$ meter. Therefore, 1 nM $=$ 1 mμ.

tion maxima for carbon monoxide hemoglobin are shifted slightly to the right (blue end of spectrum), being at approximately 570 and 535 mμ. Therefore, from the absorption spectrum, carbon monoxide hemoglobin is very difficult to identify in cases of carbon monoxide poisoning, particularly since 20% to 50% of the oxyhemoglobin may still be present in the blood in severe or even fatal cases of carbon monoxide poisoning (p. 613). The absorption spectrum of methemoglobin, on the other hand, is quite characteristic and is commonly used for the qualitative detection of this pigment. There are *four* absorption bands for methemoglobin with maxima at approximately 634, 575, 540, and 490 mμ, respectively. The characteristic absorption band used in the detection of methemoglobin is in the red portion of the spectrum at 634 mμ (p. 606).

This method has various practical applications in the recognition of a number of derivatives of hemoglobin. In Fig. 19-5 are shown the absorption spectra of some of the compounds.

Chemical structure of heme   Heme, the prosthetic group of hemoglobin, is a chelate of ferrous iron, while protoporphyrin, a porphyrin, is a union of four pyrrole groups. For this reason, the heme of hemoglobin is sometimes called protoheme.

$$
\begin{array}{ccc}
\text{HC} & \!\!\!\!\!\!\!\!-\!\!\!\!\!\!\!\! & \text{CH} \\
\| & & \| \\
\text{HC} & & \text{CH} \\
\backslash & & / \\
 & \text{N} & \\
 & \text{H} &
\end{array}
\qquad \textbf{Pyrrole}
$$

Heme may be represented by the following structural formula, with its attachment to globin indicated:

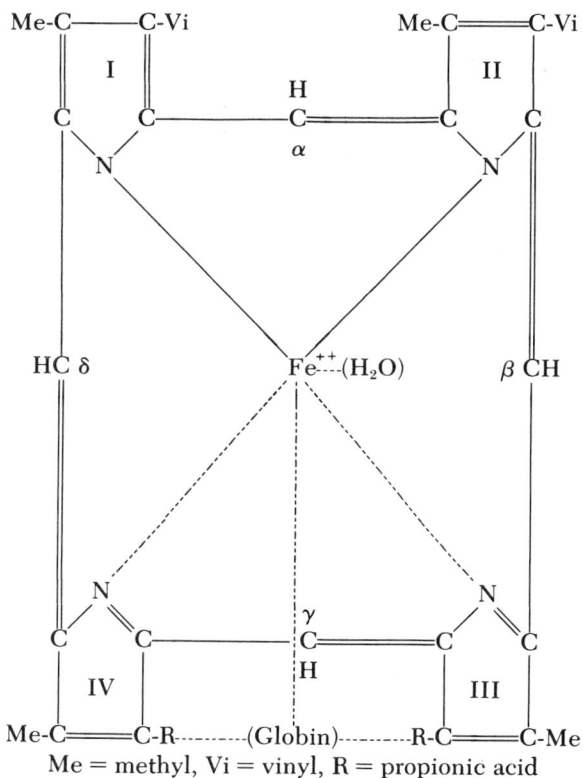

Me = methyl, Vi = vinyl, R = propionic acid

The arrangement of the double bonds varies in the different pyrrole groups. For each heme group, at least one of the coordination valences of the iron is believed to be connected to one of the imidazole nitrogens of a histidine in the peptide chain of the subunit. There is some evidence that each heme iron coordinates to two imidazole nitrogens of histidine, probably at positions 58 and 87 in the α-chain and 63 and 92 in the β-chain. Corwin believes that one of the imidazole ligands (probably with His-58 in the α-chain and His-63 in the β-chain) is reversibly displaced by oxygen rather than by water during oxygen transport. The other two linkages to the α- or β-chains are postulated to be combined with the two propionic acid groups present in heme.

Several types of heme occur in different hemoproteins. Hemoglobin contains protoheme, as mentioned. Certain cytochromes contain heme-C, in which the two vinyl groups appear with sulfhydryl groups linked to cysteine of the protein moiety of the molecule. Heme-A has different alkyl groups replacing the two vinyl groups.

Biosynthesis of heme. Our knowledge of the synthesis of heme in the body has been extended materially by the use of isotopically labeled compounds. Not only can the animal as a whole synthesize the pyrrole unit, but heme can be synthesized in vitro by mammalian reticulocytes and by the nucleated red blood cells of birds. Rittenberg, Shemin, and co-workers demonstrated these phenomena and determined the sources of the individual parts of heme in a brilliant series of experiments (Fig. 19-6). The initial findings demonstrated that glycine and succinate are concerned with the atoms of the porphyrin. The nitrogen of glycine is utilized for both types of pyrrole rings, i.e., those that have vinyl groups and those that have propionic groups. The carboxyl carbon of glycine is not used for heme formation, but the α-carbon is. Of eight such α-carbons of glycine that go into each porphyrin molecule, four are the source of the methene bridge carbon atoms, and four others go, one each, into comparable positions of each pyrrole unit. The remaining carbons are derived from succinyl-CoA, a member of the tricarboxylic acid cycle (p. 263).

Several discoveries have further extended our knowledge of the pathway

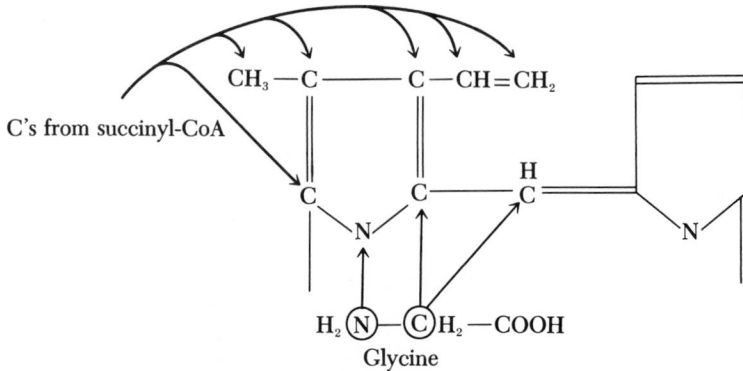

Fig. 19-6. Diagram of part of heme molecule indicating sources of N and C atoms. The α-C of glycine is shown as the source of the methene bridge C as well as of one pyrrole C, whose exact position in the ring is probably as shown.

of the biosynthesis of heme. One of these was the finding that δ-aminolevulinic acid (ALA) serves as an extremely active precursor of heme in nucleated erythrocytes. From its formula, evidently ALA can be synthesized by the combining of glycine with succinic acid (or succinate), as postulated by the Shemin succinate-glycine cycle.[42] Another important discovery was the isolation and crystallization of porphobilinogen and the determination[43] of its chemical structure, as shown below:

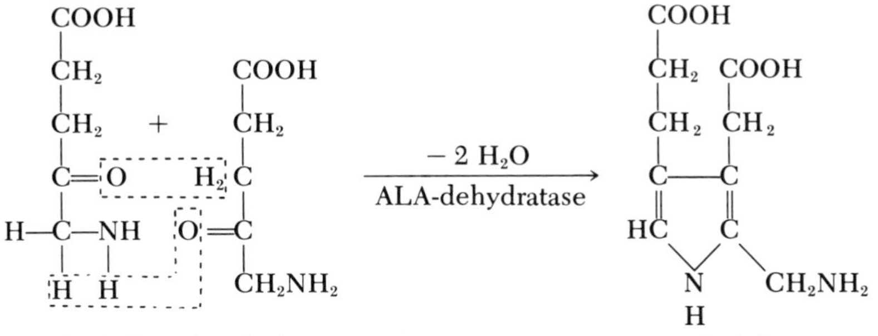

ALA (2 molecules)   Porphobilinogen

For a number of years, porphobilinogen has been known to occur in the urine of patients with a disease called *acute porphyria*. It was believed even then that this substance might be an intermediate in porphyrin and heme formation. Finally, an enzyme, ALA-dehydratase, that converted two molecules of δ-aminolevulinic acid to porphobilinogen was prepared from beef liver,[44] and an enzyme extract that converted porphobilinogen to porphyrins was obtained.[45]

During the past few years, work by several groups of investigators[46] has elucidated most of the remaining steps of the biosynthesis of heme and related compounds. The necessary enzymes were prepared in somewhat purified form and several of the cofactors required were identified. The rather wide distribution of certain enzymes required for heme synthesis is of interest; e.g., coproporphyrinogen oxidase is found in detectable amounts in most tissues and in relatively high concentrations in liver, bone marrow, intestinal mucosa, nucleated erythrocytes, and kidney. A summary of current knowledge of the biosynthetic pathway of heme is given in Fig. 19-7. Note that a portion of the process takes place in the mitochondrion, at least in liver cells, and apparently also in a particulate fraction of nucleated (chicken) erythrocytes.[47] However, the conversion of ALA to porphobilinogen and then to uroporphyrinogen and coproporphyrinogen (type III) apparently occurs only in the nonparticulate portion of the cell, since the necessary enzymes are found there. Thus, as a result of the intracellular compartmentation of the enzymes involved, Granick and his co-workers[48] believe that the biosynthesis of protoporphyrin (and heme) may be controlled by the permeability of the of the mitochondrial membrane to ALA. Bruns and London[35] obtained evidence from studies in rabbit reticulocytes that heme itself inhibits heme synthesis by a feedback mechanism. Heme appears to act as a corepressor (p. 129), combining with the aporepressor-operator mechanism to control the rate at which the structural gene transcribes messenger RNA for the synthesis of the rate-limiting enzyme, ALA-synthetase (Fig. 19-7).

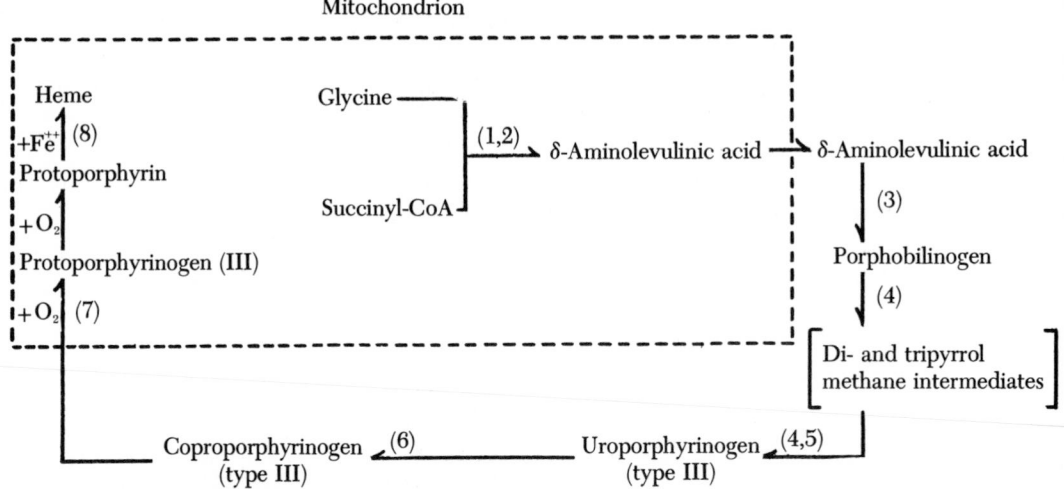

Fig. 19-7. Biosnythetic pathway of heme in the liver cell. *1*, Pyridoxal-P⁼; *2*, δ-aminolevulinic acid synthetase; *3*, aminolevulinic acid dehydrase; *4*, uroporphyrinogen synthetase; *5*, uroporphyrinogen-III cosynthetase; *6*, uroporphyrinogen decarboxylase; *7*, coproporphyrinogen oxidase; *8*, Fe^{++}-protoporphyrin chelatase (or ferrochelatase). (Adapted from Sano, S., and Granick, S.: J. Biol. Chem. **236:** 1173, 1961.)

The heme thus formed is used not only for blood hemoglobin but also for muscle hemoglobin (p. 562), the cytochromes (p. 247), and other heme pigments in the body. Recent studies further demonstrated the remarkable fact that the chlorophyl of plants and vitamin B_{12} of certain microorganisms are synthesized by the same pathway as heme, except, of course, for the terminal phase.

The normal human adult excretes small amounts of coproporphyrin (types I and III) and traces of uroporphyrin (types I and III) in the urine and feces daily. These may be regarded as waste products produced by the oxidation of small amounts of uroporphyrinogens and coproporphyrinogens (types I and III). Type III porphyrinogens are, of course, normal intermediates in the biosynthesis of heme and related substances, e.g., the cytochromes. Type I porphyrinogens probably represent the small amount not formed by way of the enzyme uroporphyrinogen III–cosynthetase. A temporary increase in the amount of porphyrins, particularly coproporphyrin, excreted in the urine occurs in alcoholism, in lead and certain other types of poisoning, and in several infectious diseases. This is termed porphyrinuria.

Considerably larger amounts of the type I isomer of uroporphyrin and coproporphyrin are excreted in the urine and feces of patients having the rather rare hereditary disease of porphyrin metabolism known as congenital *porphyria*. Several other forms of porphyria (acute intermittent, *cutanea tarda*) have been described.[49] Congenital porphyria appears to result from a deficiency of isomerase (uroporphyrinogen-III cosynthetase) (Fig. 19-7), which is necessary for the formation of the type III porphyrins used in heme synthesis.

Type I porphyrinogens and the type I porphyrins formed from them by oxidation cannot be used by the body and are excreted. Significant amounts of these may also be deposited in the tissues, particularly the bones and teeth. This fact accounts for the pinkish color and intense vermillion-colored fluorescence in ultraviolet light of the teeth of these individuals. The urine may show a similar color and fluorescence. Congenital porphyria also occurs in domestic animals, particularly in highly inbred strains of cattle and pigs.[50]

Another remarkable hereditary disease of porphyrin metabolism, acute intermittent porphyria, is more frequently found than the congenital type. It is characterized by severe abdominal pain, neurologic symptoms, and sometimes a red-colored urine, especially after exposure to light. Porphobilinogen is found in the urine. The disease is thought to be due to an increased production, or activity, of the enzyme δ-aminolevulinic acid synthetase.[51] If this is the case in man, acute porphyria is a unique hereditary disease, one resulting from an excessive formation of an enzyme rather than a deficient formation as is usually found.

An interesting recent article[52] cited evidence indicating that the British royal family of the 1700's, and particularly King George III, who reigned at the time of the American Revolution, suffered from an acute intermittent type of porphyria. His recurring abdominal pain, diagnosed at the time as "biliary concretions in the gall duct," darkening of the urine, neurologic symptoms, and delirium are all classic symptoms of this hereditary metabolic disease. He was generally believed to be insane at the time. The same historical study indicates that three royal houses, including the Hanoverian and Prussian royal lines, were affected. Apparently Mary Queen of Scots (1542–1587) was the first known to be afflicted. Modern history records a number of such examples of this hereditary metabolic disease.

Significant recent investigations by Granick and his group,[48] using chick embryo liver cultures, demonstrated that certain steroids induce the biosynthesis of porphyrins and heme. Steroids, e.g., pregnanolone (p. 503), of the 5-β-androstane or 5-β-pregnane type with alcohol or ketone substituents at carbons numbered 3, 17, 20, and possibly 11 are active inducers. Steroids such as the androgens, estrogens, cortisol, and aldosterone have little or no activity. Glucuronide conjugates, even of the most potent 5-β-H steroids, are likewise inactive. Steroids affect the biosynthesis of heme apparently by serving as an inducer of the formation of ALA-synthetase, the key enzyme of the biosynthetic chain. Granick[48] believes the steroids block or displace heme from its binding site on the aporepressor protein of the Jacob-Monod model (p. 105), thus rendering the repressor mechanism inoperative. This leads to increased ALA-synthetase formation, with the resultant increased production of δ-aminolevulinic acid, porphyrins, and heme.

Certain drugs, e.g., dicarbethoxydihydrocollidine, sedormid, hexachlorobenzene, sulfonylureas, and certain barbiturates, are also active as inducers of ALA-synthetase formation and porphyrin-heme synthesis.

Some chemical properties of hemoglobin. The iron in reduced hemoglobin is in the ferrous state. In oxyhemoglobin it is still in the ferrous state, but oxygen is attached. The oxygen is assumed to be linked loosely to the ferrous

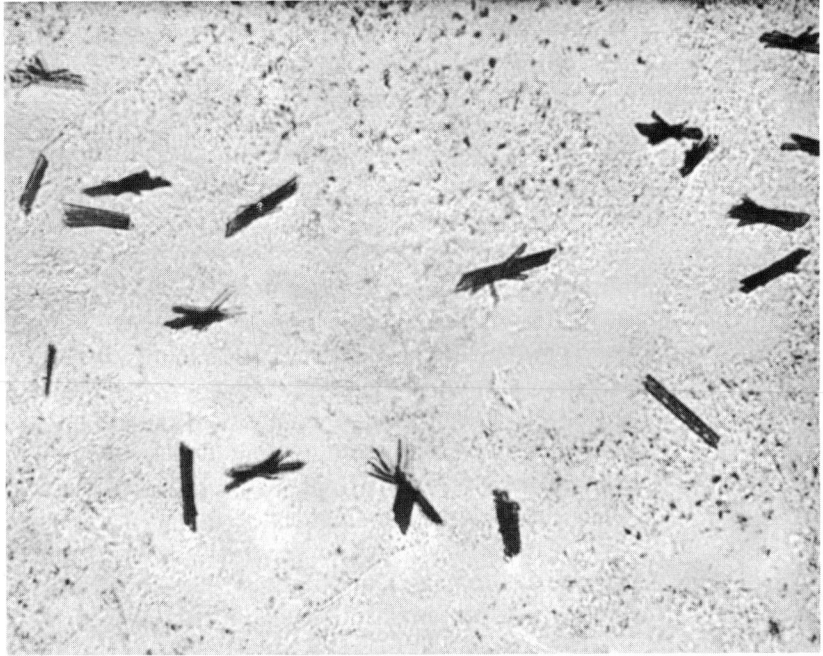

Fig. 19-8. Hemin crystals from human blood.

iron by a residual valence force, probably by sharing the unpaired electrons of ferrohemoglobin with those of molecular oxygen.

A *hemochromogen* is a compound of heme with any nitrogenous substance. Hence, hemoglobin and most of its derivatives are hemochromogens, as are also the respiratory pigments of the invertebrates, as well as the cytochromes. Heme and hemoproteins react with pyridine to form pyridine-hemochromogen. This reaction has been employed in the determination of total hemoproteins in samples.

Heme may be oxidized to hematin, which contains a hydroxyl group. This group may be substituted by a chloride ion, forming hemin. Hemin crystallizes out in characteristic brown crystals, which may be easily recognized under the microscope (Fig. 19-8). This procedure is used as a test for blood. A droplet of blood is placed on a microscope slide and warmed with acetic acid and sodium chloride. This warming under suitable conditions of acidity and salinity causes the heme to be split off from the hemoglobin and to be oxidized and permits the reaction with chloride ion. Dilute alkali similarly splits off the heme groups to form alkali hematin.

Since each molecule of hemoglobin has four heme groups, it contains four ferrous ions. Each heme group unites with one molecule of oxygen. We may accordingly represent reduced hemoglobin as globin (ferroheme)$_4$, and the reaction whereby it performs its respiratory function as:

$$\text{Globin (ferroheme)}_4 + 4\ O_2 \quad \rightleftarrows \quad \text{Globin (ferroheme-}O_2)_4$$
Reduced hemoglobin   **Oxyhemoglobin**

Usually, however, in discussions concerning this reaction, a less exact expression is used:

$$Hb \quad + \quad O_2 \quad \rightleftarrows \quad HbO_2$$

Reduced   **Oxyhemoglobin**
hemoglobin

Most of the oxygen present in arterial blood is held in this loose chemical combination with hemoglobin.

Peisach and co-workers[53] believe that the oxygenation of hemoglobin involves the migration of an electron from ferrous heme iron to the oxygen molecule. The heme iron atoms of oxyhemoglobin are thus formally in the ferric low-spin state. The ease with which this union can be brought about and broken may be demonstrated in the laboratory. Blood that has been rendered nonclotting may be poured from one vessel to another a few times and it becomes bright crimson (oxyhemoglobin). Addition of a mild reducing agent changes its color to a very dark red (reduced hemoglobin), after which it may be oxygenated again as before. These changes may be followed spectroscopically if the blood is suitably diluted. Of interest in this connection is the fact that there is a distinct displacement of the β-chains of Hb-A when oxygen combines with it.[23] This phenomenon will be considered further in Chapter 20. In addition to the oxygen combined with hemoglobin, there is a small amount held in solution in the plasma. The tension or pressure of oxygen in the plasma, together with other factors, determines the degree of dissociation of oxyhemoglobin into oxygen and hemoglobin. The partial pressure of the oxygen in atmospheric air at the barometric pressure of 760 mm. Hg is 159 mm. Hg (i.e., 20.9% O_2 × 760 mm. Hg). If blood is placed in contact with oxygen at this pressure, the hemoglobin becomes completely converted to oxyhemoglobin. Increase of oxygen pressure can add no more oxygen to the hemoglobin but can force more oxygen into solution in the plasma. Lowering the partial pressure of oxygen causes dissociation to occur; but even at 102 mm. Hg, which is the partial pressure of oxygen in arterial blood, the hemoglobin is 95% saturated. Still lower pressures, such as obtain in the tissues, cause further dissociation or release of atmospheric oxygen near the site of tissue oxidations. This discussion will be continued when the chemistry of respiration is taken up (Chapter 20).

Carbon monoxide hemoglobin. Carbon monoxide combines with the heme portion of hemoglobin to form carbon monoxide hemoglobin, also called carboxyhemoglobin and carbonylhemoglobin. This is a much firmer combination than the one between oxygen and hemoglobin. The affinity of hemoglobin for carbon monoxide is about 210 times that for oxygen. If, therefore, carbon monoxide is in the inspired air, it forms this firm combination to a greater extent than its proportion in the air would seem to warrant. Consequently, if enough carbon monoxide is present, the blood does not have sufficient oxyhemoglobin for respiratory purposes and asphyxiation occurs.

Carbon monoxide hemoglobin has a cherry red color that is not changed readily by reducing agents. Its absorption spectrum resembles that of oxyhemoglobin, but the two bands are slightly nearer the violet end of the spectrum.

Their centers are at 570 and 535 mμ. Carbon monoxide hemoglobin may also be detected by chemical tests. The simplest is to dilute the suspected blood greatly, after treating it with a little sodium hydroxide, and compare the color with normal blood similarly treated. Normal blood shows a greenish hue after such treatment, whereas carbon monoxide blood remains pink.

Poisoning by carbon monoxide is a common danger of modern life. Carbon monoxide is particularly lethal for two reasons: (1) it is odorless and colorless and, consequently, cannot be readily detected; and (2) its action is insidious and rapid. The victims frequently become unconscious in a few minutes, and death often follows quickly.

This gas is found wherever incomplete combustion of carbonaceous materials occurs—in automobile exhaust gas (4% to 7%), in chimney gases and smoke, and in blasting gases. It is also a constituent of manufactured illuminating gas (derived from coal or oil), in which its presence varies from 4% to 40%, depending on the source materials and the method of manufacture. Natural gas contains no carbon monoxide.

Poisoning may be either acute or chronic. Both are important from the standpoint of public health. Deaths resulting from the inhalation of automobile exhaust gas have increased alarmingly in the past few years. An automobile engine emits 1 cubic foot of carbon monoxide per minute per 20 horsepower. In a small individual garage with no ventilation, this amount may be fatal to a person in 5 minutes. Therefore a door or window of a garage must always be open, even in coldest weather, when the engine is running. Vehicular tunnels are also hazardous because of the possible accumulation of carbon monoxide from automobile exhaust gas in the atmosphere. The adequate ventilation of such tunnels is consequently of utmost importance.

National Safety Council figures show that in 1966 more than 843 Americans died from automobile exhaust fumes. The actual figure is probably considerably higher if deaths from carbon monoxide from other sources (faulty stoves, chimneys, heating systems, etc.) are included.

Several factors determine the degree of toxicity of carbon monoxide, but all relate to one point, i.e., the rate of absorption of this gas. The chief factors are (1) concentration of carbon monoxide in the air respired, (2) duration of exposure, and (3) rapidity of respiration. Rapidity of respiration depends on the activity of the individual, his age and size, and the temperature and humidity of the atmosphere. The symptoms produced depend on the percentage of hemoglobin combined with carbon monoxide and thus rendered physiologically useless, at least for the time being. Following are the symptoms that occur with the percentages of hemoglobin saturated with carbon monoxide:

Percent	Symptoms
0 to 10	Usually none
10 to 20	Possibly slight headache
20 to 30	Headache, throbbing in temples
30 to 40	Severe headache, weakness and dizziness, dim vision, nausea, vomiting, possibly collapse
40 to 50	Like the above but with greater possibility of collapse, increased pulse and respiration

Percent	Symptoms
50 to 60	Unconsciousness, coma with intermittent convulsions, Cheyne-Stokes respiration (periodic type of respiration)
60 to 70	Like the above, but with depressed heart action and respiration, possibly death
70 to 80	Weak pulse, respiratory failure, death

The proportion of carbon monoxide in the air necessary to produce such saturation figures depends on the factors first mentioned, but in a general way, if the respired air contains the following percentages:

Percentages	
0.01	Symptoms after a few hours
0.04	Perhaps safe for only about an hour
0.10	Uncomfortable and may be dangerous in 2 hours
0.30	Dangerous in 30 minutes
0.60	Dangerous in 10 to 15 minutes
1.30	Dangerous in 1 to 3 minutes

The treatment in cases of carbon monoxide poisoning is (1) rapid removal from the poisoned atmosphere, (2) artificial respiration, using an oxygen and carbon dioxide mixture, if available, and (3) blood transfusion, if necessary.

Methemoglobin. Methemoglobin is a derivative in which the iron is in the ferric state. It is produced by the oxidation of hemoglobin, as, for example, when potassium ferricyanide is added to blood. It is quite different from *oxygenated* hemoglobin, i.e., oxyhemoglobin, in which the oxygen is united loosely with *ferrous iron.* In methemoglobin, the iron is oxidized to the *ferric* condition and, in fact, oxygen is liberated, leaving the methemoglobin devoid of this gas; but, since there is now an additional positive charge, methemoglobin unites with a negative group, presumably a hydroxyl. Although hemoglobin may be oxidized to methemoglobin, oxyhemoglobin cannot be. Thus the following relationship may exist:

$$HbO_2 \quad \underset{\longleftarrow}{\overset{Oxygenation}{\longrightarrow}} \quad Hb \quad \underset{\longleftarrow}{\overset{Oxidation}{\longrightarrow}} \quad MetHb$$

A small amount of methemoglobin develops very slowly in shed blood. Its reduction to hemoglobin also occurs spontaneously, which reduction seems to be bound up with glycolytic reactions in the erythrocyte. After the administration of certain drugs or exposure to certain poisons, e.g., chlorates, acetanilid, nitrites, nitrobenzene, antipyrine, iodine, phenacetin, sulfonal, trional, and, perhaps most important, the sulfonamide drugs, methemoglobin is likely to be present in the circulating blood. Moreover, methemoglobin occurs in considerable amounts in the blood of certain individuals as a familial disease or inborn error of metabolism, familial methemoglobinemia, which is due to a lack of the enzyme methemoglobin reductase. Methemoglobinemia may also be found in individuals with hemoglobin-M and certain other types of abnormal hemoglobins (p. 602).

Although methemoglobin is an oxidized substance, it does not carry oxygen as oxyhemoglobin does; hence hemoglobin that has been changed to methemoglobin is unable to function as a respiratory pigment since its iron is in the ferric form. However, it slowly changes over to hemoglobin in the body. The relationship among hemoglobin, oxyhemoglobin, methemoglobin, and carbon monoxide hemoglobin is shown at the top of p. 616.

615

Pyrrole   Pyrrole
\\   /
Fe*—(H₂O)
/   \\
Pyrrole   Pyrrole
Hemoglobin

Pyrrole   Pyrrole
\\   /
Fe*—(O₂)
/   \\
Pyrrole   Pyrrole
Oxyhemoglobin

Pyrrole   Pyrrole
\\   /
Fe†—OH
/   \\
Pyrrole   Pyrrole
Methemoglobin

Pyrrole   Pyrrole
\\   /
Fe*—(CO)
/   \\
Pyrrole   Pyrrole
Carbon monoxide hemoglobin

° Ferrous.

† Ferric.

In some industries, poisons that cause methemoglobinemia are produced. Nitrobenzene is used in the manufacture of shoe dyes, floor polishes, cosmetics, and explosives. Workers in these industries may be acutely or chronically poisoned if nitrobenzene is absorbed in sufficient amounts, and in such cases methemoglobin is found to be present in the blood. The fumes from carbon arcs contain nitrous oxide, which reacts with atmospheric oxygen to form nitrogen dioxide. If this gas is breathed in high concentrations, methemoglobin may be produced. Motion-picture operators are constantly exposed to such a hazard, but it is believed to be of little danger because the projection booths are usually adequately ventilated. One method of combating this state is to inject glucose or methylene blue intravenously, which helps to reduce methemoglobin (Fe^{+++}) to hemoglobin (Fe^{++}), the pigment thus becoming again available for oxygen transport. Another procedure is to administer ascorbic acid, which also has a marked reducing action. Methemoglobin, in alkaline solution, has an absorption spectrum quite similar to that of oxyhemoglobin; but in acid solution, there is a characteristic band toward the red end of the spectrum with its center at about 634 mμ.

Interesting recent work[54] has shown that the use of silver nitrate solution in the treatment of burn patients can cause toxic methemoglobinemia. The mechanism believed to be involved is the conversion of nitrate anion to nitrite by skin bacteria. Nitrite then converts hemoglobin to methemoglobin.

Much work has been done on the toxic effects of methemoglobin. A concentration of 10% to 20% in blood may cause a mild cyanosis as the only symptom. Twenty percent to 40% levels of methemoglobin result in visible cyanosis and mild fatigue and dyspnea with activity. A 40% to 60% blood level produces severe cyanosis, serious cardiopulmonary symptoms, tachycardia, tachypnea, and depression. Levels of methemoglobin above 60% cause ataxia, loss of consciousness, and death.

Clinical methemoglobinemia is due to metabolic or structural failure in the normal reconversion of methemoglobin to hemoglobin or to a more rapid production of methemoglobin (by certain drugs, oxidants, etc.) than normal cellular mechanisms can cope with. The normal mechanism for the reconversion of methemoglobin to hemoglobin is shown schematically on p. 617. The amount of methemoglobin present in blood of normal human adults is about 1.7% of the total hemoglobin (approximately 0.3 gm. per 100 ml. blood):

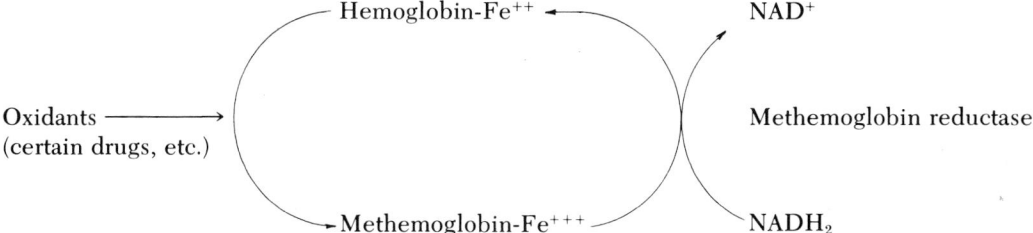

Glutathione (p. 566) and ascorbic acid, reducing substances present in significant amounts in erythrocytes, may also be involved in the reduction of methemoglobin to hemoglobin.

Other derivatives of hemoglobin. Hydrogen sulfide reacts with hemoglobin to give a compound having a characteristic absorption spectrum.

Hydrocyanic acid and cyanides, however, do not react directly with hemoglobin but do react with methemoglobin to form cyanmethemoglobin. The principal toxic action of the cyanides lies in their combination with cytochrome oxidase (p. 248). Therefore, the treatment of cyanide poisoning is based on the production of methemoglobin, in order to remove the cyanide from this important enzyme. Sodium nitrite and sodium thiosulfate are injected intravenously. The former induces the production of methemoglobin, which quickly combines with the cyanide. Methemoglobin and cyanmethemoglobin, although not useful respiratory pigments, are, in themselves, nontoxic. Cyanmethemoglobin is slowly converted to hemoglobin and cyanate, which is also nontoxic. The sodium thiosulfate reacts with cyanide, yielding thiocyanate, an innocuous salt, which is readily excreted.

A different type of combination is that of hemoglobin with carbon dioxide to form carbaminohemoglobin. In this case the combination is with the globin rather than with the heme. An amino group is responsible, in part at least:

$$\underset{\text{Hemoglobin}}{HbNH_2} \quad + \quad CO_2 \quad \rightleftarrows \quad \underset{\text{Carbaminohemoglobin}}{HbNHCOOH}$$

This is a normal and constant physiologic reaction and accounts for 2% to 10% of the carbon dioxide transported by the blood. Mechanisms for the transport of carbon dioxide are discussed in detail on pp. 648 to 653.

LEUKOCYTES

The white blood cells, or leukocytes, are much fewer in number than the red cells, and they have a lower specific gravity. Consequently, when whole blood is centrifuged, they form a narrow whitish layer above the red cells. Normally there are from 5000 to 10,000 leukocytes per cubic millimeter. The different types and variations in number cannot be considered here. Suffice it that in leukemias and in many infections and inflammatory conditions leukocytes are greatly increased in number; whereas in typhoid fever and in some other abnormal states, a leukopenia, i.e., decreased number of white cells, develops. Such a condition is agranulocytosis, which may be due to an infection or to the use of certain drugs, e.g., amidopyrine, acetophenetidin, dinitrophenol, arsphenamine, the sulfonamides. Since the leukocytes are typical cells, they contain water, nucleoproteins, albumin, globulin, and other proteins, lipids (especially cholesterol and phospholipids as well as fat), glucose, and other soluble organic substances and inorganic salts. They also possess a variety of enzymes and, undoubtedly, hormones and vitamins.

PLATELETS

Platelets are cytoplasmic fragments of the megakaryocytes found in bone marrow. In the peripheral blood, they are 2μ to 3μ in diameter, and there are 100,000 to 300,000 of them in every cubic millimeter of blood. They contain 86% to 88% water. Nineteen percent of their dry weight is lipid (phospholipids, neutral fat, cholesterol, cholesterol esters), and 57% is protein. Some of the electrolytes present are sodium, potassium, manganese, iron, copper, magnesium, and calcium. They contain enzymes, e.g., glucuronidase, catalase, amylase, phosphomonoesterase, cholinesterase, lecithinase, histaminase, trypsin, acid phosphatase, and others. They also contain agglutinogens apparently comparable to those of the red cells, and they may agglutinate or clump for that reason. It is also common for platelets to undergo morphologic changes or associate with each other. Common phrases applied to these phenomena are viscous metamorphosis, platelet "stickiness," or platelet clumping. The phenomena may occur at a "rough" spot created by injurious substances placed on blood vessel walls, on foreign bodies (e.g., a thread placed in the bloodstream), on glass surfaces, etc. Such clumps have a white appearance and are sometimes called white thrombi. Clumping is of importance for the physiology of hemostasis because the platelet mass serves as an obstruction to the flow of blood. Platelets also contain serotonin, a vasoconstrictor agent that has many functions, including a role in hemostasis and possibly also in clot retraction (p. 632). Certainly the platelets themselves or their derivatives are necessary for clot retraction, and for that phenomenon plasma factors are also involved. Platelets contain ATP and an actomyosinlike protein that may account in part for the chemical mechanisms underlying clot retraction.

Platelets are the center where blood coagulation begins, if tissue extracts, trypsin, snake venoms, and the like are excluded. Furthermore, they are stimulated by a variety of conditions. The main contribution of platelets to the clotting process seems to be the lipids. However, many other factors are also found in these formed elements, and it is customary to give the platelet factors arabic numbers. Platelet factor 1 is an accelerator globulinlike activity. Platelet factor 2 is a fibrinoplastic substance, possibly an enzyme, that alters fibrinogen so that the fibrinogen is more readily clotted by thrombin. Platelet factor 3 is very likely a lipoprotein that can be regarded as the main component for coagulation chemistry. Platelet factor 4 is an antiheparin factor. The next number (5) designates a clottable substance, very nearly like fibrinogen, while platelet factor 6 is an antifibrinolytic substance. There are different opinions about platelet factors. Some authors believe they are plasma materials adsorbed on the surface of the platelet; however, extensive washing of platelets does not remove all of them. Platelets contain a transglutaminase that is activated by thrombin and forms cross-linked fibrin. Many other substances are also found in platelets, including ADP, which has much to do with platelet aggregation.

BLOOD COAGULATION

Hemostasis, the arrest of an escape of blood, is achieved by the body via three mechanisms. There is (1) a vascular reaction, a contraction of the severed ends of small blood vessels; (2) the formation of a platelet thrombus at the site of the damage (p. 632); and (3) blood coagulation or clotting. The platelet thrombus or "white clot" disintegrates, liberating serotonin, which aids in the vascular reaction. While these events are occurring, the blood that has already escaped begins to coagulate.

The ultimate reaction in blood coagulation is the conversion of the soluble protein fibrinogen, present in colloidal solution, to the insoluble fibrin. This reaction, of course, does not occur normally in circulating blood, although most of the factors are present. Blood does not clot in a section of a blood vessel if the section is carefully tied off and removed from the body. This phenomenon indicates that the motion of the blood is not the cause of its continuing fluidity. However, the experiment is successful only if the ligatures do not crush the vessel wall and thus prevent seepage of tissue juice into the ligated vessel segment. The addition of tissue juice induces intravascular coagulation.

As mentioned previously, the coagulation may be prevented if ionized calcium is removed from blood; and the coagulating power is restored when these ions are again added in sufficient amount.

The chemistry of blood coagulation consists of three main basic reactions that are accelerated in special ways. The three fundamental biochemical events[55] are:

1. Formation of autoprothrombin-C
   (F-X_a, thrombokinase, Stuart factor)
2. Formation of thrombin
3. Formation of fibrin

The principal sequence of events in the coagulation of blood initiated by alterations of platelets following the shedding of blood thus is as follows:

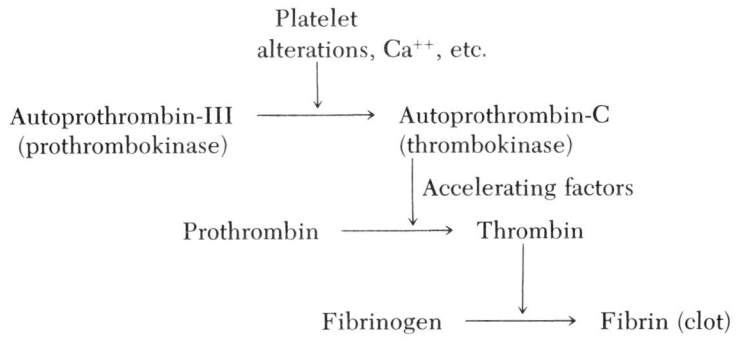

A delicate balance obviously must exist between the rapid clotting of blood when the vascular system is damaged and the fluidity of blood when the vascular system is intact. Also, once the damaged area is sealed, some mechanisms for the rapid inactivation of the clotting factors must be available to return the system to its initial state. Intensive research in recent years has clarified considerably the mechanisms involved. Current knowledge in this area will be considered next. Several names for certain of the factors concerned will be mentioned since multiple terminology in the field may lead to some confusion.

Fibrin formation In the interaction of thrombin and fibrinogen, the main alterations are with fibrinogen. This is a unique protein, resembling the globulins in its solubilities, and it can be isolated by a salting-out procedure. The addition of an equal volume of saturated ammonium sulfate solution to oxalated plasma precipitates fibrinogen, which may be purified by dissolving in dilute sodium chloride solution and reprecipitating with saturated ammonium sulfate. Fibrinogen has a molecular weight of about 340,000 and an isoelectric point of pH 5.5, contains practically all the known amino acids, and is normally found in plasma to the extent of 350 mg.%. In the presence of thrombin, fibrinopeptides of low molecular weight arise by cleavage of fibrinogen[55]:

$$\text{Fibrinogen} \xrightarrow{\text{Thrombin}} \text{Fibrin} + \text{Fibrinopeptides}$$

This leaves a protein with uneven electric charge distribution. These electric charges function to align the molecules laterally and, end to end, to form the fibrin gel. The rate of the above reaction is directly proportional to the thrombin concentration. The fibrin so formed in laboratory experiments happens to be soluble in concentrated urea solution, whereas the fibrin of a natural blood clot is not. To change the urea-soluble clot to a urea-insoluble clot, calcium ions and a plasma globulin, called the *fibrin-stabilizing factor,* are necessary. The influence of calcium ions is also manifested by an increase in the rate of thrombin-fibrinogen interaction. This rate is also augmented by platelets, and the latter play an important role in the phenomenon of clot retraction, which is associated with the properties of fibrin.

$$\text{Fibrin} \xrightarrow[\text{Fibrin-stabilizing factor}]{\text{Ca}^{++}} \text{Fibrin clot}$$

Returning to the interaction of purified fibrinogen and purified thrombin in laboratory experiments, it is interesting to note that not only do relatively large amounts of thrombin form a fibrin gel but in time the gel dissolves. Fibrin may thus, under proper conditions, be a mere transition state of more extensive changes associated with thrombin; and thrombin may be a special kind of proteolytic enzyme. Thrombin has been studied in connection with synthetic substrates. The proteolysis at the beginning of the fibrinogen-thrombin reaction is followed by polymerization.

The fibrinogen molecule has an α-polypeptide chain to which is attached the short A-fibrinopeptide chain that is removed by thrombin. There is also a β-chain with a B-peptide attached, and a third γ-chain, from which thrombin does not remove a peptide. These three main polypeptide chains are duplicated as a dimer. The formula for half a fibrinogen molecule (bovine) can be written: α (A) β (B) γ. For the whole molecule this would be $(\alpha\,[A]\,\beta\,[B]\,\gamma)_2$. After thrombin removes peptides A and B, the fibrin monomer $(\alpha\,\beta\,\gamma)_2$ remains and forms fibrin polymer $([\alpha\,\beta\,\gamma]_2)_n$. In the presence of the fibrin stabilizing factor, which is a plasma transglutaminase, cross-linked fibrin polymers form. This is indicated as $([\alpha\,\beta\,\gamma]_2)_n^x$. It is interesting that thrombin removes peptide-A very rapidly while peptide-B is removed slowly; and for the polymer to form, it is not even necessary to remove the B-peptide. Certain snake venoms produce fibrin without removing peptide-B, and this fibrin is designated as $([\alpha\,\beta\,\{B\}\,\gamma]_2)_n$. The amino acid sequence of peptide-A has been determined for many species. In man the A-chain sequence is known through 50 or more residues. To consider some interesting aspects, let us first write the sequence:

Ala Asp Ser° Gly Glu Gly Asp Phe Leu Ala Glu Gly Gly Gly Val

Arg (thrombin) Gly Pro Arg°° Val Val Glu Arg His . . . etc.

The word *thrombin* has been inserted to indicate where this enzyme removes peptide-A. In all species, thrombin splits an Arg-Gly bond. In the A-chain, Arg (no. 19) is marked with a double asterisk (°°). It is the third residue from the bond split by thrombin. In a case of congenital dysfibrinogenemia, the fibrinogen, known as fibrinogen Detroit, was found to have serine (Ser°) in place of arginine. Dysfibrinogenemia is thus associated with an altered amino acid sequence. From species to species, the amino acid sequence of fibrinopeptide-A can vary; however, phenylalanine is always found as the ninth residue from the bond split by thrombin, and presumably this residue is important for enzyme substrate combinations that occur during the reaction. It is also interesting that the peptides for man and monkey are identical, except that the latter has threonine as the fourteenth residue from the Arg-Gly bond split by thrombin.

In the fibrin cross-linking reaction, plasma transglutaminase (F-XIII) creates new peptide bonds. The amide acceptor is a glutamyl residue and the donor is an ϵ-amino group of lysine. This is outlined at the top of p. 622.

Fig. 19-9 represents an attempt to correlate the three basic reactions and is supposed to account for the accessories required for accelerating these reactions. The same chart is again drawn, but with additional details (Fig. 19-10) related to the inactivation of procoagulants and the fibrinolytic system. A third chart (Fig. 19-11) serves as a basis for learning the basic information for the chemical reactions and relating them to irregularities that are known to occur in clinical abnormalities of blood clotting.

Thrombin zymogen The thrombin zymogen has been obtained in three main forms by isolation procedures. One of these is referred to as *prothrombin complex*. It contains the thrombin precursor and autoprothrombin-C precursor. The amount of the latter is about 3% to 4% of the total weight. This complex, when infused in dogs, corrects the hemostatic defect produced with bishydroxycoumarin. Prothrombin complex develops thrombin activity with the two-stage analytic reagents. It also converts to thrombin and autoprothrombin-C in 25% sodium citrate solution, because in that medium autoprothrom-

$$\text{Lysyl donor} \quad
\begin{array}{c}
\text{O} \quad\quad \text{O} \\
\| \quad\quad\quad\quad \| \\
-\text{C}-\text{N}-\text{CH}-\text{C}-\text{N}- \\
\quad\; | \quad\; | \quad\quad\; | \\
\quad\; \text{H} \;\; \text{CH}_2 \quad\; \text{H} \\
\quad\quad\quad\; | \\
\quad\quad\quad\; \text{CH}_2 \\
\quad\quad\quad\; | \\
\quad\quad\quad\; \text{CH}_2 \\
\quad\quad\quad\; | \\
\quad\quad\quad\; \text{CH}_2 \\
\quad\quad\quad\; | \\
\quad\quad\quad\; \text{NH}_2
\end{array}$$

$+$

$$\text{Glutaminyl acceptor} \quad
\begin{array}{c}
\text{H}_2\text{N} \quad\; \text{O} \\
\quad\;\backslash \quad \text{\textbardbl} \\
\quad\quad\; \text{C} \\
\quad\quad\; | \\
\quad\quad\; \text{CH}_2 \\
\quad\quad\; | \\
\quad\quad\; \text{CH}_2 \\
\text{O} \quad\;\; | \quad\quad\; \text{O} \\
\| \quad\quad\; | \quad\quad\; \| \\
-\text{C}-\text{N}-\text{CH}-\text{C}-\text{N}- \\
\quad\; | \quad\quad\quad\quad\; | \\
\quad\; \text{H} \quad\quad\quad\quad \text{H}
\end{array}$$

$\xrightarrow{\text{Ca}^{++} \;\; \text{Factor XIII}}$

$$
\begin{array}{c}
\text{H} \quad\quad \text{O} \\
| \quad\quad\quad\; \| \\
-\text{C}-\text{N}-\text{CH}-\text{C}-\text{N}- \\
\| \quad\quad\; | \quad\quad\; | \\
\text{O} \quad\quad \text{CH}_2 \quad\; \text{H} \\
\quad\quad\quad\; | \\
\quad\quad\quad\; \text{CH}_2 \\
\quad\quad\quad\; | \\
\quad\quad\quad\; \text{CH}_2 \\
\quad\quad\quad\; | \\
\quad\quad\quad\; \text{NH} \\
\quad\quad\quad\; | \\
\quad\quad\quad\; \text{C}{=}\text{O} \\
\quad\quad\quad\; | \\
\quad\quad\quad\; \text{CH}_2 \\
\quad\quad\quad\; | \\
\quad\quad\quad\; \text{CH}_2 \\
\text{H} \quad\quad\; | \quad\quad \text{O} \\
| \quad\quad\quad\; \nearrow \\
-\text{C}-\text{N}-\text{CH}-\text{C}-\text{N}- \\
\| \quad\quad\quad\quad\quad\; | \\
\text{O} \quad\quad\quad\quad\quad\; \text{H}
\end{array}
\quad + \text{NH}_3
$$

$$\text{Zymogen} \xrightarrow[\text{Cothromboplastin}]{\substack{\text{Ca}^{++} \\ \text{Thromboplastin}}} \text{Autoprothrombin-C}$$

$$\text{Zymogen} \xrightarrow[\text{Platelet cofactor}]{\substack{\text{Ca}^{++} \\ \text{Platelet lipids}}} \text{Autoprothrombin-C}$$

bin-C forms spontaneously and then converts the thrombin zymogen to thrombin. A second form of the zymogen is called *DEAE-prothrombin* or simply *prothrombin*. The former term indicates the kind of chromatography by means of which it was obtained. This zymogen is free of autoprothrombin-C zymogen. A third form of thrombin precursor is called *prethrombin*. It is obtained free of autoprothrombin-C precursor. It does not form thrombin in the two-stage analytic reagents. A small amount of prethrombin is found in plasma. Presumably the prothrombin of plasma is mainly in a form combined with autoprothrombin-C precursor by weak bonds that are easily broken. In certain isolation procedures that do not disrupt the bonds, the aggregate holds together and has been obtained in crystalline form. Another possibility is that they are quite independent of each other. Recent evidence indicated that the thrombin molecule occurs as a dimer in prothrombin complex and in DEAE-prothrombin.

Autopro-thrombin-C zymogen   Mention has just been made of the association of autoprothrombin-C with the thrombin precursor. The terms autoprothrombin-III, prothrombokinase, F-X, and Stuart factor are applied to the zymogen. It has many physical chemical properties closely resembling those of the thrombin zymogen. The plasma transglutaminase must first be activated by thrombin, and ultimately

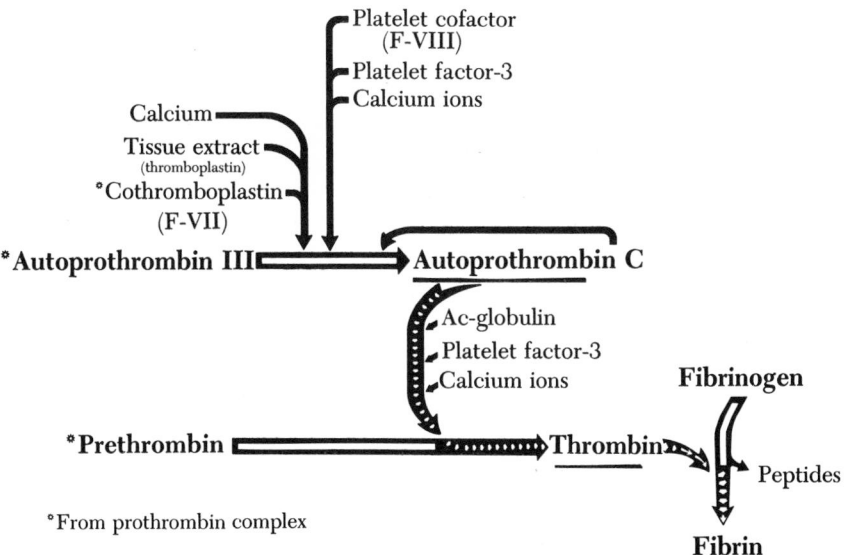

Fig. 19-9. Blood-clotting mechanisms. This represents the simplified view of the three basic reactions and takes into account the accessory factors required to accelerate these reactions. (Courtesy W. H. Seegers.)

neither the zymogen nor the enzyme is found in serum. The enzyme papain also modifies fibrinogen so that fibrinogen polymerizes and becomes cross-linked to form urea-insoluble fibrin. Liver tissue contains a transglutaminase that forms cross-links in fibrin. In lobster blood, clotting consists of gel formation only through the mechanism of cross-link formation. Thrombin is not found in that species but presumably is a later development in evolution.

Thrombin Thrombin is derived from its zymogen by a recently recognized enzyme **formation** variously called autoprothrombin-C, Stuart factor, thrombokinase, and $F-X_a$. In the activation process at least two peptides are formed:

$$Zymogen \xrightarrow{\text{Autoprothrombin-C}} Thrombin + Peptides$$

Thrombin formation by autoprothrombin-C alone is very slow and is accelerated by calcium ions by phospholipids, and Ac-globulin (F-V). The latter is a plasma protein to be discussed more extensively below.

$$Zymogen \xrightarrow[\substack{Autoprothrombin-C}]{\substack{Ca^{++} \\ Phospholipids \\ Ac-globulin}} Thrombin + Peptides$$

The rapid production of thrombin requires the enzyme to split peptides from the zymogen, and this enzyme needs two accessories. The two accessories are in two anatomic compartments, namely, the platelets (phospholipids, lipoproteins) and the plasma (Ac-globulin). When injury occurs, the platelets are stimulated. They undergo disintegration, and then the Ac-globulin and the phospholipids can function together. Either alone does not

623

influence the enzyme. As far as acceleration is concerned, the molecular requirement is thus a dual one, and this makes possible a trigger mechanism set off by injury. The injury brings the two accessories together.

Under optimum conditions the enzyme and macromolecular cofactor (Ac-G) are present in about a 1:1 molar ratio, while the lipids are effective in the micelle state. It takes numerous molecules to constitute a micelle. Detergents that destroy lipid micelles also nullify the procoagulant activity of the micelles. Presumably a complex consisting of enzyme, lipid, and Ac-globulin is held together by calcium ions. Although the lipids must be of a special composition, their primary function seems to be to supply structure for proper stereochemical requirements. Ac-globulin can be regarded as a cofactor. Recently it was found that the lipids can be replaced by certain bile salts, e.g., the conjugated sodium salt of taurocholic acid, sodium cholate, sodium dehydrocholate. These were effective in concentrations in which they form micelles. Sodium dehydrocholate does not form micelles and was ineffective.

Autopro-thrombin-C formation We started with the last basic reaction and can now consider the first one, which is the formation of autoprothrombin-C. The purified zymogen slowly develops activity spontaneously, and this process is accelerated by the addition of purified autoprothrombin-C.

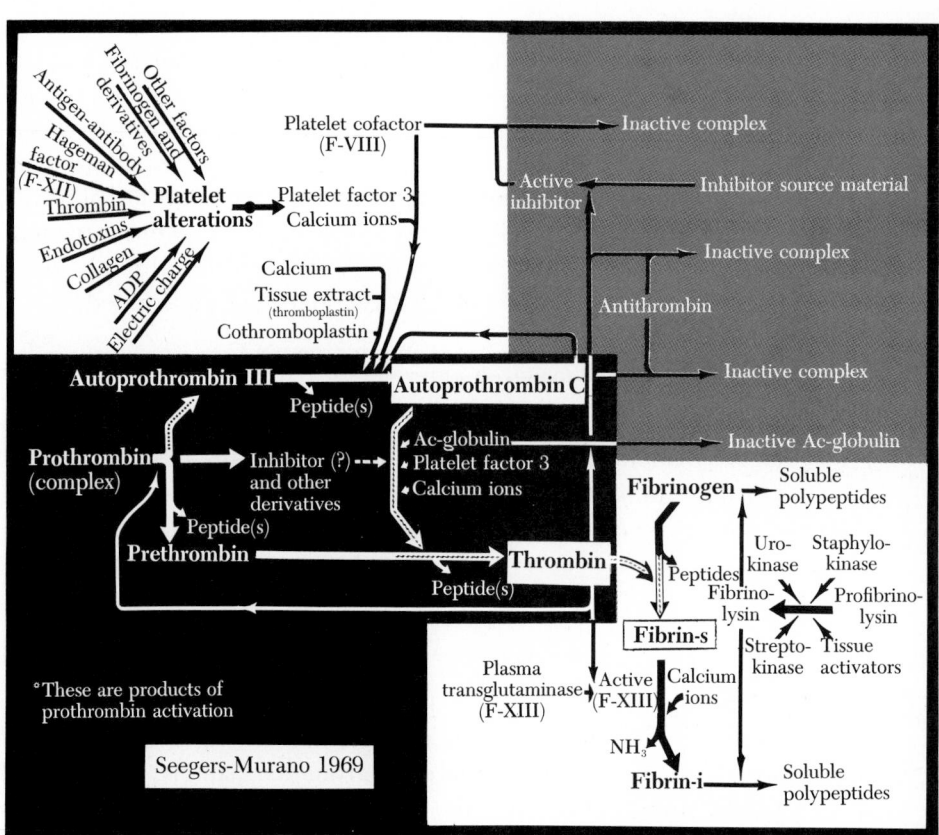

Fig. 19-10. For legend see opposite page.

$$\text{Zymogen} \xrightarrow{\text{Autoprothrombin-C}} \text{Autoprothrombin-C}$$

The spontaneous, but slow formation of autoprothrombin-C is not sufficient for physiologic requirements. The rate of formation is accelerated by accessories. Rapid generation of autoprothrombin-C occurs with calcium ions and thromboplastin. The latter itself may undergo rapid activation in the presence of cothromboplastin–(F-VII).

Additionally autoprothrombin-C formation is regulated by intrinsic mechanisms involving platelets and platelet cofactor (F-VIII, antihemophilic factor). Such a condition would prevail when a clean venipuncture is done. With platelets and platelet cofactor together and calcium ions, the rate of autoprothrombin-C formation is accelerated. In this arrangement the phospholipids and lipoproteins of platelets become available on stimulation of platelets (viscous metamorphosis and related phenomena). The basic plan for the integration thus involves two types of molecules stored in two anatomic com-

---

Fig. 19-10. Blood-clotting mechanisms. The clotting of blood consists of three main reactions:

1. Formation of autoprothrombin-C (F-X_a, thrombokinase, Stuart factor)
2. Formation of thrombin
3. Formation of fibrin

For the formation of fibrin, only thrombin is necessary. For the formation of thrombin, only autoprothrombin-C is necessary, but the formation of autoprothrombin-C can occur spontaneously and autocatalytically. The rate of thrombin formation by autoprothrombin-C is regulated by plasma Ac-globulin and lipids of platelets. The rate of autoprothrombin-C formation is regulated in two ways: Rapid formation occurs with tissue thromboplastin, which is activated by cothromboplastin (F-VII). Slow activation occurs with the lipids of platelets functioning synergistically with platelet cofactor (F-VIII, AHF). The regulatory mechanisms for zymogen activation require Ca^{++}. Each one of the two molecules needed to govern the rate of thrombin or autoprothrombin-C formation comes from a separate anatomic compartment (platelets and plasma or tissues and plasma); consequently, injury brings them together and accelerates the clotting process. Platelets are especially labile and respond to a variety of stimuli. Even without injury, the clotting mechanisms are in operation at an imperceptible level. Prothrombin complex and prethrombin are found in the plasma.

After the removal of peptides from fibrinogen by thrombin, the fibrin polymerizes, and in a cross-linking reaction, due to thrombin-activated plasma transglutaminase, ϵ-lysine (γ-glutamyl) bonds form, with the liberation of NH_3.

The powerful procoagulants generated during the forward phase of clotting are neutralized by inhibitors, and the product of clotting (fibrin) can be lysed by the fibrinolytic mechanisms and by cellular phagocytosis. Heparin accelerates the neutralization of thrombin by antithrombin and the neutralization of autoprothrombin-C by antiprothrombin. Thrombin first activates and subsequently inactivates plasma Ac-globulin. Thrombin indirectly inactivates platelet cofactor. Very little thromboplastin and very little transglutaminase are found in serum. The amount of residual autoprothrombin-C zymogen in serum is inversely related to the rate of clotting. (Courtesy W. H. Seegers.)

partments. Upon injury, conditions prevail for the two molecules to function together.

Certain snake venoms rapidly produce autoprothrombin-C from the zymogen. Trypsin also is an activator. Urine also contains a procoagulant that, together with calcium ions, functions effectively in the formation of autoprothrombin-C. Cathepsin is also effective. The main conditions are the two that generally function.

Calcium   Calcium ions are required, and normal plasma contains about 10 mg.% of calcium, about half of which is ionized. This is approximately the optimal concentration for coagulation. Even in severe tetany due to extremely low blood-calcium concentrations, the calcium level is sufficiently high for clotting. Thus the body always has enough calcium present for the formation of thrombin, and attempts to improve clotting conditions therapeutically by raising the blood calcium level are of little value.

Ac-globulin   Ac-globulin is found in plasma in trace quantities and plays an important role in the activation of prothrombin. Although powerful concentrates have been prepared in the laboratory, it has not been obtained in sufficient purity for chemical study. It appears to have a molecular weight of about 99,000. A small amount of thrombin greatly changes the properties of Ac-globulin so

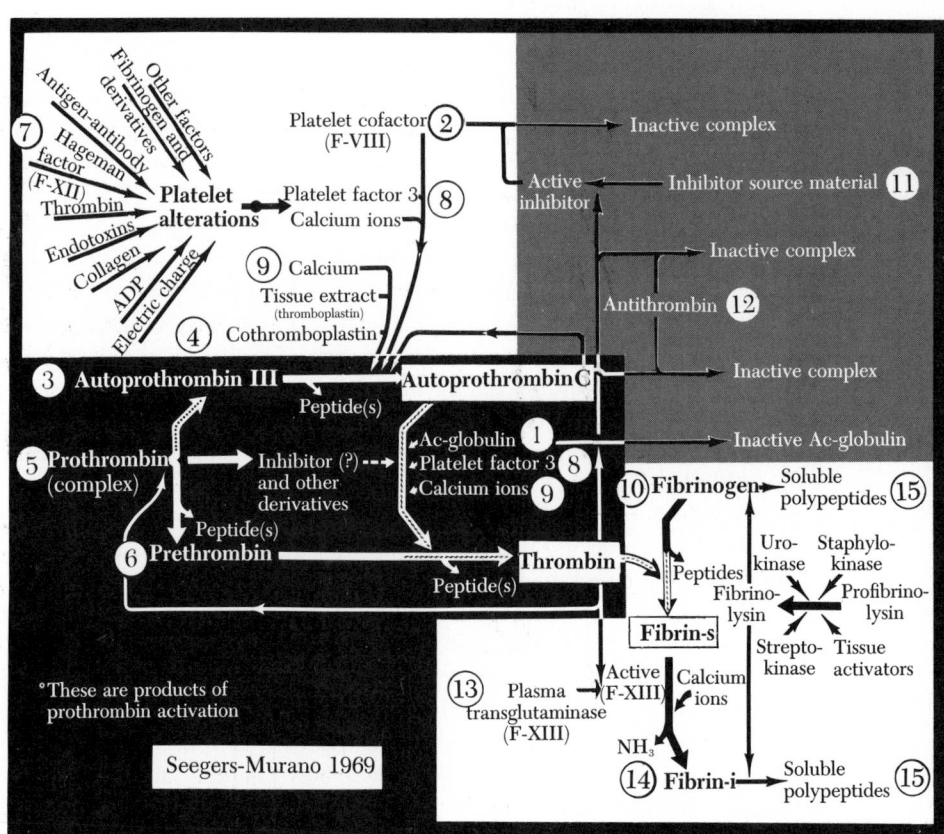

Fig. 19-11. For legend see opposite page.

that the latter becomes an accelerator of prothrombin activation. This change has been represented as follows:

$$\text{Plasma Ac-globulin} \xrightarrow{\text{Thrombin}} \text{Serum Ac-globulin}$$

The nature of the change of plasma Ac-globulin to serum Ac-globulin is not known. However, an excess of thrombin is associated with the change and ultimate disappearance of serum Ac-globulin activity. In human serum, Ac-globulin is stable for only a matter of minutes, so serum is practically devoid of Ac-globulin activity.

$$\text{Serum Ac-globulin} \xrightarrow{\text{Thrombin}} \text{Inactive Ac-globulin}$$

In oxalated human plasma, as commonly stored in a blood bank, plasma Ac-globulin is not stable. With citrate as anticoagulant, however, its activity

---

Fig. 19-11. Irregular blood clotting. (1) Deficiency (functional or absent) of Ac-globulin (F-V) is called parahemophilia; poor clotting, because any autoprothrombin-C (F-X_a, active Stuart factor, thrombokinase) that forms is ineffective without Ac-globulin; (2) ineffective in classic hemophilia (hemophilia-A) due to an inhibitor; some authors say it is due to absence of the cofactor (F-VIII); plasma concentration diminished in some patients with von Willebrand's disease; (3) abnormality in auto-prothrombin-III activation in hemophilia-B; some postulate a special factor, IX; question is what function it would have and why no one has obtained it in pure form; deficiency (functional or absent) in Stuart plasma; (4) perhaps same as factor VII; decreased or abnormal in factor VII deficiency; required to interact with thrombo-plastin before the latter functions in autoprothrombin-III activation; species specific; (5) contains thrombin and autoprothrombin-C zymogen; corrects hemophilia-B plasma-clotting defect; corrects factors VII– and X–deficient plasma; (6) low concentration in normal plasma; temporary increase in plasma when warfarin and indanedione drugs are given; (7) plasma protein, activation surface dependent; diminished in Hageman trait; not found in avian plasma; (8) low concentration in thrombocytopenia; not released or absent in certain forms of thrombocytopathy; (9) plasma levels not diminished to levels where clotting is impaired; removed by chelating agents (citrate, EDTA) or precipitating agents (oxalates); serves to form complexes with lipids; (10) afibrinogenemia and hypofibrinogenemia or dysfibrinogenemia (abnormal mole-cule); (11) possibly diminished in factor XI or PTA deficiency; (12) heparin increases rate of autoprothrombin-C and thrombin inactivation by antiprothrombin (heparin cofactor); heparin retards or blocks autoprothrombin-C formation and thrombin forma-tion; low concentration associated with clotting tendency – thrombophilia; (13) low activity in plasma associated with bleeding tendency and possibly poor wound healing; (14) urea-insoluble fibrin; cross-linked fibrin polymer due to formation of ε-lysine (γ-glutamyl) bonds; (15) competitive inhibitors of thrombin activity; interfere with normal fibrin polymerization. (1,2,3,5,7,10,12,13) Diminished appreciably and in some instances reduced to zero activity, in serum and in some patients with dis-seminated intravascular clotting (consumption coagulopathy); disseminated intra-vascular clotting creates a serum mimetic condition; it may be initiated via platelets and/or tissue extract thrombpolastin. (3,4,5,6) Synthesized by liver parenchymal cells; synthesis dependent on vitamin K; vitamin K function inhibited by warfarin and in-danedione drugs. (Courtesy W. H. Seegers.)

remains for a few days. The fundamental reason for the greater stability of Ac-globulin in citrated plasma as compared with oxalated plasma is not known. It may be due to oxidation mechanisms, since oxygen bubbled through plasma samples tends to destroy Ac-globulin activity. The Ac-globulins take part in prothrombin activation. When Ac-globulin is absent from the blood, there is a bleeding tendency and the patient is said to have parahemophilia, in accordance with the suggestion of Owren, who first described and studied the disease in detail. Besides the fact that this fact or (also called factor-V) is known to be a globulin, not much more can be said definitely about it. Sulfhydryl groups are essential for its action.

Thrombin   The most active bovine thrombin preparation obtained to date was only recently described by Seegers and co-workers.[56] This thrombin has a specific activity of 8230 units per milligram dry weight. In other words, a milligram is sufficient to clot over 8 liters of standardized fibrinogen solution in 15 seconds. Some physical constants are: with the ultracentrifuge, $S^0_{20w} = 3.2$, molecular weight $= 22,900$; with p-toluenesulfonyl-L-arginine methyl ester as a substrate, $K_M = 9.5 \times 10^{-5}$. When this thrombin is acetylated, fibrinogen no longer is a substrate, but the esterolytic activity is retained and K_M equals 4.85×10^{-4} for the acetylated thrombin. Clearly the requirements for limited proteolysis of fibrinogen are very special. Bovine thrombin was found to contain 1.7% sialic acid, 5.0% orcinol-reactive carbohydrate, 0.69% glucosamine, and 0.46% galactosamine. The thrombin molecule is found as a dimer in the zymogen. In the ultracentrifuge, molecular association and aggregation are observed. Thrombin is readily inactivated by diisopropyl-fluorophosphate and by phenylmethanesulfonyl fluoride; this fact is taken as an indication that thrombin activity is dependent on an active serine residue. In this region of the molecule, the amino acid sequence has been reported to be Gly-Asp-Ser-Gly-(Glu-Ala), thus resembling trypsin in that respect. Most likely, a histidine residue is also important for the catalytic activity, because thrombin is inactivated by 1-chloro-3-tosylamido-7-amino-2-heptanone. Kinetic studies also point to that conclusion.

The N-terminal amino acids at the end of two polypeptide chains are threonine and isoleucine. A preliminary report by Magnusson, in Stockholm, indicated that work on the amino acid sequence of thrombin is progressing rapidly and that the primary structure of thrombin will soon be known.

Acetylated thrombin has unusual pharmacologic properties. When it is infused intravenously in dogs, there is a decrease in fibrinogen concentration and a lowering of the platelet count. There is a lowering followed by an increase in leukocyte count. With rapid infusion, the pulse pressure drops and there may be arrhythmia. Blood drawn from the dog's veins clots and then may completely lyse in an hour or so. This lysis is thought to be due to the physiologic activation of the animal's fibrinolytic mechanisms. Thus far, it has not been possible to get acetylated thrombin to produce antibodies.

Autoprothrombin-C   Autoprothrombin-C can be detected in picogram quantities. It makes prothrombin refractory to the two-stage analytic reagents, and through its proteolytic action it splits peptides from the zymogen to yield thrombin. Its molecular weight is in the 25,000 range, and preliminary indications are that this is about the weight of the zymogen form. Most likely the enzyme is present as a dimer in the zymogen. It hydrolyzes p-toluenesulfonyl-L-arginine methyl ester. Autoprothrombin-C is inactivated by diisopropylfluorophosphate and by phenylmethanesulfonyl fluoride; but to be effective, these inhibitors must be used in higher concentrations than are needed for the inactivation of thrombin. Soybean trypsin inhibitor inactivates the enzyme. The purified enzyme loses its activity on freezing, but in 50% glycerol solution at −20° C. the activity has been fully preserved for 3 years.

Prothrombin derivatives For more than a half century, theories of blood coagulation practically all described thrombin as the sole substance derived from prothrombin. Work with purified prothrombin preparations has, however, shown that other derivatives besides thrombin are possible. Several have been found, and they all have the characteristic of being refractory to transformation to thrombin by any of those agents that transform prothrombin to thrombin. In a sense, the derivatives can be regarded as "inactive" or "inert" prothrombin. One of these derivatives is an inhibitor of blood clotting. Others may be procoagulants.

Neutralization of thrombin and autoprothrombin-C. There occurs in plasma a substance that can neutralize the activity of thrombin and is called *antithrombin*. It can destroy all the thrombin activity derived from prothrombin, and even thereafter much antithrombin remains in the serum. This is remarkable because there is potentially 150 times more thrombin available from the prothrombin in one volume of plasma than is needed to clot an equal volume of blood in 15 seconds. Antithrombin is a plasma protein. In addition to the antithrombin activity of plasma, a small amount of thrombin disappears by adsorption on fibrin. The natural antithrombin activity of plasma is destroyed by ether extraction. Antithrombin also neutralizes autoprothrombin-C activity and, in the presence of heparin, destroys thrombin and autoprothrombin-C activity very rapidly. In that way the autocatalytic function of these two enzymes is stopped and the result is that heparin blocks the activation of the respective zymogens.

Inhibitors of prothrombin activation. The concept of inhibitors of prothrombin activation was introduced by Howell, and heparin is perhaps the best known of this group of substances. Heparin is a mucoitinsulfuric acid. The amino sugar is glucosamine, and the uronic acid is glucuronic. If heparin is present in normal blood, it must be so in small amounts. On the other hand, it is abundantly present in the mast cells, from which it is released under special circumstances, e.g., anaphylactic shock, peptone shock.

Heparin acts as a powerful anticoagulant in conjunction with a cofactor presumed to be a plasma protein. This cofactor is required, since heparin alone does not inhibit the activation of purified prothrombin. As brought out in the preceding section, heparin also requires a cofactor to act as an antithrombin. Whether the two cofactors are the same is not known.

There are also some lipids present in blood that have anticoagulant power. This activity is associated with a variety of unidentified phosphatide-like materials and seems to be due to the colloidal and acidic nature of the lipids. Probably these lipids are inhibitors of prothrombin action as well.

629

Hemophilia　　In some individuals, clotting occurs at a very slow rate. The condition is called hemophilia, and the sufferers from it are termed *hemophiliacs* or, commonly, "bleeders." Hemophiliacs must be extremely careful not to experience even very minor wounds and injuries since these may result in severe and even fatal hemorrhages. The cause of the incoagulability of the blood in hemophilia is not known definitely. Apparently all the clotting factors are present, and even the platelets are normal, but there is a delay in the formation of thrombin. One explanation is that the equilibrium of coagulant and anticoagulant substances, or the release of these substances into the circulation, is disturbed. There may be some other component of plasma lacking that has not yet been identified. In favor of this explanation is the fact that normal human plasma globulin, when added to hemophilic blood or when injected intravenously, brings about normal coagulation. The assumption is that this unidentified factor, called the antihemophilic factor, is associated with the globulins. Consequently, transfusion of blood from a normal individual into a hemophiliac is sometimes indicated. Many other possibilities for pathology are indicated in Fig. 19-11.

Reactions involved in prevention of coagulation. Consideration may now be given to the reasons for the action of various coagulation preventives. Whipping or defibrinating blood really causes coagulation around a foreign object and therefore is not a method of preventing coagulation. Oxalates, citrates, and fluorides, of course, take calcium ions out of solution. Bile salts are inhibitors of thromboplastin. The action of heparin has been discussed above. Both heparin and hirudin prevent blood coagulation in vivo as well as in vitro. Polypeptides (peptones), however, act as anticoagulants only after injection into the living animal. They apparently stimulate the production of heparin by the body. The use of paraffined cannulas and receiving vessels and the application of cold seem to owe their virtues as preventives of coagulation to the fact that they tend to slow down the activation of prothrombin to thrombin by thromboplastin. The reason why the blood in a section of a carefully doubly ligated blood vessel does not coagulate is that no thromboplastin has been released. If some damage to the integrity of the vessel wall is caused by the ligature or by the action of bacteria, thromboplastin is produced or enters the segment from the walls and the surrounding matrix of the injured vessel, and coagulation ensues. Platelets clump or clot around the injury and then disintegrate and serve as coagulation centers. This agglutination of platelets does not depend on fibrin formation and is mainly brought about by globulins. These platelet agglutinant factors are present in tissue juice, and thus the agglutination of platelets at the site of vascular injury can be explained.

Coagulation time, bleeding time, and prothrombin time. Coagulation time, bleeding time, and prothrombin time are determined in clinical laboratories to aid in diagnosis or to ascertain the state of the blood prior to surgical operations. Several methods are available for each. For *coagulation time,* one method employs fine capillary glass tubes. These are filled from a large drop of blood that has exuded from a deep cut in the skin. At short intervals, pieces are broken off and the moment of coagulation is evidenced by the appearance of a thread of fibrin between the fragments as they are slowly separated. This test, although still popular, is not accurate because the admixture of tissue juice may accelerate considerably the coagulation time of whole blood. Methods employing venipuncture are now advocated. If *bleeding time* is desired, the blood exuding from a small cut is removed at 10- to 15-second intervals by touching the cut with filter paper. When no spot of blood is seen on the paper, bleeding has stopped; the time is noted, and this is called the bleeding time. *Prothrombin time* is an indirect and inverse measure of the amount of prothrombin present in blood; i.e., an increased prothrombin time means a lower level of prothrombin. In the method of Quick, blood is oxalated and centrifuged under standard conditions. To the oxalated plasma is added an excess of thromboplastin (usually an emulsion of rabbit's brain) and then calcium chloride. The time required for clotting to occur after the addition of the calcium chloride is taken as the prothrombin time.

Coagulation time of whole human blood is normally from 2 to 10 minutes at 37° C. Increase in coagulation time or bleeding time may be due to diminution in the amount of any one of the diversified clotting factors, but bleeding time involves not only these but also the amount of platelet agglutinant substance present in the cut tissues. The bleeding time is terminated primarily by a platelet agglutination thrombus. This clot may be mixed with a coagulation thrombus, in which fibrin may have precipitated or in which the blood has gelated. This clot, which is designated as wound thrombus, is actually a clot that seals numerous capillary vessel wounds. Moreover, in bleeding time determinations, the character of the clot plays a role, since a poorly adherent clot will be washed away by the flow of blood as rapidly as it is formed. Bleeding time also depends, in a measure, upon the degree of vascularity, the condition of the blood vessels, the elasticity of the tissues, and blood pressure. In determining coagulation time, the character of the clot is not noted—merely the time required to form any clot. By the prothrombin time technique, since an excess of thromboplastin and calcium ions are added and fibrinogen is always present, about the only variable is prothrombin.

There is little relation among these determinations. The one condition in which coagulation time is prolonged is hemophilia. Therefore a normal coagulation time is not of much significance, whereas an increased one is. In hemophilia, the bleeding time is usually not prolonged. In purpuras, on the other hand, bleeding time is usually lengthened. Prothrombin time is generally normal in hemophilia, in the purpuras, and in many types of jaundice; but in obstructive jaundice and in conditions of marked involvement of the liver, there is a low prothrombin level. Hemorrhage in the newborn infant and conditions leading to a diminished absorption of vitamin K also have lengthened prothrombin time. When the *concentration of prothrombin* falls below 30% of normal, the prothrombin time rises above 20 second, but *coagulation time* is likely to remain normal until the prothrombin falls below 20% of normal. This is why a patient with obstructive jaundice may have normal coagulation time before an operation and suddenly have uncontrollable hemorrhages after the operation.

Serum prothrombin consumption test. The normal clotting process results in a serum containing no prothrombin; i.e., all prothrombin originally present is consumed, having been converted to thrombin. However, in hemophilia and certain other abnormal conditions, prothrombin is not all consumed. The serum, therefore, contains prothrombin, and the determination of serum prothrombin time is a quantitative measure of the original thromboplastin. Thus, normally, the *serum* prothrombin time (serum prothrombin consumption test) is over 30 seconds, whereas in these abnormal cases it is less than 20 seconds. Hemophiliacs are likely to have 14 to 15 seconds as their serum prothrombin time.

Thrombi and emboli. Despite the intricate mechanism that nature has devised to prevent blood from clotting until it is shed, this sometimes fails and clotting does occur within the blood vessels. Such intravascular clots, called thrombi, may arise if the blood vessel is damaged or if platelets or red blood cells agglutinate. A local excess of thromboplastin may thus arise from the tissue fluid of the vessel wall. Platelets are agglutinated by tissue juice. Such platelet agglutination thrombi may serve as coagulation centers and initiate fibrin formation and blood gelation. A diminution in the rate of blood flow, or other conditions, may also contribute to thrombus formation. A thrombus may completely block a vessel at first, but as syneresis occurs, the retraction may permit the flow of blood past the clot. If the clot is not detached, it may eventually be organized or absorbed by aid of fibrinolysin (p. 633), with no harm resulting. However, if it is detached and is swept to some other location, it becomes an embolus. Emboli are often dangerous and even fatal, depending on the site of the obstruction, the vessels of the heart and brain being particularly important from this standpoint. The administration of heparin or bishydroxycoumarin (Dicumarol) clinically to prevent thrombosis is a recent development. It appears to lower the incidence of thrombosis after operative procedures. In certain types of vascular surgery, heparin is extremely useful.

Oral administration of heparin is ineffective. The anticoagulant must be given parenterally and, because of the transient effect of single doses, it may be given either by means of a continuous intravenous drip or intramuscularly. This results in the maintenance of a lengthened coagulation time. Heparin has been crystallized, and no toxic effects have been experienced with the purified crystalline material. The great danger is the possibility of hemorrhage during an extreme prolongation of the coagulation time. Since heparin is expensive and must be given parenterally, bishydroxycoumarin, which is inexpensive and can be given orally, represents a great advance. When given by mouth or when the sodium salt is injected intravenously, it prolongs the prothrombin time. Its effect is slow, requiring from 1 to 3 days after the start of treatment, and frequent determinations of prothrombin time must be made in order to control the dosage correctly.

Bishydroxycoumarin (Dicumarol) was discovered by Link and associates. They found that it is the causative agent of the hemorrhagic disease of cattle. It was identified and synthesized. It is a colorless crystalline solid, almost insoluble in water, acids, and most organic solvents. It forms soluble salts with strong alkalies. In spite of its insolubility in water, this anticoagulant is readily absorbed from the gastrointestinal tract. It has no effect on blood clotting in vitro, and the mechanism of its action is unknown. However, its action is antagonized by vitamin K, and therefore it is suggested to act as a structural analogue of vitamin K, inhibiting the vitamin, and thus either depressing the synthesis of prothrombin or causing the synthesis of an altered prothrombin (p. 621). Various analogues of this compound have been prepared and tested, and some have been found to be even more useful than bishydroxycoumarin. One of these, warfarin sodium (Coumadin), is very soluble in water, in contrast to Dicumarol. It is unique in being an effective hypoprothrombinemic agent when administered orally, intravenously, intramuscularly, or rectally. In this respect Coumadin has properties not shared by other coumarin derivatives. Its great solubility accounts for a shorter latent period between administration and appearance of depressed prothrombin activity of the plasma, as well as the greater ease in maintaining a lowered prothrombin activity of plasma for long periods. Because of varying nutritional states, particularly with reference to vitamins K and C, there are individual differences in response to initial hypoprothrombinemia-inducing doses. Individuals with varying degrees of liver injury may be more sensitive to the hypoprothrombinemia-inducing drugs. Overdosage is readily counteracted by vitamin K, which may be regarded as a physiologic antagonist.

Bishydroxycoumarin
3,3'-Methylenebis-
(4-hydroxycoumarin)

Warfarin sodium
3-(α-acetonylbenzyl)-4-Hydroxycoumarin

Lysis of blood clots. Although clots are quite stable, they can be removed or dissolved very slowly. The mechanism involved bears some resemblance to the clotting mechanism. A substance in plasma called profibrinolysin or *plasminogen* is activated by fibrinokinase, present in many tissues. The resulting agent is an enzyme, *fibrinolysin*, or "plasmin," which can dissolve fibrin. Fibrinokinases have also been obtained from certain bacteria. Fibrinolysin can be inactivated by normal plasma. The antifibrinolysin, which causes this inactivation, is increased in amount in various pathologic conditions. Fibrinolysin and streptokinase are being extensively studied clinically for their possible effectiveness in dissolving intravascular clots in patients.

$$\text{Profibrinolysins} \xrightarrow[\text{streptokinase}]{\text{Fibrinokinase or}} \text{Fibrinolysins}$$

$$\text{Fibrin} \xrightarrow{\text{Fibrinolysin}} \text{Peptides}$$

$$\text{Fibrinolysin} \xrightarrow{\text{Antifibrinolysin}} \text{Inactive fibrinolysin}$$

633

ANEMIAS

Those conditions in which the number of erythrocytes or the amount of hemoglobin is reduced below normal are termed anemias. There are a number of types of anemias, which can be only briefly considered here. Anemias are due to (1) loss of blood, (2) destruction of blood, or (3) defective formation of blood. The first group includes acute and chronic hemorrhage. Destruction of erythrocytes is brought about by hemolytic agents, which may be of bacterial or metabolic origin, or they may be due to the absorption of industrial poisons. Anemias of the third group include hypochromic anemias, pernicious anemia, and aplastic anemias.

A hypochromic anemia, i.e., one in which the erythrocytes contain less hemoglobin than normal, may be experimentally induced in animals by feeding them exclusively on milk. The lack of iron and copper in this food is undoubtedly the cause of the anemia, for otherwise milk is a superior food. Similarly, in man an iron-deficient diet may give rise to an anemia (hypochromic anemia) in which the hemoglobin content of the blood is reduced to a greater extent than the number of erythrocytes. The red cells not only contain less hemoglobin but may also be reduced in size. A similar anemia of infants is not uncommon. As stated before, the infant comes into the world with a rich store of iron. However, this store is accumulated toward the latter part of gestation. Hence a prematurely born baby may not have enough iron to tide him over the period during which the diet is exclusively milk, and anemia may result. In young women, anemias may occur due to a combined effect of malnutrition and menstrual bleeding. This type, called *chlorosis,* is not as common now as it formerly was. Other conditions in which hypochromic anemias sometimes develop are pregnancy and various infectious diseases. Hypochromic anemias are treated mainly by the administration of inorganic iron salts.

Pernicious anemia is due to an inability to form erythrocytes, not to any difficulty in synthesizing hemoglobin. There results a great diminution in the number of erythrocytes and consequently in the percentage of hemoglobin. The mean corpuscular hemoglobin concentration, however, is high and the blood picture is quite abnormal. The red bone marrow is greatly increased in volume, displacing the yellow marrow and sometimes even invading the true osseous tissue. This greater amount of unused hemoglobin causes a rise in iron and bilirubin in blood plasma, the latter apparently as bilirubin glucuronide (p. 682), since a direct van den Bergh reaction is observable. There is invariably a lack of hydrochloric acid in the gastric juice, a fact of great importance in aiding the diagnosis and of interest in explaining the mechanism of this condition.

As might be expected, administration of iron salts to patients with pernicious anemia is of no avail. The treatment is based on the results of brilliant experimental work of a number of investigators. The first step was the work of Whipple. He produced a severe anemia in dogs by repeated bleedings and studied the influence of diet on blood regeneration. It was discovered that beef liver is the most effective food in this respect. The discovery led Minot and Murphy[57] to administer liver in large amounts to patients with pernicious anemia. These workers noted remarkable improvement. This was followed by the successful use of various liver extract preparations, and ultimately by the discovery that the active substance in liver is vitamin B_{12} (p. 823).

In following the effect of treatment, the physician observes the proportion of reticulated erythrocytes in the blood. These *reticulocytes* are formed by overstimulated marrow and are so called because their protoplasm shows a delicate network or reticulum that stains with basic dyes. Reticulocytes represent immature stages of development of the erythrocytes, and their numbers furnish an index of the rapidity of blood regeneration. This index enabled Castle to estimate the curative influence of a number of preparations, and his work threw light on the mechanism of liver action. These experiments were performed on patients with pernicious anemia. Raw lean beef fed to patients with pernicious anemia had no effect on the anemia. However, when raw beef digested with normal human gastric juice was administered to the patient through a stomach tube, the effect was comparable to feeding liver. Gastric juice alone had no beneficial effect. These and other experiments seemed to indicate that normal gastric juice contains a factor, termed the *intrinsic* factor, that reacts with the *extrinsic* factor, found in foods, to produce the antianemia or hemopoietic principle. The existence of this principle may be linked to the fact that another symptom of pernicious anemia is a lack of both hydrochloric acid and pepsin in the gastric juice due to atrophy or degeneration of the fundic portion of the gastric mucosa. It is known that this portion of the stomach, which atrophies in pernicious anemia, normally produces the intrinsic factor. The intrinsic factor is thermolabile and is considered by Glass to be a mucoprotein of the gastric juice, or a substance closely related to it. The extrinsic factor is found in various foods, notably beef muscle, beef heart, rice polishings, and wheat germ. It is thermostable and is now known to be identical with vitamin B_{12} (p. 823).

Vitamin B_{12} is far more effective when given parenterally than when given orally, unless normal human gastric juice is also administered orally. Therefore, the intrinsic factor either facilitates the absorption of vitamin B_{12} or in some way increases the activity of the vitamin or protects it from destruction. Furthermore, there may be no *antianemic* factor formed in the liver by the interaction of the extrinsic and intrinsic factors, but, instead, vitamin B_{12} may be the effective antianemic principle through its effect in converting folic acid to folinic acid, and the intrinsic factor (in gastric juice) is necessary for its absorption (see also pp. 825 to 826). Vitamin B_{12} is highly effective in relieving not only the anemic phase but also the lingual and neurologic symptoms. This is not true of folic acid, which benefits only the anemic phase. Folic acid, however, is also efficacious in the treatment of the anemic phase of the macrocytic anemias of pellagra, pregnancy, and sprue. These anemias are nutritional in origin, partially at least, and constitute a group that is not amenable to treatment with iron.

Sickle-cell anemia is a hemolytic anemia of a hereditary nature. It occurs only in the Negro race. About 8% of American Negroes have the sickle-cell trait, but only about one in 40 of these develops the severe chronic anemia. In this disease the erythrocytes undergo reversible changes in shape to crescent and other forms in response to variations in the partial pressure of oxygen. Pauling and associates[37] showed that this is due to an abnormality of the hemoglobin itself, located in the globin portion of the molecule (hemoglobin-S, p. 604). Those individuals who have the trait, but not the anemia, possess some of this abnormal and some of the normal hemoglobin.

Anemias may also result from toxic inhibition of the bone marrow by certain chemical, bacterial, or physical agents or from replacement of the bone marrow by tumorous or fibrous growths or by leukemia.

POLYCYTHEMIAS

Those conditions in which there is an increase in the number of erythrocytes in the peripheral blood are termed polycythemias. A *primary* type of polycythemia of uncertain etiology, called polycythemia vera, occurs infrequently in man. Erythrocyte counts as high as 12,000,000 cells per cubic millimeter of blood have been recorded. Hemoglobin values are correspondingly increased, up to as much as 20 to 25 gm. per 100 ml. of blood. *Secondary* polycythemias are more common. They are usually compensatory to some other environmental condition or to some disease process. Tissue hypoxia (chronic), due to some impairment in oxygen transport, is frequently the underlying cause. Examples are the polycythemia occurring in individuals living at high altitudes and that found in persons having certain types of abnormal hemoglobins (p. 603).

Cobalt salts administered in small amounts to experimental animals for several weeks produced a remarkably severe true polycythemia.[58]

BLOOD TRANSFUSION AND BLOOD SUBSTITUTION

Loss of blood as a result of hemorrhage or shock is treated by blood transfusion or by injection of a substitute for blood. Blood transfusion, or infusion of a substitute, sometimes preceded by the removal of blood, has been used in a number of conditions other than hemorrhage and shock. In general, the purpose is to restore blood volume, to increase the colloidal osmotic pressure, or to provide nutritive or immunologic factors.

Whole blood, either citrated or heparinized, is, of course, the material most approved, being most physiologic. Care must be taken that the blood used is not only from a healthy human being but also compatible with that of the recipient. As regards plasma or fractions of plasma, we would expect that serum is the best blood substitute since no anticoagulant need be added to it. This is not the case, however. Blood serum frequently produces marked reactions. Plasma albumin has some value. It makes up about 62% of the blood proteins and exerts about 85% of the colloidal osmotic pressure of the plasma. Because of its great solubility, it may be given in concentrated form.

Blood plasma has proved to be a practical blood substitute and, in fact, is more effective than whole blood in most conditions of loss of blood *fluid* — not, of course, if there is loss of whole blood. Blood of normal human beings known to be *free of viral hepatitis* is collected and citrated, all under rigidly aseptic conditions. It is then centrifuged at from 2° to 4° C. It may be preserved in the liquid condition, if properly refrigerated, or it may be frozen or dried. The modern method of drying is the most practical and most widely used. It consists of rapidly freezing the plasma in rotating bottles. This fixes the solid plasma as a "shell." The plasma is then dried, while frozen, under greatly reduced pressure, which procedure is called the lyophilizing process. The proteins are not denatured to any great extent and the immunologic properties are essentially unchanged. The lyophilized, dry, flaky plasma is kept in sterile containers under vacuum until needed. All that is necessary for use is the addition of the required amount of sterile distilled water.

Great progress was made by Cohn[19] in fractionating the proteins of plasma so that they might be studied and put to clinical use. The methods of separation are based on complex physicochemical principles. For example, some proteins form dissociable complexes with each other, with smaller dipolar ions, with complex organic molecules, or with certain heavy metal and alkali earth ions. These characteristics of ethanol lead to considerable differences in solubility of proteins, and low temperatures are employed. By utilizing these properties, there have been separated from human plasma a series of protein products, each a stable white powder responsible for a different natural function. The fractions, with their uses, include the following:

1. Albumin, which is being used instead of dried whole plasma for the reasons mentioned
2. Immune globulin or γ-globulin, which has proved of value in the prevention and treatment of measles
   Recently it has been found to give temporary safeguard against poliomyelitis or to lessen the crippling effects of that disease.
3. Agglutinins, for blood typing
4. Fibrinogen, obtained in pure form, which can be made into plastics that have application in surgery
5. Thrombin, which, together with fibrinogen, of course, yields fibrin
   Fibrin films that can substitute for natural membranes have been prepared, and fibrin foams can be used with thrombin to accelerate blood clotting in operative work.

The infusion of plasma or plasma proteins has been recommended for many conditions, some of which may be mentioned briefly. It is usually agreed that in shock there is loss of plasma through the capillary walls into the tissue spaces. This leads to a decrease in blood volume, hemoconcentration (i.e., concentration of formed elements), and lowered colloidal osmotic pressure. In severe and extensive burns there is a great loss of proteins from the blood because of transudation of fluid at the site of the burn. At the same time there is believed to be an absorption of toxic substances formed at the burned tissue. These toxins cause an increase in capillary permeability throughout the body and more plasma is lost. After extensive burns, the loss of blood plasma may be even greater than in shock. When hypoproteinemia occurs, as it does in a number of clincial syndromes, plasma may be administered. Loss of blood as a result of hemorrhage, although best replaced by whole blood, may also be replaced by plasma, and this is perhaps the most general use of plasma.

The treatment of shock by the intravenous injection of whole blood, plasma, blood proteins, or other colloids is not accepted by all investigators as the correct method. Foremost among this group, Allen insists that large volumes of physiologic saline solution give as good results.

All these procedures are, in a sense, emergency measures. The best way, the most physiologic way, to replace blood is by enabling the organism to replenish it in the normal manner. A regimen to accomplish this should follow all transfusion methods. Blood proteins contain large amounts of histidine, lysine, and threonine. Hence proteins rich in these three essential amino acids should have a prominent place in the diet. To administer a mixture of amino acids themselves orally or parenterally to hasten the formation of natural blood proteins may also be advisable. Other dietary measures, including the administration of iron and vitamin supplements, should be taken.

BLOOD PRESSURE – VASOACTIVE PEPTIDES

Goldblatt demonstrated some time ago that mechanical interference with the blood flow through the renal arteries of a dog results in the development of a permanent hypertension. Apparently, slowing the circulation causes some substance that produces vasoconstriction to be formed. Such a substance has been demonstrated in the blood coming from such ischemic kidneys. The mechanism seems to be the following: an enzyme, *renin*, is formed in the kidney and is released into the blood; it is a proteinase and acts on an α_2-globulin, present in the systemic blood; a decapeptide, called *angiotensin-I*, is split off; this peptide, in turn, is acted on by a peptidase present in normal serum to form an octapeptide, called *angiotensin-II*. The amino acid sequence of these two peptides was recently determined by Page and associates[59] and is shown in Fig. 19-12. Angiotensin-I has only a slight effect on blood pressure, whereas angiotensin-II is the most powerful pressor agent now known, having an activity about 200 times that of norepinephrine. The pressor activity of angiotensin-II appears to be dependent on the presence of (1) the aromatic ring, (2) the free carboxyl group of phenylalanine, (3) the phenolic group of tyrosine, (4) the presence of proline in the seventh position in the peptide sequence, and (5) a hexapeptide structure with specific three-dimensional features. Angiotensin-II appears to exert its pressor effect by constricting arterioles and increasing the heartbeat.

Another peptidase, termed *angiotensinase*, produced by the kidney and, to a lesser extent, by other tissues hydrolyzes angiotensin-II and thus serves as a balancing antipressor agent.

The foregoing relations can be shown diagrammatically as follows:

$$\text{Angiotensinogen} \xrightarrow{\text{Renin}} \text{Angiotensin-I} \xrightarrow{\text{Peptidase}} \text{Angiotensin-II}$$

Angiotensinogen
(an α_2-globulin
of plasma)

$\downarrow$ Angiotensinase
Inactive products

Various other names for the above substances have been used in the literature. Angiotensinogen has been called renin activator, hypertensinogen, and renin substrate. Angiotensin-II has been termed angiotonin and hypertensin.

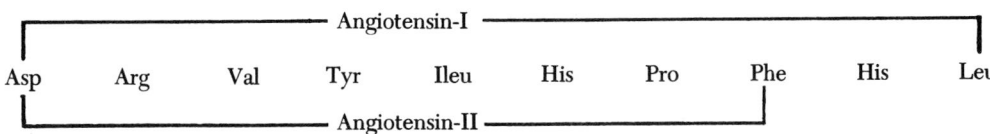

Fig. 19-12. Amino acid sequence of angiotensin-I and angiotensin-II.

The inactivating peptidase has been named angiotensinase and hypertensinase. Thus far, renin has not been found in excess in patients with chronic renal hypertension. According to Shorr, the ischemic kidney also forms, in its cortical portion, vasoexcitor material (VEM). This may act as a neutralizing agent for the hepatic vasodepressor material (VDM), which has been claimed to be identical with ferritin (p. 420).

Substances that lower blood pressure have also been obtained from kidney extracts. They have not been isolated in pure form but give promise of therapeutic usefulness in cases of hypertension. The use of low-sodium diets in hypertension is discussed on pp. 870 and 871. In this connection, it may be remarked that the use of the rauwolfia drugs for hypertension is said to be enhanced by low-sodium diets.

It has long been known that after blood coagulates it possesses vasoconstrictor properties. In 1948, the active agent was isolated and crystallized by Page and called *serotonin* (p. 380).

Another group of vasoactive peptides, the kinins, have been studied extensively during the past few years.[60-62] *Kinin* is the generic name for a group of peptides with potent biologic activities in causing smooth muscle contraction, vasodilatation, lowering of blood pressure, increasing blood flow and microvascular permeability, and inducing the emigration of granulocytic leukocytes. They thus have some activities similar to and some different from other vasoactive peptides, e.g., oxytocin, vasopressin (pp. 486, 487), angiotensin, eledoisin. Bradykinin and kallidin are typical examples. They are formed from a plasma (or serum) precursor, kininogen, apparently an α_2-globulin containing about 18% carbohydrate, by certain proteolytic enzymes, notably kallikrein and trypsin. Bradykininogen has been found in the tissues of a number of species of animals. Heart contains the most, followed by liver, kidney, and brain. Blood contains about 6 to 8 μg. per milliliter. The kinins have marked pharmacologic effects, often in nanogram amounts.

Chemically, the kinins, are small peptides of nine to 11 amino acids, similar in respect to angiotensin-I and vasopressin (p. 486), and oxytocin (p. 486). The active core of the kinins appears to be the following nonapeptide, found in bradykinin:

Arg Pro Pro Gly Phe Ser Pro Phe Arg (C-terminus)

Kallidin, a decapeptide, contains lysine in addition on the N-terminal end, and plasma kinin contains Met-Lys, in addition, also on the N-terminal end.

The kinins appear to be formed in the plasma from the α_2-globulin precursor, kininogen, by a series of interdependent reactions shown schematically in Fig. 19-13.

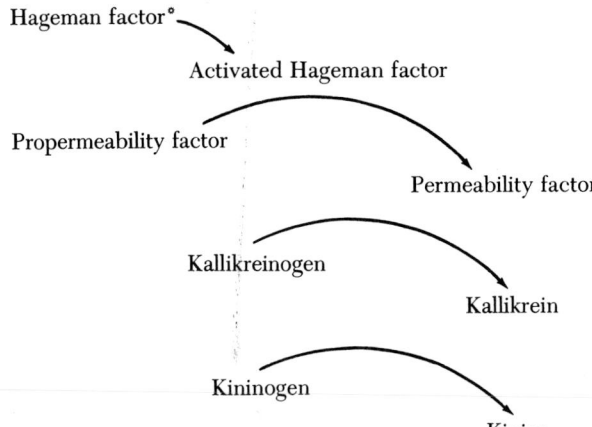

Fig. 19-13. Schematic representation of a series of interdependent reactions proposed for the in vivo formation of kinins.
*A plasma protein is activated by a glass surface or certain chemical agents and initiates blood clotting. This protein was found to be congenitally missing in the blood of Mr. Hageman. (See Fig. 19-11.)

The kinins are rapidly inactivated by the *kininases* of tissues. The "half-life" of bradykinin in blood has been estimated as less than 1 minute.[63]

The biologic significance of the kinins is not clear at the present time. Kinins appear to be the chemical mediators of inflammation. They may be involved in certain types of shock because of their powerful hypotensive properties. They also may play a role, similar to that of histamine (p. 380), as an important mediator of the sequelae of infection, injury, and foreign-body reactions.

MEDICOLEGAL TESTS FOR BLOOD

Red blood cells, if still fresh, can sometimes be seen microscopically. They can also be seen spectroscopically, because the absorption spectrum of hemoglobin is quite specific. The various tests for the catalytic oxidizing effect of heme, e.g., the guaiac, benzidine, and reduced phenolphthalein tests, are helpful but are not specific for blood. Blood reacts after it is heated, because of the catalytic action of iron, as well as before, because of the enzyme peroxidase. Raw milk, pus, saliva, and other biologic materials contain peroxidases, which react similarly, but no reaction is seen after heating. Certain salts also give the guaiac test. If hemin crystals can be prepared, they are indicative of blood; this is Teichmann's test (Fig. 19-8).

However, none of these tests are diagnostic of the species. An immunologic reaction is necessary if the species is to be determined. The test is based on the fact that blood serum of an animal into which has been injected repeatedly the blood serum of an animal of another species gradually acquires the property of producing a precipitate when mixed with serum of an animal of the species whose serum was injected. This precipitin reaction is performed essentially as follows for the detection of human blood: increasing amounts of human blood serum are injected every 4 days into a rabbit until from 25 to

35 ml. have been administered; 4 or 5 days later the rabbit is bled and the serum obtained; this is preserved in sterile containers until a test is to be made. Such serum forms a precipitate if mixed with blood serum of human beings.

References

GENERAL

Antibodies, Sympos. Quant. Biol. **32**:1, 1967.

Bishop, C., and Surgenor, D. M.: The red blood cell, New York, 1964, Academic Press, Inc.

Braunitzer, G.: Hemoglobins of various species of animals, J. Cell. Physiol. **67**: suppl. 1, 1966.

Chance, B., Estabrook, R. W., and Yonetani, T., editors.: Hemes and hemoproteins, New York, 1966–1968, Academic Press, Inc.

Dayhoff, M. D.: Atlas of protein sequence and structure, Silver Spring, Md., 1969, National Biomedical Research Foundation.

Falk, J. E.: Porphyrins and metalloporphyrins, New York, 1964, American Elsevier Publishing Co., Inc.

Fisher, J. W., editor: Erythropoietin, Ann N.Y. Acad. Sci. **149**:1, 1968.

Greenberg, D. M., editor: Metabolic pathways, vol. 4, Metabolism of porphyrins and corinoids, ed. 3, New York, 1967, Academic Press, Inc.

Harris, J. W.: The red cell, Cambridge, Mass., 1963, Harvard University Press.

Henry, R. J.: Clinical chemistry—principles and technics, New York, 1964, Harper & Row, Publishers.

Hsia, D. Y.: Inborn errors of metabolism, ed. 2, Chicago, 1966, Year Book Medical Publishers, Inc.

Ingram, V. M.: Hemoglobin and its abnormalities, Springfield, Ill., 1960, Charles C Thomas, Publisher.

Jacobson, L. O., and Doyle, M., editors: Erythropoiesis (a review of erythropoietin), New York, 1962, Grune & Stratton, Inc.

Johnson, S. A., and Seegers, W. H., editors: Symposium—Physiology of hemostasis and thrombosis, Springfield, Ill., 1967, Charles C Thomas, Publisher.

Kabat, E. A.: Structural concepts in immunology and immunochemistry, New York, 1968, Holt, Rinehart, & Winston, Inc.

Killander, J., editor: Gamma globulins—structure and control of biosynthesis, New York, 1968, John Wiley & Sons, Inc.

Lascelles, J.: Tetrapyrrole biosynthesis and its regulation, New York, 1964, W. A. Benjamin, Inc.

Lehmann, H., and Huntsman, R. G.: Man's hemoglobins, Philadelphia, 1966, J. B. Lippincott Co.

Mammen, E. F.: Physiology and biochemistry of blood coagulation. In Bang, N. U., Beller, F. K., Deutsch, E., and Mammen, E. F., editors: Thrombosis and bleeding disorders—a laboratory manual, New York, 1970, Academic Press, Inc.

Porphyrin metabolism and the porphyrias, Seminars Hemat. **5**:1, 1968.

Putnam, F. W., editor: The plasma proteins, New York, 1960, Academic Press, Inc.

Schultze, H. E., and Heremans, J. F.: Molecular biology of human proteins, New York, 1966, American Elsevier Publishing Co., Inc., vol. 1.

Seegers, W. H., editor: Blood clotting enzymology, New York, 1967, Academic Press, Inc.

Seegers, W. H.: Prothrombin, Cambridge, Mass., 1961, Harvard University Press.

Sunderman, F. W., and Sunderman, F. W., Jr.: Hemoglobin—its precursors and metabolites, Philadelphia, 1964, J. B. Lippincott Co.

Wintrobe, M. M.: Clinical hematology, ed. 6, Philadelphia, 1967, Lea & Febiger.

SPECIAL

1. MacCallum, A. B.: Physiol. Rev. **6**:316, 1926.
2. Phillips, R. A., et al.: J. Biol. Chem. **183**: 305, 331, 349, 1950.
3. Dancis, J., et al.: J. Clin. Invest. **36**:398, 1957.
4. Alpert, M. E., et al.: New Eng. J. Med. **278**:984, 1968.
5. Isaacs, A.: Endeavour **22**:96, 1963.
6. J. Immunochem. **1**:145, 1964.
7. Schultz, J.: Advances in chemistry series, no. 44, Washington, D. C., 1964, American Chemical Society, p. 1.
8. Schachman, H. K.: Biochemistry **2**:887, 1963.
9. Miller, F., and Metzger, H.: J. Biol. Chem. **240**:3325, 1965.
10. Tomasi, T. B.: New Eng. J. Med. **279**: 1327, 1968.
11. Putnam, F. W.: Science **163**:633, 1969.

12. Tanford, C.: Accounts Chem. Res. 1:161, 1968.
13. Gottlieb, P. D., et al.: Proc. Nat. Acad. Sci. 61:168, 1968; Rutishauser, U., et al.: Proc. Nat. Acad. Sci. 61:1414, 1968.
14. Gershoff, S. N., et al.: J. Nutr. 95:184, 1968.
15. Whipple, G. H., et al.: Ann. N.Y. Acad. Sci. 47:317, 1946.
16. Miller, L. L., et al.: Advances in chemistry series, no. 44, Washington, D. C., 1964, American Chemical Society, p. 17.
17. Barnhart, M. I.: Amer. J. Physiol. 199:360, 1960.
18. Tiselius, A.: Trans. Faraday Soc. 33:524, 1937.
19. Cohn, E. J., et al.: J. Amer. Chem. Soc. 72:465, 1950.
20. Auger, H. O., and Van Dyke, D. C.: Science 144:1587, 1964.
21. Orten, A. U., and Orten, J. M.: J. Nutr. 26:21, 1943.
22. Dajani, R. M., and Orten, J. M.: J. Biol. Chem. 231:913, 1958.
23. Perutz, M. F.: Science 140:863, 1963; Sci. Amer. 211:64, 1964.
24. Perutz, M. F., et al.: Nature 219:29, 131, 1968.
25. Schroeder, W. A.: Ann. Rev. Biochem. 32:301, 1963.
26. Ingram, V. M.: Nature 189:704, 1961.
27. Hill, R. L., and Buettner-Janusch, J.: Fed. Proc. 23:1236, 1964.
28. Rudloff, V.: Proc. 6th Int. Congr. Biochem. 32:208, 1964.
29. Zuckerkandl, E.: Sci. Amer. 212:110, 1965.
30. Margoliash, E., and Smith, E. L.: Proc. Nat. Acad. Sci. 50:672, 1963; Proc. 6th Int. Congr. Biochem. 32:206, 1964.
31. Bishop, J., et al.: Proc. Nat. Acad. Sci. 46:1030, 1960.
32. Werner, J. R., et al.: Proc. Nat. Acad Sci. 49:122, 1963.
33. Hammel, C. L., and Bessman, S. P.: J. Biol. Chem. 239:2228, 1964.
34. Doehr, S. A., and Orten, J. M.: Fed. Proc. 28:849, 1969.
35. Bruns, G. P., and London, I. M.: Biochem. Biophys. Res. Commun. 18:236, 243, 1965.
36. Gribble, T. J., and Schwartz, H. C.: Biochim. Biophys. Acta 103:333, 1965.
37. Pauling, L., et al.: Science 110:543, 1949; Harvey Lect. 49:216, 1953–1954.
38. Perutz, M. F., and Lehmann, H.: Nature 219:902, 1968.
39. Childs, B., and Der Kaloustien, V. N.: New Eng. J. Med. 279:1205, 1968.
40. Ingram, V. M.: Nature 180:326, 1957.
41. Schneider, B. G., et al.: New Eng. J. Med. 280:739, 1969.
42. Shemin, D., and Russell, C. S.: J. Amer. Chem. Soc. 75:4873, 1953.
43. Westall, R. G.: Nature 170:614, 1952; Cookson, G. H., and Rimington, C.: Nature 171:875, 1953.
44. Dresel, E. I. D., and Falk, J. E.: Nature 172:1185, 1953.
45. Bogorad, L., and Granick, S.: Proc. Nat. Acad. Sci. 39:1176, 1953.
46. Burnham, B. F.: Seminars Hemat. 5:296, 1968; Nandi, D. L., et al.: J. Biol. Chem. 243:1224, 1968; Nandi, D. L., and Shemin, D.: J. Biol. Chem. 243:1231, 1236, 1968.
47. Sardesai, V. M., et al.: Amer. J. Physiol. 208:1270, 1965.
48. Kappas, A., et al.: Seminars Hemat. 5:323, 1968; Granick, S., and Kappas, A.: Proc. Nat. Acad. Sci. 57:1463, 1967.
49. Watson, C. J.: Advances Intern. Med. 6:235, 1954.
50. Ellis, D. J., et al.: J. Hered. 49:125 1958.
51. Granick, S.: Trans. N.Y. Acad. Sci. 25:53, 1962; Granick, S., and Urata, C.: J. Biol. Chem. 238:821, 1963.
52. Macalpine, I., and Hunter, B.: Sci Amer. 221:38, 1969.
53. Peisach, J., et al.: J. Biol. Chem. 243:1871, 1968.
54. Strauch, B., et al.: New Eng. J. Med. 281:257, 1969.
55. Seegers, W. H.: Fed. Proc. 23:749, 1964; Laki, K., and Gladner, J. A.: Physiol. Rev. 44:127, 1964.
56. Seegers, W. H., et al.: Arch. Biochem. 128:194, 1968.
57. Minot, G. R., and Murphy, W. P.: J.A.M.A. 87:470, 1926.
58. Orten, J. M. et al.: J. Biol. Chem. 96:11, 1932; Amer. J. Physiol. 114:414, 1936.
59. Page, I. H., et al.: Chem. Eng. News 38:44, 1960.
60. Schacter, M.: Fed. Proc. Sympos. 27:49, 1968.
61. Pierce, J. V.: Fed. Proc. Sympos. 27:52, 1968.
62. Kellermeyer R. W., and Graham, R. C.: New Eng. J. Med. 279:859, 1968.
63. Sardesai, V. M.: Canad. J. Physiol. Pharmacol. 46:77, 1968.

CHAPTER 20

CHEMISTRY OF RESPIRATION AND ACID-BASE BALANCE

Respiration is that physiologic function that involves the exchange of gases between the body and the air. In the lungs oxygen passes from the air into the blood, and carbon dioxide from the blood into the air. These are the two ends of the process, but in between these ends occur many phenomena that are surprising in character. They include physical, chemical, and "nervous" changes. It is often difficult to set forth the stages in consecutive fashion, because the reactions are intricate and closely interrelated and are occurring simultaneously.

After the blood receives oxygen from the air, it is carried to the tissues, where the oxygen is utilized in metabolic processes. The end products include inorganic and organic acids—carbonic, phosphoric, sulfuric and uric, lactic, etc. The acids are largely neutralized by bases in the blood and tissue fluids, chiefly sodium bicarbonate, and thereby salts and carbon dioxide are formed. Most of the salts and acids are excreted by the kidney, and almost all of the carbon dioxide by the lungs. The mechanisms of the processes involved are the subject of this chapter.

Flow of respiratory gases At this point it is pertinent to suggest that the gas laws be reviewed. From these laws we know that a given gas tends to flow from a high partial pressure or tension to a lower one, regardless of whether it is in gaseous form or is dissolved in a liquid. First, the composition of the gases present in inspired and expired air and in the air present in the alveoli will be considered (Table 20–1).

The oxygen tensions (or partial pressures of oxygen) of these mixtures of gases are found by multiplying the total pressure by the percentage of oxygen in each case. Consequently, the partial pressure of oxygen in inspired or atmospheric air is 20.9% of the total pressure, i.e., 159 mm. Hg if the total pressure is assumed to be 760 mm. Hg. Similarly the partial pressure of the oxygen in expired air is 124 mm. Hg, and of alveolar air, 108 mm. Hg. Thus we see that the direction of the flow of oxygen is toward the alveoli. Why do the alveoli have less oxygen than inspired air? The reason, obviously, is that oxygen must have been removed in the lungs, and the reason for this is that the venous blood brought to the lungs has a low oxygen tension, namely, only

643

Table 20-1. Average composition of dry respiratory air reduced to standard temperature and pressure (0° C., 760 mm. Hg)

	Oxygen (percent)	Carbon dioxide (percent)	Nitrogen, argon, etc. (percent)
Inspired air	20.94	0.04	79.02
Expired air	16.3	4.0	79.7
Alveolar air	14.2	5.5	80.3

40 or 50 mm. Hg. Blood circulates through the capillaries of the lungs at astonishing speed. The combined thickness of the respiratory epithelium and capillary wall, which separates the blood from the air, is not over 0.004 mm. Every corpuscle is thus brought almost into actual contact with the alveolar air, and conditions are excellent for the rapid diffusion of gases. There is the added factor of the peculiar affinity of hemoglobin for gases. Consequently, oxygen flows from the partial pressure of 108 mm. in the alveoli toward the 40 to 50 mm. in the venous blood, building it up almost instantaneously to about 100 mm., the partial pressure of oxygen in *arterial blood*, the state in which it leaves the lungs.

Arterial blood, loaded with oxygen, at a partial pressure of about 100 mm., is carried to the muscles, spleen, heart, and other parts of the body. There, in the capillaries, it is separated from the tissue fluids by thin capillary walls, and from the cells by their thin walls. The partial pressures of oxygen of tissue fluids are as low as 20 to 50 mm., and those of the cell contents about the same or less. Hence, the oxygen by physical forces alone would tend to flow out from the blood into the tissues. However, other factors lead in the same direction, factors that serve to dissociate oxyhemoglobin and to combine with the oxygen. As a result, the blood comes out of the tissue capillaries and into the veins depleted of much of its oxygen, with a partial pressure of oxygen of 40 to 50 mm., and goes back to the lungs for more oxygen.

To summarize the flow of oxygen in relation to partial pressures: oxygen in *atmospheric air* (159 mm.) flows toward *alveolar air* (108 mm.) and diffuses into *venous blood* (50 mm.); this is rapidly built up with the aid of hemoglobin to *arterial blood* (100 mm.), which gives oxygen to the *tissues* (50 mm.), becoming venous blood of about the same partial pressure (50 mm.), and thence back to the *alveoli of the lungs*.

Since carbon dioxide forms carbonic acid with water and reacts chemically with bases, its distribution is not entirely a physical matter. However, the direction of its flow is also from higher to lower pressures, as can be seen from the following figures: In venous blood the partial pressure of CO_2 is 46 mm. Hg, and in alveolar air it is 40 mm.; therefore the tendency is to pass from the venous blood, into the alveoli, to the expired air (20 mm.), to the atmospheric air (0.30 mm.); after the venous blood has lost CO_2, the partial pressure is down to 40 mm., at which level arterial blood goes to the tissues; here the

CO_2 is high, with estimated partial pressures of 50 to 70 mm.; consequently, CO_2 flows into arterial blood as it courses through the capillaries, bringing the partial pressure up from 40 to about 46 at the same time that the partial pressure of O_2 is going down; the venous blood now passes to the lungs again to unload CO_2.

It may be added that there are about 2.5 to 3 vol.% of nitrogen in blood. Nitrogen is present in physical solution in the plasma and is ordinarily inert. It may, however, create a problem in individuals who are subject to marked, rapid changes in atmospheric pressure, e.g., as high-altitude flyers, on the one hand, or deep-sea divers or workers in pressurized caissons, on the other. In the latter case, increased amounts of nitrogen dissolve in the plasma of workers subjected to increased pressures in caissons used in deep excavations, tunnels, etc. If decompression when these workers leave the caisson is too rapid, bubbles of nitrogen are released from the plasma and may accumulate in the joints and adipose and other tissues. This can cause intense pain, loss of function, and even intravascular clotting, a condition known as the "bends" or caisson disease. Decompression must be gradual in order to prevent the occurrence of this condition. The same situation results if ascent to high altitudes is made too rapidly, unless, of course, the person is protected by a pressurized space suit with oxygen mask or by a pressurized cabin.

TRANSPORT OF OXYGEN

If arterial whole blood is analyzed for its content of oxygen, it is found to contain from 18 to 20 vol.%, when corrected to 0° C. and 760 mm. Hg. If the plasma is analyzed apart from whole blood, its oxygen content is about 0.3 vol.%; i.e., 100 ml. of whole blood carry from 18 to 20 ml. of oxygen, whereas if blood contained no corpuscles, it could carry only 0.3 ml. The oxygen capacity of whole blood is thus 60 or more times greater than that of plasma because of the presence of erythrocytes with their hemoglobin. If blood contained no hemoglobin, Barcroft says, we would have to have over 150 kg. of plasma in our blood system. This would mean the vascular system alone had to amount to more than twice the weight of the body and the organism would be unable to cope with the weight of its own blood. Hemoglobin thus is a truly remarkable substance. Its power of combining with oxygen and of releasing the oxygen is not the only role played by this ferroprotein, but it is the most important. The percentage of saturation with oxygen varies with several factors and is shown in dissociation curves, since this is a reversible reaction:

$$Hb \quad + \quad O_2 \quad \rightleftarrows \quad HbO_2$$
Deoxyhemoglobin $\qquad$ Oxyhemoglobin
(reduced hemoglobin)

Fig. 20-1 is a series of such curves. The oxygen association-dissociation curves are sigmoid in shape rather than linear. This is believed to be due to the so-called *heme-heme interaction,* which phenomenon, although not yet fully understood, seems to occur when oxygen is taken up and the conformation of the four subunits of hemoglobin, or more specifically the β-chains, is altered. There is then some separation of the subunits, which, in turn, in-

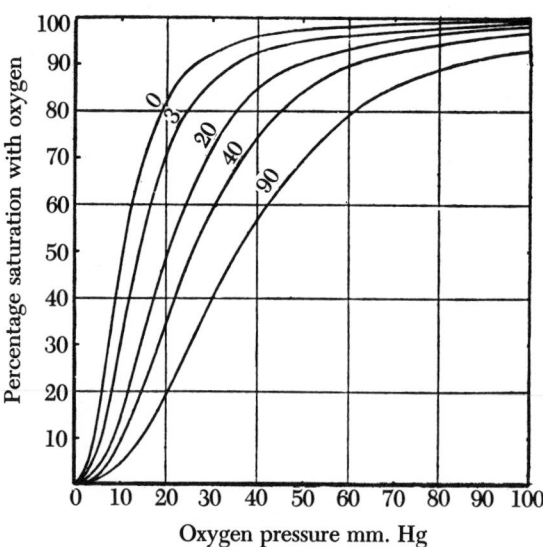

Fig. 20-1. Dissociation curves of human blood exposed to 0, 3, 20, 40, and 90 mm. CO_2. Ordinate: percentage saturation with O_2. Abscissa: O_2 pressure. (From Barcroft, J.: In Bard, P.: Medical physiology, St. Louis, 1956, The C. V. Mosby Co.)

creases the rate of uptake of oxygen by the four heme groups. Apparently the uptake of oxygen by one or more accessible (?) heme groups increases in a stepwise manner the induced affinity of the remaining three heme groups for oxygen. This phenomenon is of great physiologic advantage to the organism. Of interest, though unexplained, is the fact that hemoglobin-H (p. 602), a hemoglobin containing four β-chains, does not show such an effect or change in structure upon oxygenation.

The curves in Fig. 20-1 also show the influence of different carbon dioxide pressures in the dissociation of oxyhemoglobin of human blood. Thus, if curve *0* is followed from right to left, when no carbon dioxide is present, the blood is fully saturated with oxygen at 100 mm. oxygen pressure; at 40 mm. oxygen pressure it is about 96% saturated; at 20 mm., it is 83% saturated; and at 0 mm., it contains no oxygen. In other words, when the oxygen tension increases, the above reaction proceeds to the right and more oxyhemoglobin is formed, as in the lungs. When the oxygen tension decreases, as in the tissues, the reaction goes toward the left and more oxygen is liberated. As the carbon dioxide tension, or partial pressure, is increased, the dissociation curves are shifted to the right. This means that if more carbon dioxide is present the hemoglobin can hold less oxygen, a phenomenon known as the *Bohr effect,* after its discoverer. A definitive explanation of the Bohr effect is still not available. The decrease in oxygen saturation with an increase in carbon dioxide pressure may result from some change in the conformation of the α- and/or β-chains of the globin moiety of hemoglobin. Such a conformational change may be due more directly to an increase in hydrogen ion concentration associated with the increase in carbon dioxide tension. Interesting, but still not satisfactorily explained, is the fact that neither fetal hemoglobin nor myoglobin (muscle hemoglobin) shows the Bohr effect.

Comparing the same curve (curve 0) with no carbon dioxide and the one at 40 mm. carbon dioxide (curve 40), we see that, at 100 mm. oxygen pressure, both are practically completely saturated with oxygen; i.e., the hemoglobin is almost all present as oxyhemoglobin. At 90 mm. oxygen pressure, which is the pressure in the arteries, they are still nearly the same, curve 0 being about 99% and curve 40 about 95% saturated. At 40 mm. oxygen pressure (oxygen pressure of venous blood), the 0 curve still shows about 95% saturation, whereas curve 40 is down to 72% saturation; i.e., the presence of 40 mm. carbon dioxide has caused the oxyhemoglobin to dissociate 23% of its oxygen. Arterial blood has an approximate carbon dioxide tension of 40 mm., and venous blood about 45 mm., as stated. The high venous carbon dioxide pressures of the tissues (50 to 70 mm.) would cause the oxyhemoglobin to dissociate still more easily. Other acids have similar effects. Thus, the effect of carbon dioxide pressure is just opposite that of oxygen pressure, and both have a desirable physiologic effect. In the tissues with low oxygen and high carbon dioxide tensions, oxyhemoglobin dissociates more readily and oxygen is available for tissue needs. In the alveoli the oxygen tension of the air is high and there is no difficulty in forming oxyhemoglobin despite the high carbon dioxide pressure (see tops of all curves). It should be recalled at this point that oxygen is transported by hemoglobin loosely linked to its ferrous iron, probably by sharing unpaired electrons (p. 612). This combination is easily reversible under the conditions described on p. 613.

Some other important factors affecting the transport of oxygen by hemoglobin are pH, temperature, and the presence of electrolytes. Slight decreases in pH (more acidic) increase the dissociation of oxyhemoglobin. Thus the slightly more acid pH in tissues due to carbon dioxide favors the release of oxygen to the tissues. The slight increase in temperature in the tissues has a similar effect on the dissociation of oxyhemoglobin. The presence of physiologic amounts of electrolytes is necessary for the transport of oxygen by hemoglobin.

A recent finding implicates still another factor in the transport of oxygen by hemoglobin. The Beneschs[1] found that certain organic phosphate compounds, mainly diphosphoglyceric acid, have a marked effect on the oxygen-binding power of hemoglobin. The higher the concentration of 2,3-diphosphoglycerate (DPG) in the erythrocyte, the more readily hemoglobin gives up oxygen. Conversely, when DPG concentrations are low, oxygen is more tightly bound and therefore more slowly released.

This was shown in a classic experiment in which hemoglobin solutions were dialyzed. The oxygen dissociation curve shifted far to the left, meaning that hemoglobin increases its oxygen affinity at a given oxygen tension. Also it releases its oxygen less readily. The addition of physiologic concentrations of DPG to the dialyzed hemoglobin fully restored normal oxygen saturation characteristics. ATP has the same effect but the amounts required are well above levels normally occurring in erythrocytes. The effects of ATP and DPG were additive, however. You will recall that DPG is formed in erythrocytes from glucose and phosphate (p. 201).

In further work,[2] the Beneschs found that DPG is actually bound to hemoglobin, but *only* to deoxyhemoglobin not oxyhemoglobin. The binding is of surprising magnitude, one mole of deoxyhemoglobin binding one mole of DPG. Therefore, the mechanism of action of DPG appears to be one of shifting the following reaction to the *right*.

$$HbO_2 + DPG \quad \underset{\longrightarrow}{\longleftarrow} \quad Hb \cdot DPG + O_2$$

An interesting extension of this work is the fact that fetal erythrocytes have a lower content of DPG than do adult red blood cells, hence a higher oxygen affinity, which may explain how the fetus is able to obtain oxygen from the maternal blood supply.

A further application of the *DPG effect* is the inverse relation between the levels of erythrocyte-DPG and hemoglobin in human blood.[3] For example, under identical living and environmental conditions (a prison), the levels of erythrocyte-DPG in Negro males are some 10% to 15% higher than in white males, whereas the hemoglobin levels in Negro males are proportionately lower. Apparently the Negro is thus able to transport oxygen as efficiently with less hemoglobin.

It is conceivable that some aberrations in oxygen transport may be found to result from lowered erythrocyte-DPG levels due, in turn, to some impairment in carbohydrate metabolism in erythrocytes, hence in DPG formation.

Studies of the affinities of various hemoproteins for oxygen have shown that important differences exist. The oxygen affinity of cytochrome oxidase is greater than that of myoglobin, which, in turn, is greater than that of blood hemoglobin. This means, then, that oxygen is removed from the transporting blood hemoglobin, first, by muscle hemoglobin for storage, and, second, by cellular cytochrome oxidase, for biologic oxidations in the cell itself, thus ensuring the efficient transfer of oxygen from the lungs to the individual cells of the organism for the ultimate biologic function of oxygen, i.e., cellular oxidation for energy, as was described earlier (p. 249).

TRANSPORT OF CARBON DIOXIDE

Carbon dioxide tends to flow from the tissues to the venous blood and from the venous blood in the lungs into the alveoli. But the carriage and elimination of carbon dioxide in the expired air are not entirely a question of pressure. In fact, pressure is one of the least important factors. Of the 50 to 60 volumes of carbon dioxide per 100 ml. of blood, only 2 to 3 ml., about 5%, are in solution and exerting a pressure. This is often written in the hydrated form, H_2CO_3, although over 99% of dissolved carbon dioxide is not in this form. If all of it were in simple solution in an aqueous medium, the pH would be about 4.0, which is far on the acid side, and would mean death to the tissues. Since the pH of the plasma varies only from 7.3 to 7.5 normally (and but little more abnormally), evidently the major part of the carbon dioxide must be in combined form. Most of it—over 90%—is in the form of bicarbonate, some in the red cells and some in the plasma and tissue fluids. Only about 0.5% is present as carbonate. Another fraction, about 3% or 4%, is present as carbamino compounds, formed with proteins, whose free amino groups react with carbon dioxide.

$$\text{Prot-NH}_2 + \text{CO}_2 \rightleftarrows \text{Prot-NH} \cdot \text{COOH}$$

By far, the major portion of this fraction is in the red cells, because hemoglobin is the most abundant protein in blood. The resulting carbamino compound of hemoglobin is often called carbaminohemoglobin.

$$\text{HbNH}_2 \quad + \quad \text{CO}_2 \quad \rightleftarrows \quad \text{HbNH} \cdot \text{COOH}$$
Hemoglobin   **Carbaminohemoglobin**

The direction of this reaction is determined almost entirely by the proportion of oxyhemoglobin present in blood, not by the level of the carbon dioxide tension. Oxyhemoglobin is a more acid substance than reduced hemoglobin. When more oxyhemoglobin is present, the reaction goes to the left; i.e., more carbon dioxide is released. On the venous side, when hemoglobin is in the less-oxygenated, less-acid state, more carbon dioxide is combined. Hence the blood can carry more carbon dioxide as carbaminohemoglobin on the venous side. At the instant of oxygenation in the lungs, the more acid oxyhemoglobin forces the carbaminohemoglobin to unload some of its carbon dioxide into the alveoli. This, however, is only a small part of the carbon dioxide story.

Chloride shift   An important mechanism in the transport of carbon dioxide is the chloride shift. A few factors that play important roles must be mentioned first. Although we know that the reaction $H_2O + CO_2 \rightleftarrows H_2CO_3$ takes place readily in both directions, the rapidity with which this occurs in the body in certain sites has led biochemists to wonder whether it might be catalyzed by some enzyme. This was found to be so. Meldrum and Roughton[4] discovered that an enzyme that catalyzes the above reaction is present in high concentration in red cells. The enzyme was given the name *carbonic anhydrase*. Thus carbonic acid can be formed with extreme speed, and it can be decomposed equally rapidly by the enzyme under appropriate conditions. Another factor is the permeability of the erythrocyte, which is impermeable to hemoglobin and the plasma proteins but is permeable to water, carbon dioxide, HCO_3^-, Cl^-, OH^-, Na^+, K^+, and H^+. Most of the sodium ions are in the plasma, and most of the potassium ions are in the cells. In the erythrocytes a great deal of the hemoglobin is combined with potassium, the amount fluctuating in different parts of the cycle. With these facts in mind, let us follow the courses of oxygen and carbon dioxide, into and out of the erythrocytes and through the various parts of the respiratory cycle.

I. In the lungs:

1. Oxygen enters the erythrocyte due to the higher pressure of oxygen in the lungs. Reduced hemoglobin becomes oxyhemoglobin as shown:

$$\text{HHb} + O_2 \longrightarrow \text{HHbO}_2; \quad \text{HHbO}_2 + \text{KHCO}_3 \longrightarrow \text{KHbO}_2 + H_2CO_3$$

Because oxyhemoglobin ($HHbO_2$) is a stronger acid than reduced hemoglobin (HHb), the equilibrium point is shifted toward the right, converting bicarbonate (HCO_3^-) to carbonic acid (H_2CO_3). Thus an increased proportion of potassium ions becomes paired with oxyhemoglobin. The increase in acid strength of hemoglobin on oxygenation (or the reverse on deoxygenation), without change in blood pH, is called the *isohydric change*.

2. The decrease in bicarbonate (HCO_3^-) concentration in the erythrocyte leads to diffusion of bicarbonate from the plasma, where its concentration is higher, into the erythrocyte.

3. To preserve electroneutrality, i.e., the equality in the number of positive and negative charges, some negative ion must leave the erythrocyte for each bicarbonate ion entering it. Since the cell is permeable to chloride ions, which are present in sufficient amount, chloride ions diffuse out of the erythrocyte. The total cation content (i.e., K^+, Na^+) of the erythrocyte remains essentially constant.

4. The carbonic acid formed quickly decomposes, in the presence of the carbonic anhydrase (*C-A*) of the erythrocyte, to carbon dioxide and water thus:

$$H_2CO_3 \xrightleftharpoons{\text{C-A}} H_2O + CO_2$$

5. The low carbon dioxide pressure in the lungs, compared with that of the blood arriving at the lungs, favors the escape of carbon dioxide from the erythrocyte and plasma into the lungs, thereby shifting the above reaction and, consequently, the first reaction to the right. (Because there are fewer osmotically active particles in the erythrocyte after CO_2 escapes, some H_2O leaves the erythrocyte.)

II. In the tissues:

1. Because of the low oxygen pressure of the tissues, as compared with that of the lungs, the oxyhemoglobin of the erythrocyte gives up oxygen to to the tissue fluids and becomes reduced hemoglobin, as shown:

$$KHbO_2 + H_2CO_3 \xrightarrow{\quad} HHbO_2 + KHCO_3; \quad HHbO_2 \xrightarrow{\quad} HHb + O_2$$

Reduced hemoglobin (*HHb*) is a weaker acid than oxyhemoglobin; consequently, the equilibrium is shifted toward the right, converting carbonic acid to bicarbonate. As a result, an increased proportion of potassium ions now become paired with bicarbonate ($K^+HCO_3^-$).

2. Now the increase in bicarbonate concentration in the erythrocytes leads to diffusion of these ions from the erythrocytes into the plasma.

3. Again a shift of the chloride ions in exchange for the bicarbonate ions occurs, but this time a chloride ion must enter the cell for each bicarbonate that leaves it. The total cation content of the red blood cell continues to remain essentially unchanged.

4. Carbon dioxide diffuses from the tissues, where it is being formed in oxidative processes, into the plasma and then into the erythrocyte. Here in the presence of C-A some carbonic acid is formed, as the increase in carbon dioxide shifts the reaction to the left (although the equilibrium constant favors the existence of much more CO_2 than H_2CO_3):

$$H_2CO_3 \xrightleftharpoons{\text{C-A}} H_2O + CO_2$$

5. The shifting of the reaction (4) on p. 650 toward the left results in a shifting of the other reaction (1) toward the right. Because there are more osmotically active particles in the erythrocyte after CO_2 enters it, some water now enters the red cell.

Each phase of this cycle takes place with great rapidity. Therefore, a catalyst such as carbonic anhydrase must be present and conditions must be optimal for rapid diffusion of gases. The extremely thin membranes, the small bore of the capillaries, allowing in parts of the system for only a single erythrocyte to pass through at a time, and the temperature all contribute to this end.

The phenomenon is known as the Hamburger phenomenon or chloride shift and is summarized diagrammatically in Fig. 20-2. Carbonic acid (or CO_2 gas) and chloride ions always move in a direction opposite that of bicarbonate in the Hamburger shift. The differential distribution of electrolytes between the red blood cells and the plasma, as described here, is also partially explainable by the Gibbs-Donnan equilibrium, but only insofar as the erythrocyte membrane is semipermeable.

The increased acidity of hemoglobin on oxygenation acts as though acid had been added to the red cell, liberating carbon dioxide. Conversely, in the tissue capillaries, deoxygenation decreases the acidity of hemoglobin, which therefore accepts hydrogen ions from the carbonic acid entering the red cell. This allows most of the carbon dioxide (or H_2CO_3) from the tissues to be carried in the blood as bicarbonate (K^+ or $Na^+HCO_3^-$). The chloride-bicarbonate shift subsequently permits about 60% of the carbon dioxide from the tissues to be carried to the lungs as bicarbonate *in the plasma*. Venous blood has 4% to 10% more total carbon dioxide than does arterial blood, i.e., 2 to 5 more volumes percent, or 1 to 2 millimoles more per liter. About three fourths of this extra carbon dioxide in venous blood is carried as K^+ or $Na^+HCO_3^-$. Twice as much K^+ or Na^+ for HCO_3^- formation arises from the isohydric change of hemoglobin as is available from the ordinary buffering action of hemoglobin and plasma proteins on the invading carbon dioxide (H_2CO_3). The former does not change the pH of the plasma, whereas the latter lowers it slightly. The remaining one fourth of the extra carbon dioxide is carried as carbaminohemoglobin and as physically dissolved carbon dioxide gas. The pH of venous plasma is 0.02 to 0.04 unit lower than that of arterial plasma, but venous plasma has about 1 or 2 millimoles more $Na^+HCO_3^-$ per liter than does arterial plasma.

Hemoglobin is the most important buffer against any pH change that would result from carbon dioxide entering the blood, mainly because the isohydric change of oxyhemoglobin to hemoglobin results in the conversion of most of the invading carbon dioxide to bicarbonate.

Chemical regulation of respiratory movements. The control of respiratory movements is considered in detail in textbooks of physiology, and only a few words will be devoted to it here. There is some degree of voluntary control, but the regulation is chiefly involuntary and depends on afferent impulses to the respiratory center, which thereupon sends its impulses to the various muscles involved. Chemical influences have much to do with some of these mechanisms. Excess carbon dioxide (H_2CO_3) in the blood stimulates the

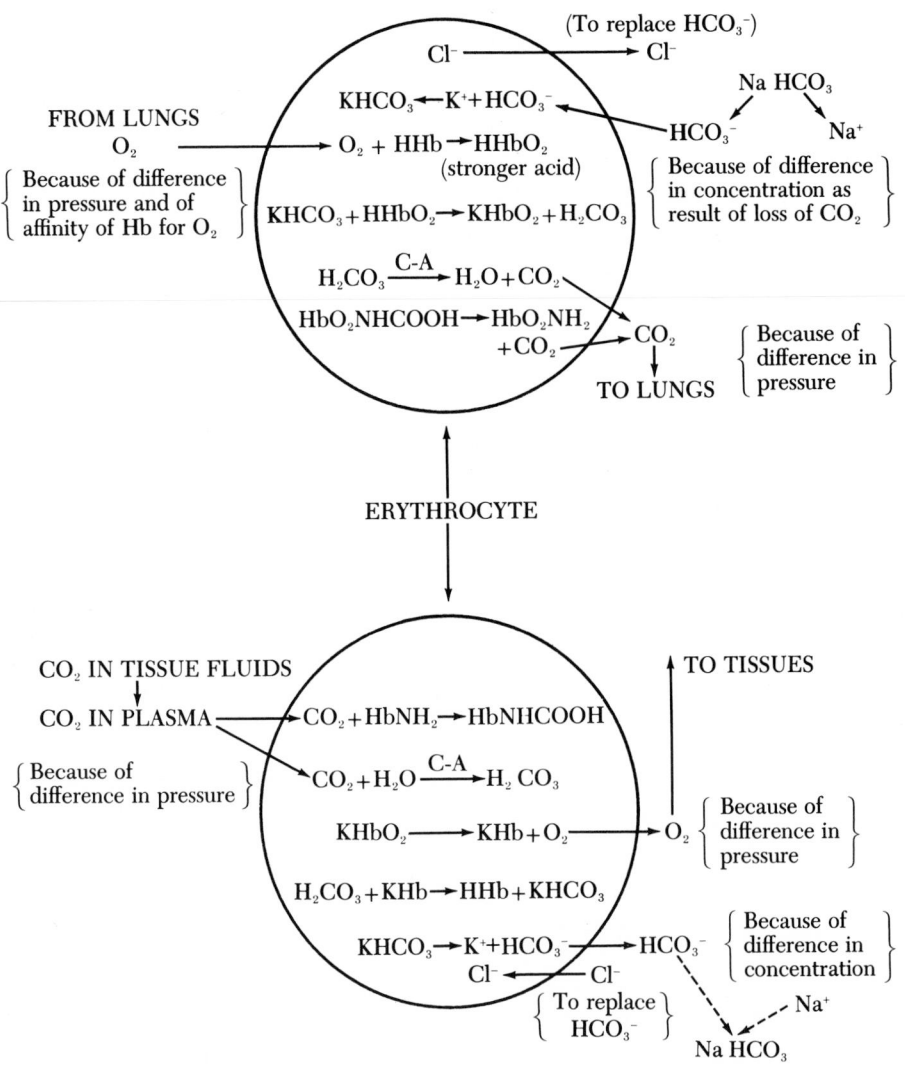

Fig. 20-2. Diagrammatic representation of O_2 and CO_2 transport and the chloride shift.

center directly, and, since fixed acids have the same effect, presumably the response is due to a slight increase in hydrogen ion concentration (or decrease in OH^- and HCO_3^-) at the site of the center. Increased carbon dioxide of the inspired air raises the rate and depth of respiration, and the result is a remarkable constancy in the percentage of carbon dioxide in the alveolar air (about 5.5%). Air or oxygen given for resuscitation should contain about 5% carbon dioxide to stimulate the respiratory center. Lack of oxygen has little effect unless it is very great. In that case, respiration is increased, because of the responses of the carotid and aortic bodies, acting as emergency mechanisms.

Under basal conditions, i.e., when the subject is at mental and physical rest, the concentration of the carbon dioxide in the expired air (collected over a period of from 5 to 25 minutes) is constant for normal subjects. The range in a large number of determinations was found to be from 18.0 to 22.5 mm., and an average partial pressure of about 20.0 mm. is an acceptable clinical standard for both sexes and for all ages.

Low concentrations of carbon dioxide in the expired air, indicating respiratory stimulation, would be expected in subjects with circulatory failure, acidosis, severe anemia, and certain forms of pulmonary disease. High concentrations would be expected in alkalosis and in depression of the respiratory center, as occurs after morphine or barbiturate administration. In cardiac patients a definite relation between degree of cardiac failure and carbon dioxide concentration in the expired air has been found. Patients with slight limitation of physical activity had an average carbon dioxide of 18.55 mm., those with marked limitation of physical activity had an average of 15.81 mm., and those who were unable to carry on any physical activity whatever without discomfort averaged 13.44 mm.

Cellular oxidations. It has been seen that hemoglobin combines with oxygen during the brief interval the red cell spends in the capillaries of the lungs. About 95% of the hemoglobin is united with oxygen when the arterial blood speeds to the tissues. In the tissue capillaries, because of the high carbon dioxide tension and the low oxygen tension, the dissociation of oxyhemoglobin is accelerated and oxygen flows into the plasma and diffuses through the walls of the capillaries into the tissue fluids and into the cells themselves. In and around the cells there occur those vital reactions whereby the digested and, in some cases, partly resynthesized food products, as well as fragments of protoplasm, are oxidized. In these processes energy is released and carbon dioxide and water are formed as final products of some of these reactions (Chapter 10).

Carbon dioxide utilization in animal tissues. In the past it was commonly accepted that only plants utilize carbon dioxide in photosynthetic and other processes but that in animals carbon dioxide is produced in the course of metabolism, is not utilized at all, and is excreted as an end product. In recent years this idea has had to be modified in view of the increasing evidence that carbon dioxide (as HCO_3^-) can enter into synthetic reactions in the animal body. The incorporation of the carbon of sodium bicarbonate into glycogen has already been mentioned (p. 192). A number of other reactions have been demonstrated, usually with the aid of isotopically tagged compounds. Evans showed that carbon dioxide can be fixed by pigeon liver, by addition to pyruvic acid. The product is oxaloacetic acid.

$$^{13}CO_2 + CH_3 \cdot CO \cdot COOH \;\rightleftarrows\; ^{13}COOH \cdot CH_2 \cdot CO \cdot COOH$$

The enzyme that catalyzes this reaction is oxaloacetate-β-carboxylase, and ATP is a cofactor for the reaction. A similar reversible reaction by aid of a specific enzyme occurring in heart muscle, and also in liver, converts α-ketoglutaric acid to oxalosuccinic acid.

$$COOH \cdot CH_2 \cdot CH_2 \cdot CO \cdot COOH + CO_2 \quad \rightleftarrows \quad COOH \cdot CH_2 \cdot CH \cdot CO \cdot COOH$$

COOH

α-Ketoglutaric acid   Oxalosuccinic acid

You may also recall (p. 310) that, in the biosynthesis of fatty acids by the cytoplasmic system, *active* carbon dioxide is incorporated into acetyl-CoA to form malonyl-CoA, which, in turn, reacts with additional acetyl-CoA to form fatty acids.

In bacterial metabolism, many other carbon dioxide fixations have been found to occur, and these presage the discovery of similar enzyme systems in mammalian tissues.

ACID-BASE BALANCE

As has been described in previous chapters, the oxidation of metabolites in the living organism results in the formation of a variety of acids and bases. Protons, for example, may originate from the ionization of various organic acids that are intermediates in the metabolism of glucose, fatty acids, and amino acids. These include pyruvic, lactic, acetoacetic, and β-hydroxybutyric acids. Uric acid from the catabolism of purines (p. 402) is another source of protons, as is sulfate from the oxidation of cystine-cysteine and methionine sulfur. In general, these metabolic protons are oxidized to water in the process of biologic oxidations (p. 249) and thus disposed of. Likewise, carbon dioxide, although excreted primarily by the lungs as just described, may be hydrated to form carbonic acid and retained to some extent in the tissues and body fluids. This ionizes to a limited degree and becomes still another source of protons.

Bases, too, can arise during the catabolism of certain metabolites. The formation of ammonia from the deamination of amino acids (Chapter 13) is an important example. The formation of anions such as bicarbonate, biphosphate, and acetate are other examples. The alkalinizing effect of certain basic salts, e.g., citrates of citrus fruits, is still another example.

Thus during normal metabolic processes, both acids and bases are formed; usually, however, acidic substances predominate. These substances may enter the blood plasma and other extracellular fluids for metabolic, excretory, or other forms of disposal. In a variety of pathologic conditions, to be discussed, excessive amounts of metabolic or exogenous acids or bases may accumulate in the cells and tissues of the body, leading to disturbances of acid-base balance. The remaining part of this chapter will consider mechanisms for the biochemical regulation of acid-base equilibrium in the body.

The blood and body fluids remain at the remarkably constant level of pH 7.3 to 7.5—usually 7.35 to 7.45—during health.* For the accomplishment of this, the body has four lines of defense: (1) the buffer systems of the blood, tissue fluids, and cells, as well as mineral salts of bones; (2) the excretion or retention of carbon dioxide by the lungs; (3) the excretion of an acid or al-

---

* These pH values are determined at body temperatures, 37° to 38° C., at which the neutrality point is 6.8, since $K_W = 10^{-13.6}$ at this temperature.

kaline urine; and (4) the formation and excretion of ammonia or organic acids. Thus the body's internal environment is maintained at a rather constant hydrogen ion concentration, which enables the various enzyme systems to operate under proper conditions, particularly in relation to each other.

At this point, a few words are in order concerning the meaning and use of the term *base* as it is ordinarily applied to the subject of acid-base balance. According to current concepts (e.g., the Brønsted) (see also p. 884), a base is any substance that combines with protons (H^+ ions). An acid is any substance that gives off protons. Accordingly, bases would usually be such anions as OH^-, HCO_3^-, $HPO_4^=$, CH_3COO^-, etc. Also, ammonia and the amino group would be classed as bases because they can accept protons. Traditionally in the medical and allied sciences, however, the term "base" has been applied to sodium and potassium ions and sometimes even to calcium ions and other cations. Actually, of course, they are not bases in the sense of being proton acceptors. Their salts with weak acids are basic because on hydrolysis the weak acid and the conjugate base are formed, giving a net excess of free hydroxyl ions. Such forms of sodium and potassium ions are probably more accurately termed "alkalies." In this discussion sodium or potassium may be called bases or alkalis in the sense that they serve as cation carriers or conjugates of strongly basic ions such as OH^-, HCO_3^-, $HPO_4^=$, and CH_3COO^-. (All salts, strong acids, and strong bases are virtually completely ionized; thus $KHbO_2$ is $K^+HbO_2^-$, HCl is H^+Cl^-, and $NaOH$ is Na^+OH^-.)

Buffer systems of the blood   In the Appendix (p. 885) it is shown that the hydrogen ion concentration of a solution of a weak acid, HA, and its salt, B^+A^-, is

$$[H^+] = K \frac{[HA]}{[B^+A^-]}$$

where K is the dissociation constant, and $[H^+]$, $[HA]$, and $[B^+A^-]$ or $[A^-]$ the concentrations of hydrogen ions, of the acid, and of the salt, respectively. The hydrogen ion concentration of such a buffer pair remains constant if the ratio of the numerator to the denominator remains constant. Slight additions of acid or base to buffers (or subtractions of either) have very little effect for reasons outlined previously, but large changes, of course, make a decided difference. These relations should be kept in mind.

In logarithmic form, the relation (Henderson-Hasselbalch equation) is as follows:

$$pH = pK' + \log \frac{[B^+A^-]}{[HA]}$$

For carbonic acid, the pK' is 6.1; for $B^+H_2PO_4^-$, it is 6.8. Therefore, to keep the pH at 7.4, the ratios of these acids to their salts must be kept constant. Substituting in the Henderson-Hasselbalch equation (p. 885):

$$\text{For } H_2CO_3 \quad 7.4 = 6.1 + \log \frac{BHCO_3}{H_2CO_3} \quad \text{or} \quad 1.3 = \log \frac{BHCO_3}{H_2CO_3}$$

and since antilog of 1.3 = 20

$$\frac{B^+HCO_3^-}{H_2CO_3} = \frac{20}{1} \text{ (at pH 7.4)}$$

655

This ratio, namely, 20:1, will be referred to later in this chapter.

$$\text{For } B^+H_2PO_4^-, \quad \frac{B_2^+HPO_4^=}{B^+H_2PO_4^-} = \frac{4}{1} \text{ (at pH 7.4)}$$

The principal buffers of the blood are:

$$\frac{Na^+HCO_3^-}{H_2CO_3} \quad \frac{Na_2^+HPO_4^=}{Na^+H_2PO_4^-} \quad \frac{Na^+ \text{ Protein}}{H \text{ Protein}} \qquad \text{(plasma)}$$

$$\frac{K^+HCO_3^-}{H_2CO_3} \quad \frac{K^+Hb^-}{HHb} \quad \frac{K^+HbO_2^-}{HHbO_2} \quad \frac{K_2^+HPO_4^=}{K^+H_2PO_4^-} \quad \text{(red cells)}$$

The buffer pairs in the first line are chiefly or wholly in plasma and extracellular fluids, and those of the second are chiefly or wholly in the red cells. The sodium and potassium are not confined exclusively to the plasma or red cells, respectively. In the blood, of course, these buffers are all in equilibrium with each other. Therefore the estimation of any one buffer pair would be an index of acid-base equilibrium. Of all the pairs enumerated, the $\dfrac{B^+HCO_3^-}{H_2CO_3}$ is the most important, insofar as action against fixed, i.e., nonvolatile, acids is concerned. The phosphate pair, although more efficient as a buffer, is actually less effective, because of its low concentration in plasma. Plasma proteins play a greater buffering role than phosphates but much less than hemoglobin. The bicarbonates neutralize more than 50% of all acids stronger than carbonic. Finally, in such neutralization carbon dioxide is again formed and is readily eliminated as a gas by the lungs. An increase in $[H^+]$ or $[H_2CO_3]$ stimulates the respiratory centers to increase the rate and depth of respiratory ventilation. Similarly, an increase of $[OH^-]$ or $[CO_3^=]$ depresses respiratory ventilation. The lungs thus play a leading role in the minute-to-minute regulation of the pH of the blood and extracellular fluids.

Examples of acids that can alter the acid-base balance include sulfuric, phosphoric, uric, lactic, acetoacetic, and β-hydroxybutyric. Their formation has been discussed in previous chapters.

As acid enters the blood, one of the buffer reactions that occur is as follows:

$$2 \, Na^+HCO_3^- + H_2^+SO_4^= \rightarrow 2 \, H_2CO_3 + Na_2^+SO_4^-$$

Here a strongly dissociated acid is transformed into the weakly dissociated acid (H_2CO_3), thus changing the hydrogen ion concentration but little, i.e., only as much as carbonic acid is dissociated. This slight decrease in the ratio $\dfrac{BHCO_3}{H_2CO_3}$, due to an increase in the denominator, can be rapidly brought down to normal because of the easy disposal of carbonic acid via the lungs. Carbonic acid is over 99% carbon dioxide gas. Thus any nonvolatile acid stronger than carbonic can be buffered by $BHCO_3$ as long as any bicarbonate is present. Consequently the plasma bicarbonate is a measure of the base remaining after all acids stronger than carbonic have been neutralized. It represents the reserve of alkali available for the neutralization of such strong acids. Hence it was termed the "alkali reserve" by Van Slyke and Cullen.[5] However, hemoglobinate plays an important role in buffering fixed acids, although not as great a one as bicarbonate. It is not, however, directly measured when the alkali reserve (CO_2 combining power) is determined by the procedure described on p. 661, but a decrease in plasma alkali reserve generally parallels a depletion of the reserve of buffering power represented by hemoglobinate.

Again it must be pointed out that the other buffers are in equilibrium with the bicarbonate pair and will react with acids (or bases), but to a lesser extent, because of their lower concentrations. For example:

$$Na\ Protein + HCl \rightleftharpoons H\ Protein + NaCl$$
$$Na_2HPO_4 + HCl \rightleftharpoons NaH_2PO_4 + NaCl$$
$$2\ KHbO_2 + H_2SO_4 \rightleftharpoons 2\ HHbO_2 + K_2SO_4$$
$$Na_2CO_3 + H_2CO_3 \rightleftharpoons 2\ NaHCO_3$$
$$HHb + KOH \rightleftharpoons KHb + H_2O$$

In every case, the strong acid or base is transformed to a weak one, and consequently the pH of the blood fluctuates very little. However, the acid formed in largest amounts in the body is carbonic acid or its anhydride carbon dioxide, and this cannot be buffered by bicarbonates. It can be buffered by serum proteins and by phosphates:

$$H_2CO_3 + Na\ Protein \rightleftharpoons NaHCO_3 + H\ Protein$$
$$H_2CO_3 + Na_2HPO_4 \rightleftharpoons NaHCO_3 + NaH_2PO_4$$

Both these factors are of minor consequence. The most important buffer for carbonic acid is hemoglobin. Table 20-2 gives estimates of supplies of buffers in the various compartments of the body.

Role of the kidney   The kidney contributes to the maintenance of the alkali reserve and to a constant level of blood pH by reabsorbing, secreting, and excreting acidic or basic substances, as the case may be.[6] Moreover, although the lung can help excrete acid, it cannot restore the alkali reserve ($BHCO_3$)—something the kidney can do. Although phosphates are present in only small concentrations in the blood, they are concentrated by the kidney and are the principal buffers in urine as excreted. In acid urines there is a relative excess of BH_2PO_4,

Table 20-2. Buffers of body fluids*

Estimated percent buffering of invading fixed acid or alkali	Chief buffers present	Location of buffer depots
40	Partly $BHCO_3$ Partly unknown	Tissue cells
30	$BHCO_3$	Extracellular fluid except blood
13	BHb and $BHbO_2$	Blood
17	$BHCO_3$	

*From Van Slyke, D. D., and Cullen, G. E.: J. Biol. Chem. 30:289, 1917.

and in alkaline urines, B_2HPO_4. There is also a considerable amount of $BHCO_3$ in alkaline urines—notably potassium bicarbonate from the metabolism of fruits and vegetables. Organic acids, carbonic acid, and salts of organic bases contribute to the urinary pH. In quite a different way, the kidney has another effect on acid-base balance. It is the site of the formation of ammonia, which is secreted probably as ammonium bicarbonate by the kidney tubules because of the omnipresence of carbon dioxide (H_2CO_3) in the carbonic anhydrase–rich kidney. This results in the conservation and restoration of $B^+HCO_3^-$ or alkali reserve in the following manner: if a strong acid, H^+A^-, has been thrown into the blood, resulting in the replacement of some of the $B^+HCO_3^-$ by B^+A^-, then the following occurs in the kidney to restore $B^+HCO_3^-$ of the blood:

$$B^+A^- \;+\; NH_4^+HCO_3^- \;\rightleftarrows\; B^+HCO_3^- \;+\; NH_4^+A^-$$

Filtered	Secreted	Reabsorbed	Excreted
through	in	in tubule	in urine
glomeruli	tubule		

in acidosis the urinary ammonia rises considerably as a result of increased formation in the kidney; all the ammonium ion produced and excreted in this way takes the place of an equivalent amount of the cations Na^+, K^+, Ca^{++}, or Mg^{++}, which are reabsorbed, paired with the HCO_3^- anion; the undue loss of these cations in the urine is prevented while the level of the bicarbonate anion in the body fluids is restored; the fixed acid anion (A^+), which had disturbed the constancy of the internal enviornment, is excreted in the urine paired with the NH_4^+ ion.

The mechanism of ammonia formation by the kidney is discussed on p. 362. The method whereby an acid urine is formed from a slightly alkaline blood plasma deserves some consideration. Urinary acidification is necessary to provide for the excretion of fixed acids and acid salts and to restore alkali reserve. There are several current theories to account for the phenomenon of a glomerular filtrate of pH 7.4 being converted to a urine having a pH as low as 4.8. Some of these concepts are illustrated in Fig. 20-3 and may be summarized as follows: According to the *phosphate reabsorption theory*, the glomerular filtrate contains as its significant constituents sodium dihydrogen phosphate and disodium phosphate. The dibasic phosphate is reabsorbed by the renal tubule and returned to the blood, whereas the monobasic (acidic) salt remains in the tubule and becomes the titratable acid of the urine. The *carbonic acid filtration theory* maintains that the glomerular filtrate contains carbonic acid and sodium bicarbonate in addition to the two types of phosphate. There is also the assumption that the tubules can remain impermeable to carbonic acid (CO_2) as they actively reabsorb sodium bicarbonate. Thus the equilibrium $Na_2HPO_4 + H_2CO_3 \rightleftarrows NaHCO_3 + NaH_2PO_4$ is moved to the right as bicarbonate is removed, leaving dihydrogen phosphate in the urine. If the tubules are considered permeable to carbon dioxide (H_2CO_3), the carbonic acid available from surrounding areas serves as an almost endless source of bicarbonate, through the above equilibrium reaction, which is moved to the right as the bicarbonate is reabsorbed. This mechanism, the *carbonic acid filtration-diffusion theory*, can account for a greater urinary acidity than the

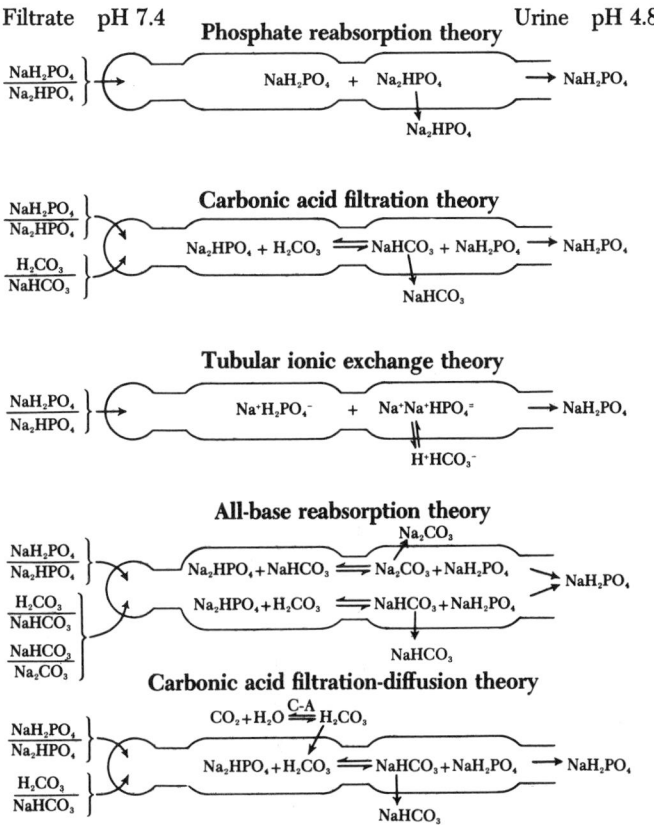

Fig. 20-3. Theories to account for the acidification of urine. (Upper three parts from Pitts, R. F., and Alexander, R. S.: Amer. J. Physiol. **144**:239, 1945.) (See also Pitts, R. F.: Physiology of the kidney and body fluids, Chicago, 1963, Year Book Medical Publishers, Inc.)

preceding theory, which is limited by the amount of carbon dioxide (H_2CO_3) filtered. The *tubular ionic exchange theory* postulates that the hydrogen ions are actively transported by the tubular cells into the urine in exchange for sodium (and K^+) ions of the glomerular filtrate, thus converting disodium phosphate to dihydrogen phosphate, and bicarbonate to carbonic acid, the last escaping from the tubular lumen into the cells as carbon dioxide.[7,8] In all these theories, carbonic anhydrase in the tubular cells assures the rapid conversion of carbon dioxide ($+H_2O$) to carbonic acid.

According to the *all-base reabsorption theory*, the absorption of alkaline compounds, notably sodium carbonate, followed by sodium bicarbonate, can completely explain any urinary acidity reported.[5] As carbonate is reabsorbed, the equilibrium $Na_2HPO_4 + NaHCO_3 \rightleftarrows Na_2CO_3 + NaH_2PO_4$ is moved to the right, converting the disodium phosphate to dihydrogen phosphate. Subsequent reabsorption of the bicarbonate completes the acidification process by converting more disodium phosphate to dihydrogen phosphate as sodium bicarbonate reabsorption moves the following equilibrium to the right:

$$Na_2HPO_4 + H_2CO_3 \rightleftarrows NaHCO_3 + NaH_2PO_4$$

659

Over three times as much bicarbonate as carbonate is reabsorbed in this postulated mechanism. (H_2CO_3, present in the carbonic anhydrase–rich kidney, readily reacts with reabsorbed Na_2CO_3, Na_2HPO_4, Na_3PO_4, or $NaOH$.)

In all the acidifying mechanisms cited, B^+ instead of Na^+ might be used.

The kidney also protects the organism against an excess of alkali. An alkaline ash diet results in the production of potassium bicarbonate and biphosphate. The kidney produces an alkaline urine by excreting, i.e., not reabsorbing, alkaline bicarbonate and disodium phosphate. It might here reabsorb alkaline dihydrogen phosphate. When excreting an alkaline urine, the kidney also excretes much more organic acid, notably citric, essentially in the salt form, at this pH range. Gamble and associates[9] demonstrated, in human subjects, that citric acid is the only acid of the citric acid cycle that increases in the urine in response to alkali administration. Similar increases in urinary citrate excretion were found in respiratory alkalosis due to hyperventilation and during the alkaline tide after meals. A decrease in urinary citrate was found in a case of severe diabetic acidosis. Thus citric acid appears to be a physiologic acid in the same sense that ammonia serves as a physiologic base.

Since the ingestion or formation of fixed acids results (by interaction with $BHCO_3$) in the formation of volatile carbon dioxide, which is readily eliminated by the lungs, whereas no base can be exhaled in a similar manner, and since the kidney can form and excrete much ammonia, the organism is better equipped to combat the invasion of acid than alkali.

The most rapid response to changes in the acidity or alkalinity of the blood is that of the blood buffers and the respiratory mechanism. The next is the acidification or alkalinization of the urine. The production and excretion of ammonia in the urine takes a longer time to begin and end.

ACIDOSIS AND ALKALOSIS

Peters and Van Slyke defined acidosis as "an abnormal condition caused by the accumulation in the body of excess acid or by the loss from the body of alkali." Similarly alkalosis is "an abnormal condition caused by the accumulation in the body of excess alkali or by the loss of acid." Ordinary amounts of acid or alkali are taken care of by the mechanisms just considered; i.e., ordinarily the ratio $\dfrac{B^+HCO_3}{H_2CO_3}$ of the equation $pH = pK + \log \dfrac{[B^+HCO_3^-]}{[H_2CO_3]}$ is constant at about 20/1, and since this is in equilibrium with all the other sets of buffers, the pH remains at 7.3 to 7.5. In acidosis or alkalosis the ratio may almost be kept constant. If the acidosis is due to an increase of the denominator, a concomitant and sufficient increase in the numerator holds the ratio almost constant. If it is due to a loss of alkali, i.e., diminution of the numerator, a simultaneous decrease in the denominator has the same effect. Similarly an alkalosis arising from an increased amount of alkali may be compensated for by an increased retention of carbonic acid, and a decrease in the denominator may be followed by a decrease in the numerator. In all these four conditions the pH scarcely changes. Such courses of events result in compensated acidosis or alkalosis. When the ratio actually changes and the pH is outside of the normal range, the term "uncompensated" is used. However, long before any abnormally great deviation in the pH occurs, the bicarbonate content changes. This is easily detected by determining the carbon dioxide combining power of blood plasma.

The normal concentration of alkaline bicarbonate in plasma is about 0.025 mole or 25 millimoles per liter. Plasma carbonic acid (mainly CO_2 gas) is about 1.2 millimoles. Plasma alkaline carbonate is 0.1 millimole. The total carbon dioxide (mainly bicarbonate) is thus about 26 millimoles. When measured in the laboratory by the addition of acid to plasma, the amount of carbon dioxide liberated from the plasma represents mainly alkaline bicarbonate or the alkali reserve and is reported in volumes percent—the number of milliliters of carbon dioxide that would be liberated from 100 ml. of plasma. From the gas laws we know that 22.4 ml. of a perfect gas represent 1 millimole of the gas. If 1 ml. of plasma gave 0.224 ml. of carbon dioxide on acidification, it would be reported as 22.4 vol.% and would mean that there are 10 millimoles of total carbon dioxide in 1 liter of plasma. To convert volumes percent to millimoles per liter, divide by 2.24.

Carbon dioxide combining power of blood plasma. The principles involved in the determination of carbon dioxide combining power of plasma are as follows: the blood is taken from a vein by syringe and is transferred to an oxalated centrifuge tube; after centrifuging, the plasma is placed in a separatory funnel and is exposed to an atmosphere whose carbon dioxide tension is approximately that of alveolar air; a measured volume of this saturated plasma is then placed in a Van Slyke carbon dioxide apparatus, acidified, and subjected to negative pressure (this treatment liberates the carbon dioxide from bicarbonate as well as the carbon dioxide in solution); the bubble is returned to the calibrated part of the apparatus and measured at atmospheric pressure (normal blood plasma combines with from 50 to 70 ml. of carbon dioxide per 100 ml.); if the buffering power is depleted because acids have been thrown into the blood in excessive amounts (acidosis), less carbon dioxide can be taken care of and the carbon dioxide combining power is, of course, lower. In alkalosis more carbon dioxide can be combined. If a patient has received sodium bicarbonate, a false picture may result because this increases the volume of carbon dioxide itself, although the fundamental metabolic condition of the patient may be unchanged, and this possibility must be kept in mind. In general a carbon dioxide combining power of over 70 ml. per 100 ml. indicates alkalosis; 50 to 70 ml., normal; 41 to 50 ml., mild acidosis; 31 to 40 ml., moderate acidosis; 30 ml. or less, severe acidosis. For details of this procedure, refer to laboratory manuals.

Disturbances in acid-base balance   If you remember that acid-base balance depends on the ratio $\dfrac{B^+ HCO_3^-}{H_2CO_3}$, you can see that there are nine possible states that may occur in the blood. They are, in the first place, a normal relationship. Then there are excesses of either numerator or denominator and deficits of either; i.e., there are four deflections from the normal, and since each may be compensated or uncompensated, they total eight. If the ratio $\dfrac{B^+ HCO_3^-}{H_2CO_3}$ remains within normal limits, i.e., about 16/1 to 25/1, corresponding to pH 7.3 and 7.5, the situation is compensated.

Primary alkali deficit. In primary deficit of alkali, the bicarbonate is diminished as a result of increased production, ingestion, or retention of acid. The increased production occurs in diabetes mellitus, in starvation, and in certain other metabolic disturbances. Such acids as β-hydroxybutyric are not utilized in the normal manner and they therefore make inroads on the alkali reserve. The ingestion of mineral acids, as might occur from the administration of hydrochloric in gastric disturbances, has the same effect. Infantile diarrhea may result in loss of base. In nephritis the kidney may not excrete acids in sufficient amounts and retention therefore occurs. Except in the case of retention, a primary alkali deficit leads to increased elimination of acid in the urine. There is also a rise in urinary ammonia. Respiration is increased in order to get rid of carbon dioxide faster. All these compensatory mechanisms tend to reduce carbonic acid (denominator). If the reduction is sufficient to keep the pH in the normal range, a *compensated acidosis* results. If not, the acidosis is *uncompensated,* the pH falls, and the patient may go into coma. Primary alkali deficit has also been called *metabolic acidosis.*

Primary alkali excess. The ingestion of excessive amounts of sodium bicarbonate is about the only example of increasing the bicarbonate fraction in an absolute manner. However, removing acid from the body has the same result, relatively. An example of the latter is excessive vomiting as it occurs in pyloric obstruction, with consequent loss of gastric hydrochloric. The physiologic mechanisms for combating this are an increased excretion of alkali by the kidney and, at the same time, a diminished formation of ammonia. Respiration is depressed so that loss of carbon dioxide is very low. If these physiologic efforts are successful in keeping the pH below 7.5, again there is a compensated condition of alkalosis with few, if any, untoward symptoms. However, if it is uncompensated and the pH rises to an abnormal level, the alkalosis is grave and tetany may occur. Tetany is a condition that may arise from other causes besides severe alkalosis. Neuromuscular excitability is the chief symptom in man, and even convulsive seizures occur in children as they do in lower animals. *Metabolic alkalosis* is another term applied to this type. It is usually minimally compensated, the pH being above 7.45 as a rule when the alkaline bicarbonate is above 30 millimoles per liter.

Primary carbon dioxide excess. A primary excess of carbon dioxide is caused by any obstruction to respiration or depression of it. The former may occur in penumonia or emphysema, and the latter from depression of the respiratory center as a result of toxic doses of morphine or other respiratory depressants. Under these conditions usually the lack of oxygen (anoxia) is more to be feared than the acidosis. However, it is an acidemia, and the compensatory mechanisms are an increase in the renal reabsorption of bicarbonate and a rise in urinary acid and ammonia. This leads to high alkaline bicarbonate with acidemia. Again this may be either compensated or uncompensated. Primary carbon dioxide excess has sometimes been designated *respiratory acidosis* despite the high alkaline bicarbonate.

Primary carbon dioxide deficit. A loss of carbon dioxide may occur when respiration is stimulated in some abnormal manner. Examples of this are more common than are usually believed. Fever and hot baths were the two most usual instances formerly cited, but two others have more recently been brought to the attention of observers. One is the lack of oxygen existing at high altitudes. When this is very great, it increases the rate of respiration and carbon dioxide is eliminated more rapidly. A second factor is anxiety or hysteria. Such a mental state results in hyperventilation also, and the two factors may operate together in airplane passengers. In the Army the hyperventilation anxiety syndrome was said to be a rather common condition in hospitalized cases in wartime. It is often difficult to recognize. Primary carbon dioxide deficit is, of course, an alkalemia that usually becomes compensated by a reduction of urinary ammonia formation and increased excretion of bicarbonate. A common term for primary carbon dioxide deficit is *respiratory alkalosis*, despite the low alkaline bicarbonate.

From a consideration of these conditions it must be evident that the determination of the alkali reserve alone will not always give a true picture of the condition. Sometimes a pH determination is also needed. For instance, in an uncompensated carbon dioxide deficit there is an alkalemia, due to a loss of volatile acid. In the attempt to compensate for the reduction in carbonic acid, there is, as stated, an increased excretion of bicarbonate. Thus we have a lowered blood bicarbonate with an alkalemia. On the other hand, in an uncompensated carbon dioxide excess, the attempt of the body to compensate is the production and hoarding of bicarbonate. The blood actually is more acid (acidemia) despite the presence of increased bicarbonate. These, of course, are extreme cases, but their implications are important. A good clinical history to determine the cause of the disturbance is most helpful. Acidemia or alkalemia refers to low or high pH, respectively.

References

GENERAL

Barcroft, J.: The respiratory function of the blood, Cambridge, 1928, Cambridge University Press.

Christensen, H. N.: Diagnostic biochemistry, New York, 1959, Oxford University Press, Inc.

Davenport, H. W.: The ABC of acid-base chemistry, ed. 4, Chicago, 1958, University of Chicago Press.

Ellington, J. R., and Danowski, T. S.: The body fluids, Baltimore, 1955, The Williams & Wilkins Co.

Frisell, W. R.: Acid-base chemistry in medicine, New York, 1968, The Macmillan Co.

Gamble, J. L.: Chemical anatomy, physiology and pathology of extracellular fluid, ed. 6, Cambridge, 1958, Harvard University Press.

Muntwyler, E.: Water and electrolyte metabolism and acid-base balance, St. Louis, 1968, The C. V. Mosby Co.

Peters, J. P.: Water balance in health and disease. In Duncan, G. G., editor: Diseases of metabolism; detailed methods of diagnosis and treatment, ed. 3, Philadelphia, 1952, W. B. Saunders Co.

Peters, J. P., and Van Slyke, D. D.: Quantitative clinical chemistry, Baltimore, 1932, The Williams & Wilkins Co., vol. 1.

Pitts, R. F.: Physiology of the kidney and body fluids, ed. 2, Chicago, 1968, Year Book Medical Publishers, Inc.

Welt, L. G.: Clinical disorders of hydration and acid-base equilibrium, Boston, 1955, Little, Brown & Co.

SPECIAL

1. Benesch, R., et al.: Proc. Nat. Acad. Sci. **59**:526, 1968.
2. Benesch, R., and Benesch, R. E.: Science **160**:83, 1968.
3. Eaton, J. W., and Brewer, G. J.: Proc. Nat. Acad. Sci. **61**:756, 1968.
4. Meldrum, N. V., and Roughton, F. J. W.: J. Physiol. **75**:15P, 1932.
5. Van Slyke, D. D., and Cullen, G. E.: J. Biol. Chem. **30**:289, 1917.
6. Lotspeich, W. D.: Science **165**:1066, 1967.
7. Pitts, R. F., et al.: J. Clin. Invest. **27**:48, 1948.
8. Smith, H. W.: The physiology of the kidney, New York, 1937, Oxford University Press.
9. Gamble, W., et al.: J. Appl. Physiol. **16**:593, 1961.

CHAPTER 21

OTHER SPECIALIZED BODY FLUIDS AND SECRETIONS

As was discussed in Chapter 15, the total amount of fluid in the human body is approximately 70% of body weight. About 70% of the total body fluid is intracellular, about 20% is interstitial (lymph, etc.), and 7% is in the blood plasma. The remaining 3% is present in the intestinal lumen, cerebrospinal fluid, and other compartments. There are similarities, and yet marked differences, in the chemical composition of these major compartments of body fluids. As shown in Fig. 15-7, the protein content of intracellular fluid is nearly four times that of the blood plasma, which, in turn, is much greater than that of interstitial fluid. Marked differences also exist in the electrolyte composition. Potassium and magnesium are the predominant cations in intracellular fluid, whereas sodium predominates in blood plasma and interstitial fluid. Likewise, phosphate and sulfate are the major anions in intracellular fluid, whereas chloride and bicarbonate predominate in plasma and interstitial fluid. Differences in the concentrations of nonelectrolytes (glucose, urea, etc.) also exist in the different compartments. These general differences are due to differing membrane permeabilities, active transport mechanisms, and metabolic activities in the different areas. There are significant differences in the composition of various body fluids as adaptations to functions, as is true of tissues (Chapter 18).

The chemical composition of blood plasma as a major body fluid was discussed in Chapter 19. The composition of other specialized body fluids will now be considered. Also a consideration of major fluid secretions, those of the gastrointestinal tract, milk, tears, sweat, etc., will be included. Similarities, yet distinctive chemical differences, will be evident, especially in electrolyte and protein content.

It is important to keep in mind, at the outset, that the compositions of the various body fluids and secretions may vary somewhat from time to time depending on environmental, physiologic, and pathologic situations, as discussed in Chapter 15. However, they tend to readjust gradually back to a physiologic norm for that body fluid when average conditions are reestablished—the state that will be emphasized in the following pages.

Considerable progress has been made in determining whether the various body fluids are dialysates (ultrafiltrates) of blood plasma or true secretory products. In accordance with the Donnan equilibrium, an ultrafiltrate has a different distribution from plasma of the electrolytes whereas the nonelectrolytes, e.g., glucose, urea, are in the same concentrations. This is true of lymph, pleural fluid, peritoneal fluid, synovial fluid, and pericardial fluid. In cerebrospinal fluid and in the aqueous humor of the eye, analyses indicate that simple dialysis is supplemented by some selective secretion. For instance, glucose is lower in cerebrospinal fluid than in the blood, even in hyperglycemia, and the other nonelectrolytes vary in their concentrations from those of the blood plasma. The protein content of all these fluids is lower than that of blood plasma, and the ratios of the various proteins differ.

Some fluids, e.g., synovial fluid, vitreous humor, on dilution and acidification yield a fibrous clot, the so-called mucin clot. These clots are polar complexes formed by the basic group of the protein and the carboxyl group of hyaluronic acid. The hyaluronic acid occurs in these fluids as a dissociated complex that can interact with protein or with itself, forming loose complexes of ill-defined nature.

Lymph Since the lymphatic capillaries drain the tissue (interstitial) spaces, the fluid present in both is similar. These fluids resemble blood plasma in composition, the chief difference being that blood plasma contains a higher percentage of protein than does lymph and tissue juice. This was mentioned before as the reason for the colloidal osmotic pressure of plasma being higher than that of tissue fluids, whereas the crystalloidal osmotic pressure is about the same. The albumin:globulin ratio is higher in lymph than in plasma. This is so because albumin, with a smaller molecule, diffuses from plasma into lymph more readily than does globulin although neither diffuses freely. A smaller amount of fibrinogen is present, as well as some prothrombin, and many leukocytes. It clots very slowly. The lymph of the thoracic duct has a higher concentration of protein than that of the lymphatic capillaries but lower than that of plasma; in other respects, during the fasting state, it also tends to resemble plasma. Since it drains the abdominal viscera, however, its composition changes with the state of digestion. After a meal, the fat content rises, since more than half the fat absorbed goes by this route. In fact, the lymph or chyle is decidedly milky if the food contains much fat.

Cerebrospinal fluid. Normal cerebrospinal fluid is a clear, colorless fluid, having a specific gravity of from 1.004 to 1.008. It has an extremely low protein content with no fibrinogen and, as already stated, differs considerably from plasma in its concentration of nonelectrolytes. Its pH, however, is about the same as that of blood, namely, pH 7.35 to 7.40.

Pathologically the fluid may be increased in amount and, as a consequence, may be under great pressure. In many of these conditions, the protein content increases appreciably. It is usually referred to in clinical tests as the globulin fraction, since this seems to be the chief constituent to show an increase. Besides various quantitative and qualitative procedures of the usual type, Lange's colloidal gold test is also employed. The exact nature of the substances responsible for this reaction is unknown, but the substances are probably of a protein nature. The procedure consists in mixing cerebrospinal fluid in progressively increasing dilutions with a colloidal gold solution. Nor-

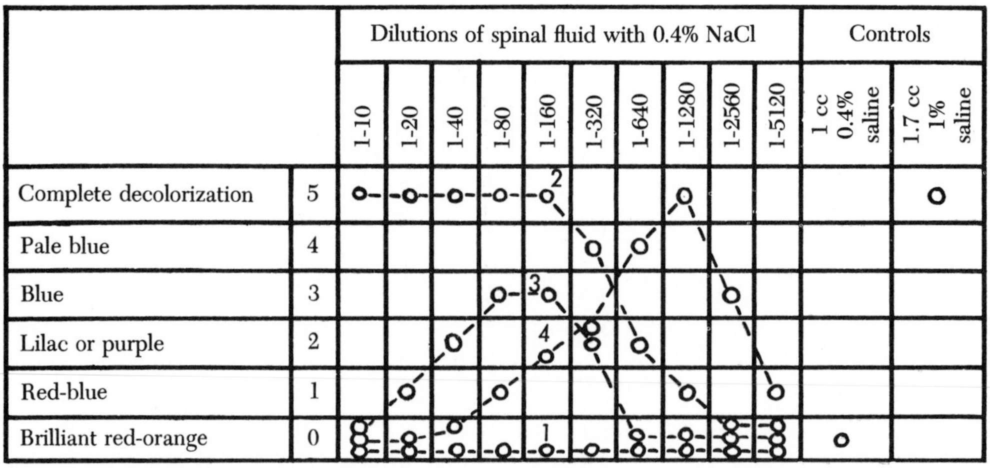

		Dilutions of spinal fluid with 0.4% NaCl										Controls	
		1-10	1-20	1-40	1-80	1-160	1-320	1-640	1-1280	1-2560	1-5120	1 cc 0.4% saline	1.7 cc 1% saline
Complete decolorization	5												
Pale blue	4												
Blue	3												
Lilac or purple	2												
Red-blue	1												
Brilliant red-orange	0												

Fig. 21-1. Types of reactions in the colloidal gold test. *1*, Normal cerebrospinal fluid (no reaction); *2*, paretic type; *3*, syphilitic or tabetic type; *4*, meningitic type. (From Todd, J. C., and Sanford, A. H.: Clinical diagnosis by laboratory methods, Philadelphia, 1944, W. B. Saunders Co.)

mal fluid causes no change in the appearance of this orange red–colored solution. Fluids from certain pathologic conditions produce changes in this color, depending on the particular condition and the dilution. When the results are plotted, they produce curves that are rather characteristic and thus aid in diagnosis. In Fig. 21-1 are shown some of the curves obtained by this test.

Semen. The study of the composition of semen has assumed greater interest in recent years because of its possible bearing on the problem of infertility. Most of the work has been done on seminal plasma, the fluid in which the spermatozoa are suspended. The spermatozoa are constituted largely of nucleoproteins, which differ in various species as regards their isoelectric points, amino acid makeup, etc.

Human seminal plasma is a mixture of the secretions of a variety of glands and tubular epithelial linings. This may account for the great differences in analytic figures reported in the literature. The pH is about the same as that of blood plasma, as is the carbon dioxide content. Chloride and cholesterol are much lower, whereas phosphorus and lactic acid are much higher. The high phosphate is undoubtedly of importance in buffering any acid present in the female secretions. Calcium, urea, and sugar are about twice as high in semen as in blood. It is interesting that the sugar present is fructose rather than glucose. The analyses of proteins are most discordant, both qualitatively and quantitatively, but most of the work by electrophoretic methods indicates that the protein fractions are qualitatively identical with those of blood serum. From these facts it would appear that seminal plasma is not an ultrafiltrate; and, indeed, its derivation from so many sources would lend support to this hypothesis.

Transudates and exudates. The fluid formed by passage through a membrane is called a transudate. A fluid deposited in or on a tissue is known as an exudate, e.g., nasal and vaginal mucus secretions. Actually the difference between a transudate and an exudate is difficult to define. If inflammation exists, the fluid is an exudate. Thus a transudate may be a normal fluid, e.g., lymph, or it may be a pathologic fluid, e.g., some sterile ascitic fluid such as peritoneal. From a physical and chemical standpoint, transudates have a low specific gravity (below 1.015) and a low protein content and clot more slowly than do exudates, if at all. Exudates have a higher specific gravity (above 1.018) and a higher protein content (above 3%) than have transudates and clot rapidly. However, in some rare instances in which these physical and chemical features tend to merge, transudate is difficult to distinguish from exudate.

Electrophoresis is being used to aid in determining the origin of these fluids. Constant and distinct patterns are produced as a result of a different distribution of the proteins; e.g., ascites due to hepatic disease may be differentiated from that due to malignant disease by this procedure.

Synovial fluid. As might be predicted, the characteristic constituent of synovial fluid is mucopolysaccharide formed by the cells of the synovium. Synovial fluid contains about 0.9% hyaluronic acid (p. 174). This gives synovial fluid its high viscosity, which is essential to its function in the lubrication of joints and other moving parts. The protein content of synovial fluid is much lower than that of blood plasma, about 1 gm. per 100 ml. The albumin concentration is relatively higher than in plasma, however, the albumin: globulin ratio being approximately 4:1. Little or no fibrinogen is present. The glucose concentration is variable, lipids are usually present in only trace amounts, and the amounts of nonprotein nitrogenous (NPN) substances are somewhat less than those in plasma. Electrolytes and other easily diffusible substances apparently exchange readily with those in plasma.

Tears. The composition of tears is similar, in general, to that of interstitial fluid. Tears have a lower protein content than plasma, somewhat less than 1 gm. per 100 ml. The lipid content is low. The electrolyte and NPN constituents are present in concentrations similar to those of plasma.

A distinctive constituent of tears is the enzyme lysozyme, which is also found in nasal and bronchial secretions, milk, and egg white. Its function in tears appears to be to protect the cornea from infection by hydrolyzing the mucopeptide of the polysaccharide cell walls of many microorganisms.

Sweat. Sweat is produced continuously by the sweat glands but at a low rate at moderate temperatures so that no visible perspiration is apparent. This *insensible perspiration,* amounting to some 300 to 700 ml. per day, plays an important role in body temperature regulation by cooling by evaporation. At higher temperatures or with vigorous activity the production of sweat is increased and visible perspiration occurs. Values as large as 10 to 14 liters per day have been reported. This can create a severe problem in the maintenance of water and electrolyte balance (p. 439) since the concentrations of the major cations (Na^+, K^+, Mg^{++}, etc.) and anions (Cl^-, HCO_3^-, etc.) are similar to those found in plasma.

The pH of perspiration varies considerably, usually between 5.2 and 7.3. Glucose is present in very small amounts whereas the concentration of urea is four to six times that of blood plasma. Apparently only traces of protein and lipid are present. Significant amounts of several amino acids have been reported in sweat. The amount of lactic acid in sweat is far greater than that in blood or urine, suggesting that some active transport mechanism may be present.

The excessive loss of sodium chloride in perspiration under extremely hot or humid conditions may result in miners' or stokers' cramps or be a factor in heat prostration. Small amounts of salt should be added to the drinking water under such conditions.

SECRETIONS OF THE GASTROINTESTINAL TRACT

The constituents of gastrointestinal secretions are proper enzymes for the hydrolysis of foodstuffs, electrolytes to provide a favorable environment for the activity of the enzymes, and mucus for mechanical lubrication and protection. The digestive action of the various secretions of the intestinal tract was discussed in earlier chapters on the metabolism of carbohydrates,

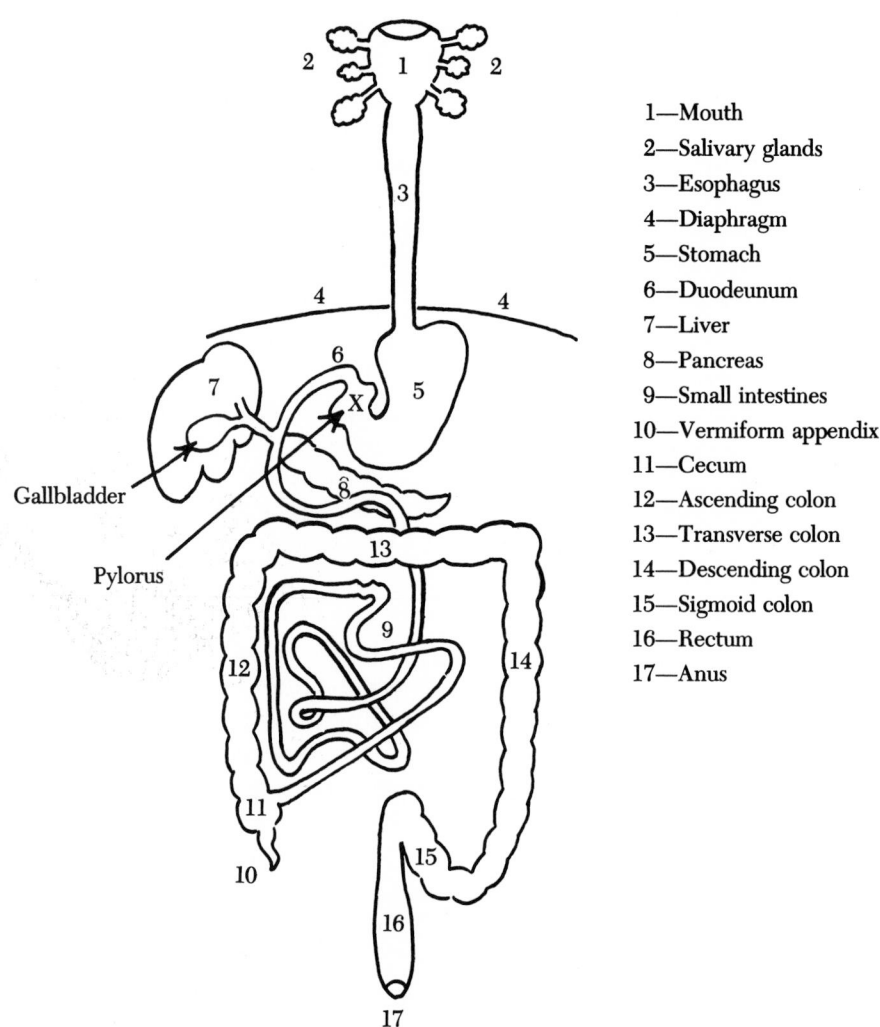

1—Mouth
2—Salivary glands
3—Esophagus
4—Diaphragm
5—Stomach
6—Duodeunum
7—Liver
8—Pancreas
9—Small intestines
10—Vermiform appendix
11—Cecum
12—Ascending colon
13—Transverse colon
14—Descending colon
15—Sigmoid colon
16—Rectum
17—Anus

Gallbladder
Pylorus

Fig. 21-2. Diagram of the alimentary tract. (Modified from Mottram, V. H.: Physiology, New York, 1928, W. W. Norton & Co., Inc.)

lipids, and proteins. Consideration should now be given to the chemical composition of the secretions themselves.

Under normal conditions, the water and electrolytes of the digestive secretions, as will be discussed, are reabsorbed and little is lost by way of the feces. However, in certain diseases in which either excessive vomiting or diarrhea occurs, fluid and electrolyte loss, particularly potassium, may cause serious derangements of acid-base, electrolyte, or water balance. Knowledge of the composition of the fluids lost, therefore, is essential to rational therapy.

The secretions of the gastrointestinal tract are produced by the salivary glands, the epithelial cells of gastrointestinal mucosa, the pancreas, and the liver. The relations of these various structures are shown diagrammatically in Fig. 21-2.

SALIVA

Saliva is the mixed secretion of the parotid, submaxillary, sublingual, and buccal glands. It contains 99.3% to 99.7% water and has a specific gravity of 1.002 to 1.008. Some 1500 ml. are believed to be the approximate daily secretion in man. The secretion of saliva is entirely under the control of the nervous system. A variety of stimuli cause an increased flow by reflex stimulation. This is true whether the stimulus is psychic (sight, smell, or thought of food), mechanical (chewing), or chemical (action of acids, salts, etc. on the taste buds). There seems to be no hormonal control of salivary secretion. There is no secretion by the parotid or sublingual glands during sleep and very little by the submaxillary glands.

Saliva is almost colorless and rather viscid, and if a quantity of saliva in a vessel is exposed to air, the surface becomes covered with an incrustation consisting of calcium carbonate with a small proportion of organic matter. The reaction of the saliva of a given individual is not constant. Resting saliva is slightly acidic, pH 6.4 to 6.9, whereas saliva obtained during active stimulation of the glands is neutral to slightly alkaline, pH 7.0 to 7.3.

The solid constituents of saliva comprise albumins, globulins, mucins, enzymes, urea, uric acid, and inorganic salts. The salivary mucins consist of mucoproteins and mucoids. They yield over 10% carbohydrate on hydrolysis. This includes sialic acid (p. 175). The protein portion appears to be a globulin, rich in threonine, with a low isoelectric point, about 3.5. This material has a relatively high viscosity and a high degree of hydration, which, in part, account for the protective and lubricating functions described below. The inorganic components differ markedly in concentration from those of blood serum, but the NPN constituents (urea, uric acid, NH_4^+ salts) appear to bear some relation to these same constituents in the blood. Amino acids and glucose occur in extremely small amounts in the saliva of healthy individuals (11 to 30 mg. glucose per 100 ml.). Both salivary cholesterol and lipid phosphorus values are very low as compared with blood. The salivary glands, therefore, appear to be quite selective in secretory action.

The chief inorganic ions present are K^+, $PO_4^\equiv$, and Cl^-, with smaller amounts of Na^+, Ca^{++}, and $SO_4^=$. Some of these may combine to form insoluble precipitates. This may be aided by changes in the pH brought about by decomposing food material left between the teeth or by evaporation of carbon dioxide, held in solution in the saliva, as soon as it meets atmospheric conditions. Thus tartar may be formed. This consists chiefly of calcium carbonate and phosphate. Salivary calculi sometimes are formed in the ducts and are similar in composition to tartar (namely, $Ca_3[PO_4]_2$ or $CaCO_3$). It is usually stated that a clump of bacteria or a foreign body establishes a nucleus around which the precipitation of these salts occurs. However, calcium oxalate may be the precipitated salt, which, together with mucin and globulin, may form the calculus. Increased acidity is necessary for oxalate calculus formation.

Functions Saliva has a digestive function due to the enzymes present, but it also has other functions. It moistens and lubricates the food, permitting it to be swallowed easily. Saliva holds the taste-producing substances in solution and so brings them in contact with the taste buds. It dilutes salts, acids, etc., thereby protecting the mucosa and, to some extent, the teeth. It also has a cleansing action on the teeth, gums, and buccal mucosa. It owes its viscous and lubricating property to its content of mucin. This protein is present as an alkaline salt, which is soluble at the pH of saliva but is precipitated on acidification. It is one of the chief buffers present in saliva. A major function of epithelial mucins in general is the protection of the mucosal lining of the mouth, the gastrointestinal tract, and the inner surfaces of other body cavities. They form water-soluble films. In the stomach the acidity probably results in the formation of insoluble gels, and although the mucins are not completely resistant to proteolytic enzymes, the action is slow and thus there is considerable protection. Some authorities maintain that saliva has an excretory function, since certain elements and drugs are found in it after administration. Among these are mercury, lead, and potassium iodide. Any part of these lost in expectoration could be considered excreted, but some of the part swallowed may be reabsorbed. Hence it is difficult to see how these elements can be called a true excretion. The same is true of the traces of urea, uric acid, and ammonium salts ordinarily found in saliva.

The parotid and submaxillary salivary glands have been implicated in the deiodination of the hormone thyroxine and hence in the regulation of the thyroxine level of the blood. The iodine thus released is excreted in the saliva and is reabsorbed in the small intestine for reuse, completing an iodine cycle.

Enzymes The principal enzyme of human saliva is an amylase, *ptyalin*. There are also present a maltase, a catalase, a lipase, a urease, a protease, and numerous others. The saliva of the lower animals is not comparable with that of man, since the same enzymes may not be present. No amylase is found in the saliva of the sheep, goat, dog, or cat. The role of ptyalin in the digestion of food starches was discussed earlier (p. 182).

Pigman and Reid[1] maintain that an important function of salivary amylase is as a cleansing agent for the oral cavity; i.e., it digests starch particles or pastes left in or near the teeth.

GASTRIC JUICE

Gastric juice consists of water (99.4%), hydrochloric acid, mucins, and the enzymes pepsin and lipase. The hydrochloric acid is secreted by the parietal cells and the pepsin by the chief cells. According to Glass and Boyd, the gastric mucous substances comprise (1) the mucoid of the visible gastric mucus, secreted by the surface epithelium, (2) dissolved mucoproteose, a digestion product of the visible gastric mucus, and (3) glandular mucoprotein, secreted by the neck mucous cells of the gastric glands. Glandular mucoprotein is considered by these authors to be the main carrier of the intrinsic factor of human gastric juice (p. 825).

Early experiments on gastric juice. Réaumur (1683–1757) experimented chiefly on a bird, the kite. He caused the bird to swallow perforated metallic containers of food and discovered that the food was dissolved out. The same type of experiment was repeated and extended by Abbé Spallanzani (1729–1799). Using himself as the experimental animal, he swallowed sponges attached to strings, withdrawing them and squeezing out the gastric juice, and demonstrated the solvent power of gastric juice outside the body. He also discovered that it prevents putrefaction, but he failed to recognize the acid character of this fluid. Carminati, at about the same time, declared that it was not acid after fasting but became acid after partaking of food. Werner, in 1800, and others confirmed Carminati's observation, but in 1812, Montegre, who was able to vomit whenever he wished, declared that gastric juice contained no acid, was not a food solvent, and was probably only swallowed saliva. In 1824, an English scientist, Prout, proved that gastric juice is acid and that the acidity is due to hydrochloric acid. This was independently discovered by Tiedemann and Gmelin. It is evident that knowledge of gastric physiology was chaotic at the beginning of the nineteenth century. In fact, Magendie, who was one of the leading physiologists of that time, stated in his textbook that gastric juice was without digestive power outside the body, and the general opinion was that any digestion taking place in the stomach was due to mechanical, rather than to chemical, action. It was an American Army surgeon, Beaumont, who brought order out of chaos in this field. In 1822, an accidental discharge of a shotgun near the upper abdomen of a young French-Canadian, Alexis St. Martin, resulted in a permanent gastric fistula. For many years Beaumont was able to make observations and to obtain human gastric juice through this opening. He confirmed the facts of the acidity of gastric juice and its solvent power and studied the temperature, movements, and appearance of the interior of the stomach. Among his numerous physiologic observations was the fact that the presence of certain foods in the stomach stimulates secretion and that intense emotions inhibit it. He studied the relative digestibility of different common foods; and nutritionists agree that his conclusions were, in the main, thoroughly sound. In fact, there are very few of his observations that have not stood the test of time, and they have become the foundation of modern gastric physiology.

Beaumont maintained that there must be some principle present with digestive activity. In 1836, the actual discovery of pepsin was made by Schwann, who showed that boiled gastric juice, although still acid, has no digestive power. He gave this active principle the name *pepsin*, from a Greek word meaning "digestion."

Later, Heidenhain devised, and more recently Pavlov improved, methods for producing accessory stomachs in experimental animals. These involved detaching a flap from the stomach, everting this in such a way that it formed a pouch with an opening through the body wall and skin of the animal. Blood and nerve supply had to be unharmed, and consequently a flow of pure gastric juice, under the same nervous and vascular conditions as the main stomach, uncontaminated by food, could be obtained. Using such "Pavlov pouch" dogs, scientists have made many contributions to the physiology and biochemistry of gastric juice and digestion.

Control of secretion The secretion of gastric juice is said to be continuous in man, but this fact is not certain. Gastric secretion is intermittent in animals in which experimental conditions are carefully controlled. If it is continuous in man, it is probably at an extremely slow rate.

Stimulatory influences. The factors that increase the flow of gastric juice will be discussed from the following standpoints: cephalic, gastric, and intestinal phases.

Cephalic phase of secretion. Psychic stimuli have long been known to produce an increase in gastric secretion. The thought, smell, or taste of food or even an action related to food (the conditioned reflex of Pavlov, e.g., the ringing of a dinner bell) all reflexly cause an increased flow of gastric juice. The production of low blood sugar in man by the injection of insulin is followed by an increased secretion of gastric juice, rich in both hydrochloric acid and pepsin. The low blood sugar is believed to be the stimulus for the parietal cell, brought about by a central stimulation of the vagus.

Gastric phase. When food is present in the stomach, gastric juice continues to be secreted longer than would be expected from psychic stimuli alone. Beaumont declared that mechanical stimulation of the mucosa would cause secretion. This was denied by Pavlov, but, in 1925, Ivy showed that it is true. Application of a distending force to the antrum produces a flow of gastric juice after some time. Certain foods and, indeed, specific constituents of the foods are powerful stimulants, e.g., meat extractives and products of protein digestion, the polypeptides (so-called proteoses and peptones). These secretagogues probably act indirectly; i.e., in some way they cause the formation of a hormone in the mucosa of the pyloric antrum (which secretes no hydrochloric acid) that is absorbed into the bloodstream and carried back to the gastric glands and stimulates them to secrete. This hormone, discovered by Edkins, is called *gastrin* (p. 457). He found that when the pyloric mucosa is ground up and extracted with peptones, or other of the stimulating substances, a fluid that, on intravenous injection, has a powerful secretory effect is obtained. Histamine has a similar but less powerful secretory effect. However, histamine-free gastrin has been obtained from a hydrochloric acid extract of pyloric mucosa, and further evidence for the existence of gastrin has been furnished.[2] Dilute ethyl alcohol also stimulates gastric secretion and is often used as a test meal. Alcohol may produce its action by liberating histamine. Dragstedt found that removal of the antrum of the stomach causes a profound reduction in the secretion of gastric juice by the rest of the stomach. If the antrum is transplanted to the abdominal wall so that it does not come in contact with food, the same decrease in gastric secretion is observed; but transplantation into the duodenum, as a diverticulum, restores the gastric secretion to its normal value. The factor involved is presumably gastrin. The secretion of gastrin is stopped when the acidity of the antral contents reaches pH 1.5.

Intestinal phase. When the products of gastric digestion leave the stomach and enter the duodenum, they have a stimulating effect on gastric secretion. The mechanism of this action is not at all clear but it is probably due to substances present in the foods. These are absorbed and, perhaps, stimulate nervous structures.

Inhibitory influences. The activity of the gastric glands may be inhibited by depression of the formation of secretagogues. This may occur during the cephalic phase, as well as during the gastric and intestinal phases, whenever digestion or propulsion of food is impaired. Fat has a definite inhibitory effect on gastric secretion. The common belief that greasy foods are "hard to digest" rests on a solid foundation. All three secretory phases, cephalic, gastric, and intestinal, seem to be similarly depressed, as is also the motility of the stomach. The quantity, acidity, and enzymic potency of gastric juice are all reduced, but the mechanism is rather obscure. It has been shown that fat causes the production of an inhibitory hormone, enterogastrone, in the intestinal mucosa. Enterogastrone has been purified sufficiently to be tested on human beings in certain pathologic conditions. It is believed to be a mixture of a secretion inhibitor and a motility inhibitor that can be separated from each other. Another inhibiting effect is that of the hydrochloric acid secreted. This is termed acid inhibition. When the gastric contents reach a certain threshold, perhaps 0.03 N in human beings, secretion begins to slow up, and at about 0.10 N the acid-forming cells are almost completely inhibited. The intestinal phase of gastric secretion is similarly affected. Acid inhibition is probably brought about also by the enterogastrone mechanism (p. 458).

Inhibitors of carbonic anhydrase have also been shown to have a depressant effect on the secretion of gastric hydrochloric acid. This enzyme undoubtedly plays some role in the formation of hydrochloric acid by the gastric mucosa (see below), and its inhibition would be expected to decrease the secretion of the acid.

Gastric emptying. The stomach does not retain its contents until gastric digestion is completed. Soon after food has reached the stomach, some material is ejected into the duodenum, and intestinal digestion and absorption begin. There are a number of factors[2] that influence gastric emptying. The propulsive force lies chiefly in the antrum. Extragastric factors are mainly inhibitory, e.g., enterogastrone. The result is to keep the duodenal lumen within certain limits so that damage to the mucosa of the small intestine is minimized and its functions may be maintained.

Hydrochloric acid The secretion of a strong mineral acid by the gastric mucosa is almost unique from a biologic standpoint. At the instant of secretion by the parietal cells, the hydrochloric acid has a concentration of about 0.17 N and a pH of 0.87. Pure parietal secretion apparently contains no phosphate, neutral chloride, or combined acid. It is practically free of ions other than chloride and is approximately isotonic with blood plasma and body fluids. According to Hollander, it is of remarkably constant composition. How, then, does the parietal cell manufacture such a strong acid from fluids, e.g., blood plasma and tissue fluid, that are neutral or slightly alkaline (pH 7.3)? There have been a number of theories to account for this phenomenon, but only one will be outlined here. It was formulated by Hollander and takes into account the fact that the parietal cells contain a high concentration of carbonic anhydrase, which catalyzes the following reaction:

$$CO_2 + H_2O \rightleftharpoons H_2CO_3 \rightleftharpoons H^+ + HCO_3^-$$

This is a reaction that, as is well known, proceeds in either direction by itself, but the enzyme hastens it enormously. The scheme in Fig. 21-3 illustrates this hypothesis, which may be summarized as follows:

Since uncontaminated parietal secretion is entirely devoid of cations other than hydrogen and of anions other than chloride, the membrane of the intracellular canaliculus is assumed to be permeable only to these ions and to water. On the other hand, the cell membrane separating the parietal cell from the interstitial fluid must be permeable to a variety of ions, including sodium, bicarbonate, chloride, and lactate, and to carbon dioxide and oxygen. The actual formation of hydrogen ions occurs in the canalicular wall by the dissociation of water:

$$H_2O \rightleftharpoons H^+ + OH^-$$

This reaction proceeds to the right because of the selective permeability of the membrane, whereby hydrogen ions are passed into the gastric juice along

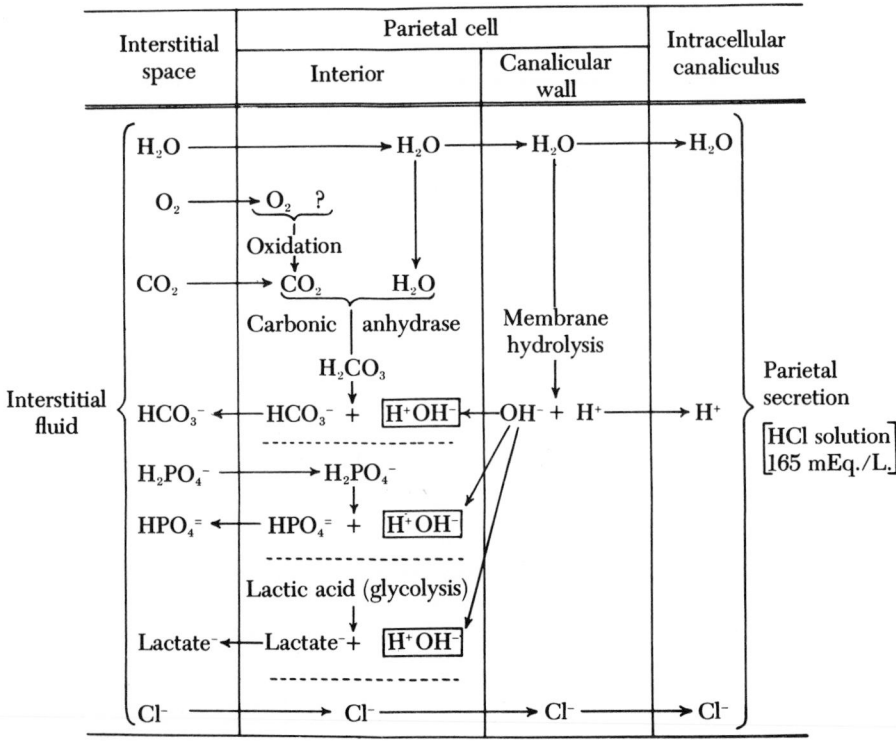

Fig. 21-3. Chemistry of HCl formation by the parietal cell. (Courtesy F. Hollander.)

with chloride ions, and because the hydroxyl ions may immediately be com-bined with the hydrogen ions formed by the dissociation of the carbonic acid. The formation of this acid is accelerated by the carbonic anhydrase in the cytoplasm of the parietal cell. The carbon dioxide, which gives rise to it (on combination with water), is derived from that diffusing into the cell or result-ing from oxidation due to metabolic processes. Phosphates and lactates also yield hydrogen ions to neutralize the hydroxyls formed. If not buffered, this base might well injure the tissue and be the cause of ulcers.

Blood plasma ultimately receives alkaline factors during or after acid gastric secretion. This fact harmonizes with analyses of the blood at such times and also with the fact that usually soon after meals the urine secreted is alkaline. The so-called *alkaline tide* is one of the mechanisms for keeping hydrogen ion concentration of the blood quite constant.

Functions of hydrochloric acid and factors decreasing its strength. The hydrochloric acid of gastric juice initiates the conversion of the zymogen pepsinogen to active pepsin (p. 112) and provides a favorable pH for the activity of pepsin. Besides these most important functions, it serves other purposes. It has some physical action on the proteins, swelling some and making them more easily digested. It has a slight hydrolytic action, perhaps more on the disaccharides than on other foodstuffs, but even in the case of disaccharides, it is not of great significance. Another action of hydrochloric acid is to convert the colloidal ferric hydroxide, found in some foodstuffs, to monomolecularly dispersed ferric ions. Then these and any other ferric ions present are more readily reduced to ferrous ions at pH 5 or lower by ascorbic acid, cysteine, or the sulfhydryl groups of proteins, which may be in the food. The strong acid also has a strong antiseptic action. Alvarez says, "Contrary to popular belief, there is rarely any fermentation in the stomach. Its con-tents are too acid and the food does not remain long enough for gases to be formed. . . ."

Gastric acidity may be decreased by various factors. These include the following:

1. Variations in the rate of parietal secretion (the composition is constant but the rate may vary)
2. Dilution by the secretions of the other cells, especially mucus
3. Dilution and buffering by food
4. Dilution and buffering by the saliva that is swallowed
5. Regurgitation of duodenal fluid and bile
6. Dilution and neutralization by a distinct dilution secretion

The dilution secretion may be formed by the cuboidal cells. It is possibly produced in order to dilute the stomach contents to proper concentration and consistency. The secretion of mucus is undoubtedly of great value. It has a high buffering power and must aid in slowing the acidification of stomach contents.

Enzymes   *Pepsin.* Pepsin, a powerful proteinase, is present in the chief cells as the zymogen pepsinogen. The conversion of pepsinogen to pepsin and its role in the digestion of proteins were discussed earlier (p. 339). Pepsinogen is stable up to pH 9, at which point it is reversibly denatured; but at pH 12 or higher the denaturation of pepsinogen is irreversible. Since pepsin is more sensitive to alkali than is pepsinogen, the fact that pepsin exists in the inactive form can be readily demonstrated (Langley's experiment). A neutral extract of gastric mucosa is divided into two parts. Part A is acidified and can be shown to digest protein; it contains pepsin. Part B is treated with an equal amount of water; it does not digest protein in neutral solution and presumably contains pepsinogen. Both are now made alkaline (pH 8.3); then they are neutralized and acidified to pH 2 or less. Part A now is incapable of digesting protein, whereas part B, the pepsinogen, has been unaffected by the alkali and now has proteolytic power.

About 99% of the pepsinogen elaborated in the gastric mucosa is secreted into the lumen of the stomach. The 1% remaining is secreted into the tissue fluid, then carried in the bloodstream to the kidney, and excreted in the urine. It is called uropepsin. This small amount can be determined in the urine, and, since the rate of excretion of uropepsin varies directly with the rate of secretion of pepsinogen into the stomach, this determination may become a useful method in clinical studies of gastric secretion.[3]

Estimation of pepsin. There are a number of methods for measuring the amount of pepsin in gastric contents. The most accurate methods are not adapted to clinical use, and great accuracy is not needed. The classic procedure is that of Mett. In this method, small glass tubes are filled with egg albumin and then boiled to coagulate the protein. They are then placed in definite amounts of the gastric fluid for a number of hours, and the length of the columns of digested protein, which can easily be seen because the columns become transparent, is measured in millimeters. A simple calculation gives the amount of pepsin. A quicker and easier method is based on the milk-clotting power of pepsin. Cow's milk diluted with a buffer of pH 5 is used as a substrate. The gastric fluid is diluted in a definite way and the smallest amount of this that will clot 10 ml. of buffered milk in 10 minutes is determined. The calculation of the number of clinical units present is simple. In patients having peptic ulcers there is usually a high pepsin value, whereas in pernicious anemia, cirrhosis of the liver, and various chronic gastric ailments a low pepsin content is found. According to Gray, pepsinogen may be absorbed into the bloodstream and is excreted as uropepsin in the urine. The amount of uropepsin parallels gastric peptic activity.

Rennin. Some textbooks include rennin, another proteolytic enzyme, among the gastric enzymes, but this is incorrect. Rennin occurs in the fourth stomach of the calf and probably of other young ruminants. Its action is to clot milk. This it does by a slight digestive action on casein as described later (p. 707).

Gastric lipase. The lipase of gastric juice is less important than the pancreatic lipase because it is present in very small amounts. It is probably secreted in the active form, not as a zymogen, and is a tributyrase, having almost no action on fats containing long-chain fatty acids.[4] The optimum pH is about 7.8 but in the presence of calcium ions is shifted to the acid side. A further discussion of gastric lipase is given on p. 293.

Gastric analysis. The clinical procedures for testing various gastric functions include the administration of a test meal or of alcohol or the injection of histamine or insulin and the withdrawal by a stomach tube of the gastric contents for analysis. The routine use of test meals is practically abandoned. Fifty milliliters of 7% ethyl alcohol are sometimes administered on an empty stomach and removed either after 1 hour or at regular intervals. Histamine given subcutaneously is a powerful gastric secretory stimulant. However, histamine produces other physiologic effects that may be highly undesirable and an invariably effective dose of histamine has heretofore not been advisable. To overcome this difficulty, the augmented histamine test has been devised. An antihistaminic is first given. This antagonizes all histamine effects save that on gastric secretion. Then a large dose of histamine is administered, and its effect on gastric secretion observed. Recently, the drug betazole hydrochloride has been introduced as a substitute for histamine. It has minimal side effects. The stimulating action of insulin apparently depends upon its hypoglycemic effect. A low blood sugar stimulates the vagus centers in the brain, resulting in increased gastric secretion. The value of the insulin test is chiefly to ascertain the effectiveness of vagotomy in patients with ulcer.

Qualitative tests include those for butyric acid, lactic acid, occult blood, bile, and perhaps trypsin. The presence of the first two acids would point to yeasts or other microorganisms in the gastric secretions and, hence, a lack of free hydrochloric acid. If blood is present, ulcers, hemorrhages, or other pathologic states would be indicated. In testing for blood, a meatless test meal is imperative. Either bile or trypsin is evidence of regurgitation of intestinal contents; this is a frequent normal occurrence. A microscopic examination is also usually made.

The quantitative procedures are gradually being changed to conform to modern chemical ideas. The total acidity comprises the acidity contributed by hydrochloric acid, organic acids, and acid salts, neutralized or buffered by various constituents of the gastric juice and the foodstuffs. With the use of various indicators, a rough idea of the relative amounts of these fractions may be obtained. This is not usually done today. From a clinical standpoint determination of pH or titration of free acid is probably sufficient.

The clinician usually wishes to ascertain whether there is hyperacidity or hypoacidity, high or low pepsin, large or small volume secreted, as well as whether abnormal constituents are present. The absence of hydrochloric acid is termed *achlorhydria*. Achlorhydria may occur in pernicious anemia, in gastric carcinoma, and in a number of other conditions. If hydrochloric acid is not entirely absent but is below normal, the condition is called hypoacidity. Hypoacidity frequently accompanies gastric carcinoma, as well as many gastrointestinal ailments, e.g., gastritis and constipation, secondary anemia, chronic debilitative diseases. Many normal pregnant women have low gastric acidities. Of the conditions in which the acidity is elevated (hyperacidity), perhaps the most noteworthy are duodenal ulcer and gallbladder disease. It should be emphasized that the acidity can never exceed a certain value (pH 0.87) since the parietal cells secrete a fluid of constant composition.

Gastric acidity may be determined without intubation by means of a cation exchange resin treated with quinine, or with a dye, such as azure-A. The acid (H^+) of the gastric juice replaces the quinine that is excreted in the urine and may be determined photometrically. With appropriate techniques, the procedure may be made semiquantitative and is useful for some clinical purposes.

PANCREATIC JUICE

The pancreatic duct joins with the common bile duct to form the ampulla of Vater; thus pancreatic juice and the bile empty into the duodenum at the same point. The total volume of pancreatic juice secreted daily in man has been estimated at about 500 ml., but this is little more than a guess. The solids present amount to about 1.3% to 1.4%; the specific gravity is about 1.007; and the fluid is alkaline, with a pH of about 8. The alkalinity is due to sodium bicarbonate. Since carbonic anhydrase is present in pancreatic tissue and since the administration of an inhibitor of this enzyme has been shown to decrease the bicarbonate content of pancreatic juice, most of the bicarbonate ion is probably produced according to the following reactions:

$$CO_2 + H_2O \xrightarrow[\text{anhydrase}]{\text{Carbonic}} H_2CO_3 \rightarrow H^+ + HCO_3^-$$

Enzymes. Pancreatic juice, as secreted, contains a number of powerful digestive enzymes, some in their inactive, zymogen forms. The list includes trypsinogen, chymotrypsinogen, elastase (as zymogen), two carboxypeptidases, a lipase (steapsinogen), an amylase (amylopsin), two polynucleotidases (ribonuclease, deoxyribonuclease), lactase, sucrase, possibly a maltase, several esterases, and an alkaline phosphatase. The properties and specific digestive functions of each of these enzymes have been discussed earlier (Chapters 7, 9, 12, 13, and 14).

Control of secretion. The secretion of pancreatic juice is controlled by two principal mechanisms, hormonal and nervous by way of the vagus nerve. Two hormones, secretin (p. 457) and pancreozymin (p. 457), stimulate the secretion of pancreatic juice. Acid chyme discharged from the stomach into the duodenum plays a role in causing the pancreas to begin its secretory activity. Bayliss and Starling found that a hydrochloric extract of intestinal mucosa, upon intravenous injection, accelerates pancreatic secretion. They claimed that an inactive substance in the mucosa is converted to an active one by hydrochloric acid. The first was termed *prosecretin*, and the second, *secretin*, but secretin is now known to occur in the mucosa as such and in some way be liberated by the action of the hydrochloric acid of the chyme. It is absorbed into the circulation and carried to the pancreas, where it stimulates the secretion of pancreatic juice, which is rich in bicarbonate but not in enzymes. Pancreozymin causes a stimulation of the secretion of enzymes by the pancreas. It is found only in the upper intestinal mucosa, whereas secretin is found also in the gastric mucosa.

Pancreatic function test. The fact that secretin stimulates the flow of pancreatic juice has been made use of in a test of external pancreatic function. The preparations now available are free of histamine, cholecystokinin, and many other contaminants but are really mixtures of secretin and pancreozymin. A double-lumen tube, with sections of unequal length, is passed so that the longer end reaches the third portion of the duodenum and the shorter end remains in the stomach. Continuous aspiration with negative pressure of 20 to 30 mm. of mercury prevents the overflow of gastric juice into the duodenum and sucks out both gastric juice and duodenal contents into separate containers. After a basal flow has been obtained, the secretin is injected intravenously and the volume of flow and bicarbonate concentration are measured. Sometimes the enzymes are also determined.

Shortly after the injection of secretin, there occurs an outpouring of pancreatic juice. The duodenal fluid therefore loses its biliary color under normal conditions; but if this bile color remains, a nonfunctioning gallbladder is indicated. The total volume varies normally from 135 to 250 ml. in 1 hour, and the bicarbonate, from 90 to 130 mEq.

The test is of value in detecting disease of the pancreas when all other tests have failed. In pancreatitis with extensive destruction of parenchymal structures, there is usually a diminution in the volume of pancreatic juice and bicarbonate output. In less severe pancreatitis about half the cases show these effects. The influence on the enzymes has not been consistent enough to justify the determination of the enzymes. In pancreatic malignancy there is a lowering of the volume response, with less change in the bicarbonate.

INTESTINAL JUICE—SUCCUS ENTERICUS

The secretion of the intestinal mucosa is at least partly under the control of the nervous system. Mechanical stimuli reflexly cause a flow of this fluid. Secretin probably exerts a hormonal effect for this secretion as well as for pancreatic secretion and for bile secretion. There is also a specific hormone, enterocrinin[9] (p. 458), secreted by the intestinal mucosa, that stimulates the mucosal glands. Both the volume of fluid and the content of enzymes are increased by enterocrinin. Intestinal juice is not as definite an entity as gastric or pancreatic juice, because it varies at different levels of the intestinal tract and because its composition is not nearly as constant at different periods. Moreover, there seem to be two different types of secretion; one has digestive powers and the other, secreted periodically at about 2-hour intervals, contains mucoprotein and excretory products. Intestinal juice is usually quite turbid because of the presence of leukocytes, epithelial cells, and mucus. The total solids amount to about 1.5%, about half of which is sodium chloride, sodium bicarbonate, and other inorganic salts. It has a pH of about 8.3. The pH of intestinal contents, on the other hand, is slightly acidic. The acid chyme from the stomach is partially neutralized by the alkaline pancreatic juice, bile, and succus entericus so that the pH of the lower duodenal contents in man ranges from 4.5 to 5.1. When the ileum is reached, its contents range in pH from 5.9 to 6.5.

Grisolia and Schloerb[5] believe, however, on the basis of theoretic as well as experimental evidence, that the base (HCO$_3^-$, etc.) content of the pancreatic juice, bile, and succus entericus is insufficient to neutralize gastric juice to this degree. They suggest that intestinal exchange and transfer are responsible for the major portion of gastric acid neutralization.

The organic material of intestinal juice comprises mucoprotein and a number of different enzymes. Some of these enzymes are undoubtedly not actually secreted but are present in the leukocytes and epithelial cells, which disintegrate and liberate their enzymes. Moreover, since intestinal juice is difficult to obtain most studies have been on extracts of the mucosa. Hence we are not sure whether all the enzymes ascribed to intestinal juice are actually secreted or are in the mucosa or in desquamated epithelial cells, where they do their work as intracellular enzymes.

Enzymes. An important carbohydrase present in the intestinal mucosa of the hog, and presumably in that of other mammals, is oligo-1,6-glucosidase. This splits the α-1 bonds of the products of digestion of amylopectin, resulting chiefly in maltose.

The saccharidases maltase, sucrase (or invertase), and lactase split the disaccharides maltose, sucrose, and lactose, respectively, into their constituent monosaccharides. These enzymes are almost entirely intracellular.[6] Enterokinase is the enzyme that transforms trypsinogen to trypsin. A number of peptidases are present in the intestinal mucosa cells and/or their secretion. These include a group of *aminopeptidases* and a group of *dipeptidases.*

A lipase, which is activated by bile salts, is reported to be present in the succus entericus of several species of animals, but it is apparently not of high activity. An amylase also occurs in the intestinal juice.

Three enzymes that decompose nucleic acid to its constituents are present here, also. They are the nucleases, phosphatases, and nucleosidases. The nucleases attack nucleic acids, releasing the mononucleotides in each (Chapter 15). The phosphatases, which are not specific for nucleotides, hydrolyze them to phosphoric acid and purine or pyrimidine nucleosides. The nucleosidases complete the digestion of the nucleosides to purines, pyrimidines, and sugar.

BILE

The bile is secreted, probably continuously, by the liver and passes into the hepatic ducts and into the common duct. It fills the gallbladder, via the cystic duct, and tends to distend all ducts and the gallbladder between digestive periods. The bladder wall, during these intervals, absorbs water from the bile contained in it, thus producing a highly concentrated bladder bile and making more space for the liver secretion. It also absorbs bicarbonate, chloride, and sodium ions and perhaps other inorganic ions. Although bladder bile by this process is four or more times as concentrated as hepatic bile, both have the same osmotic effect as that of blood serum. Gallbladder bile becomes slightly acid in the process of concentration. The other constituents of bile do not appear to be absorbed to any appreciable extent by the normal gallbladder.

The hepatic secretion is not under nervous control. It can be accelerated by various substances; secretin and bile salts are notable examples, bile salts being by far the more effective. These are usually referred to as cholagogues.

It has been suggested, however, that they be termed *choleretics*, the word cholagogue being reserved for substances that stimulate the gallbladder to contract and thus bring about the flow of bile into the duodenum. The gallbladder is under nervous, hormonal, and food control. Ordinarily the sphincter at the junction of the common duct and the duodenum is closed. The ducts are kept filled with bile by hepatic secretion, and upon increase of pressure the bile passes into the gallbladder. Although the gallbladder wall is very thin and has few muscle fibers, it probably does contract feebly and perhaps the sphincter of Oddi relaxes simultaneously. There seems to be a nervous mechanism for controlling this phenomenon, but just how it acts is not clear. With regard to hormonal control, Ivy obtained an acid extract of intestinal mucosa that on intravenous injection causes contraction of the gallbladder. The hormone involved is not secretin but is apparently similar to it. It has been named *cholecystokinin* (p. 457). The two hormones can be separated by absolute alcohol extraction; secretin is thereby removed. Even more effective than the hormone as a stimulus for the discharge of bile is fatty food. Protein and carbohydrate have little effect, but emulsified fats like cream and egg yolk call forth a profuse discharge of bile. No explanation for this has been given.

Composition Human bile as secreted by the liver is clear, golden or brownish yellow in color, but sometimes olive green. It has a bitter taste and is a viscid slimy fluid. It is alkaline, with a pH of from 7.8 to 8.6, but bladder bile may be even as acid as pH 6.5. The daily volume has been variously estimated at from 500 to 1100 ml. In a case of biliary fistula there was an output of 525 ml. in 24 hours. Bile contains the following characteristic substances: bile pigments, bile salts, and cholesterol. There are, in addition, variable quantities of proteins, lecithin, inorganic salts, and urea. The proteins include mucin, the usual serum proteins, and a unique protein that migrates electrophoretically more rapidly than the blood proteins. Hepatic bile contains about 2.5% to 3.5% solid matter, and bladder bile as much as 17%. The high solid content of the latter is due to the absorption of water; at the same time small quantities of inorganic salts are absorbed. The net result is a fluid with about the same osmotic properties and pH. The specific gravity of the bile in the gallbladder may be as high as 1.040, whereas bile secreted by the liver has a specific gravity of about 1.010.

In Table 21-1 is given the range of various constituents in bile as found by several investigators.

Bile pigments. The bile pigments, bilirubin and biliverdin, give bile its color and are excretory products. Bilirubin predominates. Oxidation and reduction produce a series of varicolored compounds, some of which have received definite names.

$$\underset{\text{(brown)}}{\text{Urobilin}} \xleftarrow{-\text{H}_2} \underset{\text{(colorless)}}{\text{Urobilinogen}} \xleftarrow{+4\text{H}_2} \underset{\text{(red)}}{\text{Bilirubin}} \xleftarrow{+\text{H}_2} \underset{\text{(green)}}{\text{Biliverdin}} \xrightarrow{-\text{H}_2} \text{(blue, yellow, etc.)}$$

The Gmelin test is based on this color reaction. Concentrated nitric acid, if overlaid with urine or other fluid that may contain bile pigments, oxidizes them at the junction of the two fluids, producing a rainbow of colors as a positive reaction.

Table 21-1. Composition of bile

Constituent	Bladder bile (percent)	Liver bile (percent)
Water	82.3–89.8	96.5–97.5
Solids	10.2–17.7	2.5–3.5
Bile salts	5.7–10.8	0.9–1.8
Mucus and pigments	1.5–3.0	0.4–0.5
Cholesterol and other lipids	0.5–4.7	0.2–0.4
Inorganic salts	0.6–1.1	0.7–0.8

The bile pigments are derived from the heme of hemoglobin from worn-out red blood cells and from other heme proteins, e.g., myoglobin, catalase, cytochromes, peroxidase, and others. The hemoglobin escapes into the plasma and is captured by *haptoglobin*, a colorless α_2-globulin. Each molecule of haptoglobin binds two hemoglobin molecules stoichiometrically. This complex is removed from the bloodstream by the reticuloendothelial system. The transformation of heme to the bile pigments occurs in the reticuloendothelial cells. There are cells of the reticuloendothelial system in the liver, the von Kupffer cells, and consequently a portion of bilirubin originates in the liver itself. Some bile pigment, however, is produced by the reticuloendothelial cells in other parts of the body, whence it is transported to the liver for excretion. Since the bile pigment is water insoluble, it is carried in the plasma in combination with plasma proteins. Involved in the formation of bile pigment are (1) denaturation of the globin of hemoglobin, (2) splitting off of the denatured globin, (3) oxidation and loss of the α-methene carbon atom as carbon monoxide[7] and opening of the tetrapyrrole ring at this point, and (4) removal of iron (Fig. 21-4). The iron removed is utilized for the manufacture of new heme or stored temporarily as ferritin.

Biliverdin is next reduced to bilirubin by the addition of two hydrogen atoms at the double bond attached to the central γ-methene group.

The conversion of heme to bilirubin apparently is enzymatic, involving a mixed-function oxygenase (p. 242) present in liver microsomes.[8] The oxygenase system has an absolute requirement for $NADPH_2$ and molecular oxygen. The system is inhibited by carbon monoxide, as might be expected. The hepatic microsomal heme oxygenase system also converts other hemoproteins to bilirubin. The latter hemoproteins may be responsible for the so-called early peak in isotopically labeled bile pigments found after the administration of labeled precursors of heme synthesis.[8] Blood hemoglobin is responsible for the late peak, appearing some 120 days after the labeled precursors are given.

The free bilirubin thus formed in the reticuloendothelial system from hemoglobin and other hemoproteins is transported to the liver in the plasma loosely associated with plasma albumin. In the liver, the bilirubin is conjugated with glucuronic acid to form bilirubin diglucuronide, which is water

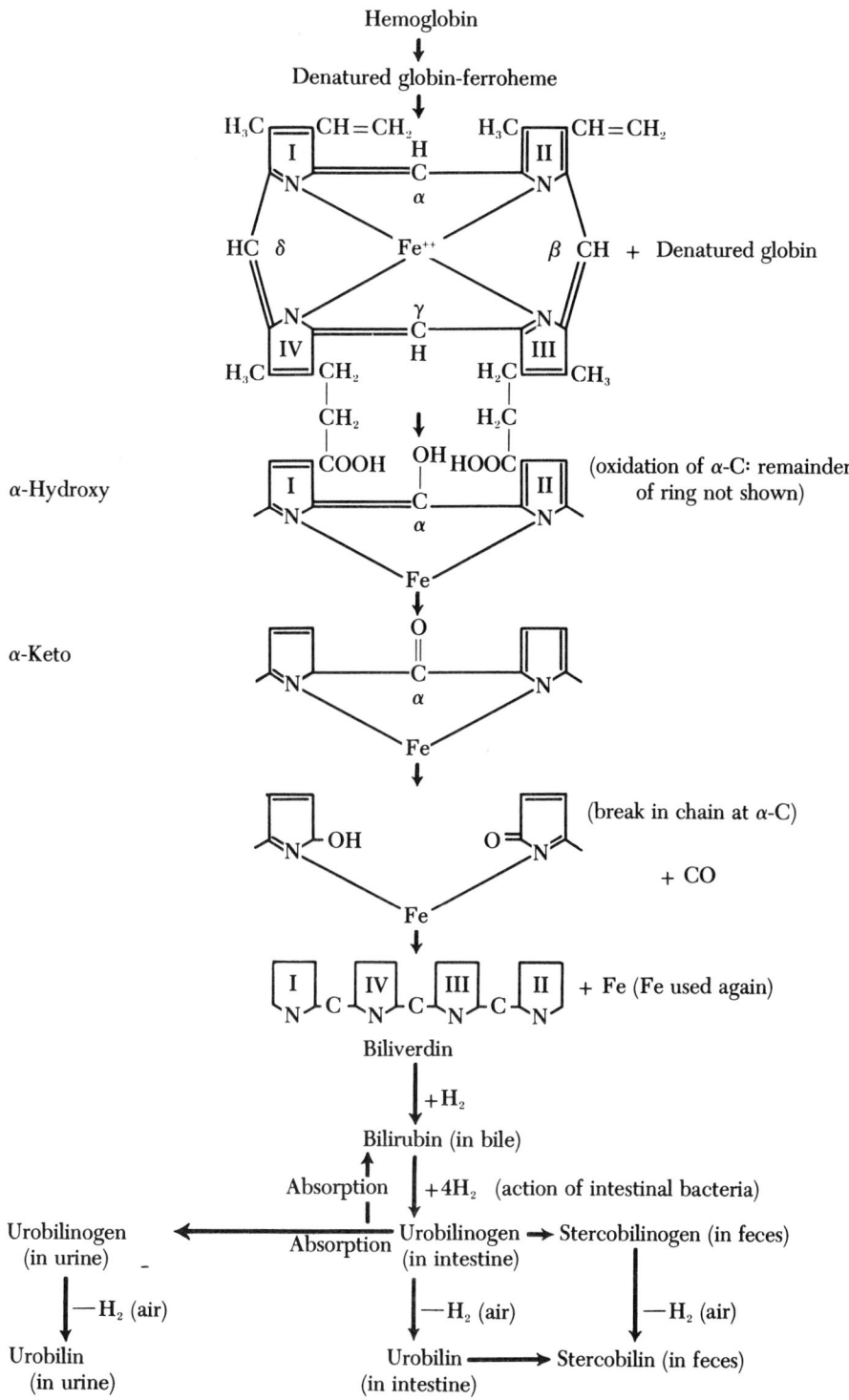

Fig. 21-4. Origin of bile pigments. The diagrammatic structure for biliverdin shown above does not include the various side groups of the pyrrole rings. (Modified from Granick, S., and Gilder, H.: Advances Enzym. **7**:305, 1947.)

soluble and is therefore readily excreted via the bile into the intestine and eliminated in the feces. The conjugation of bilirubin with glucuronic acid involves the formation of a diester with the two propionic acid groups of bilirubin and the carbon-1 hydroxyl groups of two moles of glucuronic acid. The reaction is catalyzed by the hepatic microsomal enzyme, bilirubin-UDP-glucuronyl transferase.

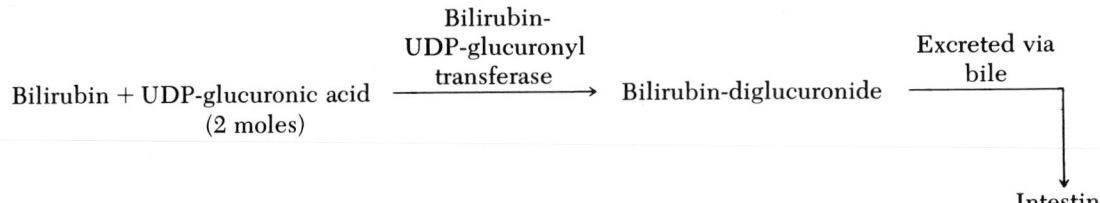

A small amount of bilirubin is conjugated with sulfate, as active sulfate (3'-phosphoadenosine-5'-phosphosulfate, or PAPS, p. 385) and involving an appropriate enzyme (sulfokinase). The sulfate ester of bilirubin is also water soluble and is excreted in the bile.

After the bile passes into the duodenum, the glucuronic acid (and sulfate) groups are hydrolyzed off and the bilirubin is reduced by the bacterial flora of the intestine. The product is the colorless urobilinogen (mesobilinogen), in which four hydrogens are attached at the two double bonds of the chain and four more are used to convert the two vinyl groups to ethyl groups. Urobilinogen, on contact with air, is oxidized to urobilin (mesobilin). Another alleged reduction product is stercobilinogen, which is oxidized to stercobilin. However, current evidence indicates that these are identical with urobilinogen and urobilin, respectively. The two latter compounds are excreted in the feces. Indeed, this is the fate of most of the urobilinogen. Amounts up to 240 mg. of urobilinogen per day are excreted in the feces. Some of the urobilinogen is absorbed by way of the portal circulation and is mostly eliminated again by way of the bile, after reconversion to bilirubin, but a small amount of it (4 mg. or less) is excreted unchanged by the kidneys. In the urine this urobilinogen may be reoxidized, on standing, to urobilin. These reactions are shown schematically in Fig. 21-4.

An elevation of the amount of bilirubin in the plasma may occur in several types of jaundice. There are three principal types, based on the clinical cause:

1. *Hemolytic,* in which excessive erythrocyte destruction results in the formation of bilirubin in amounts exceeding the conjugating ability of the liver and hence its excretion in the bile

   This type of jaundice is sometimes termed nonobstructive or retention jaundice. Free bilirubin increases in the plasma as a result.

2. *Obstructive,* due to the partial or complete blocking of the bile ducts, either inside or outside the liver

   This type is also referred to as hepatic or regurgitative jaundice. Conjugated bilirubin is prevented from being excreted into the intestine and consequently appears in increased amounts in the plasma.

3. *Hepatocellular,* in which damage to the liver by toxins, poisons, cardiac failure, or acute or chronic disease impairs the liver's capacity to conjugate circulating bilirubin and hence excrete it

Enlargement of the liver, as in acute hepatitis, may also cause an internal bile duct obstruction, resulting in an increase in both unconjugated and conjugated bilirubin in the plasma of the patient. This type of jaundice may also occur in Wilson's disease.

An elevation of serum bilirubin may also be found in patients in whom there is a hereditary deficiency of the hepatic enzyme, bilirubin-UDP-glucuronyl transferase, required for the conjugation of bilirubin[9] (Gilbert's disease).

Likewise, hyperbilirubinemia is frequently encountered in newborn children, especially when premature. This may develop into the serious condition kernicterus if the serum bilirubin levels become sufficiently high. Brain damage and neurologic disorders, and often death, may ensue. The elevation in serum bilirubin in this condition is due to the unconjugated (water-insoluble) form. Crystals of free bilirubin may be deposited in the brain. The accumulation of bilirubin apparently is caused by a relative deficiency of the conjugating enzyme in the liver. Bilirubin-UDP-glucuronyl transferase does not appear to be formed in the liver in sufficient amounts until about the normal time of birth. Hence the problem is particularly acute in the premature infant. Immaturity of the blood-brain barrier may also be a factor. The level of serum bilirubin decreases to normal values soon after birth as the synthesis of the bilirubin-conjugating enzyme increases in the liver.

Interesting recent studies indicate that the hyperbilirubinemia of the premature can be reduced by exposing the infant to fluorescent light—a so-called "bilirubin reduction lamp." Apparently the lamp rays degrade bilirubin to products, possibly di- and monopyrrole derivatives,[10] that are less toxic and can be metabolized or excreted by the infant.

The excretion or nonexcretion of bile pigments in different types of jaundice, as well as the mechanism of the direct and indirect *van den Bergh tests* for serum bilirubin, are explained as follows[11]: Free bilirubin is practically insoluble in water at a pH below 8. It is conjugated in the liver microsomes with glucuronic acid. The glucuronide is soluble in aqueous solutions and probably circulates in loose combination with a mucoprotein. A small amount may be conjugated with sulfate. The glucuronide and sulfate, being water soluble, give the *direct* van den Bergh test, whereas the free pigment must be dissolved in alcohol first and then is responsible for the *indirect* test. The conjugated water-soluble forms are readily excreted into the bile by the liver. They are also excreted by the kidneys if present in the blood. This occurs when the bile ducts are obstructed and the bile is dammed back into the liver and consequently into the circulation. Hence, in obstructive jaundice, bilirubin glucuronide is found in the plasma (direct van den Bergh reaction) and in the urine. If for any reason there is an accumulation of free bilirubin, this insoluble molecule is not eliminated by the kidneys but circulates in the blood, attached to blood proteins, chiefly albumin. Such "free" bilirubin in the plasma gives an indirect van den Bergh reaction.

In hemolytic jaundice there is an overproduction of bilirubin, in amounts greater than the ability of the liver to conjugate it. Much of this free bilirubin circulates in the blood but is not excreted by the kidney. There are also thrown into the intestine increased amounts of bilirubin glucuronide. This is reduced to urobilinogen in the normal way but in abnormally large amounts. Therefore, urobilinogen is increasingly absorbed and excreted in the urine.

There are other types of jaundice in which primarily some damage to the liver occurs. This damage may be caused by toxic agents, e.g., chloroform or arsphenamine, or by some acute or chronic liver disease. In such conditions there is not necessarily an increase in the production of bilirubin, but the damaged or incapacitated hepatic cells cannot conjugate the bilirubin or excrete it in the bile. Hence a considerable amount circulates free. No bilirubin appears in the urine, but urobilinogen does because the urobilinogen, absorbed from the intestinal tract, cannot be reeliminated via the bile by the poorly functioning liver. Excellent reviews of the metabolism of bilirubin have appeared recently.[12]

Bile salts. The bile salts are chiefly the salts of *glycocholic* and *taurocholic* acids. These acids are combinations of cholic acid with glycine and taurine, respectively, joined together by means of peptide linkages. The hydrolysis of each of these bile acids is as follows:

$$C_{23} \cdot H_{39} \cdot O_3 \cdot CO \cdot NH \cdot CH_2 \cdot COOH + H_2O \rightarrow C_{23} \cdot H_{39}O_3 \cdot COOH + NH_2 \cdot CH_2COOH$$

Glycocholic acid   **Cholic acid**   **Glycine**

$$C_{23} \cdot H_{39} \cdot O_3 \cdot CO \cdot NH \cdot CH_2 \cdot CH_2 \cdot SO_2 \cdot OH + H_2O \rightarrow C_{23} \cdot H_{39} \cdot O_3 \cdot COOH + \begin{array}{c} H_2 \cdot C \cdot SO_2 \cdot OH \\ | \\ H_2 \cdot C \cdot NH_2 \end{array}$$

Taurocholic acid   **Cholic acid**   **Taurine**

The structural relations of taurine to both cysteine and methionine are very close. Experiments in which radioactive sulfur, ^{35}S, was introduced in trace amounts into methionine showed that when this amino acid is fed to dogs its sulfur is used in part to form taurine. Cysteine, also, is converted to taurine (p. 381). Different species vary in the proportions and even in the nature of the bile salts found in their bile. In man, besides cholic acid, linked to taurine and glycine, there are also small amounts of chenodeoxycholic, deoxycholic, and lithocholic acids. Cholic acid is formed from cholesterol in the liver. The formulas show how closely they are related. The steps involved in the conversion of cholesterol to cholic acid are first the successive oxidation of rings B and C to form hydroxyl groups in the 7- and 12-positions. This is followed by the oxidation of one of the terminal methyl groups of the side chain to a carboxyl group, which is converted to its coenzyme-A (CoA) derivative, followed by α,β-dehydrogenation, addition of water, and again dehydrogenation to form a β-carbonyl group. Propionyl-CoA is finally split off the side chain, leaving cholyl-CoA. This derivative of cholic acid plus taurine or glycine forms taurocholic or glycocholic acid, respectively. Note that the three hydroxyl groups of cholic acid are in the α-position (dotted bond lines) whereas the hydroxyl group of cholesterol is in a β-position (solid bond line).

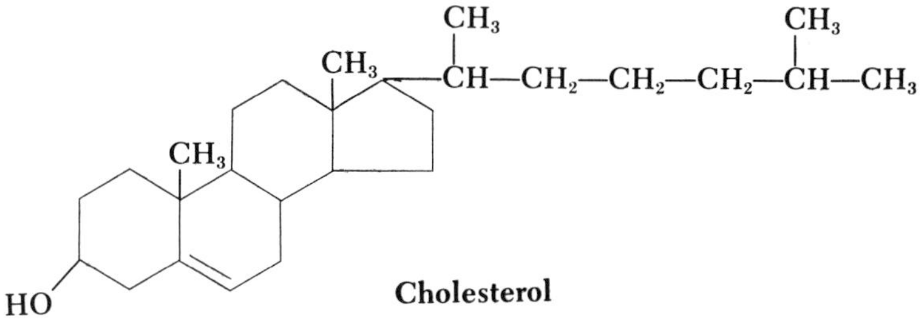

Cholesterol

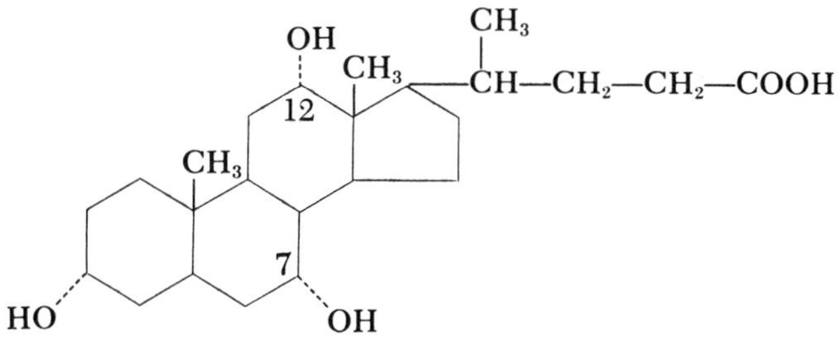

Cholic acid

Deoxycholic acid and chenodeoxycholic acid each have one less hydroxyl, and lithocholic acid has no hydroxyl at the 7- and 12-positions.

Functions. The bile salts are not excretory products. Some 5 to 15 gm. are formed in the liver daily in man and are the most useful consitutents of bile. In human bile, glycocholate predominates over taurocholate in a ratio of about 3:1. After secretion into the intestinal tract, the bile salts are absorbed almost completely and are carried by the portal blood back to the liver for resecretion. Perhaps 10% may be destroyed by bacterial action in the intestine or be lost by excretion. Several of their functions have been mentioned previously. They may be summed up as follows:

1. Bile salts accelerate the action of pancreatic lipase. This nonspecific activation transforms a relatively weak enzyme into a quite powerful one.
2. Because of their power of lowering surface tension, they aid in the emulsification of fats and tend to stabilize such emulsions. In fact, the bile salts, fatty acids, and lower glycerides are said to form one of the best emulsifying mediums for fats. This may permit the absorption of some emulsified fat and leads to the presentation of a greater amount of surface of the remainder to the lipolytic enzyme, and thus further aids its action.
3. They aid in the absorption of the fat-soluble vitamins. This is particularly important in the case of vitamin K. In the surgery of patients having biliary disease, the administeration of bile salts by mouth is necessary to aid in the absorption of vitamin K, unless the vitamin is given parenterally (p. 790).
4. It is the bile salts that keep cholesterol in solution.
5. They have great choleretic action. Thus the liver is stimulated to secrete bile as long as bile salts are absorbed. This secretion apparently

687

continues during fat digestion and the absorption of the bile salt–fatty acid complex, i.e., exactly during the period necessary for such secretion.

6. They stimulate intestinal motility.

The bile salts have an extremely bitter taste.

Cholesterol. The bile seems to be the chief vehicle for the excretion of excess cholesterol. The sources of biliary cholesterol are (1) synthesis by the liver, (2) decomposition of red blood cells, and (3) dietary cholesterol. Reabsorption of some of the cholesterol may occur but not after it has been reduced. Reduction occurs by bacterial action, and the product is *coprosterol*, the sterol of the feces. Since cholesterol is not a very soluble substance, it is not surprisingly found to precipitate out of solution from bile and form gallstones.

Functions of bile. To sum up the functions of bile, we may say that (1) it tends to neutralize the acid chyme, thus providing a more favorable hydrogen ion concentration for the enzymes secreted by the pancreas and the intestinal mucosa; (2) it aids in fat digestion in several ways; (3) it promotes the absorption of fat, the products of fat digestion, other lipids, and fat-soluble vitamins; (4) it has a choleretic action; and (5) it is an excretory channel for bile pigments, cholesterol, certain drugs, metals, etc. Bile has no antiseptic properties; in fact, bacteria grow in bile very rapidly. If bile is diverted to the exterior by a biliary fistula, the feces become clay colored, increased in amount, and greasy and they have an extremely offensive odor. The color is, of course, due to the lack of stercobilin, and the greasiness and odor, to the undigested fat, which has become rancid. Animals with such fistulas eventually develop abnormalities of the bones, associated with loss of inorganic salts, thus indicating some other function that is vital, since animals with bile fistulas do not survive very long.

Some of the nontoxic emulsifying detergents (p. 276) have been tested therapeutically in cases of biliary and pancreatic deficiency in which digestion and emulsification of fat are incomplete. The administration of these agents has been found to be helpful.

Gallstones. Gallstones or biliary calculi are composed of material that has precipitated out of bile to form masses of varying size and shape. They usually are found in the gallbladder but may form in the bile ducts. If single, the stone is generally ovoid in shape; but if multiple, they have facets formed by pressing and rubbing against each other. When many are present, the shape of most of them is cuboidal. A gallbladder may contain as many as 2000 calculi. The color, hardness, and inner structure vary with the composition of these stones. When cut in cross section, a central nucleus around which concentric layers of the constituents are deposited may be seen. Gallstones are usually classified, with regard to composition, as (1) cholesterol, (2) pigment, and (3) calcium carbonate stones. As a matter of fact, no gallstones are ever composed entirely of any one constituent. The so-called pure cholesterol stones may contain from 90% to 98% cholesterol, but there is always some bile pigment and some inorganic salt. Human gallstones are almost always of the cholesterol or pigment variety.

The mechanism of the formation of gallstones is not entirely clear. Gallstones apparently form for physical reasons when there is a change in the normal composition of the bile[13] due to:

1. Change in the relative composition of the major constituents of bile (e.g., excess cholesterol) or excess bilirubin as in hemolytic anemias, etc.
2. Presence of foreign substances or change in trace constituents, e.g., calcium-deoxycholate stones, bacterial infection in the gallbladder, etc.

A fact that was held for a long time and still is rather generally accepted is that an infection or injury to the gallbladder mucosa produces a nucleus of microorganisms or a tiny clot around which cholesterol or pigment is deposited. The proteins present in this nucleus are thought to carry an electric charge opposite those present on cholesterol, pigments, and calcium carbonate and in that way bring about a precipitation. Since the gallbladder tends to concentrate bile, conditions are favorable for further precipitation. Bladder bile is normally more acid than liver bile. This would tend to keep calcium carbonate in solution ordinarily. Infection, it has been shown, interferes with this acidification of bladder bile, leading to precipitation. A metabolic origin has been put forth as another explanation, i.e., that the high concentrations of blood cholesterol (hypercholesterolemia) are often associated with gallstones. It has also been suggested that the protective colloidal action of some protein of the bile (together with the solvent action of the bile salts on cholesterol) may be responsible for the usual nonprecipitation of gallstone constituents, and any factor that disturbs the balance is likely to initiate the formation of a concretion. A mucin or a lipoprotein may be the effective agent. Once started, the number and size of the gallstones increase more or less rapidly. Another theory is that the bile salts, in solutions of increasing concentration, show definite alterations in surface tension and conductivity; these alterations denote a change of phase, indicating ionic aggregation or micelle formation. Such concentration can, and does, occur in the gallbladder. Consequently, the cholesterol-dissolving power of the bile would be decreased and precipitation of cholesterol would be explained.

Duodenobiliary drainage. The technique of duodenobiliary drainage is used to attempt to obtain information regarding the duodenum, pancreas, liver, gallbladder, and the various ducts carrying their secretions to the intestine. A small-caliber rubber tube is passed, first, into the stomach, at which stage the gastric residuum may be obtained and examined, then, through the pylorus to the duodenum. Duodenal contents and then bile may be obtained when the tip of the tube has reached the sphincter of Oddi. The operator may assure himself of this position by use of a fluoroscope. According to the method of Lyon, the fasting duodenal contents are first removed and then a measured volume of saturated magnesium sulfate is introduced by means of a glass syringe. Part or all of it is removed by suction, and then the fluid flows by syphonage. When the bile begins to appear, it is usually seen to be light, golden yellow in color. This is designated A-bile and is considered to be the bile present in the common duct. It usually amounts to from 10 to 30 ml. When the bile begins to show a darker color, it is collected separately as B-bile. This is presumed to be gallbladder bile. When this

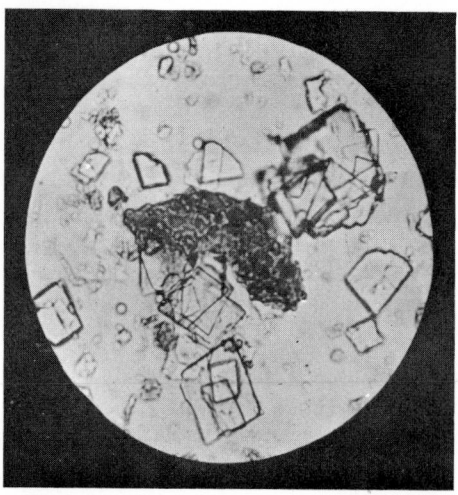

Fig. 21-5. Sediment from B-bile (×360). The combination of cholesterol and calcium bilirubinate is indicative of gallstones. (Courtesy H. Barowsky.)

changes again to a lighter shade, usually even lighter than the A-bile, it is collected as C-bile and is probably bile just as it is secreted from the liver. A-bile is usually golden yellow, B-bile is darker yellow to brown, and C-bile is lemon yellow. Abnormally they may be quite different. Olive oil is often used instead of magnesium sulfate as a relaxing agent for the sphincter of Oddi. It has the advantage of permitting a more exact determination of volume. However, it has the disadvantage of changing the surface tension, which may need to be determined as a means of estimating the amount of bile salts present. Obviously, even under the best conditions, one cannot be sure that the fluid obtained is pure bile. Duodenal fluid, gastric juice, and pancreatic juice may be mixed with it. However, even under such circumstances, certain information, e.g., the absence of bile salts or the absence of B-bile, may be of decided importance. A microscopic examination should be made and may prove to be of great value. This is particularly true of B-bile. The appearance of pus cells, bacteria, and characteristic crystals aids the clinician in diagnosis and treatment. Fig. 21-5 is a typical photomicrograph of abnormal sediment from B-bile.

LIVER FUNCTION TESTS

Many attempts have been made to devise a test that would measure, with some degree of accuracy, the amount of normal liver tissue actively functioning. Two facts have militated against such an achievement. (1) Although the liver may be quite badly damaged, it may nevertheless perform all its functions, because only a comparatively small proportion of healthy liver tissue is needed for all normal activities, i.e., the liver has a large factor of safety. (2) The functions of the liver are many and diverse in nature. Liver is concerned in protein, carbohydrate, and fat metabolism, in the production of the plasma proteins and heparin, in the secretion of bile, in storage of nutrients, in detoxication and excretion, and in a number of other activities. Often a defect in performing one function is not paralleled by a diminution in others, and the function tested may happen to be one that is not affected.

Nevertheless, if one knows their limitations, certain of these tests have considerable clinical value. Some of the procedures will be outlined, with their biochemical background when possible.

Tests for bile pigments. The *icterus index* is a crude test, but it has been of considerable service. The modifications of the *van den Bergh test* indicate whether the pigment is combined with glucuronic acid or is free. The former gives the direct test, and the latter the indirect. These have been described on p. 685. They furnish information regarding the concentration of bile pigment in blood serum. These tests, together with the determination of urobilinogen and bilirubin in the urine, aid in the differential diagnosis of obstructive and nonobstructive jaundice. Total serum bilirubin of 95% in healthy individuals is below 1.10 mg. per 100 ml. of serum. An increase is an unfavorable sign, and, if a high total serum bilirubin value decreases, it indicates a remission of liver disease or of biliary obstruction. A stabilized serum bilirubin concentration is considered highly desirable for an operation of biliary obstruction. The determination of urinary coproporphyrin is also of value as an index of liver function in certain conditions.

Other tests. In Chapter 9 the importance of the liver in various phases of carbohydrate metabolism was described. Therefore almost any procedure that measures carbohydrate metabolism would be, indirectly at least, a liver function test. The glucose tolerance tests (p. 228) are the most commonly used.

Other liver function tests include the hippuric acid test for the detoxication function. This is described on p. 733. There are several dye-secretion tests in which a nontoxic dye that is excreted almost exclusively by the liver is injected, and the amount excreted, and hence the functional capacity of the liver to eliminate it, is determined.

CHEMICAL CHANGES WITHIN THE LARGE INTESTINE

Although the large intestine does not secrete any significant amount of body fluid but is rather a reabsorptive and an excretory structure, biochemical processes occuring in its lumen can perhaps be appropriately considered at this point.

The biochemical processes that go on in the large intestine are due mostly to the activity of the myriads of microorganisms that live and die there. These enter the tract with food and saliva and may survive passage through the stomach since the hydrochloric acid is not always present in bactericidal concentration. Consequently, some living microorganisms pass into the small intestine and begin to multiply as the reaction becomes favorable. However, even near the ileocecal valve the intestinal contents do not contain large numbers of such organisms. At this point are present some undigested food residues, unabsorbed secretions, e.g., bile and pancreatic juice, and cell detritus. Analysis of this material shows it to have about the same amounts of nitrogen, fat, and carbohydrate (based on dry weight) as normal feces, but it is not like feces. The pH is about 5.9 to 6.5.

Feces   In the large intestine, such materials as just described are transformed into feces. A number of enzymes are possibly present in the secretion of the mucosa of the large gut, but digestion by them is generally believed to be of little importance. This secretion is alkaline and viscid and undoubtedly tends to bring the contents over to the alkaline side. The conditions for bacterial growth (particularly anaerobic) are excellent: there are warmth, darkness, little oxygen, an almost neutral medium, and food material in a semisolid condition. The organisms flourish, utilize the food materials, transform them into their own protoplasm, multiply, and die. In fecal material, from one fourth to one half of the dry matter is made up of living and dead bacteria. Water is absorbed by the mucosa and the characteristic consistency results.

In the newborn infant the first fecal discharge is termed meconium. This is a dark brownish green semisolid material. It consists of intestinal and biliary secretions that have accumulated in the large intestine from the fourth fetal month on. Meconium continues to be passed for the first 3 or 4 days after birth and accounts for much of the loss of weight that occurs during this period. Usually, with the ingestion of milk, a gradual change to the usual type of infant feces is seen. These are soft, golden yellow to greenish yellow in color and have an acid reaction. The odor is slightly "sour" but not unpleasant. The approximate general composition of stools of the infant and of the adult is given in Table 21-2. In the feces of infants, there is very little of the milk protein but rather large amounts of fat, fatty acids, and soaps.

Adult fecal material is normally brown, varying in color with fat and water, which lighten the color, and bile pigments, which darken it. About 80 to 170 gm. of feces are eliminated per day. The composition varies greatly, and not much significance can be attached to analytic findings. This is easily understood when we realize that feces contain undigested, indigestible, and unabsorbed food residues, secretions of the gastrointestinal tract, bile constituents, and desquamated epithelial cells. Included in the unabsorbed food may be rather large amounts of iron compounds, since the intestine does not absorb more than a limited amount of iron ingested. There is also a variable amount of phosphate, depending on the precipitation of this ion in insoluble form. A large amount of calcium is found in feces, either as the phosphate or the oxalate. In fact, more calcium is present in feces than in urine. Lipids of various types are also present and comprise about one third of the dry weight.

The bile derivatives in feces are *urobilin* (stercobilin), a transformed bile pigment, which gives the stool its brown color, and *coprosterol*. Coprosterol

Table 21-2. General composition of stools (in percent)

	Stool of breast-fed infant	*Stool of adult*
Water	85	75
Organic solids	13	20
Ash	1	5

is a reduced sterol, coming partly from the cholesterol of the bile and partly from any unabsorbed food cholesterol.

The pH of the stools of healthy adults on a mixed diet varies from 7.0 to 7.5. Common laxatives, even magnesium oxide, tend to change this to the acid side, but whether the contents of the large intestine can be changed to an acid reaction by feeding acid-producing bacteria is questionable. This was the rationale of feeding fermented milk products, e.g., acidophilus milk, etc. The belief was that by implanting such organisms in the large intestine, an acid flora that would have a favorable effect on health could be established.

Intestinal gases. The volume of gas present in the gastrointestinal tract of the human being is variable but averages about 1 liter daily. Since some of this is absorbed, the total volume expelled in the course of a day is somewhat less than a liter but may be as much as 2600 ml. or as little as 12 ml. The components of the mixed gases vary with the diet. On a high-milk diet the predominant gas is hydrogen; on a vegetable diet, methane; and on a meat or mixed diet, nitrogen. In all cases, these gases, as well as carbon dioxide and usually hydrogen sulfide, are present. The nitrogen is derived from swallowed air, from air dissolved in food and drink, and from that which diffuses out of the blood in the blood vessels of the gut. It is in solution in the blood, having passed into the blood during respiration. A typical analysis of the intestinal gases obtained from a normal man showed nitrogen, 59.4% by volume; methane, 29.6%; carbon dioxide, 10.3%; and oxygen, 0.7%. In intestinal obstructions gases of somewhat similar composition accumulate, except that there seems to be less methane and traces of hydrogen and hydrogen sulfide. The amount of hydrogen sulfide depends on the presence of the sulfur-containing amino acids and the type of decomposition they undergo. The concentrations of carbon dioxide and hydrogen sulfide are low because these gases are quite soluble in the aqueous medium and therefore are absorbed rather easily.

Intestinal gas may cause considerable distress because of distention of the abdominal viscera. This is increased when atmospheric pressure is diminished, e.g., at high altitudes, and serious symptoms may result.

Action of microorganisms on carbohydrates and lipids Bacteria, yeasts, and other organisms in the large intestine probably act on carbohydrates present, producing butyric, lactic, and perhaps other organic acids, ethyl alcohol, carbon dioxide, methane, and hydrogen. How much absorption of any of these takes place in the human being is not known. In the rat, at least half the cellulose fed is converted to fatty acids and other metabolic products.

The action of intestinal organisms on fats is probably simple hydrolysis and saturation of part of the unsaturated fatty acids. There is also some synthesis of lipids by microorganisms.

From lecithin and sphingomyelin, choline is split off and is converted to neurine by anaerobic organisms.

$$(CH_3)_3\overset{+}{N}-CH_2CH_2OH \quad \rightarrow \quad (CH_3)_3\overset{+}{N}-CH=CH_2$$

Choline   **Neurine**

Both choline and neurine are toxic to animals.

From one cephalin, serine is derived, and this on decarboxylation yields aminoethyl alcohol, which is a derivative of another cephalin (p. 286). Amino-ethyl alcohol is also called colamine.

$$\text{HO—CH}_2\text{—CH—COOH} \quad \rightarrow \quad \text{HO—CH}_2\text{—CH}_2\text{NH}_2$$

$$\underset{\text{Serine}}{} \quad \underset{}{\overset{|}{\text{NH}_2}} \qquad\qquad \underset{\text{Colamine}}{}$$

Colamine is only slightly toxic, but aminoethyl mercaptan has a marked hypotensive effect and this is formed during the bacterial decomposition of cysteine.

Fecal lipids Normally the main portion of the fecal fatty acids and fatty acid derivatives represents (1) unabsorbed and unaltered fatty acids of dietary fat, e.g., stearic acid, which may be present as esters, soaps, and free fatty acids; (2) saturated fatty acids, soaps, or glyceryl esters, derived from unsaturated fatty acids of the diet, apparently by action of the intestinal flora; and (3) fats synthesized by intestinal flora. Increases may be due to blockage of the bile ducts, the pancreatic ducts, or both; to failure of the pancreas to secrete pancreatic juice; or to imperfect absorption (e.g., when there is increased motility of the upper intestine and the food rushes through too rapidly). Conditions in which the feces contain large amounts of fat, fatty acids, and soaps are called *steatorrheas*. Part of this "fat" may be actually secreted into the intestinal tract.

The normal values for fat and its derivatives in feces vary widely. On a fat-free diet they amount to 0.5 to 1 gm. of fatty acid, or fatty acid derivatives, per day. On diets containing the ordinary amounts of food fats, about 5 gm. or more will be excreted per day. Most of this increase represents unabsorbed dietary fat, some of which has been made more saturated by action of the intestinal flora. The range of total fatty acid in normal feces is from 7% to 25% of the dry weight. A figure of over 25% is considered abnormal and requires more detailed study. If the neutral fat is high, one should suspect deficient fat digestion; and if the total split fat (i.e., sum of soaps and free fatty acids) is above its usual percentage, probably some abnormality in the absorptive process is occurring. In this way a fractional fecal analysis may aid in diagnosing obscure gastrointestinal conditions.

In steatorrheas, lesions of the bones similar to those seen in rickets, sometimes dwarfism, are found. A low serum calcium is usually present and sometimes tetany, from an excessive loss of calcium in the feces along with the fat, results. This must be due to a lowered absorption of calcium from the intestinal tract, which may be accounted for in one of three ways: (1) The excess of fat in the tract holds the fat-soluble vitamin D there and prevents its absorption; vitamin D is concerned in the absorption of calcium from the gastrointestinal tract. (2) The intestinal wall may be impermeable to calcium ions in these conditions. (3) The fatty acids form insoluble soaps with the calcium and these are excreted in the feces as such. There is some evidence for each of these three possibilities.

In addition to neutral fats, fatty acids, and soaps, there are always found various sterols in feces. They are true secretions eliminated by way of the bile or through the intestinal wall. There are also dihydrocholesterol and coprosterol, the reduction products of cholesterol, formed by the action of microorganisms, and unabsorbable plant sterols as well as any excess cholesterol of the diet that has escaped absorption or reduction.

Action of microorganisms on proteins   *Putrefaction.* The decomposition of proteins by anaerobic organisms is termed putrefaction. The nitrogenous materials that reach the large intestine may be undigested or partly digested food residues, unabsorbed amino acids, or cellular detritus. In addition, there are the proteins of dead bacteria. The action of microorganisms on this varied assortment begins with a digestive action. There may be proteases, e.g., trypsin, that have not been destroyed, proteases from disintegrated epithelial or bacterial cells, or the active enzymes of the living bacteria. Proteolysis results, of course, in the formation of free amino acids, and since little or no absorption takes place in the large intestine, they are attacked by the microorganisms to a varying degree and in two general ways: decarboxylation and deamination. Oxidations, reductions, and hydrolyses also occur. These reactions are all results of the appropriate enzymes. If deamination occurs first, acids are formed, whereas amines result from decarboxylation. The simpler amino acids yield simple organic acids or amines, as the case may be. Thus alanine forms propionic acid or ethylamine.

$$CH_3CHNH_2COOH \xrightarrow{\text{Deamination}} CH_3CH_2COOH \text{ (Propionic acid)}$$

Alanine

$$CH_3CHNH_2COOH \xrightarrow{\text{Decarboxylation}} CH_3CH_2NH_2 \text{ (Ethylamine)}$$

The amino acid tyrosine may undergo decomposition along two routes also.

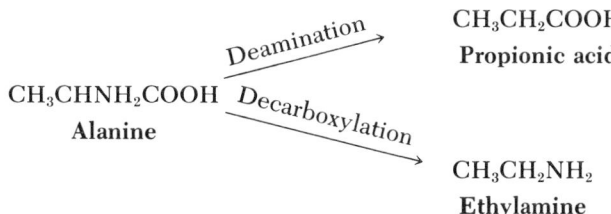

695

Phenol is the ultimate product of both series of reactions, but the first series converts the amino acid to an acidic intermediary, whereas the second is through a basic one, an amine.

The two types of action on cysteine are as follows:

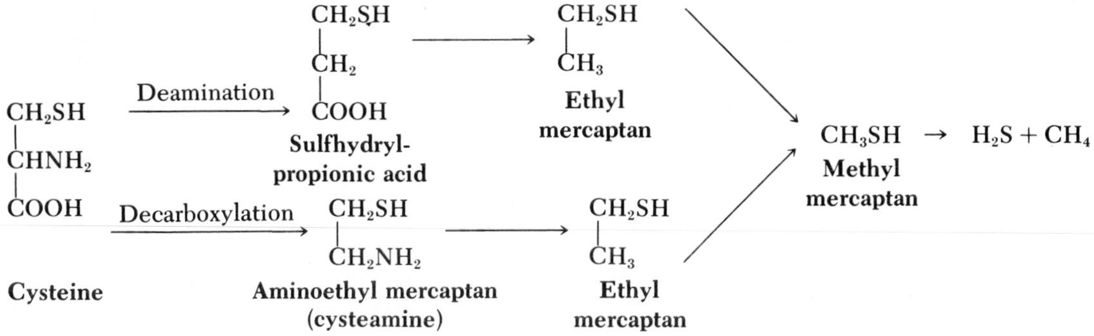

This indicates how, by (1) first deaminating and then decarboxylating and (2) first decarboxylating and then deaminating, different intermediate products are formed, which, if further attacked by the bacterial enzymes, yield finally the same products.

The products of tryptophan deamination are quite important.

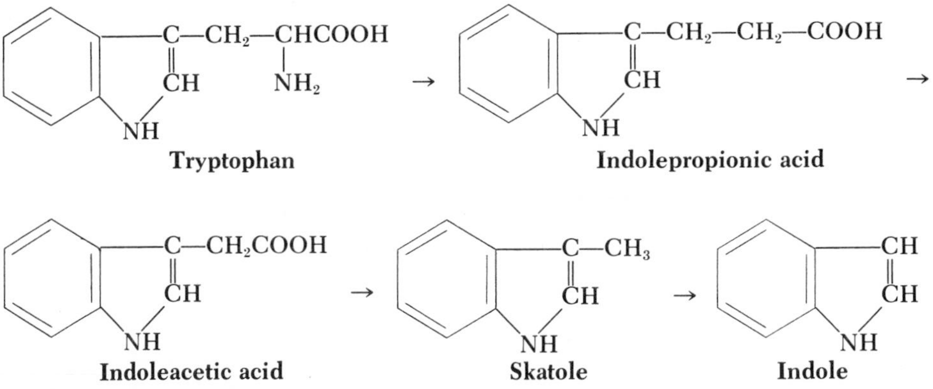

Indole and skatole are the two substances that give the characteristic foul odor to feces. If first decarboxylated, tryptophan yields tryptamine. This and other amines that may be formed in the large bowel are as follows:

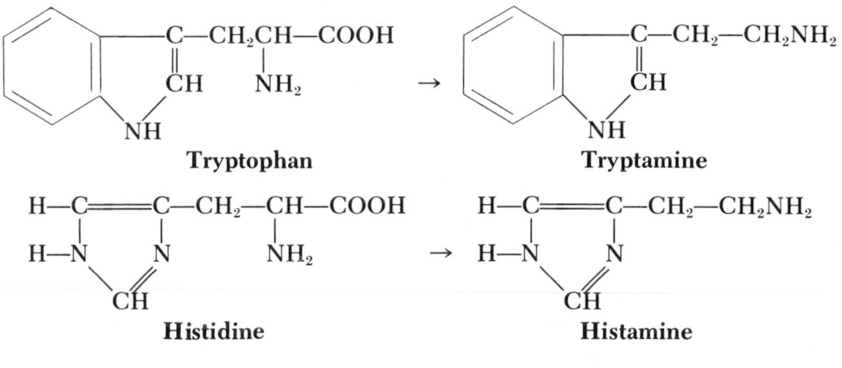

$$CH_2NH_2—CH_2—CH_2—CH_2—CHNH_2—COOH \quad \rightarrow \quad CH_2NH_2—CH_2—CH_2—CH_2—CH_2—NH_2$$

Lysine   Cadaverine

$$CH_2NH_2—CH_2—CH_2—CHNH_2—COOH \quad \rightarrow \quad CH_2NH_2—CH_2—CH_2—CH_2NH_2$$

Ornithine   Putrescine

Most of the amines, when introduced into the bloodstream in appropriate dosage, have marked pharmacologic effects. Histamine, as has been seen, stimulates the gastric glands and, especially in large doses, lowers blood pressure. This depressant action is shared by several other amines produced in the large intestine, e.g., putrescine, cadaverine. On the other hand, tyramine raises blood pressure. This is particularly interesting in view of its structural relation to epinephrine, the hormone of the adrenal medulla, which has a pronounced hypertensive action. Tryptamine also raises blood pressure after a preliminary depressor action.

Tyramine   Epinephrine

Autointoxication   Diarrhea may result from an overabundance of some of the products of intestinal putrefaction, particularly the acidic compounds. The question arises, however, as to whether the other toxic products, the amines, the choline derivatives, the mercaptans, etc., are harmful in other ways. The idea that the absorption of some of these products of bacterial activity is the cause of many of the ills of mankind has long been prevalent, even among medical men. There is no question that some of the products are somewhat toxic when administered orally and even more so if given parenterally, i.e., by any route other than the mouth. It is doubtful, however, if large enough amounts are ever absorbed to produce harmful effects. For example, the total amount of indole in the feces is seldom over 60 to 70 mg., and yet 1 gm. of indole given by mouth produces no ill effects and 2 gm. cause only a slight headache and dizziness. Small amounts of indole and skatole are often absorbed, as evidenced by the excretion of their detoxication product, indican, in the urine. They are therefore fully detoxicated. Sherwin reported that the amines produced in putrefaction may be introduced into the gastrointestinal tract in amounts much greater than occur in constipation without the appearance of unusual symptoms. Regarding other toxic products formed by bacteria in the large intestine, they are (1) not absorbed in appreciable quantities, (2) destroyed by the mucosa of the intestine, or (3) detoxicated in the liver or some other organ.

What is the basis, then, for autointoxication, the symptoms of which often accompany constipation—mental laziness, malaise, headache, dullness, coated tongue, poor appetite, and "biliousness"? Evidently the old idea that

697

these symptoms are caused by absorption of toxic materials from the sluggish intestine is untenable. Alvarez is of the opinion that most of these symptoms result from mechanical distention and irritation of the rectum by the fecal masses and their effects are caused by reflex action. Many of the symptoms can be reproduced by simply packing the rectum with cotton. Probably small waves of contraction originate at such packed locations and travel in a reverse direction up the intestinal tract (antiperistalsis) and thus give rise to foul breath, coated tongue, and other symptoms. It is not to be assumed that absorption of toxic products from the intestine never occurs. Probably it does, but the symptoms usually associated with constipation and with what has been termed autointoxication in the past are not caused by products absorbed from the large intestine. Absorption of toxins is more likely to occur in diarrheal conditions; but even in these cases the toxic action of the substances is of little moment.

Food poisons. A number of toxic products have been classed together as ptomaines. These include muscarine, neurine, cadaverine, and putrescine. If food, particularly meat or fish, decomposes under the influence of putrefactive organisms, these compounds are formed. Usually this decomposition results from inadequate refrigeration of food or storage for too long a time. If such spoiled foods are eaten, they are likely to cause food poisoning. Possibly this type of poisoning results because these toxic products are absorbed more readily from the small intestine than from the large. However, the body can detoxify (p. 747) fairly large quantities of toxic substances. Usually food poisoning means an infection carried by infected food into the gastrointestinal tract, and the pathologic effects can be explained by assuming the continued formation and absorption of the toxic products plus specific toxins elaborated by the bacteria.

A different type of food poisoning is botulism. *Clostridium botulinum,* growing in food, elaborates a group of neurotoxins, stated to be "the most poisonous poison." Type-A toxin is a crystallizable protein. Although it is digestible by proteolytic enzymes, minute amounts escape digestion and are absorbed by the intestinal mucosa in some unaccountable manner and produce violent effects. As little as 0.25 μg. of the pure toxin may be lethal for man.

Probably the most common cause of food poisoning in this country, however, is from staphylococcal toxin from foods contaminated with certain species of staphylococci. These types of toxin are highly incapacitating though rarely fatal. They may develop in foods, particularly custards, potato salads, and similar foods, kept unrefrigerated for too long a time in hot weather.

Pathologic constituents of feces. In order to detect abnormal constituents, the stools may be examined macroscopically, microscopically, and chemically. Each of these methods may yield valuable information. For example, simple observation, after mixing with water, and straining through cheesecloth, may enable one to find gallstones, undigested food residues, mucus, epithelial shreds, and, rarely, intestinal concretions. Intestinal concretions are chiefly inorganic, usually ammonium magnesium phosphate, with some admixture of calcium phosphate, calcium carbonate, calcium sulfate, protein, or calcium or magnesium soaps. They always have a nucleus of some indigestible substance, e.g., hair or even a gallstone.

Microscopically one may see crystals that might indicate the presence of salts or organic compounds that are ordinarily absorbed. Undigested food (fat globules, meat and vegetable fibers, starch granules, etc.) is often observed.

Chemically the quantitative estimation of fat, fatty acid, and soaps is sometimes required, but a strict control of the intake is then important. A qualitative test for unchanged bile pigments is rarely positive, except in severe diarrhea, when the intestinal contents are rushed through the tract. Ordinarily they are converted to stercobilin and stercobilinogen. The most important chemical determination is the qualitative one for blood. Among other determinations, this aids in the diagnosis of gastrointestinal ulcers and malignancies. A chemical test is often necessary because the colors that blood imparts to feces vary from bright red to black. A small amount of reddish black in the brown feces is indistinguishable by the naked eye. The color of blood in the feces depends on the length of time the blood remains in the small intestine, not on the site of the hemorrhage. Blood from the duodenum stains feces red if it moves through the small intestine fast enough, because the darkening mechanism requires time and takes place solely in the small intestine.

It is, therefore, often necessary to test for *occult* blood, i.e., blood that is not macroscopically evident. This may be done most simply by suspending a small amount of feces in 5 ml. of water, boiling to inactivate the oxidizing enzymes, and then applying to the cooled fecal suspension any of the standard tests for blood, e.g., benzidine, reduced phenolphthalein, orthotolidine. If a positive reaction is obtained with a patient on a mixed diet, the test should be repeated after he has been on a meat-free diet for a sufficient length of time.

MILK

Milk is the fluid secreted by the mammary gland for use as food by the young mammal. Consequently, milk may be considered from two standpoints: (1) as a secretion and (2) as a food.

Secretion of milk. Milk is secreted by the alveoli of the mammary gland. These are not present in either sex in early childhood. In the female, at puberty, proliferation of the tubules and development of the alveoli occur, and the gland, of course, increases in size. These changes result from the liberation of ovarian and other hormones. During pregnancy the estrogens and progesterone stimulate an increased growth of the breasts and cause functional changes, but the estrogens tend to suppress lactation until after delivery. The actual secretion of milk does not occur until the end of pregnancy. The initiation of lactation may result from a sudden removal of the placenta and from other factors. The chief hormone involved is prolactin, a pituitary factor. One of the posterior pituitary hormones, oxytocin, causes milk ejection. Nervous stimulation induced by suckling is believed to cause the secretion of the hormones that have their continuing secretory effect upon the mammary gland. For further discussion see p. 488.

Composition and factors modifying it   In addition to being used as the food of the very young, milk, particularly cow's milk, has been adopted as a nutrient for all ages. It is the most complete food found in nature, and for a long period it is the only food of the young mammal. The first secretion of the mammary gland postpartum differs a great deal from true milk. It is called *colostrum*. It is a yellowish, alkaline, and slightly viscid fluid. It has a higher content of total solids, the components of which are not exactly the same as those of milk. Colostrum coagulates on heating, whereas milk does not. The lipids present in colostrum have a higher content of cholesterol and lecithins, and the fat has a higher iodine number. Colostrum seems to have a laxative action and thus may aid in bringing about evacuation of the meconium. The amount of colostrum secreted by the human being is rather small, about 150 to 300 ml. in 24 hours. About the third or fourth day, true milk begins to be secreted and the colostrum qualities diminish steadily. For 1 or 2 weeks, however, human milk continues to retain some of the characteristics of colostrum. This is reflected in the changing composition of milk (p. 701).

Milk is an oil-in-water type of emulsion stabilized by complex phospholipids and proteins adsorbed on the surface of fat globules. It contains proteins in colloidal dispersion, lactose in true solution, and a number of minerals, particularly calcium and phosphorus. There are also present some organic acids or their salts, vitamins, enzymes, and some undetermined constituents, including antibodies and substances called lactenins that have antibacterial properties against certain streptococci. In human milk there are present one or more bifidus factors, which aid the growth of certain microorganisms found

Table 21-3. Average composition of milk of different species*

Species	Water (percent)	Protein (N × 6.37) (percent)	Fat (percent)	Lactose (percent)	Ash (percent)	Fuel value per pound (kilocalories)
Man	87.4	1.4	4.0	7.0	0.2	316
Cow	87.1	3.4	3.9	4.9	0.7	310
Goat	87.0	3.3	4.2	4.8	0.7	318
Sheep	82.6	5.5	6.5	4.5	0.9	447
Reindeer	63.7	10.3	19.7	4.8	1.5	1,078
Buffalo (Indian)	82.2		7.5	4.8	0.8	
Zebra	86.1	3.0	4.8	5.3	0.7	
Camel†	87.1	3.5	4.8	4.7	0.7	
Mare‡	87.1	1.8–3.0	1.1	5.9	0.4	
Ass	90.1		1.4	6.2	0.5	
Pig‖	80.1	5.8	8.2	4.8	0.9	

* Data, in part, from Farmer's Bulletin no. 363, 1909; no. 1705, 1933.
† Data from Kheraskov, S. G.: Chem. Abstr. **58:**2779, 1963.
‡ Data from various sources.
‖ Data from Braude, R., et al.: Brit. J. Nutr. **1:**64, 1947.

in the breast-fed baby's intestine (p. 705). It is not a fluid of constant composition, a number of influences tending to vary it. Some of these factors are species differences, individual variations within the species, age, period of lactation, diet, physical and mental condition, time of day, and fraction of single nursing.

Species. It is well known that different animals have milk of different composition. Table 21-3 is a comparison of the milk of a variety of mammals, and Table 21-4 shows how, in a general way, the proportion of protein and salts parallels the rate of growth. Animals that grow faster have milk containing more protein, for soft tissue building, and more inorganic salts, for bone building. Moreover, within a given species there are differences, e.g., in the composition of milk of various breeds of cattle. Holsteins produce a milk with lower fat content than that of Jerseys and Guernseys.

It will be noted that goat's milk has about the same composition as cow's milk. The proportion of lactalbumin is slightly higher, and the amounts of thiamine and riboflavin are stated to be higher also than the corresponding values for cow's milk. The curd tension, i.e., toughness, is lower; this fact and also the somewhat greater resemblance to the distribution of proteins in human milk have led to many claims of superiority of goat's milk over cow's milk for infant feeding. However, about the only practical indication for its use is for babies who are allergic to the proteins of cow's milk.

Individual variations, age. There is some individual variation in the milk of cows of the same breed and of the same cow from day to day. Consequently, the mixed milk from a herd is bound to be more uniform in composition than the milk of individual cows. Furthermore, the effect of any deleterious change in composition of the milk of a single cow, as a result of any factor whatever, is minimized by mixing with the milk of many others.

Table 21-4. Protein and ash content of milk of different species as related to rate of growth[*]

Species	Time in which body weight of newborn animal is doubled (days)	Protein (percent)	Ash (percent)	Calcium (percent)	Phosphoric acid (percent)
Man	180	1.4	0.2	0.0328	0.0473
Horse	60	2.0	0.4	0.124	0.131
Cow	47	3.4	0.7	0.160	0.197
Goat	19	3.3	0.8	0.210	0.322
Pig	18	5.2 [†]	—	0.250[‡]	0.537[‡]
Sheep	10	5.5	0.9	0.272	0.412
Dog	8	7.1	1.3	0.453	0.493
Cat	7	9.5	—	—	—

[*] Data chiefly from Bunge, G.: Text-book of physiological and pathological chemistry, ed. 2 (English), Philadelphia, 1902, P. Blakiston's Son & Co.
[†] Data from Sheffy, B. E., et al.: J. Nutr. 48:103, 1952.
[‡] Data from Braude, R., et al.: Brit. J. Nutr. 1:64, 1947.

Table 21-5. Composition of human milk at different periods*

Time	Number of cases	Protein			Sugar			Fat		
		Minimum (percent)	Maximum (percent)	Average (percent)	Minimum (percent)	Maximum (percent)	Average (percent)	Minimum (percent)	Maximum (percent)	Average (percent)
5 days	88	1.45	2.83	2.00	4.62	7.37	6.42	0.9	8.2	3.2
9 days	88	1.12	2.65	1.73	4.76	7.65	6.73	1.6	7.1	3.7
3–4 wk.	35	1.03	1.79	1.37	6.17	7.89	7.11	1.4	6.1	3.6
5–6 wk.	32	0.98	1.57	1.30	5.97	8.33	7.11	1.3	7.6	4.0
7–8 wk.	14	1.04	1.40	1.21	6.25	7.83	7.11	1.1	7.0	4.0

* From Bell, M.: J. Biol. Chem. 80:239, 1928.

The same individual variations occur among human beings. Some mothers produce milk of poor quality or small volume, although most women are quite capable of nursing their babies adequately. The total volume secreted depends on the demands of the infant and the secretory capacity of the mammary glands. In some instances, wet nurses have been found to secrete more than a gallon of milk a day. Young mothers, as a rule, secrete more milk than older ones; this does not appear to be related to the fact that there are more primiparas (women who have had only 1 birth) among the young mothers but is probably because of youthful health and vigor. Milk secretion is under hormonal control. Undoubtedly this accounts for some of the normal variations, particularly that variation due to age. Pronounced effects on lactation are observed in certain types of endocrine dysfunction. For example, milk secretion may persist for an exceptionally long period after childbirth in cases of acromegaly.

Period of lactation. Since the early secretion, colostrum, has quite a different composition from true milk and since it is known that milk retains some of the characteristics of colostrum for 1 or 2 weeks, analyses of milk during the first 2 weeks would be expected to be variable. In fact, human milk continues to change for at least 8 weeks. Table 21-5 gives the results of an investigation of this subject; the same results compared with the average change in the weights of the infants are shown in Fig. 21-6. After the third week, the lactose content remains constant and a little later the fat also levels off. The first colostrum secreted is extremely high in protein, diminishing considerably during the next few days, and the amount of essential amino acids available is correspondingly high. The infant's need for protein is most acute during its first 2 weeks. Later it requires and obtains a higher percentage of the energy-forming foods — fats and carbohydrates.

Diet. The diet of the mother, or other lactating animal, has some influence on the amount and quality of the milk but not as much as we would expect. Feeding more liberally than the accepted standards results in slight changes

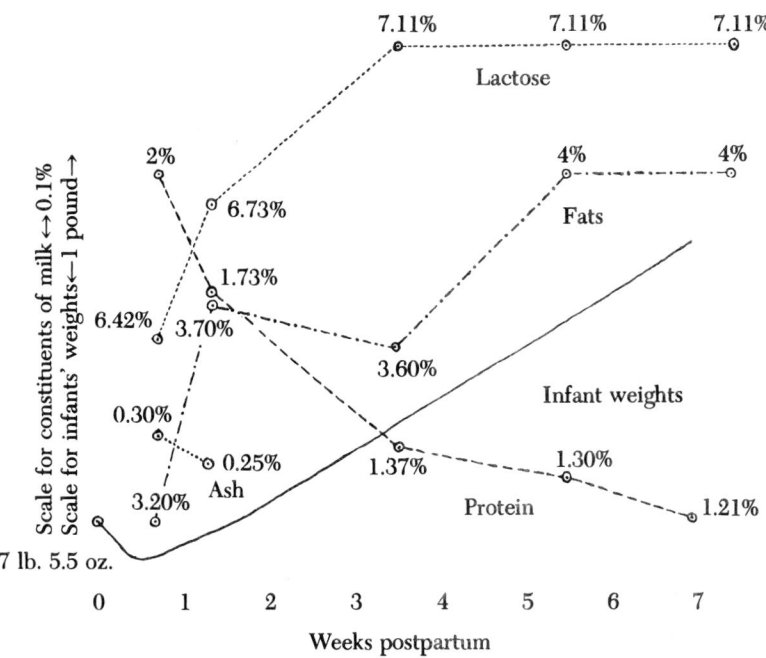

Fig. 21-6. Average composition of human milk at different periods compared with the average weight curve of infants. The different constituents are plotted on different base lines, but the scale is the same in all cases. (From Bell, M.: J. Biol. Chem. **80:** 239, 1928.)

in volume and composition. During the early days of lactation, a higher carbohydrate diet tends to increase the volume somewhat and also the lactose. High protein also increases the volume secreted, whereas a high-fat diet forces the fat up and the volume down. However, these changes are not of great significance. The vitamin content may be improved by feeding larger amounts; this is particularly true in the case of vitamin D. A poor nutritive condition of the mother influences the quantity of the milk secreted. Inadequate diets result in fluctuations of the inorganic constituents, calcium and magnesium being decreased usually, while potassium, sodium, chlorine, and phosphorus are irregularly influenced. In other respects, however, no marked changes have been noted.

Physical and mental conditions. A poor state of health is reflected in an inadequate milk secretion. Either the quality or the quantity may suffer. If the mother is in good health, her milk usually "agrees with" the baby. This does not mean that the milk is necessarily adequate nutritionally. The most usual difficulties are too low or too high fat content, insufficient vitamins in the mother's diet and, consequently, in her milk, and a sensitivity to certain proteins in the milk that are traceable to the mother's diet.

The amount of milk secreted is diminished by excessive physical work, and emotional disturbances have a similar effect, e.g., excitement, worry, fear. There is a greater volume secreted at night than during the day. The most characteristic analytic figures are said to be obtained at 9 or 10 A.M.

703

Fractions of a single nursing. During a single nursing the mammary gland begins by secreting milk richer in proteins and poorer in fats. As secretion continues, the protein content diminishes and fat increases so that the last fraction has a composition just opposite the first. Consequently, if the physician wishes to get an accurate quantitative idea of the composition of a mother's milk, the entire contents of one breast should be obtained. If this is not practicable, 1 ounce should be obtained before and 1 ounce after nursing and the two should be mixed.

Comparison of human and cow's milk   Table 21-6 shows a comparison of the composition of human and cow's milk in two ways: (1) the range of values ordinarily found and (2) the round numbers, which represent the usual approximate values. The outstanding differences are a greater concentration of lactose in human than in cow's milk, with lower concentrations of total protein and ash. The percentage of fat is about the same in cow's and human milk, but cow's milk generally comes to a constant composition of about 3.9% at the dairy where the milk is pooled and analyzed. The legal requirement is usually 3.25%.

Besides these variations in general composition, several special points should be noted. The distribution of the three milk proteins is quite different. In cow's milk the casein is greater in amount than the albumin-globulin fraction, whereas in human milk the albumin-globulin fraction is slightly greater. The inorganic constituents are about the same qualitatively but not quantitatively. Although human milk contains slightly more iron than cow's milk, this is not sufficient for the baby's day-to-day needs. Nature has provided for this inadequacy by having the infant come into the world with a store of iron in the liver and as extra hemoglobin and erythrocytes—enough to last until the infant can obtain iron from foods other than milk. The calcium and phosphorus are sufficient to provide for bone growth and tissue requirements, but they are not present in excessive amounts.

One unfavorable effect of human milk is the fact that hyperbilirubinemia may occur in very young infants who are breast fed. This seems to be due to the presence of pregnanediol in the milk.[14] It is known that this hormone occurs in the serum of pregnant women and has an inhibitory (competitive) effect on bilirubin conjugation.

Table 21-6. Comparison of human and cow's milk

	Total protein (percent)	Lactose (percent)	Fat (percent)	Ash (percent)
Human milk				
Range	1.0–2.8	4.6–8.3	0.9–8.2	0.25–0.30
Round numbers	1.4	7.0	4.0	0.25
Cow's milk				
Range	2.1–6.4	2.1–6.1	1.7–6.5	0.35–1.21
Round numbers	4.0	5.0	4.0	0.75

Physical characteristics and reaction. Milk is a white to yellowish white fluid having a specific gravity varying from 1.026 to 1.036 (cow's and human). Since the specific gravity of fat is less than 1.000, a high fat (cream) content tends to lower the specific gravity. Watering the milk (diluting with water), of course, has the same effect. Consequently, the determination of specific gravity aids very little in estimating the composition of milk. The reaction is usually faintly acid, with a pH of 6.6 to 6.9. The color is due partly to the calcium salt of casein, which is bluish white in solution, and partly to the emulsified fat. The yellowish color often observed is derived from pigments in the food that dissolve in the fat. These are carotene and xanthophyll, chiefly the former. They cannot be synthesized, and, if absent from the diet, similar pigments present in the body fat may be drawn upon. By changing feed, many degrees of color may be observed in butterfat, from almost colorless to a very deep yellow. The yellowish color of whey, the fluid remaining after casein has been precipitated out, is probably due to the presence of riboflavin.

Lactose. Lactose apparently occurs only in milk. Moreover, galactose is not found free in nature but is found in combination. However, not enough galactans or other galactose-containing substances may be ingested by the lactating mother to furnish the requisite amount of galactose to form lactose. Therefore lactose must be synthesized by the lactating mammary gland. This means that one molecule of glucose must be converted to one of galactose and joined to another of glucose. This occurs as a result of two enzyme reactions: (1) uridine diphosphate-D-glucose (p. 215) is converted to UDP-D-galactose by an epimerase and (2) UDP-D-galactose and -glucose are linked by galactosyl transferase to form lactose and UDP. Isotope experiments have shown that blood glucose is the principal source of both the glucose and galactose of lactose (see also p. 215). Furthermore, a soluble protein, presumably an enzyme, from the lactating guinea pig mammary gland catalyzes the synthesis of lactose from glucose-1-phosphate and starch or glycogen. For this reaction no magnesium or phosphate ions or ATP are needed.

If milk is permitted to stand long enough at ordinary temperatures, it sours. This is called lactic *fermentation* or lactic acid production. It is brought about by certain bacteria and the reaction may result in (1) about 50% production of lactic acid or (2) about 100% depending on the type of organism present. The reactions would be, perhaps, as follows:

$$C_{12}H_{22}O_{11} + H_2O \rightarrow C_6H_{12}O_6 + C_6H_{12}O_6$$

$$\text{Lactose} \qquad\qquad \text{Galactose} \quad \text{Glucose}$$

$$2\ C_6H_{12}O_6 + H_2O \rightarrow 2\ CH_3 \cdot CHOH \cdot COOH + CH_3COOH + C_2H_5OH + 2\ CO_2 + 2\ H_2$$

$$\text{Galactose} \qquad\qquad \text{Lactic acid} \qquad\quad \text{Acetic} \quad\ \text{Ethyl}$$
$$\text{acid} \qquad \text{alcohol}$$

$$C_6H_{12}O_6 \rightarrow 2\ CH_3 \cdot CHOH \cdot COOH$$

$$\text{Galactose} \qquad \text{Lactic acid}$$

In human milk there occur growth factors for *Lactobacillus bifidus* var. *Penn,* an organism that grows in the intestinal tract of breast-fed infants. These factors consist of a group of N-acetylglucosamine– and sialic acid–containing oligosaccharides and polysaccharides. They are grouped together and are termed the *bifidus factor*. One of them appears to be a tetrasaccharide composed of N-acetylglucosamine, D-glucose, D-galactose, and L-fucose, a methyl pentose. Another, bifidus factor 2, contains a peptidelike component and hypoxanthine (p. 32). Two other sugars have been found in milk, namely, gynolactose and allolactose. Gynolactose contains nitrogen and may very well be one of the components of the bifidus factor. The same possibility holds for glucosamine and galactosamine, which have also been reported in human milk. The significance of the bifidus factor is not clear, but the factor may be needed to establish or maintain the growth of a favorable flora in the intestinal tract of infants.

Although lactose is the natural milk sugar and is peculiar to milk, the question arises, does it have special advantages in infant nutrition? The spatial configuration of lactose, and especially of its constituent galactose, may give it unique nutritional properties. The sugar level in milk tends to vary directly with the weight of the adult brain. Man has the largest brain, in proportion to the body weight, of all animals, and human milk has the highest percentage of milk sugar. The concentration of milk sugar may be related to the glycolipids of brain, which, you remember, usually contain galactose. Moreover, glucose is the only fuel normally used by the brain in its activities, and, conceivably, during brain formation the more stable galactose, being less easily oxidized, is more suitable as a building material. Infants may be less able to synthesize galactose than adults; hence its presence in their food may be highly desirable from this standpoint. There is considerable evidence that lactose has a special relation to calcium absorption and metabolism. Probably other sugars have the same effect, but lactose appears to be digested less readily than other disaccharides and to be absorbed very slowly and probably to a very slight extent. It increases the retention of dietary calcium, apparently by improving the utilization of calcium already absorbed, and increases the mineral content of bone. There is no good explanation for this phenomenon. The lactose molecule may take part in biochemical processes fundamentally concerned in calcium metabolism. In infant feeding it has a special advantage in helping to maintain the natural flora seen in the breast-fed infant, and this results in fewer gastrointestinal upsets. Galactose metabolism is discussed further on p. 215.

Proteins. The proteins of milk are the caseins, the lactalbumins, and the lactoglobulins. These proteins, especially the caseins, are peculiar to milk. They are manufactured by the mammary glands. The sources of the chief milk proteins are the amino acids present in the blood. The fatty acids, glucose, and bicarbonate contribute in greater or smaller amounts to the carbon skeleton of proteins. This was shown by the intravenous injection into lactating rabbits or cows of the precursor, labeled with ^{14}C, and finding the labeled carbon in the milk proteins. Inorganic phosphate, labeled with ^{32}P, when injected into a cow's udder, was incorporated into casein, and there is evidence that casein synthesis in the cow occurs in the udder. Immune globulins and any serum albumin present come directly from blood, although a portion of the globulins may be synthesized in the udder. The loss of protein during lactation has no deleterious effect on the mother's blood proteins, which are maintained at normal levels. Of course, the lactating mother must have a plentiful supply of proteins of good quality in her diet in order to provide the amino acids necessary to build these proteins.

Casein is a phosphoprotein. It is insoluble at its isoelectric point, pH 4.6, but since the pH of milk is nearly 7.0, it is undoubtedly present as a salt, calcium caseinate. On acidification casein precipitates.

$$\text{Ca-casein} + 2\ \text{HCl} \rightarrow \underline{\text{Casein}} + \text{CaCl}_2$$

In souring of milk, the same reaction occurs. Rennin also precipitates casein. However, this is not quite true because a partial digestion takes place, some fragment of the protein molecule being split off. It further differs from acid precipitation in that the precipitate contains calcium. In fact, in the absence of calcium, the precipitation does not occur. Thus:

$$\text{Ca-caseinate} \xrightarrow{\text{Rennin}} \underline{\text{Ca-paracaseinate}} + \text{Peptide}$$

but

$$\text{Casein} \xrightarrow{\text{Rennin}} \text{Paracasein} + \text{Peptide}$$

The paracasein remains in solution until calcium ions are added:

$$\text{Paracasein} + \text{Ca}^{++} \longrightarrow \underline{\text{Ca-paracaseinate}}$$

This can be demonstrated by adding some oxalate to milk and obtaining by filtration the decalcified milk. Rennin, if added to this decalcified milk, does not clot it, whereas it does clot the untreated milk in a few minutes. The subsequent addition of a soluble calcium salt, in excess, brings down a clot. If rennin is added to boiled or evaporated milk, there is no clot formed because the heating has caused the calcium to be precipitated as calcium phosphate. Clotted milk or junket is frequently used in the American diet. Under suitable conditions other proteolytic enzymes can cause milk to clot in this way, but rennin, the enzyme present in the fourth stomach of the calf, is especially effective and apparently its action is limited to this digestion.

Casein is not a single protein but a group of three or more proteins. These have been designated α-, β-, γ-, κ-, and λ-. κ-Casein is the protein that stabilizes the micelle, preventing the precipitation of the entire complex. An attack by a proteolytic enzyme on this protective colloidal protein renders the protein incapable of protecting the other two, and if calcium ions are present and pH and temperature favorable, they precipitate then as calcium paracaseinate. The various caseins differ chiefly in their phosphorus content.

Lactalbumin, like casein, is not a single entity but consists of three proteins, β-lactoglobulin,* α-lactalbumin, and blood serum albumin. It is even sug-

---

*The apparent confusion in nomenclature here, i.e., placing β-lactoglobulin in the albumin fraction, stems from the decision of milk chemists[15] to designate as albumins those proteins soluble in a saturated solution of magnesium sulfate, and as globulins, those insoluble in that solution.

gested that these may be multiple in nature. The β-lactoglobulins make up the bulk of the lactalbumin fraction and have some globulin properties; e.g., they are insoluble in water. The lactoglobulins include euglobulin and pseudoglobulin. About 5% of the noncasein proteins are in this group, but colostrum contains much more. They carry the immunologic properties of milk and protect the young animal until it can acquire immune systems of its own. Lactalbumins and lactoglobulins are coagulable proteins and coagulate when isolated from milk by suitable separation methods. As present in milk, they do not coagulate on heating because the pH is not favorable, but they are undoubtedly denatured by heat.

Interesting recent studies[16] indicate that α-lactalbumin has activity as lactose synthetase, along with a second protein.

$$\text{UDP-galactose} + \text{Glucose} \xrightarrow[\substack{\text{synthetase} \\ \text{Protein}}]{\text{Lactose}} \text{Lactose}$$

The synthesis of lactalbumin appears to be under hormonal control, the lactogenic hormone and insulin stimulating it and progesterone inhibiting it. Increased progesterone levels during pregnancy apparently repress the formation of lactalbumin. At parturition, decreased levels of plasma progesterone with increasing prolactin secretion cause an increased α-lactalbumin synthesis.

The sequence of the 123 amino acid residues of α-lactalbumin is partially known. Interesting is the finding that 40 residues in the amino acid sequence are identical with those of lysozyme (129 amino acids) (p. 137). This suggests a common genetic ancestry of the two proteins.

All the proteins are excellent biologically, containing a wide assortment of amino acids. The combined milk proteins yield the known amino acids, essential and nonessential. Table 21-7 indicates the content of the essential amino acids in the proteins of cow's milk, as well as the amounts present in 1 quart. When compared with the recommended daily intake of these amino acids, a quart of milk provides a large proportion of the adult's daily requirement of essential amino acids. From a consideration of the amino acid content alone, human milk proteins are not nutritionally superior to the proteins of cow's milk. The difference in the proportion of albumin to casein explains why cow's milk forms heavy tough curds and human milk soft fine curds. Such soft fine curds are much more easily and rapidly digested.

Very small amounts of free amino acids are also present in milk. These represent about 4 and 6 mg. of nonprotein nitrogen per 100 ml. of cow's and human milk, respectively. In this connection, it is interesting to note that the objectionable flavor that milk acquires on exposure to sunlight for periods of a half hour or more has been found to be due to photolysis of methionine, aided by the vitamin riboflavin.

Lipids. The fat of milk is in the form of very small globules. There is no appreciable difference in the size of the fat particles in human as compared with cow's milk, although there may be slight variation in the fat globules obtained from different individuals. Most of the fat of cow's milk consists of

Table 21-7. Essential amino acids in cow's milk

Amino acid	Percent in milk proteins[°]	Recommended daily intake for man[†] (grams)	One quart of milk contains	
			Grams[°]	Percent of recommended daily intake
L-Tryptophan	1.4	0.5	0.45	90
Total aromatic amino acids	10.0		1.06	
Phenylalanine	4.9	2.2	1.54	70
Tyrosine[‡]	5.1		1.62	
L-Lysine	7.9	1.6	2.47	154
L-Threonine	4.7	1.0	1.46	146
L-Valine	7.0	1.6	2.18	136
Total sulfur amino acids	3.4		1.06	
Methionine	2.5	2.2	0.78	36
Cystine[‡]	0.9		0.28	
L-Leucine	10.0	2.2	3.11	141
L-Isoleucine	6.5	1.4	2.02	144
L-Histidine[§]	2.7			

[°]Food and Nutrition Board, National Academy of Sciences, Washington, D.C., 1968.
[†]Rose, W. C., Wixom, R. L., Lockhart, H. B., and Lambert, G. F.: J. Biol. Chem. **217**:987, 1955.
[‡]Related dispensable amino acid.
[§]Not required for adults but may be for children.

the triglycerides of palmitic, oleic, stearic, myristic, and other higher fatty acids, but a small amount, about 10%, is composed of the triglycerides of butyric, caproic, caprylic, and other fatty acids with short carbon chains. The latter include several volatile fatty acids; in this respect, milk fat differs from other fats formed in the body. Small amounts of cholesterol, phospholipids, and free fatty acids are present. Human milk fat differs from bovine in that few or none of the fatty acids present have chains shorter than 10 carbons. Oleic acid occurs in largest amount, palmitic next, lauric, myristic, stearic, octadecadienoic in smaller amounts, and still smaller quantities of a considerable number of long-chain fatty acids. The fat of human milk resembles human body fat much more than it does typical milk fat of other species. In fact, the milk fat of most mammals except ruminants has a composition similar to that of the remainder of their body fat. The fat of cow's milk contains a variety of triglycerides of fatty acids, of which about two thirds are saturated and one third is unsaturated, and there is a large proportion of short-chain fatty acids. The unsaturated fraction includes a small but appreciable amount of the essential fatty acids linoleic and arachidonic as well as the related linolenic acid. Furthermore, cow's milk contains traces of fatty acids having odd numbers of carbon atoms, i.e., 7, 9, 11, 13, 15, and 17 carbon atoms. As regards the source of milk fat, isotope experiments indicate that, in the lactating cow, injected acetate gives rise chiefly to the fatty acid fraction of the fat of milk whereas glucose furnishes more of the glycerol. Recently it has been shown that all the ester classes of lipids are readily synthesized in the mammary gland.

Since the fat globules are lighter than water, they rise to the top to form cream. Commercially, the fat of milk is its most valuable constituent, being marketed as cream and butter and entering into the composition of cheese and being largely responsible for the pleasing flavor of these foods as well as of others into which they enter. The percentage of fat in milk often determines the price of milk to the farmer. It is also an index of the nutritional value of milk. Consequently, the analysis of milk for fat is of considerable importance to farmers and dairymen, as well as to food and health authorities and, of course, to the physician. There are many methods of determining fat content in milk, but the quickest, easiest, and almost universally adopted method is the Babcock procedure. This can be used not only for cow's milk but, with modifications, also for cream, skimmed milk, ice cream, human milk, etc.

The amount of cholesterol in cow's milk is approximately 11 mg. per 100 ml., all of which is free cholesterol. The cholesterol content of the milk does not seem to bear any relation to the level of this lipid in the cow's blood serum.

Ash. The inorganic salts of milk include chiefly calcium, potassium, and sodium salts of hydrochloric and phosphoric acids. Potassium is present in

Table 21-8. Composition of ash of mature human and cow's milk*

	Human milk (milligrams per 100 ml.)	Cow's milk (milligrams per 100 ml.)
Total ash	210	710
Calcium	34	126
Chlorine	43	106†
Magnesium	4	13
Phosphorus	16	90†
Potassium	55	160†
Sodium	15	51†
Sulfur	14	30
Bromine	0.91	0.02
Copper	0.04	0.03
Iodine	0.01‡	0.05†
Iron	0.21	0.13
Rubidium	1	Trace
Zinc	0.66	0.35
Aluminum, barium, boron, chromium, lead, lithium, manganese, molybdenum, silver, strontium, titanium, vanadium	Traces	Traces

*Data from Macy, I. G., Kelley, H., and Sloan, R.: Bull. Nat. Res. Council, no. 119, 1950.
†Data from Rusoff, L. L.: Borden Rev. Nutr. Res. 25:17, 1964.
‡Skimmed milk.

larger amounts than sodium. Other elements present in milk include magnesium, sulfur, iron, copper, iodine, and zinc (Table 21-8). Although some elements are present only in traces, it must not be assumed that they are of no value. Only minute amounts of copper, for instance, are needed for hemoglobin formation. Iron, it is true, is present in too small an amount in milk to warrant the exclusive use of this food in later childhood. Iron-containing foods must supplement the diet. Milk is, however, the most practical and adequate source of calcium and phosphorus. Both of these are needed by all cells, but particularly by bones and teeth.

Vitamins. Milk contains most of the vitamins in greater or lesser amounts. The fat-soluble vitamins A, D, E, and K and the precursors of A and D are carried in the lipid fraction, while the water-soluble vitamins are found in the aqueous fraction. It is quite deficient in ascorbic acid and vitamin D and rather low in the B vitamins, except riboflavin and pantothenic acid, although human milk is richer in ascorbic acid than cow's milk. In order to enrich the milk with vitamin D, this factor must be taken just prior to or during lactation. Macy's group showed that the content of vitamins A and C also can be increased in human milk if the lactating woman is fed large amounts

Table 21-9. Vitamin contents of fresh mature human and cow's milk*

Vitamin	Concentration per 100 ml.	
	Human milk	Cow's milk
Vitamin A, μg.	54	37
Carotenoids, μg.	32	39
Vitamin D, U.S.P. units	0.4 to 10[†]	0.5 to 4[†]
Vitamin E (α-tocopherol), mg.	0.66	0.06
	0.10–0.48[‡]	
Vitamin K, Dam-Glavind units	26	100
Ascorbic acid, mg.	4.4	1.8[§]
Biotin, μg.	0.4	3.5
Choline, mg.	9	13
Folic acid (pteroylglutamic acid), μg.	0.01–0.22[‖]	0.02–0.4[‖]
Inositol, total, mg.	39	13
Nicotinamide, μg.	172	85
Pantothenic acid, μg.	203	350
Pyridoxine, μg.	11	48
Riboflavin, total, μg.	46.9	158[§]
Thiamine, total, μg.	15	42
Vitamin B_{12} (cyanocobalamin), μg.	0.01–0.16[‖]	0.32–1.24[‖]

*Data, except where otherwise noted, from Macy, I. G., Kelley, H., and Sloan, R.: Bull. Nat. Res. Council, no. 119, 1950.
[†]Data from Lawrence, J. M., Herrington, B. L., and Maynard, L. A.: Amer. J. Dis. Child. **70:**194, 1945.
[‡]Data from Harris, P. L., Quaife, M. L., and O'Grady, P.: J. Nutr. **46:**459, 1952.
[§]Very large losses of ascorbic acid and riboflavin may occur during the processing and delivery of cow's milk. Small losses of thiamine may also occur. The other vitamins are known to be stable.
[‖]Data from Collins, R. A., Harper, E. E., Schreiber, M., and Elvehjem, C. A.: J. Nutr. **43:**313, 1951.

of these vitamins in a multiple-vitamin supplement. Milk is an excellent source of vitamin A, riboflavin, and pantothenic acid. Babies usually are given orange juice or tomato juice, or ascorbic acid itself, to furnish additional C, and there are various methods of increasing their vitamin D intake. Pregnant and lactating women on high-milk diets also require additional vitamins C and D as well as the B complex. Table 21-9 gives a comparison of the vitamin contents of human and cow's milk. Since the amounts of the different vitamins vary with diet, exposure to sunlight, and other factors, these figures are to be considered as typical rather than absolute values.

Enzymes. A catalase, a peroxidase, and a phosphatase are present in milk. It is doubtful whether these have any significance, but the presence of any active enzymes is evidence that the milk has not been pasteurized or sterilized.

Sterilization and pasteurization It is practically impossible to obtain sterile milk from the mammary gland of a cow or of a woman unless bacteriologic technique is employed and the first portion obtained, which washes out the organisms present in the ducts of the nipple, is discarded. Modern dairy practice, with extreme emphasis on cleanliness and the use of sterile containers, has reduced the bacterial count greatly. Nevertheless, public health authorities do not recommend raw cow's milk for human consumption. Milk is seldom sterilized for ordinary sale and use but is commonly rendered safe by pasteurization. In pasteurization the milk is heated to 60° to 63° C. and is held at that temperature for 30 minutes or is kept at 72° C. for 15 seconds. It is then cooled rapidly and kept cold until delivered. Pasteurized milk is free of pathogenic bacteria, although it usually contains other microorganisms. The pathogenic organisms that cause tuberculosis, undulant fever, diphtheria, the streptococcal diseases, septic sore throat, scarlet fever, typhoid fever, dysentery, and others are destroyed by this treatment. Pasteurization, of course, is not insurance against subsequent contamination. In order to prevent bacteria from multiplying, all milk should be kept at 10° C. or below. In pasteurization some precipitation of calcium phosphate occurs and about 10% of thiamine and 30% of ascorbic acid are destroyed. Boiling raw milk from 1 to 3 minutes is somewhat more effective than pasteurization insofar as the bacteria are concerned. It has the same effect on the vitamins and produces a film that contains a small amount of the nutritive constituents. The flavor of boiled milk is different from pasteurized and is not relished by some people. True sterilization of milk usually requires heating to 100° C. on several successive days or a single application of heat at 120° C. for 30 minutes under 15 lb. pressure.

Film formation. When milk is heated to about 60° C., a film forms on the surface. Upon removing the pellicle, cooling, and reheating, a second film forms. If the heating is done in a closed vessel, no such skin forms even at 100° C. The film consists of proteins, calcium phosphate, and some enmeshed fat globules. The mechanism of this phenomenon is rather complicated. At the air-liquid interface there occurs a concentration of the proteins, because the water evaporates faster than it can be replaced by diffusion. The proteins thus form a semisolid layer in which fat globules are enmeshed. This retards the diffusion of water still more. There then occurs an irreversible precipitation of proteins, the casein micelles being destabilized and the albumin and globulin being denatured or coagulated to some degree. If the boiled milk is to be used for infant feeding, the film may be removed and discarded. The loss in nutritive value is slight.

Passage of foreign substances into milk. It is well known that cow's milk acquires distinctive and often unpleasant flavors if the cow feeds on some strong-tasting food, e.g., turnips, onions, garlic, wild carrots. The volatile oil or other flavor of the food is absorbed and finally passes through the mammary gland. The same is true of human milk, and the possibility of ingestion of toxic substances by the infant via the mother's milk should be mentioned. Among the substances known to get into human milk after they have been administered to the mother are opium, morphine, alcohol, barbiturates, ergot, cascara, thiouracil, salicylates, iodides, bromides, arsenic, bismuth, antimony, zinc, lead, mercury, and iron. However, few of these have been found in high enough concentrations to be injurious to the infant. Barbiturates, iodides, and bromides are among the latter. Thiouracil is the only substance known to appear in milk at a higher level than in blood or urine. Nicotine does not pass through the mammary gland under moderate smoking conditions, and the amounts of alcohol and caffeine that may be present are of no importance. In cases of jaundice, neither bile pigments nor bile salts are found in the milk.

Milk products   From a commercial standpoint, the fat of milk is the most valuable constituent of milk. This is concentrated in cream and butter. If milk is allowed to stand, the cream rises and may be poured or skimmed off. Centrifuging is the commercial procedure for doing this. The fluid remaining is *skimmed milk.* From Table 21-10, it may be seen that skimmed milk has almost the same composition as whole milk except for a low fat content. In diets designed to reduce body weight, skimmed milk is useful in providing calcium and good proteins, while at the same time limiting the caloric intake. It must be remembered, however, that skimmed milk is deficient in vitamin A but contains the same amount of water-soluble vitamins as whole milk. Cream contains the same constituents as milk but in different proportions. Ordinarily, cream is sold in two grades: 20% fat in thin cream and 40% in thick or whipping cream. Butter is produced by churning or agitating milk or cream. Usually the milk or cream is first soured by lactic acid bacteria in order to permit the fat globules to coalesce more easily. Since the vitamins A and D of milk are dissolved in the fat, cream and butter are much better sources of these vitamins than is milk.

The fluid left after milk is churned in butter-making is called *buttermilk.* It differs very little in food value from skimmed milk, but since it has been soured, some of the casein may be precipitated. Buttermilk is the most popular fermented milk used in the United States, but frequently that purchased is really cultured buttermilk. This is made by treating raw or pasteurized milk (skimmed or whole milk) with lactic acid bacteria cultures and then breaking up the curd into fine particles. Such milk may have almost the same food value as whole milk. Various other types of fermented milk are used here and abroad. Kefir, kumiss, and yoghurt are widely used in central Asia

Table 21-10. Composition of dairy products*

	Protein (per-cent)	Fat (per-cent)	Carbo-hydrate (per-cent)	Water (per-cent)	Cal-ories (per 100 gm.)	Calcium (per-cent)	Phos-phorus (per cent)	Iron (per-cent)
Milk, whole fresh, cow's	4	4	5	87	69	0.120	0.093	0.0002
Milk, skimmed fresh	4	<1	5	91	36	0.122	0.096	0.0002
Cream, 20%	3	20	4	73	192	0.086	0.067	0.0002
Cream, 40%	2	35	3	59	337	0.086	0.067	0.0002
Buttermilk, churned from cream	4	1	5	91	37	0.105	0.097	0.0003
Buttermilk, cultured skimmed	4	<1	5	91	36	0.105	0.097	0.0003
Milk, condensed, sweetened	8	8	55	27	327	0.300	0.235	0.0006
Milk, evaporated unsweetened	7	8	10	74	139	0.316	0.244	0.0007
Milk, kumiss	3	2	6	90	265			
Milk, malted, dry	15	9	71	3	418			
Milk, powdered, skimmed	36	1	52	4	359	1.220	0.960	0.0030
Milk, powdered, whole	26	27	38	4	496	0.900	0.696	0.0017
Milk, whey	1	<1	5	93	27	0.044	0.035	
Butter	1	81	<1	16	733	0.015	0.017	0.0002
Cheese, cottage, skimmed milk	19	1	4	74	101	0.124	0.177	0.0003
Cheese, Swiss	29	31	2	34	404	1.086	0.812	0.0013
Ice cream, average commercial	3	15	18		219	0.08	0.06	0.002

The figures in the first five columns are given to the nearest whole number.
* Data from Hawley, E. E., Carden, G., and Munves, E.: The art and science of nutrition, ed. 4, St. Louis, 1955, The C. V. Mosby Co.

and Turkey; acidophilus milk is marketed in the United States. These fermented-milk products, containing as they do, tremendous numbers of lactic acid–producing bacteria, are believed by some people to replace the intestinal bacteria with lactic acid organisms. This, it is assumed, is favorable to health. No doubt, the fine soft curd of these fermented milk products is more easily digested than the tough curd that usually forms when cow's milk reaches the stomach, but whether this curd promotes growth of a more favorable flora in the large intestine is still an open question.

When milk is clotted by rennin or acid, it becomes *curds* and *whey*. The whey, which is the fluid that may be pressed or squeezed out, carries with it a large portion of the lactose, some of the albumin and globulin, and part of the water-soluble vitamins and minerals. The solids or curds become *cottage cheese*. Cheese may be made from cream, whole milk, or skimmed milk. The various types and flavors of cheeses depend on the type of milk, the method and degree of curing or aging, and the various organisms that bring about curing. Some particular varieties are prepared only in certain localities where, it is asserted, the required organisms thrive. Cheese is an excellent source of protein and usually a good source of fat, calcium, and other minerals.

Homogenization is the process of reducing the size of the fat globules of milk by physical means. This is accomplished by forcing the milk through very small apertures under high pressure. The fat globules of *homogenized milk* are approximately one sixth their original diameter. Such fat does not rise as cream when the milk stands. Having a greater surface area, the fat of homogenized milk is more rapidly digested by lipases. Furthermore, with such an increased fat surface, the amount of protein encasing the globules is increased. This tends to make less protein available in solution when clotting occurs and a softer curd is formed. Cream may be homogenized also.

The large amount of water in milk, over 85%, has led to several methods of concentration in order to have less bulk for transportation and at the same time to improve the milk's keeping qualities. *Evaporated milk* is cow's milk that has had about 60% of the water removed and is then homogenized and sterilized in hermetically sealed cans. It contains no added substance. *Condensed milk* is reduced to about the same concentration as evaporated milk, but sugar, which acts as a preservative, is added. Evaporated milk is heated to a higher temperature than condensed milk to ensure preservation.

Dry milk contains no added substance. It may be prepared from whole, half-skimmed, or skimmed milk. The two principal methods of drying are the roller process and the spray process. In the former, thin layers of milk pass over heated rollers in vacuo and the dried milk is scraped off the rollers. In the spray process the partially evaporated milk is sprayed into warm drying chambers. Some dried milk products are irradiated to increase their vitamin D value. The food values of the concentrated and dried milks are comparable to the milks from which they were obtained, the only loss being in the heat-labile vitamins. The flavors of these products vary somewhat but are agreeable to most people. The high sugar content of condensed milk must be remembered in advising its use in infant feeding and for diabetics.

The small amount of vitamin D in milk produced by cows on ordinary rations and the fact that many physicians consider vitamin D to be best assimilated when dispersed in milk have created a demand for *vitamin D milk*. This is pasteurized, pasteurized-homogenized, evaporated, condensed, or dried milk that has been enriched with vitamin D. To meet the requirements of acceptance by the Council on Foods and Nutrition of the American Medical Association, vitamin D milk must contain not more than 400 U.S.P. units of vitamin D per quart. Vitamin D milks may be produced by (1) mixing into the milk a purified concentrate of natural vitamin D or a pure crystalline vitamin D_3 or D_2, (2) irradiating the milk, or (3) feeding irradiated material (usually yeast) to the cow. The latter two methods are rapidly disappearing from commercial practice. The first method makes possible a milk with a vitamin D content of 400 U.S.P. units per quart. The vitamin D content of milk may be increased by adding two activated sterols: 7-dehydrocholesterol, found in animal fats, or ergosterol, found in plants. The 7-dehydrocholesterol is changed to vitamin D_3 (cholecalciferol) when irradiated; the ergosterol is changed to vitamin D_2 (ergocalciferol). Many pediatricians, though not all, prefer vitamin D_3 to vitamin D_2 perhaps because calciferol (D_2), in large doses, has been found to be slightly more toxic in animal experiments.

Nutritive importance of milk Although the nutritive importance of milk has been stressed frequently in this chapter, a few additional points may be taken up. Milk is the ideal food for the infant, an excellent food for the growing child, and a very good food for the adult. Its proteins are among the best biologically, and its carbohydrate and fat are easily digested and assimilated. It also contains 0.1% to 0.2% citrate, the significance of which is not known. Regarding minerals, it is a dependable source of calcium and phosphorus. Vitamin A and riboflavin are present in large amounts and other vitamins to a lesser extent. Nutritionists generally agree that growing children and adults should drink some milk every day. If 1 quart of milk is included in the daily diet, more than the usual calcium requirement is provided as well as two thirds of the phosphorus, one third of vitamin A, and the full quota of riboflavin. A pint per day very nearly meets requirements and should be the minimum daily intake of each individual.

However, milk should not be the sole article of diet for adults or even for infants or children. To meet the energy requirements of an adult, a very large volume would be needed, putting an undue strain upon heart and kidney. It would also provide an unnecessarily large amount of protein. Furthermore, forcing children to drink inordinate amounts of milk is likely to curb their appetites to such an extent that they cannot ingest the required amounts of other essential foods. On the other hand, the belief that milk impairs prolonged athletic performance is not true. Milk has no effect one way or the other. It is deficient in some of the vitamins, but its greatest defect is a low iron content. Weanling rats fed an exclusive milk diet develop a nutritional anemia as a result of the deficiency of iron and also of copper. The addition of small amounts of these two minerals to the milk either cures or prevents the anemia. Breast-fed babies occasionally develop this type of anemia, the nutritional anemia of infancy, particularly those prematurely born.

Considerable interest has developed in the past few years regarding the nutritional value of *filled* and *imitation* milks, which have appeared on the market. The fat apparently used in many of these products appears to be hydrogenated coconut oil, a fat notably high in saturated fatty acids and low in essential unsaturated fatty acids. The use of this type of fat for infants and children, and perhaps also for adults on fat-modified diets, appears to be open to question. Also, in some filled milks, isolated proteins are added in unspecified amounts. These points should be carefully considered before contemplated use of imitation milks in place of natural milk, with its recognized balance of nearly all nutrients now known to be essential to man.

References

GENERAL

Botelho, S. Y., Brooks, F. P., and Shelley, W. B.: The exocrine glands. Symposium of the XXIV International Congress of Physiological Sciences, Philadelphia, 1968, University of Pennsylvania Press.

Cowie, A. T., and Kon, S. K., editors: Milk:

its physiology and biochemistry, New York, 1961, Academic Press, Inc.

Folley, S. J.: The physiology and biochemistry of lactation, Springfield, Ill., 1961, Charles C Thomas, Publisher.

Gray, C. H.: Bile pigments in health and disease, Springfield, Ill., 1961, Charles C Thomas, Publisher.

Macy, I. G., Kelley, H., and Sloan, R.: The composition of milks, Bull. Nat. Res. Council, no. 119, 1950.

Myer, J. S.: Life and letters of Dr. William Beaumont, St. Louis, 1912, The C. V. Mosby Co.

Rusoff, L. L.: The role of milk in modern nutrition, Borden Rev. Nutr. Res. **25**:17, 1964.

Schiff, L., Carey, J. B., and Dietschy, J., editors: Bile salt metabolism, Springfield, Ill., 1969, Charles C Thomas, Publisher.

With, T. K.: Bile pigments, New York, 1968, Academic Press, Inc.

SPECIAL

1. Pigman, W., and Reid, A. J.: J. Amer. Dent. Ass. **45**:325, 1952.
2. Woodward, E. R., and Dragstedt, L. R.: Physiol. Rev. **40**:490, 1960.
3. Janowitz, H. D., and Hollander, F.: Gastroenterology **17**:591, 1961.
4. Davenport, H. W.: Ann. Rev. Physiol. **21**:183, 1959.
5. Grisolia, S., and Schloerb, P. R.: Physiol. Chem. Phys. **1**:251, 1969.
6. Miller, D., and Crane, R. K.: Amer. J. Clin. Nutr. **12**:220, 1963.
7. Engsted, L.: Acta Med. Scand. **159**:suppl. 332, 1957.
8. Schmid, R., et al.: Proc. Nat. Acad. Sci. **61**:748, 1968.
9. Black, M., and Billing, B. H.: New Eng. J. Med. **280**:1266, 1969.
10. Lester, R., and Troxler, R. F.: New Eng. J. Med. **280**:779, 1969.
11. Schmid, R.: Bull. N.Y. Acad. Med. **35**:755, 1959.
12. Lester, R., and Schmid, R.: New Eng. J. Med. **270**:779, 1964; Feingold, D. S., and Parris, E. E.: New Eng. J. Med. **279**:143, 1968; Gartner, L. M., and Arias, I. M.: New Eng. J. Med. **280**:1339, 1969.
13. Small, D. M.: New Eng. J. Med. **279**:588, 1968.
14. Arias, I. M., et al.: J. Clin. Invest. **42**:913, 1963.
15. Samuelson, E. P.: Int. Dairy Fed. Ann. Bull. part 2, p. 27, 1962.
16. Turkington, R. W., and Hill, R. L.: Science **163**:1458, 1969.

CHAPTER 22

URINE

The main function of the kidneys is the excretion of urine. Kidneys possess certain other functions also — the formation of ammonia to aid in the neutralization of acids and the secretion of some physiologically active compounds. Primarily, however, the kidney is an excretory organ.

The functional unit of the kidney is the *nephron*, which consists of a glomerulus, a convoluted and collecting tubule, and blood vessels (Fig. 22-1). The afferent arteriole goes to the glomerulus, carrying blood to the tuft of capillaries that supply it, then continues on as an efferent arteriole. It breaks up into capillaries again, which are the sole means of blood supply to the tubules. The afferent arteriole enters the glomerulus, and the glomerular filtrate is formed. This is a fluid, very low in protein, formed by the process of ultrafiltration. The concentration of solutes in the glomerular filtrate is similar to the arterial plasma except for the protein. As a result of this filtration, the blood is more concentrated when it leaves the glomerulus in the efferent arteriole. Its protein content is consequently increased, and, therefore, its osmotic pressure is greater. This blood surrounds the tubules as the glomerular filtrate flows through them. Most of the filtrate is now reabsorbed through the tubule cells. About 90% of the water is reabsorbed as a result of the difference in pressure. Glucose is reabsorbed after enzymic phosphorylation in the tubular epithelial cells. Sodium, potassium, amino acids, and other substances are also reabsorbed, apparently by specific transport mechanisms. Carbonic anhydrase controls the carbon dioxide–bicarbonate transfer. Urea, creatinine, uric acid, and certain other compounds are not absorbed proportionally to the fluid. At the same time, certain solutes are added to the fluid by an excretory function of the tubules. Among these are hippuric acid, other derivatives of benzoic acid, and still other organic waste products. Of the 10% of water remaining, much is reabsorbed as a result of the action of ADH, elaborated by the posterior lobe of the pituitary gland, except for 1% to 2%. This small fraction, 1% or 2% of the glomerular filtrate, flows into the urinary bladder as urine. Since an adult excretes from 1000 to 1800 ml. in 24 hours, evidently the total glomerular filtrate must be in the neighborhood of from 50,000 to 180,000 ml. The end result, urine, is generally a fluid having an osmotic pressure effect greater than that of the body fluids. In this way the

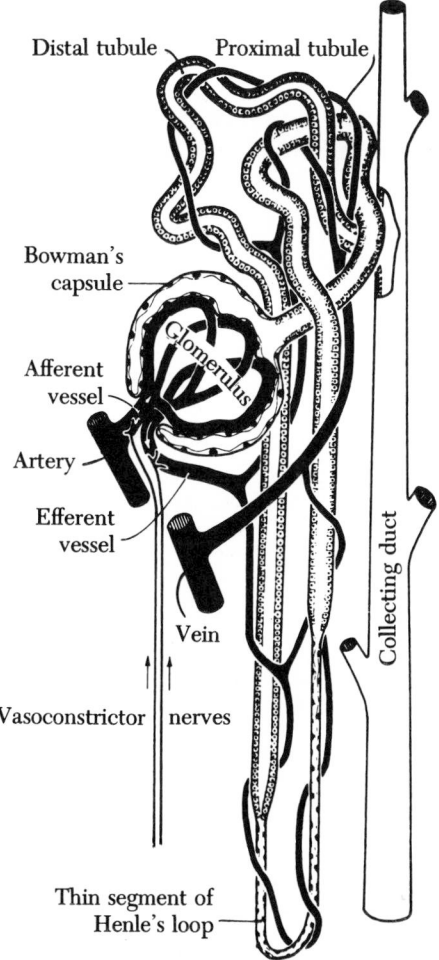

Fig. 22-1. Diagram of a single nephron. (From Amberson, W. R., and Smith, D. C.: Outline of physiology, Baltimore, 1939, The Williams & Wilkins Co.)

kidney conserves water. However, the kidney may also produce a more dilute urine. The tubular cells may actively reabsorb most of the solutes of the glomerular filtrate. This occurs, for example, after the ingestion of large quantities of water and leads to *water diuresis*, with the formation of an extremely dilute urine.

The plasma electrolytes pass through the glomerulus, but some potassium leaves the blood by way of the tubules, perhaps by active secretion. Sodium and chloride ions predominate in the glomerular filtrate just as they do in the plasma. As the glomerular filtrate flows through the tubules, the electrolytes are reabsorbed into the blood along with the water. They, like the water, are not absorbed completely, however. Part of the absorption of sodium chloride is brought about through the influence of hormones of the adrenal cortex, aldosterone and deoxycorticosterone. The tubules are the more particular site of action of these hormones.

Diuresis, the increased secretion of urine, is brought about chiefly by a failure of the tubules to reabsorb their usual quota of the glomerular filtrate. Sodium salts and urea exert diuretic effects. After they filter through the glomerulus, they increase osmotic pressure to such an extent that less filtrate is reabsorbed by the tubules. There are some diuretics, e.g., organic mercurial compounds, that may exert their action on the enzymes in the tubular cells, preventing the absorption of sodium salts and hence of water.

Recent studies[1] indicate that sodium- and potassium-activated adenosine triphosphatase, in the renal medulla and cortex, plays an important role in the urine-concentrating mechanism. If the enzyme is inhibited with *digoxin*, impaired concentrating ability with natriuresis occurs.

The urine thus formed carries off (1) water and salts in such amounts as to maintain the normal equilibria between the extracellular and intracellular fluids, (2) acids or bases to maintain a normal acid-base balance, (3) waste products, (4) toxic and detoxicated substances, and (5) other substances that are present in the blood in excessive amounts, if they can be so excreted.

GENERAL CHARACTERISTICS

Although it is frequently desirable to obtain and analyze casual specimens of urine, or the excretory output for short periods, it is usually customary to examine 24-hour specimens in order to have a "yardstick" for comparison and study. The physical characteristics usually noted in examining such a specimen are volume, turbidity, color, odor, specific gravity, and reaction.

Color. The color of normal urine is amber yellow, which is a difficult color to reproduce artificially in a fluid or to determine colorimetrically, because it results from a mixture of natural pigments that are not always produced in the same proportion. The principal pigment is *urochrome*, which is yellow. This is a compound of urobilin and urobilinogen with a peptide. Small amounts of *uroerythrin, coproporphyrin* and *uroporphyrin* are usually present. Uroerythrin, which is possibly derived from the melanins, is red; uroporphyrin and coproporphyrin are brownish red iron-free pigments arising from heme metabolism. *Riboflavin* and one of its metabolic products, *uroflavin*, may be present and give a greenish fluorescence to the urine.

On standing, urine usually deepens in color, a result of colorless chromogens changing to colored compounds. Thus urobilinogen and urochromogen on oxidation yield urobilin and additional urochrome, respectively.

Abnormally, excessive amounts of some of the normal pigments, notably coproporphyrin and uroporphyrin may be excreted. The color may also be changed by the appearance of hemoglobin, urobilin, bile pigments, or melanins. Foreign pigments, e.g., dyes, occasionally are found following their administration. Among the chromogens that are not normal is homogentisic acid, which occurs in that inborn error of metabolism known as alkaptonuria. In this condition the urine, when passed, is of normal color but assumes a smoky or blackish hue on standing. The darkening begins at the top, from exposure to oxygen, and travels downward. Homogentisic acid is a product of the incomplete metabolism of tyrosine and phenylalanine, as shown previously (p. 373). Porphyrinuria occurs in porphyria, an unusual hereditary disorder of heme metabolism. In addition to excessive porphyrin excretion in this disorder, there are clinical manifestations involving the cutaneous, gastrointestinal, and nervous systems. This state is to be distinguished from simple porphyrinuria seen in toxic and disease conditions, e.g., lead poisoning, chronic liver disease. The urine may be pink to brown, or at times it may have a normal color when voided and darken only on exposure to light. The specimens exhibit a characteristic pink to red fluorescence when exposed to ultraviolet light. Porphyrins are present in normal urine but in such small amounts that they are not detectable in ultraviolet light and do not contribute to its color.

Volume. The rate of secretion of urine is not constant and depends on a number of factors. Normally more urine is secreted during the day than at night, but this is reversed in the case of night workers. The food and fluid intake, the temperature and humidity of the atmosphere, and exercise are the chief influences. Young children excrete more urine in proportion to their weight than do adults. Emotional excitement also increases the volume secreted. The total output in a 24-hour period in the northern part of the United States averages from 1000 to 1500 ml.; in the South it is likely to be somewhat less. This difference is, of course, related to climate. In summer a day's output may be as low as 600 ml. because of the diversion of water to the skin and lungs. Exercise results in a similar diminution, for the same reason. Loss of large quantities of water in diarrheal discharges also lowers the volume of urine.

Foods contain varying amounts of water, and some water arises in the oxidation of foodstuffs. Salty and spicy foods, as a rule, induce diuresis, and certain beverages, e.g., beer, have a decidedly diuretic influence. Among the diuretic drugs is caffeine, so coffee and tea have this property. Urea has the same effect; hence a high-protein diet results in a larger output of urine.

Pathologically the volume of urine is increased as a result of injury to the posterior pituitary gland. Diabetes insipidus is a disease in which there is a deficient secretion of this gland. In diabetes insipidus, enormous volumes of urine are eliminated, with resulting intense thirst. An increased urinary output is designated *polyuria*. Polyurias are also seen in diabetes mellitus, because glucose is a diuretic; in malnutrition; in certain endocrine imbalances; and in some renal conditions. In fact, an increased flow of urine at night is frequently one of the earliest symptoms of chronic kidney disease. This is called *nocturia* and is defined as the passage of a volume of over 500 ml. of urine having a specific gravity below 1.018 during a 12-hour night period. This polyuria of the early stages of chronic glomerulonephritis is believed by some authorities to be an effort on the part of the kidney to compensate for the smaller number of healthy functioning renal units. Others, however, consider it to be a definite diminution of the ability of the tubules to reabsorb the water from the urine that has filtered through the glomerulus, even if this water is normal in quality and quantity. In later stages, because of the involvement of the glomerulus, urine volumes decrease. This is usually also the state of affairs in acute glomerulonephritis. A diminished excretion of urine is termed *oliguria*, and a cessation is known as *anuria*. Oliguria also occurs in fevers, cardiac conditions, and diarrhea. In fevers the explanation is that there is a shift in the water balance, much of the water of the blood going into the tissues temporarily. From a concentrated blood (anhydremia), the kidney cannot remove water. With a weakened heart action the kidney is not supplied with a sufficient quota of blood and therefore does not secrete urine efficiently. In diarrhea the loss of fluid results in anhydremia, with consequent diminution in the secretion of urine. Other causes of dehydration, e.g., persistent vomiting, excessive sweating, similarly cause oliguria.

Specific gravity. The normal range of specific gravity is from 1.008 to 1.030, but usually it is within the limits of 1.015 to 1.025. In a general way, specific gravity varies inversely with the volume of urine excreted. In diabetes insipidus the specific gravity is very low, approaching 1.000, whereas in fevers, in which a small volume is excreted, the urine is concentrated and has a high specific gravity. An exception to the inverse ratio is diabetes mellitus. Here the volume is usually large and the specific gravity is high because of the glucose present.

Normally urine secreted at night has a higher specific gravity than that secreted during the day. A considerable variation also is seen from hour to hour throughout the day. In fact, a constancy or fixation of the specific gravity over any appreciable length of time is considered a sign of abnormal renal function. The principle involved is used in several concentration and dilution tests. In each of these, under a fixed set of conditions as regards the kind and amount of food and water taken, the urine is collected at specified intervals and the volume and specific gravity are determined. In the concentration tests, relatively dry food and little drink are given; a highly concentrated urine should be eliminated if the kidneys are normal. On the other hand, normal kidneys are able to secrete a large volume of urine of extremely low specific gravity when a considerable quantity of water is taken, as in the dilution tests. Abnormal kidneys cannot meet the same demands. Moreover, normally the specific gravity is not constant. For example, in the Mosenthal test, specimens are collected every 2 hours. The specific gravities of these samples show a difference of at least 10 points between the lowest and the highest in normal individuals. These tests are excellent criteria of the qualitative detection of renal dysfunction, but they do not give information regarding the extent of damage to the kidneys.

The specific gravity affords a method of estimating the total solids excreted in the urine. Actual determination of the total solids is time consuming and, because of volatile substances present, not very accurate. Consequently, a rough method based on a simple calculation is often used. The figure 2.6 (Long's coefficient) multiplied by the last two digits of the specific gravity at 25° C. is taken as the total solids in grams *per 1000 ml. of urine.* The adult usually excretes about 60 gm. of urinary solids in 24 hours. About 35 gm. of this are organic and 25 gm. inorganic.

Acidity. Normal human urine may be neutral, acid, or alkaline, having a pH range of from 4.8 to 7.5. It is usually acid, with an average pH of 6.0. The reaction is dependent on the many different inorganic ions as well as organic compounds of acid and basic character present in urine.

Protein diets give rise, in general, to highly acidic urine. This is chiefly due to the sulfur of the sulfur-containing amino acids, which is oxidized to sulfuric acid. The phosphoproteins, in addition, yield phosphoric acid, as do the nucleic acids and the phospholipids. Meats, therefore, are most productive of acid because of their high content of proteins, nucleic acids, and phospholipids. Alkaline urines are excreted when there is a predominance of vegetables and fruits in the diet, since, in general, these have an alkaline ash (p. 860). Thus the proportions of the various foods influence the reaction of the urine. There is another factor that plays an important part. It is the production of ammonia by the kidney, and this modifies the amount of titratable acidity. The total titratable acidity usually is equivalent to 150 to 500 ml. of 0.1 N acid per day.

Specimens of urine taken at intervals usually vary a great deal in their acidity. Soon after meals the urine secreted is quite alkaline for a while. This "alkaline tide" is explained by the fact that hydrogen ions are secreted in great quantity in the gastric juice. This would result in an alkaline blood if the kidneys did not secrete a preponderance of base at that particular time.

Urine must not be permitted to decompose during or after the collection of a 24-hour sample. If microorganisms begin to grow, they convert the urea to ammonia carbonate and the urine becomes ammoniacal. In addition to having an unpleasant odor, ammoniacal urine indicates a change in the distribution of the nitrogenous constituents, with some loss of nitrogen as volatile ammonia. To avoid this, the urine may be kept cold, or a preservative, e.g., toluene with thymol, may be added to the container at the start of the collection period.

Odor. Freshly voided urine or urine that has not been permitted to spoil has a not unpleasant odor, sometimes described as "aromatic." If urine does not have such an odor soon after it is passed, it may be in a pathologic state. A putrid or strongly ammoniacal smell points to decomposition by bacteria, probably occurring in the urinary bladder. Other odors arise from foods eaten, e.g., the unpleasant odor of methyl mercaptan after partaking of asparagus. Oil of sandalwood, cubebs, and other drugs give rise to characteristic odors in the urine. Oil of wintergreen (methyl salicylate) gives rise to a strong odor of evergreens (conifers). Perhaps the most important odor, and one that sometimes aids in diagnosis, is the fruity aroma observed when a large amount of acetone is present.

Turbidity. Normal urine is almost always perfectly clear and transparent when voided. On standing there is likely to separate out a faintly cloudy flocculence, believed to be nucleoprotein or mucoprotein, which is present only in traces, together with some epithelial cells. Turbidities may be of several types. Ammonium urate may precipitate from alkaline urine, whereas other urates are found only in acid urines. The former dissolve on acidification; the latter, on warming. Calcium phosphate and ammonium magnesium phosphate (triple phosphate) are seen only in alkaline urines, or they may form a cloudy precipitate from an alkaline urine on warming. They dissolve on acidification. It is, therefore, quite essential to be sure that a urine sample is slightly acidified when making a test for heat-coagulable proteins. Furthermore, the isoelectric points of most proteins that may appear in the urine

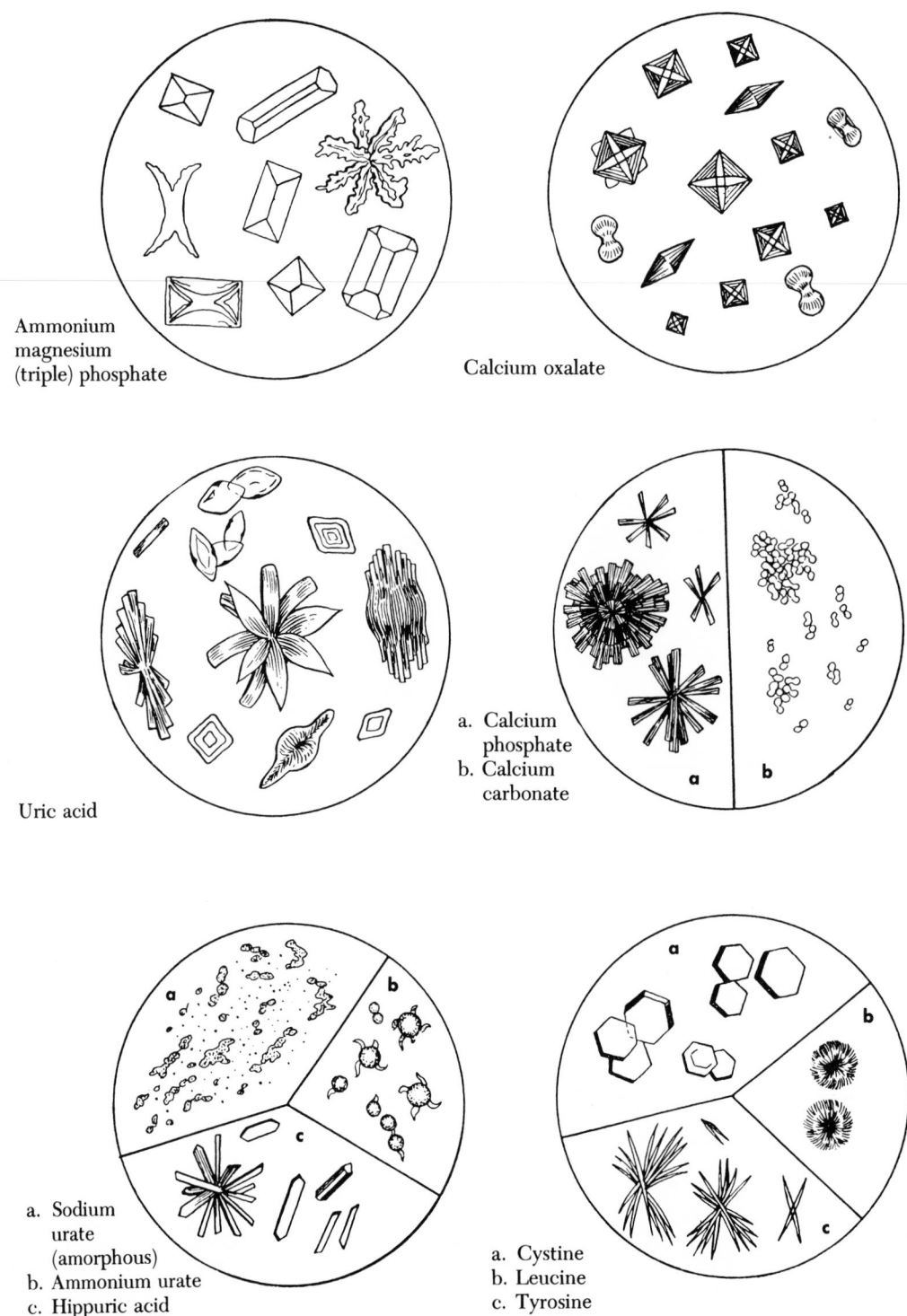

Fig. 22-2. Crystalline constituents found in urinary sediments. (From Myers, V. C.: Laboratory directions in biochemistry, St. Louis, 1942, The C. V. Mosby Co.)

are slightly acidic. Hence, adjustment of the pH also facilitates detection of these proteins, especially if only small quantities are present. If a clear urine is acidified slightly without heating and a precipitate is formed, the precipitate is either a mucoprotein or a nucleoprotein, since these proteins come down at an acid pH. A sediment in urine that does not dissolve on adding acid or on heating is most likely made up of cellular matter, i.e., pus, epithelial cells, or microorganisms.

A microscopic study of the sediment present in urine is often of great assistance to the clinician in diagnosis. Both crystalline substances and cells afford many clues that an expert microscopist can utilize to advantage. A number of these crystals sketched from typical fields are shown in Fig. 22-2. A small number of leukocytes are always, or almost always, present. Only an increase is pathologic, and the accumulation is then called *pus*. Pus is usually accompanied by protein and may arise from an inflammation of any part of the genitourinary tract. The presence of a small or moderate number of epithelial cells in the urine also is an ordinary occurrence, but a great number is abnormal. However, in the female, catheterized specimens are required for careful diagnostic work because fairly large numbers of erythrocytes and leukocytes and vaginal epithelial cells are likely to be present in uncatheterized urine.

GENERAL COMPOSITION

Normal urine is composed of the following: (1) water, (2) inorganic salts, (3) nitrogenous organic compounds, and (4) nonnitrogenous organic compounds.

The inorganic ions include the following:

Cations—Na^+, K^+, Ca^{++}, Mg^{++}, NH_4^+; traces of Fe^{++}, Fe^{+++}, Cu^{++}, Zn^{++}
Anions—Cl^-, $PO_4^=$, $SO_4^=$; traces of NO_3^-, HCO_3^-, SiO_2^-, Fl^-; also minute traces of many inorganic compounds

The nitrogenous organic compounds excreted in the urine are, with few exceptions, waste products. The most important ones are urea, uric acid, creatinine, creatine, hippuric acid, indican, purines other than uric acid, peptides, and amino acids.

Nonnitrogenous organic substances are less in amount and include traces of glucose, glucuronic acid, cholesterol, and the ketone bodies; oxalates and salts of other organic acids, including six members of the citric acid cycle, namely, citric, aconitic, α-ketoglutaric, succinic, fumaric, and malic, and organic sulfur compounds.

Sulfur of urine Most of the sulfur of our diet is protein sulfur—from the amino acids cystine, cysteine, and methionine. Some enters the body also as chondroitin sulfate, and there are small amounts in other forms. It is excreted as sulfate and as neutral sulfur. Sulfates are both organic and inorganic. The former is called *ethereal sulfate*. There is no definite proportion among the three forms, the inorganic, ethereal, and neutral, but on an ordinary mixed diet from 79% to 84% of the total sulfur is excreted in the form of inorganic sulfate. The remainder is divided between the ethereal sulfates and the neutral sulfur; about 4% to 7% is ethereal sulfate and 16% to 21% is neutral sulfur.

The sulfur of the amino acids is mostly oxidized to sulfate, which combines with inorganic bases, for the most part, and, to a lesser extent, with organic compounds. These may be phenols, cresols, indoxyl, skatoxyl, or other compounds. Some are toxic, and the formation of the conjugated sulfates transforms them into easily excreted products. The reactions are analogous to that shown for the formation of indican from indoxyl on p. 735. Since the sulfates are derived from the sulfur-containing amino acids, the amount of total sulfate excreted is, in a general way, an index of the amount of protein metabolized, although not as accurate an index as the total nitrogen excretion. Hence the total sulfate and the total nitrogen of the urine generally run parallel.

The remaining fraction of urinary sulfur, the neutral sulfur, includes a variety of compounds having the sulfhydryl, sulfide, and thiocyanate groups. It would, accordingly, include sulfur-containing amino acids, e.g., cystine and any peptides containing them. Also in this fraction would be thiosulfates, taurine, ergothioneine, urochrome, and the thiazole part of thiamine. The amount excreted is largely independent of protein intake but is related to cellular protein catabolism.

Pathologically, sulfate excretion is increased when tissue protein catabolism is speeded up, as in acute fevers. Neutral sulfur excretion rises in cases of poisoning by cyanides and nitriles, because of the transformation of these compounds into thiocyanates and their excretion in that form. Chloroform and other anesthetics also increase the excretion of neutral sulfur. In cystinuria, naturally, this fraction is greatly increased.

Phosphorus The only phosphorus compounds found in urine in appreciable amounts are the derivatives of phosphoric acid. The total amount of phosphate eliminated in the urine varies with the amount of phosphorus in the food and the amount absorbed. Food phosphorus is contained in the phosphoproteins, phospholipids, nucleoproteins, and preformed phosphate. If calcium or magnesium ions are present in the intestinal tract in abundance at the same time as phosphate ions, insoluble calcium or magnesium phosphate is formed but is not absorbed. Other insoluble phosphates are also possible, and, consequently, the urinary phosphate may represent only 50% to 70% of the food phosphate. Most of the remainder goes through into the feces. The determination of the amount of phosphorus in urine is therefore of little value.

Certain major fluctuations of the urinary phosphorus that are of interest occur, however. In acidosis, phosphate excretion may rise (unless the kidney is incapable of secreting it, as may be the case in nephritis). This is a direct effort of the organism to get rid of hydrogen ions, preserve its base as far as possible, and maintain the normal pH. An increased elimination of phosphate is one of the first events in hyperparathyroidism, or after the administration of parathyroid hormone. Low urinary phosphate is likely to be associated with diarrhea, because the intestinal contents are hurried through the tract; with acute infections and nephritis, because of failure of the kidneys to function adequately; with pregnancy, as a result of the fetal requirement for phosphate; and with rickets and other bone diseases, in which there is a diminished absorption or increased intestinal elimination of phosphate. When insulin is administered, there is an increased requirement of phosphate for the formation of hexose phosphates. This results in a diminished urinary phosphate for a time, often followed by an increase.

Chloride   About 10 to 15 gm. of chloride (as NaCl) are ingested per day. Normally the amount eliminated in the urine is almost equal to that taken in. Next to urea, the chlorides of the urine are the chief solid constituents. Acid-base balance and water balance are intimately associated with the distribution and elimination of sodium chloride. As has been seen, the sodium may be retained in times of stress, to conserve base. This is evident in the last stages of such a condition as pyloric obstruction.

It should also be remembered that, as the filtrate formed by the glomerulus of the kidney is reabsorbed, much of the sodium chloride is absorbed. Sodium chloride is one of the threshold substances needed by the body and is therefore retained in fairly definite concentrations. Table 22-1 gives a number of the common constituents of blood and urine with their relative concentrations. Sodium, calcium, and chloride ions have about the same concentrations in both urine and blood, which indicates that these are retained normally through the reabsorption mechanism of the kidney. In the case of sodium and chloride, the evident result of this retention is a very large contribution to the osmotic pressure of the blood.

Deprivation of salt, as in salt-poor diets or in starvation, leads to a marked decrease in the volume of urine. It is the amount of chloride in the interstitial fluid that largely determines chloride and water excretion. Ordinarily the addition of salt to a diet results in the elimination of the excess within 48

Table 22-1. Relative concentrations of constituents of urine and blood*

Substance	Concentration in urine (milligrams percent)	Concentration in blood (milligrams percent)	Concentration ratio	Concentration in blood in renal insufficiency
Urea	2,000	30	67	Increased
Uric acid	60	2	30	Increased
Creatinine	75	2	37	Increased
Indican	1	0.05	20	Increased
Phosphate	150	3	50	Increased
Sulfate	150	3	50	Increased
Potassium	150	20	7.5	Slightly increased
Chloride	500	350	1.4	Not increased
Sodium	350	335	1	Not increased
Calcium	15	10	1.5	Not increased
Water			1	Not increased

*From Fishberg, A. M.: Hypertension and nephritis, ed. 5, Philadelphia, 1954, Lea & Febiger, p. 70.

hours. After a period of salt deprivation, such an excess will be retained until the volume and salt content of the interstitial fluid have been reconstituted.

An excessive loss of sodium chloride by way of the urine occurs in adreno-cortical insufficiency (Addison's disease). A clinical diagnostic test (Cutler's) is based on this fact. With a low-sodium and high-potassium diet for 3 days, the excretion of sodium by normal individuals averages 22 mg. per 100 ml. of urine on the third day, whereas that of patients having Addison's disease averages 206 mg. per 100 ml.

During the formation of the exudate in pneumonia, salt is removed from the other body fluids. Less salt is available, therefore, to the interstitial fluid, and both blood and urine chlorides drop. When the exudate is reabsorbed, the condition is reversed and larger quantities of chloride reappear in the urine.

Cations   Ammonium, sodium, and potassium ions leave the body chiefly by way of the urine. Calcium and magnesium are excreted both through the intestinal tract and through the urine, chiefly perhaps by the former route. Ammonium salts will be considered among the nitrogen compounds.

Urea   Urea is the diamide of carbonic acid and, as such, is represented by the formula $CO(NH_2)_2$. This simple formula is in accordance with many of the reactions of urea, including its preparation from ammonia and carbonic acid in vitro. Ammonia is caused to react with carbon dioxide, yielding ammonium carbonate. This is heated under pressure, liberating water and producing urea:

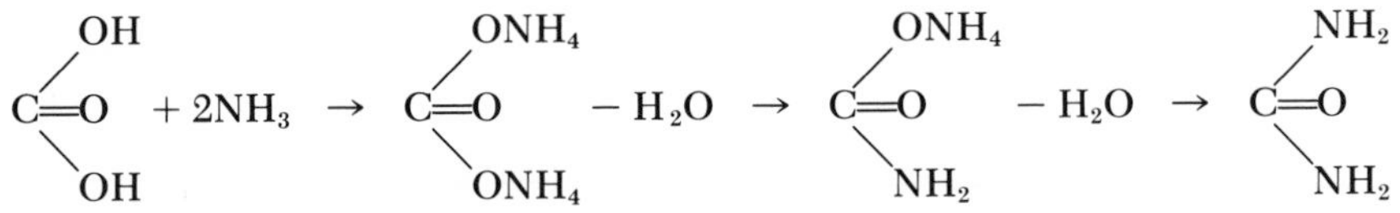

$$
\begin{array}{cccc}
\underset{\substack{\text{Carbonic} \\ \text{acid}}}{\overset{\text{OH}}{\underset{\text{OH}}{\text{C=O}}}} + 2NH_3 \rightarrow &
\underset{\substack{\text{Ammonium} \\ \text{carbonate}}}{\overset{\text{ONH}_4}{\underset{\text{ONH}_4}{\text{C=O}}}} - H_2O \rightarrow &
\underset{\substack{\text{Ammonium} \\ \text{carbamate}}}{\overset{\text{ONH}_4}{\underset{\text{NH}_2}{\text{C=O}}}} - H_2O \rightarrow &
\underset{\text{Urea}}{\overset{\text{NH}_2}{\underset{\text{NH}_2}{\text{C=O}}}}
\end{array}
$$

This formula, however, does not explain all the properties and reactions of urea, and a number of others have been suggested. Some of these are shown in the following diagram[*]:

Carbamide (Dumas)   Isocarbamide (Butlerov)

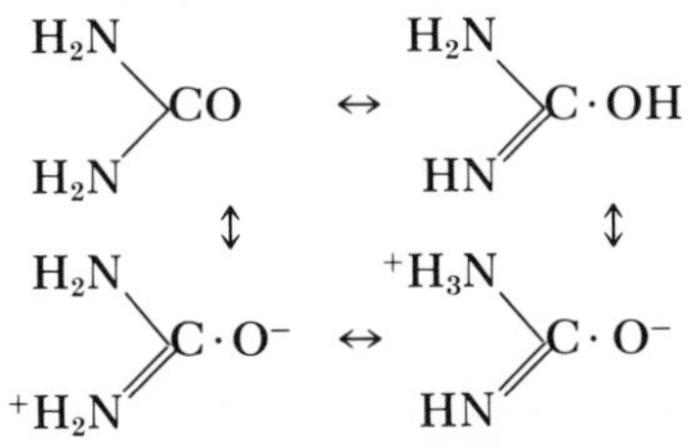

Mesocarbamide   Dipolar urea (Werner)

---

[*] From Fearon, W. R.: An introduction to biochemistry, ed. 2, St. Louis, 1940, The C. V. Mosby Co.

728

Urea is a white solid; it is odorless but has a bitter, salty flavor. It crystallizes in long prisms. Although urea is neutral, it reacts with acids as a monobasic amide. Urea nitrate and oxalate form characteristic crystals insoluble in excess of the acid. Urea is soluble in water and alcohol but not in ether or chloroform. The enzyme urease, which occurs in the jack bean and soybean, accelerates its conversion to ammonium carbonate:

$$CO(NH_2)_2 + 2\ H_2O \quad \rightarrow \quad (NH_4)_2CO_3$$

This is the basis for the quantitative determination of urea in blood, urine, or other fluids. The ammonium carbonate formed is easily measured in a number of different ways.

If dry urea is heated above its melting point, biuret is formed with the evolution of ammonia.

As has been seen, urea is the chief end product of protein metabolism and is formed in the liver (p. 359). It is excreted in the urine in larger amounts than any other substance (about 30 gm. per day) and makes up from 85% to 92% of the total nitrogen on a medium- or high-protein diet. On a low-protein diet the proportion (as well as the actual amount) of urea nitrogen is lower. It may be as low as 60% of the total nitrogen. The reason for this is that the urea output parallels protein metabolism whereas the nonurea fraction depends only in part on protein metabolism and in part on other factors. Fig.

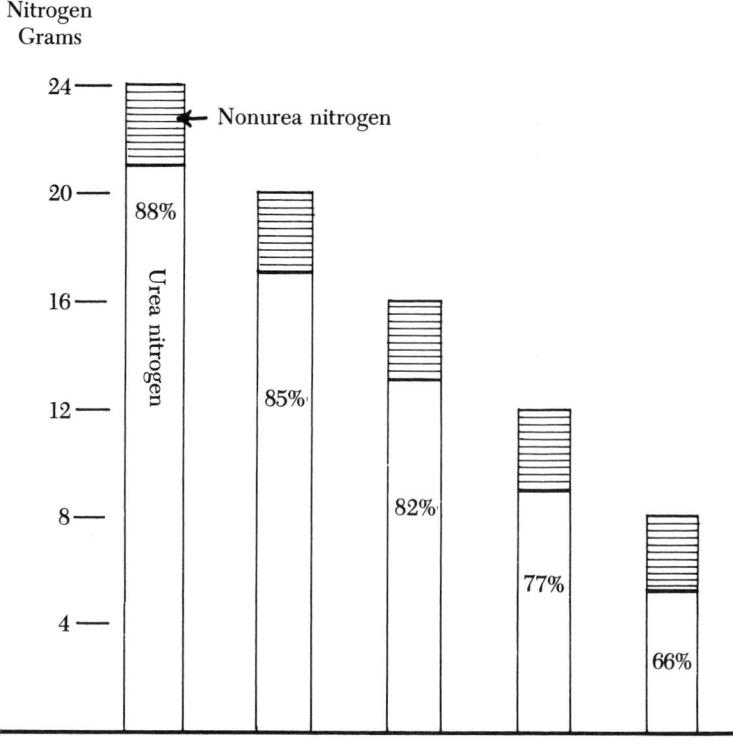

Fig. 22-3. Relation of urea nitrogen of urine to nonurea nitrogen at various nitrogen levels.

22-3 is an indication of how, with a decreasing total nitrogen, the urea nitrogen assumes a smaller and smaller proportional part of the total nitrogen.

Urea is nontoxic even when present in the blood in relatively large amounts. Consequently, high concentrations are regarded with concern not because of any inherent danger from the urea itself but rather they indicate inadequate excretory function. Indeed, in neurosurgery, hypertonic solutions of urea are sometimes administered to reduce intracranial pressure and brain volume. This procedure is also used in the treatment of glaucoma. Hyaluronidase facilitates absorption. Urea is a diuretic. It freely passes the glomerular filter and is passively reabsorbed to the extent of about 50% under normal conditions. *Passively* indicates by physical rather than by active physiologic means. Thus, urea diffuses from the relatively higher concentration in the tubules (due to the simultaneous reabsorption of water) to the lower one in the blood plasma.

Ammonia   The total amount of urinary ammonia, as ammonium salts, is approximately 0.7 gm. per day (0.5 to 0.8 gm.). It is formed in the kidney; its precursors have been discussed in Chapter 13. The production of ammonia aids in the neutralization of acids, about 67% to 75% of the hydrogen excreted in the urine being as ammonium (see text by Pitts, cited at end of chapter). By so doing, it conserves sodium and potassium, which are essential for important physiologic activities, e.g., buffer action. Thus, when an acid like acetoacetic (H^+A^-) is produced in large amounts, it passes into the blood, where it is buffered by sodium bicarbonate. Thus:

$$H^+A^- + Na^+HCO_3^- \rightleftarrows H_2CO_3 + Na^+A^-$$

Acetoacetic
acid

The H_2CO_3 is excreted in the lungs. To restore the lost $Na^+HCO_3^-$, the following occurs in the kidney:

$$Na^+A^- + NH_4^+HCO_3^- \rightleftarrows Na^+HCO_3^- + NH_4^+A^-$$

| Filtered through glomerulus | Secreted by tubule | Reabsorbed into blood | Excreted in urine |

Normally the urinary ammonia nitrogen comprises about 2.5% to 4.5% of the total nitrogen. In acidosis the amount rises above 5%. At one time this was the method of determining the presence and degree of acidosis clinically (p. 362). Since urea is easily decomposed and converted to ammonium carbonate, ammonia determinations must be made on fresh or sterile urine.

Acidified urine, on standing, shows a reddish crystalline deposit of uric acid. In fact, the normal acidity may be enough to permit this deposition to take place. The crystals assume a variety of shapes, e.g., wedges, prisms, dumbbells, rosettes (Fig. 22-2). The impure uric acid may be purified by dissolving in concentrated sulfuric acid and pouring into a large volume of cold water. Pure uric acid, or nearly pure, crystallizes out in white rhombic plates under these conditions. These crystals are odorless, tasteless crystalline substances that are insoluble in alcohol and ether, slightly soluble in boiling water, but quite soluble in alkalies and alkali carbonates. Their alkaline solutions have some reducing power on silver salts, copper salts, phosphomolybdates, and phosphotungstates. The reduction of phosphotungstate is utilized in the Folin method for the determination of uric acid.

When uric acid crystals are oxidized in alkaline solution, allantoin is formed; but in acid solution, alloxan is the product:

(lactam form)   Uric acid   (lactim form)
(2,6,8-trioxypurine)

Oxidation in OH⁻   Oxidation in H⁺

Allantoin   Alloxan

Allantoin is an end product of purine metabolism in many animals but not in man. Alloxan is of interest as a substance that can produce diabetes experimentally (p. 225).

The murexide test is a color test for uric acid and other purines in a dry state. The dry material in a small porcelain evaporating dish is treated with a drop or two of concentrated nitric acid and is then dried on a boiling water bath. A bright red color is produced in the presence of uric acid, which changes to purple if a drop of ammonium hydroxide solution is added at one side and to violet if sodium hydroxide is touched to another portion. This is a useful test in analyzing urinary calculi.

Although uric acid has no carboxyl groups, it acts as a weak, dibasic acid, because of the enolization of the three hydroxyl groups as shown in the above lactim form. This should be tribasic, but apparently the third hydrogen is not dissociated. Thus, we have salts of the type $C_5H_3NaN_4O_3$ and $C_5H_2Na_2N_4O_3$. Of the alkali salts, the ammonium are the least soluble; then, in increasing order of solubility, come sodium, potassium, and lithium. The fact that lithium urate is the most soluble gave rise to the use of "lithia waters" in the treatment of pathologic conditions ascribed to an excess of uric acid or uric acid deposits. The lithium was expected to expedite the elimination of uric acid as the more soluble lithium urate.

The total amount of uric acid eliminated per day is approximately 0.7 gm. The determination of uric acid in urine, however, is of little clinical value. Since uric acid is an end product of purine metabolism, it, of course, normally fluctuates directly with the purine intake. Diets rich in nucleoproteins, e.g., meats, particularly glandular meats, meat extracts, and legumes, lead to an increased excretion of uric acid. Caffeine, theophylline, and theobromine are not converted to uric acid. On a purine-free diet some of the acid is constantly excreted, amounting to about 0.2 to 0.5 gm. per day for an adult. This fraction is referred to as *endogenous* uric acid. If it is determined for a given individual, the excess above this figure, which he excretes on a purine-containing diet, is termed *exogenous*. Endogenous is supposed to refer to the metabolism of the body cells, and exogenous to the metabolism of food. Although metabolism cannot be divided in such an arbitrary way, the terms are often useful and are frequently employed. The uric acid excreted on a purine-free diet must arise from synthesis. This was discussed in Chapter 14.

The intensity of nuclear metabolism is frequently reflected in the uric acid output. Thus in leukemia, in which there is a high degree of nuclear catabolism, the uric acid excretion is markedly increased. However, it must be remembered that nucleoproteins occur in the cytoplasm as well as in the nuclei.

Creatine and creatinine In Chapter 13 the relation of creatine to creatinine was discussed in detail. Creatinine is a constant normal constituent of urine, whereas creatine is an inconstant one. Indeed, very little creatine is present in the urine of normal males. Creatinine is easily determined by a colorimetric method, based on Jaffe's reaction. This is the production of a red-colored substance when a creatinine solution is treated with picric acid and alkali. Creatine may be estimated, after it is transformed to creatinine, by the same reaction. This gives creatine plus creatinine. The transformation is accomplished by long boiling in acid solution or by heating in an autoclave at from 115° to 120° C. for 20 minutes. However, a simpler method is now available. It is based on the fact that ninhydrin forms an addition product with creatine that is highly fluorescent.[2]

Creatinine also yields a deep red color when a few drops of fresh sodium nitroprusside solution are added and the fluid is made alkaline. This color disappears after acidification with acetic acid. The importance of this test lies in the fact that acetone, a pathologic constituent, gives a similar color under the same conditions, which is not dispelled by acid.

The amount of creatinine eliminated varies chiefly with the weight of the individual, unless he is obese, i.e., it has some relation to the muscular mass. The creatinine coefficient for men is about 18 to 32 mg. per kilogram of body weight; for women, 9 to 26 mg. per kilogram. A round number for the daily excretion is a total of about 1.5 gm.

Amino acids Small amounts of amino acids, both free and combined, are excreted in the urine. Normal adult women excrete more amino acids than do men. The free amino acid amounts to about 1.4 mg. per kilogram for men and 2.3 mg. per kilogram for women, and there is some evidence for the existence of individual patterns of amino acid excretion. In other words, one person tends to excrete more of one amino acid and less of another than does another person. The sex difference does not hold for children, who excrete somewhat less than adults; infants and prematurely born babies excrete about four times as much per kilogram as do older children. Growing children excrete higher levels of hydroxyproline than do adults, reflecting an increased metabolism of collagen. Increased excretion of amino acids may occur pathologically. It is frequently observed in wasting diseases and in diseases affecting the parenchyma of the liver, presumably because of the inability of the liver to deaminate the amino acids. Thus, in acute yellow atrophy of the liver, the amino nitrogen level may rise to 40 mg. per 100 ml. urine. Even greater amounts have been found in the urine of a patient having hepatolenticular degeneration, a disease in which there is cerebral degeneration accompanied or followed by cirrhosis of the liver. Alanine, glutamic acid, and aspartic acid have been identified. The aminoaciduria of this condition (Wilson's disease) is now believed to be secondary to an abnormality in copper metabolism (excessive deposition of copper particularly in the liver and kidneys). An increased number of amino acids are excreted by patients suffering from muscular dystrophy and by their mothers and siblings. Among these are methionine or valine, isoleucine or leucine, methionine sulfoxide or sarcosine, methylhistidine, and cysteic acid. A generalized hyperaminoaciduria commonly occurs in lead intoxication and indicates damage to the renal tubules. Other abnormalities in which amino acids appear in urine in increased quantities include cystinuria, homocystinuria, histidemia, Hartnup's disease, tyrosinosis, and phenylpyruvic oligophrenia. These were discussed in Chapter 13.

Increased elimination of those amino acids normally present in urine is seen in the Fanconi syndrome, a condition in which there is a defect in renal tubular reabsorption. As a result there may be an increased output of any of a variety of substances, including amino acids, other organic acids (e.g., lactic), ketone bodies, glucose, ammonia, and phosphates.

More than 1 gm. of peptides is excreted daily by the average normal human adult, which accounts for about half the urinary amino nitrogen and about 2% of the total nitrogen.

Large quantities of β-aminoisobutyric acid are excreted in the urine of a small proportion (about 5%) of otherwise normal people. It has also been found in various pathologic states, sometimes with other amino acids. It is apparently due to a disturbance in the metabolism of thymine and dihydrothymine, which are precursors of this amino acid.

Hippuric acid   Hippuric acid is so called because it was first found in the urine of horses. It is benzoylglycine, a compound of benzoic acid and glycine.

| Benzoic acid | Glycine | Hippuric acid |

This is a physiologic metabolic reaction that results in the detoxication of benzoic acid and benzoates. The latter occur in vegetable foods or are derived from the oxidation of aromatic substances. About 0.7 gm. of hippuric acid per day is eliminated on the average diet, but deviations from this are to be expected, depending on the amount of precursors in the diet. Glycine is usually present in sufficient amounts to combine with any quantity of benzoates that are likely to be ingested. Cranberries contain from 0.05% to 0.09% benzoic acid, and other fruits and berries, smaller amounts. Some foods, e.g., catsups, are permitted by law to have 0.1% sodium benzoate added as a preservative. This is, of course, also converted to hippuric acid.

Hippuric acid can easily be isolated from urine containing considerable amounts of it by concentrating and then acidifying. Both uric and hippuric acids crystallize out, but they can be separated by the use of hot water, in which hippuric acid is more soluble than uric acid. After again concentrating and acidifying, the hippuric acid crystallizes out in long, rhombic prisms.

In man the synthesis of hippuric acid takes place almost entirely in the liver. It is accomplished by the action of hippuricase, an amidase that also hydrolyzes hippuric acid to its constituents. Both ATP and coenzyme-A are required for this biosynthesis. The synthetic action of these compounds has been used as a test for liver function but evidently is a test for only this particular liver function—not for all. Nevertheless, subnormal values have been claimed in patients with various types of hepatitis and other liver conditions but not in those with uncomplicated obstruction of the common bile duct; i.e., it may aid in differentiating between hepatic and obstructive jaundice.

The test consists of administering by mouth 5.9 gm. of sodium benzoate in 30 ml. of water 1 hour after a breakfast of toast and coffee. One half glass of water is then taken, the bladder is emptied, and the urine is collected hourly for 4 hours. Although the hippuric acid may be determined in each specimen, the total amount excreted is the most significant fact. During the 4 hours, a normal person excretes about 3 to 3.5 gm. of hippuric acid, whereas one with a poorly functioning liver does not form that amount. There are several methods of determination, the simplest one being to acidify with hydrochloric acid, filter off the hippuric acid, and dry and weigh it; or liver function may be estimated by titration with standard alkali. A correction must be made for the amount of hippuric acid remaining in solution.

Indican* Indican is the salt or salts of indoxyl sulfate. It is derived from indole, which, in turn, arises from the action of putrefying bacteria on tryptophan or of proteins containing it. This occurs in the large intestine. If any indole is absorbed, it undergoes a series of detoxication transformations, probably in the liver, and indoxyl is formed. This is conjugated with sulfate and neutralized to yield a salt. Indican is detected in the urine by oxidizing it to indigo blue. Obermayer's reagent, which is concentrated hydrochloric acid containing a small amount of ferric chloride, is a good oxidizer for this purpose. Chloroform is then added and, after shaking gently, the blue dye is taken up by the

---

*The term "indican" is employed here in the usual clinical sense. This is not accurate from the organic chemical standpoint, according to which, indican is a colorless glucoside, a combination of indoxyl with glucose, and is found in the indigo plant. This is hydrolyzed by enzymes to glucose and indoxyl. The indoxyl is then oxidized by the air to indigo. The clinical indican is more properly designated *indoxyl sulfate*, but long usage warrants the term "indican."

chloroform. The formation of indican and its oxidation to indigo blue are shown below:

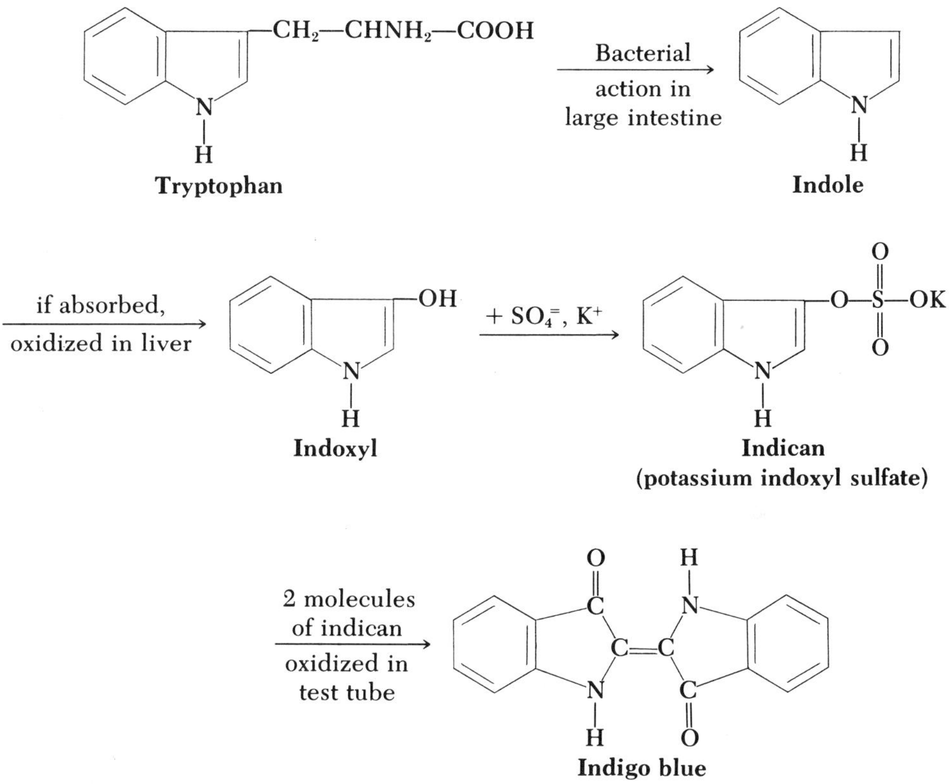

Tryptophan → (Bacterial action in large intestine) → Indole

Indoxyl → (+ SO$_4^=$, K$^+$) → Indican (potassium indoxyl sulfate)

if absorbed, oxidized in liver

(2 molecules of indican oxidized in test tube) → Indigo blue

The steps between tryptophan and indole are not known, but they are thought to occur in the manner shown on p. 379. It should be remembered that indole is not formed in the normal metabolism of tryptophan in the body. It is a product of putrefaction, usually in the intestine, but possibly in other locations. Normally from 4 to 20 mg. are excreted daily, but a qualitative reaction may not be positive for this amount. An increase in urinary indican is found when there is increased putrefaction, provided the products are absorbed. Putrefaction, you will remember, is the anaerobic bacterial decomposition of proteins. Among the pathologic conditions in which this is likely to be observed are hypochlorhydria, because of diminished bactericidal action of the gastric juice; intestinal obstruction and paralytic ileus, because peristaltic movement is inhibited; and obstructive jaundice, because the absence of bile produces voluminous feces with higher nutritive value for the bacteria. Indicanuria is rather rare in simple constipation and rather common in diarrheas. Furthermore, some individuals showing no gastrointestinal symptoms excrete large amounts of indican continually, whereas others, with or without such symptoms, have no indican in their urine. It is thus an index of absorption of putrefactive products but does not necessarily have any other significance.

If putrefaction occurs elsewhere than in the intestinal canal, indole is produced and absorbed and follows the same course. The bacterial decomposition of tissue proteins or of the proteins of body fluids, e.g., exudates, occurs in gangrene, abscesses, empyema, etc. and may lead to a marked indicanuria.

Nonnitrogenous organic compounds Small but variable amounts of a number of other organic compounds are found in the urine. The range of glucose in the urine of normal individuals is from 0.01% to 0.10%, but the quantity of glucose is in the lower part of that range, and a negative Benedict test is almost invariably observed in normal urines. Glucuronides are formed after the administration of camphor, chloral, menthol, phenol, morphine, aspirin, and other drugs. Some of these, you remember, also combine with sulfate, forming ethereal sulfates. The conjugated glucuronides reduce alkaline copper solutions and rotate the plane of polarized light to the left but are not fermented by yeast. The sex hormones are excreted as conjugated glucuronides; they are more soluble in water than the uncombined hormones.

The ketone bodies or acetone bodies are present in normal urine in very small amounts, less than 0.1 gm. in 24 hours. They consist of β-hydroxybutyric acid, acetoacetic acid, and acetone. These substances arise in normal fatty acid catabolism in the liver and are carried by the blood to the extrahepatic tissues, where their further degradation occurs. Their concentration in the blood is normally less than 1 mg. per 100 ml.

Oxalates are probably excreted constantly in minute amounts. If present in sufficient concentration, they unite with calcium to form insoluble calcium oxalate. This forms characteristic crystals of two types: dumbbell and octahedral (Fig. 22-2). An abnormally great amount of oxalates in urine, hyperoxaluria, seems to be an inborn metabolic error involving a failure to degrade glyoxylate normally, in consequence of which the excess of glyoxylate is converted to oxalate. There is some evidence[3] that tryptophan is a precursor of oxalates, particularly if a deficiency of pyridoxine exists.

Citrate also is a normal constituent of urine. About 0.2 to 1.2 gm. are found in adult urine in a 24-hour output under ordinary circumstances. It is increased following the administration of alkali or during a high-carbohydrate, high-fat dietary regimen. This extra citrate does not come from the citrate present in the bones but arises metabolically. The output of citrate also is related to changes in the steroidal reproductive hormones, but this may be an indirect effect. The significance of these facts is not apparent. Undoubtedly other organic acids occur in urine in small amounts, but, because they do not crystallize out or give characteristic reactions, they have not been studied extensively.

Vitamins, hormones, and enzymes The water-soluble vitamins are excreted by the kidneys in variable amounts. If excessive quantities are present in the diet, some, but not necessarily all, of the excess is eliminated. For certain vitamins the determination in urine has been used as a measure of deficiency; e.g., on an adequate diet the excretion of thiamine amounts to 90 μg. or more in males and 60 or more in females; on a deficient diet it is 66 and 43, or less, respectively. Sometimes saturation experiments have proved valuable, i.e., the response to the administration of a large dose of the vitamin. The excess eliminated reflects the degree of saturation previously present. However, the excess is not always eliminated quantitatively. Nicotinamide and its derivatives are found in the urine normally to the extent of from 1 to 2 mg. together with 5 to 15 mg. of the physiologically inert trigenelline, a methylated derivative. Only 27% to 42% of administered nicotinamide is eliminated in urine. On a normal average diet, there is ordinarily excreted from 15 to 28 mg. of ascorbic acid in 24 hours. In an avitaminosis, as would be expected, the excretion of the particular vitamin involved is diminished.

As mentioned previously, the sex hormones are secreted in the urine conjugated with glucuronic acid. A great deal of research has been done regarding the variations in excretion of the individual hormones normally and under various conditions; but a consideration of the subject is beyond the scope of this work. The urine of pregnant women contains a hormone, sometimes called the anterior pituitary–like substance (APL), that is secreted by the chorionic cells of the placenta. Urine containing this hormone, when injected into an immature female mouse, causes marked changes in the ovaries, and the procedure, known as the Aschheim-Zondek test, is used as a diagnostic test for pregnancy. A modification, the Friedman test, employing adult female rabbits, is now more generally used.

The enzymes present in urine are small in amount and of little significance. The enzymes of the blood are not likely excreted in appreciable quantities. Those found in urine probably arise from the disintegration of leukocytes and epithelial cells, which always occur in urine. An exception is diastase, which is found in the urine in fairly high concentration in acute pancreatitis. Another exception is urinary pepsinogen, which seems to vary directly with the secretion of gastric pepsin.

ABNORMAL CONSTITUENTS

Glucose. The term *glycosuria* is normally used for "glucose in the urine," although it really should mean "sugar in the urine," and *glucosuria* is a more accurate word in this connection. The other kinds of glycosuria include *pentosuria, lactosuria, galactosuria,* and *fructosuria.*

Perhaps mention should be made at this point of the availability of a more specific test for detecting glucose in urine by an enzymatic glucose oxidase procedure. This test is apparently not affected by the presence of other carbohydrates tested.[4] However, glucose oxidase–impregnated test papers may fail to detect glucose in certain types of abnormal urine,[5] e.g., from alkaptonuric or jaundiced patients. Epinephrine and ascorbic acid may also interfere with the reaction.

More than a trace of glucose in a 24-hour specimen of urine is pathologic Easily detectable amounts may be found in specimens voided soon after a high carbohydrate intake, but this alimentary glycosuria seldom gives a positive Benedict test when the entire day's output is pooled and analyzed. In diabetes mellitus the urine is usually light colored, with a higher specific gravity than the color would seem to warrant and a glucose content of from a few tenths of 1% up to 12% or 15%. Values as high as 250 gm. of glucose per day, nearly the entire carbohydrate intake for a 24-hour period, have been recorded in the literature.

The severity of the condition cannot be gauged by the percentage alone, since this can be modified by varying the volume of fluid ingested. It is the actual amount in grams excreted in 24 hours that is important. If the preformed and potential dietary carbohydrate is calculated and the amount of glucose excreted is subtracted from it, the remainder is the amount in grams of glucose utilized. This gives the physician a basis for determining what diet to prescribe and whether insulin is necessary. The blood sugar must also be determined and taken into account. Suffice it that if there is a normal renal threshold, i.e., the blood sugar does not rise above 160 mg. per 100 ml. before glucosuria results, the urinary output is a very good guide for treatment. In certain renal conditions—glomerulonephritis, nephrosclerosis, nephrosis, and renal glucosuria or "renal diabetes"—glucosuria may occur. This seems to result from a lowered renal threshold and is thus probably not due to any derangement in carbohydrate metabolism.

In addition to diabetes mellitus, glucosuria, as a result of high blood sugar, accompanies about a fourth to a third of the cases of hyperthyroidism. Hyperpituitarism and hyperadrenalism belong in the same category. Ether anesthesia, asphyxia, acidosis, and a variety of other conditions also lead to hyperglycemia and glucosuria.

Lactose. Lactose may be found in the urine of a considerable proportion of lactating women. *Lactosuria* seldom occurs during normal pregnancy. However, *glucosuria* is present in from 10% to 15% of all normally pregnant women, with no accompanying hyperglycemia. Since it usually disappears later, it is frequently assumed to be lactosuria. No such assumption is justified, and the urine should be analyzed carefully to determine what sugar is present. Sometimes an early diabetes is not diagnosed because no differential analysis or blood sugar determination is made. Lactose may easily be distinguished from glucose in that it is not fermented by baker's yeast, gives a positive mucic acid test, yields lactosazone, and reacts negatively with Barfoed's reagent. The amount of lactose eliminated is usually small.

Pentoses. An alimentary *pentosuria,* as a result of ingesting large amounts of prunes, plums, cherries, grapes, or their juices, is likely to be noted in normal individuals. Like alimentary glucosuria, it is temporary and has no significance. The excretion of a pentose in the urine has been reported in cases of morphine addiction. However, the most interesting type of pentosuria is the chronic type. This is an inborn error of metabolism, a recessively inherited anomaly that occurs in persons of all age groups. There apparently is a deficiency of the enzyme L-*xylulose dehydrogenase.* The individual is born with the condition, and no cure for it is known. However, the utilization of other carbohydrates is not impaired, the mortality rate of such individuals is not lowered, and the only danger to the person having this derangement is that it *might be mistaken for diabetes mellitus.*

The urinary pentose, L-xylulose (L-xyloketose), may be detected in urine by several methods. A rapid procedure is to add 0.5 ml. of benzidine in glacial acetic acid (1:25) to 0.1 ml. of urine. After heating to boiling, the test tube is cooled and 1 ml. of distilled water is added. A rose-pink color is positive for pentose. Lasker[6] showed that L-xylulose reduces Benedict's qualitative reagent more rapidly than does glucose. If 1 ml. of urine and 5 ml. of this reagent are mixed in a test tube and placed in a bath at 55° C., a yellow precipitate appears in 10 minutes in the presence of 0.1% or more of the pentose. Fructose gives the same reaction since it also is a ketose. These two can be easily distinguished from each other because fructose is fermented by yeast and forms glucosazone with phenylhydrazine. L-Xylulose is sometimes present in minute amounts in normal human urine.

Ribosuria has been observed in patients with progressive muscular dystrophies, myotonia congenita, and amyotonia congenita but not with myasthenia gravis or progressive neuropathic atrophy. A provisional test for ribose is a positive Benedict qualitative test (in the absence of other sugars) after 45 minutes' heating.

Other sugars. *Galactosuria* has been observed in nursing infants suffering from congenital galactosemia (p. 215) and also in adults, as well as infants, with hepatic disease. Galactose detection includes (1) reduction of alkaline copper solutions, (2) slight if any fermentation by baker's yeast, (3) positive Barfoed's test, and (4) positive mucic acid test. *Fructosuria* is said to occur occasionally in association with glucose, in severe cases of diabetes mellitus. There is also a rare condition, known as *essential* fructosuria or levulosuria, in which no other carbohydrate is involved. It may be regarded as another inborn error of metabolism, because persons are afflicted from birth. Insulin does not help the patient to utilize fructose. The site of the difficulty is believed to be the liver, where fructose normally is stored as glycogen. There appears to be a deficiency of the enzyme *fructokinase* or of *fructose-1-phosphate aldolase* in this condition. No other symptoms are peculiar to this condition, which does not lead to diabetes mellitus or to any change in the utilization of other carbohydrates. The method of detecting fructose was mentioned under pentosuria.

A seven-carbon sugar, D-mannoheptulose, appears in the urine of normal individuals after eating large amounts of avocado. Although some of this sugar is utilized, enough is excreted to be a possible source of confusion in diagnosis.

Fat. Alimentary *lipuria* may be observed when a large amount of fat has been ingested. Cod-liver oil in great quantity is an example. The urine is opalescent, or turbid, or even milky when voided. After standing, a peculiar creamy layer is seen at the top in those rare instances in which the fat content of the urine is high. The high blood fat (lipemia) that sometimes occurs in diabetes mellitus and lipoid nephrosis may lead to lipuria. The same results may be observed following fractures of the long bones with injury to the bone marrow, which is rich in fat, and any injuries to the subcutaneous layer of fat. Other conditions in which fatty urines may be seen are pyelitis, pyonephrosis, lipoid nephrosis, and alcohol or phosphorus poisoning.

Chyluria is the term applied to the condition resulting from an obstruction to the thoracic duct. This is even more infrequent than lipuria. The lymph vessels of the urinary tract become distended and burst, allowing lymph to pass directly into the urine. The appearance of the urine in chyluria is milky rather than opalescent.

Proteins. The amount of protein that is excreted in normal urine is insignificant. It probably consists of serum albumin, serum globulin, and muco-protein from the blood. A relatively small amount of a glycoprotein, termed the Tamm-Horsfall protein, is also found. It is secreted by the mucous glands of the normal genitourinary tract. It has a molecular weight of about 300,000. Apparently it serves to protect the epithelial membranes of the tract. Normal urine does *not* give positive reactions with any of the ordinary protein tests.

Abnormally, proteins appear in urine in varying amounts. The condition is commonly known as *albuminuria,* although the albumins seldom are found alone, and consequently the term *proteinuria,* which is being more and more generally employed, is to be preferred. The proteins that are found in the urine in kidney conditions are commonly believed to be plasma proteins that pass the damaged renal epithelium. The albumins, with the smallest molecules, pass most easily, globulins next, and fibrinogen least readily. How-ever, some authorities are of the opinion that the plasma proteins undergo a slight change and therefore are, in a sense, foreign proteins. Since foreign proteins are promptly eliminated by the kidney, these are eliminated in the same way.

Proteinurias may be grouped in two general classes: functional and organic. Functional proteinurias are those that are not related to a diseased organ. The amount of protein excreted is usually small, and the condition is ordinarily temporary. Violent exercise is an example. Soldiers, after long marches, and athletes, after strenuous contests, frequently have proteinuria. Here there may be a slight kidney damage to account for it, but the condition almost al-ways clears up. Cold bathing, leading to constriction of renal blood vessels and anoxia, is another cause, and occasionally an alimentary proteinuria oc-curs after excessive protein ingestion. In all of these, the subjects may be of any age. Orthostatic or postural proteinuria occurs chiefly in children or ado-lescents, usually 14 to 18 years of age. In these young people, the urine con-tains protein when they are in the upright position only. When they are lying down, it is free from protein. This is not an evidence of kidney disease but is probably due to some disturbance in the blood supply to the kidneys, leading to venous stasis and consequent anoxia. These benign proteinurias usually disappear within a few years, but sometimes they continue into adult life. Proteinuria is frequently associated with pregnancy, probably as a result of pressure interfering with the return of blood in the renal veins.

There are many pathologic conditions that cause organic proteinuria, which may be classed conveniently as (1) prerenal, (2) postrenal, and (3) renal.

The prerenal conditions causing proteinuria are those that are primarily not related to the kidney. In most cases, however, they affect the kidney in such a way as to render it more permeable to the protein molecule. For ex-ample, cardiac disease, by affecting the circulation of the kidney, leads to proteinuria. Any abdominal tumor or mass of fluid in the abdomen does the same, by exerting pressure on the renal veins. Fevers, convulsions, anemias, other blood diseases, liver diseases, and many other pathologic states belong in this category. An increased amount of urinary mucoproteins generally ac-companies elevated serum mucoprotein levels. These have been observed in patients with cancer, with highest values when the carcinomatous invasion was most widespread. Collagen disease and inflammatory conditions also have high mucoprotein levels.

Postrenal proteinurias are sometimes called *false* proteinurias, all others being *true*, because these are conditions in which the protein does not pass through the kidneys. They may be due to some inflammatory, degenerative, or traumatic lesion of the pelvis of the kidney, the ureter, bladder, prostate, or urethra. Bleeding into this tract, of course, contributes proteins. Urine containing pus also contains protein, since the exudate that accompanies the pus is rich in protein.

Proteinuria accompanies various types of kidney diseases. These are the *renal* proteinurias. In acute glomerulonephritis, protein is always found in the urine. In the chronic form of this disease, proteinuria is seen in the early stages but may disappear later as the kidney becomes more and more impaired. In nephrosclerosis, albuminuria is frequently but not always found, and the same is true of tuberculosis and carcinoma of the kidney. There are several types of nephrosis—conditions characterized by degenerative lesions of the renal parenchyma. Protein is almost always excreted in nephroses, varying from small to large amounts. Lipoid nephrosis is a form of chronic kidney disease in which lipid deposits occur in the tubules. It is, however, considered to be an affection of the glomerulus. In this disease, large quantities of albumin are lost in the urine, and since albumin is derived from the blood, the concentrations of the blood proteins, particularly serum albumin, fall considerably. A number of investigators believe that lipoid nephrosis is merely a modified glomerulonephritis—not an entirely different condition. This view is supported by evidence that in some cases of definite chronic nephritis the character and quantity of proteins in the urine are the same as those found in the urine of patients with nephrosis.

Polypeptides, the so-called proteoses and peptones, sometimes are excreted in the urine. This may happen in pneumonia, diphtheria, carcinoma, and other conditions and is due to some protein-containing material, e.g., an exudate, or a tissue mass or pus undergoing autolysis (self-digestion). If any soluble products of proteolysis with molecules too large for direct utilization or deamination get into the circulation, they are excreted as foreign bodies.

A peculiar protein is eliminated by some patients having multiple myeloma, a tumorlike hyperplasia of the bone marrow, and also in some other diseases of the bone marrow, and sometimes in leukemia. This is the Bence Jones protein. It precipitates when the urine is warmed to 40° to 60° C. but dissolves almost completely when the temperature is raised to 100° C. It is believed to be a globulin of comparatively low molecular weight, i.e., about 37,000. An increased protein diet does not seem to be followed by a greater output of Bence Jones protein. One study[7] indicated that the Bence Jones protein is really more than one protein, i.e., the proteins excreted by various patients differ from each other in the proportions of amino acids present, electrophoretic mobility, isoelectric point, stability in acid or alkaline solution, etc. More recent investigations (p. 585) indicate that the Bence Jones protein represents the urinary excretion of an excess of the light-chain moiety of immunoglobulins.

Nucleoproteins are found in the urine in inflammation of the urinary epithelia (e.g., pyelitis, cystitis) and even in nephritis, at times. Since these proteins precipitate in the cold on addition of mineral acids, they have frequently been designated mucoproteins, which have the same property.

Hematuria is the occurrence of blood in urine i.e., whole blood, including erythrocytes, and is a result of hemorrhage. Sometimes the shade or appearance gives a clue as to the site of bleeding. The hemorrhage may be due to any of a variety of causes, including benign or malignant neoplasms of the kidney or urinary tract, physical injury to the kidney, violent exercise, infection of the urinary tract, or administration of certain drugs (salicylates, methenamine, sulfonamides, barbiturates, anticoagulants). Allergic reactions and low prothrombin levels also cause hematuria, further indicating the difficulty of determining the etiology of this clinical sign. *Hemoglobinuria* refers to the excretion of hemoglobin and follows a hemoglobinemia. Excessive hemolysis precedes hemoglobinemia; i.e., the red cells are laked by some hemolytic agent. It appears as pink or light red oxyhemoglobin in alkaline urine and as brown methemoglobin or brownish reduced hemoglobin in acid urine. However, there is a renal threshold for hemoglobin, and normally a reabsorption from the renal tubules. When this threshold is exceeded, hemoglobinuria results. Apparently hemoglobin, when it is in solution in the blood plasma, is treated by the body as a foreign substance and is excreted into the urine. If the kidneys are normal, the threshold is a concentration of about 155 mg. per 100 ml. of blood plasma, but it may be lower when the kidneys are damaged. When the threshold is exceeded and hemoglobin is excreted into the urine, the hemoglobin may precipitate in the tubules if the urine is acid in reaction. Hence, in the treatment of hemoglobinuria, e.g., following incompatible blood transfusions, the administration of alkalies may prove to be helpful. In attempting to differentiate between hematuria and hemoglobinuria, you should remember that the red cells may disintegrate, especially if the reaction is alkaline, and the hemoglobin dissolves out. Myohemoglobin or myoglobin also may be found in human urine. It is difficult to diagnose spectroscopically, but there is a chemical test for it.[8]

Ketone bodies. The ketone bodies are acetoacetic acid, β-hydroxybutyric acid, and acetone. The first two are normal products of fatty acid catabolism (Chapter 12). They are formed in the liver and are destroyed or utilized by the extrahepatic tissues. If these two activities balance, there is no excess in the blood, i.e., no *ketonemia*. If the formation by the liver is too rapid for the extrahepatic tissues to keep pace with it, ketonemia results, followed by *ketonuria*. Acetone is generally believed to be a secondary product; i.e., it results from the decomposition of acetoacetic acid.

$$CH_3 \cdot CO \cdot CH_2 \cdot COOH \rightarrow CH_3 \cdot CO \cdot CH_3 + CO_2$$

Acetoacetic acid   **Acetone**

Ordinarily a normal person on a mixed diet excretes less than 0.1 gm. of ketone bodies in 24 hours. In *ketosis*, as the condition of excessive ketone production is termed, values as high as 100 gm. per day, or even higher, have been reported. Ketonuria may be expected to occur in the acidosis of diabetes mellitus and starvation, in normal and toxic pregnancies, after ether anesthesia, and often in alkalosis. It is, therefore, not necessarily a sign of acidosis, although the most severe ketoses, with marked ketonuria, are seen in severe cases of diabetic acidosis.

Acetone and acetoacetic acid are easily detected by qualitative color tests. However, the common Gerhardt test for acetoacetic acid, which is the appearance of a Bordeaux red color upon the addition of ferric chloride, may be masked if salicylates or certain other compounds are present. If this is suspected, a portion of the urine may be boiled and then tested. A positive test before boiling, followed by a negative one after boiling, is definite evidence that the color is caused by acetoacetic acid. However, a positive test before and after boiling leaves one in doubt as to whether acetoacetic acid is present in addition to the disturbing drug. In such an event, the acetoacetic acid may be extracted from the urine and tested separately. β-Hydroxybutyric acid can best be detected by polarimetric examination. If glucose is also present, it must first be removed by fermentation. After clarification the fermented urine is examined in the polarimeter, and if levorotation is observed, the presence of β-hydroxybutyric acid is indicated. Glucuronates are also levorotatory, but they have reducing power, whereas β-hydroxybutyric acid does not.

In order to detect phenylketonuria early (p. 375), it has been suggested[9] that every child's urine be tested for phenylpyruvic acid at the age of 21 days or before. To a fresh specimen of urine is added a little 5% ferric chloride solution. A green coloration, reaching a maximum within 5 minutes and then fading slowly, constitutes a positive result. The urine should not be acidified. If the test is positive, the blood level of phenylalanine should be determined (p. 375) and dietary procedures should be instituted.

Bile and its derivatives. Both bile pigments, or their derivatives, and bile salts may be found in urine in pathologic states. If there is a stasis or damming back of bile, the bile invariably enters the bloodstream and is excreted in the urine. Both the pigments and the salts are detectable, but only the pigments are tested for ordinarily. In obstructive jaundice, relatively large amounts of bilirubin diglucuronide may be found in the urine. In hemolytic and in toxic jaundice, on the other hand, little or no bilirubin passes into the urine. The reason is that bilirubin glucuronide can be readily excreted by the kidney if it is present in the circulating blood, as it is in obstructive jaundice. Free bilirubin (p. 684) is present in the blood in high concentration in hemolytic and toxic jaundice. The kidney cannot excrete it easily, since the kidney threshold for this large molecule is relatively high.

Urobilinogen, you will remember, is formed from bilirubin in the intestine by bacterial action. Urobilinogen may be absorbed from the gut and either be excreted by way of the bile after having been reconverted to bilirubin or be excreted by the kidneys. The presence of urobilinogen in urine, therefore, is dependent on the passage of bilirubin into the intestine. Thus, practically no urobilinogen is found in the urine in obstructive jaundice, but in hemolytic and in toxic jaundice it occurs in appreciable quantities.

Urobilinogen may be detected by either Ehrlich's or Schlesinger's test. The former consists of adding to a few milliliters of urine a few crystals of *p*-dimethylaminobenzaldehyde and acidifying definitely with hydrochloric acid. In the presence of abnormal amounts of urobilinogen, a cherry red color is seen. Normal urines give a negative test or a positive test only after heating. Watson changed this into a quantitative procedure. Urobilin is first reduced to urobilinogen with ferrous hydroxide. The color is then developed with the Ehrlich reagent under definite conditions, and a colorimetric estimation is made, using a phenolsulfonphthalein standard for comparison. The Schlesinger test is performed as follows: to 10 ml. of urine are added a few drops of Lugol's solution to transform urobilinogen to urobilin. An equal volume of a saturated alcoholic solution of zinc acetate or zinc chloride is then added. The presence of urobilin is evidenced by a greenish fluorescence. This is best seen if the tube is placed in direct sunlight with a black background. If bile pigments are also present they should be removed first by adding about one fifth of a volume of 10% calcium chloride solution and filtering off the precipitated calcium-pigment compound.

Urinary calculi. The less soluble constituents of the urine sometimes precipitate out in the urinary tract. They may form minute particles or masses and be passed readily, or they may become larger aggregates, varying in size from "sand" or "gravel" to good-sized "stones." The substances of which they are composed are the same as those that may form sediments in the urine on standing, namely, uric acid and urates, calcium oxalate, calcium phosphate, calcium carbonate, and, very rarely, cystine, xanthine, and others.

These substances are ordinarily held in solution at body temperature in urine. Undoubtedly some of them are in a supersaturated state, and it is probable that they are kept in solution because certain urinary colloids exert a protective colloidal action. The colloids may be the urinary pigments, the traces of certain proteins, or other undetermined compounds. The crystalloids are assumed to become insoluble either because of a change in the quantitative relations (i.e., not enough protective colloid available) or because of a change in the degree of dispersion of the protective colloid. On the other hand, there is some evidence that certain urinary mucoproteins have a great affinity for calcium, with which they precipitate out of solution. These precipitates may become centers of stone formation as solids are added to them little by little until the concretion becomes macroscopic. The change from a soluble to an insoluble state may well depend on the hydrogen ion concentration of the urine. Calcium phosphate, for example, is far less soluble in neutral urine than in acid and is still less soluble at pH 8.0. Infection and diet may easily tend to change the pH of urine, and stasis may also be a factor in promoting the precipitation of salts.

Certain other factors have been suggested as contributing to the formation of urinary calculi. Among them are hyperparathyroidism, hypervitaminosis D, avitaminosis A, and avitaminosis B_6. Kidney stones are quite prevalent in tropical countries; hence the suggestion that the overproduction of vitamin D by sunlight is a causative factor. The effect of high vitamin D in producing a calcium imbalance coupled with a possible low vitamin A intake might induce the formation of calcium stones. An avitaminosis A regularly produces bladder stones in rats. Vitamin B_6 deficiency causes increased urinary oxalate excretion in some animals and in man.[10] Feeding large amounts of glycine or tryptophan causes increased oxalate excretion that can be corrected only by prolonged parenteral administration of vitamin B_6. Therefore a diet low in oxalates and oxalate precursors and supplemented with this vitamin is recommended in oxaluria.[11] Urinary calculi are often associated with hyperparathyroidism, which results in a removal of calcium salts from bone, with a rise in blood calcium and urinary calcium. However, many types of urinary calculi contain no calcium.

The relative frequency of occurrence of the different varieties of kidney stones is indicated by a series of 510 cases reported by Stillman. About 44% were alkaline earth stones, i.e., composed largely of calcium carbonate, calcium phosphate, or ammonium magnesium phosphate. These are "infectional stones," i.e., secondary to an infection, and are whitish gray and may be either rough or smooth. Calcium oxalate stones comprised about 49% of the total. These are associated with a high calcium content of urine and are dark brown to black, exceedingly hard, and usually rough, particularly the larger ones. This roughness is due to the protrusion of the sharp octahedral crystals. A small type is termed the "hempseed" calculus and may have a smooth surface. The majority of stones found in the kidney at operation are either oxalate or phosphate concretions. These two groups, making up over 90% of all urinary stones, are radiopaque. *Metabolic* stones include uric acid concretions (6%) and cystine calculi (0.8%). Uric acid calculi are always colored, being yellow to reddish brown, and usually, but not always, have a smooth surface. The nuclei or centers of urinary concretions of other types are often composed of uric acid or urates.

Cystine calculi may occur in cases of cystinuria. They are white, yellow, or greenish yellow and rather soft. They are very rare. Even rarer are xanthine calculi. These, however, are harder than cystine stones and are brown to red in color.

Investigations[12] have indicated that an *organic matrix* appears to be the one essential component of all urinary calculi. This matrix is a mucoid, containing about 65% protein, 14% carbohydrate, 12% inorganic ash, and 10% "bound" water. The carbohydrate portion may contain glucose, galactose, mannose, rhamnose, fucose, deoxypentose, and hexosamine. The precursor of the matrix is believed to be *uromucoid*, a protein found in small amounts in all human urine. Uromucoid seems to be quantitatively increased in the urine of patients who are actively forming calculi. Its origin is as yet unknown, but it may be derived from depolymerized renal tubular ground substance or possibly from bone matrix. The exact mechanisms by which uromucoid is transformed into the matrix and by which it accretes organic or inorganic crystals to form organized urinary calculi are also unknown at the present time. Certain nutritional deficiencies and a number of pathologic states appear to trigger the matrix-forming mechanism and thus the formation of urinary calculi.

Inborn errors of metabolism   A condition of deranged metabolism that exists at birth and persists throughout life is known as an inborn error of metabolism. In all instances the abnormality is a hereditary condition, a defect in one of the genes as discussed earlier (Chapter 4, 6, and 13). The individual is unable either to utilize a certain type of nutrient or to produce from the ordinary foodstuff a particular physiologically important substance. As a result, certain of these substances appear as abnormal constituents of the urine. Some of these have already been discussed (Chapter 13).

Alkaptonuria is a disturbance in the intermediary metabolism of phenylalanine and tyrosine (p. 373). Homogentisic acid is excreted in the urine. Upon exposure to the oxygen of the air, this becomes very dark. Frequently ochronosis and arthritis occur as the patient matures. Ochronosis is a blackening of the cartilages of the individual. Alkaptonuria is a rather rare condition.

Cystinuria occurs in various degrees of severity. Mild cases are not uncommon, but the very severe condition is quite rarely seen. Cystine itself, when fed to patients with cystinuria, is metabolized apparently normally, but cysteine and methionine are excreted as cystine. Persons suffering from cystinuria are likely to have renal cystine calculi, which sometimes must be removed surgically (p. 382).

Fructosuria is a very unusual state. Free or combined fructose of the diet is not converted to glycogen but is excreted. It seems to produce no harmful effects (p. 214).

In galactosemia (p. 215) there is also a galactosuria and sometimes an aminoaciduria and a ketonuria.

Pentosuria is another condition in which a sugar is excreted. Here the sugar is L-xyloketose (L-xylulose). The amount excreted seems to bear no relation to the diet, and again we have an apparently harmless abnormality (p. 216).

Phenylketonuria was discussed on p. 375. Phenylpyruvic acid and increased quantities of phenylalanine are eliminated in the urine.

Hyperoxaluria is a condition in which a superabundance of oxalates is found in the urine (p. 736).

Maple syrup urine disease is a hereditary condition resulting from the failure to decarboxylate oxidatively leucine, isoleucine, and valine. The urine acquires an odor resembling that of maple sugar (p. 371).

Porphyrins are sometimes found in urine, giving it a red color if sufficient amounts are present. The urine may fluoresce a brilliant vermillion color in ultraviolet light. Porphyrins are found in urine in the porphyrias, congenital diseases in the biosynthetic pathway of heme (p. 610). Porphyrins may also appear in the urine temporarily following the administration of certain drugs, e.g., sulfonamides and sulfonal, or in alcoholism or lead poisoning, or following excessive exposure to ionizing radiations. The porphyrinuria in these instances usually disappears with the cessation or removal of the causative agent.

Tyrosinosis is an exceedingly rare anomaly in which the aromatic amino acids are eliminated as tyrosine or hydroxyphenylpyruvic acid (p. 373).

A summary of some of the more common or biochemically unique hereditary metabolic disorders is given in Table 22-2 (see also Table 13-4). Where known, the specific enzyme defect and the characteristic metabolite appearing in the urine in abnormal amounts are also given. Obviously the list does not include those metabolic derangements in which there is a *tissue* accumu-

Table 22-2. Some hereditary metabolic disorders with enzyme defect (where known) and characteristic metabolite excreted in urine

Hereditary metabolic disorders	Enzyme defect	Characteristic urinary metabolite
Albinism	Tyrosinase	Tyrosine
Alkaptonuria	Homogentisic acid oxidase	Homogentisic acid
Cystathioninuria	Deficient amount of cystathionase in liver	Cystathionine
Cystinuria	? Renal reabsorption of Cys	Cystine (also Lys, Arg, ornithine)
Diabetes mellitus	? Insulin	Glucose
Diabetes, renal	? Renal reabsorption of glucose	Glucose
Fructosuria	Fructokinase (or fructose-1-P-aldolase)	Fructose
Galactosemia	Galactose-1-P-uridyl transferase	Galactose
Gout	? Excessive synthesis	Uric acid
Hartnup's disease	Tryptophan pyrrolase	Tryptophan
Histidinemia	Histidase	Histidine
Homocystinuria	Cystathionine synthetase	Homocystine
Hyperbilirubinemia, congenital	UDP-glucuronate transferase	Bilirubin
Hyperoxaluria	? Defect in glycoxylate metabolism	Oxalate
Maple syrup urine disease	Decarboxylases or Leu, Ileu, Val	Keto acids of Leu, Ileu, Val
Multiple myeloma, etc.	? Varied	Bence Jones protein
Orotic aciduria	Orotidine-5'-pyrophosphorylase	Orotic acid
Pentosuria	L-Xylulose dehydrogenase	L-Xylulose
Phenylketonuria	Phenylalanine hydroxylase	Phenylpyruvate
Porphyria, congenital	Porphobilinogen isomerase	Uro- and coproporphyrins, type I
Porphyria, acute intermittent	Excess ALA-snythetase	δ-Aminolevulinic acid and porpholinogen
Wilson's disease	Decrease in ceruloplasmin; defective renal reabsorption	Various amino acids
Xanthinuria	Xanthine oxidase	Xanthine

lation of a metabolite rather than an increased urinary excretion. As discussed earlier, hereditary disorders of this type include the glycogen storage diseases (p. 195), the various lipidoses (p. 335), and those in which there are alterations in the biosynthesis of body proteins (e.g., the hemoglobinopathies and aberrations in the formation of various plasma proteins).

DETOXICATION

It was stated in Chapter 21 that the quantities of toxic products absorbed from the large intestine are not very great, and even these small amounts are detoxified. The process is commonly called detoxication and is appropriately considered at this point because the detoxified products are excreted mainly in the urine. The term "detoxication" is a misnomer, from one point of view at least. The detoxified product is sometimes more toxic than the original substance. "Biotransformation" has been suggested as a preferable term.

The primary purpose of the detoxication process is to convert the toxic substance to a more *polar* compound, which is thus *less lipid soluble*. The object is to decrease the permeability of the polar compound through lipid membranes, thus protecting the cell interior; the object is also, if possible, to increase the water solubility and hence the excretion of the compound in the urine or bile or intestinal secretions.

A summary of the typical pathways for the hepatic detoxication of a variety of classes of chemical compounds is presented in Table 22-3. As stated previously, the detoxified substance is excreted primarily in the urine. This desirable result is effected by mechanisms that the body ordinarily uses in its normal metabolic processes; i.e., detoxication mechanisms are probably not specific in regard to toxic substances absorbed from the bowel nor indeed for any substances simply because of their toxicity, but rather they are directed toward particular types of substances that arise in cellular activities. Some of these substances happen to be harmful and may be rendered less so by the chemical transformations resulting from the usual activities of enzymes on definite chemical groups or linkages. Hence it is not surprising to note, on the one hand, that these detoxication systems operate against poisonous substances of whatever origin or however introduced and, on the other hand, that the operation of some of these detoxicating systems does not necessarily imply or guarantee that a nontoxic or even a less toxic substance will be produced.

Detoxication reactions have a direct bearing on the pharmacologic reactions of drugs. Because of this, it is important to list several factors that influence the detoxication process: (1) the specific chemical structure of the compound being acted on, (2) the dose of the compound in relation to the weight of the organism, and (3) the species of the animal metabolizing the compound. A realization of this last factor is of prime importance in the pharmacologic evaluation of a drug. It emphasizes that drugs tested on animals cannot be administered to the human being with absolute assurance of safety since detoxication routes may vary in different animal species (including the human being). Thus phenylacetic acid is detoxified by conjugation with glycine in the rabbit and dog, by conjugation with ornithine in the bird, and by glutamine in man and the chimpanzee. Other factors are age, sex, environmental conditions, e.g., temperature and barometric pressure, heredity (alkaptonuria), concurrent administration of other compounds, and the physiologic state of the organism. Further details can be obtained from textbooks on pharmacology.

Most detoxications occur in the liver.

Oxidation Oxidation usually occurs first and sometimes is followed by conjugation. Indole is an example (p. 735). It is first oxidized to indoxyl, which is then conjugated with sulfate. Some substances can be completely decomposed by oxidation. Ethyl alcohol, in moderate amounts, can be oxidized by the body to carbon dioxide and water. The fact that methyl alcohol yields intermediate toxic products, formaldehyde and formic acid, in the same kind

748

Table 22-3. Typical pathways of hepatic detoxication*

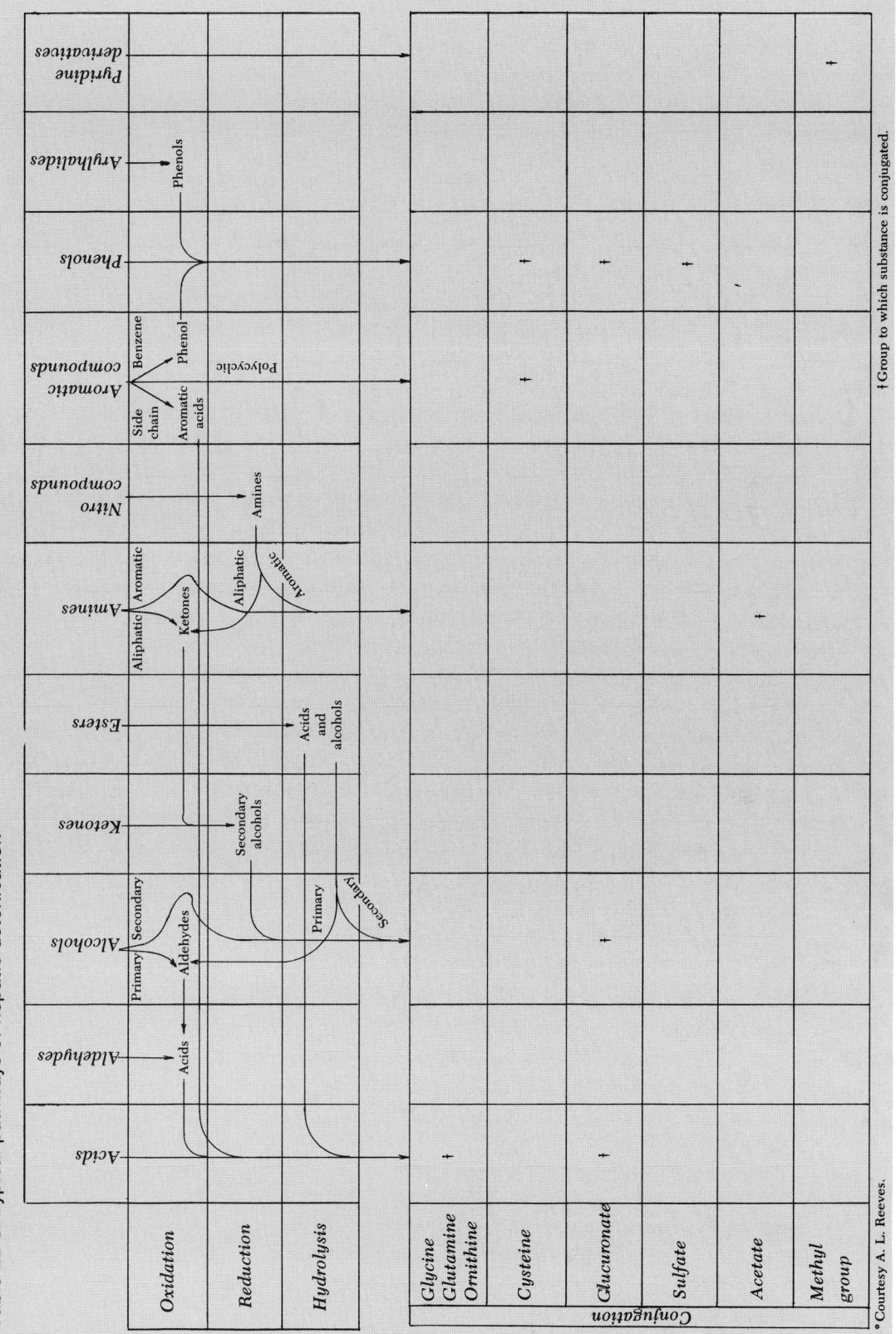

*Courtesy A. L. Reeves.

†Group to which substance is conjugated.

of combustion, emphasizes the fact that these reactions are general metabolic mechanisms that may fall short of total detoxication.

Aliphatic amines are completely oxidized by the body. An enzyme, amine oxidase, that accomplishes this has been found to occur in brain and other tissues. In the case of butylamine, a product of the reaction is acetoacetic acid, which is, of course, a normal metabolite. There is present in liver, intestine, and other tissues a similar enzyme that catalyzes the oxidative deamination of epinephrine and related amines.

The reaction is as follows:

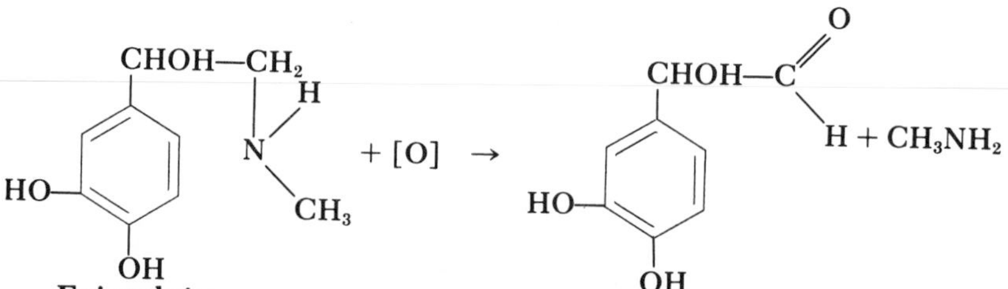

Epinephrine

It was pointed out on p. 306 that phenyl-substituted fatty acids are oxidized by β-oxidation, losing two carbons at a time in the process. The final products are phenylacetic acid, if the chain contains an even number of carbons, and benzoic acid, if an odd number of carbons. Both phenylacetic acid and benzoic acid are then conjugated with glycine to yield phenaceturic acid and hippuric acid, respectively. In man, however, phenylacetic acid is conjugated with glutamine, as will be shown later. Benzene itself is slowly oxidized in the presence of enzymes to phenol and other products, including muconic acid, which involves splitting the ring. Benzene derivatives with a single side chain usually have this side chain oxidized. Thus toluene (or methylbenzene) and benzaldehyde are oxidized to benzoic acid.

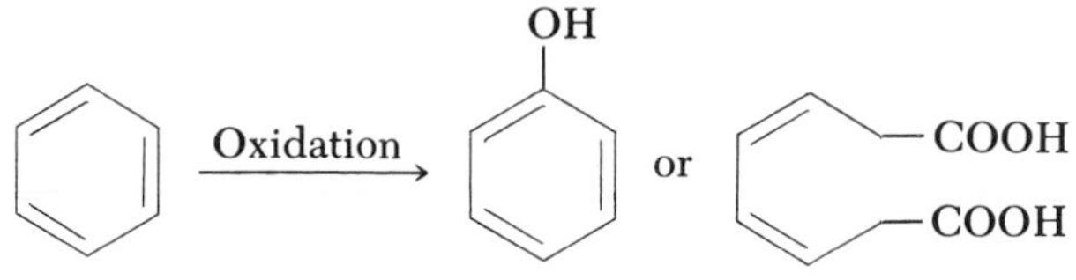

Benzene   **Phenol**   **Muconic acid**

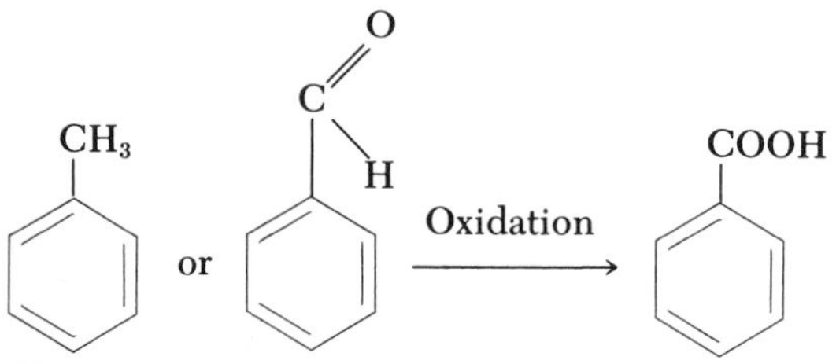

Methylbenzene   **Benzaldehyde**   **Benzoic acid**

In all these instances the final products are more acidic than the parent substance.

When two side chains are attached to the benzene ring, only one is oxidized. This is very unfortunate because the aliphatic dicarboxylic acids are injurious to the kidney. The simplest member of this series, oxalic acid, is a notable example and, as is well known, may give rise to calcium oxalate crystals in the kidney or urinary tract. Oxalic acid is present in various foods, e.g., rhubarb, spinach, chard, beet leaves, cocoa, tea.

Reduction   Reduction is less common and apparently less important than oxidation. We have seen that bile pigments are reduced to urobilin and urobilinogen in the intestinal tract. This is generally ascribed to bacterial action; hence it can scarcely be termed a physiologic mechanism. There are, however, some reductions that are accomplished metabolically.

Picric acid is converted to picramic acid:

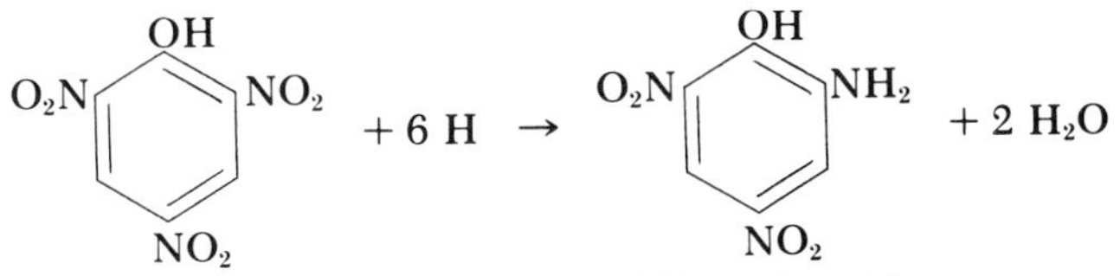

Picric acid $+ 6$ H $\rightarrow$ Picramic acid $+ 2$ H$_2$O

Chloral is reduced to trichloroethyl alcohol:

$$CCl_3 \cdot CHO + 2 \ H \rightarrow CCl_3 \cdot CH_2OH$$
Chloral   **Trichloroethyl alcohol**

Quinone is reduced to hydroquinone:

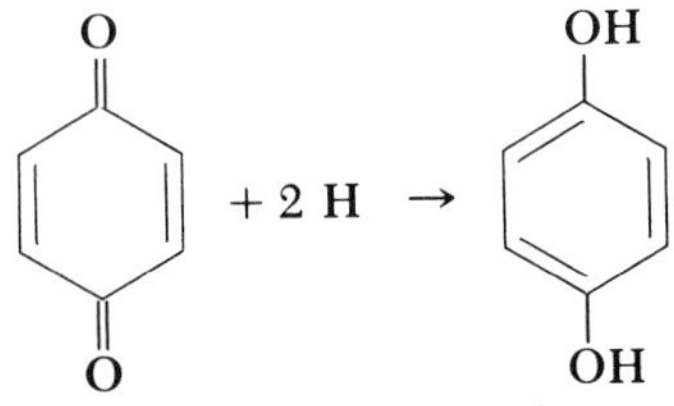

$+ 2$ H $\rightarrow$

p-Benzoquinone   Hydroquinone

By conjugation, we mean the synthetic union of one compound with some other. The most common conjugating agents (Table 22-3) are glycine, cysteine, glutamine, glucuronic acid, and acetic acid, with sulfate as the best example of an inorganic agent. Methylation is also resorted to.

Conjugation   *Glycine.* The classic example of conjugation with glycine is its union with benzoic acid to form hippuric acid (p. 733). Many of the derivatives of benzoic acid are conjugated with glycine in this way, but the presence of a group ortho to the carboxyl inhibits this type of action. Conjugation with glycine is not limited to members of the aromatic series; many other acids are handled in the same way, including, to some extent, niacin. The formation of glycocholic acid, of the bile, by the union of cholic acid with glycine is probably another example of this normal metabolic reaction, which is available for detoxication purposes. There is created a peptide linkage; to accomplish this, the presence of ATP and specific enzymes are required. The type reaction is shown at the top of p. 752.

751

Glutamine. An interesting example of the employment of glutamine in conjugation reactions is the union of phenylacetic acid with this compound. The reaction occurs only in man and other primates. In other animals, glycine or ornithine is conjugated with it. Here again a peptide linkage is formed.

Phenylacetic acid   Glutamine   Phenacetylglutamine

Ornithine. Ornithine does not appear to be important in human detoxication processes. The ornithine conjugation, however, serves to emphasize the importance of species specificity in determining the pathways of the detoxication process. As mentioned above, phenylacetic acid is detoxified by ornithine in birds. Thus:

Phenylacetic acid   Ornithine   Diphenylacetylornithine

Cysteine. Bromobenzene, chlorbenzene, and iodobenzene, when fed to animals, are converted to mercapturic acids by conjugation with cysteine and acetylation.

Bromobenzene   Cysteine   Acetic acid   *p*-Bromphenylmercapturic acid

752

Naphthalene, anthracene, benzyl chloride, and a number of other substances are known to be handled similarly by animals. Stekol showed that mercapturic acid formation occurs also in man. The administration of some of these substances to animals results in an inhibition of growth if the protein intake is low. The explanation is that the cysteine required for growth is used in the detoxication process.

Acetic acid. It has just been seen that acetic acid is used, together with cysteine, in the formation of mercapturic acids. However, conjugation of acetic acid alone with other substances having an amino group is a common occurrence. One notable example is the acetylation of the sulfa drugs. This occurs after absorption or parenteral administration, and the efficacy of the drugs as bacteriostatic agents is thereby decreased. Coenzyme-A is, of course, required for these acetylations.

We would expect the vitamin *p*-aminobenzoic acid to be handled similarly.

Incidentally, *p*-aminobenzoic acid (PABA) itself is a detoxicant. Symptoms of hydroquinone poisoning can be overcome by the oral administration of this substance. PABA can also detoxicate certain phenylarsonates, which are trypanosomicides, when these are given in toxic doses. Such actions of PABA differ from the others discussed since they are not metabolic reactions of the cells of the body but are brought about by the *administration* of a compound, even though it be a physiologic compound.

Sulfate. Phenol, cresol, indole, and skatole, formed by the action of intestinal bacteria on some of the amino acids in the large intestine, are transported to the liver, where they are conjugated with sulfate. These processes have been followed on pp. 696, 725, and 734. The resulting ethereal sulfates appear to be less toxic than their precursors and, because they are more acidic, are more easily excreted by the kidney.

Conjugation with sulfate appears to be accomplished by way of active sulfate, which is transferred to the substance to be detoxified by the enzyme sulfokinase. Active sulfate seems to be phosphoadenosine phosphosulfate (PAPS) (p. 385).

Glucuronic acid. Glucuronic acid is an oxidation product of glucose in one of the paths of metabolism of glucose and glycogen (p. 217). Perhaps 150 to 200 mg. per day is found in the urine of a normal man. This is combined with the number of products of normal metabolism and is increased, sometimes to a considerable extent, after the administration of various drugs.

Glucuronic acid participates in detoxication reactions as its UDP-derivative. This is formed from glucose-1-phosphate as described on p. 217. A transfer enzyme is also required here. The detoxication of bilirubin as an example is shown diagrammatically as follows:

$$\text{Bilirubin} \xrightarrow[\text{UDP-glucuronic acid transferase}]{+ \text{ UDP-glucuronic acid}} \begin{array}{c} \text{Bilirubin glucuronide} \\ + \text{ UDP} \end{array}$$

The linkages with glucuronic acid are of two types: glucosidic and ester. Alcohols and phenols are combined in glucosidic linkage, and acids in ester linkage. For example:

Phenol   β-Glucuronic acid   Phenylglucuronide

Benzoic acid   β-Glucuronic acid   β-Glucuronic acid monobenzoate

The products of sex hormone metabolism are, in a number of instances, known to be excreted as glucuronides. Morphine, menthol, camphor, chloral hydrate, borneol, salicylic acid, acetanilid, pyramidon, creosote, vanillin, PABA, sulfapyridine, and bilirubin are representatives of a long list of compounds that are excreted in one or the other of these two forms.

It will be noted that several of the compounds cited, e.g., benzoic acid, phenol, PABA, and the sulfa drugs, have been shown to be handled by other mechanisms, again indicating that the body uses more than one method of detoxication.

Methylation Methylation and transmethylation have been discussed on p. 352, and the importance of the methyl group in the formation of methionine and creatine was indicated. Although these are not detoxications in the original sense, they are syntheses, and analogous methylations are known to occur in the body. Nicotinamide is an important example. It is metabolized in part as follows:

| Nicotinamide | N^1-Methylnicotinamide |

Hydrolysis Aspirin, acetylsalicylic acid, is a good example of hydrolytic action within the body. The acetic acid formed is either oxidized or used for synthesis of physiologic compounds, and the salicylic acid is excreted by the kidney, combined partly with glucuronic acid. Glucosides are, in many cases, hydrolyzed to the sugar and the aglycone, each of which is treated by the body according to its particular nature.

Thiocyanate detoxication The animal organism normally excretes thiocyanates. Human saliva contains an average of 0.01%; normal human blood contains about 1.31 mg. potassium thiocyanate per 100 ml. Habitual smokers have values much higher. The formation of thiocyanate is said to be affected by an enzyme rhodanese, which is believed to act on small quantities of cyanide formed during the course of normal metabolism.

$$HCN + S \xrightarrow{\text{Rhodanese}} HSCN$$

In vitro the sulfur can be obtained from thiosulfate, but its source in the body is unknown.

KIDNEY FUNCTION TESTS

The body has a considerable factor of safety in renal as well as hepatic tissue. One normal kidney can do the work of two, and if all other organs are functioning properly, less than a whole kidney may suffice. On the other hand, there are extrarenal factors that interfere with kidney function, particularly circulatory disturbances. Therefore, methods that appraise the functional capacity of the kidneys are very important. Such tests have been devised but, as in the case of liver function, no single test can measure all the kidney functions, although the kidney is not so versatile an organ as the liver. Consequently, more than one test is usually indicated. These procedures throw light on the functional capacity of the kidney as related to the general physiology of the patient, not on the extent of any lesion or pathologic process in the patient. Many renal function tests have been proposed and are being used, but only a few can be given space here.

A stepwise increase in three nitrogenous constituents of blood is believed by some authorities to parallel a deteriorating kidney function. Uric acid usually rises first, later urea, and finally creatinine. By determining all three in blood, an estimate of kidney function can be made. However, gout and certain other conditions also result in a high uric acid.

Concentration and dilution tests for renal function are also used. There are a number of variations, but all are based on the principle that the normally functioning kidney is capable of secreting a dilute urine if a large volume of fluid has been ingested and a concentrated urine if the individual has been deprived of fluid.

Phenolsulfonphthalein test. Phenolsulfonphthalein is a harmless dye that, after parenteral administration, is eliminated only by the kidneys. It is easily detected and estimated by colorimetric methods. Under standard conditions, it appears in the urine normally in about 10 minutes, and, within the first hour thereafter, from 40% to 50% is eliminated; in 2 hours, a total of from 60% to 70% is eliminated. In renal insufficiency, the amount secreted in 2 hours is much reduced, sometimes to even a trace. In very early nephritis, an excessively high elimination may be found because of irritation to or a compensatory hyperactivity of undamaged kidney tissue. In such cases, other tests must be used to aid in diagnosis. The phenolsulfonphthalein test is widely used because it is easy to perform and has given valuable information in many instances.

Blood urea clearance test. The concentration of urea in the blood rises in nephritis and in other conditions of deficient kidney function. However, urea concentration is subject to great fluctuations and is not, by itself, a good index of the ability of the kidney to excrete nitrogenous waste. Ambard was the first to study the concentration of urea in the blood and relate it to the rate of excretion in the urine, and *Ambard's coefficient* was, for a while, the subject of much clinical study. At present, the blood or, better, the plasma urea clearance test of Van Slyke is widely used. By *plasma urea clearance*, we mean the rate at which plasma is cleared of urea while passing through the kidneys. As a matter of fact, the plasma is not completely cleared of urea. Only about 10% of the urea is removed. Consequently, if 750 ml. of plasma pass through the kidney per minute and 10% of the urea is removed, this is equivalent to completely clearing 75 ml. of plasma per minute.

The data required are the plasma urea concentration, the urine urea concentration, and the rate of urinary flow. When the volume of urine secreted is large, the rate of urea excretion is directly proportional to the concentration of urea in the blood. When the volume of urine is small, this simple relationship does not hold. Therefore, two different formulas are required for calculating the urea clearance:

Maximum clearance (Cm), when 2 ml. or more urine are secreted per minute:

$$Cm = U/B \times V$$

Standard clearance (Cs), when the urinary secretion amounts to less than 2 ml. per minute:

$$Cs = U/B \times \sqrt{V}$$

Where U = mg. urea N per 100 ml. of urine
B = mg. urea N per 100 ml. of plasma
V = urine volume in ml. per minute

The technique of a typical test, with illustrative figures, is as follows:

7:00 A.M.   Patient receives a light breakfast; later, one glass of water
9:00 A.M.   Bladder emptied and urine discarded
9:50 A.M.   Sample of blood taken
10:00 A.M.   Bladder emptied and urine saved
11:00 A.M.   Bladder emptied and urine saved

(Exact 1-hour specimens are not necessary, but the exact periods to which they correspond must be known.)

Plasma urea N:	15 mg. per 100 ml.
First urine specimen:	48 ml., 770 mg. urea N per 100 ml.
Second urine specimen:	52 ml., 730 mg. urea N per 100 ml.
Average:	50 ml., 750 mg. urea N per 100 ml.

Since the volume of urine is 50 ml. per hour or 0.83 ml. per minute, the standard formula is used:

$$Cs = 750/15 \times \sqrt{0.83} = 45.5 \text{ ml. of plasma cleared of urea per minute}$$

The average normal Cs is 54 ml. of plasma cleared per minute. Therefore, this case showed 45.5/54 or 84% of normal. A figure of 75% or more is considered normal. In maximum clearances the average normal is 75 ml. of plasma cleared per minute.

Inulin, iodopyracet, and p-aminohippuric acid clearance tests. Inulin and iodopyracet have been used in clearance tests because they are selectively secreted. Inulin is removed from the blood only by the glomeruli, whereas iodopyracet is excreted almost entirely by the tubules. Inulin, as previously stated, is the polysaccharide yielding fructose on hydrolysis. Iodopyracet is a complex organic iodine compound (3,5-diiodo-4-pyridine-N-acetic acid diethanolamine). It is opaque to roentgen rays and is therefore also used for roentgenologic examination of the urinary tract. By determining the amount excreted and the plasma content under standard conditions, either the inulin or the iodopyracet clearance can be determined, and thus the functional activity of the glomeruli or tubules may be estimated. By doing simultaneous iodopyracet and inulin clearance tests, the active mass of renal tissue, the tubular excretory mass, can be ascertained. Recently the p-aminohippuric acid test has largely superseded the iodopyracet test because (1) p-aminohippuric acid does not penetrate the erythrocytes, (2) it is not bound by plasma proteins to the same extent, and (3) its quantitative determination is simpler.

References

GENERAL

Aldridge, W. N., editor: Mechanisms of toxicity, Brit. Med. Bull. 25:suppl. 3, 1969.

Cantarow, A., and Trumper, M.: Clinical biochemistry, ed. 5, Philadelphia, 1955, W. B. Saunders Co.

Hoffman, W. S. The biochemistry of clinical medicine, ed. 3, Chicago, 1964, Year Book Medical Publishers, Inc.

Lonsdale, K.: Human stones, Sci. Amer. 214:104, 1968.

Oser, B. L., editor: Hawk's physiological chemistry, ed. 14, New York, 1965, Blakiston Division, McGraw-Hill Book Co.

Pitts, R. F.: Physiology of the kidney and body fluids, ed. 2, Chicago, 1968, Year Book Medical Publishers, Inc.

Smith, H. W.: Principles of renal physiology, New York, 1956, Oxford University Press, Inc.

Stanbury, J. B., Wyngaarden, J. B., and Fredrickson, D. S.: The metabolic basis of inherited disease, ed. 2, New York, 1966, McGraw-Hill Book Co.

SPECIAL

1. Martinez-Maldonado, M., et al.: Science 165:807, 1969.
2. Conn, R. B., Jr.: Clin. Chem. 6:537, 1960.
3. Ludwig, G. D.: Ann. N.Y. Acad. Med. 104:465, 1963; Faragelle, F. F., and Gershoff, S. N.: Proc. Soc. Exp. Biol. Med. 114:602, 1963.
4. Adams, E. C., et al.: Science 125:1082, 1957.
5. Naganna, B.: Clin. Chim. Acta 17:219, 1967.
6. Lasker, M., and Enklewitz, M.: J. Biol. Chem. 101:289, 1933; 110:443, 1935.
7. Putnam, F. W., and Miyake, A.: Science 120:848, 1954.
8. Blondheim, S. H., et al.: J.A.M.A. 167:453, 1958.
9. Woolf, L. I., et al.: Arch. Dis. Child. 33:31, 1958.
10. Andrus, S. B., et al.: Lab. Invest. 9:7, 1960; Calhoun, W. K., et al.: J. Nutr. 67:237, 1959.
11. Zinsser, H.: J.A.M.A. 174:2062, 1960.
12. Boyce, W. H., and King, J. S., Jr.: J. Urol. 81:351, 1959.

CHAPTER 23

FAT-SOLUBLE VITAMINS

At about the turn of the century, students of nutrition considered that a well-balanced diet need contain only a suitable amount of each of the "proximate principles": proteins, carbohydrates, fats, inorganic salts, and water. Many investigations based on this premise were undertaken to determine the quality or amounts of these several ingredients or to vary their proportions. According to McCollum,[1] the first person to publish the results of a study of this question in man was Dumas. In 1871, he described the effects of substitute foods on the infants of Paris during the siege, necessitated by the shortage of food, and especially milk. The effects were disastrous, although many formulas, "all reproducing an albuminous liquid with sugar and an emulsion of a fatty body," were employed. Apparently unrecognized nutrients were lacking.

However, even earlier reports suggested that certain diseases in man were due to a "lack of something in food." Jacques Cartier and other sea voyageurs in the 1500's stated that the "scurvy" of sailors could be prevented by an "infusion of pine needles." James Lind, in 1753, successfully treated scurvy with citrus fruits.

Later animal experiments were undertaken. Magendie, in 1816, found that animals fed a purified protein, carbohydrate, fat, and mineral diet grew poorly and died. Lunin, in Bunge's laboratory in 1880, fed young mice on the purified proteins, sugar, fats, and salts of milk and found that they did not grow. He expressed the opinion that some "unknown substances" must be present in milk without which normal health and growth cannot be maintained. This work was soon forgotten.

Theobald Smith, in 1895, reported his classic experiments on the production of scurvy in guinea pigs by a diet deficient in the factor later found to be vitamin C. In 1897, Eijkman, a Dutch physician working in Java, came to the conclusion that the disease beriberi resulted from an imperfect diet that consisted chiefly of polished rice. This was also experimentally proved on fowls. When chickens or pigeons were fed for some time on polished rice, they developed a polyneuritis. Both patients and birds could be cured by adding the polishings of the rice to the diet. Eijkman explained this by assuming that white rice contained a toxin that could be neutralized by an anti-toxin present in the husk of the rice. When Eijkman returned to Holland, the investigation was taken up by Grijns, in 1901, who repeated and enlarged on it. He was not able to extract a toxin from polished rice; but he showed that there is actually a protective and curative substance in the polishings and also in other foods. Grijns was probably the first to have a clear concept of a deficiency disease and to attempt to isolate an active protective principle from foods.

These experiments led Pekelharing to again perform experiments with purified foodstuffs. He fed them to mice and found that, although at first they ate well and seemed healthy, after about 4 weeks all died. However, if milk, or even whey, was given instead of water, the mice throve upon the diet. He concluded that "an unrecognized substance occurs in milk which is of paramount importance for nutrition, even in minute quantities." This was published in a Dutch journal in 1905 and did not become widely known. The same type of experiment was performed independently by Osborne and Mendel in the United States, and the same conclusion was reached. They were studying the nutritive values of highly purified proteins isolated from various cereals. They also could obtain no growth, or even maintenance of weight, in young rats unless "protein-free milk" was added to the diet. These experiments were done in 1911, and McCollum, in the United States, and Hopkins, in England, made similar observations at about the same time. Also in 1911, Funk isolated from rice polishings a crystalline substance that was effective in preventing or curing polyneuritis in pigeons. His analyses indicated that it contained nitrogen in a basic form and that it was probably an amine. Since it appeared to be essential to life, he named it "vitamine." The spelling has since been changed to "vitamin" and has been applied to a whole series of such substances found in foods, without regard to their chemical structure.

The history of vitamin D and its relation to rickets, rheumatism, and other diseases is most interesting. The medicinal value of cod-liver oil was recognized as early as 1771 but was forgotten and rediscovered several times.[2] The medical profession usually refused to believe that this ill-tasting oil could have curative properties. More of this absorbing chapter of biochemical history cannot be detailed here, nor can the names of other brilliant investigators in the field even be listed. The interested reader may consult the references at the end of this chapter.

By 1948, at least 14 different vitamins had been isolated in crystalline form, their structures had been determined and proved by synthesis, and their biochemical functions had been partially established. Today, investigations continue to determine the precise structure of the metabolically active forms and the metabolic functions of vitamins at a molecular level, and the search goes on for other possible, still unknown, vitamins.

The experimental animal hitherto most widely used in vitamin work is the white rat. This animal has been bred and studied in many laboratories, and its normal average growth curves and vital statistics are available. Moreover, the rat responds in very characteristic fashion to many food deficiencies.

Other animals have been used, partly because the rat does not seem to need to ingest all nutritional factors and partly because substantiating or supplementary evidence is required. Thus the guinea pig is used in vitamin C studies because the rat apparently can synthesize this vitamin in its liver and therefore does not require much, if any, in its food. Pigeons are the classic test animal for demonstrating the polyneuritis caused by lack of thiamine, and dogs, mice, ducks, chickens, hamsters, roaches, and particularly microorganisms are used for other vitamin studies.

One method of demonstrating a vitamin deficiency is to feed a group of animals a diet adequate in all nutritive factors except the single substance in question. A control group must be fed the same diet plus a sufficient amount of the substance omitted from the diet of the experimental group. All animals are weighed at regular intervals and their physical condition is carefully observed. After a time, the animals on the deficient diet may stop gaining weight and later they may lose weight; if the vitamin needed is not restored to their diet in time, they may die of malnutrition. Sooner or later, after they start to lose weight, they begin to develop symptoms or signs characteristic of the particular avitaminosis (vitamin deficiency) concerned. Often these symptoms may be alleviated by administering the required vitamin, but in prolonged avitaminoses the pathologic lesion may have become so fixed that it is irreversible. This general method, the biologic method or *bioassay*, is the one originally used to determine whether a given food contains a given vitamin, and it can be made fairly precise. The biologic method usually requires weeks before an answer is obtained.

Now that the chemical structure and chemical and physical properties of probably all the individual vitamins are known, quantitative chemical methods are used; but some authors claim that biologic assay is the only correct way to determine the vitamin content of any food because a vitamin may be present and react chemically but still be unavailable nutritionally. The chemical methods depend, of course, on some outstanding chemical property of the vitamin, such as the production of a color, lending itself to colorimetric estimation, or the reducing activity, that can be rather accurately measured. Nowadays microbiologic methods are being used also because of their rapidity and economy. The principle of these methods is the same as that of the microbiologic methods for the determination of amino acids, described on p. 62. In this case, all the amino acids and all other nutritional factors, except the vitamin studied, are included in the medium, and the amount of growth depends on the amount of vitamin in question in the added *unknown*. Of course, the particular organism used must be susceptible to a lack of the nutritional factor being assayed.

Intestinal organisms play a role in the vitamin quota available to the animal or man. They may synthesize vitamins in significant amounts. Vitamin K is an important example of a vitamin synthesized by intestinal organisms. Folic acid, nicotinic acid, pyridoxine, biotin, thiamine, and riboflavin are other examples. These may be absorbed to varying extents and utilized. This fact renders rather inaccurate the figures for "daily requirements" of the different vitamins, so it is recommended that everyone ensure an adequate intake of each vitamin and rely very little on intestinal synthesis. Certain organisms have the opposite effect; i.e., they destroy vitamins. Adding certain antibiotics and sulfa drugs to the feed of domestic animals benefits growth; this increased growth may be due to a selective bacteriostatic action upon the organisms that destroy vitamins (p. 826).

Definition A vitamin is a naturally occurring essential organic constituent of the diet that, in minute amounts, aids in maintaining the normal activities of the tissues. The vitamins differ from the hormones in that they are supplied to the body chiefly from the food eaten, whereas hormones are synthesized by the body's own glands. Most vitamins and some hormones are involved directly or indirectly in enzyme systems in order to effect their physiologic functions. Some vitamins are known to be coenzymes, and their structure and action have been ascertained.

Early in their study, vitamins were classified as to their solubilities. It was at first thought that there was only one "vitamine" and later that there were two: a fat-soluble A and a water-soluble B. Then B was differentiated from C, both being water-soluble entities, components of the earlier "B." Then "A" was found to be a mixture of two fat-soluble substances, which were named A and D. As their curative powers came to be recognized, they were given the subtitles indicative of their action in this respect: vitamin A, fat-soluble A, the antixerophthalmic vitamin; vitamin C, water-soluble C, the antiscorbutic vitamin; and so on. Some of the materials proved to be mixtures, and individual factors having different effects from the main action of the original extract were isolated. An example is the B vitamin group. In other instances a series of compounds, closely related chemically, proved to have similar effects, so that, for example, one should not speak of vitamin D but of the vitamins D, since there are several of them. The structures of all the commonly known vitamins have been worked out, and some of them are manufactured on a large scale, either by chemical or fermentation processes. Others are still obtainable only from natural sources.

Avitaminoses —deficiencies of vitamins As will be discussed in some detail for the individual vitamins, a lack of one or more vitamins (multiple deficiencies being the more usual in man) produces rather characteristic symptoms. These have been extensively studied in experimental animals as well as in man. The avitaminosis may be *primary* or direct, due to a deficient intake resulting from chronic alcoholism, dietary fads, etc. This is usually discovered from the dietary history of the individual. The avitaminosis may be *secondary*, a "conditioned deficiency" due to other factors such as gastrointestinal disorders, poor teeth, anorexia, allergies, malabsorption, increased excretion, imbalance, and others to be discussed later. Avitaminosis from any cause, if prolonged, leads to (1) a gradual decrease in tissue levels of the vitamin or vitamins deficient, (2) a biochemical lesion, and, in time, (3) an anatomic lesion and, finally, cellular pathology and disease. This sequence is shown schematically in Fig. 23-1.

Although avitaminoses may not be common in the United States, they occur rather frequently in certain other parts of the world for socioeconomic reasons. Therefore, consideration must be given to their characteristic features and underlying biochemical causes.

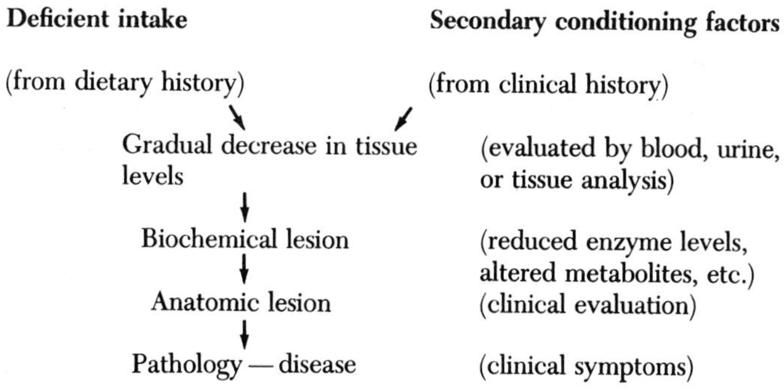

Deficient intake	Secondary conditioning factors
(from dietary history)	(from clinical history)

Gradual decrease in tissue levels   (evaluated by blood, urine, or tissue analysis)

Biochemical lesion   (reduced enzyme levels, altered metabolites, etc.)

Anatomic lesion   (clinical evaluation)

Pathology — disease   (clinical symptoms)

Fig. 23-1. Schematic representation of the sequence of events occurring in a typical avitaminosis.

Biochemical functions
The biochemical functions of most of the vitamins have been discussed in earlier chapters since the primary roles of vitamins appear to be as coenzymes in a variety of metabolic reactions. Therefore, the main emphasis in this chapter will be placed on the chemical structures and properties of the vitamins, their sources, their recommended daily allowances, their active cofactor forms, a summary of their principal metabolic functions, and the primary effects of their deficiency.

Nomenclature
Although the terms "vitamin A," "vitamin B," "vitamin C," etc. are still used and probably will be for some time, the International Union of Pure and Applied Chemistry has formulated definitive rules for the nomenclature of vitamins. Wherever possible, the correct chemical name or a good descriptive trivial name is recommended, for example, cholecalciferol (vitamin D_3), retinol (vitamin A), and thiamine (vitamin B_1). Derivatives, e.g., alcohols and aldehydes, have been given the terminations -*ol* and -*al*. Both the letter system and the official system will be employed in the following discussion, which begins with the fat-soluble vitamins A, D, E, and K.

VITAMIN A

Properties. Vitamin A, *retinol*, is soluble in fats and in fat solvents. It is stable at rather high temperatures, except when the conditions are favorable for oxidation, and in ordinary cooking or canning operations it is harmed but little. Retinol is destroyed by exposure to ultraviolet light. It is available to the human organism either in the form of the vitamin itself or of a precursor or provitamin, one of a series of carotenoid pigments, commonly called *carotenes*. The carotenes form part of the pigments of many green and yellow vegetables. After absorption they are converted to the vitamin in the intestinal wall. The carotenoids themselves do not possess vitamin A activity and are not all equally potent in their ability to form retinol. It is therefore not surprising that the sources of the vitamin itself are of animal nature. β-Carotene is the most effective provitamin since, as can be seen from the formula, it is a symmetric compound, each half of which is convertible to a molecule of the vitamin. Other members of this group that lead to the formation of vitamin A, but only half as much as does β-carotene, are α-carotene, γ-carotene, and cryptoxanthine. Retinol has a characteristic absorption spectrum, which in chloroform solution has a maximum (λ_{max}) at 328 nm. — quite different from that of carotene, which has an absorption maximum at 335 nm.* It also gives a beautiful color reaction, an intense blue (λ_{max} 620 nm.) when treated with antimony trichloride. Carotene under the same conditions yields a greenish blue color. This chemical reaction has been used for quantitative determination of the vitamin. Recently retinol in aqueous dispersions has been recommended for clinical use since it is claimed to be more rapidly absorbed than its oil solutions.

Structure. Vitamin A is a complex primary alcohol, with the empiric formula $C_{20}H_{29}OH$. The terminal hydroxyl is ordinarily esterified. This alcohol was isolated in 1931, by Karrer, and was synthesized in 1946, by Milas. It contains a β-ionone ring:

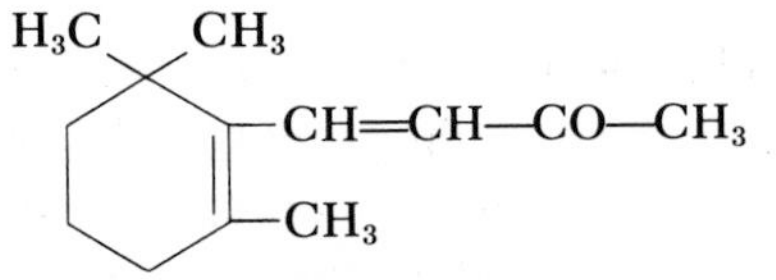

$$H_3C \quad CH_3$$
$$-CH{=}CH{-}CO{-}CH_3$$
$$-CH_3$$

β-Ionone

β-Carotene has two such rings and no alcohol groups. The other pigments mentioned each have one β-ionone ring and one group similar to it. We can thus see why they yield only half as much vitamin A as β-carotene does. The structures of β-carotene and vitamin A were worked out by Karrer. There are actually two vitamins A, known as vitamin A_1, or retinol, and vitamin A_2, or 3-dehydroretinol. Vitamin A_1 predominates in the livers of the cod and other saltwater fish, and A_2 in those of freshwater fish. The physiologic activity of both seems to be the same qualitatively, and both are justifiably called "vitamin A," although A_2 is much less active in promoting the growth of rats

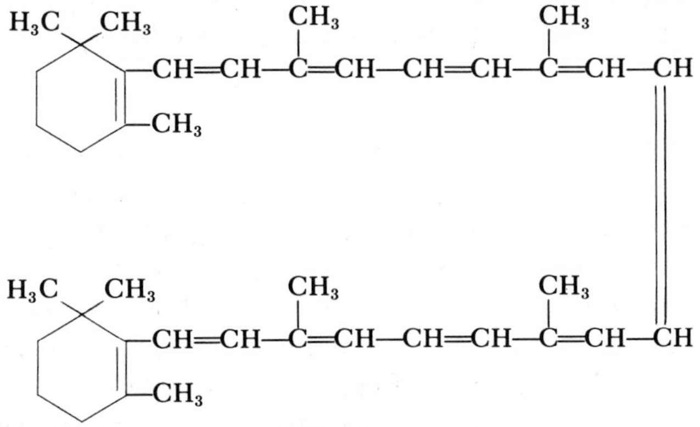

$$H_3C \quad CH_3 \qquad CH_3 \qquad CH_3$$
$$-CH{=}CH{-}C{=}CH{-}CH{=}CH{-}C{=}CH{-}CH$$
$$-CH_3$$

$$H_3C \quad CH_3 \qquad CH_3 \qquad CH_3$$
$$-CH{=}CH{-}C{=}CH{-}CH{=}CH{-}C{=}CH{-}CH$$
$$-CH_3$$

β-Carotene
(provitamin A)

than is A_1. Vitamin A_2 has the following ring structure, possessing an extra double bond in the 3,4-position:

* The designation λ_{max} is now commonly used as the symbol for the wavelength maximally absorbed by a pigment and its derivative. The abbreviation *nm.* (nanometer) is now preferred to $m\mu$ (millimicron).

3-Dehydroretinol

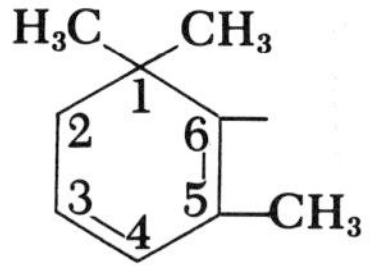

It is thus seen that the β-ionone ring is not absolutely essential for vitamin A action and that certain modifications, but not others, may allow of biologic activity. Moreover, there are eight possible stereoisomers of retinol, namely, all-*trans*, 9-*cis*, 13-*cis*, 9:13-di*cis*, and four hindered (less probable) configurations, 11-*cis*, 9:11-di*cis*, 11:13-di*cis*, and 9:11:13-tri*cis*. All-*trans* has a straight side chain; all other *cis-trans* isomers are bent at one, two, or three of the double bonds:

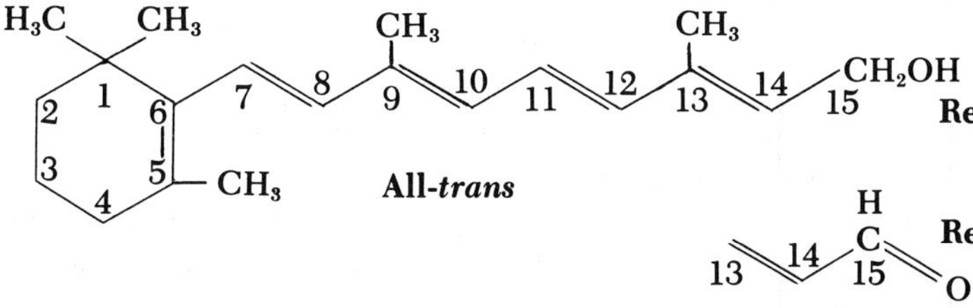

Retinol

All-*trans*

Retinal

Although a hindered configuration, the 11-*cis* aldehyde appears to be the one uniquely required for the biosynthesis of the photopigments used in vision:

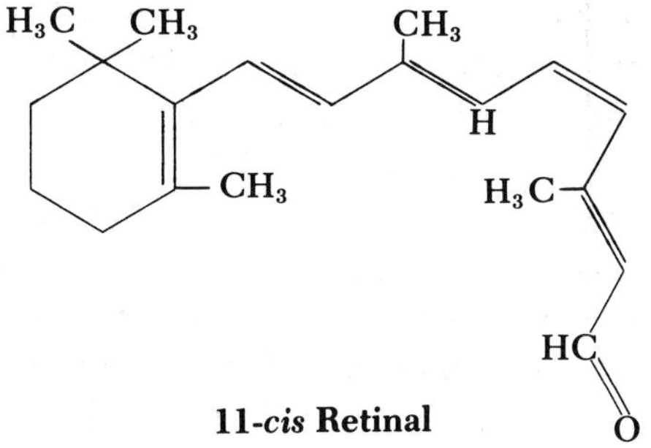

11-*cis* Retinal

The configuration of 11-*cis* retinal brings the hydrogen of carbon-10 into proximity with the methyl group of carbon-13, causing *hindrance*. An unhindered isomer, 9-*cis*, appears in retinal extracts as a by-product of photolysis of the visual pigment rhodopsin:

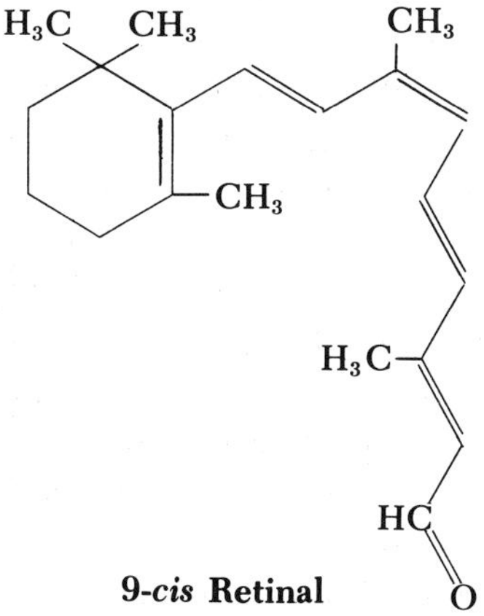

9-*cis* Retinal

The biologically active form of vitamin A apparently differs from any of the foregoing. The active form has been isolated[4] chromatographically from the liver of rats given ^{14}C-labeled retinoic acid and differs from the known vitamin A compounds. It is highly active in stimulating growth in vitamin A–deficient rats.

Occurrence. The best sources of vitamin A are cod-liver oil and other fish-liver oils, fish roe, the flesh of oily fish, the livers of other animals, butter, eggs, and cheese. The provitamin occurs most abundantly in carrots and other yellow vegetables, e.g., squash, sweet potatoes, and many green vegetables, particularly broccoli, spinach, and beet greens. In fish-liver oils retinol is present as esters of fatty acids, chiefly stearic, palmitic, and higher unsaturated acids. When the liver oil is ingested by man or animal, the retinol esters are hydrolyzed by pancreatic esterases and the vitamin rapidly absorbed into the intestinal mucosa. In those conditions in which the individual is unable to hydrolyze esters, e.g., celiac disease and tropical sprue, severe deficiencies of vitamin A may occur. The esters cannot be absorbed, unhydrolyzed, in the way that a part of the fats apparently is. The vitamin is recombined with fatty acids *characteristic of the host* (not of the diet) immediately after passage through the gut wall. The vitamin esters are then conveyed by the portal vein to the liver, where they are stored in ester form. From the liver, vitamin A is redistributed to the various organs, by way of the bloodstream, in the form of a protein complex. The carrier protein has been isolated and characterized. The principal fatty acids present in the retinol esters of the retinas of various animals are palmitic, stearic, and oleic.[5]

For the absorption of the provitamins from the intestinal tract, bile salts are necessary. The conversion to the vitamin is not well understood. However, there is evidence to indicate that it occurs primarily in the intestinal wall and, to some extent, in the liver. The actual process may be either hydrolytic or oxidative. Each molecule of provitamin yields either two molecules or one molecule of retinol, depending on whether the provitamin is β-carotene or one of the others, respectively. Man, as well as the experimental animal, is an inefficient converter of carotene to retinol. On the average, about four times as much carotene is required as retinol to maintain normal dark adaptation in adults, and in some cases there are even more marked individual variations. We might expect one molecule of β-carotene to yield two retinol molecules, but since it is only about half as active biologically, the β-carotene molecule is apparently split in an unsymmetric manner. The other carotenoid precursors of vitamin A are even less active biologically since each molecule can form only one of retinol. This inefficiency of conversion may not be real but may be due to the fact that carotene is not absorbed as easily as retinol and a considerable amount is lost in the feces. As stated above, carotene apparently requires the presence of bile salts and fat in the intestine for its absorption, whereas bile does not appear to be necessary for the absorption of vitamin A, although it is helpful. Consequently, in cases where there is a stoppage of bile, bile salts or desiccated bile should be administered in order to be sure that the provitamin is taken up. Another practical point is the fact that carotene is soluble in mineral oil, which has been shown to remove much of the carotene present in the digesting food and thus cause a deficiency of the vitamin if the mineral oil is taken repeatedly shortly after a meal. This may also be true of retinol. For individuals using mineral oil constantly, such a danger should be recognized. Vitamin E seems to have a sparing action on vitamin A (p. 788).

Neither retinol nor the provitamins pass the placenta into the fetus very readily, although the vitamin is more easily transferred. Consequently, new-born infants have low stores of both. The milk of well-fed mothers, however, contains ample amounts of this vitamin, mostly in ester form, for the nursing infant's needs.

Effect of deficiency. In the experimental animal a lack of vitamin A is manifested by a slowing or stopping of growth in the young. This effect, however, is not peculiar to vitamin A, since lack of other vitamins or other essential nutritive factors has similar results. The most manifest specific effect of retinol deficiency is on the eye. This is shown in animals by an avoidance of light (photophobia) and by the occurrence of *xerophthalmia* and *keratomalacia.* Xerophthalmia is an eye disease characterized by drying of the eyes. The cells of the lacrimal glands become keratinized and stop secreting tears. The external surfaces thus become dry and have a dull appearance. Ulcers form; bacteria are not washed away; the eyelids swell and become sticky and scaly. Frequently there are bloody exudates and severe eye infections. If not treated in time, blindness results; but in most instances the animals die of respiratory infections before this occurs. The reason for this is that retinol deficiency has an effect upon other epithelial structures as well as those of the eye. In other words, the eye affection is only one manifestation of the specific influence which this vitamin has upon many epithelial structures. This deficit results in "the substitution of stratified keratinizing epithelium for the normal epithelium in various parts of the respiratory tract, alimentary tract, eyes and paraocular glands, and the genito-urinary tract."[*] One of the results of this keratinization is the loss of cilia in the respiratory epithelium. These ordinarily tend to sweep upward bacteria-laden foreign particles and thus combat infection.

Pertinent in this connection is the current report[6] that germ-free rats fed a vitamin A–deficient diet survived as long as 272 days whereas litter-mate weanling germ-free rats transferred to a conventional animal room and fed the same vitamin A–deficient diet died within 23 to 54 days. This important investigation leaves little doubt that the early death of rats fed a vitamin A–deficient diet must be a consequence of bacterial infection.

In rats, vitamin A is definitely necessary for reproduction and lactation. In fact it is just as essential as vitamin E, the "antisterility" vitamin, and must be given in greater amounts than are needed for optimal growth, if normal reproduction and lactation are to occur. Another interesting effect of a deficiency of vitamin A was reported in recent studies; this is a loss of normal taste acuity in vitamin A–depleted rats. Both the intensity and the quality

---

[*] From Wolbach, S. B.: Pathologic changes resulting from brain deficiency, J.A.M.A. **108**:7, 1937.

of taste are affected. There are distinct histologic changes in the taste buds and surrounding tissue.

In man, deficiencies in vitamin A result in epidermal lesions and ocular changes. The appellation, "anti-infective," which was formerly given to this vitamin, may not be justified. As stated, however, a lack of the vitamin may contribute to infection, and there is no doubt that a lowered resistance to bacterial invasion is brought about.

Extreme cases of vitamin A deficiency in man are rare at the present time in Western civilization, although in Eastern countries they are still seen. Livingstone's party suffered from it in 1857 during their African explorations as a result of a deficient diet, and many instances have been described since. In 1904, there was a report of 1400 cases of xerophthalmia among Japanese children. During and after World War I, many cases of the same condition occurred in Denmark, because of the fact that butterfat was shipped out of that country in large amounts and substitutes containing no retinol were used. Xerophthalmia, of course, results from a total or nearly total lack of retinol, and seldom does a person today subsist on a diet of this type.

Less serious subclinical symptoms are frequently found in human beings because of a diet containing less retinol than the required minimum. Night blindness or *nyctalopia* is often encountered. This is an inability to see in dim light or to adapt to a decrease in intensity of light. Both the rods and the cones of the retina contain substances that depend on retinol for their formation and regeneration. The rods are particularly involved in dark adaptation, and vitamin A, or retinol, is especially needed for this function. Night blindness and slowing down of dark adaptation are frequently associated with cirrhosis of the liver and other liver conditions, which may indicate that the liver has something to do with the activity of retinol, in addition to the storage and absorption of the vitamin. The most important chronic disease in which carotene cannot be transformed easily into retinol is diabetes mellitus. If diabetic subjects are on restricted diets without insulin and try to satisfy their hunger with large amounts of green and yellow vegetables, their skin may acquire a yellow tinge due to the deposition in it of carotene. Night blindness is likely to occur under such conditions, but the addition of the vitamin itself to the diet quickly brings a return to normal vision. Perhaps even earlier than night blindness is the occurrence of *xerosis conjunctiva*, minute dry spots, which may be detected with biomicroscopic examination. Both night blindness and the other eye symptoms are treated by administration of carotene or, better, of retinol itself. Fairly large doses are given, but there is a limit to the amount that can be absorbed, or put to work, in healing the damage present. Usually results are noted in a short time.

Skin conditions frequently result from an inadequate retinol intake. Dryness and scaliness of the skin are often seen as early stages of retinol deficiency. Sometimes small pustules, termed *follicular hyperkeratosis*, appear around the hair follicles or extensor surfaces of the upper and lower extremities, on the shoulders, neck, back, lower abdomen, and buttocks. They are hard and pigmented and are surrounded by a zone of pigmentation (Fig. 23-2). In other instances the pimples resemble those of acne except that there is

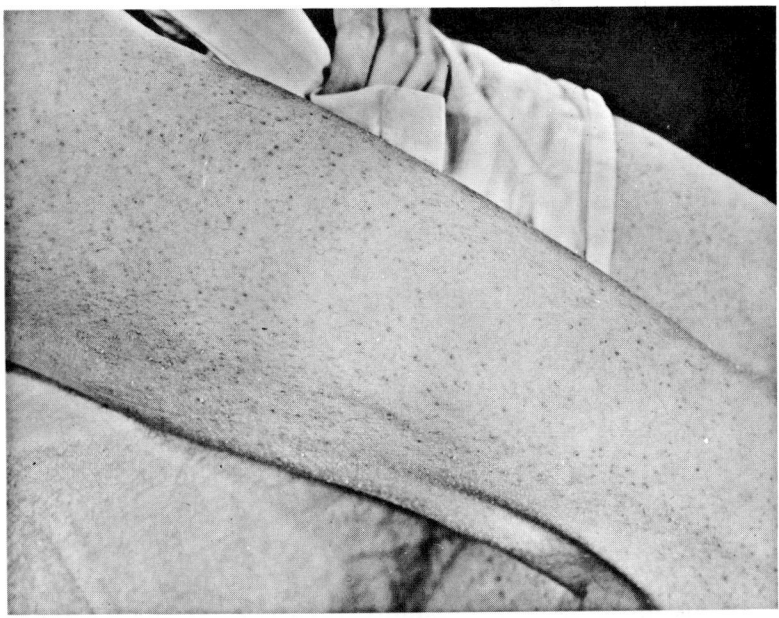

Fig. 23-2. Follicular hyperkeratosis due to vitamin A deficiency. (From files of Therapeutic Notes; courtesy O. D. Bird.)

seldom any pus. Large doses of retinol are required over a period of many weeks to cure these conditions. Although the epithelium of the mucous membranes is often keratinized in animals, whether similar pathologic changes occur in man is not certain. Another finding in animals with retinol deficiency is urinary calculi, and here again whether the same result follows in man is uncertain.

Retinol is an important factor in tooth formation. This is probably related to the fact that the enamel layer is an epidermal structure. As a result of retinol deficiency, there is a defective formation of enamel, with the consequent possible exposure of the dentin. Sound teeth, of course, cannot be expected under such circumstances.

Retinol deficiency has been asserted to result in paralysis and nerve degeneration. The explanation possibly lies in the fact that such a deficiency may retard bone growth and, in particular, the formation of endochondral bone while the central nervous system, as well as other soft tissues, continues to grow at a nearly normal rate. If this occurs at an early age, it has an effect on the nervous system. Because the skull does not grow rapidly enough, there may be overcrowding of the cranial cavity, with distortion of the brain and pressure on the spinal cord and nerve fibers. Therefore, the nervous lesions may be entirely mechanical in origin. These results have been seen to occur in laboratory animals, but whether they occur in man is not certain. The retardation of endochondral bone formation must be specific because bone matrix (osteoid) formation continues.

Other effects that have been attributed to an avitaminosis of this vitamin are atrophy of the testes and disturbances of the female genitals. Retinol has also been shown[7] to be essential to vision in invertebrates since the common housefly is dependent on it in this respect.

Mode of action. As mentioned previously, retinol deficiency has a deleterious effect on epithelial structures in general. Hence a general function of this vitamin is the maintenance of epithelial tissues in a normal condition. How this is accomplished is not well understood, but certain structural proteins of tissues appear to be stabilized by combination with retinol or its derivatives and to deteriorate in the retinol-deficient state, which helps to explain the role of this vitamin in the chemistry of vision, where it plays a direct and special role.[8]

Effect on vision. The light receptors of the eye are the rod and cone cells of the retina. The outer segments of both kinds of receptor contain light-sensitive pigments that require vitamin A for their formation and proper functioning. The rod and cone outer segments are surrounded by pigment epithelium cells that store vitamin A. The pigment contained in the outer segments of the rods, *visual purple* or *rhodopsin,* is a conjugated protein, consisting of a protein, *opsin,* linked to a prosthetic group, the red-colored aldehyde of 11-*cis* vitamin A$_1$, also called *neo-b retinene,* or *11-cis retinal.* Rhodopsin is extractable from the rods by mild detergents, e.g., bile salts or digitonin, with which it forms a soluble complex; but it is insoluble in the usual protein solvents. It has been estimated as having a molecular weight of about 40,000. Its absorption spectrum is maximal at about 500 nm., corresponding to the wavelength for minimal threshold of the eye in dim light. It is sensitive to light and, when illuminated, changes from red to orange to yellow and, on prolonged exposure, to colorless retinol and opsin. The eye becomes less sensitive to light during the bleaching of rhodopsin (light adaptation). In the dark, rhodopsin is regenerated and the sensitivity of the retina is restored (dark adaptation). The recovery is rapid or slow, according to the wavelength and the intensity and duration of the pre-exposure to light. If there is a deficiency of retinol in the retina, regeneration is incomplete and the patient is night blind.

Rhodopsin is the prototype of some 190 visual pigments identified in about 150 animal species.[9] Visual pigments and their derivatives are characterized by the shape of their rather broad (about 200 nm.) absorption spectra and particularly by their absorption maxima. Two interconvertible pigments with widely separated absorption maxima are readily converted back and forth by irradiating at appropriate wavelengths. Since the nomenclature of photopigments has become very involved, Dartnall proposes that each pigment be identified by its λ_{max}.[9] Table 23-1 is presented to assist in identification of pigments discussed in the literature under different names.

The scheme shown in Fig. 23-3 presents the probable in vivo rhodopsin cycle of cattle and human retinas. The cycle may be conveniently divided into three stages: photothermal, thermal degradation, and thermal regeneration.

Photothermal stage. Rhodopsin, composed of one molecule of the chromophore 11-*cis* retinol bound by a Schiff-base linkage to the ε-amino groups of lysyl residues and by forces involving sulfhydryl groups to one molecule

Table 23-1. Visual photopigments and photoproducts in primate and ox retinas

Current names	λ_{max} in nanometers	Other identities
Rhodopsin	497 ± 2	Visual purple
11-*cis* Retinal opsin		11-*cis* Vitamin A_1 aldehyde opsin
11-*cis* Retinaldehyde opsin		neo-b Retinene opsin
Isorhodopsin	487 ± 6	
9-*cis* Retinal opsin		
9-*cis* Retinaldehyde opsin		
N-Retinylidene opsin	365	Alkaline indicator yellow
NH-Retinylidene opsin	440	Acid indicator yellow
all-*trans* Retinal	385	Vitamin A_1 aldehyde
all-*trans* Retinaldehyde		Retinene
all-*trans* Retinol	325	Vitamin A_1 alcohol
		Visual white
11-*cis* Retinal	376.5	11-*cis* Vitamin A_1 aldehyde
11-*cis* Retinaldehyde		neo-b Retinene
11-*cis* Retinol	319	11-*cis* Vitamin A_1 alcohol
		neo-b Vitamin A_1
Prelumirhodopsin	543 ⎫	Along with N-retinylidene opsin, these
Lumirhodopsin	497 ⎬	are successive stages in the thermal
Metarhodopsin (transient	479 ⎭	weakening of linkages of all-*trans*
orange?)		retinal to opsin

of colorless opsin, upon absorbing 1 photon or quantum of light, is isomerized to the all-*trans* configuration prelumirhodopsin. This is unstable and quickly breaks down to lumirhodopsin and then to metarhodopsin. Note, in Table 23-1, that these changes are accompanied by an increase in λ_{max} from 497 to 543, followed by a decrease to 497 and then to 479, indicating a rise in energy level followed by two successive falls. This is typical of photochemical reactions, as shown by Ciamician in 1912.

A fourth but thermostable product, isorhodopsin (9-*cis* retinal opsin), is formed by isomerization of any of the three orange, all-*trans* intermediates. At low temperatures, where thermal degradation is almost halted, all of the substances mentioned so far, including rhodopsin, under steady illumination are freely interconverted and enter a photosteady state in which the proportion of each participant is determined by the wavelength of light, in accordance with the several absorption maxima of the participants. This also occurs at body temperature during very brief flashes of light before the slower thermal reactions have made much progress toward removal of metarhodopsin.

Thermal degradation stage. Once rhodopsin has been photoisomerized to prelumirhodopsin, all subsequent changes proceed in light or in darkness. The portion of metarhodopsin not reverting to lumirhodopsin or isomerized

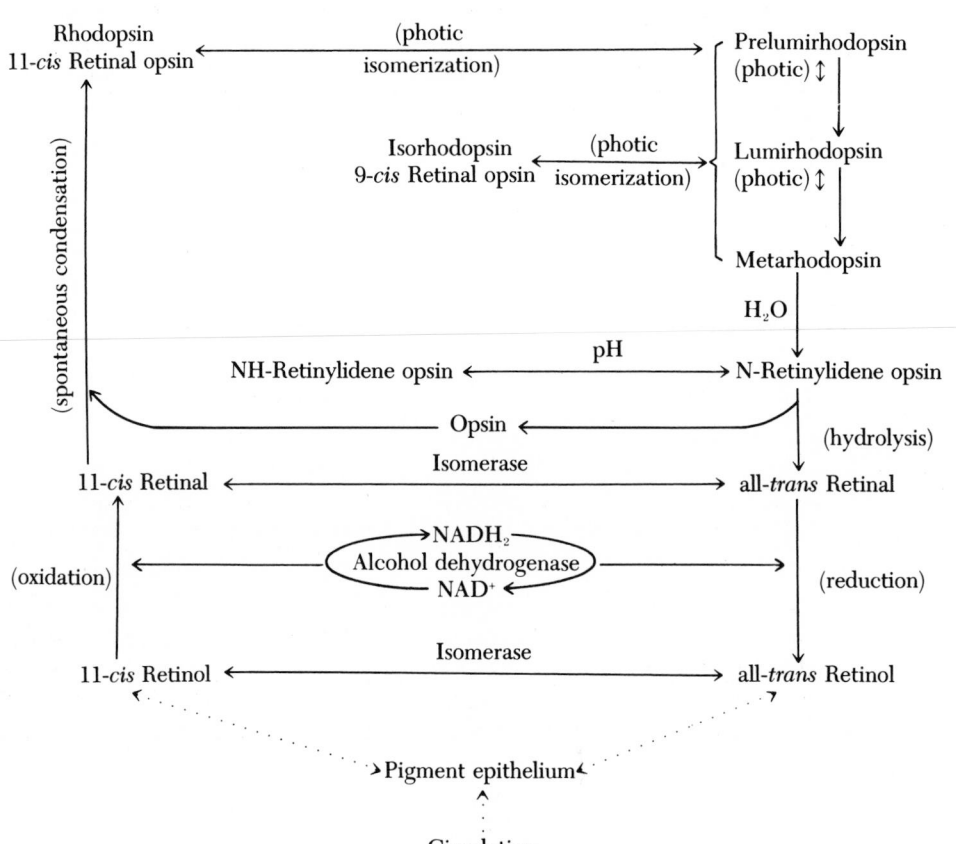

Fig. 23-3. Principal transformations occurring in the retina during the visual cycle. Arrows not labeled *photic* indicate thermal reactions uninfluenced by light. (Courtesy C. Haig, Northampton College of Advanced Technology, London, England.)

to isorhodopsin is converted to N-retinylidene opsin, the acid form of which is NH-retinylidene opsin. Collins found that all-*trans* retinal and opsin are bound by a Schiff-base linkage between the aldehyde group of retinal and an amino group of opsin.[10] This yields the pH-sensitive system:

$$C_{19}H_{27}CH{=}H\overset{+}{N}R \; \leftrightharpoons \; C_{19}H_{27}{=}NR + H^+$$

In the above reaction, R is opsin. In this all-*trans* configuration the additional electric forces are weak; in rhodopsin, which is 11-*cis*, they are strong and the compound is stable. N-Retinylidene opsin, however, is readily hydrolyzed to all-*trans* retinal and free opsin. Some all-*trans* retinal is immediately isomerized (by isomerase produced by the pigment epithelium) to 11-*cis* retinal, which spontaneously combines with opsin to form rhodopsin. The rest of the all-*trans* retinal is reduced to all-*trans* retinol by the action of alcohol dehydrogenase and NADH₂. Some all-*trans* retinol leaves the outer rod segments and is temporarily stored in the pigment epithelium. The rest of the all-*trans* retinol is isomerized to 11-*cis* retinol.

Thermal regeneration stage. The regeneration of rhodopsin requires reconversion of all-*trans* retinol to 11-*cis* retinal, which spontaneously condenses with opsin to form rhodopsin. We have seen that a proportion of 11-*cis* retinal is formed by isomerization of some all-*trans* retinal as soon as it is released from combination in N-retinylidene opsin. Some arrives preformed from the circulation via the pigment epithelium. The remainder is derived from all-*trans* retinol that has been temporarily stored in the pigment epithelium. The latter all-*trans* retinol is isomerized to the 11-*cis* configuration, which is then oxidized by NAD^+ to 11-*cis* retinal. The equilibrium point of the latter reversible reaction is well over toward reduction but is displaced toward oxidation by the trapping of 11-*cis* retinal by opsin to form rhodopsin. Since rhodopsin is a principal structural component of retinal rods, this trapping action is a perfect example of the general role of vitamin A in the stabilization of structural proteins.

This, then, is the cycle that operates in the retinal rods in the presence of dim light to give us night vision. If the light intensity is held constant, the entire system enters a *steady state*, rhodopsin being regenerated as fast as it is bleached. As the light intensity is raised or lowered, the rhodopsin concentration is decreased or increased to sustain higher or lower steady states; i.e., when light intensity is raised, the rhodopsin concentration is decreased and night vision sensitivity becomes reduced, and vice versa.

Color vision. While vision in dim light is mediated by rhodopsin of the *rod* cells, color vision is mediated by three different retinal-containing pigments in the *cone* cells.[8] The three pigments are called *porphyropsin, iodopsin,* and *cyanopsin* and are sensitive to the three essential colors red, green, and blue, respectively. Thus, when light strikes the retina, it bleaches one or more of these pigments, depending on the color quality of the light. The pigments are converted to all-*trans* retinal; and the protein moiety, opsin, is released as in the case of rhodopsin. This reaction gives rise to the nerve impulse that is read out in the brain as color—red, if porphyropsin is split, green, if iodopsin, or blue, if cyanopsin. If mixtures of the three are converted, the color read out in the brain depends on the proportions of the three split.

We might ask at what point in the cycle the nerve fibers associated with the rod or cone cells of the retina are stimulated. The answer to this question is not known with certainty, but from our knowledge of the time constants of visual phenomena, the stimulation probably takes place immediately after isomerization of rhodopsin by light, when electrically charged groups on opsin have been exposed owing to the poor fit of the all-*trans* configuration.

Experiments on patients and normal controls have established the fact that retinol is required by the cone pigments as well as by rhodopsin. In fact, probably the only chemical difference between the rod and cone pigments is in the protein components.[8,9] Thus, if we substitute cone opsins for rod opsin, the scheme in Fig. 23-3 describes the chemistry of cone vision. The light intensities required, however, are much higher and the absorption maxima are different, in accordance with the requirements of day vision and of color vision.

There is evidence that color blindness is due to a congenital deficiency of the red- or green-sensitive cone pigments, porphyropsin or iodopsin. Apparently a sex-linked recessive mutation is involved since the defect is rare in females. The two genes for the red- or green-sensitive pigments probably lie close together on the x-chromosome. Blue color blindness, due to a lack of cyanopsin, appears to be very rare. However, a small portion of the central part of the normal fovea of the retina lacks cyanopsin in the cone cells. Hence, this area is *blue blind.*[8] Trichromatic vision is restricted to a portion of the cone cells in the central part of the retina (20 to 30 degrees). Dichromatic vision, red or green blind, occurs in the next portion of the retina (70 to 80 degrees). The peripheral part of the retina shows only monochromatic vision. Hence, there appears to be a definite pattern of distribution of the retinal opsin pigments in the normal retina.[8]

Effect on other processes. We have seen that vitamin A has other functions in the body besides those related to vision. Animals on a vitamin A–deficient diet frequently die without any serious eye symptoms.

Retinol appears to be involved in mucopolysaccharide biosynthesis at an enzymatic level according to recent work.[11] Vitamin A increased the incorporation of ^{35}S- and of ^{14}C-glucose into chondroitin sulfate in homogenates of rat colon from vitamin A–deficient rats. The effect may involve sulfate formation or activation, which could explain the damage to mucus-secreting epithelial tissues manifested as xerophthalmia, and dryness and keratinization of the skin and epithelium of the gastrointestinal and genitourinary systems in vitamin A deficiency. Maintenance of epithelial tissue is a second major function of retinol, as emphasized previously. Retinol may have some relation to nucleic acid metabolism, since there is a decrease in the DNA content of several organs during vitamin A deficiency, which is remedied by administration of this vitamin. Retinol may also be involved in electron transport systems.

Storage. Most of the carotene and retinol absorbed goes to the liver, where it is stored. A sufficient amount of this vitamin can be "hoarded" to last a long time, but when a vitamin A–deficient diet is given to rats, the liver stores begin falling immediately. The plasma level remains constant until the liver is almost depleted, the rhodopsin level in the retina remaining normal until the blood vitamin A is depleted. At this point, night blindness begins. When rhodopsin is about 50% depleted, the protein opsin begins to decline and the rod cells of the retina to degenerate.[8]

Excretion and secretion. Neither vitamin A nor provitamin A is excreted in the urine. Either may appear in the feces but probably as an unabsorbed portion. Even this happens to only a slight extent, the unused material being destroyed by bacteria. Amounts in liver and other tissues in excess of the normal storage capacity or requirement must also be destroyed, but how this happens is still unknown. Both carotene and the vitamin are secreted by the mammary gland. Human colostrum has two or three times as much as early human milk, and the latter has from five to 10 times the vitamin A activity of cow's milk.

Human requirements. In measuring human requirements of vitamin A, as well as of other vitamins, certain units have been used. These were at first rather arbitrarily fixed and were often based on the amount necessary to prevent avitaminosis in animals under standard conditions. In time, as the vitamins were synthesized, it became possible to base the unitage on the weight of carefully purified and standardized preparations. For vitamin A, the World Health Organization has chosen as one international unit the activity of 0.000344 mg. (0.344 μg.) of synthetic vitamin A–acetate, which is equivalent to 0.300 μg. of retinol.

The minimum daily allowance of vitamin A recommended (1968 revision, Food and Nutrition Board, National Academy of Sciences–National Research Council) is about 5000 units for men and women (Table 25-1). For pregnant and nursing women, from 6000 to 8000 units daily are recommended. Infants and growing children require 1500 to 5000 units daily, depending on age. The well-balanced dietary of most Americans contains this amount under normal conditions, but it is more than possible that the underprivileged do not get the minimum. It is also possible that some individuals require more than the minimum because of either faulty absorption or some other reason. Therefore, the addition of supplements may be indicated, especially since a moderate excess seems to be nontoxic.

Toxic effects. Overdosage with vitamin A may produce hypervitaminosis and toxic effects, presumably because this vitamin, like vitamin D (p. 786), is not readily excreted and consequently tissue levels may build up to dangerous concentrations. Excessive amounts of vitamin A, especially in children, may cause loss of appetite, weight loss, irritability, fissuring at the corners of the mouth, and cracking and bleeding of the lips. Later, loss of hair, liver enlargement, and bone and joint pains may occur.

VITAMIN D

Vitamin D is the vitamin that is related to rickets and is therefore spoken of as the *antirachitic* vitamin. It is necessary for normal calcium and phosphorus metabolism and consequently for healthy bone and tooth development.

Discovery and properties. In the early days of the vitamins, "fat-soluble A" was considered a single substance, the vitamin that was capable of curing both xerophthalmia and rickets. In 1922, McCollum bubbled oxygen through cod-liver oil for several hours at 120° C. and found that the resulting oil was ineffective against xerophthalmia but was capable of curing rickets. Vitamin A had been destroyed by this procedure, and the factor remaining was called vitamin D, the antirachitic factor. Other evidence was brought forward to prove the same point. For example, it was found that a small amount of dehydrated spinach would cure xerophthalmia in rats in a few days but huge amounts of the same dried spinach could not prevent rickets produced in rats that had been fed a rachitic diet.

Vitamin D is a white crystalline substance, soluble in fats and fat solvents. It is fairly heat resistant and also relatively resistant to oxidation. However, pharmaceutic preparations such as calciferol and 7-dehydrocholesterol should be stored in hermetically sealed containers under nitrogen. It is not affected in mild acids or alkalies. When cod-liver oil is saponified, the vitamin is found in the nonsaponifiable fraction. It is a sterol.

Relation to radiant energy. From the time of Herodotus, the health-giving effects of sunlight have been emphasized, but the particular relation of lack of sunshine to rickets did not begin to be recognized until the last century. It was seen that underprivileged children, living in dark, crowded quarters, were likely to be victims of this disease. There was a greater incidence in winter than in summer, which was considered to be due to the differences in the length of the days. In 1822, a Polish physician, Sniadecki, maintained that exposure of the body to direct sunlight had both a preventive and a curative effect for rickets. Much later, Palm, an Englishman, as a result of correspondence with medical missionaries all over the world, revealed the absence of rickets, in spite of poor sanitary conditions, in those regions where sunlight was most abundant and definitely concluded that rickets was mainly caused by a lack of sunlight. However, demonstrations of the curative action of ultraviolet rays by modern methods of x-ray diagnosis were lacking. In 1919, Huldschinsky, using such methods, proved that exposure to ultraviolet rays would cure rickets, and Hess duplicated this success with sunlight. Later it was shown that animals fed a diet deficient in vitamin D but containing a sufficiency of calcium and phosphorus would not acquire rickets if they were irradiated with ultraviolet light. The final chapter in this story was the announcement that cholesterol-containing inactive foods could be given antirachitic properties by irradiating them with ultraviolet light. Dried milk and other foods can be irradiated on a commercial basis. A potent antirachitic agent, ergocalciferol, is produced by the irradiation of ergosterol, a sterol derived from ergot and from yeast.

The explanation of these phenomena is that ultraviolet irradiation causes a change in the molecular structure of certain sterols that, unless so changed, are inactive. If the irradiated sterols are taken by mouth, they act just the same as the naturally occurring vitamin D; if they are produced in or on the skin by the irradiation of the inactive sterols present there, they are absorbed and find their way into the circulation and behave similarly to orally administered vitamin D. These inactive sterols are the provitamins of vitamin D. One of them, 7-dehydrocholesterol, can be synthesized by animals, including man.

Interesting recent observations[12] suggest that the rate of synthesis of cholecalciferol from 7-dehydrocholesterol in the skin (stratum granulosum) is regulated by the amount of pigmentation and keratinization in the overlying stratum corneum. This regulates the amount of solar ultraviolet radiation, especially at 290 to 320 nm., that penetrates into the stratum granulosum and forms vitamin D. Thus, white skin, which contains little pigment and keratin, allows maximal ultraviolet penetration. Yellow skin, which contains more keratin, permits less ultraviolet penetration; whereas black skin, which is more pigmented, permits still less. These differences are apparently a genetic adaptation to climate. Hair or fur in animals is a still further regulatory mechanism. Vitamin D synthesis is thus maintained within physiologic limits, estimated to be 0.01 to 2.5 mg. cholecalciferol per day. Skin pigmentation also may correct for seasonal variations, e.g., *tanning* in the summer months in northern latitudes.

Structure. At least 10 different compounds are known to have antirachitic properties and are designated D_1, D_2, etc. Five of them are rather well defined as chemical compounds, but only two are of great importance, D_2, of vegetable origin, now called *ergocalciferol*, and D_3, or *cholecalciferol*, of animal origin. The common vitamin D of fish-liver oils is D_3. This is probably the form also present in milk and eggs and is produced on irradiation of the skin and when

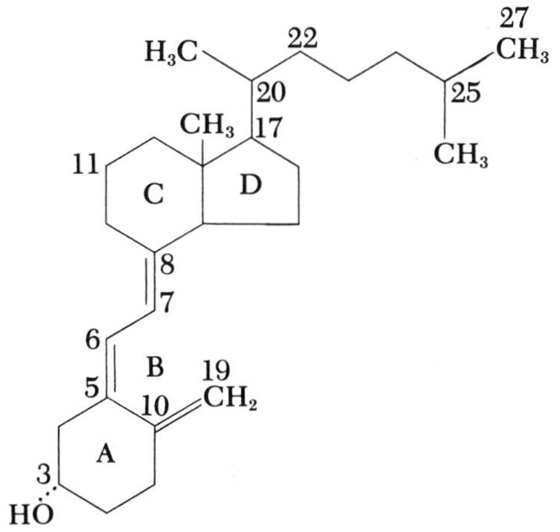

Cholecalciferol (vitamin D_3)
(Courtesy L. F. Fieser)

7-dehydrocholesterol is irradiated. Vitamin D_2 is derived from ergosterol. The formula shows that the effect of irradiation is the opening of ring *B*.

Ergocalciferol (D_2) has the same structure as cholecalciferol (D_3), with the exception of the side chain, which is as follows:

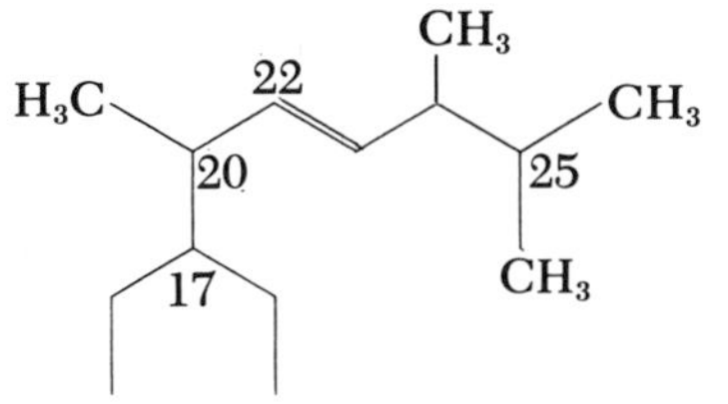

Both forms of the vitamin have about the same degree of activity in the human being. In nature, these vitamins occur as esters.

The above structure of cholecalciferol differs from that given in the last edition of this book and from those presented in most other textbooks on the subject. However, it now seems established.[13] X-ray analysis has shown that the triene system is *trans*oid and coplanar. Supporting evidence has come from studies of the ultraviolet absorption spectrum and from partial synthesis and degradation. For this reason, the present structure more accurately depicts the actual configuration of vitamin D_3 and has therefore been adopted. An accurate knowledge of the conformation of vitamin D_3 is, of course, essential to ultimately understanding the biochemical function of this vitamin.

Recent investigations[14] indicate, however, that the biologically active form of cholecalciferol has a slightly different structure. It is a more polar compound, having an additional hydroxyl group in the carbon-25 position. Its structure, therefore, is as shown on p. 780.

779

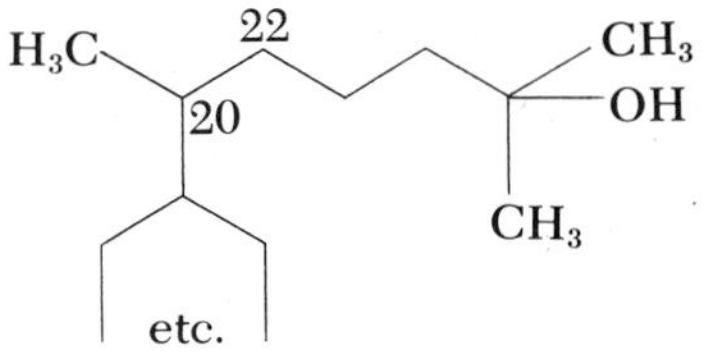

25-Hydroxycholecalciferol (active form of vitamin D_3)

The active form of cholecalciferol was isolated chromatographically as a pure compound from the plasma of hogs fed large amounts of vitamin D_3. Its structure was established as 25-hydroxycholecalciferol (as shown above). It is the major if not sole biologically active metabolite of cholecalciferol. It has about 50% more activity than cholecalciferol in curing rickets in rats, in increasing bone ash in vitamin D–deficient chicks, and in increasing the transport of calcium across the intestinal mucosa of vitamin D–deficient rats. As little as 0.25 μg. of 25-hydroxycholecalciferol injected intravenously into vitamin D–deficient rats increased calcium absorption from the intestine.[14] The addition of 2.5 μg. via an arterial blood perfusate to cholecalciferol-deficient rats increased calcium transport to normal levels within 2 hours.[14] 25-Hydroxycholecalciferol also produces an earlier rise in serum calcium resulting from bone resorption in vitamin D–deficient rats than does cholecalciferol in a similar dose. These observations, taken as a whole, are strong evidence that 25-hydroxycholecalciferol is, indeed, the metabolically active form of vitamin D_3.

Occurrence. Cod-liver oil and other fish-liver oils are the best natural sources of vitamin D. The flesh of oily fish, e.g., sardines, salmon, herring, are also excellent sources. Egg yolk and liver of the commonly slaughtered animals contain amounts that depend on the food of the animal from which they are derived, but mammalian liver is not very rich in this vitamin. Milk contains little vitamin D unless enriched in one of the three ways described below, and vitamin D milk is now a common article of the American dietary. Many of our ordinary foods, among them the green plants, contain small quantities; and mushrooms contain slightly greater amounts. In general, this vitamin is not widely distributed, but the fact that it can be provided in three ways should make its deficiency rather uncommon in the future. These three ways of providing vitamin D are (1) by furnishing the vitamin as it occurs naturally in foods or by enriching the food by the addition of vitamin D; (2) by irradiating foods containing precursors of the vitamin; and (3) by irradiating the skin of the individual with ultraviolet light or sunshine.

Absorption. Absorption of vitamin D from the intestinal tract requires the presence of bile. Here, again, mineral oil acts as a hindrance, because the vitamin is soluble in it and consequently is carried through the intestine into the feces. After absorption, calciferol is apparently transported in the plasma, tightly bound to an α_2-globulin.

Effects of deficiency. A deficiency of vitamin D leads to rickets in children (Fig. 23-4) and to osteomalacia in adults, a condition that might be termed "adult rickets." Rickets usually develops in infancy or early childhood, although juvenile or late rickets is seen in India, x-ray–detectable rickets

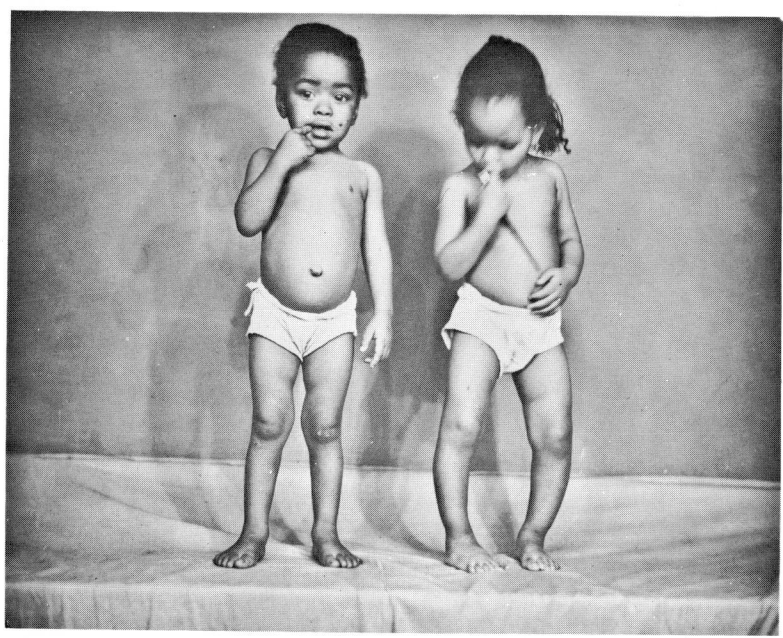

Fig. 23-4. Rachitic children, showing knock-knees on left and bowlegs on right. (From files of Therapeutic Notes; courtesy T. D. Spies and O. D. Bird.)

being frequently observed up to the age of puberty in that country. Defective ossification is the result of this avitaminosis. The bones become soft and pliable, and a number of different deformities may ensue: bowlegs, knock-knees, enlargement of the ends of bones (epiphyses), rows of beadlike swellings at the rib junctions (the "rachitic rosary"), contracted pelvis, and the development of bosses on the temporal bones. X-ray photographs of the bones reveal that ossification is not normal; the shadows cast are less dense and the ends of the bones less sharply defined (Fig. 23-5). Chemical analysis of the bones reveals a lower content of inorganic constituents and a higher content of organic substances and water. However, the *ratio* of calcium to phosphorus remains constant, indicating that the type of bone salt laid down is normal, although the amount is insufficient. In the blood serum there is usually, but not always, a normal content of calcium, but the phosphate is decreased. Howland and Kramer, who first discovered this, stated that, if the product of the serum calcium content and the serum phosphate, both expressed as milligrams per 100 ml., equaled or exceeded 40, rickets did not develop whereas a product of below 30 always led to rickets. There is also a marked increase in serum phosphatase in rickets and a decrease when recovery is brought about as a result of vitamin D treatment. The exact significance of this is not known. Some authors believe that the increased serum phosphatase in rickets (and in other bone diseases) is a result of overproduction in the bone in a vain attempt at bone formation. Others consider it a result of the bone's increased capacity for cellular activities because of the absence of true bone which is relatively inactive.

A vitamin D–resistant form of rickets in children has been described

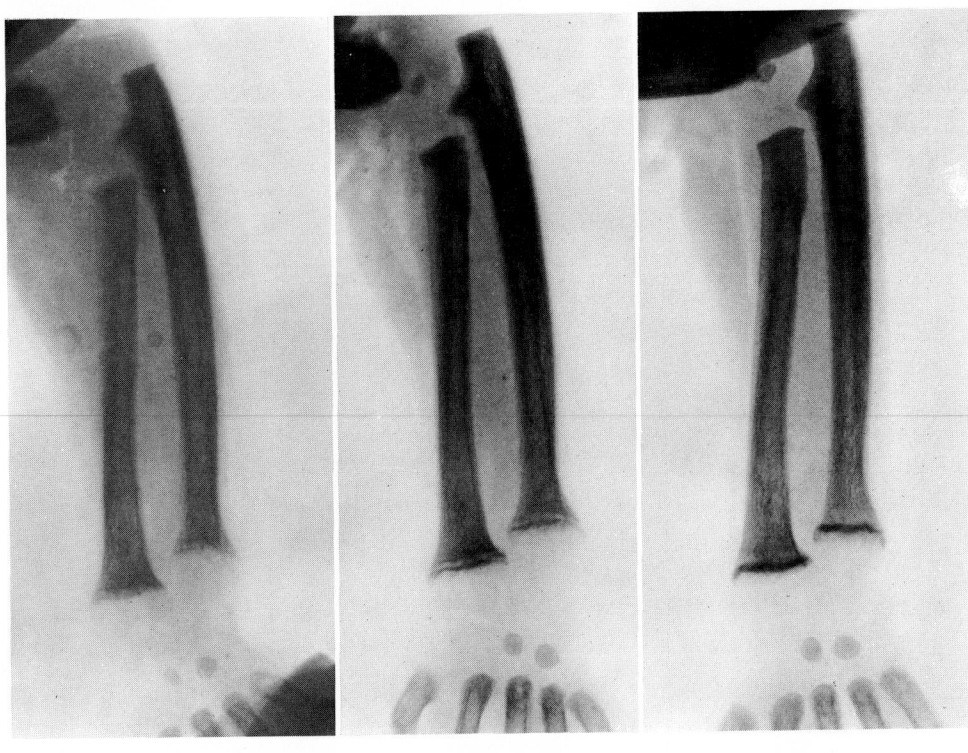

A   **B**   **C**

Fig. 23-5. X-ray films of the forearms of a rachitic child, showing the effect of treatment. **A,** Feb. 11, Marked trabeculation of the radius and ulna, particularly in the cortical portion of the bone, with slight periosteal thickening. The end of the bone is slightly mushroomed and cupped and shows distinct fringing. The cartilage is swollen. The distal epiphyses of the radius are absent. There are two small centers of ossification in the wrists. **B,** March 11, A new center of ossification has appeared in the distal epiphysis of the humerus. The centers of ossification at the wrists are still two in number but larger and more distinct in outline. There is a fresh line of calcium deposition at the ends of the radius and ulna in the zone of provisional cartilage (line test). A clear area is present between this new calcification and the shaft (submetaphyseal rarefaction). Cupping, fringing, and stippling are present, and spur formation is also noted outlining the swollen cartilage at the distal epiphysis of the ulna (beginning healing). **C,** March 24, Healing is now advanced. The shaft shows calcification of subperiosteal osteoid at the outer aspect of the radius, giving the bone a greater width. Calcification of the provisional zone in the metaphyses is much more distinct and the submetaphyseal area is filling in.

Case history. Diagnosis: Rickets and infantile tetany. Admitted Feb. 9, because of carpopedal spasm of 6 hours' duration. Had never had cod-liver oil. Had 3 oz. of orange juice daily for 1 month (6 months old upon admission). Physical examination on admission: Carpopedal spasm, separation of the sagittal and lambdoid sutures, with marked occipitoparietal craniotabes. Thorax: Flaring of the lower ribs with enlargement of the costochondral junctions. Chvostek's sign, positive. Laboratory data: Serum CO_2, 41 vol.%; Ca, 4.6; P, 5.6 (mg. in 100 ml.); Ca × P, 25.7; phosphatase, 57.2 units (Bodansky). Treatment: Calcium gluconate, 10 ml. of a 10% solution, intramuscularly at 10 P.M. and 12 P.M. $CaCl_2$, 1 dram q. 4 h. (1 gm.). Orange juice, 2 oz. daily. Vitamin D preparation, 10 drops daily, i.e., approximately 2500 I.U. vitamin D. Feb. 20, $CaCl_2$ discontinued.

repeatedly in the literature and is the subject of a recent study.[15] This condition is hereditary and characterized by a low serum phosphate level and high serum alkaline phosphatase. The chief clinical manifestation is shortness of the legs, which may be bowed, rather than of the trunk of the body. Treatment with massive doses of vitamin D does not change the height or deformity or improve the hypophosphatemia, but it does lower the level of alkaline phosphatase. Roentgenographic evidence of improvement in bone structure is usually found. Vitamin D therapy entails the risk of vitamin D toxicity, however. Treatment with phosphates or with human growth hormone have proved of uncertain value.

The pathogenesis of the disease is unknown. There is no demonstrated renal disease and no dietary vitamin D insufficiency. The rickets, however, is clinically similar to the form caused by vitamin D deficiency. The disease may be due to a renal tubular defect in the reabsorption of phosphate, to a decreased intestinal absorption of calcium, resulting in secondary hyperparathyroidism, or to an abnormal metabolism of or resistance to vitamin D.

It now appears[16] that patients with familial vitamin D–resistant rickets may lack the ability to convert cholecalciferol to 25-hydroxycholecalciferol, the active form of the vitamin. They have been found to respond satisfactorily to treatment with the 25-hydroxy–vitamin D derivative.[16]

In rickets there is commonly a delay in dentition. The first tooth in rachitic babies seldom appears between the sixth and ninth month, at which time it has appeared in about half the number of normal babies. This would be expected in view of the close relation of bones and teeth. Lady Mellanby showed also that lack of vitamin D leads to hypoplasia, i.e., poor structural development, of teeth in dogs. This may predispose to dental caries since a hypoplastic tooth is less effectively protected by enamel. The question as to whether healthy human teeth are likely to be more carious if vitamin D is lacking is still unsettled, as is also the companion question of the effect of a high vitamin D intake in preventing caries. Much work has been done on both these problems, and results indicate that vitamin D probably reduces the incidence of caries indirectly, i.e., by improving the general health and nutrition of the individual.

Osteomalacia presents a somewhat different picture from rickets, although the action on the bones is essentially the same. The bone becomes softer than rachitic bone and the ratio of calcium to phosphorus is changed. The loss of calcium is greater than that of phosphorus, and there is a relative gain in magnesium. This softness of the bones leads to diverse types of deformities. Osteomalacia occurs rarely in America or Europe, except in old age, but is common in India and China, particularly among women because of the custom that confines them indoors. Thus they are deprived of exposure to sunshine, and their diet is also deficient in vitamin D and calcium. In osteomalacia the serum calcium is reduced, sometimes to such an extent that tetany ensues. Tetany is a state of muscular twitching that may be brought about by low blood calcium.

Another clinical condition indirectly associated with a lack of cholecalciferol is celiac disease, also known as idiopathic steatorrhea and nontropical sprue. Here, as in osteomalacia, there is a demineralization of the bones, which may result in deformities or dwarfism. Here, too, a low serum calcium and low serum phosphorus are found, with possible manifestations of tetany. Celiac disease is *indirectly* a vitamin D deficiency because the primary abnormality seems to be, in part, a fatty diarrhea. The fat in the intestinal canal is not absorbed normally and carries with it into the stools calcium salts (soaps) and vitamin D.

In all the conditions mentioned, the administration of vitamin D in therapeutic doses, or ultraviolet irradiation, or both, produces good results. Deformities cannot be rectified by this means, but further malformation may be checked. Serial x-ray photographs of rachitic bones before and during treatment show this effect in a striking manner (Fig. 23-5).

Mechanism of action. Vitamin D has a regulatory power on calcium and phosphorus metabolism. Both calcium and phosphorus must be present in the diet in order to have the complex calcium salt deposited in bone. However, no matter how great an amount of these minerals is available, normal calcification does not take place in the absence of this vitamin. On the other hand, if the supply of calcium and phosphorus is practically at starvation levels, an optimum amount of cholecalciferol can enable them to be utilized and deposited in a nearly normal manner. "Vitamin D not only acts as a regulator of the metabolism of these elements; it permits the body to operate with greatly increased economy" (McCollum). It does this by apparently influencing two different functions.

In the first place, it causes an increased absorption of calcium and phosphorus from the intestinal tract. The Harrisons[17] studied the effect of vitamin D on the absorption of calcium from the intestinal tract by the *everted sac* technique of Wilson and Wiseman. The transfer of ^{45}Ca across the membrane of everted segments of small intestine of rats was measured. In the presence of vitamin D, the rate of passage of ^{45}Ca across the intestinal mucosa was greatly increased. There was an active transport (i.e., against a concentration gradient) in the proximal portion of the small intestine that was dependent on the energy of oxidative metabolism. Vitamin D also increased the rate of diffusion (passive transfer) of calcium along the entire length of the small intestine. Currently, using the same technique, these investigators have found that ergocalciferol likewise increases the absorption of phosphate. They suggested that vitamin D increases the intestinal absorption of calcium and phosphorus by increasing the permeability of the mucosal cell surface to these ions.

There is evidence that actinomycin-D, which inhibits protein synthesis at the RNA level (p. 54), inhibits vitamin D action. The injection of this antibiotic into rats completely prevented both the rise in serum calcium normally induced by vitamin D and the increased transport of calcium by everted sacs of small intestine. Injection of parathyroid hormone did not alter this result, thus eliminating the possibility that the inhibition of vitamin activity was due to blocked hormone synthesis. Actinomycin-D inhibited the action of a subsequent dose of vitamin D_3 in increasing calcium absorption from the intestine. It was suggested that vitamin D may therefore influence the absorption of calcium by controlling somehow the biosynthesis of a protein component of the calcium-transport system.

This suggestion has been strongly supported by recent evidence. Vitamin D increases the incorporation of ^{3}H-orotic acid into RNA of the rat intestinal mucosa.[18] Furthermore, a vitamin D–dependent calcium-binding protein from the chick intestinal mucosa has been prepared in purified form by gel filtration and disc electrophoresis.[19] The amount of this protein in the intestinal mucosa decreases in vitamin D deficiency and increases when cholecalciferol is administered. The administration of estrogens and certain other steroids has no effect on its concentration. The amount of the calcium-binding protein is largest in the duodenal mucosa, the primary site of calcium absorption, and is progressively less in the jejunum and ileum. It is absent in mucosa from the colon.

The foregoing current investigations thus strongly indicate that a major function of cholecalciferol, or more probably its active metabolite form, 25-hydroxycholecalciferol, is inducing the biosynthesis of a calcium-binding protein essential to the active transport of calcium through the intestinal mucosa. This would increase the plasma level of calcium and thus increase the availability of calcium for deposition in the bones; these are the major effects of vitamin D in the body.

Cholecalciferol and, more particularly, 25-hydroxycholecalciferol also increase bone resorption in the rat, producing a rise in serum calcium. The mechanism involved is uncertain but may entail an effect on a calcium-transport system in bone analogous to that occurring in the intestinal mucosa. Vitamin D was believed to have some relation to the actual deposition of calcium in bone by earlier investigators.

The effect of cholecalciferol on plasma and bone phosphate levels is apparently indirect, resulting from the direct effect of cholecalciferol on calcium transport.

Tests for vitamin D. In experimental animals there are several tests for vitamin D deficiency and recovery. X-ray photographs of the distal ends of the ulna and radius show a characteristic indistinctness. When healing occurs, the entire bone assumes a more homogeneous appearance and the cupped ends fill out (Fig. 23-5). The *line test* is used in experimental studies in ascertaining at autopsy the degree of healing. The split bone is treated with silver nitrate, which stains the provisional zone of recalcification, leaving the uncalcified rachitic tissue unstained. Another method is to analyze the bone for total ash. In rickets, the total ash is low, although the calcium:phosphorus ratio remains normal.

Human requirements. The calcium-phosphorus requirements of normal infants and children depend partly on the amount of ultraviolet light to which the children are exposed. It should be remembered that the effective ultraviolet rays do not penetrate ordinary glass. Therefore exposure to sunshine coming through window glass is of little value. Smoke also impedes the progress of these rays, and consequently city sunshine is not always beneficial. For this and other reasons, some vitamin D should be included in the food. The recommended amount is 400 International Units for infants daily. The same amount is advised for women in the latter half of pregnancy and during lactation. For other adults and for older children, probably 400 units are sufficient (see Table 25-1). One International Unit (I.U.) is equivalent to the biologic activity of 0.025 μg. of pure crystalline vitamin D_3.

Toxic effects. After administration of an excess of vitamin D to a mammal, the vitamin can be found in the circulating blood for months. It is undoubtedly stored in several organs but not to a great extent in the liver, as is the case in fish. Any excretion is by way of the bile. Since the distribution of this factor in foods is quite uncertain and exposure to sunshine is often inadequate for long periods of time, the inclusion of moderate amounts of vitamin D in adults'—as well as in children's—diets is recommended. This is particularly true for older people. The use of enormous doses of vitamin D for therapeutic purposes is not without danger, however. Severe and even fatal effects have been noted. The toxic manifestations caused by excess dosage include nausea, anorexia, weakness, headache, digestive disturbances, and polyuria. Irreversible damage to the kidneys, as well as calcification of other soft tissues, results. The threshold of toxicity seems to be about 20,000 to 25,000 units per kilogram of body weight per day. Such doses are not ordinarily employed.

The reason for the toxicity of vitamin D is the difficulty of excretion of this vitamin, rather than its storage in the liver. Any excretion is gradual, by way of the bile. Excess cholecalciferol injected into animals remains in the circulation for several months. In contrast, the *water-soluble* vitamins, if given in excess, are excreted promptly in the urine and are therefore nontoxic.

VITAMIN E — α-TOCOPHEROL

The possibility that reproductivity might be dependent on a vitamin was first suggested by Mattill, in 1920. The actual discovery of such a vitamin was announced 2 years later by Evans and by Sure. They fed rats a diet of purified foodstuffs plus cod-liver oil and yeast. Such a diet was assumed to contain all the vitamins necessary for the rat. However, although the animals grew at a normal rate, they did not bear young. Addition of a variety of vegetable foods rectified this condition. The factor contained in these foods was termed vitamin E, the *antisterility* vitamin or fertility factor. Numerous subsequent investigations resulted in the isolation of vitamin E in crystalline form, the determination of its structure, and finally its synthesis. It was given the name tocopherol (from the Greek, meaning child-bearing, plus -*ol*, for an alcohol).

Properties and structure. Vitamin E is a fat-soluble, water-insoluble, light yellow oil, stable to heat and acids, rather unstable to alkalies, that is slowly oxidized. It is found in the nonsaponifiable fraction of the vegetable oils.

α-Tocopherol

Like vitamins A and D, there is more than one form of vitamin E. We now distinguish several different tocopherols. α-Tocopherol is the most potent, has been synthesized, and is commercially available. Its structure is shown on p. 786. The other tocopherols differ in the number and position of the methyl groups attached to the benzene ring.

Occurrence. The tocopherols are widely distributed in plant and animal tissues and differ from vitamin A in not being concentrated chiefly in the liver. Particularly good sources are cottonseed oil, corn oil, peanut oil, and wheat germ oil, but not olive oil. Green lettuce leaves and orange peels also have a high content, and nearly all green-leaved plants have some of this vitamin. It is also present in meat, butter, milk, eggs, and fish-liver oils. Vitamin E activity is displayed by many other organic compounds, some of them quite unrelated structurally to the vitamin. A number of phenols, quinones, coumarins, etc. show some vitamin E action. Slight changes in the structure of the active tocopherols, e.g., shortening the side chain, may reduce or even abolish the physiologic effects of these compounds.

Absorption. Absorption of the tocopherols is not efficiently accomplished, but it is believed to occur similarly to that of the other fat-soluble vitamins. Bile salts and the presence of fats are thought to be useful if not entirely essential. However, rancid fats destroy this vitamin by oxidation (p. 277).

If the mother is fed an adequate diet, the fetus absorbs through the placenta sufficient tocopherol for its needs but not enough for storage. This must be supplied to the young animal (and presumably to the infant) by the milk. Storage occurs in various tissues but chiefly in adipose tissue.

Water-soluble forms are available. The water-soluble disodium phosphate ester of α-tocopherol, when administered to rabbits intramuscularly, has a more rapid and constant effect than the oil-soluble vitamin administered orally.

Effects of deficiency. In rats, a lack of α-tocopherol results in damage to the reproductive system of both males and females. There is a degeneration of the germinal epithelium that cannot be remedied, after it is once established, by feeding the vitamin. If the female on a vitamin E–free diet does become pregnant, the embryo dies and is resorbed. In mice, deprivation of vitamin E does not cause testicular degeneration in the male; in pregnant females, the same resorption of the fetus takes place as in rats.

At the present time, it cannot be definitely stated that man requires vitamin E for reproduction. Many clinical investigations have been reported in which vitamin E concentrates were used to attempt to remedy sterility, habitual abortion, and various abnormalities of premature infants, but results are doubtful. However, the National Academy of Sciences has incorporated α-tocopherol in its list of recommended dietary allowances. The need of man for this vitamin is thus recognized.

Besides having effects on the reproductive system, vitamin E is also necessary for the structural and functional maintenance of skeletal muscle, cardiac muscle, smooth muscle, and the peripheral vascular system in a variety of laboratory animals. Indeed, the present opinion is that the effects on muscle are of greater importance than are the effects on fertility. Muscular dystrophy and morphologic changes in various tissues are caused by a vitamin E deficit and are accompanied by increased oxygen consumption of the muscle and by alterations in chemical composition and functional behavior. Creatine elimination then is increased (p. 396). This latter effect is believed to be due to an inability of the skeletal muscle to utilize creatine.

Recent investigations[20] demonstrated that a type of muscular dystrophy can be produced in lambs by the feeding of a raw kidney bean–hay ration. The condition can be prevented by administering α-tocopherol *plus selenium* (p. 430). The unheated beans are believed to contain a heat-labile, antivitamin E or antiselenium factor, or both.

Probably the factors responsible for fertility and muscular dystrophy are somewhat different. α-Tocopherylhydroquinone has no antisterility activity but does have a curative effect on muscular dystrophy in rabbits. The hydroquinone is an antidystrophic factor, whereas the tocopherol has chiefly an antisterility action. In chicks, a vitamin E deficiency results in injury to the nervous system due to an impairment of the blood vessels in the brain. In all these conditions, there seems to be no comparable effect on human beings.

In rabbits, vitamin E deficiency causes derangement of nucleic acid metabolism. This is shown by a higher output of allantoin and a change in the content of tissue nucleic acids.

Vitamin E has a sparing action on vitamin A and carotene; e.g., vitamin A and carotene are more effective in curing their deficiency symptoms if vitamin E is administered at the same time. Ingestion of extra amounts of α-tocopherol increases the storage of vitamin A in the liver of rats; and many other examples of the close connection between these two vitamins could be cited. This biologic relation undoubtedly has a chemical basis. Vitamin E is an antioxidant; i.e., it can prevent the oxidation of various other easily oxidized substances, notably fats (p. 277) and vitamin A. For this reason it is often added to foods to prevent oxidation. Possibly this protection is effective even within the cells. Vitamin A, you will remember, is also essential for reproduction. Although the beneficial action of vitamin A is primarily on ectodermal and endodermal tissues and that of E is on the mesoderm, quite likely vitamin E indirectly influences all three layers of the embryo by preventing the too rapid destruction of A. The antioxidant properties of E are enhanced by certain other substances, many of which are also antioxidants. Phenols and ascorbic acid are notable examples.

Other recent work[21] suggests the involvement of vitamin E in combatting certain human nutritional anemias. Serum α-tocopherol levels have been found to be low in some types of anemia, particularly in infants. The anemia is a macrocytic type and responds favorably to vitamin E therapy. The erythrocytes appear to be less resistant to hemolysis, resulting in a hemolytic type of anemia. The vitamin E may protect unsaturated fatty acids in the erythrocyte cell membrane from oxidative destruction and hence prevent hemolysis of the cell. Further studies into the biochemical nature of the effect are needed, however.

Mechanism of action. Although the mechanism of action of vitamin E has not been clearly elucidated, there is some evidence that the vitamin may serve as a cofactor in the electron-transfer system, probably functioning between cytochromes b and c. Horwitt[22] believes α-tocopherol acts primarily as an antioxidant for preserving the physiologic lipid configuration of cell membranes, protecting especially linoleic acid and perhaps other unsaturated fatty acids.

Human requirements. For the first time, the Food and Nutrition Board of the National Research Council has included vitamin E in its 1968 revision of recommended daily allowances (p. 841). The recommended allowance for adults is 30 International Units for men and 25 I.U. for women. The amount for women is increased to 30 I.U. during pregnancy and lactation. For infants and children, 1 to 1.25 I.U. per kilogram body weight are recommended. The amounts of vitamin E needed apparently increase when the amounts of dietary polyunsaturated fatty acids increase.[22]

One International Unit (I.U.) of dl-α-tocopherol is defined as the biologic activity of 1.1 mg. of the pure compound (or 0.67 mg. d-α-tocopherol).

VITAMIN K

Dam, a Danish investigator, in 1929, discovered a hemorrhagic disease in chicks due to the lack of a food factor that he later (1934) called "Koagulations Vitamins." From this, came the term vitamin K. A deficiency of vitamin K leads to a slowing of the rate of blood clotting. More specifically, there is an increased *prothrombin time* (p. 630). This factor, therefore, appears to be necessary for the production of a normal amount of prothrombin. It is a fat-soluble substance found in various food oils and is of considerable importance from a medical and surgical standpoint.

Properties. The naturally occurring vitamin K, or *phylloquinone*, is fat soluble and stable to heat and to reducing agents. It should be kept in dark bottles since it is sensitive to light. The activity is also abolished by irradiation, alkalies, strong acids, and oxidizing agents.

Structure. Vitamin K_1, obtained from the alfalfa leaf, is 2-methyl-3-phytl-1,4-naphthoquinone. Vitamin K_2, produced by bacterial synthesis, is 2-methyl-3-difarnesyl-1,4-naphthoquinone, called *farnoquinone*. Both these natural types have the same general activity. Many vitamers (synthetic products with similar structures) having antihemorrhagic effects have been prepared. Some of these are water soluble, but only one is more potent (weight for weight) than vitamin K_1. This is 2-methyl-1,4-naphthoquinone, which has been given the name *menadione*. It is soluble in oil, sparingly soluble in water, and stable to air when protected from light. Its diphosphate ester is water soluble and is widely used clinically.

Vitamin K_1 (phylloquinone)
(2-methyl-3-phytyl-1,4-naphthoquinone)

Vitamin K₂(farnoquinone)*
(2-methyl-3-difarnesyl-1,4-naphthoquinone)

Menadione
(2-methyl-1,4-naphthoquinone)

Occurrence. As mentioned, vitamin K₁ is obtained from alfalfa. A rich source of K₂ is putrefied fish meal. Other excellent sources are cabbage, cauliflower, kale, spinach, and other green vegetables. Good sources include tomatoes, cheese, egg yolk, and liver. The vitamins is also found in a number of bacteria and is undoubtedly synthesized by microorganisms in the intestinal tract and is thus available to the host.

Absorption. The natural vitamins K are fat soluble and require bile in order to be absorbed. Consequently, absorption occurs in the upper parts of the small intestine where bile salts are present. A vitamin K deficiency is likely to occur whenever bile is prevented from entering the intestinal tract. This is true of most of the fat-soluble vitamins, but it is particularly important in the case of vitamin K because of its bearing on blood clotting. Thus, when there is an obstruction of the bile channels and jaundice ensues, clotting is delayed. This is not due to the occurrence of bile in the blood, as was formerly thought, but to a deficiency of vitamin K. As in the case of fatty acids, probably the bile acids can be ascribed the specific function of absorption of fat-soluble vitamins. Consequently, whenever vitamin K is given per os, the presence of bile is essential, and if there is a deficient bile flow, a bile or bile salt preparation should be administered. The parenteral administration of one of the vitamers, e.g., menadione, obviates this necessity. The water-soluble analogues may be given orally without the use of bile or bile salts. Excess vitamin K can be stored to a moderate degree, but in which tissues this occurs is not known.

Effects of deficiency. Animals suffering from vitamin K deficiency have a remarkable tendency to bleed profusely from minor wounds, and slight bruises result in extensive subcutaneous hemorrhages. Blood withdrawn from such animals clots very slowly; in some cases, it may remain fluid for hours. This is a result of lack of prothrombin. In rats, the female is much less

---

*Recent evidence indicates that the side chain of vitamin K₂ has seven isoprene units rather than the six indicated and is therefore 2-methyl-3(all-*trans*–farnesyldigeranyl)-1,4-naphthoquinone.

susceptible to vitamin K deficiency than the male. This is due to hormonal influences. Newly hatched chicks on a vitamin K–free diet show a gradual diminution in the concentration of prothrombin in the blood. Their intestinal flora produces some farnoquinone but not enough to prevent avitaminosis without additions from the diet. Administration of the vitamin brings the clotting time of their blood up to normal levels within a few hours. The vitamin does not form part of the prothrombin molecule but has some influence on the production of prothrombin by the liver. Hepatectomized animals show a rapid decline in the blood-clotting power due to lowered prothrombin, and administration of vitamin K does not raise it. Vitamin K treatment is ineffective if the liver is so badly damaged that it cannot produce prothrombin or if the intestine is incapable of absorbing the orally administered vitamin.

In human beings the same effects are attributable to lack of vitamin K. In normal newborn infants the prothrombin level is low. It continues to fall, reaching the minimum on the third day of life. This is undoubtedly due to a lack of vitamin K. Apparently the vitamin passes from the mother to the fetus with great difficulty, especially toward the end of pregnancy, and, since the intestine of the newborn infant is sterile, there is no opportunity for synthesis by bacteria for a while. However, the prothrombin level may reach normal by the end of the first week, probably as a result of bacterial synthesis of vitamin K, concomitant with the ingestion of milk, and the establishment of the normal intestinal flora. Hemorrhagic disease of newborn infants is a frequent cause of infant mortality, and the high incidence of hemorrhage in the newborn infant is thus easily accounted for. Often an intracranial hemorrhage may result in brain injury and, if the infant survives, imbecility or some other mental and nervous condition. Prophylactic treatment is recommended by many clinicians. The expectant mother is given vitamin K supplements for several days before delivery is expected. If this has not been done, the infant is given such treatment soon after birth.

In adults, *available* vitamin K is seldom lacking. It is either present in the food in sufficient quantity or is produced by bacterial activity in the intestinal tract. A deficiency in the system may usually be referred to one of three fundamental causes: (1) There may be faulty absorption of the vitamin due to lack of bile in the intestine because of an insufficient secretion of bile salts, obstruction of the bile duct, intestinal lesions or obstruction, or surgical procedures in the intestine. (2) This and other fat-soluble vitamins may be swept into the feces, particularly if the intestinal contents are unusually greasy. This has been experienced in diarrheal diseases, e.g., ulcerative colitis, sprue, celiac disease, or following excessive use of mineral oil. (3) The administration of sulfaguanidine, succinylsulfathiazole, or other intestinal antiseptics may cause a deficiency by limiting the production of farnoquinone by the intestinal flora. The surgeon about to operate on a patient known to have any of the conditions mentioned gives vitamin K before the operation in order to avoid excessive hemorrhage during or after the operation. Bile or bile salts may be irritating and produce vomiting; therefore, instead of the natural vitamin, the water-soluble substitutes may be given by mouth, or these or some of the others may be given parenterally. It should be remembered that vitamin K is not always indicated when there is prothrombin deficiency, which may also result from various liver diseases that render the liver incapable of producing prothrombin. Intake of vitamin K cannot restore this function.

Physiologic function. The role of vitamin K in the synthesis of prothrombin in the liver is well established. Studies employing the fluorescent antibody technique[23] demonstrated that this effect occurs in the liver parenchymal cell and may be observed within a few hours after vitamin K is administered intravenously. Another function ascribed to vitamin K, probably in the form of *coenzyme-Q* (a polyisoprenoid derivative of 2,3-dimethoxy-5-methylbenzoquinone), is as a component of the electron-transfer system and in oxidative phosphorylation (p. 252) as an electron acceptor.[24]

Recent studies indicated that vitamin K has a genetic action in inducing RNA formation for the synthesis of blood-clotting proteins. The evidence for this is supported by the work of Olsen and Phillips,[25] who showed that actinomycin-D inhibits the vitamin K–induced prothrombin formation in chicks deficient in vitamin K. The inhibition involves hepatic RNA formation from ATP, as detected by the use of adenine-8-^{14}C.

Other recent work,[26] however, indicates that the site of function of vitamin K is not at the transcription level but rather is at a late stage in the translation of prothrombin mRNA to form a functional prothrombin molecule. Further investigations will be necessary to fully elucidate the precise biochemical role of vitamin K (phylloquinone, etc.) in the biosynthesis of prothrombin.

Table 23-2. Summary of fat soluble vitamins

Vitamin	Best food sources	Recommended dietary allowances[*] (1968)	Active cofactor form
Retinol (A) Retinal (aldehyde form) (precursors, carotenes)	Butter, whole milk, fortified margarine, egg yolk, green and yellow vegetables, yellow fruits	5000 I.U.	(A_1) Uncertain (A_2) Rhodopsin and other visual pigments
Cholecalciferol (D_3) Ergocalciferol (D_2)	Fish-liver oils, fortified or irradiated milk	400 I.U.	25-Hydroxycholecalciferol
D-α-Tocopherol (E)	Vegetable oils	30 I.U. (20 mg.)	Not identified
Phylloquinone (K_1) Farnoquinone (K_2)	Green leafy vegetables, liver	(probably met by bacterial synthesis in intestine)	Not identified

[*] For American men, 22 to 35 years of age, of average activity.

Human requirements. It is difficult to produce a deficiency of vitamin K in mammals or human beings by dietary methods alone. As mentioned, there is seldom a lack of sufficient vitamin K. Consequently, no standard requirement has been set.

Antagonists. The effect of heparin and bishydroxycoumarin in inhibiting blood clotting was discussed on pp. 632 and 633. These anticoagulants act as antagonists to vitamin K since their action is to diminish the amount of available prothrombin. The salicylates also are antagonistic to vitamin K. Consequently, when any of these are administered over a long period of time, supplements of the vitamin may be required to enable the liver to restore the prothrombin level to normal.

COENZYME-Q

The coenzyme-Q group has been classed as vitamins by some investigators[27] because of the ability of these compounds to cure or protect against vitamin E deficiency in several species of animals. Some of the coenzymes are also active in electron transport and/or oxidative phosphorylation (p. 252).

ANTISTIFFNESS FACTOR

Another alleged fat-soluble vitamin is the antistiffness factor, stigmasterol. It is a plant sterol with a formula quite similar to that of ergosterol. Its absence causes stiffness of the wrists and elbows of guinea pigs. The muscles atrophy and become streaked with bundles of fine white lines of calcium de-

Principal metabolic functions	Major clinical manifestations of deficiency
(A_1) Formation and maintenance of epithelial tissues (A_2) Constituent of visual pigments; toxic in large amounts	Nyctalopia, xerophthalmia, keratinization of epithelium and other epithelial tissues; faulty tooth formation
Induces synthesis of transport protein for Ca in intestinal mucosal cells and (bone?); intestinal and renal absorption of phosphate; toxic in large amounts	Rickets (children) Osteomalacia (adults)
Antioxidant; protects vitamin A and unsaturated fatty acids	Hemolytic anemia, degenerative changes in muscle; sterility in rats
Essential for prothrombin formation in the liver; possibly involved in electron-transport and oxidative phosphorylation mechanisms	Hemorrhagic disease in newborn and in biliary disease; Anemia

posits. Calcium phosphate is found under the skin, in the joints, and elsewhere. Cod-liver oil accelerates the onset of the condition and intensifies it. Stigmasterol is found in fresh kale or alfalfa and in fresh cream. It has now been isolated in crystalline form, and its administration, in doses of 0.1 μg. per day for 5 days, cures the above conditions.

SUMMARY

Table 23-2 summarizes the best food sources, the 1968 recommended dietary allowances, the active cofactor forms, the principal metabolic functions, and the major clinical manifestations of deficiencies of the fat-soluble vitamins just discussed.

References

GENERAL

Baker, H.: Clinical vitaminology, New York, 1968, Interscience Publishers, Inc.

Dyke, S. F.: The chemistry of the vitamins, New York, 1965, Interscience Publishers, Inc.

Goldsmith, G. A.: Nutritional diagnosis, Springfield, Ill., 1959, Charles C Thomas, Publisher.

Harris, L. J.: Vitamins in theory and practice, New York, 1955, Cambridge University Press.

Marks, J.: The vitamins in health and disease, Boston, 1969, Little, Brown & Co.

McCollum, E. B., Orent-Keiler, E., and Day, H. G.: The newer knowledge of nutrition, ed. 5, New York, 1939, The Macmillan Co.

Mendel, L. B.: Nutrition—the chemistry of life, New Haven, 1923, Yale University Press.

Neisser, U.: The process of vision, Sci. Amer. **211**:204, 1968.

Present knowledge of nutrition, ed. 3, New York, 1967, Nutrition Foundation, Inc.

Roels, O. A.: Present knowledge of vitamin A, Nutr. Rev. **24**:129, 1966.

Sebrell, W. H., Harris, R. S., Szent-Györgyi, P., and Pearson, W. H.: The vitamins. Chemistry, physiology and pathology, ed. 2, New York, 1967–1968, Academic Press, Inc.

Strobecker, R., and Heming, H. M.: Vitamin assay: tested methods, Cleveland, 1967, The Chemical Rubber Co.

Symposium: Recent developments in the fat-soluble vitamins, Fed. Proc. **28**:1670, 1969.

Williams, S. R.: Nutrition and diet therapy, St. Louis, 1969, The C. V. Mosby Co.

Wohl, M. G., and Goodhart, R. S., editors: Modern nutrition in health and disease, Philadelphia, 1968, Lea & Febiger.

SPECIAL

1. McCollum, E. V.: Science **118**:632, 1953.
2. Guy, R. A.: Amer. J. Dis. Child. **26**:112, 1923.
3. J. Amer. Chem. Soc. **82**:5575, 1961.
4. DeLuca, H. F., and Zile, M.: Chem. Eng. News **43**:34, 1965.
5. Futterman, S., and Andrews, J. S.: J. Biol. Chem. **239**:81, 1964.
6. Bieri, J. G., et al.: Science **163**:574, 1969.
7. Goldsmith, T. H., et al.: Science **146**:65, 1964.
8. Wald, G.: Science **162**:230, 1968.
9. Dartnall, H. J. A.: In Davson, H., editor: The eye, New York, 1962, Academic Press, Inc.; Dartnall, H. J. A., and Lythgoe, J. N.: Vision Res. **5**:81, 1965.
10. Collins, F. D.: Nature **171**:469, 1953.
11. Gloor, U., and Wiss, O.: Ann. Rev. Biochem. **33**:313, 1964.
12. Loomis, W. F.: Science **157**:501, 1967.
13. Fieser, L. F., and Fieser, M.: Steroids, New York, 1955, Reinhold Publishing Corp., p. 148.
14. DeLuca, H. F., et al.: Proc. Nat. Acad. Sci. **61**:717, 1968; Science **165**:405, 1969.
15. McNair, S. L., and Stickler, G. B.: New Eng. J. Med. **281**:511, 1969.
16. Pak, C. Y. C., DeLuca, H. F., et al.: Clin. Res. **17**:291, 1969.
17. Harrison, H. E., and Harrison, H. C.: Amer. J. Physiol. **199**:265, 1960; Fed. Proc. **20**:292, 1961.
18. DeLuca, H. F., et al.: Biochemistry **6**:1304, 1967.
19. Wasserman, R. H., et al.: J. Biol. Chem. **243**:3978, 3987, 1968.
20. Gardner, R. W., and Hogue, D. E.: J. Nutr. **93**:418, 1967.
21. Oski, F. A., and Barnes, L. A.: J. Pediat. **70**:211, 1967.
22. Horwitt, M. K.: Fed. Proc. **24**:68, 1965.
23. Barnhart, M. I.: Amer. J. Physiol. **199**:360, 1960.
24. Green, D. E., and Hartefi, Y.: Science **133**:13, 1961.
25. Olson, R. E., and Phillips, G. R.: Science **158**:533, 1967.
26. Johnson, B. C., et al.: J. Biol. Chem. **243**:3930, 1968.
27. Roels, O. A.: Nutr. Rev. **25**:97, 1967.

CHAPTER 24

WATER-SOLUBLE VITAMINS

The individual water-soluble vitamins bear no closer resemblance to each other chemically than do the fat-soluble vitamins. However, they are conveniently grouped together merely because of their solubility in water. This characteristic was the first basis for their classification. It also becomes of some importance from nutritional and clinical aspects, i.e., vitamin deficiencies are likely to be multiple in nature and often may be mixed fat-soluble or mixed water-soluble vitamin deficiencies. The water-soluble vitamins include ascorbic acid, thiamine, niacin, riboflavin, pyridoxine, pantothenic acid, biotin, folic acid, and cobalamin. *p*-Aminobenzoic acid, inositol, α-lipoic acid, and choline are frequently included in this list, but these are believed by many nutritionists to be not true vitamins, although deficiencies of them in the diet of experimental animals cause characteristic symptoms to develop. None of them, with the possible exception of α-lipoic acid, appears to be a coenzyme or a part of one.

ASCORBIC ACID—VITAMIN C

Scurvy was probably the first disease to be definitely associated with a food deficiency. It was common in Europe in the fifteenth century and must have been known long before that. It frequently occurred among sailors on long voyages when fresh food was not available. An instance of this was the voyage of Vasco da Gama around the Cape of Good Hope. He lost more than half his crew from scurvy. In 1535, Cartier's men were stricken with this disease during their explorations in Canada. Several died and the remainder were saved by drinking an extract of the leaves of an evergreen tree, as instructed by a friendly Indian. Scurvy was long the dread of Arctic explorers who had to provide food for months in advance and were, of course, unable to take along fresh foods. It is said that Dutch mariners, as early as the fifteenth century, knew of the efficacy of fresh vegetables and citrus fruits in the cure of this condition. In 1747, Lind, a British naval surgeon, treated a number of scorbutic sailors on his ship with different medicaments, including fruit juices. He observed dramatic recovery in those partaking of lemons and oranges and recommended lemon juice as a standard part of the ration. It was not until 1795 that his advice was heeded and the government had limes put into the ration of the British sailor. From this practice is derived the sobriquet "limey." In 1843, Pereira referred to lemon juice as "one of our most valuable antiscorbutic foods."

In scurvy there occur anemia, pains in the joints, and hemorrhages from the mucous membranes of the mouth and gastrointestinal tract, skin (Fig. 24-1), muscles, and subperiosteal tissues. The gums are particularly affected, showing swelling, tenderness, gingivitis, redness, ulceration, and even gangrene. Weakness and emaciation are seen in later stages. There are definite defects in skeletal calcification without much disturbance in mineral metabolism. For example, x-ray examination of the bones in scurvy shows a white line on the outside of the shaft, a line not seen in normal bone. The pathologic change leading to all these symptoms is a weakening in the endothelial wall of the capillaries, *because of a reduction in the amount of intercellular substance.* The body normally produces intercellular material, absorbs it, and replenishes it continually. This new formation of cementing

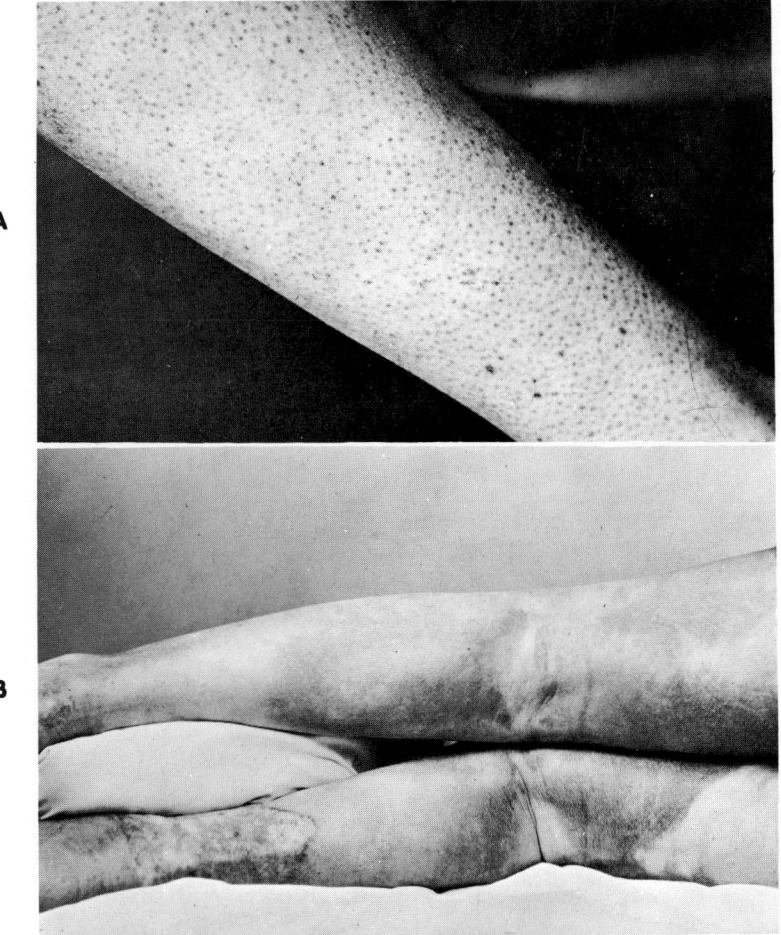

Fig. 24-1. **A,** Perifollicular hemorrhages of early scurvy. **B,** Ecchymosis of scurvy. (From Merck Report, May, 1956, Merck & Co., Inc., Rahway, N.J.)

and supporting material does not occur in the absence of vitamin C. The deficiency in supporting material may extend to the cartilage, bone, muscles, and other tissues and is responsible for the symptoms mentioned. We thus see that ascorbic acid is essential for the production of intercellular material (p. 543) and that it is necessary for the healing of wounds and fractures of bones.

Properties. Ascorbic acid is water soluble and insoluble in fats and oils. It is very sensitive to oxidation, particularly in the presence of copper but not of aluminum. Therefore, foods prepared in copper vessels or with copper utensils lose ascorbic acid quickly. This factor is also rapidly destroyed by alkalies but is fairly stable in weakly acid solutions. Consequently, baking soda has a harmful effect, but cooking in steam has little destructive action on the ascorbic acid of foods, if they are neutral or slightly acid. Drying vegetables usually results in a loss of ascorbic acid, but many attempts have been made to provide desiccated foods containing all the vitamins, including ascorbic acid, unchanged. Freezing has no deleterious effect on the vitamin. Because it is so easily oxidized, ascorbic acid is a strong reducing agent.

Occurrence. From a nutritional standpoint, the citrus fruits and tomatoes are the best sources of ascorbic acid. Other natural sources may be richer in it, but they are either inedible or are not consumed in considerable amounts. For example, both green peppers and parsley are richer than oranges in this vitamin, but they do not enter into the diet to any great extent. Spinach and other greens are good sources of it also, but they lose their vitamin C content progressively on storage at room temperature. Citrus fruit juices and tomato juice may be canned with but slight loss of the antiscorbutic factor. However, they should not be permitted to be in contact with air for a long period of time because of loss by oxidation. Cantaloupes, strawberries, cabbage, and turnips, when raw, are all about equivalent to tomatoes, but the two latter lose some vitamin C in cooking. Potatoes, fresh peas, asparagus, and lettuce are good sources also.

Plant polyphenols apparently play an important part as antioxidants in protecting ascorbic acid from oxidative destruction.[1] A number of polyphenols, especially rutin, quercetin, and related flavonols, have this property. The effect is believed to be indirect, due to the chelation of heavy metal ions (Cu^{++}, etc.) that catalyze the oxidative degradation of ascorbic acid. The vitamin C–like action of the so-called bioflavonoids is attributed to this protective action. Bioflavonoids thus decrease oxidative losses of ascorbic acid from foods, etc. during storage or in the intestinal tract, especially in individuals in achlorhydria or hypochlorhydria.

Ascorbic acid occurs to some extent in animal tissues. In 1928, Szent-Györgyi found a "hexuronic acid" with high reducing power in the adrenal cortex and later showed that it had antiscorbutic properties. However, the adrenal gland is of no importance as a food source of the vitamin because of the almost insignificant quantity of tissue involved. The same is true of corpus luteum, which is said to have a high content of ascorbic acid. Most fresh animal tissues have small amounts of vitamin C. Liver is the best animal source, although fish roe and milt are also rather rich in it.

Cow's milk contains small amounts of ascorbic acid, which vary with the cow's fodder. In summer, when the cows are in the pasture, their milk is relatively high in ascorbic acid; but in winter, or whenever fresh food is unavailable to the cow, the milk has little antiscorbutic value. Human milk has a somewhat higher vitamin C content, but this, too, is dependent on the quality of the food. Pasteurizing milk is somewhat destructive of vitamin C. Accordingly, babies should have supplements of orange juice or tomato juice at least until they receive a varied diet.

Effects of deficiency. The guinea pig is the standard animal for demonstrating vitamin C deficiency and it has been used in the biologic assay of foods for this vitamin. At first, there is good growth on the vitamin C–free diet, but in about 2 weeks growth ceases and symptoms begin to appear. The joints become swollen and tender, and the animals show signs of pain when these are present. The animals may lie on their sides or assume a peculiar "scurvy" position, lying flat with hind legs sprawled. They may be excitable at first but soon become very quiet and not easily disturbed. There may also be enlargements of the junctions of the ribs with cartilage, as well as other bone lesions. Hemorrhage of the gums and loosening or breaking of the teeth may occur. Small amounts of orange juice change the picture even at a late stage, and animals may be brought back to an almost normal condition quite rapidly. Pertinent in this connection is the fact that recent work has shown that injected ascorbic acid in the guinea pig tends to concentrate in skin, muscle, and bone, and after injury in the scar tissue of the wound and callus of the fracture.

It has been thought that rats and mice require no ascorbic acid in their diets. However, these animals cannot entirely dispense with the vitamin, and their ability to get along with exceedingly small amounts is due to the fact that they synthesize it in their tissues.

In man an extreme deficiency results in scurvy, as already described; but in our ordinary life such marked deficiencies seldom occur. There do occur, however, deficiencies of various grades, due either to a subnormal intake of the vitamin or to an increased requirement. These deficiencies may result in slow healing of wounds and decreased ability to combat infections and to metabolize amino acids, especially tyrosine, as well as in the scorbutic symptoms already mentioned.

Investigations have shown that vitamin C is a threshold substance; i.e., it is not excreted by the kidney until the ascorbic acid level in the blood exceeds a certain value, which in turn depends on the degree of saturation of the body tissues. Vitamin C is not stored in the way that vitamin A and D are. As will be seen, there are methods of determining vitamin C chemically that are much quicker than biologic assay. The degree of saturation of the tissues with ascorbic acid can be easily estimated by the aid of such methods. One clinical test is the determination of the concentration of ascorbic acid in blood plasma. The normal range is 0.6 to 2.5 mg. per 100 ml., but subnormal values have been found in some cases during pregnancy and lactation and in all cases of scurvy.

Some other conditions in which low values have been found are infectious disorders, congestive heart failure, kidney and liver diseases, gastrointestinal disturbances, purpura, endocrine cases, and malignancies. In none of these conditions is the lack of vitamin C a primary causative factor, but the fact that the vitamin C blood level is found to be reduced in many pathologic states may be significant. This reduction is probably a result of an increased requirement for the vitamin or a lowered threshold for its excretion, but nevertheless it may contribute to the pathologic condition of the patient. After burns, fractures, or extensive surgery, there is also a marked diminution of plasma ascorbic acid.

Another clinical test depends on the amount of vitamin C excreted in the urine after a test dose of ascorbic acid has been administered. If the tissues are well supplied with the vitamin, a larger amount is eliminated. If they are in need of it, more is retained. Another interesting test is the ability of the tissues to bleach a dye, sodium-2,6-dichlorophenol indophenol. This is the same dye as is used to determine vitamin C quantitatively in blood, urine, and foods. The dye is injected under the skin and forms a blue spot. If no ascorbic acid is present, the color remains, but with increasing concentration of vitamin C in the tissues the spot disappears more and more rapidly. Children on normal diets, except for citrus fruits and tomatoes, quickly develop a lack of vitamin C, as shown by this test or by blood analysis, even though no gross clinical symptoms may be present.

Structure. Ascorbic acid is a hexose derivative. Its formula, together with the formulas of two closely related compounds, is given below. In fact, glucose, labeled at any one, or all, of its carbons, is converted, in the rat, to the correspondingly labeled ascorbic acid.[2]

| L-Ascorbic acid | Dehydro-L-ascorbic acid | 2,3-Diketo-L-gulonic acid |

As seen from these formulas, L-ascorbic acid and dehydro-L-ascorbic acid are lactone derivatives of the diketogulonic acid. The acidity of ascorbic acid is derived from the dissociation of the enolic hydroxyl groups. When ascorbic acid is oxidized, it loses two hydrogen atoms and becomes the dehydro derivative, which may be reduced to the original ascorbic acid form. The reduced form, L-ascorbic acid, predominates in the plasma and also apparently in tissues at a ratio of about 15(or more):1 of the oxidized form, dehydroascorbic acid. Both of these are biologically active, but the stereoisomer, D-ascorbic acid, is not. When dehydro-L-ascorbic acid is hydrated, it changes to 2,3-diketo-L-gulonic acid, which not only is inactive biologically but cannot be converted back to either of the active forms in the body. Since this hydration takes place spontaneously in neutral or alkaline solution, the oxidation of ascorbic acid frequently means its biologic inactivation.

Since L-ascorbic acid is so easily oxidized to its dehydro derivative and vice versa, this is believed to occur in the tissues. Ascorbic acid may be a part of one of the important respiratory enzyme systems. It can be oxidized and reduced by glutathione, which may also be a part of the system. Thus:

$$\text{Ascorbic acid} \quad \overset{\overset{\text{GS-SG}}{\xrightarrow{\hspace{1.5cm}}}}{\underset{\text{2 GSH}}{\xleftarrow[\hspace{1.5cm}]{+ \text{ Enzyme}}}} \quad \text{Dehydroascorbic acid}$$

The importance of ascorbic acid today is reflected by the fact that some 12 million pounds of pure crystalline ascorbic acid are used annually. A manufacturing plant capable of producing 17 million pounds annually is being constructed in the United States. In addition to its use in foods and pharmaceutics, ascorbic acid is used in poultry feeds to increase eggshell strength, in plastics to retard yellowing, as an initiation of polymerization in polyvinyl and related types of plastics, and as a spray for fruit trees to facilitate mechanical harvesting.

Mechanism of action. From the various effects of vitamin C deficiency seen in man and experimental animals, evidently a major function of ascorbic acid is the formation of tissue collagen or *intercellular cement substance.* Recent investigations have, indeed, supported this view. In addition, ascorbic acid, with ferrous iron, has been shown to catalyze the hydroxylation of proline and possibly lysine in collagen formation (p. 545). Ascorbic acid appears to be essential to the activity of the enzyme collagen proline hydroxylase, which catalyzes the conversion of proline to hydroxyproline. The latter is vital in maintaining the tertiary structure of collagen (p. 545). The tissue levels of collagen proline hydroxylase have been reported to be lower in scorbutic guinea pigs than in normal animals. Higher concentrations of the enzyme, and of ascorbic acid (p. 545), are found in injured tissues in which wound healing and scar tissue or callus formation are occurring. The precise biochemical role of ascorbic acid in collagen formation has not been clearly elucidated as yet, however.

Ascorbic acid also is involved in biologic oxidations in some manner not completely understood at the present time. Apparently its link into the mitochondrial electron-transport chain (p. 249) is at the stage of cytochrome-c. Thus the oxidation of a metabolite through one mole of ascorbic acid would yield one mole of ATP via oxidative phosphorylation (p. 252). An involvement of ascorbic acid in biologic oxidations is a predictable function because of the readily reversible conversion of ascorbic to dehydroascorbic acid.

Ascorbic acid may also be involved in the metabolism of tyrosine (p. 374). Alkaptonuria in guinea pigs results when they are fed a diet deficient in vitamin C but containing an excess of tyrosine. This may be due to the fact that ascorbic acid normally protects the enzyme that oxidizes p-hydroxyphenylpyruvic acid, a metabolic product of tyrosine. The subsequent administration of ascorbic acid reduces and even abolishes the output of p-hydroxyphenylpyruvic acid. Although ascorbic acid does not have the same effect in alkaptonuria in man, premature infants excrete p-hydroxyphenylpyruvic and p-hydroxyphenyllactic acids in the urine if ascorbic acid is not present in sufficient amounts in the diet.

Recent studies indicate that another function of ascorbic acid is its role in the conversion of folic acid to a physiologically active form, tetrahydrofolic acid (p. 822).

Ascorbic acid also appears to act as a regulator of cholesterol metabolism. The rate of conversion of labeled acetate to cholesterol in the adrenal glands was found to be heightened in scorbutic animals as compared with normal ones.

In view of the fact that anemia occurs in scurvy, ascorbic acid not surprisingly aids in the absorption, and possibly the utilization, of iron in the nutritional anemia of infants and children.

Human requirements. As little as 10 mg. of ascorbic acid per day are sometimes sufficient to prevent scurvy. This is by no means the optimal amount necessary to ensure normal physiologic function for children or adults. The exact requirement is uncertain, but for men and (during pregnancy and lactation) for women, the recommended dietary allowance (Table 25-1) is 60 mg. Infants should have 35 mg. per day, and, as the child gets older, a gradually increasing amount is required until a maximum need is reached at adolescence, 55 to 60 mg. daily for boys and 50 to 55 mg. for girls. Conditions requiring larger quantities of ascorbic acid are thyrotoxicosis, achlorhydria, diarrhea, rheumatic fever, rheumatoid arthritis, infections, and after physical trauma and surgery. In such instances 200 mg. per day or more may be administered.

• • •

When the vitamins were first designated *fat-soluble* A and *water-soluble* B, only one active principle was thought to be present in each. Water-soluble B had growth-promoting properties for the rat and cured the polyneuritis that had been produced in pigeons by feeding them polished rice. In man, the disease beriberi was found to result from a deficiency of vitamin B and to yield to treatment with it. Later, pellagra was shown to be due to a deficiency of some other factor present in vitamin B preparations. The designation *P-P* (pellagra-preventive) was at first assigned to it. Additional factors were separated, at first on the basis of varying biologic reactions, using different sources and different species, and later on the basis of adsorbability by Fuller's earth and other physical or chemical properties.

Two systems of nomenclature were used: one giving each factor a different letter, (e.g., vitamin B, vitamin G) and the other naming them vitamin B_1, B_2, B_3, etc. Although the latter system is used more than the former, there is a growing tendency to abandon both for the definite names of the compounds as soon as they are isolated, in conformity with the official recommendation (p. 841). Thus the group includes thiamine (B_1), riboflavin (B_2), pantothenic acid (B_3), niacin (B_5), pyridoxine (B_6), biotin (B_7), folic acid (pteroylglutamic acid) (B_9), lipoic acid, and cobalamin (B_{12}).

THIAMINE – VITAMIN B₁

Vitamin B_1 or thiamine has been called the antineuritic or antiberiberi factor; in Europe it is also designated *aneurin*.

Effects of deficiency. A marked deficiency of thiamine in the diet results in the following:

1. Arrested growth of young animals

   There is a specific effect on growth not due to the inhibitory influence on appetite, which this vitamin also exerts.

2. Polyneuritis in animals

   Birds develop acute polyneuritis after several weeks and are unable to fly, walk, or even stand. Death occurs unless the vitamin is given. Rats develop, among other symptoms, a bradycardia (slowing of the heart rate). The curing of both the polyneuritis of pigeons and the bradycardia of rats has been used in methods of biologic assay.

   Recent studies[3] demonstrated that there is malfunction of the blood-brain barrier in experimental thiamine deficiency in rats. The evidence is from the labeling patterns of glutamic acid from brain tissue of rats injected with sodium pyruvate-2-^{14}C, which normally does not pass the blood-brain barrier directly but only after conversion to glucose by gluconeogenesis. The results indicate that the alterations in selectivity of the blood-brain barrier permit pyruvic acid to enter the brain directly. Altered metabolic pathways in the brain, therefore, must occur; these, in turn, may be responsible for the polyneuritis that develops.

3. Beriberi in man

   This disease is common in the Orient but also occurs in other parts of the world. In the adult it is characterized by polyneuritis, with muscular atrophy, cardiovascular changes, and edema (Plate 1). At first there is weakness and fatigue, followed by headache, insomnia, dizziness, loss of appetite and other gastrointestinal symptoms, and tachycardia. Later the major symptoms may follow chiefly one of the following patterns: (a) nervous symptoms (*dry beriberi*); (b) symptoms associated with edema and serous effusions (*wet beriberi*); (c) symptoms of heart involvement (*acute pernicious beriberi*). Often the symptoms are characteristic of more than one of these three classes and are called *mixed beriberi*. Although beriberi is a thiamine deficiency disease, it is almost always accompanied by deficits of other vitamins. This is true of all vitamin B complex–deficiency conditions in man, and perhaps of other vitamin deficiencies as well.

   Beriberi in infants results when their diet is restricted to the milk of mothers suffering from beriberi and undoubtedly is due to a lack of thiamine in the milk. It occurs suddenly. The symptoms include rigidity of the body, constipation, diminished flow of urine (oliguria), a peculiar whining, weakness, edema, enlargement of the heart, cyanosis, and a rapid, irregular pulse.

Properties. Thiamine is a white, crystalline compound, readily soluble in water, slightly soluble in ethyl alcohol, but insoluble in ether and chloroform.

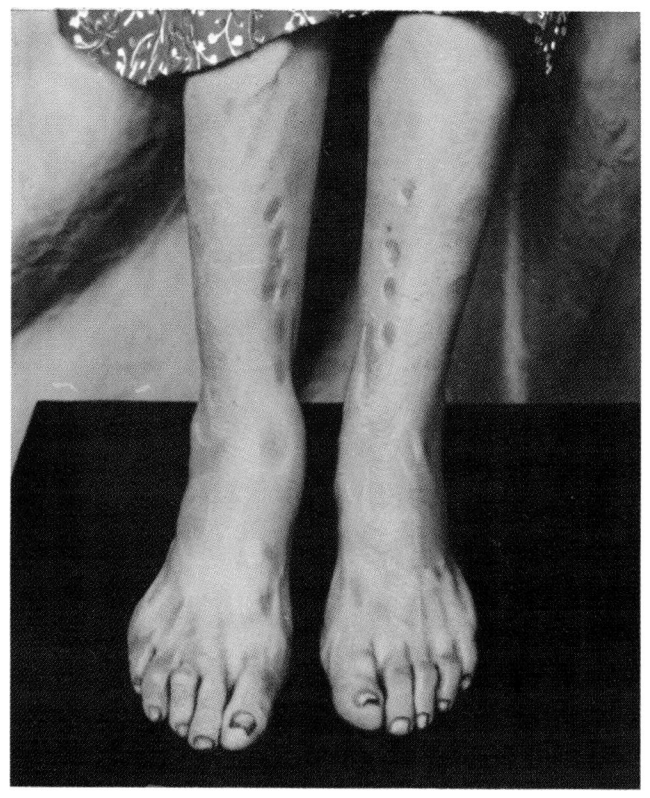

Plate 1. Pitting edema of the leg in thiamine deficiency. (Courtesy T. D. Spies.)

It has the odor and flavor characteristic of yeast. The aqueous solution has an acid reaction and is optically inactive. In dry heat, it is relatively stable up to 100° C. but is slowly destroyed by moist heat. Acid retards and alkali hastens this destructive action. In cooking, thiamine is not destroyed to any great extent if the temperature is not much above 100° C., provided the reaction is not alkaline and heating is not continued for too long a time.

Occurrence. Vitamin B_1 is present in many plant and animal foods. Whole grains, legumes, beef, pork, liver, nuts, and yeast are the best sources; fair sources are eggs, fish, and many vegetables. Although the vitamin is widely distributed, many foods have such small amounts present that partial thiamine deficiencies can easily occur. The milling of wheat flour has lowered the thiamine content more than 80%; as a consequence, enrichment of white flour or of white bread with thiamine is widely practiced. Furthermore, because of its solubility in water, much vitamin B_1 may be lost if the water in which foods are cooked is discarded. The desirability of utilizing these "cook waters" for soups, gravies, and sauces is evident.

Foods may be classed, in general, into three groups as to their thiamine content:

1. Foods highest in thiamine: whole cereals, lean pork, heart, kidney, although none of these is rich to the same degree as are some foods in vitamins A, C, and D

2. Foods high in thiamine consumed in relatively small amounts, e.g., yeast, and foods low in thiamine but consumed in relatively large amounts: meats other than those mentioned in group 1, milk, fresh fruits, vegetables

    The liver and roe of fish are reasonably good sources of thiamine, as well as of the other vitamins of the B complex.

3. Foods quite deficient in thiamine: white flour (not enriched), polished rice, white breakfast cereals, spaghetti, macaroni, refined cane sugar, molasses

Structure. The structure of thiamine has been determined to be as follows:

(pyrimidine)   (thiazole)

Thiamine (hydrochloride)

It has been synthesized, and the synthetic vitamin is frequently used in medicine. It occurs in nature either as the free vitamin or as the pyrophosphate. Note that the structure of thiamine contains a pyrimidine (p. 32) and a thiazole ring. No other natural compound contains the thiazole group, with the exception of penicillin, which has a hydrothiazole nucleus. The pyrimidine is also unique in that it is the only natural pyrimidine having an alkyl group in position-2. Plants can use a mixture of pyrimidine and thiazole compounds in place of thiamine itself, whereas animals require the complete vitamin. An apparent exception is polyneuritic pigeons, which may be cured by being fed large doses of a mixture of these intermediates. Perhaps a preliminary synthesis is brought about by microorganisms in the intestinal tract of the pigeons.

The three-dimensional conformation of thiamine pyrophosphate is being studied by x-ray analysis.[4] Knowledge of its conformation should provide new insight into the biochemical mechanisms involved in reactions catalyzed by this vitamin.

Mechanism of action. Thiamine is involved in the intermediary metabolism of carbohydrates in all the cells of the body. Several oxidative phenomena have been shown to depend on it, and probably they are related to each other. Brain tissue from pigeons having severe thiamine deficiency takes up oxygen at a lower rate than normally. This rate can be increased by adding thiamine to the tissue. Such tissue is also found to have an excess of lactate and pyruvate; and the suggestion has been made that neuritic symptoms may be a result of excess of pyruvate. The vitamin, linked to two molecules of phosphoric acid, becomes thiamine pyrophosphate (TPP) or diphosphothiamine (DPT). This is a coenzyme, *cocarboxylase*. Each coenzyme requires a protein apoenzyme. Carboxylases are present in yeast and other microorganisms, and oxidative carboxylases, e.g., pyruvic dehydrogenase, are found in animal tissues. Thiamine pyrophosphate takes part in the decarboxylation of α-keto acids, notably pyruvic and α-ketoglutaric (Chapter 9). Thiamine is also involved in transketolation (p. 210). Usually the content of cocarboxylase in blood parallels that of thiamine. However, in diabetes mellitus there is a high thiamine content with a low cocarboxylase.

Thiamine as the pyrophosphate thus functions primarily as a coenzyme in the decarboxylation of α-keto acids, including pyruvic and α-ketoglutaric. It is a component of the multienzyme complex pyruvic dehydrogenase. It apparently serves to transfer the decarboxylated intermediate on carbon-2 of the thiazole ring. In the case of pyruvic acid, this intermediate is active acetaldehyde, α-hydroxyethylthiamine pyrophosphate (see also p. 204).

The biochemical role of thiamine pyrophosphate in the decarboxylation of α-keto acids, together with other factors required for the conversion of these acids to acyl-CoA, may be shown schematically as follows:

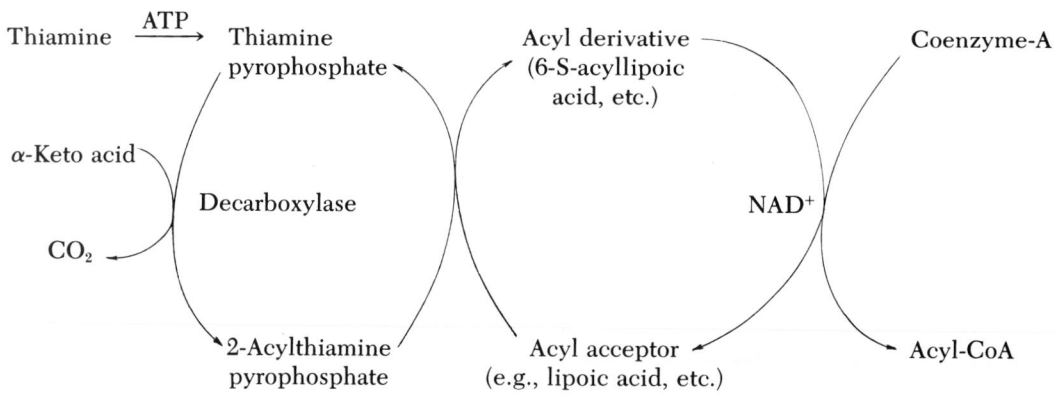

In the case of pyruvate, the acyl derivative of thiamine pyrophosphate would be 2-α-hydroxyethylthiamine pyrophosphate:

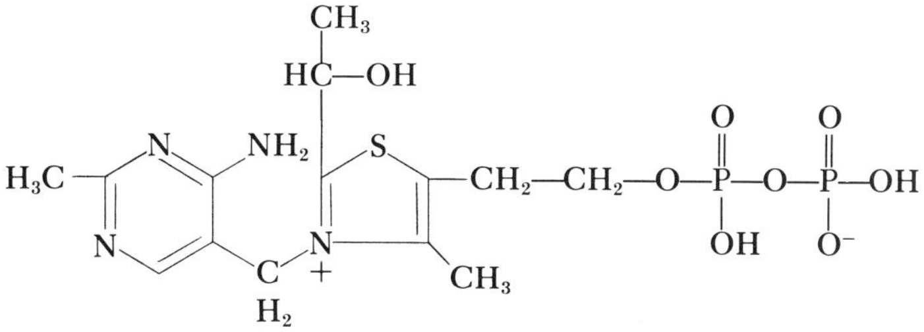

Active acetaldehyde (2-α-hydroxyethylthiamine pyrophosphate)

Human requirements. Thiamine is not stored in the tissues to any great extent, and loss of this water-soluble substance continually occurs by way of the urine. Apparently the thiamine content of tissues varies somewhat with the amount in the food, and, consequently, following a period of overabundance, a temporary reserve sufficient to accomodate the needs of the individual for a few weeks is built up. Ordinarily, however, any loss must be made good soon after it occurs. There are various factors that influence the requirement,[5] and all may be related to the amount of carbohydrate metabolized: (1) age—children require more per kilogram of body weight than adults; (2) activity—thiamine needs vary with caloric requirements; (3) pregnancy and lactation—greater amounts must be provided for the fetus or the suckling infant; (4) diet—high carbohydrate increases the need for thiamine. Substitution of fat for carbohydrate decreases the thiamine requirement, whereas protein seems to have no specific effect. The recommended allowances are 1.2 to 1.4 mg. daily for adult men and 1.0 mg. for women, increasing to 1.1 to 1.5 mg. during pregnancy and lactation (Table 25-1). This is about 0.5 mg. for each 1000 calories for adults and adolescents on ordinary levels of calorie intake, but when the calorie intake is lower, the thiamine provision should not fall below 1.0 mg. daily. During pregnancy the need for thiamine is increased. The thiamine requirement of the infant in relation to calories and to carbohydrate content of the diet is similar to that of the adult. In absolute figures it is between 0.2 and 0.5 mg. daily.

In view of its limited distribution in foods, thiamine is almost the only vitamin that may be lacking even in a fairly good diet. In patients on a restricted diet or with a diuresis leading to a rapid loss, the deficiency may be appreciable. Administration of thiamine under these circumstances is widely practiced.

If raw clams, or certain other raw seafood, are included in the diet, a thiaminase present may destroy enough thiamine to produce a deficiency. The enzyme action is a cleavage between the pyrimidine and thiazole rings. Horses and cattle that consume large amounts of fern sometimes become ill of "fern poisoning." This has been shown to be another type of thiamine antagonism, not enzymic in nature, since heated ferns are just as toxic. Several possible explanations have been offered, among them the idea that an inhibitory structural analogue, e.g., pyrithiamine, may be present in this plant.

Other clinical applications. Clinically the administration of thiamine has met with considerable success in a number of conditions besides frank beriberi. As might be expected, other types of neuritis have been treated with thiamine. Alcoholic neuritis and pregnancy neuritis seem to be due to a lack of this vitamin, and definite improvement is usually seen upon treatment with thiamine alone, or, preferably together with other constituents of the vitamin B complex. If the neuritis is not associated with a thiamine avitaminosis, the administration of thiamine does not help, nor does it help if permanent destruction of nervous tissue has taken place.

In various forms of nutritional deficiency there are symptoms of cardiovascular disturbance. Weiss showed that vitamin B_1 administration usually ameliorates these symptoms even though the patient is suffering from a lack of several vitamins. Gastrointestinal disorders also have been ascribed to thiamine deficiency. Lack of appetite and loss of muscular tone of the stomach and intestine were first shown in animals. To correlate a vitamin deficiency with gastrointestinal symptoms in man is more difficult because of the great number of other factors that influence the condition. However, several investigators believe that a certain group of symptoms are frequently caused by lack of thiamine. These include loss of appetite, low gastric hydrochloric acid, atony of the stomach and intestines, constipation, and a marked tendency toward the development of intestinal inflammatory processes. Treatment of gastrointestinal conditions with thiamine (and other vitamins) may require parenteral administration since the intestinal disturbance may operate to prevent absorption of the vitamin.

Although thiamine is ordinarily nontoxic, it has occasionally produced anaphylactic shock symptoms after repeated intravenous injections. The explanation for this is not known.

• • •

A number of different vitamins have been found to comprise the heat-stable fraction of the vitamin B complex. These are riboflavin, niacin, pyridoxine, pantothenic acid, and biotin. Choline, p-aminobenzoic acid, and inositol are also of nutritional importance but are not considered to be true vitamins. They will, however, be discussed in this chapter.

RIBOFLAVIN

No recognized disease is associated with an exclusive deficiency of riboflavin; but in pellagra, which is due to a lack of niacin, there is usually also a lack of riboflavin. In rats a riboflavin-free diet causes, besides a cessation of growth, vascularization of the cornea, frequently a loss of hair, and scaliness of the skin (with pediculosis); later, cataracts may develop. Dogs also develop cataracts if deprived of riboflavin. There may be nervous manifestations in animals suffering from a lack of this vitamin. In the human being, whether cataract is a result of this deficiency is doubtful. In man there is cheilosis, a condition characterized by inflammation of the lips, fissures at the corners of the mouth, scaliness, greasiness, and fissures in the folds of the ears and nose. Some initial trauma or infection is likely to be followed by a skin lesion if a riboflavin deficiency is present. There may be ocular disturbances like inflammation of the cornea, bloodshot eyes, photophobia, dimness of vision, and itching, burning, and dryness of the eyes with redness of the conjunctiva. The increase in the blood supply to the eye may be an attempt to furnish oxygen by means of oxyhemoglobin to tissues that ordinarily depend more on the respiratory functions of the vitamin than on the respiratory pigment of the blood.

Properties. Riboflavin is an orange-yellow crystalline compound. It is water soluble and heat stable, especially in acid solution, but is easily decomposed by exposure to light. Its water solution exhibits a yellow-green fluorescence. It is a pigment consisting of dimethylisoalloxazine attached to a D-ribityl group. In nature it may occur as the free pigment, as riboflavin phosphate, or as a constituent of flavoproteins. Its structural formula is as follows:

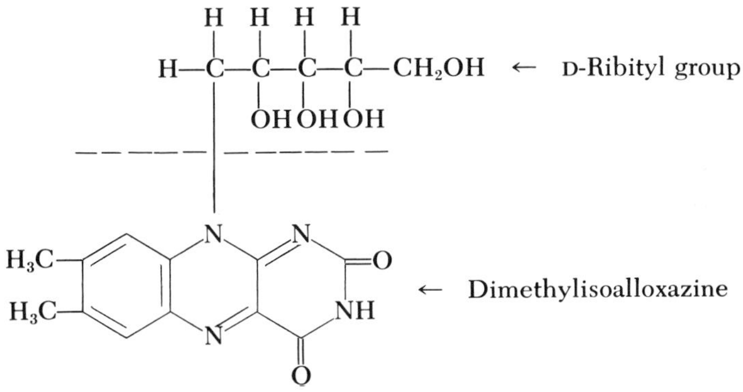

Riboflavin

Distribution. Riboflavin occurs widely in nature. Milk is an important source of it. Lactoflavin, one of the pigments of milk, is identical with riboflavin. Other excellent sources are meats, especially liver and kidney, fish, and eggs. Leafy vegetables are richer in riboflavin than they are in thiamine. Fruits and most root vegetables contain moderate quantities. Whole grains, cereals, and milled flour are not good sources.

Mechanism of action. The flavoproteins, i.e., combinations of riboflavin with proteins, are enzymes that function in tissue respiration as components of the electron-transport system and in a number of enzymes including Warburg's "yellow enzyme," L- and D-amino acid oxidases, xanthine oxidase, cytochrome-c reductase, and certain dehydrogenases. The flavin prosthetic group is usually FAD (flavin adenine dinucleotide, p. 246), but in some instances it may be FMN (flavin mononucleotide). The flavoproteins thus form a varied and important group of intracellular enzymes involved in oxidation-reduction reactions. This fact emphasizes the necessity of adequate riboflavin supplies in the diet.

The formation of the active cofactor forms of riboflavin and their participation in biologic oxidations may be shown schematically. (See p. 808.)

The positions at which the hydrogen atoms are added when FMN or FAD is reduced are shown in the structural formulas on p. 246.

Requirements. The recommended dietary allowances of riboflavin per day vary from 0.6 to 1.7 mg. for children and adults or 0.6 mg. per 1000 calories

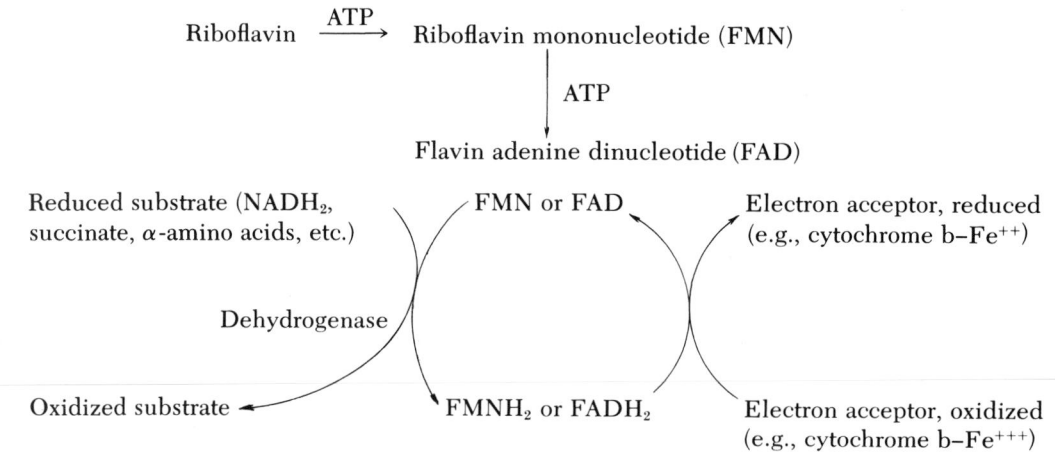

(Table 25-1). A well-diversified dietary should furnish these amounts, but, as has been pointed out, appetite alone may lead the individual to select food with a distinct deficiency in riboflavin.

Excretion. Riboflavin is excreted predominantly in the feces and, to a lesser extent, in the urine. During riboflavin avitaminosis, this small urinary fraction diminishes greatly. Riboflavin is excreted mostly in the free form but in varying amounts as the phosphate ester. Another flavin, uroflavin, is also found in the urine. It is similar chemically to riboflavin but appears to be more soluble in water and to contain more oxygen. It is probably derived from riboflavin.

NICOTINAMIDE (NIACIN OR NIACINAMIDE)

Pellagra is a disease that was long prevalent in southern Europe and in the southern United States. Most cases occurred in the low-income groups, where diet was restricted to a few cheap foodstuffs. Concurrent with monotony of diet was the crowded unsanitary housing of the poor. This coincidence of circumstances led early investigators to two hypotheses concerning the disease: it was due to (1) a nutritional defect or (2) an infection. The latter hypothesis had many supporters but was, with great difficulty, finally set aside in favor of the nutritional nature of the disease. Goldberger and his colleagues in the United States Public Health Service were chiefly responsible for the settlement of this issue. They conducted a long series of investigations, the most interesting of which was the prison farm experiment. Twelve convicts were promised pardons if they would agree to subsist on a diet of cornmeal, cornstarch, sweet potatoes, rice, syrup, and pork fat for a year. This was the diet that Goldberger knew was typical of diets consumed by pellagrous families. One of the subjects found the diet so much worse than the regular prison farm fare that he refused to continue. The others kept on with the diet, under the same sanitary conditions as existed for other prisoners on regular prison fare. Before the year was up, more than half the subjects showed symptoms of pellagra, whereas no such symptoms appeared among the prisoners on the usual diet.

At first, an amino acid deficiency was thought responsible. Later it was considered purely a vitamin deficiency, and finally, in 1926, Goldberger discovered that yeast, heated to destroy its thiamine, still had curative action on pellagra. This agent was provisionally called the *pellagra-preventive* (P-P) factor. Elvehjem[6] and co-workers proved that nicotinic acid (niacin) and its amide were capable of curing blacktongue, a deficiency disease of dogs, and soon niacin was shown to be identical with the P-P factor.

Relation to tryptophan. However investigators were confronted with a number of facts about pellagra that could not be explained by a purely vitamin theory. One of these was that for the cure of pellagra not only nicotinamide was needed but also adequate amounts of good-quality protein foods, such as milk, which is low in nicotinamide. Another fact was that a diet composed largely of corn led to the development of pellagra, even though an *apparently* sufficient amount of nicotinamide was present. Animal experiments substantiated this and later led to the observation that addition of casein to the diet has an effect that counteracts the effect of the corn. Soon the amino acid tryptophan was found to be the factor, lacking in corn proteins but present in casein, that simulates nicotinamide.[7] The explanation of this nicotinamide tryptophan relationship is as follows:

Tryptophan can be transformed into nicotinamide by the body tissues and thus contributes to the body's supply of the vitamin. This could occur in the following manner. Tryptophan is normally converted to kynurenine (p. 377); this may be oxidized in the liver and kidney to hydroxyanthranilic acid, which has been shown to substitute in animals for nicotinic acid.

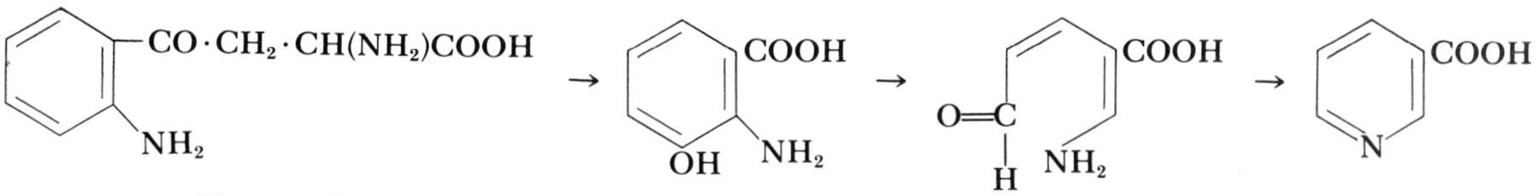

$-CO \cdot CH_2 \cdot CH(NH_2)COOH$ NH_2	$\rightarrow$ COOH OH NH_2	$\rightarrow$ COOH $O=C$ H NH_2	$\rightarrow$ COOH N
Kynurenine	**Hydroxyanthranilic acid**		**Nicotinic acid**

For this transformation the presence of pyridoxine seems to be necessary. From extensive studies in human subjects, it has been found that approximately 60 mg. of tryptophan are equivalent to 1 mg. of nicotinamide.

In pellagra there occur patches of dermatitis, soreness and inflammation of the tongue and mouth, alimentary disorders (achlorhydria and diarrhea), and pigmentation and thickening of the skin (Plate 2). There is usually a rash that appears symmetrically on the sides of the body and backs of the hands and arms. The pigmentation of the skin may persist for years after the dermatitis has healed. Nervous disorders and mental disturbances occur, particularly in the later stages. Some of the mental symptoms seen in chronic alcoholism have been ascribed to a nicotinamide avitaminosis, at least in part, since the diet of many alcoholics is deficient in B vitamins. Although these are the typical pellagrous symptoms and the administration of nicotinamide relieves them, generally other symptoms accompany them; also, generally the administration of nicotinamide does not entirely cure the patient. The reason is that, together with the deficiency of nicotinamide, there is usually a deficiency of riboflavin and thiamine as well. Often other food factors are missing so that other vitamins may have to be administered. A well-rounded and complete diet must be insisted on in order to prevent the recurrence of the symptom complex.

Properties. Although nicotinamide was discovered as a vitamin comparatively recently, the compound was known long before the "vitamin era." Since it could be produced by the oxidation of nicotine, it was known as nicotinic acid. This name was considered misleading by some authorities, so the terms niacin and niacinamide, respectively, were coined for the acid and its amide; now the "official" names are again nicotinic acid and nicotinamide. When pure, nicotinamide occurs as white, needlelike crystals. It is water soluble and stable in air and also in heat. There is little loss in cooking unless the cooking water is discarded.

Structure. The structural formulas of the acid and the acid amide are as follows:

| Nicotinic acid | Nicotinamide |

Occurrence. Nicotinamide is found in largest amounts in meats, especially liver. Fish and eggs are also good sources, as are some cereals and vegetables, notably whole wheat and unpolished rice, and peanuts. However, a number of our staple vegetable articles of diet are not particularly rich in nicotinamide, and therefore vegetarian diets may be lacking in this vitamin. Although whole wheat is an excellent source of nicotinamide, most of this vitamin, like thiamine, is lost in the milling process. Thus, nicotinamide is now one of the substances used to enrich white flour.

Effects of deficiency in animals. The dog, pig, and monkey are the only experimental animals that exhibit symptoms as a result of nicotinamide deficiency. Chittenden and Underhill, in 1917, described a condition in dogs known as blacktongue. This is characterized by a sudden refusal to eat the deficient diet, apathy, and lesions in the mouth. The inner surfaces of the lips and cheeks become covered with pustules, and the mucous lining comes away in shreds. Intense salivation and bloody diarrhea are additional symptoms, and there may be pustules on the thorax and upper abdomen. In monkeys the chief symptoms are tender bleeding gums, leading to ulceration and necrosis of the gum tissues. Vincent's infection is likely to set in, and, if nicotinamide is not provided, monkeys die usually in from 2 to 6 weeks.

Mechanism of action. Nicotinamide has been shown to be a part of two important coenzymes, NAD$^+$ and NADP$^+$, also called DPN and TPN and coenzymes I and II, respectively. The Enzyme Commission of the International Union of Biochemistry recommended that they be renamed NAD$^+$ and NADP$^+$, from their chemical constituents, nicotinamide adenine dinucleotide and its phosphate derivative, respectively. This corresponds with the terminology used for most other coenzymes, e.g., FAD, FMN. These are nucleotides; their structural formulas are shown on p. 246. They are members

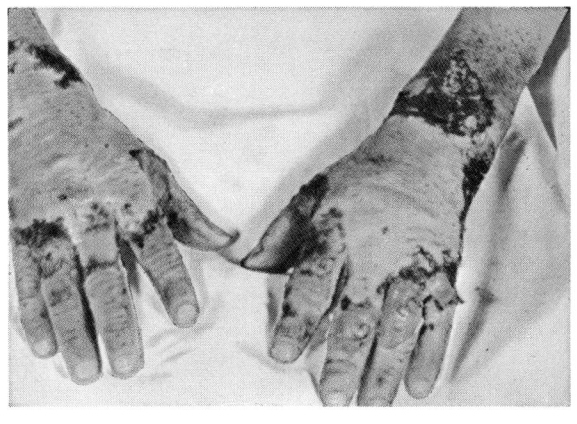

A

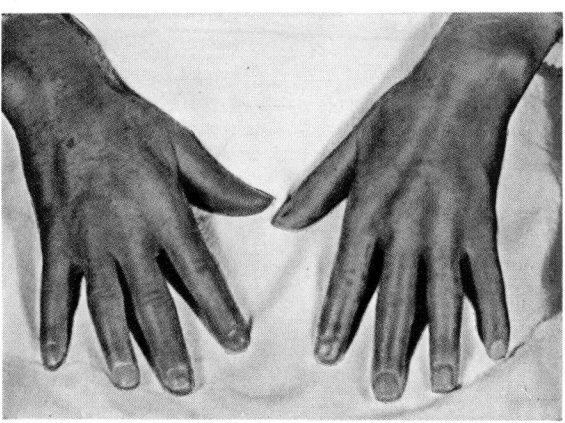

B

Plate 2. Results of severe niacin deficiency. **A,** Lesions of the hands in pellagra. **B,** Same patient after treatment with nicotinamide. (Courtesy T. D. Spies.)

of enzyme systems involved in cellular respiration as components of the electron-transport system. As has been seen (p. 249), nicotinamide and riboflavin are intimately associated in these reactions.

The pathway for the synthesis of the active coenzyme forms of nicotinamide and the role of NAD^+ in biologic oxidation are shown schematically below:

Nicotinamide + 5-Phosphoribosyl pyrophosphate +

Glutamine + 2 ATP $\rightarrow$ Nicotinamide-D-ribose-

diphospho-D-ribose-adenine or NAD

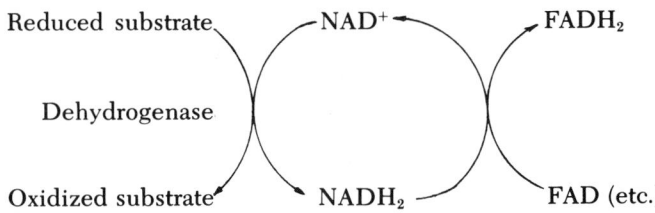

The positions at which the hydrogen atoms from substrates being oxidized are added to the NAD^+ molecule are shown in the structural formulas on p. 245.

The triphospho derivative, $NADP^+$ (p. 244), plays an important role in a microsomal system for biologic oxidations (p. 251) and, as $NADPH_2$, also in many biosynthetic reactions, e.g., the biosyntheses of fatty acids (p. 310) and various steroids (p. 326).

Human requirements. The recommended dietary allowance of nicotinamide for children is from 8 to 15 mg. per day, and for adults, from 13 to 18 mg. Active muscular work, pregnancy, and lactation increase the requirements to some extent (see Table 25-1). Large doses of nicotinic acid or its amide are not toxic. Up to 2 gm. per kilogram of body weight have been given to human beings, without any toxic effects.

PYRIDOXINE

Pyridoxine (vitamin B_6) is another pyridine derivative that belongs to the heat-stable B complex. In pyridoxine deficiency in rats there is a swelling of the ears and dermatitis of the paws and of the nasal region, followed by incrustation (Fig. 24-2). Other species that show symptoms when deprived of pyridoxine are the chick, dog, pig, and rhesus monkey. These symptoms include epileptiform seizures in rats, dogs, and pigs along with a characteristic anemia in dogs. In the monkey an arteriosclerosis apparently develops, but whether this has any relation to the disease in human beings is not known.

Properties. Pyridoxine is water and alcohol soluble and is slightly soluble in fat solvents. It is sensitive to light, ultraviolet irradiation, and alkali. Although pyridoxine itself is resistant to heat, its derivatives, pyridoxal and pyridoxamine, are destroyed rapidly at high temperatures.

Structure. In addition to pyridoxine, two derivatives, pyridoxal and pyridoxamine, also have B_6 activity. Pyridoxal is the aldehyde, and pyridoxamine the amine form. All three are found in foods in varying proportions. Pyridoxine can be converted to either of the other two, but neither of them can

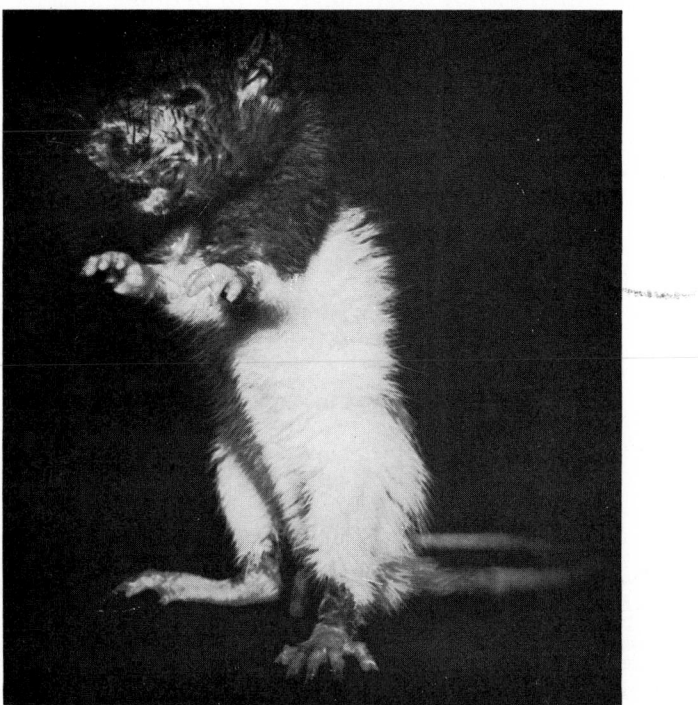

Fig. 24-2. Pyridoxine (vitamin B_6) deficiency in a rat, characterized by dermatitis of the extremities, beginning with swelling of the ears, nasal region, and paws, and followed by crust formation on these areas. (Courtesy Research Laboratories, S.M.A. Corporation, Chagrin Falls, Ohio.)

be changed to pyridoxine. All three are found in the urine after ingestion, but 4-pyridoxic acid is quantitatively the most important excretion product. The formulas and relationships of these substances are shown below:

Pyridoxine and derivatives

Functions. A major function of pyridoxine is as a coenzyme for the transaminases, as discussed earlier (p. 315). The change from pyridoxal to pyridoxamine, and vice versa, is required in transamination reactions (p. 352). Pyridoxal phosphate is the coenzyme for the decarboxylases that act on a number of amino acids and for two enzyme systems involved in the metabolism of sulfur-containing amino acids. Vitamin B_6 is essential for the dehydration and desulfhydration of amino acids. It also appears to be essential for the normal metabolism of tryptophan (p. 378). In its absence, large amounts of xanthurenic acid, a product of the incomplete metabolism of tryptophan, are excreted in the urine. For the conversion of tryptophan to nicotinamide, pyridoxine is also needed. Another function of pyridoxine is that in its aldehyde form, pyridoxal, it increases the rate of transport of amino acids and of potassium into cells against a gradient. In rats, pyridoxine and magnesium are necessary for the prevention of excessive oxalate formation, but whether this applies to man has not been determined. Pyridoxine is also believed to be involved in the metabolism of the unsaturated fatty acids.

Occurrence. The foods that are richest in pyridoxine are egg yolk, meat, fish, and milk, among animal sources, and whole grains, cabbage, and legumes.

Effects of deficiency in man. Although pyridoxine is undoubtedly required by man, symptoms of pyridoxine deficiency in adult human beings are difficult to produce. Long periods of deprivation are required before any effects are noted. These include a fall in the hemoglobin and alteration of the leukocyte relationships, depression, and mental confusion. By the use of a structural antagonist, however, skin lesions can be produced in a shorter time. These resemble the ones that occur in riboflavin and nicotinic acid deficiencies.

Since increased amounts of xanthurenic acid are excreted during and shortly after pregnancy, tryptophan metabolism is apparently altered at these times. Extra pyridoxine should be given to women during the second half of pregnancy to correct this abnormality. Recent clinical reports showed that an apparent pyridoxine deficiency occurs in patients receiving the drug isonicotinic acid hydrazide (INH). This is an antitubercular remedy and sometimes produces a peripheral neuritis. This condition results from an abnormal vitamin B_6 metabolism and can be prevented or cured by the administration of pyridoxine.

Reports of a curious syndrome in infants appeared in various parts of the United States in 1953. There were general irritability, abdominal distention, vomiting and diarrhea, and convulsions. All the babies with these symptoms were being fed the same proprietary liquid food. A change to a different food produced a dramatic cure. Evidently the sterilization procedure had lowered the vitamin B_6 content to a dangerous level. Since pyridoxine added to milk prior to processing is resistant to heat destruction, probably either *pyridoxal* or *pyridoxamine*, or both, had been affected by the sterilization process, because both are heat labile.

Human requirements. In the cases described above, symptoms developed when the milk contained 60 μg. or less per quart, and none developed when the food contained 100 μg. per quart. Current pediatric procedure recommends the addition of 2 mg. of pyridoxine daily to the diet of an infant. The recommended dietary allowance (Table 25-1) for men and women has been set by the National Research Council (1968) as 2.0 mg. per day. Since the requirement is closely related to protein metabolism, this amount has been established to allow for a daily intake of 100 gm. or more of protein to provide a reasonable margin of safety. The recommended dietary allowance for infants and children is from 0.2 to 1.2 mg. daily, depending on age. During pregnancy and lactation 2.5 mg. daily is recommended.

PANTOTHENIC ACID

Pantothenic acid (B_3) was at first called the *filtrate factor* and was given its present name by its discoverer, R. J. Williams. Pantothenic acid was so called because of its widespread occurrence.

Effects of deficiency. A deficiency of pantothenic acid causes dermatitis in the chick and graying of the hair in black rats (Fig. 24-3). This, however, is not the only antigray hair factor. Rusting of the hair and porphyrin caking of the whiskers have been observed in white rats; and in the rat are also seen dermatitis, inflammation of the nasal mucosa, and "spectacled eye" condition (which is more characteristic of biotin deficiency). Atrophy of the adrenal cortex, with necrosis and hemorrhage, occurs in many pantothenic acid–deficient animals, particularly if stress has been experienced. Corneal changes consisting of vascularization, thickening, and opacity are seen. Interference with sexual function and reproduction also is noted in various species, and there are neurologic lesions in chicks and pigs.

There seems to be no evidence of a pantothenic acid–deficiency disease

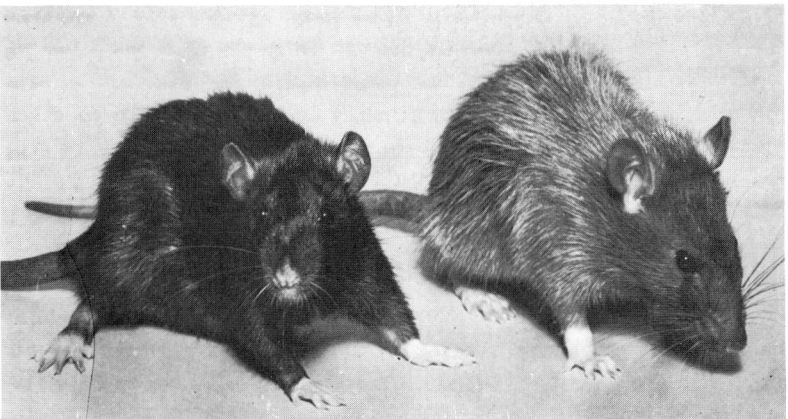

Fig. 24-3. Pantothenic acid deficiency in a rat. These rats were litter mates, both originally black. Their diet, after weaning, contained no pantothenic acid, but the rat on the left received 100 μg. of this vitamin daily. After 3 weeks on this diet, the animal on the right showed evidences of graying, which gradually became more pronounced. Other deficiency symptoms included scaly dermatitis, inflammation of the nasal mucosa, and hemorrhages in various organs, particularly the adrenal cortex. (Courtesy Research Laboratories, S.M.A. Corporation, Chagrin Falls, Ohio.)

in man. The vitamin is widely distributed, and consequently even on restricted diets no actual deficiency seems to have occurred. However, such a
deficiency has been produced experimentally. Human subjects were given a
synthetic diet to which was added every known essential mineral and vitamin except pantothenic acid. Although this resulted in lowered blood cholesterol and altered response to corticotropin, no clinical signs of deficiency
were evident. Then, to the synthetic diet was added a pantothenic acid antagonist (thiopanic acid), designed to still further deplete the system of this vitamin. Now definite signs appeared. The men became easily fatigued, had
cardiovascular disturbances, and, later, had gastrointestinal symptoms. There
were numbness and tingling of the extremities, and a number of other distressing conditions, including mental depression and upper respiratory infections, appeared. Administration of fluids intravenously and cortisone,
together with dietary supplementation, restored the subjects to normal
health.

Occurrence. In the first rank of dietary contributors of pantothenic acid
may be placed liver, kidney, eggs, lean beef, skimmed milk, buttermilk,
molasses, peas, cabbage, cauliflower, broccoli, peanuts, sweet potatoes, kale,
and yeast. In the second rank are white potatoes, tomatoes, wheat bran, whole
milk, and canned salmon. Many other animal and vegetable foods have a
moderately high content of this vitamin. The average amount of pantothenic
acid in the daily American diet is about 10 mg. This appears to be adequate.
No official figure as a recommended dietary allowance for man has been
adopted at the present time.

Properties and structure. Pantothenic acid is a water-soluble, yellow viscous oil, stable to moist heat and to oxidizing and reducing agents. It is destroyed by dry heat and by heating in an alkaline or acid medium. It is a
β-alanine derivative, possessing a peptide linkage, and has the following
formula:

$$\text{H-}\underset{\underset{\text{H}}{|}}{\overset{\overset{\text{OH}}{|}}{\text{C}}}\text{---}\underset{\underset{\text{CH}_3}{|}}{\overset{\overset{\text{CH}_3}{|}}{\text{C}}}\text{---}\underset{\underset{\text{H}}{|}}{\overset{\overset{\text{OH}}{|}}{\text{C}}}\text{---}\overset{\overset{\text{O}}{\parallel}}{\text{C}}\text{-N-}\underset{\underset{\text{H}}{|}}{\overset{\overset{\text{H}}{|}}{\text{C}}}\text{-}\underset{\underset{\text{H}}{|}}{\overset{\overset{\text{H}}{|}}{\text{C}}}\text{-}\overset{\overset{\text{O}}{\diagup}}{\underset{\diagdown\text{OH}}{\text{C}}}$$

Pantothenic acid

Functions. Pantothenic acid forms a part of coenzyme-A, the coenzyme in
acylation reactions. All cellular pantothenic acid, whether of animal or vegetable origin, is accounted for by the coenzyme. Consequently, coenzyme-A
(CoA) represents the only functional form of this vitamin. The structure
of CoA has been worked out by a number of investigators. It is an atypical
dinucleotide (p. 35), the usual mononucleotide being replaced by phos-
phopantetheine. *Pantetheine* is pantothenic acid, joined to β-mercaptoethy-
lamine through a peptide linkage. At the other end, pantothenic acid is joined
by a pyrophosphate bridge to an adenylic acid group. This adenylic acid
(p. 35) consists of adenine, D-ribose, and phosphate, but the phosphate is
linked onto the carbon-3 of the ribose.

In order to effect an acetylation, CoA must be present in the form of acetyl-
CoA. This is what was known as active acetate until its identity was estab-

$$HS—CH_2—CH_2—NH—\overset{\displaystyle O}{\overset{\|}{C}}—CH_2—CH_2—NH—\overset{\displaystyle O}{\overset{\|}{C}}—\overset{\displaystyle OH}{\underset{\displaystyle H}{C}}—\overset{\displaystyle CH_3}{\underset{\displaystyle CH_3}{C}}—\overset{\displaystyle H}{C}—H$$

Structural formula of coenzyme-A

lished. It may arise in various ways, among them the following: CoA, in the presence of adenosine triphosphate (ATP, p. 35), acetate, and a suitable enzyme, is converted into acetyl-CoA. The overall reaction, which was worked out in Lipmann's laboratory, can be shown in three steps.

ATP + Enzyme ⇄ Adenylic acid–Enzyme + Pyrophosphate

Adenylic acid–Enzyme + CoA ⇄ CoA-Enzyme + Adenylic acid

CoA-Enzyme + Acetate ⇄ Acetyl-CoA + Enzyme

The acetyl group may be transferred to an acetyl acceptor in the presence of a suitable enzyme. This occurs in two ways. The acetyl group is attached to the accepting group at the carbonyl end (head reaction) or at the methyl end (tail reaction):

$$\overset{*}{C}H_3CO\text{-}CoA + (CH_3)_3—N^+—CH_2CH_2OH \xrightarrow{OH^-} (CH_3)_3—N^+—CH_2CH_2O—\overset{*}{C}O—CH_3 + CoA$$

Acetyl-CoA   **Choline**   **Acetylcholine**

$$\overset{*}{C}H_3CO\text{-}CoA + \begin{matrix} COCOOH \\ | \\ CH_2COOH \end{matrix} + H_2O \rightarrow HO—\overset{\overset{\displaystyle *}{\overset{\displaystyle CH_2COOH}{|}}}{\underset{\displaystyle CH_2COOH}{C}}—COOH + CoA$$

Acetyl-CoA   **Oxaloacetic acid**   **Citric acid**

The asterisk indicates, in each instance, the carbon attached. Other functions of CoA are discussed in other chapters.

Reactions of this nature have been shown to result in the synthesis of (1) acetoacetic acid from two molecules of acetic acid and (2) citric acid from the acetylation of oxaloacetic acid. The products of these reactions enter into carbohydrate and fat metabolisms, as were brought out earlier. Furthermore, the acetylation of sulfanilamide and related compounds is an example of the importance of acetyl-CoA in detoxication reactions (p. 753).

Another interesting possibility is that the physiology of skin and hair pigmentation is in some way dependent on both the adrenal cortex and CoA. This is indicated by the fact that graying of the hair (achromotrichia), which develops in rats as a result of pantothenic acid deficiency, may be reversed by the removal of the adrenal glands.

BIOTIN

Biotin (B_7) is a food factor that for a long time was known to be necessary for the development of microorganisms. Biotin deficiency cannot be readily induced in animals by feeding biotin-free diets, nor is such a deficiency seen in man. It is produced by feeding large quantities of raw egg white. If rats are fed such a diet, they develop a characteristic group of symptoms including an extensive dermatitis, with "spectacled eye," hair loss, and involvement of the nervous system (Fig. 24-4). The condition can be prevented by adding yeast

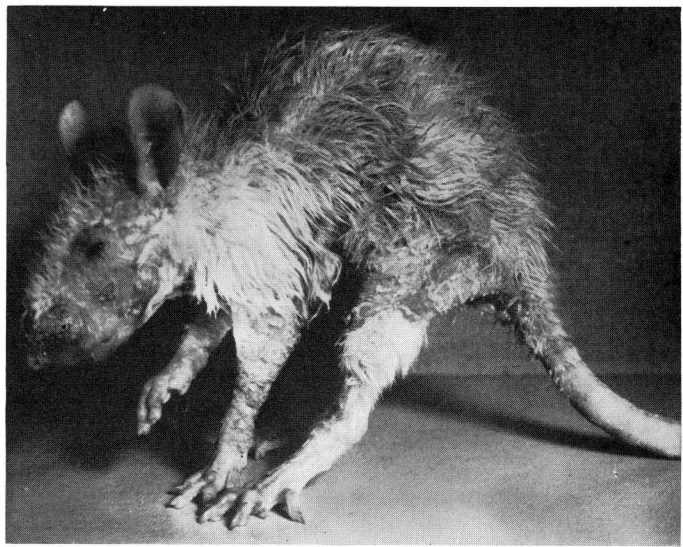

Fig. 24-4. Biotin deficiency in a rat. This animal had been on a diet containing 35% uncooked dried egg white as the sole source of protein. Alcoholic extract of yeast supplied vitamin B complex. Although not biotin free, the uncooked egg white combined with the biotin, making this vitamin unavailable to the animal. Such a deficiency is characterized by swelling and redness of the lips, denuded areas, and brown scaliness of the skin with extensive dermatitis. Later the eyes become gummed shut, the edema of the paws increases, and nerve involvement is shown by progressive spasticity. In advanced cases the rat exhibits the so-called "kangaroo posture" as seen here. (Courtesy Research Laboratories, S.M.A. Corporation, Chagrin Falls, Ohio.)

or other food rich in biotin. The explanation for these facts is that uncooked egg white contains a protein, called *avidin,* that is responsible for the egg white injury. Avidin combines with biotin in a firm linkage to form a compound that cannot be absorbed by the body and is therefore excreted. Thus an induced biotin deficiency, or egg white injury, results. The heating of egg white denatures avidin and destroys its ability to bind biotin.

Similarly, biotin deficiency has been produced in man by a low-biotin diet containing large amounts of raw egg white. This was done experimentally in the case of four volunteers and was also observed in one patient who had for years subsisted on a diet that included 4 to 6 dozen raw eggs a week. The chief symptom that occurred was a fine scaly desquamation of the skin without pruritus. Other symptoms included anemia, anorexia, nausea, lassitude, and muscle pains. Apparently, under ordinary conditions, the intestinal bacteria synthesize sufficient biotin for the body needs.

Properties and structure. Biotin crystallizes in long needles and is soluble in water and ethyl alcohol but is insoluble in ether and chloroform. It is heat stable. The structure of this compound was worked out by du Vigneaud[8] as follows:

$$
\begin{array}{c}
\text{O} \\
\parallel \\
\text{C} \\
\diagup \quad \diagdown \\
\text{H—N} \qquad \text{N—H} \\
| \qquad\qquad | \\
\text{H—C}\text{————}\text{C—H} \\
| \qquad\qquad | \\
\text{H}_2\text{C} \qquad \text{CH—CH}_2\text{—CH}_2\text{—CH}_2\text{—CH}_2\text{—COOH} \\
\diagdown \quad \diagup \\
\text{S}
\end{array}
$$

Biotin

Biotin is said to occur in both the free and the combined states in foods. The combined form is easily liberated by the action of proteolytic enzymes, and therefore the linkage is believed to be of a peptide nature.

Occurrence. Biotin is widely distributed in both the animal and the vegetable kingdoms. Excellent food sources are liver, kidney, milk, and molasses. There is some evidence that biotin vitamins, which do not combine with avidin, also occur. Apparently, much of the biotin absorbed is synthesized by the intestinal flora. Therefore a definite requirement for man is difficult to set; and a deficiency is hardly likely to occur.

Function. The role of biotin is primarily of carbon dioxide fixation, or carboxylation, as occurs in the conversion of pyruvic to oxaloacetic acid (p. 205). Biotin is also essential for a number of other carboxylation reactions, including the conversion of acetyl-CoA to malonyl-CoA in the biosynthesis of fatty acids (p. 311) and of propionyl-CoA to methylmalonyl-CoA (p. 828). The carbon dioxide is carried as a carboxyl group attached to one of the ureido-nitrogen atoms of biotin, as shown at the top of the following page.

Biotin was found to be a component of crystalline pig heart propionyl-CoA carboxylase by Kaziro and associates.[9] The enzyme has a molecular weight of about 700,000 and contains four moles of biotin per mole of protein.

$$
\begin{array}{c}
\overset{\displaystyle O}{\underset{\displaystyle \|}{C}} \\
\overline{O}OC-N \qquad NH \\
HC \!\!-\!\!-\!\!-\!\!-\!\!-\!\! CH \\
H_2C \qquad CH-CH_2-CH_2-CH_2-CH_2-CONH-Enzyme \\
S
\end{array}
$$

N-Carboxybiotin complex

Recent studies by Meister and his co-workers on *E. coli* indicate a new role for biotin, as a component of the enzyme carbamyl phosphate synthetase (p. 359). Apparently, the biotin-containing enzyme reacts with bicarbonate, glutamine, and ATP in a four-step reaction to form carbamyl phosphate, glutamate, and ADP. The reaction is inhibited by avidin, and added biotin restores activity. Biotin is present in highly purified enzyme preparations. It probably is also present in mammalian (rat liver) carbamyl phosphate synthetase. These observations thus implicate biotin in the biosynthesis of arginine and pyrimidines (nucleic acids).

Human requirements. Biotin is an essential nutrient for man. The adult requirement is supplied by the average American diet and is estimated to be 150 to 300 μg. per day. No recommended dietary allowance value has been established by the National Research Council as yet.

FOLIC ACID (PTEROYLGLUTAMIC ACID, FOLACIN)

The discovery of the folic acid group of vitamins is the result of many different investigations. The research proceeded along two chief lines, however. Certain substances were found to be essential to the growth of microorganisms, particularly *Lactobacillus casei* and *Streptococcus lactis* R. Other investigations dealt with factors found to be necessary in the nutrition of chicks, guinea pigs, monkeys, and other species of higher animals. Since these substances were not the same as the known vitamins, they were given new names as their functions became apparent. Not until 1941 was it evident that the chick vitamin and the bacterial growth factor were probably a single substance.

The vitamin to which all of these are related is folic acid (or pteroylglutamic acid, PGA). This is the *Lactobacillus casei* factor, isolated from liver, first shown to be a factor necessary for the growth of that organism. A number of other compounds, isolated from other sources, and having similar or even different biologic properties, have been found to be closely resembling substances. In other words, liver *L. casei* factor, fermentation *L. casei* factor, folic acid, vitamin B_c (Hogan), vitamin M (Day), factors R, S, and U, and yeast norite eluate factor are all vitamins of the same group. All are related to folic acid, also known as folacin. The structure and synthesis of this compound were soon determined. Pteroylglutamic acid is composed of three main parts: (1) a two-ringed nitrogenous compound called a *pteridine*, which is a yellow pigment first isolated from butterflies' wings, (2) p-aminobenzoic acid, and (3) glutamic acid. Its structure is as shown on p. 820.

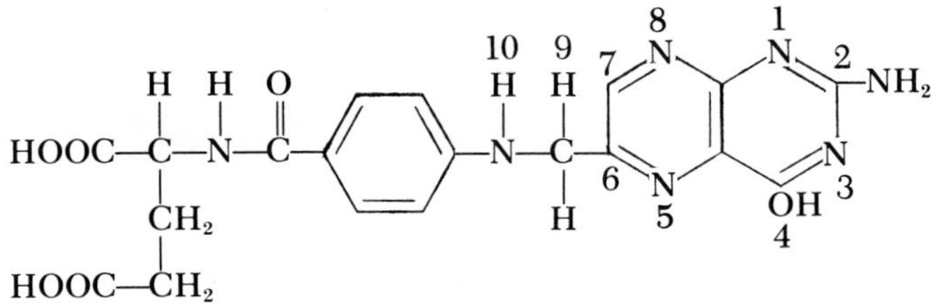

Folic acid
(pteroylglutamic acid)

The related vitamins differ in two respects. The first difference is the number of glutamic acid groups present, the additional glutamic acid molecules being conjugated in peptide linkages. The commonly occurring ones are the monoglutamate (PGA), the triglutamate (fermentation factor), and the heptaglutamate. The conjugates, i.e., those compounds having more than one glutamic acid in the molecule, are ineffective for some species that do not possess *conjugase*, the enzyme necessary to release the free vitamin. Normally a conjugase is present in the intestinal mucosal cells.[10]

The second difference is the structure of one of the rings, which occurs when folic acid is converted to folinic acid, the citrovorum factor (CF). This is so called because it supports the growth of *Leuconostoc citrovorum*, which the other members of this group are unable to do. The important fact to remember, however, is that folic acid can be converted to the CF, which is perhaps a thousand times more active biologically. Vitamin B_{12} (also ascorbic acid) is involved in this conversion of PGA to CF either directly or indirectly. The CF, folinic acid, or, to a much less degree, folic acid, is concerned in the production of an agent that stimulates the formation of normal red blood cells. If the *p*-aminobenzoic acid–glutamic acid portion of PGA is represented by R, the formula for the CF, folinic acid, 5-formyl derivative of 5,6,7,8-tetrahydrofolic acid, is as follows:

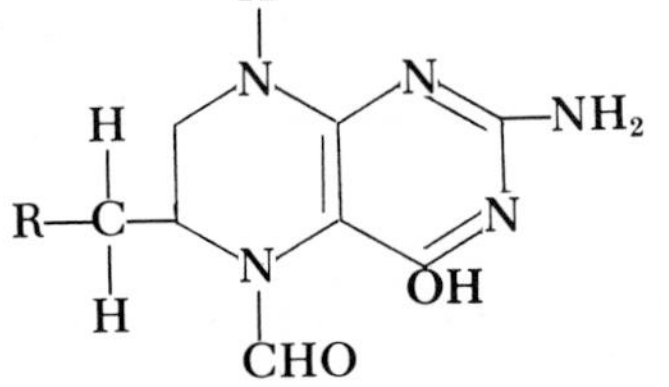

Folinic acid

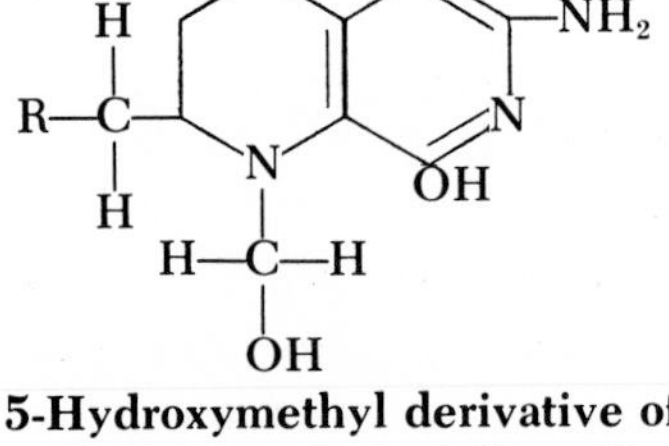

5-Hydroxymethyl derivative of
5,6,7,8-tetrahydrofolic acid

Mechanism of action. The difference in the formulas of folic acid and folinic acid gives a clue to the biochemical role of this group of vitamins. They are involved in *one-carbon* metabolism in somewhat the same way as CoA is involved in *two-carbon* metabolism. Folic acid is first converted to tetrahydrofolic acid (THFA) in the presence of $NADPH_2$ and ascorbic acid. THFA then acts as an acceptor of a one-carbon unit from either formate or formaldehyde. If formate is the donor, the product is probably the 5-formyl derivative of 5,6,7,8-tetrahydrofolic acid, the *citrovorum factor.* If formaldehyde is the donor, however, the end result probably has a hydroxymethyl group in place of the formyl and is 5-hydroxymethyl-5,6,7,8-tetrahydrofolic acid.

Tetrahydrofolic acid (THFA) has been shown to be involved in the transfer of the methyl group (p. 352) and in the utilization of single carbons (formate) in the synthesis of serine, thymine, purines, methionine, choline, and nucleotides, e.g., inosinic acid (Fig. 24-5). Folic acid also appears to have some relation to tyrosine metabolism, possibly in conjunction with ascorbic acid. These functions undoubtedly are involved in the role folic acid plays in nucleoprotein metabolism and erythrocyte formation.

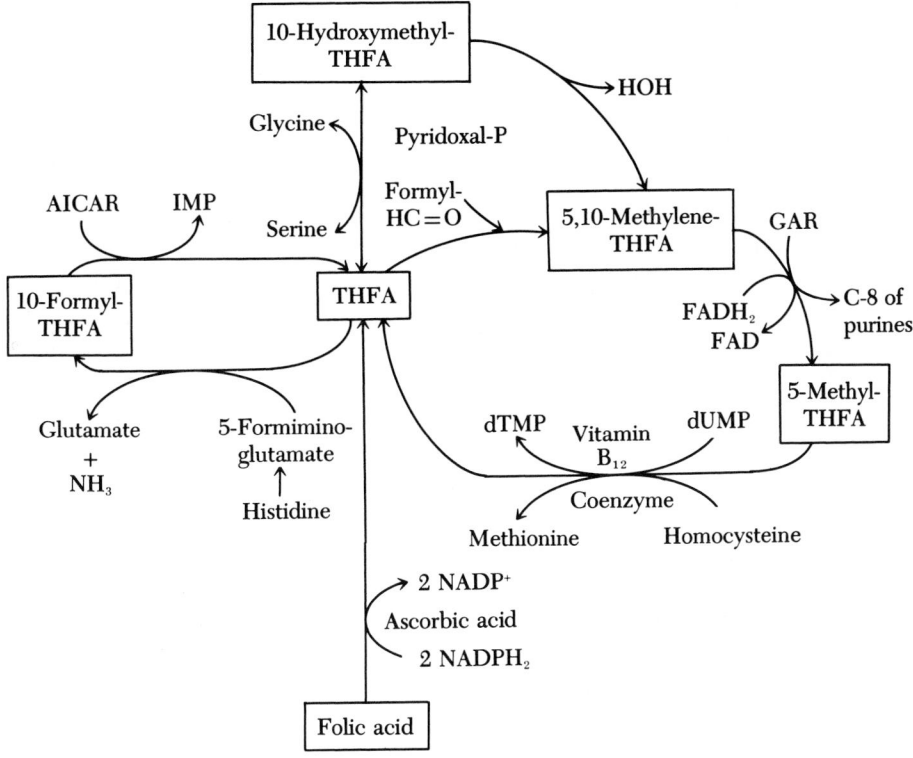

Fig. 24-5. Summary of some THFA-dependent reactions. *AICAR,* Aminoimidazolecarboxamide riboside phosphate; *IMP,* inosine monophosphate; *GAR,* glycinamide riboside phosphate; *dUMP,* deoxyuridine monophosphate; *dTMP,* deoxythimidine monophosphate. (Adapted from Loughlin, R. E., Elford, H. L., and Buchanan, J. M.: J. Biol. Chem. 239:2888, 1964.)

The formation of the active form and primary function of folic acid thus may be summarized schematically:

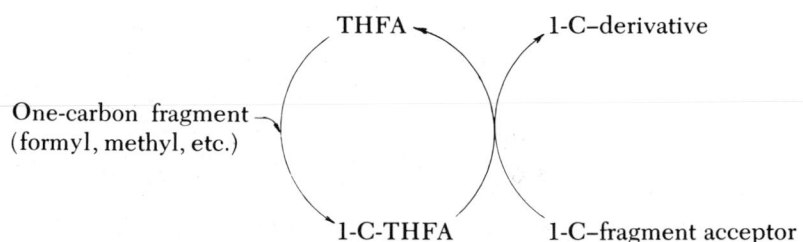

$$\text{Folic acid} \xrightarrow[\text{Ascorbic acid}]{\text{2 NADPH}_2 \quad \text{2 NADP}^+} \text{THFA}$$

THFA ⟶ 1-C–derivative

One-carbon fragment (formyl, methyl, etc.)

1-C-THFA   1-C–fragment acceptor

Properties. Folic acid is a yellow substance, only slightly soluble in water; its sodium salt is quite soluble in water, but both the acid and the salt are insoluble in lipid solvents. It is stable to heat in neutral or alkaline solution but is not stable if heated in an acid medium. It is inactivated by sunlight. A considerable loss occurs in foods stored at room temperature.

Occurrence. Folic acid is widely distributed in nature, particularly in the foliage of plants; hence the name "folic." Other good sources are yeast, cauliflower, liver, and kidney. Fair sources are beef, veal, and wheat, whereas root vegetables, tomatoes, bananas, rice, corn, sweet potatoes, pork, ham, and lamb contain little.

Most of the folic acid in foods is present as a polyglutamate, containing three to seven γ-linked glutamate residues. These are poorly absorbed. However, as mentioned, the mucosal cells of the duodenum and jejunum contain a *deconjugating* enzyme that splits off the extra glutamate residues. The monoglutamate is then readily absorbed from the normal intestine.

Effects of deficiency. In chicks a lack of this factor causes anemia as well as decreased resistance to malarial infection and impairment of the response to estrogens. Rats show achromotrichia (absence of normal pigmentation of the hair) and staining of the fur and whiskers with porphyrin, whereas monkeys respond with a macrocytic anemia, leukopenia, diarrhea, edema, and lesions of the mouth. Similarly, in man the chief symptoms of folic acid deficiency are megaloblastic anemia, glossitis, and gastrointestinal tract disturbances.

Clinical uses. Folic acid seems to be quite useful in certain macrocytic anemias, i.e., anemias that are characterized by the presence of giant red corpuscles in the blood. In fact, folic acid deficiency is the most common cause of megaloblastic anemia in the world. The deficiency may result from an inadequate intake, defective absorption, or abnormal metabolism. Among these conditions are sprue; the macrocytic anemias of pregnancy, infancy, and pellagra; and anemias following gastric resection and other intestinal dysfunctions. In such circumstances, folic acid has been found to be an effective hematopoietic factor. In sprue not only does it produce satisfactory effects on the blood picture, but it also relieves the gastrointestinal symptoms. It has been suggested as the effective agent in maintaining normal gastrointestinal absorption.

Folic acid also has a favorable effect on hematopoiesis in pernicious anemia. In fact, it has qualitatively the same effect on blood formation as does vitamin B_{12}. However, far less vitamin B_{12} is needed than folic acid; and the latter is unable to check the degenerative changes in the nervous system that take place in pernicious anemia. Because of the efficacy of folic acid in the treatment of macrocytic anemias, its careless use by patients with pernicious anemia, although improving the hematologic picture, may temporarily mask the neurologic symptoms which may appear later in an advanced stage refractory to treatment even with vitamin B_{12}. For this reason, the Food and Drug Administration (FDA) restricts the inclusion of folic acid in "one-a-day"–type vitamin preparations.

Requirements. The recommended dietary allowance for folacin, just established (1968) by the National Research Council, is 0.4 mg. per day for men and women. The recommended allowance during pregnancy and lactation is slightly higher, 0.8 and 0.5 mg., respectively. The allowance for infants and children varies with age and body weight (see Table 25-1). The dosages used in macrocytic anemias range from 10 to 30 mg., intravenously, to 200 mg., orally per day. The lethal dose for animals ranges from 125 to 600 mg. per kilogram. This is many times the therapeutic dose and indicates the relatively low toxicity of this vitamin.

VITAMIN B_{12} (COBALAMIN)

Vitamin B_{12}, called the antipernicious anemia vitamin, was isolated, purified, and extensively studied in 1949. It is the factor of liver extracts responsible for the curative effects of these extracts on pernicious anemia, and it is now believed to be identical with the "extrinsic factor" of Castle. It was isolated in 1948, independently and almost simultaneously, by Folkers and associates, in, and by Smith and his group, in England. This vitamin was soon found to be isolatable from culture broths of *Streptomyces griseus*, the strain used for the production of the antibiotic streptomycin. Indeed, various related compounds, also members of the vitamin B_{12} group, are present as by-products when other antibiotics are made, and commercial production of these vitamins utilizes fermentation by special microorganisms.

Structure. The structure of vitamin B_{12} was worked out be several teams of scientists, each made up of American and British members. A unique feature of the B_{12} compounds is the presence of the cobalt atom in the trivalent state. No other cobalt-containing organic compound has been found in nature. Cyanide is present in vitamin B_{12a}, but this is replaced by hydroxyl in vitamin B_{12b} and by nitrite in B_{12c}. These latter two may be converted to vitamin B_{12a} by treatment with cyanide. Vitamin B_{12a} is now designated cyanocobalamin; B_{12b} is aquocobalamin; and B_{12c} is nitritocobalamin. Several other members of the group also have been isolated. The empiric formula of vitamin B_{12a} is $C_{63}H_{90}N_{14}O_{14}PCo$, and the actual formula includes a portion somewhat similar to the tetrapyrrole ring structure of the porphyrins, e.g., heme and chlorophyl. The single cobalt atom is in the center of the prophyrin, like iron in heme. The structure is shown below.

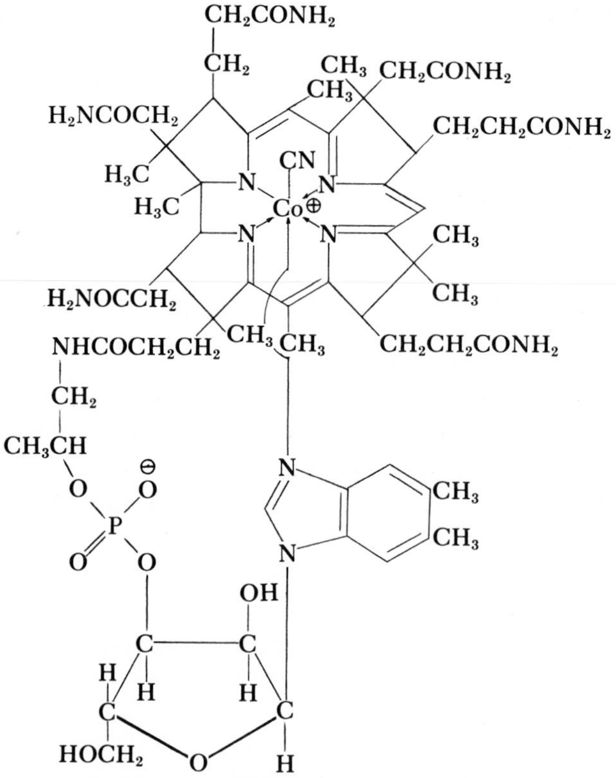

Vitamin B$_{12}$

Coenzyme B$_{12}$–5-deoxyadenosine (form in liver) replaces the cyano group on the central cobalt atom. It is thus the only known biologic compound with a direct carbon-to-metal bond. Coenzyme B$_{12}$ (cobamide coenzyme) has been called a "biologic Grignard reagent."

A series of investigations indicated that cyanocobalamin is a minor component of the total cobalamins actually present in the liver and in certain bacteria. Indeed, it may be an artifact produced by the chemical decomposition of the major component, now shown to be coenzymes B$_{12}$. Three different forms of the coenzyme have been isolated: one form crystallized from the bacteria *Clostridium tetanomorphum* and *Propionibacterium shermanii*; the other two highly purified from the liver of rabbits, chickens, sheep, and man. The three forms are termed *AC* (adenylcobamide), *BC* (benzimidazolylcobamide), and *DBC* (5,6-dimethylbenzimidazolylcobamide). In addition, the BC and DBC moieties contain one mole of *adenosine*, i.e., adenine plus the sugar deoxyribose. Cyanide is *not* present in any of the three forms. Thus the main form of vitamin B$_{12}$ in human liver is the DBC form in which the cyanide group is replaced by a 5-deoxyadenosine group to form *coenzyme B$_{12}$*.[11] BC and DBC are present in liver, comprising 48% to 72% of the total cobalamins. DBC is present in human liver.

The coenzymes B$_{12}$ are highly active as growth factors for B$_{12}$-requiring mutants of *E. coli* and for the conversion of glutamate to β-methylaspartate. Thus, the active forms of the cobalamin vitamin group appear to be the adenine-containing coenzymes B_{12}.

Occurrence. The chief source of vitamin B_{12} is liver, although the vitamin is also present in milk, meat, eggs, fish, oysters, and clams. Under certain dietary conditions this vitamin may be synthesized by intestinal organisms. In general, it is not present in vegetable foods. Pernicious anemia, which is due to a deficiency of vitamin B_{12}, must be regarded as the result of a gastric mucosal deficit rather than a dietary one, in most cases, since ample quantities of the vitamin (estimated at 3 to 5 μg. per day) are present in foods or are provided by the intestinal flora.

Vitamin B_{12} occurs in foods bound to proteins. It apparently is split off by proteolytic enzymes.

Requirements. The Food and Nutrition Board of the National Research Council set the recommended dietary allowance, in 1968, for vitamin B_{12} in men and women at 5 μg. For the adult past 55 years of age, 6 μg. daily are recommended. During pregnancy and lactation, the recommended daily intake is 8 and 6 μg., respectively. The daily dietary allowance for infants and children varies with age (Table 25-1).

Properties. Vitamin B_{12} is a deep red crystalline compound containing nitrogen, phosphorus, and cobalt but no sulfur. It is soluble in water, alcohol, and acetone but not in chloroform. It is levorotatory and is stable to heat in neutral solutions although destroyed by heat in dilute acid or alkaline solutions. It has been crystallized.

Physiologic effects and clinical uses. Vitamin B_{12} is perhaps the most potent therapeutic agent known. Only 5 μg. per day are required for satisfactory hematopoiesis in pernicious anemia. It is a powerful medicament in the parenteral treatment of megaloblastic anemias associated with a deficiency of the intrinsic factor. Apparently the intrinsic factor (p. 670), present in normal gastric juice, is necessary for the absorption of vitamin B_{12}, the extrinsic factor, from the gastrointestinal tract. Consequently, when administered by mouth, B_{12} is of little value unless normal gastric juice is present or is given at the same time; or, if administered alone, the dosage required is much greater.

The *intrinsic factor* has been isolated in highly active form,[12] along with another high-capacity B_{12}-binding protein devoid of intrinsic factor activity, from hog pyloric mucosa. Both are glycoproteins and appear to be homogeneous upon column chromatography and starch gel electrophoresis. The intrinsic factor glycoprotein is active in binding vitamin B_{12} and facilitating the absorption of B_{12} in amounts as small as 50 μg. The intrinsic factor glycoprotein contains approximately 15% reducing sugars, including galactose and glucosamine, and 33% total carbohydrate. It has a molecular weight of about 50,000 and a sedimentation coefficient of 3.7 S. It may form a dimer when complexed with one or two moles of B_{12}.

The mechanism by which the intrinsic factor enhances vitamin B_{12} absorption is still unclear. The protein may serve as a "carrier" in increasing intestinal transport, or it may "protect" the vitamin from, or render it unavailable to, intestinal bacteria. Maximal absorption of vitamin B_{12} in man occurs in the lower ileum, as determined by labeling the vitamin with ^{60}Co.

Vitamin B_{12} deficiency in man is usually due to poor absorption rather than inadequate dietary intake. Vegetarians tend to have low serum B_{12} levels but usually are not anemic.

Hereditary malabsorption of vitamin B_{12} was recently reported[13] in a case of pernicious anemia of long standing. A normal amount of active intrinsic factor was present in the gastric juice, and no detectable antibodies to intrinsic factor were found in the gastric contents. The mechanism for the malabsorption of B_{12} in this disorder is obscure.

Thus today it appears[14] that pernicious anemia, long an enigma, may be due to (1) a chronic dietary deficiency of vitamin B_{12} or (2) malabsorption of B_{12} because of a lack of intrinsic factor in the gastric juice. The latter may be caused by (a) the presence of antibodies to the intrinsic factor in the gastric juice, (b) a lack of secretion of intrinsic factor (due to gastric mucosal cell atrophy, etc.), or (c) hereditary malabsorption of uncertain nature. Pernicious anemia may, thus, frequently be an *autoimmune disorder.*

Vitamin B_{12} may also favorably influence the course of the anemias of sprue, pellagra, and infancy, but in these conditions pteroylglutamic acid may also be needed.

Effect on growth. If crude vitamin B_{12} (animal protein factor) is added as a supplement to the food of young animals, a pronounced improvement in the rate of growth is observed. Since the two main constituents of the supplement are vitamin B_{12} and streptomycin, there has been some controversy over which one is the causative agent. Other antibiotics have also been used, often with striking results (e.g., stimulating growth in plants). Although the vitamin alone has growth-promoting properties, the effect is enhanced by the antibiotics. Consequently, the effects on animals have been ascribed to (1) improvement of appetite by the vitamin, (2) diminution of the multiplication of intestinal microorganisms by the antibiotics, and (3) specific inhibitory effects of the antibiotics on oxidative phosphorylation. Whatever the mechanism, the influence of such supplements on the growth of fowl and domestic animals may be quite important from an economic standpoint. A somewhat similar effect has been seen in children, but apparently only in children who have a previous history of nutritional stress, i.e., not those in normal health. If adequate nutrients and calorie distribution are supplied, the addition of vitamin B_{12} brings these children into conformity with normal height:weight ratios.

Mechanism of action. The mechanism of action of vitamin B_{12} is being clarified. The vitamin seems to have an influence in various phases of metabolism. Among these are the synthesis of nucleic acids and the metabolic pathways of glycine, serine, methionine, and choline. Vitamin B_{12} or, more probably, coenzyme B_{12} takes part in the metabolism of methyl groups, serving as transmethylating agent (Fig. 24-5). Apparently the methyl group replaces the 5-deoxyadenosine group of coenzyme B_{12} and is transferred in this manner. Coenzyme B_{12} functions in the biosynthesis of thymine, methionine, and possibly choline in this way.

The role of vitamin B_{12} (cobalamin) as coenzyme B_{12} (cobamide coenzyme) in the transfer of methyl groups may be depicted schematically as follows:

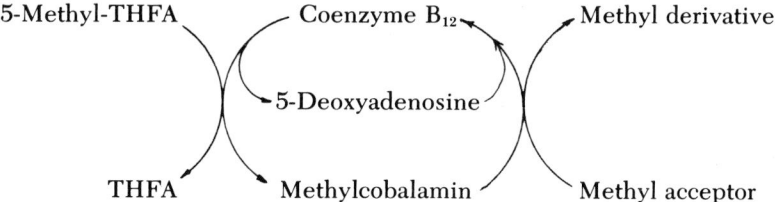

In this way, such important biochemical substances as thymine, methionine, and choline can be formed from the methyl group acceptors uracil, homocysteine, and aminoethanol, respectively.

Vitamin B_{12}, probably as coenzyme B_{12}, appears to be involved in at least seven or eight different enzyme reactions.[11] These include the following: reduction of disulfide to sulfhydryl groups; activation of amino acids for protein synthesis; conversion of methylmalonyl-CoA to succinyl-CoA; conversion of β-methylaspartic to glutamic acid, coenzyme B_{12} serving as a mutase; reduction of formate to methyl groups; reduction of ribonucleotides to deoxyribonucleotides via a ribonucleotide reductase; dismutation of vicinal diols to their corresponding aldehydes by means of a diol dehydrase reaction; anaerobic degradation of lysine. With the exception of the methylmalonyl-CoA reaction and the glutamic mutase reaction, the role of vitamin B_{12} or its coenzyme form is poorly understood.

The methylmalonyl-CoA mutase reaction has been the subject of intensive study during the past few years and is a remarkable reaction "without precedent in organic chemistry."[15] Ochoa and his associates, in 1955, discovered that methylmalonic acid plays some role in propionate metabolism in animals. In 1962, White[16] published the remarkable observation that large quantities, up to 50 to 90 mg. daily, of methylmalonic acid appear in the urine of patients with pernicious anemia. This was verified by Barness and co-workers[17] in patients and in vitamin B_{12}–deficient rats.[18]

As the result of the work of a number of investigators, including Ochoa, Wood, Lynen, and Johnson, during the past few years, the relation between vitamin B_{12} and methylmalonic acid metabolism has been clarified. Vitamin B_{12} coenzyme is a cofactor of the enzyme methylmalonyl-CoA isomerase, which catalyzes the *intramolecular* conversion of methylmalonyl-CoA to succinyl-CoA and thus facilitates the further metabolism of methylmalonyl-CoA presumably via the citric acid cycle. This reaction may be summarized as shown at the top of p. 828. The remarkable *mutase reaction* given above has been shown, by the use of various isotopically labeled (^{13}C, ^{14}C, ^{3}H) intermediates, to involve the shift of the $-\underset{\underset{O}{\|}}{C}-SCoA$ of the *b form* of methylmal-

onyl-CoA from the α-carbon to the CH_3-carbon, with a corresponding shift of the hydrogen atom in the opposite direction. The role of coenzyme B_{12} in this unprecedented type of organic reaction is as yet a matter of conjecture.

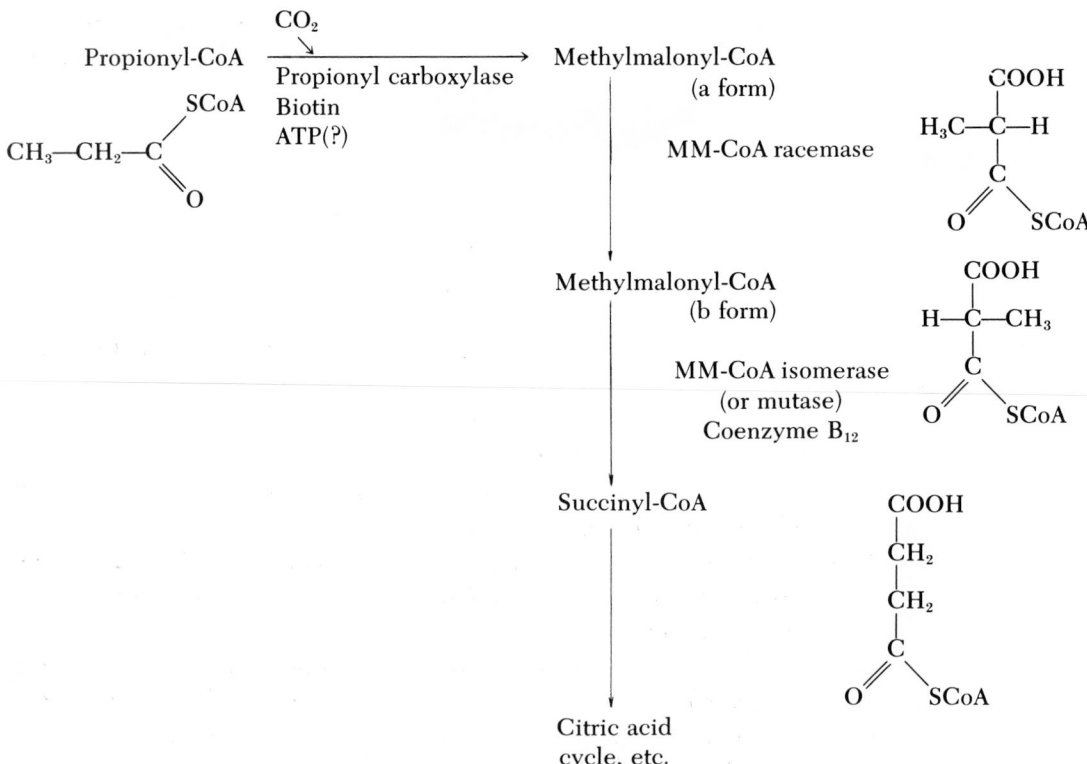

Propionyl-CoA and methylmalonyl-CoA may be derived from a variety of sources in the animal body, e.g., uracil, β-alanine, the biosynthesis of cholic acid from cholesterol, the metabolism of odd-carbon atom fatty acids, the metabolism of certain amino acids (Val, Ileu, Thr, Met), and the metabolism of thymine. Thus in vitamin B_{12} deficiency, including pernicious anemia in man, this metabolic pathway is blocked at the methylmalonyl-CoA stage and the unique metabolite appears in relatively large amounts in the urine. Methylmalonic acid recently has been suspect as related to the neurologic symptoms of pernicious anemia.

SUMMARY OF WATER-SOLUBLE VITAMINS

Table 24-1 presents a brief summary of the best food sources, the 1968 recommended daily allowances (where established), the active cofactor forms, the principal metabolic functions, and the major clinical manifestiations of deficiencies of the recognized water-soluble vitamins.

OTHER ESSENTIAL NUTRITIONAL FACTORS

Choline, inositol, p-aminobenzoic acid, the bioflavonoids, and α-lipoic acid are not considered by most authorities to be vitamins. They are, however, nutritionally important substances and will be considered here.

Choline   Choline is not a true vitamin because other naturally occurring substances can substitute for it and because it has not been shown to act catalytically. However, its importance in nutrition is unquestioned. Choline, you will remember, is a constituent of the lecithins and has the formula trimethylhydroxyethylammonium hydroxide:

$$
\begin{array}{c}
H_3C \qquad\quad CH_2CH_2OH \\
\diagdown \qquad \diagup \\
H_3C{-}N^+ \\
\diagup \qquad\quad OH^- \\
H_3C
\end{array}
$$

Choline

Effects of deficiency. Choline deficiency was discovered in the course of work on diabetic animals. In depancreatized dogs not only does diabetes occur but also a fatty infiltration of the liver. The former condition may be controlled by insulin but not the latter. Feeding raw pancreas, however, does cure the fatty liver; and the effective agent, or one of the effective agents, was found to be the choline part of lecithin present in the pancreatic tissue. This so-called *lipotropic* action of choline has been demonstrated in a number of other experimentally produced fatty livers. Choline has been shown to have several other physiologic functions.

On a low-choline diet, puppies develop a severe anorexia (lack of appetite) and fail to grow; hens do not lay eggs; rats do not have normal lactation. Together with manganese and folic acid, choline prevents perosis (slipped tendon disease) in chicks and young turkeys, and it prevents cirrhosis of the liver in rats. A low-choline diet also produces hemorrhages of the kidneys and eyes in addition to fatty livers in young rats; and if the diet is low in methionine as well, the hemorrhagic condition appears in other organs also.

This relation of methionine to choline should be noted carefully. Both compounds contain methyl groups and, with betaine, are sources of these groups in metabolism. If methionine is added to a low-choline diet, it decreases liver fat, probably because it has a methyl group to offer the system, which is lacking in such groups. A shift of the methyl groups is in some way required in fat metabolism and in other types of metabolism. This is called *transmethylation* (p. 352), and methyl groups are shifted, depending on the need for them and the dietary supply of them. Therefore, methionine or betaine may replace choline.

Best has reported a curious effect of choline deficiency. If very young rats are kept on a choline-deficient diet for 6 days and are then given a normal diet, they eventually develop high blood pressure. This may indicate that some of the systemic diseases of human adult life are due to unbalanced diets for relatively short periods during childhood.

As yet, no applications of choline to human nutrition have been definitely accepted. Possibly, alcoholic cirrhosis of the liver in man is, in large part, a result of dietary deficiency of lipotropic agents, of which choline and related substances are important examples.

Occurrence. Choline is widely distributed and no deficiency need ordinarily be expected. The most important sources in our diet are meats, egg yolk, bread, cereals, and various other vegetables, especially beans and peanuts. The human daily requirement has not been established.

Inositol Inositol is hexahydroxycyclohexane. Biologically active inositol—there are nine stereoisomers—is the optically inactive myoinositol (see p. 565 for

Table 24-1. Summary of water-soluble vitamins

Vitamin	Best food sources	Recommended dietary allowances° (1968)	Active cofactor form
Thiamine (B_1)	Pork, liver, yeast, whole or enriched grains	1.4 mg. (0.5 mg. per 1000 kcal.)	Thiamine pyrophosphate (thiamine diphosphate; co-carboxylase)
Riboflavin (B_2)	Milk, organ meats, animal protein, enriched grains	1.7 mg.	FMN (flavin mononucleotide), FAD (flavin adenine dinucleotide)
Niacin (nicotinic acid, niacin-amide) (precursor, trypto-phan)	Meat, enriched grains	18 mg. equiv. (1 mg. equiv. per 60 mg. Trp)	NAD^+ (DPN) $NADP^+$ (TPN)
Pyridoxine (B_6)	Meat, whole and enriched grains, walnuts	2.0 mg.	Pyridoxal phosphate or pyridoxamine phosphate
Pantothenic acid	Liver, meat, cereal, milk, legumes; widely distributed	–	Coenzyme-A
Biotin	Egg yolk, organ meats, yeast; widely distributed	–	Biotin
Lipoic acid	Liver, yeast	–	(constituent of lipothiamide complex?)
Folic acid (fola-cin, pteroyl-glutamic acid)	Liver, deep-green leafy vegetables; widely distri-buted	0.4 mg.	Tetrahydrofolic acid
Cobalamin (B_{12})	Animal protein, meats, milk, egg	5 μg.	Cobamide coenzymes (with 5-deoxyadenosine)
L-Ascorbic acid (C)	Citrus fruits, tomatoes, strawberries, melon	60 mg.	Not identified (cofactor, proline hydroxylase?)

° For American men, 22 to 35 years of age, of average activity.

formula). It is one of the muscle extractives and is also found in brain, erythrocytes, and tissues of the eye. It occurs widely in the plant kingdom in fruits, vegetables, whole grains, and nuts. Milk and yeast contain considerable amounts.

Inositol was included in the discussion of muscle extractives (p. 565). Possibly it is an intermediate between aromatic substances and carbohydrates. It is found in nature in at least four forms: free inositol, phytin, phosphatidylinositol, and a water-soluble, nondialyzable complex. Phytin is the

Principal metabolic functions	Clinical manifestations of deficiency
Decarboxylation of α-keto acids; transketolation	Beriberi (polyneuritis), cardiovascular—vasodilatation, tachycardia, edema; gastrointestinal—anorexia, nausea; neurologic—fatigue, apathy, neuritis, paralysis
Coenzyme of electron-transfer system	Angular stomatitis (cheilosis), seborrheic dermatitis, conjunctivitis, photophobia, glossitis
Coenzyme of electron-transfer system; dehydrogenase reactions; oxidation to produce ATP (NAD$^+$); biosynthesis of fatty acids, steroids, etc. (NADP$^+$)	Pellagra, diarrhea, scaly dermatitis, dementia, stomatitis
Coenzyme in amino acid metabolism: transamination, decarboxylation, transulfuration, tryptophan synthetase, amino acid transport	Cheilosis, glossitis, stomatitis, seborrheic dermatitis, convulsions, anemia
Acylation reactions (acetyl group transfers)	Anemia, achromotrichia; human deficiency most unlikely
Carboxylation; transcarboxylation	Dermatitis, alopecia, anemia; experimentally only in man
Transfer of acyl groups	Not known
Transfer of 1-carbon fragments (formyl); biosynthesis of purines, choline, methionine, etc.	Macrocytic and megaloblastic anemias, sprue, malabsorption, leukopenia, thrombocytopenia
Transfer of 1-carbon fragments (methyl); biosynthesis of purines, choline, methionine, etc.; mutase reactions	Pernicious anemia, neurologic lesions; sprue
Biologic oxidations; intercellular cement substance formation, collagen, capillary walls; metabolism of Tyr, Phe, folic acid; iron absorption	Scurvy, petechial hemorrhages, anemia, delayed wound healing, bone fragility

mixed calcium and magnesium salt of inositol hexaphosphate (phytic acid) and was formerly thought to be exclusively of vegetable origin. Now it is known to be a constituent of the nucleated erythrocytes of several species of animals. The inositol-containing phosphatide has been called *lipositol*. It has been isolated in pure form from soybeans and is known to be present in brain and spinal cord.

There have been a number of different types of effects produced in animals when fed a diet deficient in inositol. Among them is that inositol deficiency results in retarded growth and a peculiar hairlessness in mice (Woolley). Gavin showed that inositol has a curative action on the fatty livers produced in rats by the administration of biotin. Its significance in human nutrition is still undetermined.

p-Amino-benzoic acid   In 1941, it was found that failure of lactation occurred in rats whose diet contained all the then known B vitamins, including thiamine, riboflavin, nicotinamide, pyridoxine, pantothenic acid, and choline. The failure to lactate could be cured by yeast and other sources of the B complex. Graying of the hair of black rats also resulted when animals were fed on the deficient diet. Both effects have now been related to p-aminobenzoic acid (PABA), which had previously been shown to be necessary for growth in the rat and chick and also for bacterial multiplication. As mentioned before, pantothenic acid has also been described as an antigray-hair factor; however, the possibility that both biotin and PABA have similar properties also exists. Graying of the hair in man may sometimes be the result of a nutritional deficiency. For instance, Greeley, the Arctic explorer, became gray after a 9-month period of undernutrition. After he had eaten a normal diet for a while, his hair darkened perceptibly. Since the experimental field is still in confusion, the fact that results are not clear cut in human beings is not surprising; but neither PABA nor pantothenic acid seems to be the responsible factor in man.

p-Aminobenzoic acid blocks the bacteriostatic effect of sulfanilamide in vitro. The explanation for this is that there is competition between the two substances in some vitally important enzyme system. PABA is synthesized by the bacteria and is an essential metabolite for the bacterial cell. It takes part in some enzyme reaction necessary for the life of that cell, possibly in a phenolase system. Because of its structural resemblance to PABA, sulfanilamide (p-aminobenzene sulfonamide) takes its place in the enzyme system but does not permit the vital reaction to proceed normally. Other sulfa drugs have similar action, although they differ quantitatively. It is interesting to note that the bacteriostatic potency of each sulfa drug is directly proportional to the drug's ability to counteract the antibacteriostatic action of PABA.

PABA forms part of the folic acid molecule. This may be the point of attack by the sulfa drugs. Some investigators have questioned whether PABA itself has catalytic actions; hence they have not accepted it as a true vitamin. In view of the antagonism between the vitamin and the sulfonamide drugs, the continuous ingestion of extremely large doses of PABA is to be avoided. In itself, PABA is relatively nontoxic, but the presence of a high PABA level in blood and tissues might render sulfonamide therapy of little value.

Properties and occurrence. p-Aminobenzoic acid is a crystalline white compound, slightly soluble in cold water but quite soluble in hot water and in alcohol. It is widely distributed in nature but is more concentrated in liver, yeast, rice bran, and whole wheat.

Bioflavonoids In 1936, Szent-Györgyi and associates reported the existence in lemon peel of a material that they called *citrin*; it consisted of a mixture of flavonoids and was shown to have physiologic activity associated with the maintenance of normal capillary permeability and fragility. The active principle in citrin was found to be hesperidin, which was shown to have similar physiologic activity exerted by a number of compounds of like structure, including flavanones, flavones, and flavonols.

Flavanone Flavone Flavonol

Chalconization (opening of the ring system at the 1,2-position) does not affect this biologic activity, nor, within fairly wide limits, do the types and positions of ring substituents. Thus hesperidin (5,3'-dihydroxy-4'-methoxy-7-rhamnoglucosidoflavanone), its aglycone hesperitin, rutin (5,7,3',4'-tetra-hydroxy-3-glucorhamnosidoflavone), and its aglycone, quercetin, all have comparable actions, as do other compounds of the same basic structure. The term "vitamin P" (for permeability) was at first assigned to this group of compounds. They are now more commonly referred to as bioflavonoids, to indicate their structural characteristics and the fact that they show physiologic activity.

The mechanism by which the flavonoids exert their influence on capillary permeability and fragility has been extensively investigated; and compounds of this type have been found capable of interacting with various metabolites and enzyme systems that can affect the vascular system.

Bioflavonoid deficiency has been produced in animals; it results in a syndrome characterized by increased capillary permeability and fragility. In man, although the deficiency syndrome has not been observed, the bioflavonoids have been utilized clinically, with good results, in the treatment of diseases in which vascular abnormality is a factor.

Recent investigations,[1] mentioned earlier (p. 797), indicate that the principal action of the bioflavonoids is as an antioxidant (chelating of heavy metal oxidative ions?), thus protecting ascorbic acid from oxidative destruction. Their effect on the maintenance of normal capillary permeability would thus be indirect, via ascorbic acid.

The various members of this group are widely distributed in nature. They occur in the juice, peel, or pulp of citrus fruits, in tobacco leaves, in buckwheat, and in currants and many other fruits and vegetables. Whether the bioflavonoids can properly be considered to act as vitamins has not been firmly established; daily requirements are not known.

α-LIPOIC ACID

α-Lipoic acid is a relatively newly discovered factor. Its formula and that of its reduced form are as follows:

$$\text{CH}_2\text{—CH}_2\text{—CH—(CH}_2)_4\text{—COOH} \quad \rightleftharpoons \quad \text{CH}_2\text{—CH}_2\text{—CH—(CH}_2)_4\text{—COOH}$$

$$\underset{\text{S}\text{————————}\text{S}}{|\qquad\qquad|} \qquad\qquad \underset{\text{SH}\qquad\quad\text{SH}}{|\qquad\quad|}$$

α-Lipoic acid **Reduced α-lipoic acid**
(6,8-dithiooctanoic acid)

It appears to be necessary for oxidative decarboxylation of pyruvic acid and α-ketoglutaric acid (p. 204) by certain microorganisms and is probably a coenzyme or part of a coenzyme, sometimes called lipothiamide pyrophosphate (LTPP), for this reaction. It is found in many biologic materials, including yeast and liver, and is also called the pyruvate oxidation factor (POF). α-Lipoic acid has not been shown to be a dietary requirement for mammals.

BIOSYNTHESIS OF VITAMINS

Many vitamins are synthesized to a greater or less extent in the body. This may occur as a result of bacterial growth in the intestinal tract or by metabolic transformations within the body's cells. For example, bacteria produce large amounts of vitamin K, while an instance of metabolic synthesis is seen in the tryptophan-niacin transformation (p. 809). The continued use of antibiotics per os has been found to result in vitamin deficiency signs in many cases. This is due to the destruction of vitamin-elaborating organisms in the gastrointestinal tract.

TOXICITY OF THE VITAMINS (HYPERVITAMINOSIS)

With the exceptions of vitamins A and D, as described on pp. 765 and 777, there is little danger of toxic manifestations from the usual amounts of vitamins either in the diet or in the ordinary vitamin concentrates. For example, the minimal lethal dose of niacin is about 6 gm. per kilogram of body weight. For a person weighing 60 mg., this would amount to 360 gm., i.e., over 12 ounces, obviously an amount no person would be at all likely to ingest. The ratio of the amount required daily for optimal nutrition to the toxic or lethal dose is about as follows: vitamin D, 1:2000; niacin, 1:5000; vitamin A, 1:7500; thiamine, 1:25,000; pyridoxine, 1:60,000; vitamin B_{12}, 1:100,000. In view of the fact that enormous doses of some vitamins have been recommended and used clinically, we should note that there is a danger zone, even though it is far above the usual level of intake. The toxicity of the liver of the polar bear and of the Arctic fox is said to be associated with these animals' high content of vitamin A. There seems to be no information regarding the possible toxicity of riboflavin, pantothenic acid, p-aminobenzoic acid, or ascorbic acid. The feeding of 1000 mg. of ascorbic acid per day to human beings for as long as 3 months, without harmful effects, has been reported. However, there have been some instances of toxic and even fatal manifestations following *repeated parenteral* large doses of thiamine.

CONDITIONED VITAMIN DEFICIENCIES

The term "conditioned vitamin deficiency" is used to indicate those disorders that arise not because of a lack of vitamins in the diet but because of an interference with the ingestion, absorption, or utilization of these vitamins. Some examples have been mentioned previously in various connections and are now summarized.

Decreased intake. Persistent vomiting from whatever cause may lead to a diminished intake of vitamins. Any mouth deformities, e.g., cleft palate, loss of teeth, may have a similar effect. In chronic alcoholism there is also a diminished ingestion of all food, including vitamins. In cases of long-standing organic disease, either the appetite may be poor or the individuals may be unable to utilize their food properly.

Decreased absorption. Under the heading decreased absorption comes loss of vitamins due to their being (1) rushed through the enteric tract by diarrheas or (2) dissolved in undigested "grease," as in celiac disease or after the administration of mineral oil, and then being eliminated. Defective absorption because of any damage to the epithelium or diminution in the area of absorptive surfaces as a result of surgery also should be noted.

Impaired utilization. Examples of impaired utilization of vitamins are sulfonamide therapy and malignancy.

Increased elimination. Diuresis as a result of saline infusions or other causes leads to an excessive and rapid loss of the water-soluble vitamins. Excessive perspiration and diarrhea have similar effects, and lactation, a physiologic activity, may deplete the mother while benefiting the baby.

Increased requirements. Besides those increased requirements due to physiologic needs, e.g., growth in children, pregnancy, and lactation, there are some other factors that may be mentioned. Greater utilization of carbohydrate demands greater amounts of thiamine and the other B vitamins. Thus the infusion of glucose may lead to symptoms of B complex deficiency, as may also sudden increase in carbohydrate intake with insulin administration. When glucose infusions are given, concentrates of B complex vitamins should be administered concurrently. Fever increases the rate of metabolism and hence the vitamin requirement. The administration of thyroid preparations likewise increases the requirement for the B vitamins.

Faulty bacterial synthesis. It is now known that vitamin K, several members of the B vitamins, and perhaps others are synthesized by intestinal microorganisms and may thus add a significant contribution to the vitamin intake. If the flora is not suitable or if intestinal antisepsis is practiced (as is often the case in the oral administration of some antibiotics or sulfa drugs), a vitamin deficiency is likely to occur.

Bacterial destruction. There is considerable evidence that a large number of intestinal bacteria can decompose ascorbic acid. Decomposition is rapid and complete but is inhibited by the presence of any sugar that can be fermented by the organisms. Niacin and possibly thiamine and folic acid are also susceptible to destruction by intestinal flora.

Inhibitors. The sulfonamides are direct inhibitors of *p*-aminobenzoic acid. Other *structural analogues* have been produced. Massive doses of vitamin A, or even larger doses of vitamin E, given to animals produce hypoprothrombinemia, which is counteracted by the administration of vitamin K; thus apparently vitamins A and E are antagonists of vitamin K.

Imbalance. There is some evidence that the amounts of the various vitamins in the diet bear some relation to each other. For instance, vitamin E has a sparing action on vitamin A, and instances of interdependence of the members of the B complex have also been observed.

Therapeutic diets. Therapeutic diets, of necessity, are frequently nutritionally inadequate diets, particularly with respect to vitamins and iron. If such diets are to be used for periods longer than a few days, suitable therapeutic vitamin and iron supplementation must be provided. Some diets prescribed for allergies, for peptic ulcer, and for renal disease are excellent examples.

References

GENERAL

(See also references at the end of Chapter 23.)

Burns, J. J., editor: Vitamin C, Ann. N.Y. Acad. Sci. 92:1, 1961.

Cowgill, G. R.: The vitamin B requirement of man, New Haven, Conn., 1934, Yale University Press.

Greenberg, D. M., editor: Metabolic pathways, vol. 4, Metabolism of B-vitamin derivatives, ed. 3, New York, 1969, Academic Press, Inc.

Krampitz, L. O.: Catalytic functions of thiamine diphosphate, Ann. Rev. Biochem. 38:213, 1969.

Williams, R. J., et al.: The biochemistry of the B-vitamins, New York, 1950, Reinhold Publishing Corp.

SPECIAL

1. Clemetson, C. A. B., and Andersen, L.: Ann. N.Y. Acad. Sci. 136:341, 1966.
2. Horowitz, H. H., and King, C. G.: J. Biol. Chem. 200:125, 1953.
3. Warnock, L. G., and Burkhalter, V. J.: J. Nutr. 94:256, 1968.
4. Pletcher, J., and Sax, M.: Science 154:1331, 1966.
5. Cowgill, G. R.: The vitamin B requirement of man, New Haven, Conn., 1934, Yale University Press.
6. Elvehjem, C. A.: Physiol. Rev. 20:249, 1940.
7. Krehl, W. A., et al.: Science 101:489, 1945.
8. du Vigneaud, V.: Science 96:455, 1942.
9. Kaziro, Y., et al.: J. Biol. Chem. 236:1917, 1961; 240:64, 1965.
10. Rosenberg, I. H., et al.: New Eng. J. Med. 280:1019, 1969.
11. Barker, H. A., et al.: Ann. N.Y. Acad. Sci. 112:547, 1964.
12. Ellenbogen, L., and Highley, D. R.: J. Biol. Chem. 242:1004, 1010, 1967.
13. Goldberg, L. S., and Fudenberg, H. H.: New Eng. J. Med. 279:405, 1968.
14. Editorial: New Eng. J. Med. 279:433, 1968.
15. Whitlock, H.: Ann. N.Y. Acad. Sci. 112:721, 1964.
16. White, A. M.: Biochem. J. 84:41P, 1962.
17. Barness, L. A., et al.: New Eng. J. Med. 268:144, 1963.
18. Barness, L. A., et al.: Science 140:76, 1963.

CHAPTER 25

NUTRITION

Food is needed to provide the fuel for our energy requirements, to build and rebuild tissues, and to furnish the vitamins and inorganic compounds that are indispensable to good health. Thus we eat to live, but the complementary "we live to eat" is not to be lightly regarded simply because it implies enjoyment of food. Such pleasure, we know, leads to better digestion. As a rule, it also leads to a wider choice of foods, tending to provide a diversity of all the important food factors. The gourmand never dies of a deficiency disease. However, the other extreme of overeating is equally undesirable since it may lead to obesity and its consequent perils to health.

Historical background As a result of the brilliant investigations of Osborne and Mendel and of Hopkins, in the 1920's, leading to the discovery of the essential amino acids, of W. C. Rose's classic work in the identification of the remaining 10 essential amino acids, and of the studies of Mendel, McCollum, Elvehjem, du Vigneaud, Steenbock, and many others, on the vitamins, nutrition emerged in the early 1930's as a scientific discipline in its own right. Concomitant investigations of the mineral elements, including the trace elements, and of the essential fatty acids gave additional strength to the newly recognized science of nutrition. Of course, the roots of nutrition date back much earlier than this—back to Lavoisier's classic experiments on respiration, in 1775 (p. 512), and Magendie's work, in 1816, on "accessory food factors," mentioned earlier (p. 761). But nutrition at that time was not a recognized entity. Rather, it was a branch of physiology and later of biochemistry.

In the early 1930's, with the research discoveries of great practical as well as scientific significance, national nutrition societies became established in the United States and in Europe, and separate journals of nutrition began publication. Public recognition of nutrition increased. During World War II, the United States government sponsored extensive public education programs in nutrition as related to physical fitness. The "basic seven food groups" (now the basic four, p. 839) were popularized. Nutrition became recognized, in the words of Dr. Youmans, as "the most important single environmental factor affecting human health."

Current
nutritional
problems
Today, the science of nutrition, founded on a sound biochemical base, occupies a key position in dealing with many public health problems and their control both in this country and, through the World Health Organization, in the entire world. Malnutrition, resulting in part from the current "population explosion," is currently a problem of grave concern. An estimated 50% or more of the world's population, mainly in the Orient, South America, Central America, and Africa, suffer from hunger and malnutrition. Pockets of undernutrition occur even in the United States. Paradoxically, however, another segment of the American population is overfed and, as a result, subject to a different type of nutritional disorder—obesity, with attendant cardiovascular disease, diabetes, and other related disorders aggravated by overeating.

It is predicted that unless prompt and adequate remedial steps are taken in time the world malnutrition problem will become critical by 1980 and catastrophic by 2000, when the projected world population may have more than doubled (to some 6.41 billion!).

The major nutritional problem in the underdeveloped countries is an adequate amount of *protein* of good quality. Among the some 300 million children in these areas, protein malnutrition is found in the majority and causes poor growth, small size, even a reduction of the head circumference. This may lead to impaired growth of the brain and its development and mental retardation. Malnutrition may likewise lessen resistance to infection, setting up a vicious cycle. These interrelations have been discussed recently by Scrimshaw[1] and are represented schematically below:

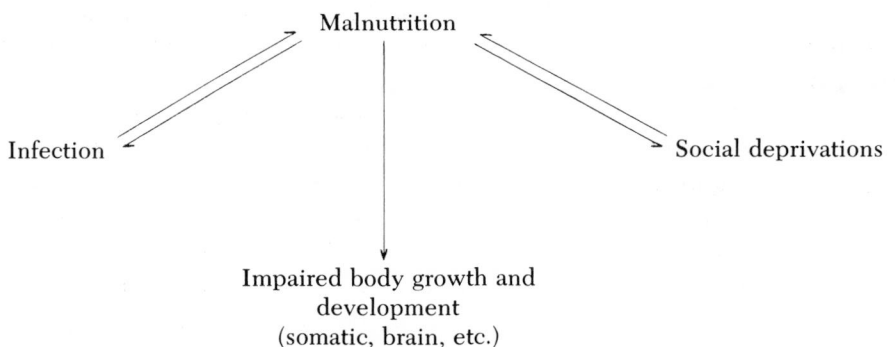

The obvious remedies to the problem recommended by authorities in the field[2,3] are (1) population (birth) control and (2) increased food production by improved (genetic) varieties, better fertilizers, and better management and distribution practices. Improvements in varieties of rice, wheat, and corn, which are the most important food crops, in that order, are essential. Also, new and increased sources of protein (fish, algae, microorganisms, leaf proteins, petroleum, etc.) are likely to become increasingly important. Education in the use of unfamiliar foods is a necessary accompaniment. Some of these questions will be considered in more detail later.

Malnutrition can be caused by factors other than a primary dietary deficiency of one or more essential nutrients, just as secondary, or conditioned avitaminoses may occur (pp. 835 and 836). These factors include faulty or impaired ingestion, digestion, absorption, and utilization or excessive catabolism caused by pathologic processes. A classic example is the magnesium deficiency syndrome seen in chronic alcoholism, in which the renal reabsorption of magnesium can be impaired.[4] Other examples have been cited in preceding pages. Some therapeutic procedures likewise may, in themselves, precipitate malnutrition. Emotional disturbance is still another factor just now being recognized as possibly interfering with nutrient utilization and inducing a *negative balance,* i.e., a state in which the output of the nutrient (or its metabolite) in the urine, feces, and sweat exceeds the amount ingested.

Recommended dietary allowances. The recognition of nutrition as a major environmental factor in human health and physical fitness during the World War II period led the federal government, in 1942, to establish a Food and Nutrition Board of the National Research Council–National Academy of Sciences. The board was composed of authorities in different specialties within the broad field of foods and nutrition. One of the primary functions of the board is to periodically review and evaluate available scientific data on human nutrient requirements, from which our official *Recommended Dietary Allowances* (RDA) are derived. The current values established in the latest (1968) revision are given in Table 25-1. The recommended nutrient values are set at levels designed to maintain good nutrition in practically all healthy persons in the United States and are now used as a guide in overall food planning and in the formulation of special diets, therapeutic ones included.

The RDA should not be interpreted as nutritional *requirements* of individuals. The latter are usually the *minimal* amounts needed to maintain a balance between the intake of a nutrient and its excretion or utilization, as has been discussed previously. Nor should the diet of an individual be called deficient if it does not contain the RDA of nutrients, since the values do not represent minimal requirements. In general, the RDA values allow a considerable margin of safety to account for individual variations in food utilization by normal persons. Similar recommended dietary allowances have been developed in other countries, appropriate for their population. In general, their values tend to be somewhat lower than ours.

Practical daily food plan. For practical convenience in planning a diet, nutritionists suggest the following food plan. It is based on four basic food groups, which, when consumed daily in the amounts suggested, supply the *normal* individual with an adequate amount, the RDA, of all food factors now known to be essential for man, with the possible exception of iron for women.

I. *Milk group:* Some milk daily:

Children	3 to 4 cups
Teen-agers	4 or more cups
Adults	2 or more cups
Pregnant women	4 or more cups
Nursing mothers	6 or more cups

Cheese and ice cream or other dairy products can replace part of the milk

II. *Meat group:* 2 or more servings daily:

Beef, veal, pork, lamb, poultry, fish, eggs, with dry beans and peas and nuts as alternates

III. *Vegetable-fruit group:* 4 or more servings daily, including the following:

A dark green or deep yellow vegetable important for vitamin A — at least every other day.
A citrus fruit or other fruit or vegetable important for vitamin C — daily
Other fruits and vegetables, including potatoes

IV. *Bread-cereal group:* 4 or more servings daily
Whole grain, enriched, restored

Each of the four food groups has been included because it contributes certain nutrients essential for a complete and balanced diet. For example, the milk group is especially important for its contribution of high-quality protein, calcium, and riboflavin. The meat group supplies excellent protein, thiamine, vitamin B_{12}, and minerals. The vegetable-fruit group contributes vitamin A (and β-carotene), ascorbic acid, smaller amounts of other vitamins and minerals, and bulk (cellulose, etc.). The bread-cereal group furnishes carbohydrate, protein, and, especially if enriched, whole grain, or restored, thiamine, niacin, riboflavin, and iron.

This food plan, then, along with some additional fats (butter, margarine, oils), forms a foundation for a well-balanced diet. Most nutritionists agree that it should form the basis not only for the diet of normal individuals but also, with suitable modifications, the diets used for therapeutic purposes.

•   •   •

The principal food factors — energy, protein, carbohydrate, fat, mineral, vitamin — will now be considered.

ENERGY FACTOR

The energy or caloric value of foods is measured in "large" calories. A large calorie, now called a *kilocalorie* (kcal.), is equal to 1000 small calories and is therefore the amount of heat required to raise the temperature of a kilogram of water from 15° to 16° C. In this discussion only the term kilocalorie will be used. The common foodstuffs yield, when oxidized in the body, approximately the following caloric values:

	Kilocalories per gram
Proteins	4
Carbohydrates	4
Fats	9

These are round (and corrected) figures. Individual members of each class have slightly different values, but these figures are usually accepted as average and reasonably accurate (p. 514).

In Chapter 17 the energy requirements of man were discussed in greater detail. The average normal man needs from 2400 to 2800 kcal. per day, and the normal woman somewhat less, usually 1700 to 2000 kcal. per day. These figures are general averages taken from the RDA values as revised in 1968 (Table 25-1).

The values are averages for normally active adults living in a temperate climate. For more precise values, the above and following figures must be

Table 25-1.

Recommended daily dietary allowances,[1] revised 1968

Food and Nutrition Board, National Academy of Sciences—National Research Council

Designed for the maintenance of good nutrition of practically all healthy people in the U.S.A.

	Age[2] Years From To	Weight kg.(lb.)	Height cm.(in.)	kcal.	Protein gm.	Fat-soluble vitamins			Water-soluble vitamins							Minerals				
						Vitamin A activity[6] I.U.	Vitamin D I.U.	Vitamin E activity I.U.	Ascorbic acid mg.	Folacin[3] mg.	Niacin mg. equiv.[4]	Riboflavin mg.	Thiamine mg.	Vitamin B_6 mg.	Vitamin B_{12} μg.	Calcium gm.	Phosphorus gm.	Iodine μg.	Iron mg.	Magnesium mg.
Infants	0 – 1/6	4 9	55 22	kg.×120	kg.×2.2[5]	1500	400	5	35	0.05	5	0.4	0.2	0.2	1.0	0.4	0.2	25	6	40
	1/6 – 1/2	7 15	63 25	kg.×110	kg.×2.0[5]	1500	400	5	35	0.05	7	0.5	0.4	0.3	1.5	0.5	0.4	40	10	60
	1/2 – 1	9 20	72 28	kg ×100	kg.×1.8[5]	1500	400	5	35	0.1	8	0.6	0.5	0.4	2.0	0.6	0.5	45	15	70
Children	1 – 2	12 26	81 32	1100	25	2000	400	10	40	0.1	8	0.6	0.6	0.5	2.0	0.7	0.7	55	15	100
	2 – 3	14 31	91 36	1250	25	2000	400	10	40	0.2	8	0.7	0.6	0.6	2.5	0.8	0.8	60	15	150
	3 – 4	16 35	100 39	1400	30	2500	400	10	40	0.2	9	0.8	0.7	0.7	3	0.8	0.8	70	10	200
	4 – 6	19 42	110 43	1600	30	2500	400	10	40	0.2	11	0.9	0.8	0.9	4	0.8	0.8	80	10	200
	6 – 8	23 51	121 48	2000	35	3500	400	15	40	0.2	13	1.1	1.0	1.0	4	0.9	0.9	100	10	250
	8 – 10	28 62	131 52	2200	40	3500	400	15	40	0.3	15	1.2	1.1	1.2	5	1.0	1.0	110	10	250
Men	10 – 12	35 77	140 55	2500	45	4500	400	20	40	0.4	17	1.3	1.3	1.4	5	1.2	1.2	125	10	300
	12 – 14	43 95	151 59	2700	50	5000	400	20	45	0.4	18	1.4	1.4	1.6	5	1.4	1.4	135	18	350
	14 – 18	59 130	170 67	3000	60	5000	400	25	55	0.4	20	1.5	1.5	1.8	5	1.4	1.4	150	18	400
	18 – 22	67 147	175 69	2800	60	5000	400	30	60	0.4	18	1.6	1.4	2.0	5	0.8	0.8	140	10	400
	22 – 35	70 154	175 69	2800	65	5000	–	30	60	0.4	18	1.7	1.4	2.0	5	0.8	0.8	140	10	350
	35 – 55	70 154	173 68	2600	65	5000	–	30	60	0.4	17	1.7	1.3	2.0	5	0.8	0.8	125	10	350
	55 – 75+	70–154	171 67	2400	65	5000	–	30	60	0.4	14	1.7	1.2	2.0	6	0.8	0.8	110	10	350
Women	10 – 12	35 77	142 56	2250	50	4500	400	20	40	0.4	15	1.3	1.1	1.4	5	1.2	1.2	110	18	300
	12 – 14	44 97	154 61	2300	50	5000	400	20	45	0.4	15	1.4	1.2	1.6	5	1.3	1.3	115	18	350
	14 – 16	52 114	157 62	2400	55	5000	400	25	50	0.4	16	1.4	1.2	1.8	5	1.3	1.3	120	18	350
	16 – 18	54 119	160 63	2300	55	5000	400	25	50	0.4	15	1.5	1.2	2.0	5	1.3	1.3	115	18	350
	18 – 22	58 128	163 64	2000	55	5000	400	25	55	0.4	13	1.5	1.0	2.0	5	0.8	0.8	100	18	350
	22 – 35	58 128	163 64	2000	55	5000	–	25	55	0.4	13	1.5	1.0	2.0	5	0.8	0.8	100	18	300
	35 – 55	58 128	160 63	1850	55	5000	–	25	55	0.4	13	1.5	1.0	2.0	5	0.8	0.8	90	18	300
	55 – 75+	58 128	157 62	1700	55	5000	–	25	55	0.4	13	1.5	1.0	2.0	6	0.8	0.8	80	10	300
Pregnancy				+200	65	6000	400	30	60	0.8	15	1.8	+0.1	2.5	8	+0.4	+0.4	125	18	450
Lactation				+1000	75	8000	400	30	60	0.5	20	2.0	+0.5	2.5	6	+0.5	+0.5	150	18	450

1. The allowance levels are intended to cover individual variations among most normal persons as they live in the United States under usual environmental stresses. The recommended allowances can be attained with a variety of common foods, providing other nutrients for which human requirements have been less well defined. See text for more detailed discussion of allowances and of nutrients not tabulated.

2. Entries on lines for age range 22–35 years represent the reference man and woman at age 22 years. All other entries represent allowances for the midpoint of the specified age range.

3. The folacin allowances refer to dietary sources as determined by *Lactobacilius casei* assay. Pure forms of folacin may be effective in doses less than one fourth of the RDA.

4. Niacin equivalents include dietary sources of the vitamin itself plus 1 mg. equivalent for each 60 mg. of dietary tryptophan.

5. Assumes protein equivalent to human milk. For proteins not 100% utilized, factors should be increased proportionately.

6. Assuming one fifth is from preformed vitamin A and four fifths is from β-carotene.

adjusted to take into account variations in body size, physical activity, age, and environmental temperature.

The current values are somewhat lower (by 100 kcal.) than those recommended in 1963. The reason is recognition of the relatively sedentary living pattern in the United States today, even among young adults. However, the Food and Nutrition Board adds: "It is likely that a better level of health would be reached if the population were more physically active. There is growing evidence that a sedentary life contributes to degenerative arterial disease as well as to obesity with its many complications."

For calculating calories and certain other nutrients for the age group 22–35 years, the Food and Nutrition Board has arbitrarily assumed the "reference" man or woman to be 22 years of age, weighing 70 kg. (154 lb.) and 58 kg. (128 lb.), respectively. The age of 22 years was adopted since weight gained after that age is believed to be primarily *unnecessary fat.*

During pregnancy and lactation, an additional 200 and 1000 kcal. per day, respectively, are recommended. Children, and adolescents have caloric needs averaging from 1100 to 3000 kcal., depending on age and sex. The recommended allowance for infants is the body weight in kilograms multiplied by 120, for the first 2 months of life; by 110, for the 2- to 6-months age period; and by 100, for ages from 6 months to 1 year.

The energy factor plays a role in growth as well as in the more apparent energy relations discussed in Chapter 17. Handler and associates[5] showed that when animals are fed a diet in which the proteins, vitamins, and minerals are adequate, but the calories severely restricted, both skeletal and generalized body growth may be inhibited even to the point of complete cessation.

Calculating energy value of a food. Few naturally occurring foods are pure protein, carbohydrate, or fat. Most are mixtures and, in addition, contain varying amounts of water. Their energy value is calculated on the basis of the actual percentages of protein, carbohydrate, and fat present multiplied by the caloric values given. For example: White bread contains 36% water, 9% protein, 2% fat, 52% total carbohydrates. A slice of this bread weighs about 25 gm. and therefore contains the following:

	$25 \times 9\%$	$25 \times 2\%$	$25 \times 52\%$
	or	or	or
	2.3 gm. protein	0.5 gm. fat	13 gm. carbohydrate
Its caloric value	$\times 4$	$\times 9$	$\times 4$
would be	9.2 kcal.	4.5 kcal.	52 kcal. = 65.7 kcal.

If the composition of the food is known, the approximate energy value can be estimated by this type of calculation. The analyses of many foods can be found in various government publications as well as in some nutrition textbooks, several of which are listed at the end of this chapter. It must be noted, however, that all foods vary considerably from time to time. Meats differ markedly in their fat content—even meats of the same grade and cut. A given vegetable— e.g., peas—shows differences in composition (both organic and inorganic), depending on variety, age, moisture availability, amount and type of fertilizer, and other variables in cultivation. Prepared foods show the widest divergence, of course, because of the variety of ingredients and methods of cooking. It is evident, therefore, that such data must be used with intelligence, and calculation to the first decimal place is unnecessary. In some tables the energy values are given *per 100 gm.* and *per pound.* In the United States Department of Agriculture Handbook no. 8, tables are arranged to give the number of grams in average portions, the size of each portion being stated, or in convenient amounts. Other tables give the number of grams per 100 gm. of edible material. Still others state the number of grams of each foodstuff per 100 kcal. The vitamin and mineral contents are similarly listed.

PROTEIN FACTOR

The question as to what is the optimum amount of protein has been discussed for many years. Indeed, at one time it was one of the most popular topics in biochemistry. The reasons for this are very evident. Protein is the most important foodstuff. The caloric needs of the body can be supplied by protein, carbohydrate, and fat, but the protein of our tissues can come only from the protein of food. Protein is required by every cell and is the basis of protoplasm. Moreover, it is the most expensive of the foodstuffs. It was, therefore, felt to be of economic as well as physiologic interest.

In the latter part of the nineteenth century, Voit studied the protein intake of many adults in Germany and found that their average consumption was 118 gm. This was set up as the standard, even as the optimum protein intake, although the only evidence for such an assumption was that it was the amount usually eaten. Chittenden, in 1904, came to quite a different conclusion. As a result of nutritional investigations on students, instructors, soldiers, and others, he found that the protein requirement was much less than Voit's figure. The general method used in these studies was to determine the nitrogen balance, i.e., a comparison between the nitrogen intake as protein and the nitrogen output in the urine and feces. If the output and intake are equal, the subject is in nitrogen equilibrium. If the output is greater than the intake, there is a negative balance, which means that the individual is not getting enough protein in his food to take care of his physiologic requirements. Chittenden's subjects could be kept in nitrogen equilibrium on from 45 to 53 gm. of protein daily. The subjects on low-protein diets (45 to 53 gm.) were able to do just as much physical and mental work as before. In fact, their general health and athletic prowess were usually improved. Chittenden came to the conclusion that Voit's "standard" of 118 gm. per day was far above the actual need of men and that the excess intake might actually lead to various pathologic states, e.g., indigestion, intestinal toxemia, liver disease, gout, rheumatism.

Many investigations have shown that the minimum protein requirement compatible with nitrogen equilibrium is much lower even than the figures set by Chittenden. In order to attain nitrogen equilibrium with a low protein intake, enough carbohydrate and fat must be eaten to provide sufficient energy for the individual's needs. If this is not done, body protein is consumed for this energy requirement, and more nitrogen is eliminated than is taken in. Consequently, carbohydrates and fats are known as "protein sparers." The

843

question has been raised as to whether a person could continue on a very low-protein diet for a considerable length of time, even if he were in nitrogen equilibrium. All experiments have necessarily been restricted to a few weeks or, at best, a few months; but could a person live for years, and live comfortably, on a minimum or near-minimum protein ration? Nutritionists today doubt whether he could. With the modern concept of essential amino acids, it becomes apparent that a person on a highly restricted diet might easily experience a lack of one or more of these vital building stones. If the protein or amino acid content of the diet could be so planned as to have all the essential amino acids in requisite amounts at about the same time, such a lack would not occur and a minimal protein diet might be the ideal one. However, this is not possible at present, even if it were demonstrated to be entirely desirable. To select foods, having exactly the same amino acid composition as human proteins, so that food protein could be converted to body protein weight for weight would be practically impossible.

Consequently, an amount of protein greater than the Chittenden figure and yet lower than the Voit figure is today considered the optimum one for good nutritive condition. Sherman and his associates[6] pointed out that the protein requirement of man is quite different from the protein allowance or standard. Total calories fed must not exceed total calories required by very much or for very long. Such excess is usually converted to fat. However, excess protein over the required minimum is not stored to any great extent and is not converted to fat, unless the total caloric value of the food is excessive. Therefore, a moderate excess of protein over and above the required amount is not only harmless but is also a common dietary habit, which constitutes a desirable factor of safety. It provides an excess of essential and semiessential amino acids (p. 349), which circulate in the blood or are temporarily stored in the tissues, ready and available for any cell in need of them.

The studies of various investigators have shown that an intake of about 0.9 gm. of protein per kilogram of body weight is adequate for all ordinary needs in the normal adult. In childhood this allowance must be increased considerably to permit growth of new tissue. The same applies in pregnancy and lactation. In elderly persons the protein intake should be maintained even though there is a somewhat lower caloric need. Negative nitrogen balances are said to be common in this population group. The recommended dietary allowance for protein for an average man is 65 gm. per day, and for an average woman 55 gm. per day. Values for other age groups for men and women are given in Table 25-1. These values, like the RDA values for calories, are somewhat lower than previously given. They have been determined on the basis that the protein nitrogen requirement equals the sum of the losses of endogenous nitrogen in the urine and feces, plus nitrogen in sweat, skin, and other integumental losses. The actual protein requirement for the average man thus calculated is approximately 35 gm. per day. Increasing this figure by 30%, to allow for individual variability within a large population, and an additional 70% to compensate for the efficiency of utilization of the average protein in the American dietary, has resulted in the present RDA values, with adjustments for growth, pregnancy, and lactation.

Heretofore it had been generally accepted that protein requirement does not run parallel to the amount of work done. Recent work, however, has thrown doubt on this.[7] Apparently, long-continued heavy muscular work does lead to an increased protein need, probably for growth and replacement of muscle tissue.

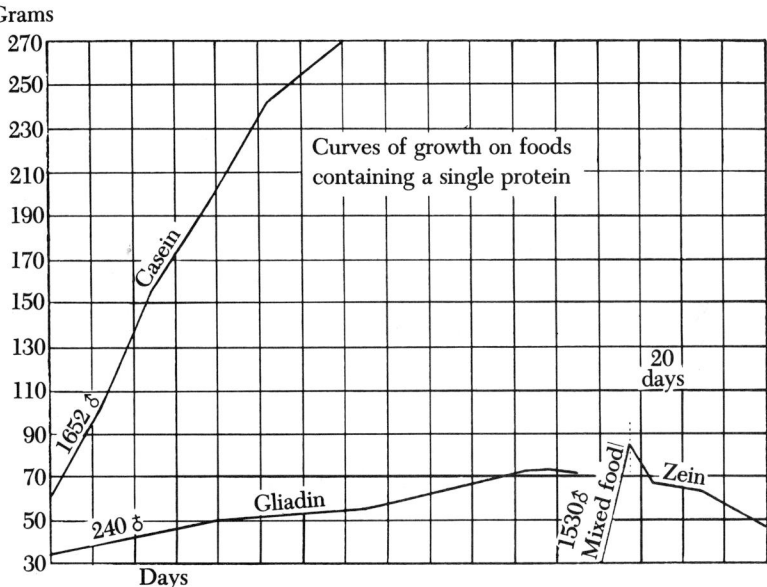

Fig. 25-1. Typical curves of growth of rats on diets containing a single protein. On the casein food (devoid of glycine), satisfactory growth is obtained; on the gliadin food (deficient in lysine), little more than maintenance of body weight is possible; on the zein food (devoid of glycine, lysine, and tryptophan), even maintenance of body weight is impossible. (From Mendel, L. B.: J.A.M.A. **64**:1539, 1915.)

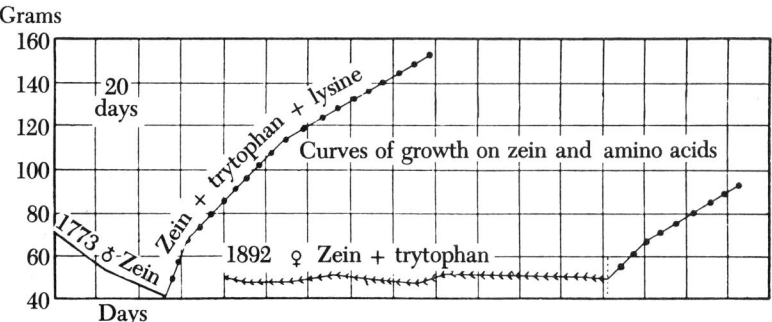

Fig. 25-2. Effect of the addition of tryptophan and lysine to zein, which is deficient in them. Addition of tryptophan permits maintenance without growth, whereas further addition of lysine enables the animals to make considerable growth. (From Mendel, L. B.: J.A.M.A. **64**:1539, 1915.)

ESSENTIAL AMINO ACIDS

Early investigators in the field of protein requirements include Osborne and Mendel, F. G. Hopkins, Sherman, and Rose. The type of earlier experiments was as follows: Young animals (usually the standard white rat) were fed highly purified foods. The diet was made up to contain all known necessary nutritional factors, the protein alone being limited in kind or in amount. At first, single purified proteins were included as the sole source of protein. Some were found to be quite satisfactory for growth; others were found capable of maintaining the animal but at a stationary weight; still others did not even permit the animal to remain at its initial weight. Figs. 25-1 and 25-2

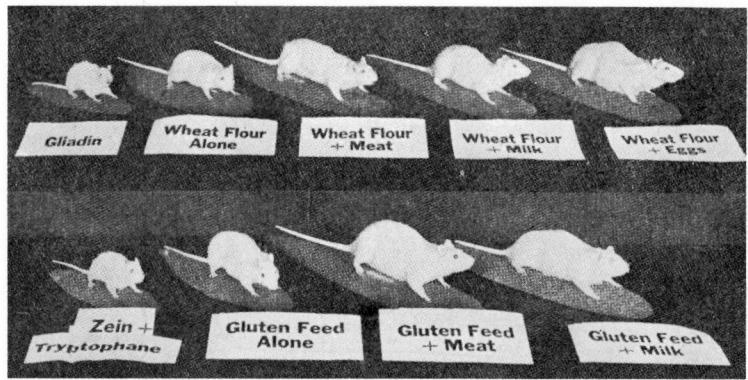

Fig. 25-3. These rats were all the same age and fed for the same length of time on diets containing the same proportion of protein. The variation in size is due to differences in chemical constitution of the proteins eaten (from experiments by Osborne and Mendel). (From Mendel, L. B.: Nutrition: the chemistry of life, New Haven, Conn., 1923, Yale University Press.)

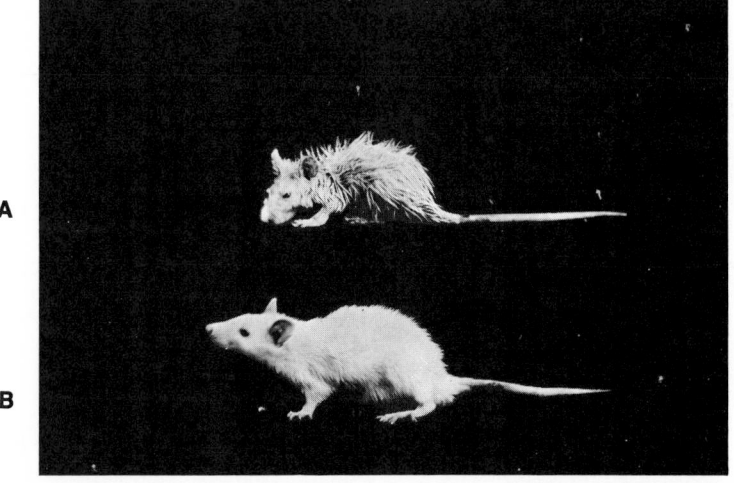

Fig. 25-4. Essential amino acid deficiency in the growing rat. **A**, Rat fed a mixture of amino acids lacking valine. **B**, Same rat after receiving valine added to the amino acid mixture. (Courtesy W. C. Rose.)

are growth curves illustrating these typical experiments with single purified proteins, and Figs. 25-3 and 25-4 are pictures of the animals. It is evident that casein is a very good protein, gliadin is not as good, and zein is very poor, when fed as the only protein. Tables 25-2 and 25-3 show that casein contains little glycine but is nevertheless suitable for growth, that gliadin is moderately low in lysine and tryptophan, and that zein is very low in glycine, lysine, and tryptophan. This would indicate that the ingestion of glycine is not essential for growth, whereas the ingestion of lysine and tryptophan is. Experiment (Fig. 25-2) bears this out. To the imperfect protein zein are added the two amino acids tryptophan and lysine. Both are needed to supplement the deficiency and permit growth of the animal. Many commonly employed foods have rather low contents of lysine, and therefore lysine or lysine-rich food protein is being added to food products for the very young and the very old, since both classes appear to be benefited by such supplements.

Other methods of experimentation have been devised. W. C. Rose intro-

Table 25-2. Approximate percentage composition of some plant proteins*

Protein	Corn gluten	Wheat gluten	Soybean proteins	Yeast proteins	Zein	Gliadin	Edestin
Nitrogen	(16.0)†	(16.0)†	(16.0)†	(16.0)†	16.1	17.7	18.7
Sulfur		1.1		0.8	0.52	1.24	0.88
Arginine	3.1	3.9	7.3	4.5	1.7	2.7	16.7
Histidine	2.1	2.2	2.9	3.0	1.3	2.3	2.9
Lysine	1.5	1.9	6.8	7.5	0	1.1	3.2
Tyrosine	6.3	3.8	4.0	3.6	5.3	3.2	4.3
Tryptophan	0.6	0.8	1.4	1.3	0.1	0.6	1.5
Phenylalanine	6.6	5.5	5.3	4.5	6.2	6.9	5.5
Cystine	1.5	1.9	1.9	1.1	0.8	2.6	1.2
Methionine	2.5	1.5	1.7	2.0	2.4	1.7	2.4
Threonine	4.0	2.5	3.9	5.5	3.5	2.1	3.9
Leucine	16.0	7.0	8.0	7.5	23.7	6.5	7.4
Isoleucine	5.1	4.2	6.0	6.0	7.3	5.4	4.6
Valine	5.7	4.1	5.3	5.8	3.5	2.7	5.7
Glutamic acid	24.5	27.0	18.4	14.7	26.9	45.7	20.7
Aspartic acid		3.7			6.6	1.3	12.0
Glycine	4.3	7.0	4.0	4.0	0.4	<0.5	5.1
Alanine		2.8	3.3		11.6	2.1	5.5
Proline		8.0	5.0		10.5	13.4	4.3
Serine		4.0	4.2		8.3	4.9	6.3
Total	84	88	89	67	120‡	105‡	113‡

* Courtesy R. J. Block.

† Calculated to a 16% nitrogen basis. The actual percentage of nitrogen is lower than 16.0. However, the percentage amino acid composition was calculated on a 16.0% nitrogen basis to make the values more comparable with those of other proteins, particularly animal proteins.

‡ The explanation for these totals of more than 100% is that in hydrolysis water is added. Therefore, if the analyses were complete, each would total over 100%. Of the substances analyzed, only zein, gliadin, and edestin are purified proteins; the others are mixtures.

Table 25-3. Approximate percentage composition of some animal proteins*

Protein	Gela-tin	Elas-tin	Horse hemo-globin	Egg albu-min	In-sulin	Pep-sin	Wool	Casein	β-Lacto-globu-lin	Beef mus-cle	Silk fi-broin
Nitrogen	18.0	17.1	16.7	15.5	15.7	15.4	16.0	15.6	15.6	16.0	18.7
Sulfur	0.5	0.17	0.58	1.83	3.33	0.94		0.8	1.68	1.1	0.0
Arginine	8.6	0.9	3.7	5.9	3.1	1.0	10.1	4.1	2.9	7.7	1.1
Histidine	0.7	<0.1	8.7	2.6	4.9	0.9	1.0	3.1	1.7	3.3	0.4
Lysine	5.0	0.5	8.5	6.5	2.5	1.6	3.1	8.2	11.3	9.0	0.7
Tyrosine	1.0	1.6	3.0	3.7	13.0	8.5	5.5	6.3	3.7	4.0	12.8
Tryptophan	0	0	1.7	1.2	0.3	2.4	1.5	1.2	1.9	1.4	0.0
Phenylalanine	2.4	5.0	7.7	7.7	8.1	6.4	4.0	5.0	4.8	5.0	3.4
Cystine	0.1	0.6	1.0	2.8	12.5	2.1	13.6	0.35	3.5	1.2	0.0
Methionine	0.9	0.3	1.0	5.3	0.3	1.7	0.7	3.4	3.2	3.2	0.0
Threonine	2.2	1.3	4.4	4.0	2.1	9.6	6.5	4.9	5.5	5.0	1.6
Serine	3.4	0.8	5.8	8.2	5.2	12.2	7.4	7.7	4.4	6.0	16.2
Leucine	3.2	8.7	15.2	9.9	13.2	10.4	8.6	9.2	15.2	8.0	0.9
Isoleucine	2.1	4.0	0.2	7.0	2.8	10.8	4.3	6.1	7.3	6.0	1.1
Valine	2.7	17.4	9.0	8.8	7.8	7.1	5.4	7.2	6.2	5.5	3.6
Glutamic acid	10.8	2.1	8.2	16.5	18.6	11.9	14.0	23.3	21.5	17.0	2.2
Aspartic acid	7.5	0.6	10.6	9.3	6.8	16.0	7.4	7.1	11.4	10.5	2.6
Glycine	29.3	29.9	5.6	3.1	4.3	6.4	6.8	2.7	1.5	5.0	43.6
Alanine	10.0	18.9	7.4	6.7	4.5		4.0	3.0	7.1	7.4	29.7
Proline	16.5	17.0	8.5	3.8	2.5	5.0	8.0	11.3	5.0	6.0	0.7
Hydroxy-proline	14.0	2.0	0	0.0	0.0			0.0	0.0	1.0	
Total	120†	112†	110†	113†	113†	114†	118†	114†	118†	112†	120†

° Courtesy R. J. Block.
† See footnote to Table 25-2 for explanation of totals over 100%(‡).

duced the method of feeding mixtures of pure amino acids, and the results obtained were valuable. From all these investigations has come the realization that certain amino acids are *essential* or indispensable; i.e., they must occur in the food if the young animal is to grow. They cannot be synthesized by the animal organism. Others are considered *semiessential*. This was explained on p. 349. At present, the amino acids are classified as essential, semiessential, and nonessential (see Table 25-4).

In addition to being required for growth, the essential amino acids are also required for the maintenance of health in adults as well as in children. Such requirements for adult maintenance are definitely lower than those for growth and vary, to some extent, with the individual amino acids. A lack of tryptophan, histidine, or phenylalanine is one cause of cataract formation in rats; other effects observed following tryptophan deficiency have been defects in teeth, alopecia, hypoproteinemia, hypochromic anemia, atrophy of the testes, and other effects on the reproductive organs.

Table 25-4. Nutritive classification of the amino acids*

Essential	Semiessential	Nonessential
Lysine	Arginine†	Glutamic acid
Tryptophan‡	Tyrosine‡	Aspartic acid
Phenylalanine	Cystine‡	Alanine
Methionine	Glycine†	Proline
Threonine	Serine†	Hydroxyproline
Leucine	Histidine	
Isoleucine		
Valine		

* Adapted from Block, R. J.: Borden Rev. Nutr. Res. 17:75, 1956.
† Arginine and glycine are essential for chicks and turkeys. Serine spares or replaces glycine.
‡ Tyrosine spares but does not completely replace phenylalanine. Cystine spares but does not completely replace methionine. Nicotinic acid spares but does not completely replace tryptophan.

Experiments have been cautiously extended to human subjects to ascertain whether the same essentiality of amino acids applies. The chief criterion has been the determination of nitrogen balance, i.e., a comparison of the amount of nitrogen excreted with that ingested (Chapter 13). Normally, the amounts are about the same. If, following the feeding of a food mixture, there is a net loss of nitrogen, the assumption is that the food is not adequate to maintain the tissues of the body. As a consequence, tissue protein is broken down and more nitrogen is lost than is taken in. Rose[8] has done much work on this problem, using pure amino acids in the ration administered to human subjects and following the nitrogen equilibrium over a considerable period of time (Fig. 25-5). From his experiments, he concludes that only eight amino acids are essential to young, healthy men: lysine, tryptophan, phenylalanine, leucine, isoleucine, threonine, methionine, valine. In these experiments neither histidine nor arginine was found to be essential; i.e., man can apparently synthesize them in sufficient amounts if they are not present already in his diet. Rose's group also determined the minimum daily requirement of the eight essential amino acids (Table 25-5). This requirement was determined on a group of healthy young men and, consequently, cannot be taken as the human standard under all conditions. For instance, infants seem to require histidine in their diets for normal growth and healthy skin,[9] whereas adults do not.

Since it is evident that no one eats purified proteins or mixtures of amino acids, we must ask ourselves how this affects us from a practical standpoint. Are the proteins of any foodstuff deficient in one or more of the essential amino acids? Whole corn is low in tryptophan and lysine, wheat gluten is low in tryptophan, lysine, and threonine, and gelatin is deficient in tryptophan, leucine, isoleucine, threonine, methionine, and valine. Except for gelatin,

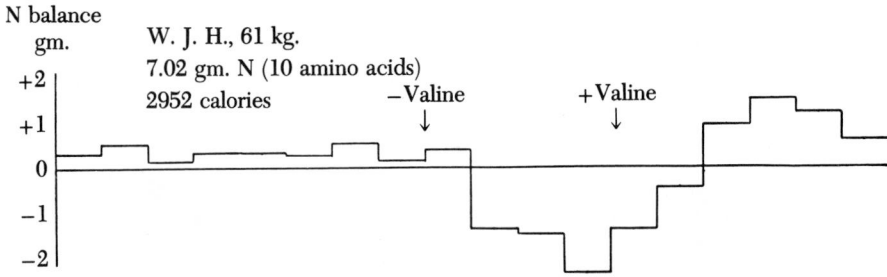

Fig. 25-5. Determination of the indispensability of an amino acid for man. The initial diet contained 6.7 gm. N in the form of a mixture of the 10 amino acids previously found to be essential for the growth of animals. The remaining N came from other components of the ration. The total N content of the diet was kept constant throughout. Valine was removed from the food at the first arrow and was returned at the second arrow. The horizontal units represent single days. (Courtesy W. C. Rose.)

Table 25-5. Minimum and recommended intakes of essential amino acids for young healthy men when diet furnishes sufficient nitrogen for synthesis of nonessentials*

Amino acid	Minimum daily requirement (grams)	Recommended daily intake (grams)	Number of subjects tested
L-Tryptophan	0.25	0.5	42
L-Phenylalanine	1.10	2.2	32
L-Lysine	0.80	1.6	37
L-Threonine	0.50	1.0	29
L-Valine	0.80	1.6	33
L-Methionine	1.10	2.2	23
L-Leucine	1.10	2.2	18
L-Isoleucine	0.70	1.4	17

* From Rose, W. C., Wixom, R. L., Lockhart, H. B., and Lambert, G. F.: J. Biol. Chem. **217**:987, 1955.

hemoglobin, and keratin, the animal proteins are, in general, well balanced in their amino acid distribution. Yeast, corn germ, wheat germ, and soybeans yield approximately the same proportions of amino acids as do the animal proteins. The analysis of many foodstuffs for amino acid content is now available.[10] A mixed diet, containing some animal protein—milk, meat, fish, eggs—ensures an adequate mixture of the essential amino acids.

The general effect of a deficiency of one or more essential amino acids, as stated earlier, is to restrict growth and protein synthesis and produce a negative nitrogen balance. However, deficiencies of specific amino acids may result in disturbances characteristic of that particular amino acid. The role of tryptophan in niacin formation is an example (p. 809). Another is the role of lysine and proline in collagen formation. The hydroxylysine and hydroxy-proline in collagen are derived from lysine and proline, respectively. These amino acids are essential in forming the characteristic tertiary structure of collagen (p. 81). The participation of ornithine and arginine in urea formation is still another important example. Thus the key roles played by the essential and, likewise, certain nonessential amino acids in metabolic processes emphasize the vital importance of adequate protein nutrition.

Dietary sources of protein. In general, the proteins of animal origin, e.g., eggs, milk, meat, fish, poultry, along with soybean protein, are best, having the highest *biologic value.* Whole eggs are ranked first. Proteins of cereals, nuts, and legumes are less adequate, although selected mixtures of grains and legumes serve very well. Cereal grain proteins alone are low in lysine, as is corn protein in tryptophan. However, when cereals are employed as mixtures with other proteins, particularly milk, meat, or eggs, an excellent source of protein results. The enrichment of wheat flour and other cereal grain products with lysine has been suggested as a means of markedly increasing the biologic value, making them, thereby, nearly equivalent to the more expensive animal protein foods. Table 25-6 gives the amino acid composition of some typical animal and vegetable proteins.

For human nutrition most of the varied dietaries of modern civilization provide adequate mixtures and amounts of the essential amino acids. Even when the cereal grains, especially wheat and rye, furnish most of the protein intake, only one amino acid, lysine, is likely to be lacking. Corn, soybean, and food yeast have been found to be a nutritionally adequate mixture, as has refined wheat flour and yeast. Such plant mixtures might conceivably be substituted for meat, in part at least, or entirely for short periods, in emergencies. Another food preparation supplying low-cost protein of good quality is composed of soybean meal fortified with vitamins and minerals. This preparation was developed by Borsook for the "meals for millions" project and was studied extensively in the United States and in India and Asia. *Incaparina,* a low-cost mixture of vegetable proteins, has been developed by Scrimshaw in his important studies in Central America. In Table 25-6 is shown the distribution of amino acids in some of the common food proteins; apparently foods vary considerably in their amino acid composition.

There are several "instant" dried skimmed milk preparations on the market that are excellent, economic sources of protein of high biologic value. These preparations may be reconstituted to supply skimmed milk or may be added to milk, soups, cereals, or other foods to increase their protein content. Dehydrated, defatted, and deodorized fish meal is also receiving considerable attention as an economic source of protein of high quality. It may be particularly important in areas where the supply of animal protein is limited, as in parts of Africa and Asia.

There is a tremendous food reserve, mainly protein and minerals, in the fish of oceans, lakes, and rivers.[11] Of the present approximate 65 million tons harvested annually, only half is consumed directly by man. The other half is converted to fish meal and used for livestock feed. A well-managed world fishery could produce four times this amount or over 200 million tons an-

Table 25-6. Approximate percentage of amino acids in some animal and vegetable proteins (calculated to 16% nitrogen)*

	Whole milk		Casein (cow's milk)	Lact-albumin (cow's milk)	β-Lacto-globulin (cow's milk)	Hen's egg (whole)	Egg white	Muscle			Gelatin	Whole grain			Potato
	Human	Cow's						Fish	Fowl	Mam-mal		Corn meal	Whole wheat	Oat-meal	
Arginine†	5.0	3.5	4.2	3.1	2.9	6.7	5.9	6.6	6.7	6.6	7.8	4.4	4.3	6.9	5.3
Histidine†	2.7	2.7	3.0	1.8	1.7	2.4	2.5	2.9	2.0	2.8	0.8	2.4	1.8	2.2	1.8
Lysine‡	7.2	8.0	8.2	9.7	11.9	6.9	6.4	10.1	7.7	8.5	4.8	2.7	2.5	4.4	5.3
Tyrosine†	5.1	4.9	6.3	3.2	4.0	4.1	4.3	2.4	2.7	3.1	0.6	4.6	3.6	3.9	2.5
Tryptophan‡	1.9	1.3	1.5	1.8	2.3	1.6	1.8	0.9	1.0	1.1	0.01	0.7	1.2	1.2	1.1
Phenylalanine‡	5.9	5.1	5.8	4.0	3.8	5.8	6.0	3.8	4.1	4.5	2.0	4.5	4.4	4.8	5.1
Cystine†	3.4	0.9	0.4	2.7	3.0	2.3	2.6	1.2	1.0	1.4	0.1	1.6	3.3	1.2	1.2
Methionine‡	2.0	2.4	3.3	1.9	3.3	3.3	4.0	2.8	2.4	2.5	0.9	1.8	1.2	1.5	2.1
Serine†		5.2	6.3	4.8	4.3	7.8	7.3	3.5		5.1	3.4	4.4	3.8	3.7	2.6
Threonine‡	4.6	4.7	4.5	5.2	5.2	5.0	4.7	4.5	4.0	4.6	1.7	4.1	3.9	3.7	3.7
Leucine‡	15.0	9.9	10.1	12.0	15.0	9.4	9.0	7.9	8.2	8.0	3.5	12.7	6.9	7.2	6.2
Isoleucine‡	5.2	6.5	6.6	6.7	7.4	6.9	6.4	5.2	4.2	4.7	1.4	4.0	4.4	4.9	5.1
Valine‡	5.5	6.7	7.4	5.3	5.8	7.4	7.8	5.5	4.1	5.5	2.7	5.3	4.5	5.3	5.9
Glutamic acid		21.7	23.6	17.7	19.8	12.6	12.8	12.0	17.0	14.6	7.8	18.4	31.4	14.3	7.4
Aspartic acid		7.5	6.5	11.1	11.7	8.2	7.6	8.6	10.5	8.0	4.9	12.3	3.8	4.1	9.8
Glycine†		2.1	2.1	2.5	1.7	3.6	3.7	5.4	5.7	5.0	15.7	3.5	3.4	3.6	1.9
Alanine		3.6	3.1	7.0	6.8			6.1		6.5	7.9	10.0	3.0	5.2	6.1
Proline		9.2	12.3	4.7	5.2	4.5	2.9	5.1		5.0	14.8	7.2	10.3	4.9	3.0
Hydroxyproline		0.0	0.0	0.0	0.0					4.7	13.3				

*From Block, R. J., and Weiss, K. W.: Amino acid handbook, Springfield, Ill., 1956, Charles C Thomas, Publisher; data on human milk from Block, R. J., and Bolling, D.: J. Amer. Dietet. Ass. 20:69, 1944.

†Semiessential amino acids; i.e., cystine can spare methionine, and tyrosine can spare phenylalamine.

‡Essential amino acids.

nually. In North America, the average amount of protein obtained from fish per capita per day is only approximately 2.5 gm., whereas, an average of 63 gm. daily come from other animal proteins and 28 gm. from vegetable proteins. A similar distribution of food proteins is seen in Europe. However, in Asia and Africa the amount of protein from animal sources other than fish is less than in North America, and that from vegetable proteins is much higher. The intake of protein from fish is about the same, although the proportion is higher since the average daily protein intake is lower.

Heat processing. Heat processing alters (generally improves) the nutritive value of proteins. Egg white is said to be more easily digested; phaseolin, a protein of the navy bean, has greater nutritive value if cooked; soybeans have a higher nutritional value after cooking, due, in part, to the inactivation and detoxication of a toxic protein, soyin.[12] As mentioned on p. 341, there is also present in soybeans a trypsin inhibitor, which is destroyed by heat. *Dry* heat, however, seems to have a deleterious effect, particularly on the proteins of cereals. Apparently lysine becomes less available, although it is not destroyed. A linkage between the ϵ-amino group and a free carboxyl group of a dicarboxylic amino acid may result in the formation of an unnatural peptide linkage that cannot be split by the digestive enzymes.[13] Other explanations have been suggested, e.g., a reaction of free amino or other groups with reducing sugars to form derivatives resistant to enzyme cleavage. This is sometimes called the "browning reaction." As a result of heating, the protein is thus so altered that the rate of release of the particular amino acids is slowed up. The delays result in less efficient amino acid mixtures. The importance of these observations lies in the widespread use of toasted and "puffed" cereals in the American dietary.

Kwashiorkor. A nutritional disease due chiefly to protein deficiency has come into prominence, although undoubtedly it has been known for centuries. Since its victims live in the Tropics, the disease has escaped detection in the presence of the great variety of tropical debilitating diseases that occur in this part of the world. Furthermore, its symptoms differ somewhat in different parts of the world. It is called kwashiorkor in Africa, and the name is now generally used for it everywhere. The disease occurs in children *after weaning* and is related to a deficiency of protein and apparently other essential nutrients. The diet of such children usually consists of high-starch foods, e.g., yams, bananas, potatoes, maize, cassava. The proteins are poor in quality, being vegetable, and low in amount. A child with this disease often has an enlarged abdomen (Fig. 25-6). A rash occurs in various sites, and the skin cracks behind the ears and at the knees and elbows. Cheilosis, stomatitis, and conjunctivitis may appear. The hair loses its black pigment and looks gray or red. Edema is rather common. The child later loses his appetite and becomes cachectic, and diarrhea occurs. A mild anemia follows, and serum proteins are lowered considerably, as is blood urea. Cholinesterase, alkaline phosphatase, and the enzymes of the digestive tract also are depressed. Many pathologic changes are seen, chiefly in the liver and pancreas. β-Aminoisobutyric acid is invariably excreted in the urine, and ethanolamine is usually excreted in this manner, as are some of the nonessential amino acids.[14]

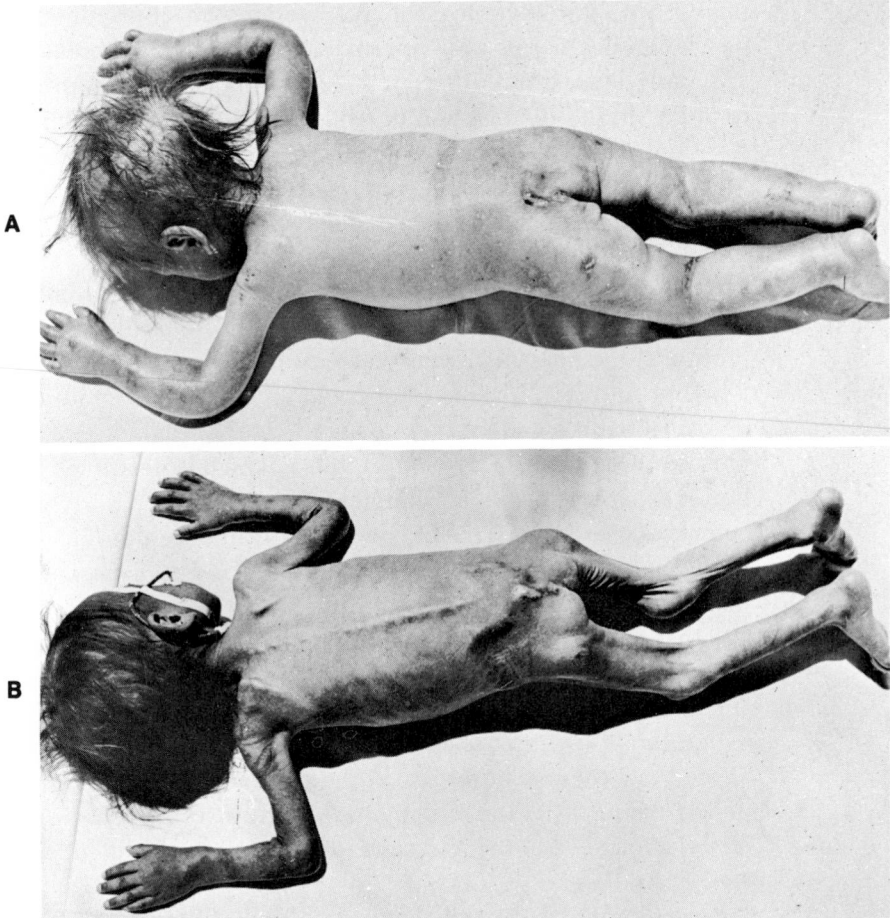

Fig. 25-6. Child suffering from kwashiorkor. **A,** Two years, 1 month, old on admission. Note the widespread distribution of skin lesions and edema. **B,** Two weeks after beginning treatment. Note the disappearance of edema and the improvement in the skin lesions. Note also the degree of muscular wasting, which had been concealed by the edema. (Courtesy Pan American Sanitary Bureau, Regional Office of WHO.)

Recent studies [15] demonstrated that morphologic changes occur in human scalp hair roots during deprivation of protein. Both the bulb and the external root sheath are affected. It is well known that the color and texture of human hair change during protein-calorie deficiency. These observations may be useful in the early diagnosis of protein-calorie malnutrition. The cells of the hair matrix normally proliferate at a rate greater than that of any other tissue, with the possible exception of bone marrow and intestinal mucosal cells. Therefore, the cells of the hair matrix have a high protein-synthesizing activity and would be expected to show effects of protein deprivation earlier than other tissues.

The changes in the hair characteristic of kwashiorkor—loss of melanin pigmentation, giving the hair a reddish appearance—are undoubtedly due to the deficiency of protein. Treatment, of course, is to administer good-quality proteins; but this is not as simple as it seems, partly because of the cost and unavailability of such foods and partly because of feeding and educational problems. Moreover such treatment is often too late to be of benefit. Prevention is much more important, and the introduction of good nutritional practice should eventually greatly lessen the occurrence of kwashiorkor.

CARBOHYDRATE FACTOR

Glucose, fructose, galactose, and, to a minor degree, mannose, as well as carbohydrates that yield these sugars on digestion, are available to the body as energy producers. The pentoses in foods seem to be of limited value nutritionally (Chapter 9). Moreover, they form a small fraction of the total carbohydrate intake. As stated before, polysaccharides or even disaccharides cannot be utilized until digested to the monosaccharide stage. When introduced directly into the bloodstream, they act as foreign bodies and are excreted, chiefly by the kidneys.

Other nonutilizable carbohydrates are the indigestible polysaccharides — cellulose, lignin, agar-agar, gums, etc. These constitute a large part of the roughage of food, the indigestible fraction that gives bulk to the feces. Food must contain such substances, for a dearth of them tends to produce constipation. The tendency in modern civilization has been toward a refinement of food, with a lessening in the amount of the indigestible parts of grains, fruits, and vegetables. On the other hand, an overabundance of roughage can lead to irritation of the intestinal mucosa. The physical presence of the indigestible material, or the distention of the colon that it causes, is not the sole factor stimulating peristalsis. Certain intestinal bacteria that are capable of decomposing hemicelluloses and mixed polysaccharides, with the production of lower volatile fatty acids, along with the hygroscopic nature of carbohydrates and of some other products resulting from the action of microorganisms, have a stimulating peristaltic effect and so induce bowel movement. Lignin and cellulose, which also escape digestion, have less effect than the hemicelluloses and mixed polysaccharides in this respect. In food tables this fraction is usually termed "fiber." Thus the total carbohydrate of a food is not available for energy by the body.

The monosaccharides utilized are converted to glucose after absorption. The glucose then is utilized either directly or indirectly after it has been converted to glycogen or to fat. It is in these two forms that excess carbohydrate is stored in a number of tissues and organs. Since a fraction of the protein molecule may be transformed into sugar, this fraction also may become part of the glycogen and fat stores of the body.

The 1968 recommended dietary allowances include no definite value for carbohydrate because of insufficient data. However, the statement is made that at least 100 gm. of carbohydrate are needed per day by the normal adult to avoid ketosis, excessive protein catabolism, and other undesirable metabolic responses. The suggestion is also made that a diet containing 100 gm. of carbohydrate, 100 gm. of protein, and 100 gm. of fat, possibly with vitamin supplementation, would be satisfactory as a reducing diet for an average normal man.[16]

FAT FACTOR

Fat furnishes a proportionally greater amount of the body energy than do the other two major foodstuffs. It is rather slowly digested, and large amounts of it in a meal tend to slow down the digestion of the other foods as well. Furthermore, fats are usually not quite as completely digested as the digestible carbohydrates and proteins. This is probably not because of any inherent indigestibility of a particular fat but because of insufficient amounts of lipase present, because the conditions for fat digestion are not entirely favorable, and because some of the fat is absorbed, undigested, in emulsified form.

There is no rule for the proportions of fat and carbohydrate in a diet. The normal person can exist equally well on a diet high or low in either fat or carbohydrate. Of course the essential fatty acids must be supplied (p. 320), but the requirement is small and these fatty acids are found in many food oils. For optimum growth of the young, Deuel[17] has recommended that about 30% of fat by weight be included in the diet. The reason for this percentage is that a diet containing a relatively large amount of fat provides for greater efficiency of utilization; i.e., there is less loss of calories than with diets that are lower in fat.

The National Research Council has set no specific amount for the recommended dietary allowance of fat in its 1968 revision, due to a lack of experimental data; nor does it recommend any specific amount of the essential unsaturated fatty acid linoleic, for the same reason. Its publication (see "General References") does, however, review the epidemiologic studies indicating a relation between the type and amount of fat with elevated serum lipids and the incidence of coronary heart disease. The possible role of this and other risk factors must be considered and judged on an individual basis.

Dietary fat has a rather high satiety value; i.e., it has the ability to satisfy hunger. However, current opinion is that 30% fat in the diet is a rather high figure, in view of statistics relating the level of fat intake to the blood cholesterol level and atherosclerosis, as discussed earlier (p. 351). Some authorities believe that 20% to 25% is a more acceptable level.

The hydrogenation of fats, which is carried on extensively to convert liquid oils to a more solid condition, results in a considerable reduction in the amount of essential unsaturated fatty acids.

It is common knowledge that carbohydrate can be converted to fat; and some of the protein may also be; but can fat be converted to carbohydrate? There is general agreement that the glycerol fraction of fat is convertible, since it is a simple three-carbon chain. For purposes of dietetic computation, this fraction is usually taken as 10% of the average fat molecule. Since fatty acids are catabolized to the two-carbon stage and then can enter the citric acid cycle and other metabolic systems, evidently the possible conversion of fatty acid to sugar is no longer a subject of controversy, as discussed in Chapter 12.

MINERAL FACTOR

The functions of the individual inorganic ions or elements were discussed in Chapter 15. In this discussion, the chief mineral elements that are of importance in foods will be pointed out. These are calcium, magnesium, sodium, potassium, phosphorus, chlorine, sulfur, iron, and iodine.

Calcium. Foods that are relatively high in calcium salts are milk and milk products, beans, leafy vegetables, shellfish, and fish of the sardine type (i.e., in which the bones are eaten). Vegetables, in general, contain more calcium than do animal foods. Some vegetables, however, have an appreciable amount of oxalic acid present (p. 736), and this forms insoluble calcium oxalate in the intestinal tract and thus lessens the absorption and utilization of some of the calcium present. Moreover, although calcium is widely distributed, it is not present in most foods in sufficiently high concentrations to prevent a deficiency of this element in our diet. A temporary deficiency or even a long-continued deficiency of calcium in the food may occur without the appearance of any symptoms attributable to a low calcium intake because the bones act as a storehouse. Under the influence of parathormone, calcium is withdrawn from the bone to maintain the calcium levels of the blood and soft tissues.

The minimal adult requirement has been found to be about 0.5 gm. of calcium per day; but, since calcium is poorly absorbed, a higher level is usually advised. The recommended amount for adults has been set at 0.8 gm., and for children, 0.7 to 1.4 gm. per day (Table 25-1). In pregnancy and lactation, an additional 0.4 to 0.5 gm. per day is recommended to provide the necessary calcium salts for the fetus and the nursing child.

The recommended dietary allowance values for calcium were determined from the sum of urinary calcium excretion (about 175 mg. per day), endogenous fecal excretion (about 125 mg. daily), and losses in sweat (about 20 mg. per day), or a total loss of 320 mg. daily. Allowing 40% absorption of calcium from the intestinal tract, the RDA is thus 800 mg. and represents the average daily amount recommended to maintain calcium balance in the adult. Since a quart of cow's milk contains about 1.2 gm. of calcium, we can see that a pint of milk a day almost provides the total calcium requirement of an adult and a quart of milk does the same for a child. The importance of milk in the diet, from this standpoint, cannot be stressed too strongly.

Phosphorus. Phorphorus is found in those foods containing phosphoproteins, nucleoproteins, phospholipids, and glycerophosphates, as well as the inorganic phosphates, chiefly calcium and sodium. Since quantitatively the greatest proportion of the phosphorus is used to form the bone salt, which is largely calcium phosphate, evidently the phosphorus intake should bear an optimal relation to the calcium intake. That is why the expression Ca:P ratio is used so often in this connection. In growing children the Ca:P ratio should be between 1 and 2; i.e., the calcium intake should be as great as the phosphorus intake, or even somewhat greater. In the adult, the need for bone formation is less and the Ca:P ratio may be lower. If the calcium intake is satisfactory, the phosphorus intake will usually also be. The foods richest in calcium are also richest in phosphorus, namely, milk, cheese, and beans. Eggs, cereals, fish, and meats are also high in this element.

Phosphorus is present in foods also as phytates. In fact, a large proportion of the phosphorus of vegetables is in this form. Although the exact structure of these salts is not known, phytates are quite insoluble mixed calcium and magnesium salts of phytic acid, which in turn is a hexaphosphate of inositol. Available evidence indicates that phytic acid and its compounds interfere with the absorption of calcium and iron from the intestinal tract. Unrefined cereals are rich in phytates, but white flour contains little. Hence the phytate problem is not serious in the United States; but in areas of the world where unrefined cereals form a large part of the diet and little calcium is consumed, the interference with calcium absorption may result in serious deficiencies of calcium, including the development of so-called "cereal rickets." The phosphate and inositol of these substances are, for the most part, unavailable nutritionally. However, slight digestion may be accomplished by gastric juice and somewhat more by intestinal phosphatases.

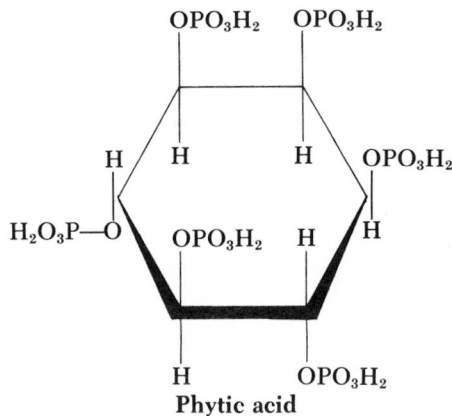

Phytic acid

As stated earlier (p. 418), the recommended dietary allowance for phosphorus is set at a 1:1 ratio with calcium, or 0.8 gm. per day for men and women. Amounts for infants and children, and during pregnancy and lactation, are given in Table 25-1.

Magnesium, sodium, and potassium. The common mixed diet contains sufficient sodium and potassium and usually, but not always, sufficient magnesium (p. 418). These elements are widely distributed in foods, and, unless too much highly refined food, e.g., white flour, is consumed, there is scarcely any likelihood of a deficiency. The same applies to chloride. Since we add sodium chloride to our foods, we ordinarily have enough of both elements. When there is excessive perspiration, as in summer, or in the case of men working at high temperatures, as at blast furnaces, there may be a need for additional sodium chloride intake. This is generally recognized by physicians and industrial experts. Magnesium is needed for bone salts, and the proper balance of sodium, magnesium, calcium, and potassium is of importance in regulating the irritability of many, if not all, cells. Chloride is required to produce gastric hydrochloric acid, and it also plays a role in the transport of gases in the blood.

Recommended dietary allowance values for magnesium were given for the first time in the 1968 revision of the National Research Council's estimates (Table 25-1). The allowance for men is 350 mg. daily, and for women 300 mg.

The requirement for sodium, potassium, and chloride is so variable, depending on activity, environmental temperature, and other factors, as well as age and weight, that it is difficult to set precisely. The requirement for sodium chloride is ordinarily easily met by the foods of a mixed diet and seasonings.

Sulfur. We obtain most of our sulfur from sulfur-containing amino acids, methionine, cysteine, and cystine. There is a small amount of organic sulfide in foods but very little sulfate. The organic sulfur is oxidized, in large part, to sulfate and as such plays a significant role in acid-base balance. One of the sulfur-containing amino acids, methionine, is considered essential. Other sulfur-containing compounds of physiologic importance are glutathione, insulin, biotin, and thiamine. The supply of sulfur in our food is chiefly dependent on the amount and quality of the protein. Therefore, an optimum protein diet will lead inevitably to an adequate sulfur intake.

Iron. Iron is, of course, a constituent of hemoglobin. It is therefore necessary in sufficient quantity whenever new hemoglobin must be produced. Children or patients who have lost blood are in greater need of iron than are normal adults, for whom the recommended dietary allowance is 10 mg. for men and 18 mg. for women.

The new recommended dietary allowance for iron for women is higher than previous values. This is because of recent studies that indicate iron stores are reduced or absent in 67% of menstruating women and in the majority of pregnant women. Since the increased recommended amounts cannot easily be met by customary diets, increased iron fortification of foods (breads, cereals) may be desirable. In fact, the Food and Nutrition Board of the National Research Council has currently recommended (April, 1970) an increase in the federal standards for iron enrichment of cereal products. The proposed increase would allow no less than 40 and no more than 60 mg. of iron per pound of flour and no less than 25 or more than 40 mg. per pound of bread. The same changes are recommended for the enrichment of corn meal, corn grits, rice, farina, and macaroni and noodle products. This increased enrichment of cereal products would enable women to get the newly recommended 18 mg. of iron daily from usual dietary sources. It would thus correct the one known remaining inadequacy in the American dietary. The additional iron would pose no problem for men.

Many foods with considerable quantities of iron are available, but there is some doubt as to what type of iron can be utilized by the body. Some authorities maintain that iron in the heme form is of no value, that it cannot be absorbed and utilized, and that only iron in the ionizable form is of physiologic value. If these theories are true, the total iron content of any food does not necessarily represent the amount available. All nutrition authorities are not in agreement on this point. Studies have shown that the iron in beef can be made available by merely heating the beef; thus, quite possibly further investigation will show that much of the iron of the heme and related forms can be rendered physiologically available in this same way.

Several factors influence the absorption of ionizable iron. Ferrous iron is generally absorbed to a greater extent than ferric iron, probably because of the greater solubility of many ferrous compounds. Therefore, the presence of ascorbic acid, sulfhydryl compounds, and other reducing agents tends to modify the absorbability of the iron present. An acid medium is also favorable for reduction. Hence a normal gastric acidity tends to aid iron absorption. Any element that forms insoluble precipitates with the ferric or ferrous ions tends to prevent the absorption of these ions. Thus, phosphate or phytate in abundance inhibits iron absorption. Conversely, a paucity of these groups or a sufficient amount of calcium ions to combine with them would increase the possibility of iron absorption. A biochemical mechanism that regulates the uptake of iron to correspond with body needs is described on p. 420. It is thus evident that iron absorption is limited. Indeed, the ingestion of foods, e.g., eggs, meat, spinach, into which radioactive iron had been incorporated, led to the conclusion[18] that, on an average, only 10% of the daily intake of iron is absorbed.

Iodide. Iodide is needed in very small amounts by man, but there is no general agreement as to the exact requirement. The estimates vary from 14 to 300 μg. per day, but even the highest figure is still a very minute amount.

The new recommended dietary allowances for iodide daily in men and women are 140 and 100 μg., respectively (Table 25-1). So as to ensure an adequate iodide intake, particularly in areas of the United States where endemic goiter exists or has existed, the continued use of iodized salt is urged. The Food and Nutrition Board has now recommended federal legislation requiring iodization of salt. The minute amounts of iodide recommended may be lacking in diets of regions remote from the ocean. Seafoods in general have a satisfactory content of iodine, and vegetables and fruits grown on the seaboard or wherever the soil contains iodide likewise are sufficiently rich in this element. In sections where a low iodide content of the diet occurs, sodium or potassium iodide is generally added to the public drinking water or to table salt (1:5000 to 1:200,000). In therapeutic diets, particularly sodium-restricted, care should be taken to assure an adequate supply of iodide.

Trace elements. As discussed earlier (p. 424), other elements are also present in minute amounts in foods: fluorine, bromine, copper, zinc, manganese, silicon, aluminum, cobalt, nickel. Copper, cobalt, zinc, manganese, and perhaps, fluorine, chromium, molybdenum, and selenium in traces are essential to man, but the others are accidental constituents and are of no particular benefit or harm. No recommended dietary allowance values have been established for the essential trace elements as yet, but estimates of requirements for some have been made (see Table 15-5).

ACID-FORMING AND BASE-FORMING PROPERTIES OF FOODS

When a food is incinerated in a crucible, the ash remaining has an acid, alkaline, or neutral reaction, depending on the proportion and type of anions and cations present and the effect of heat on them. When the same food is consumed by a person, its final products sometimes have the same reaction as the ash, but there are other factors that modify the "ash" left by vital processes. Proteins, phospholipids, and nucleoproteins yield sulfuric, phosphoric, and uric acids, respectively. These acids are neutralized by basic elements

Table 25-7. Potential acidity or alkalinity of foods

Foods having a predominantly acidic effect		Foods having a neutral or nearly neutral effect	Foods having a predominantly basic effect	
Bacon	Ham	Butter	Apples	Grapes
Baking powder	Lamb	Buttermilk	Apricots	Lemons
biscuit	Liver	Corn oil	Asparagus	Lettuce
Barley	Lobster	Cottonseed oil	Bananas	Limes
Beef	Macaroni or	Cream	Beans, lima	Oranges
Bread, rye	spaghetti	Custard	Beans, string	Peaches
Bread, white	Oysters	Fudge, chocolate	Broccoli	Pears
Cake, plain	Pastry	Honey	Brussels sprouts	Pineapple
Cake, cheese	Plums°	Ice cream	Cabbage	Potatoes, white
Chicken	Pork	Milk, whole	Cantaloupe	Potatoes, sweet
Corn	Prunes°	Olive oil	Carrots	Raisins
Crab	Sausage	Onions	Cauliflower	Raspberries
Crackers	Scallops	Pie, apple	Celery	Tomatoes
Cranberries°	Shredded wheat	Sugar	Dates	Walnuts
Duck	Shrimp	Syrups	Eggplant	
Eggs	Turkey	Tapioca	Figs	
Fish	Veal		Grapefruit	

°The ash of these foods is alkaline, but, because of the presence of benzoates, which form hippuric acid, they increase the acidity of the urine.

before excretion and thus tend to diminish the alkaline factors of blood and urine. Fruits and vegetables usually have enough positive radicals, e.g., calcium, magnesium, sodium, potassium, to balance the acid produced by proteins or with other acids. Organic acids, citric, malic, tartaric, and lactic, present in fruits and vegetables, are oxidized to carbon dioxide. Most of this gas is lost by way of the lungs, whereas the potassium salts of the above acids, also occurring in fruits, are oxidized to potassium bicarbonate, which, if present in excess, is excreted in the urine. Thus, vegetables, even acid fruits, usually have an *alkaline effect*. There are some exceptions: benzoic acid, present in cranberries, is not oxidized by the body and is excreted as hippuric acid (after combining with glycine) and thus has an acidic effect on the urine; oxalic acid, found in rhubarb, beet leaves, cocoa, and tea, is oxidized poorly and is neutralized and excreted as oxalate (Table 25-7).

VITAMIN FACTOR

Although vitamins have been discussed in some detail in Chapters 23 and 24, a few points may be added or repeated here from the standpoint of foods. It is true that under normal conditions the average varied diet contains sufficient vitamins of all kinds for normal, growing children and adults. (Babies, however, require additional vitamins C and D to supplement their milk diet.) It would seem, therefore, that little need for vitamin supplementation for individuals in good health exists. The "normal conditions" mentioned, however, mean access to a sufficient amount of fresh foods, properly cooked, and in a suitable variety. Absolutely fresh vegetables are difficult to obtain in the cities, and storage causes a progressive loss of ascorbic acid. Very often in the preparation of meals in restaurants, hotels, and hospitals, vegetables are kept on the steam table for hours. Under these conditions some of the vitamins A, B, and C may be oxidized and lost. If the vegetables are drained of the water in which they are cooked, all the water-soluble vitamins suffer some loss by being thus discarded. Even the shredding or cutting of raw vegetables served as salad results in the liberation of ascorbic acid oxidase and the oxidation of a considerable amount of ascorbic acid. Meals, therefore, have a higher content of vitamins if they are carefully prepared and served promptly.

The milling of wheat results in the production of a refined white flour, which has greater keeping qualities than whole wheat flour. The loss of the germ and bran, however, reduces the vitamin E, thiamine, niacin, riboflavin, pyridoxine, and iron content of the flour greatly, as well as the calcium, phosphorus, fat, and protein, to some extent. This is partly remedied by the enrichment of white flour, which was accomplished during World War II by federal order and is now carried out by millers under state laws and also voluntarily. Table 25-8 shows that enriched bread compares favorably with whole wheat bread in selected vitamin and mineral constituents but is still slightly deficient in protein. Since this program went into effect, vitamin B complex deficiencies have decreased considerably among patients in nutrition clinics.

Following the introduction of enriched flour, many other foods have had vitamins or minerals, or both, added to them. Among these are corn meal and grits, macaroni and spaghetti, rice, and processed cereals. Hydrogenated fats are devoid of vitamin. For this reason oleomargarine is commonly fortified with at least 9000 U.S.P. units of vitamin A per pound. Most of the milk on the market has added vitamin D. Some preparations of nonfat dried milk are now fortified with vitamins A and D.

Table 25-8. Comparison of enriched, plain white, and whole wheat breads*

	Plain white bread	Enriched white bread	Whole wheat bread
Thiamine (milligrams per pound)	0.3	1.1– 1.8	1.3
Riboflavin (milligrams per pound)	0.5	0.7– 1.6	0.7
Niacin (milligrams per pound)	3.0	10 –15	16.0
Iron (milligrams per pound)	3.9	8 –12.5	11.8
Calcium (milligrams per pound)	254	254†	272
Protein (grams per pound)	39	39	43

*From United States Department of Agriculture, Bull. AIS-39, 1954.
†Enriched bread may contain 300 to 800 mg. of calcium per pound as well as 150 to 750 U.S.P. units of vitamin D.

Some therapeutic or unbalanced diets for allergies or other pathologic conditions may also lead to vitamin deficiencies. Likewise, this may occur when an individual, because of extreme fondness or violent dislike for particular foods, constantly restricts himself to a few items of diet. If these conditions cannot easily be remedied by vitamin-rich foods, vitamin supplementation is indicated.

Condiments. Among condiments we may class table salt, vinegar, spices, catsup and other sauces, and flavoring extracts. These are the substances that add savor and zest to a meal, and thus they are valuable in enabling the individual to make good use of foods that otherwise might be less acceptable and in stimulating the flow of digestive fluids.

Some condiments have other qualities. Sodium chloride is a necessity but is present in the foods of the average diet in sufficient quantities for most individuals under ordinary circumstances. Excess of monosodium glutamate, which is present also in relatively large amounts in soy sauce, may precipitate severe gastrointestinal distress, the so-called "Chinese restaurant syndrome." Catsup and similar sauces often contain appreciable amounts of vitamins and minerals and small amounts of protein, carbohydrate, and fat. Vinegar is dilute acetic acid with minute amounts of flavoring substances. The spices contain volatile oils that give specific aromas and flavors. There are the stimulating spices, such as the peppers, mustard, and horseradish; the aromatic spices, of which allspice, anise, cinnamon, clove, ginger, and nutmeg are examples; and the sweet herbs, which include dill, marjoram, sage, and thyme. An excess of any of the spices may cause irritation of the gastrointestinal mucosa. Flavoring extracts are usually alcoholic solutions of the flavor-containing parts of plants; in these, too, volatile oils are often the active ingredients. Several synthetic products that imitate the natural ones very closely have been prepared, but usually the natural flavor has impurities that give it a fuller flavor or "bouquet." Vanilla is the most commonly used extract, but lemon, almond, wintergreen, and others are also frequently used. Although some of the special constituents have pharmacologic properties, the amounts involved in cooking, baking, etc. are usually so small as to render any such effects inconsequential.

Beverages. Coffee and tea have little value except as a source of fluid and the sugar, milk, or cream added. Both contain the purine alkaloid caffeine, which is responsible for the stimulating properties (and coffee contains from 1 to 3 mg. of niacin per cup, a not inconsiderable amount). Both coffee beans and tea leaves contain tannins, and the amount present in the beverage depends largely on the method of preparation. The distinctive flavors arise from aromatic volatile derivatives, which also have slight pharmacologic action. Cocoa and chocolate have higher food value, even without the usual additions, than do coffee and tea. Cocoa has had the saturated coconut oil removed. Both cocoa and chocolate contain theobromine, a purine alkaloid similar to caffeine but with less effect on the nervous system. The cola beverages also contain caffeine.

Extensive damage to teeth may result from the frequent use of lemon juice or beverages containing free acid. Certain cola beverages contain an appreciable amount of phosphoric acid. These acids have been found to cause a marked deleterious effect on tooth structure, particularly if the drink is ingested daily and at times other than with meals or without additional water.

The question of whether alcohol is a food is difficult to answer. It is almost completely utilized by the body when ingested in moderate amounts and yields about 7 kcal. per gram. This energy is available for heat and work and for sparing other foodstuffs. Therefore, the calories derived from alcoholic beverages can be significant and should be taken into account in calculating the caloric content of a diet. On the other side of the question is the fact that excessive amounts of alcohol have toxic properties not found in ordinary foods and may cause serious pathologic conditions. Furthermore, alcohol is habit forming.

PRESERVATION OF FOODS

That the preservation of foods is of tremendous importance needs no explanation. This has been true for centuries. The ancients stored grain in seasons of plenty to provide for times of want. Savages preserved game and fish by drying, salting, and smoking, and some of their primitive methods are still successfully used. To these were later added pickling and the making of jellies and preserves. Within the last century, refrigeration has progressed to such an extent that, with the increased cold-storage facilities for eggs, meats, and other perishable foods, it has become one of the major methods of food preservation. Canning also has become an industry of vast dimensions, and more recently the freezing and dehydration of foods, particularly vegetables, have added new conveniences and economies to food preservation and transportation. Newer forms of dried foods include skimmed milk, eggs, coffee, tea, potatoes, fruit juices, soups, coffee cream, and others. The list grows daily. These "convenience" items have proved extremely popular and useful. Preservation of foods by the addition of certain additives, e.g., antioxidants, bacteriostatic agents, is also practiced extensively.

The use of radiation for food preservation is being extensively studied. The food is exposed to radiation in a "cave" suitably constructed to prevent any hazard to personnel. The purpose is to extend the storage life of perishable foods at refrigerator temperatures without significantly altering the flavor, texture, or nutritional value. The forms of radiation employed are electron beams and γ-rays. γ-Ray sources are principally of two kinds: (1) fission products from uranium or plutonium reactors and (2) artificially made radioactive materials, e.g., ^{60}Co. The food may be either "radiopasteurized" or "radiosterilized," depending on the dosage (r.e.p.) of radiation employed. If foods contain enzymes, radiation at the sterilizing level or below does not inactivate the enzymes, which may then affect the flavor and texture of the food. Therefore some other process for inactivating the enzymes seems to be needed and this may be heat inactivation. Even so, radiation has some slight unfavorable effect on palatability. However, radiation sterilization is generally recognized as not significantly changing the nutritional values of foods.[19] Sterilization, however, may produce some unpalatability, changes in texture, and loss of nutritional value. To date, apparently only two food items have been approved for radiation sterilization for commercial use by the Food and Drug Administration (FDA), pending the completion of further animal and human feeding tests. The two foods approved are packaged bacon, to prevent molding, and potatoes, to inhibit sprouting.[20] The Canadian and other governments are conducting similar studies.

The magnitude and vital importance of the field of food preservation today, accelerated by new and improved technologies, have necessarily led to federal control by the FDA. This agency is both a scientific institution for the study of newer methods of food processing and preservation and a federal law enforcement agency. It sets standards and criteria for acceptable food additives and allowable amounts and for safe procedures and methods of food preservation. The FDA thus serves as the public's protector against contamination, fraud, impurity, and hazards in the food and food products upon which our very lives depend.

DIET THERAPY

For specific directions, diet lists, recipes, etc. in handling diets in disease, reference must be made to works on nutrition, diet therapy, and medicine. Several excellent general references are given at the end of this chapter. In this discussion, only the biochemical aspects will be considered and, in general, only the relations of foods—not other types of treatment.

Obesity. Obesity, an accumulation of excess body fat, results from an oversupply of calories, relative to the total caloric expenditure of the individual. The factors regulating this energy balance are varied and complex. The possible influence of endocrine dysfunction was discussed in Chapters 11 and 17.

Reference was made therein (p. 530) to the importance of the hypothalamus in the control of food intake. Recent studies have reaffirmed this concept.[21] There appears to be a *satiety center* in the medial hypothalamic region, which acts as an inhibitor of a *feeding center* in the lateral hypothalamus; an anatomic connection between these two areas has been demonstrated recently by the use of a special stain for axons.[21]

From a dietary standpoint, a reduction in body fat may be achieved by providing fewer calories than are needed by the individual. A corrective diet that allows for a loss of 1 or possibly 2 lb. per week and that supplies a generous amount of protein and all the essential minerals and vitamins should be prescribed. A daily multivitamin preparation, using the recommended dietary allowances as a guide, would provide a margin of safety. The normal diet should be modified based on the basic four groups. Diets containing 1200 kcal. daily for women and 1500 to 1800 kcal. daily for men are acceptable levels.

Rapid weight reduction is unphysiologic because it involves the rapid consumption of the body fat stores and is therefore equivalent to a predominantly fat diet, which often produces ketosis. Consequently, when the weight is reduced at a rapid rate, there frequently results acidosis, with its accompanying unpleasant symptoms. Since body fat is about one fifth water, a pound is equivalent to 454 gm. $\times \frac{4}{5} \times 9$ kcal./gram, or about 3200 kcal. In other words the maintenance diet for the present weight may be reduced by about

3200 kcal. per week, or from 450 to 500 kcal. per day. This should be taken out of the fat allowance primarily and carbohydrates secondarily. If reduction does not immediately occur, the diet need not necessarily be changed, because water is often held temporarily in the tissues in place of fat and is lost later; i.e., the actual fat has been utilized but this has not become apparent at once.

Sebrell[16] suggested that a diet containing 100 gm. of carbohydrate, 100 gm. of protein, and 100 gm. of fat, possibly with vitamin supplementation, would be satisfactory as a reducing diet for an average, normal man. The frequency of feedings or meals appears to exert a significant effect on the utilization of food. Carefully controlled studies on rats, for example, showed that "nibblers," when compared with animals fed only one or two large feedings daily, formed more protein, less fat, had lower blood lipid levels, and were less susceptible to experimental diabetes. Preliminary studies indicate that the same may be true in human beings. The serving of smaller meals more frequently, but *without* an increase in the daily total, may be beneficial in the prevention and therapy of obesity, hyperlipemia, and diabetes.

Increased physical activity can contribute to weight reduction. It is advised, in moderation, in order also to improve physical well-being and muscular tone.

Underweight. Underweight is frequently more difficult to combat than obesity. If no definite pathology is apparent to account for the condition, dietary measures should be advised. A good multivitamin supplement is indicated to take care of any unsuspected deficiency and to stimulate appetite. High-fat and high-carbohydrate foods of rather concentrated types are recommended if the patient can digest them. An adequate protein intake of varied nature should be provided, but an excess is to be avoided, because protein has a higher specific dynamic action than carbohydrates and fats; i.e., proteins stimulate the metabolic processes of the body in a unique manner (p. 531).

Gastrointestinal disorders. Hyperchlorhydria is a symptom that is frequently encountered. Since hydrochloric acid is secreted at a constant concentration, high acidity simply means an increased volume of gastric juice, too large to be buffered in the normal manner. One method of combating it is to eliminate highly spiced foods from the dietary since these may stimulate the flow of gastric juice. Another way is to feed a high-protein diet, since the proteins combine with hydrochloric acid to form a relatively weak acid, thus exerting a buffering effect.

In gastritis, dietary treatment is usually a bland, smooth, soft diet, whose composition depends on whether hypoacidity or hyperacidity is present. In peptic ulcer, hyperacidity, as well as high pepsin values, is usually present. This condition is quite common and can be very serious. Many special diets have been devised and recommended. In general, diets for peptic ulcer consist of frequent feedings of small quantities of liquid foods that constantly neutralize the secreted acid and prevent its accumulation as free acid; but the amount and kind of food must be regulated to satisfy all the nutritional requirements.

Flatulence or gas formation in the gastrointestinal tract occurs in both health and disease. It is most distressing after an abdominal operation, but in such a case it does not appear to have much relation to foods but to a lack of intestinal tonus or inhibition of peristalsis. In general, a lack of hydrochloric acid in the stomach may permit more microorganisms than usual to pass into the duodenum, and gas formation ensues as a result of their growth. Some foods are more productive of gas than others. Well-known examples are members of the cabbage family and also turnips, onions, peas, and beans. Melons, cucumbers, and radishes are other offenders in this respect. Various syrups also are gas producers, perhaps serving as media for yeasts in the lower part of the tract.

Diseases of the liver and gallbladder. In liver diseases a high-carbohydrate, moderately high-protein, and moderately low-fat diet is indicated. Liver cells are much more readily restored to normal function if their glycogen content is built up. A protein intake of from 70 to 100 gm. daily is recommended for several reasons: (1) it promotes repair of damaged cells; (2) it appears to have a protective function; (3) it tends to overcome hypoproteinemia, which may occur in hepatic conditions. The load of protein should not be too great because the liver is the site of protein degradation and formation of urea, and the excessive amount of protein might produce too much of a strain on its powers. The low fat is recommended because fat requires bile secretion for its digestion and absorption, and this hepatic function must be spared as much as possible. Since bile secretion is depressed, the fat-soluble vitamins will not be absorbed in sufficient amounts. For this reason, vitamin supplements are advised—in some instances even administered parenterally. Indeed, if the patient is unable to eat, intravenous feeding of amino acids, together with glucose, vitamins, and salts, may be instituted.

Table 25-9. Cholesterol content of foods*

Food	Cholesterol (milligrams per 100 gm. edible portion)	Food	Cholesterol (milligrams per 100 gm. edible portion)
Bacon	70	Liver	300
Beef	70	Lobster	200
Brain	2,000	Margarine (vegetable)	0
Butter	250	Milk, cow's, whole	11
Cheese (cheddar)	100	Milk, cow's, skimmed	3
Chicken	60	Oysters	200
Egg, whole	550	Pork	70
Egg, yolk	1,500	Sweetbreads	250
Fats (lard)	95	Veal	90
Fish	70	Vegetable oils	0
Kidney	375		

*United States Department of Agriculture, Handbook no. 8, 1963.

When either cholecystitis or cholelithiasis is present, contraction of the gallbladder may result in severe pain. Because dietary fat stimulates the gallbladder to contract, it should be kept at a minimum. During acute phases, only 20 to 30 gm. of fat daily would be indicated. In chronic cholelithiasis, foods rich in cholesterol may be restricted (Table 25-9) since gallstones usually contain significant amounts of cholesterol.

Celiac syndrome. The celiac syndrome is manifested in *classic celiac disease* and in cystic fibrosis of the pancreas. It has as its principal symptom fatty stools (steatorrhea). It occurs chiefly in children. The abdomen is greatly distended, largely because of accumulation of intestinal gas. At the same time, there is complete metabolic upset; fat stores are used up and growth is stunted. Similar conditions are nontropical sprue of adults and tropical sprue. Fatty stools are common to all these conditions, with a consequent loss also of calcium and vitamin D and other fat-soluble vitamins via the feces. Besides an inability to digest and absorb fats, there is frequently also an interference with starch digestion. So-called primary celiac syndrome or *gluten-sensitive enteropathy* (celiac disease of children, adult celiac disease) appears to result from damage to the intestinal mucosa by the toxic action of undigested N-glutamyl peptides derived from the protein gliadin, of certain cereal grains. The complete elimination of wheat, oats, barley, and rye from the diet has been used with dramatic results.

Pathologic kidney conditions. The diet in acute glomerulonephritis is planned to relieve the kidney without regard to the total nutritional needs of the patient because of the short period of time involved. A low-protein diet with little of anything else is given so that a urine low in total solids is excreted by the abnormal kidney. The total fluid intake should be adequate to dissolve the urinary constituents easily but not too great to put a heavy load on the kidney—perhaps from 1000 to 1200 ml. daily. As soon as the condition is corrected, the protein intake is restored to normal. In chronic glomerulonephritis there is a failure to secrete the nonprotein waste constituents, which results in accumulation of these constituents in the blood. There is also a loss of serum protein in the urine. In the past, both these phenomena influenced the physician to restrict protein in the diet—in the first instance, because more protein led to a greater production of urea, uric acid, etc. for the kidney to eliminate; in the second instance, because the feeding of protein was believed to lead to a greater excretion of it by the kidney. At present, the aim is to make good the loss of protein from the blood by feeding some extra protein. Furthermore, a low serum protein usually occurs or threatens to occur, and a high-protein diet tends to counteract this. Consequently, the general trend is to feed the normal requirement of protein plus an amount equal to that lost by way of the urine. Some clinicians have favored restricting the salt intake drastically, but today this is not generally accepted. A moderate restriction, e.g., to 2 gm. per day, is often advised. It also seems wise to have the diet tend more to the basic ash type. The total water intake should be nearer 1 than 2 liters. In nephrosis or degenerative Bright's disease, the same principle regarding protein is applied.

The condition called *lipoid nephrosis* may be a metabolic disturbance rather than a kidney disease. Edema, oliguria (small volume of urine), marked proteinuria, and low serum proteins occur. There is no retention of nitrogenous products in the blood. Very high-protein diets, containing from 120 to 240 gm. of protein per day, with low carbohydrate and very low fat, have been widely used. In conditions in which the proteinuria is not pronounced (nephrosclerosis), a balanced diet with moderately high protein is recommended.

The current trend in the dietary management of uremia is toward a semisynthetic diet, based on the Giovannetti diet. This is a relatively high caloric (2000 kcal.), low-protein diet (20 gm.) with essential amino acid supplementation. The latter tends to ensure maximal protein utilization and hence minimal urea formation.

Urinary calculi. Calculi that form in the kidney or urinary bladder are usually composed mainly of urates, oxalates, or phosphates. Their formation was considered when urinary constituents were discussed (p. 744). The treatment of a patient with urinary calculi is ordinarily surgical. Following surgery an attempt should be made to discover the underlying cause in order to prevent recurrence, which is frequent. Infection, hyperparathyroidism, or hypervitaminosis all suggest appropriate preventive measures. The composition of the calculus should be determined, and a diet that will tend to prevent the formation of more stones of the same sort should be planned. From the dietary standpoint, it should be pointed out that urates arise from nucleoprotein metabolism. Therefore, persons who have had urate stones should be on a low-nucleoprotein diet since urinary calculi are likely to recur. Glandular meats are richest in nucleoproteins, but nonglandular meats are relatively high, as are also the germ of grains and the actively growing parts of plants, e.g., asparagus tips, soybean sprouts, etc. Anchovies, sardines, and caviar also contain considerable quantities of nucleoproteins. The reason for greater oxalate excretion in the urine by some individuals than by others is not well understood. Undoubtedly some oxalate originates in metabolism. However, until our knowledge of the underlying reactions is better known, the only logical dietary suggestion is to avoid foods having a high preformed oxalate content. These include spinach, chard, beets, beet leaves, rhubarb, tomatoes, figs, okra, gooseberries, sweet potatoes, cocoa, chocolate, and tea. Phosphates precipitate in an alkaline urine. Therefore, the indicated diet for phosphaturia would be an acid-ash diet low in phosphorus. Phosphoproteins, nucleoproteins, and phospholipids all contain phosphorus. Hence milk, glandular foods, and eggs should be avoided, as should meat and cereals, both of which are acid forming, in increased amounts. However, in many cases acidosis tends to develop, and then a high acid-ash diet must not be used.

Gout. There is not entire agreement regarding the underlying cause of gout. A hyperuricemia accompanies the condition, and this is undoubtedly the source of the uric acid concretions or "tophi." Gout may be due to (1) the failure to excrete urates, (2) an increased transformation of exogenous or endogenous purines to urates, or (3) the excessive synthesis of inosine monophosphate over its utilization in adenine and guanine production (p. 410). Hereditary gout appears to be due to the last. An increased failure to excrete urates exists in elderly patients whose kidneys have been damaged. In patients with normal kidneys, there is, in fact, an increased excretion of uric acid. Onset of attacks has been correlated with an increase in weight, due to a diminution in insensible perspiration, which leads to a diuresis immediately before or during the actual attack. Although a severe limitation of purine foods has not been of much help in controlling the disease, the introduction of unnecessary amounts of purines into the system appears unreasonable. Hence it is best to omit from the diet foods rich in purines, e.g., sweetbreads, anchovies, sardines, liver, kidneys, brains, meat extracts. High fluid intake is important to aid in urate elimination. Body weight should be kept within normal limits. Several new drugs that are effective in reducing uric acid formation have been developed.

Cardiovascular disease. Dietary measures may be of considerable value in disorders of the heart and blood vessels as discussed earlier (p. 331). Obesity is a major obstacle in treating heart diseases. The disadvantages of obesity may be fourfold. (1) Even when the heart is unimpaired, a large body mass puts an abnormally great strain on the heart. (2) In obesity there frequently occur fat deposits on and between the cardiac muscle bundles, decreasing the heart muscle efficiency. (3) Abdominal fat may impede the movement of the diaphragm, and this in turn affects the heart movements. (4) Arteriosclerosis, which often accompanies obesity, may invade coronary vessels and in that way directly affect the blood supply of the heart. Accordingly, cardiac patients are usually advised to reduce their weight to normal or slightly below. As in all reducing regimens, this must not occur too quickly. A plentiful supply of vitamins, particularly the B complex and C, should be assured and the protein should be adequate. In arteriosclerosis and in hypertension, much the same dietary advice is given, stressing moderation and, perhaps, mild undernutrition.

The relation of cholesterol to atherosclerosis, a form of arteriosclerosis, was discussed on p. 331. Low-cholesterol (Table 25-9), low–saturated fat diets are advised in this condition.

The substitution of fats containing unsaturated fatty acids for saturated fatty acids is recommended in the diet for atherosclerosis. Although not a cure, such a modification of diet seems to lower the blood cholesterol. Therefore it is wise to limit severely the intake of animal fats and hydrogenated oils, using vegetable oils as much as possible. Weight reduction and a lowering of the total fat intake, with a shift to the unsaturated type, usually reduces the hypercholesterolemia. In familial hypercholesterolemia, however, low cholesterol diets are useful. The cholesterol concentrations of a number of common goods are given in Table 25-9. These are mainly of animal origin; plants contain little or no cholesterol.

Hypertension. Despite the general opinion to the contrary, protein foods do not cause an elevation of blood pressure. Consequently, they do not need to be reduced in the diet in hypertension unless there is serious kidney impairment at the same time. The preference for white meats over red meats also seems to be without foundation. The question of salt restriction in hypertension is controversial, but there seems to be increasing evidence that a considerable reduction in sodium intake is beneficial. The so-called "rice diet" therapy has been proposed and exerts a favorable influence in a fair percentage of cases of hypertension. The diet consists of rice, fruit, and sugar, with little else, except vitamin supplements, and essentially is a low-protein, low-salt regimen. It would appear dangerous to restrict proteins drastically for too long a time. A more palatable and acceptable diet may be made by a judicious selection of foods low in sodium and by removal of salts by water extraction. Water-soluble vitamins must, of course, be added. The results have been favorable.

Diabetes mellitus. For our present purposes, we may say that diabetes mellitus is a condition in which carbohydrate, arising from whatever source, is not utilized by the body to a greater or lesser degree. As a result, the glucose of the blood rises and may "spill over" into the urine. Treatment varies and is discussed in some detail beginning on p. 228. The amount of carbohydrate that 1 *unit* of insulin can aid the body to metabolize varies with the individual but is about 1 to 3 gm. Many patients can be controlled by dietary means alone, in which case the diet used need be little different from that of nondiabetics. However, when the diet must be strictly regulated, the patient must be taught the use of food tables, how to weigh his diet, and the calculations involved.

Addison's disease. Optimal therapeutic results in the treatment of Addison's disease require not only the administration of large amounts of sodium salts and the adrenocortical hormones but also the restriction of potassium intake. Since potassium is widely distributed and is especially high in protein foods, which the patient needs in large amounts, the problem is a difficult one. The extraction of potassium from food is likely to result in a tasteless meal, which the patient will not eat. Vegetables should be specially cooked in water with salt dissolved. The salt diffuses into the vegetables and the potassium salts dissolve out into the cook water because the latter has a low potassium concentration. This fluid is then discarded. Since the water-soluble vitamins are lost along with the potassium salts, provision must be made, of course, for the addition of appropriate vitamin supplements. A similar procedure is used for meats. By these methods the potassium content is reduced to one third or one fourth its original concentration. Foods to be avoided are soups and broths containing meat stock or meat extracts, gravies, catsup, chili sauce, mustard, dried fruits and vegetables, nuts, peanut butter, molasses, caviar, chocolate, cocoa, Postum, and spinach.

Epilepsy. With the availability of safe, effective anticonvulsant therapy today, the use of dietary measures, primarily a *ketogenic* diet, for the control of epilepsy is seldom required. To be effective, the ketogenic:antiketogenic ratio of this diet must be at least 2:1, which means that the diet must be high in fat (about 60%), high in protein (about 30%), and low in carbohydrate (about 10%). Such a diet is rather unpalatable, expensive, and difficult to maintain. It is sometimes used for children but seldom otherwise.

Phenylketonuria. Since the metabolic error in phenylketonuria is the inability of the organism to handle phenylalanine adequately, a diet low in this amino acid is required. Such a set of restrictions is doubly difficult because

(1) phenylalanine is an essential amino acid and (2) all dietary proteins are about equally rich in it. Woolf and his group[22] used as the basic food, a "milk" containing an acid hydrolysate of casein that had been passed through a column of charcoal. This removed phenylalanine, tyrosine, and tryptophan. The two latter amino acids were added to the hydrolysate together with protein-free starch, glucose, fats, and minerals. A commercial preparation, Lofenalac, in which most of the phenylalanine has been removed is available. Multivitamin and mineral supplements are given separately along with milk and a few other foods in moderation. Some phenylalanine is usually metabolized, and the tyrosine substitutes for it. With the use of this regimen at a sufficiently early age, the mentality of these retarded children improves, as does their general physical condition. The color of the hair also darkens. Later, in many infants, synthesis of the missing enzyme increases and the children are able to live a reasonably normal life.

Fevers. In fevers, metabolism is increased. DuBois calculated the total caloric requirements in fever by adding 13% of the normal basal metabolic rate for the individual for every degree of fever. To this was added an additional 10% if there was much extra protein catabolism, as there usually is in most fevers, and from 10% to 30% for the restlessness of the patient. It is thus seen that the caloric needs of a febrile patient may be very high indeed. The diet therefore should be high in carbohydrates to provide for much of this metabolic need, to spare proteins as far as possible, and to aid in combating acidosis. Proteins should be sufficiently high to maintain the patient in nitrogen equilibrium. Fats should be normal in quantity and of a type easily digested. In fevers an alkaline-ash diet is preferred, as a further safeguard against acidosis, and additions of sodium chloride to the diet, to make good the losses of salt in perspiration.

Food allergy. Many individuals are peculiarly sensitive to certain foods, just as others are to pollen or other particles in the air they breathe. The symptoms range from sneezing to vomiting, from headaches to hives, from edema to diarrhea, and many more, some minor and some quite serious. These effects are believed to be due to the release of histamine by an immunologic reaction. The same symptom, or group of symptoms, usually occurs in a given individual; but the symptoms may be caused by more than one food. Proteins have been considered the causative agents, and undoubtedly they are in most cases, but there are some assertions in the literature that fats and even carbohydrates have been found responsible. The discovery of the *allergen* in a particular case is often not an easy matter. One method consists of injecting the isolated concentrated proteins from different foods into the superficial layers of the skin or applying the proteins to a scratch made in the skin. A number of these scratches may be done by the physician at one session. A positive reaction is indicated by a wheal or hive around the applied protein. Sometimes the results are inconclusive or negative. In that event, the patient is put on successive standard elimination diets. These are standardized diets, each one eliminating certain foods or food groups. If the patient is without symptoms on one of these, he is not sensitive to the constituents of that diet. Then foods that are absent from the basic diet are added one at a time until a reaction, peculiar to the patient, is produced by one or more of them. The most usual allergens are milk, eggs, wheat, and potatoes. In conducting such an investigation, it may be necessary to add vitamin or other supplementation since the elimination diets may very well be low in one or more essential nutrients. The best treatment, after the offending food or foods is determined, is to plan an adequate diet that does not contain the allergens.

Pre- and postoperative diets. A good nutritive condition is a great asset before surgery. If an operation can be anticipated, the surgeon should exercise every care to build up his patient. If, just prior to an operation, the diet is restricted in bulk, such a restriction serves the same purpose as the old-fashioned purge, which both weakened the patient and drained off some of his much-needed body water. Fluids and carbohydrates (e.g., sugar candy) are given in fairly large amount on the preceding day and no food after the evening meal if the operation is in the morning, because an empty stomach at the time of operation is essential. Postoperative diets depend on the type of operation, condition of the patient, etc. In general, a high caloric (2800 kcal. minimum to 6000 kcal.) intake, therapeutic level vitamin supplementation, and some increase in protein intake is currently recommended. The high caloric intake is to permit maximal use of protein for tissue repair rather than for conversion to energy.

Parenteral feeding. The intravenous administration of amino acids is in extensive use today. Carbohydrates, vitamins, and salts can also be administered intravenously. During the past few years highly effective mixtures of glucose, amino acids, electrolytes, and vitamins have been developed and found to be extremely effective for parenteral feeding. These mixtures are especially useful in maintaining nutrition in patients having various types of gastrointestinal disorders, especially those requiring corrective surgery. Fat suspensions for intravenous feeding have been banned in the United States because of various toxic symptoms following their administration, e.g., dizziness, dyspnea, low back pain, chills with or without fever, blood-clotting abnormalities, hemorrhage, anemia.

It is interesting to note that infants under 2 months of age having various types of malfunction of the gastrointestinal tract that require long-term total parenteral nutrition have been maintained satisfactorily for periods up to 60 days.[23] Satisfactory weight gain and normal growth were obtained despite repeated surgical procedures, sepsis, and enteric losses during the period. The solution used for intravenous feeding was a mixture containing 20% glucose and 3.3% amino acids (as a fibrin hydrolysate) with appropriate amounts of electrolytes and vitamins added. The solution was delivered continuously with an infusion pump through an indwelling catheter placed in the superior vena cava. The solution was fat-free, and the caloric value of infusate was 0.9 kcal. per milliliter.

A large series of adult patients with chronic gastrointestinal disease also have been successfully nourished exclusively by intravenous feeding for as long as 210 days, receiving from 2400 to 4500 kcal. per day.[24] Positive nitrogen balance was maintained in all cases, with satisfactory wound healing, weight gain, and increased strength and activity occurring. Thus, as a result of the remarkable advances in the field of nutrition, tissue maintenance and synthesis in man can be achieved today by the prolonged, exclusive intravenous administration of essential nutrients. This is indeed a paramount example of the practical value of nutrition to medicine and mankind.

References

GENERAL

Albanese, A. A., editor: Newer methods of nutritional biochemistry, New York, 1963–1968, Academic Press, Inc.

Beaton, G. W., and McHenry, E. W.: Nutrition, New York, 1964–1966, Academic Press, Inc.

Bertolini, A. M.: Gerontologic metabolism, Springfield, Ill., Charles C Thomas, Publisher.

Block, R. J., and Bolling, D.: The amino acid composition of proteins and foods, Springfield, Ill., 1944, Charles C Thomas, Publisher.

Burton, B. T., editor: The Heinz handbook of nutrition, ed. 2, New York, 1965, McGraw-Hill Book Co.

Chichester, C. O., Mrak, E. M., and Stewart, G. F., editors: Advances in food research, New York, 1968, Academic Press, Inc.

Comar, C. L., and Bronner, F.: Mineral metabolism, New York, 1960–1964, Academic Press, Inc.

Eichenwald, H. F., and Fry, P. C.: Nutrition and learning, Science 163:644, 1969.

Food, United States Department of Agriculture Yearbook 1959, Washington, D. C., U.S. Government Printing Office.

Food and Nutrition Board, National Research Council: Recommended dietary allowances, Seventh revised edition, Publication no. 1694, Washington, D. C., 1968, U.S. Government Printing Office.

Goodhart, R. S., and Wohl, M. G.: Manual of clinical nutrition, Philadelphia, 1964, Lea & Febiger.

Leathem, J. H., editor: Protein nutrition and free amino acid patterns, New Brunswick, N.J., 1965, Rutgers University Press.

McHenry, E. W.: Basic nutrition, Philadelphia, 1957, J. B. Lippincott Co.

McLester, J. S., and Darby, W. J.: Nutrition and diet in health and disease, ed. 6, Philadelphia, 1952, W. B. Saunders Co.

Meister, A.: Biochemistry of amino acids, New York, 1965, Academic Press, Inc.

Meyer, L. H.: Food chemistry, New York, 1960, Reinhold Publishing Corp.

Mitchell, H. H.: Comparative nutrition of man and domestic animals, New York, 1962–1964, Academic Press, Inc.

Morgane, P. J., editor: Neural regulation of food and water intake, Ann. N.Y. Acad. Sci. 157:531, 1969.

Munro, H. N., and Allison, J. B., editors: Mammalian protein metabolism, New York, 1964, Academic Press, Inc.

Pike, R. L., and Brown, M. L.: Nutrition: an integrated approach, New York, 1967, John Wiley & Sons, Inc.

Present knowledge in nutrition, ed. 3, New York, 1966, Nutrition Foundation, Inc.

Review: Nutritional status – USA, Nutr. Rev. 27:196, 1969.

Turner, D.: Diet therapy, ed. 4, Chicago, 1965, University of Chicago Press.

Williams, S. R.: Nutrition and diet therapy, St. Louis, 1969, The C. V. Mosby Co.

Wilson, N. L., editor: Obesity, Philadelphia, 1969, W. A. Davis Co.

Wohl, M. G., and Goodhart, R. S., editors: Modern nutrition in health and disease, ed. 4, Philadelphia, 1968, Lea & Febiger.

SPECIAL

1. Scrimshaw, N. S., and Gordon, J. E., editors: Malnutrition, learning, and behavior, Cambridge, Mass., 1968, Massachusetts Institute of Technology Press.
2. Sprague, G. F.: Science 157:774, 1967.
3. Swaminathan, M.: Borden Rev. Nutr. Res. 28:1, 1967.
4. Krehl, W. A.: Nutr. Today 2:16, 1967.
5. Handler, P., et al.: J. Nutr. 34:677, 1947.
6. Sherman, H. C., et al.: J. Biol. Chem. 41:97, 1920.
7. Yoshimura, H.: Fed. Proc. 20:103, 1961.
8. Rose, W. C.: Fed. Proc. 8:546, 1949.
9. Snyderman, S. E., et al.: Pediatrics 31: 786, 1963.
10. Block, R. J., and Weiss, K. W.: Amino acid handbook, Springfield, Ill., 1956, Charles C Thomas, Publisher; Orr, M. L., and Watt, B. K.: Home Economics Report no. 4, United States Department of Agriculture, 1966.
11. Holt, S. J.: Sci. Amer. 221:178, 1969.
12. Liener, I. E., and Pallasch, M. J.: J. Biol. Chem. 197:29, 1952; Liener, I. E.: J. Nutr. 49:527, 1953.
13. Mitchell, H. H., and Block, R. J.: J. Biol. Chem. 163:599, 1946.
14. Edozien, J. C., et al.: Lancet 1:615, 1960.
15. Bradfield, R. B., et al.: Science 157:438, 1967.

16. Sebrell, W. H., Jr.: Nutr. Rev. **26**:355, 1968.
17. Deuel, H. J., Jr.: Fed. Proc. **14**:639, 1955.
18. Moore, C. V.: Amer. J. Clin. Nutr. **3**:3, 1955.
19. Read, M. S.: Fed. Proc. **19**:1055, 1961.
20. Comments: Science **161**:146, 1968.
21. Arees, E. A., and Mayer, J.: Science **157**: 1519, 1967.
22. Woolf, L. I., et al.: Arch. Dis. Child. **33**: 31, 1958.
23. Filler, R. M., et al.: New Eng. J. Med. **281**:589, 1969.
24. Dudrick, S. J., et al.: Surgery **64**:13, 1968.

APPENDIXES

PHYSICOCHEMICAL PHENOMENA OF IMPORTANCE IN BIOCHEMISTRY

LAW OF MASS ACTION

The law of mass action applies to the state of equilibrium existing in reversible reactions. This law states that the rate at which a reaction takes place, at constant temperature, is proportional to the product of the concentrations of the reacting substances. The concentrations are expressed as moles per liter, and such concentrations are represented by bracketing the symbols of the substances in question.

The reaction between ethyl alcohol and acetic acid to form ethyl acetate and water is a reversible reaction.

$$C_2H_5OH + CH_3COOH \underset{\text{Reaction II}}{\overset{\text{Reaction I}}{\rightleftharpoons}} CH_3COOC_2H_5 + H_2O$$

According to the law of mass action, the velocity of the reaction proceeding toward the right (Reaction I) depends on the product of the concentrations of alcohol and acetic acid:

$$V_1 \propto [C_2H_5OH] \times [CH_3COOH]$$

where V_1 represents the velocity of Reaction I. Therefore:

$$V_1 = k_1 \times [C_2H_5OH] \times [CH_3COOH]$$

where k_1 is a constant.

In a similar manner Reaction II proceeds at a velocity V_2, which is proportional to the concentrations of ethyl acetate and water:

$$V_2 \propto [CH_3COOC_2H_5] \times [H_2O]$$

and also

$$V_2 = k_2 \times [CH_3COOC_2H_5] \times [H_2O]$$

where k_2 is another constant. Now, at equilibrium, Reaction I must necessarily proceed at the same rate as Reaction II; otherwise it would not be in equilibrium, and

$$V_1 = V_2$$

879

or

$$k_1 \times [C_2H_5OH] \times [CH_3COOH] = k_2 \times [CH_3COOC_2H_5] \times [H_2O]$$

and, by algebraic division, we arrive at

$$\frac{[CH_3COOC_2H_5] \times [H_2O]}{[C_2H_5OH] \times [CH_3COOH]} = \frac{k_1}{k_2} = K_{equil.}$$

The new constant, K, is the equilibrium constant of the reaction. This constant is always the same for a given reaction after equilibrium has been established, no matter what the proportion of the reactants may have been at the start. There is, of course, a different constant for every reaction, and the constant varies with temperature and pressure. Here we are interested mainly in the electrolytic dissociation constants.

If K is always the same for this reaction at equilibrium, then if the equilibrium is upset by adding or removing any of the four reacting substances, the system tends to balance these substances until a new equilibrium is reached and K is reconstituted. For example, if more ethyl alcohol is added, more of it combines with acetic acid to form more ethyl acetate and water.

To make the equation more general, we may say for the reversible reaction:

$$aA + bB \rightleftarrows cC + dD$$

Using the same symbols as above:

$$V_1 = k_1[A]^a \times [B]^b$$
$$V_2 = k_2[C]^c \times [D]^d$$

At equilibrium:

$$k_1[A]^a \times [B]^b = k_2[C]^c \times [D]^d$$
$$\frac{[C]^c[D]^d}{[A]^a[B]^b} = \frac{k_1}{k_2} = K_{equil.}$$

HYDROGEN ION AND HYDROXYL ION CONCENTRATION

Pure water is only slightly dissociated. There is, however, a certain definite concentration of hydrogen ions, which, though small, must be balanced by the same concentration of hydroxyl ions. This state of affairs is reflected in the low but measurable conductivity of water. The dissociation of water may be represented by the following equation:

$$[HOH] \rightleftarrows [H^+] + [OH^-]$$

and, therefore,

$$\frac{[H^+] \times [OH^-]}{[HOH]} = K_1$$

In this equation the denominator, undissociated water, is extremely large when compared with the numerator and may be considered a constant. An analogy may be drawn between this and a ship that has sprung a leak when in mid-ocean. The amount of water pouring into the ship's hull is of great moment, even though it is an infinitesimal part of the ocean, which, for all intents and purposes, remains constant. Here the numerator is the volume of water passing into the ship and the denominator is the constant ocean. Therefore:

$$\frac{[H^+] \times [OH^-]}{K_2} = K_1$$

$$[H^+] \times [OH^-] = K_1 K_2 = K_w$$

K_w, the ionization product for water, is an extremely small value. It has been determined to be 0.00000000000001, or 1/100,000,000,000,000, or 10^{-14} at 25° C.

$$[H^+] \times [OH^-] = K_w = 1 \times 10^{-14}$$

In pure water the concentration of hydrogen ions must equal that of hydroxyl ions; therefore, since $[H^+] = [OH^-]$, it can be substituted for $[OH^-]$.

$$[H^+] \times [H^+], \text{ or } [H^+]^2 = 1 \times 10^{-14}$$

and taking the square root of both sides of the equation,

$$[H^+] = 1 \times 10^{-7}$$

In other words, the hydrogen ion concentration of water is 1×10^{-7} gm. per liter, or 1/10,000,000 gm. per liter. Either of these methods of expression is unwieldy, and, consequently, Sörensen suggested that the negative exponent with its sign changed to positive be used and be termed "pH." Another way of stating this is:

$$pH = -\log_{10}[H^+]$$

The pH of water, or neutrality, then, is 7.0. If acid is added to water, the concentration of hydrogen ions, of course, increases, and instead of 1/10,000,000 gram of H^+ per liter, there would be a greater value with a *smaller* denominator. The pH of acidic solutions, accordingly, is less than 7.0, and that of alkaline solutions is greater than 7.0. However, since the product of $[H^+]$ and $[OH^-]$ must remain constant, i.e., 10^{-14}, when $[H^+]$ is greater than 10^{-7} mole per liter, $[OH^-]$ is less than 10^{-7}.

In this connection it is well to define the corresponding term, pOH. The negative logarithm of $[OH^-]$ is pOH; and, furthermore, we can speak of the negative logarithm of K_w as pK_w. Using HCl and NaOH solutions as examples, and assuming complete ionization, the relationship of acidity and alkalinity to pH and pOH is shown in Table A-1. (In practice, pOH is seldom referred to.) Notice that the sum of pH and pOH is always 14. This is equivalent to stating:

$$[H^+][OH^-] = 10^{-14}$$

Examples of the conversion of hydrogen ion concentration to pH and vice versa are the following:

1. Given the hydrogen ion concentration $[H^+] = 0.00634$ N, find the pH as follows:

Table A-1. Relation of acidity and alkalinity to pH and pOH

Normality°	pH		pOH
0.1 N HCl	1		13
0.01 N HCl	2		12
0.001 N HCl	3	Acidity	11
0.0001 N HCl	4		10
0.00001 N HCl	5		9
0.000001 N HCl	6		8
0.0000001 N (= water)	7	Neutrality	7
0.000001 NaOH	8		6
0.00001 N NaOH	9		5
0.0001 N NaOH	10	Alkalinity	4
0.001 N NaOH	11		3
0.01 N NaOH	12		2
0.1 N NaOH	13		1

° A normal solution is one that contains 1 gm. equiv. of the substance per liter. For further discussion, see under "Titratable Acidity."

It is first convenient to express the concentration of hydrogen (or hydronium) ions as a whole number multiplied by 10 raised to the power indicated. Thus:

$$[H^+] = 0.00634 \text{ N} = 6.34 \times 10^{-3}$$

Since $pH = -\log_{10}[H^+]$, and $[H^+]$ is the molar concentration, the logarithm must first be obtained.

$$\log [H^+] = \log (6.34 \times 10^{-3}) = \log 6.34 + \log 10^{-3}$$
$$= 0.8021 + (-3) = -2.1979$$

To get the $-\log$, multiply both sides of the equation by -1.0.

$$-\log [H^+] = pH = 2.20 \text{ (pH is never expressed beyond the second decimal)}$$

2. Given the pH 2.20, determine the $[H^+]$ as follows:

$$pH = \log \frac{1}{[H^+]} = \log 1 - \log [H^+]$$
$$\log 1 = 0$$
$$pH = 0 - \log [H^+] = -\log [H^+]$$
$$[H^+] = 10^{-pH}$$
$$[H^+] = 10^{-2.20}$$
$$[H^+] = 10^{-3.0} \times 10^{+0.8}$$
$$\times = 10^{0.8}$$
$$\log \times = 0.8$$
$$\times = 6.31$$
$$[H^+] = 6.31 \times 10^{-3.0} \text{ or } 0.00631 \text{ N}$$

Hydrogen ion concentrations are determined either by electrometric methods or by the use of standard buffers and indicators. A description of the electrometric methods is beyond the scope of this volume. However, it should be pointed out that the instruments have been skillfully developed and simplified to such a degree that pH determinations of accuracy (to ±0.001 pH unit) may be made in a few minutes. For an understanding of pH and its regulation in body fluids and tissues, a brief discussion of buffers is now pertinent.

BUFFERS

A buffer solution is one that tends to maintain a constant hydrogen ion concentration when acid or alkali is added to it. A buffer system usually consists of a weakly dissociated acid and the salt of that acid, or a weak base and its salt; e.g., carbonic acid and sodium bicarbonate constitute a buffer system. If acid is added to $NaHCO_3$, the following reaction occurs:

$$NaHCO_3 + HCl \rightarrow NaCl + H_2CO_3$$

A strong acid, HCl, which might be expected to raise the hydrogen ion concentration, reacts with a weak base in such a way as to yield a weak acid, H_2CO_3, and a neutral salt. The hydrogen ion concentration has not been raised appreciably. Also, if NaOH is added to NaH_2PO_4,

$$NaOH + NaH_2PO_4 \rightleftarrows Na_2HPO_4 + H_2O$$

the weakly acid sodium dihydrogen phosphate buffers the strong alkali by yielding the weakly alkaline disodium hydrogen phosphate. Again the hydrogen ion concentration has not been changed very much. In the first instance the buffer system or buffer pair H_2CO_3 and $NaHCO_3$ results and the H_2CO_3 is effective in buffering alkalies. In the second instance, NaH_2PO_4 and Na_2HPO_4 become the buffer pair, also effective in buffering in either direction. Both these systems, and several others as well, operate in the body to prevent marked changes of hydrogen ion concentration, and they are remarkably efficient.

In such systems it is evident that a common ion effect is operative; i.e., if we add to a weak electrolyte a strong electrolyte having an ion in common with the weak electrolyte, the ionization of the weak electrolyte is diminished and the concentration of the ion not in common is also lessened. For example, if sodium acetate is added to acetic acid (*HAc*), the ionization of the acid is repressed, resulting in a decreased $[H^+]$.

$$\underline{\begin{matrix} HAc & \rightleftarrows & H^+ + Ac^- \\ \hline HAc & \rightleftarrows & H^+ + Ac^- \end{matrix}}$$
$$\text{(add)} \quad NaAc \quad \rightleftarrows \quad Na^+ + Ac^-{\uparrow}$$

The addition of the acetate ion (from the sodium acetate), which is in common with the acetate ion from the acetic acid, tends to drive the equilibrium to the left. As a result, the concentration of hydrogen ion is decreased by recombination with the acetate ion to form undissociated acetic acid.

The foregoing considerations may now be made quantitative by reviewing some concepts of acid-base chemistry. According to the Brønsted theory, an acid may be defined as any molecule or ion that dissociates to yield hydrogen ion or ions. If the acid *completely* dissociates when in dilute aqueous solution, then it is a *strong acid;* but if it only partly dissociates to give hydrogen ions, it is a *weak acid.*

Thus HCl is a strong acid since it dissociates completely to give hydrogen and chloride ions in dilute solutions.

$$HCl \rightarrow H^+ + Cl^-$$

Note that in this case the reaction is indicated by an arrow in only one direction. But acetic acid dissociates only slightly:

$$HAc \rightleftharpoons H^+ + Ac^-$$

Accordingly, arrows are shown in both directions.

The Brønsted theory continues in defining a base as any molecule or ion that reacts with hydrogen ion.

In dilute solution chloride ion cannot be considered a base, since it does not react with hydrogen ion. (If HCl completely dissociates, then Cl^- apparently has no tendency to remain combined with H^+ ion.) In concentrated solutions chloride ion associates slightly with hydrogen ion and is therefore a weak base, a fact reflected in incomplete dissociation of HCl in very concentrated solutions.

Acetate ion, however, is a strong base since it has a ready affinity for hydrogen ion. Chloride ion and acetate ion are called the conjugate bases of their respective acids, HCl and HAc. It is now apparent that the conjugate base of a strong acid is a weak base whereas that of a weak acid is a strong base.

Returning now to the above reactions, we can see that for:

$$HCl \rightarrow H^+ + Cl^-$$

an equilibrium cannot be reached and an equation of the kind found at the beginning of this chapter cannot be written. On the other hand, a true equilibrium equation can be written for acetic acid:

$$HAc \rightleftharpoons H^+ + Ac^-$$

$$\frac{[H^+][Ac^-]}{HAc} = K$$

It is evident that any increase in acetate ion concentration after equilibrium has been reached tends to increase K. But, since K must remain constant, an adjustment that somewhat decreases $[Ac^-]$ and increases HAc just enough to keep the ratio constant must be made. This happens if $[Ac^-]$ associates with $[H^+]$ to form more undissociated acetic acid. A consequence of this is a diminished concentration of $[H^+]$ or a rise in pH. The ions in any solution always act in such a way as to maintain K absolutely constant according to the laws of equilibria.

The hydrogen ion concentration of most body fluids and secretions is on the

Table A-2. pH values of human body fluids and secretions

Body fluid or secretion	pH values	Body fluid or secretion	pH values
Blood	7.4	Pancreatic juice	8.0
Milk	6.6–6.9	Intestinal juice	7.7
Bile	7.8	Cerebrospinal fluid	7.4
Urine	6.0	Saliva	7.2
Gastric juice		Aqueous humor of eye	7.2
(parietal secretion)	0.87		

alkaline side. Urine may be acid and gastric juice is very acid, but these are exceptions. Many influences tend to change this alkalinity, but the buffers present prevent marked fluctuations in hydrogen ion concentration. The pH of blood, for example, stays within the limits 7.3 to 7.5 in health. When these limits are exceeded, we have a condition of acidosis or alkalosis with alarming symptoms and, frequently, dire results. In Table A-2 are given some of the pH values for various human fluids.

It is quite difficult to keep a solution at constant pH if no buffer is present because of the influence of the CO_2 of the air or the alkali of the glass container or because of other influences. Consequently, buffers are frequently required. Various mixtures, consisting of definite amounts of the acid, or base, and its respective salt have been prepared. Since such buffer sets maintain their pH indefinitely, they are used in the indicator method of determining pH.

Henderson-Hasselbalch equation. Values of the pH of buffer solutions may be calculated if the composition of the mixture, as well as the ionization constant of the weak electrolyte, is known. For example, in the case of acetic acid:

$$HAc \rightleftharpoons H^+ + Ac^-$$

$$\frac{[H^+] \times [Ac^-]}{[HAc]} = K_{Ac}$$

$$[H^+] = K_{Ac} \frac{[HAc]}{[Ac^-]}$$

In a mixture of the acid and its salt, for instance, NaAc, most of the acid is un-ionized. Consequently the $[HAc]$ is about the same as the total acid concentration and $[H^+]$ would be extremely small. Also, since the salt is completely ionized, the value $[Ac^-]$ is approximately equal to the total salt concentration. Thus, for approximate calculation, the equation may be written as follows:

$$[H^+] = K_{Ac} \frac{Acid}{Salt} \quad or \quad K \frac{Acid}{Salt}$$

to make the equation applicable to other salts and acids. Taking the negative logarithm of this:

$$-\log [H^+] = -\log \left(K \times \frac{[Acid]}{[Salt]} \right)$$

$$= -\log K + \left(-\log \frac{[Acid]}{[Salt]} \right)$$

Since $-\log [H^+]$ is called pH, we may call $-\log K$ by the term pK. Therefore:

$$pH = pK + \log \frac{[Salt]}{[Acid]}$$

In other words, the pH of a buffer solution is determined by the logarithm of the ratio of salt to acid and by the pK (i.e., the negative logarithm of the ionization constant of the acid). This last equation is known as the Henderson-Hasselbalch equation.

It finds many uses in chemical calculation. Examples follow:

1. To calculate the pH of a buffer solution that contains 0.1 mole of sodium acetate and 0.1 mole of acetic acid at 25° C., $K_a = 1.8 \times 10^{-5}$:

$$pH = pK_a + \log \frac{[Salt]}{[Acid]}$$
$$pK_a = -\log K_a = -\log (1.8 \times 10^{-5})$$
$$= -(\log 1.8 + [-5]) = 4.74$$
$$pH = 4.74 + \log \frac{[0.1]}{[0.1]}$$
$$\log 1 = O, pH = 4.74$$

2. To calculate the pH of two solutions, one of which is unbuffered and the other buffered, before and after adding the same amount of a strong base to each:

A. Given a solution of HCl whose concentration is 0.0001 molar, determine the pH as follows:

$$[H^+] = 0.0001 = 1 \times 10^{-4}$$
$$pH = 4.0$$

Now add 0.0001 mole of NaOH. To determine the pH after this addition: Since the NaOH added exactly neutralizes the acid present,

$$pH = 7.0$$

B. Given the buffered solution of Example 1, containing 0.1 mole of sodium acetate and 0.1 mole of acetic acid, with a pH of 4.74, calculate the pH after adding the same amount of NaOH, namely, 0.0001 mole, as follows:

$$pH = 4.74 + \log \frac{0.1 + 0.0001}{0.1 - 0.0001}$$

(Because 0.0001 mole of base [numerator] has been added and the same amount of acid has been subtracted [denominator].)

$$pH = 4.74 + \log \frac{0.1001}{0.0999} = 4.74 + \log 0.1001 - \log 0.0999$$
$$= 4.74 + 0.0008, \text{ or } 4.74$$

These calculations (of Example 2) show also the resistance of a buffer to a change in the pH. A small quantity of base added to an unbuffered solution produces a change of three pH units, whereas an equivalent amount of base added to a buffered solution causes an insignificant change.

Titratable acidity The total potential acidity or alkalinity of a biologic fluid may be determined by titration. On the other hand, the hydrogen ion concentration might be termed the true acidity or alkalinity. Let us consider two different acids, hydrochloric and acetic, having the same normality. By normality, we mean the concentration as related to that of a normal solution, and a normal solution is one containing 1 gm. equiv. of a substance per liter of solution. For example, a normal solution of HCl is one that contains 36 gm. HCl per liter, i.e., one that contains 1 gm. H^+ per liter. A normal NaOH solution contains 40 gm. NaOH per liter, i.e., a solution that combines with 1 gm. H^+ per liter. Similarly a normal acetic acid solution has 60 gm. CH_3COOH per liter of solution. In the case of bivalent, trivalent, etc. acids, bases, and salts, we must divide the molecular weight by 2, 3, etc., respectively.

If we wish to combine a gram equivalent weight of NaOH with either HCl or CH_3COOH, we find, of course, that a gram equivalent weight of either of these acids is required.

$$NaOH \; + \; HCl \; \rightarrow \; NaCl \; + \; H_2O$$
$$40 \text{ gm.} \quad 36 \text{ gm.} \quad 58 \text{ gm.} \quad 18 \text{ gm.}$$

$$NaOH \; + \; CH_3COOH \; \rightarrow \; CH_3COONa \; + \; H_2O$$
$$40 \text{ gm.} \quad 60 \text{ gm.} \quad 82 \text{ gm.} \quad 18 \text{ gm.}$$

If, now, the 40 gm. NaOH in each case are dissolved and diluted to 1 liter and the 36 gm. HCl and 60 gm. CH_3COOH are each dissolved in sufficient water to make 1 liter, we have normal solutions of each. One liter of the normal HCl neutralizes 1 liter of normal NaOH; 1 liter of normal CH_3COOH neutralizes 1 liter of normal NaOH. Thus a liter of normal or N/1 HCl is equivalent to the same amount of N/1 CH_3COOH because each is potentially capable of yielding the same amount, namely, 1 gm. per liter, of hydrogen ions. The CH_3COOH is not nearly as strong an acid as HCl; i.e., it is not as greatly dissociated. However, if we add NaOH to it (e.g., the N/1 NaOH), little by little the small number of hydrogen ions is neutralized by the base and more and more acid dissociates until finally all the hydrogen ions have been displaced. This process is known as titration. A normal (N/1), tenth normal (N/10), etc. solution of any acid, then, is equivalent to any other N/1, N/10, etc. acid, volume for volume. Again, a N/10 basic solution neutralizes a N/10 acid, volume for volume.

The *stoichiometric point* in an acid-base titration is the point at which an equivalent amount of base has been added to the acid. The end point of such a titration, however, is not necessarily at a pH of 7.0. This will depend on the salt formed by the reaction. Obviously, we are interested in the pH of the solution at the point at which a maximum amount of salt is present. In the titration of HCl with NaOH, it is the exact point at which all the chloride ion is balanced by the sodium ion and we have a solution of NaCl. Since this is a neutral salt with no buffering action, many different indicators may be used to tell the end point, for one additional droplet of alkali above the equivalent amount can cause a great change in the pH. However, in the titration of a weak acid (e.g., CH_3COOH), with a strong base (e.g., NaOH), the salt formed at the stoichiometric point (CH_3COONa) will have an alkaline reaction, as seen from the following reaction generally referred to as hydrolysis:

$$CH_3COONa \rightleftharpoons Na^+ + CH_3COO^-$$
$$HOH \rightleftharpoons OH^- + H^+$$

$$\uparrow \qquad \downarrow\uparrow$$
$$NaOH \qquad CH_3COOH$$

In other words, as sodium acetate dissociates in the presence of water, the strong basic reaction overbalances the weak acidic one. Therefore, in this titration an indicator that changes at an alkaline pH, e.g., phenolphthalein, must be used. Similarly, in titrating a weak base (e.g., NH_4OH) with a strong acid (e.g., HCl), we finally get NH_4Cl at the stoichiometric point. This has an acid reaction and requires an indicator that changes on the acid side, e.g., methyl red.

$$NH_4Cl \rightleftharpoons NH_4^+ + Cl^-$$
$$HOH \rightleftharpoons OH^- + H^+$$

$$\downarrow\uparrow \qquad \uparrow$$
$$NH_4OH \qquad HCl$$

COLLOIDAL STATE

In 1861, Graham classified all substances into two categories, depending on the ability of the substances to pass through parchment and similar membranes. Since those substances that diffused readily were the ones that easily crystallized, e.g., copper sulfate, sucrose, etc., he designated them "crystalloids." Those that did not pass through, e.g., gelatin, starch paste, glue, etc., were considered to be noncrystallizable and were called "colloids," from the Greek word meaning "glue." These terms continue to be used, although we now are able to crystallize many of the colloids, and the crystalloids can be converted to a colloidal form. The modern concept of these differences is based on the size of the particles dispersed in the water or other medium. Colloidal particles are large; they cannot pass through the pores of ordinary parchment or collodion membranes. However, they are not large enough to settle out by gravity, as suspensions are, or to float at the top of the medium, as imperfect emulsions do. In true solutions, so-called crystalloidal solutions, the mixture is homogeneous; the constituents are present in the molecular or ionic state and are uniformly distributed throughout and among the molecules of water or other solvent. Colloidal systems are heterogeneous; i.e., there are two *phases*—the finely divided particles and the medium in which they are suspended. By "phase," we mean a physically distinct portion of matter. The particles are called the *dispersed phase*, and the medium, usually a fluid, is the *dispersion medium.* Both phases may be solids, liquids, or gases, with a single exception: it is not possible to have a colloidal dispersion of a gas in a gas. Smoke is a solid dispersed in a gas, fog is a liquid dispersed in a gas, and froths and foams are gases dispersed in liquids. We are more concerned with liquids dispersed in liquids, liquids dispersed in solids, and solids dispersed in liquids.

The size of the particles in colloidal systems is generally stated to be from 1 millimicron (mμ) to 100 mμ, but arbitrary limits at either end cannot be set. In fact, the tendency is to place the upper limit somewhat higher, at, for instance, 500 mμ (0.5μ). A millimicron is one millionth of a millimeter (0.000001 mm.). Particles having smaller diameters than 1 mμ are molecular or ionic, and if much above 100 to 500 mμ, they are coarse enough to settle out. The smallest colloidal particles, therefore, are but little larger than crystalloidal molecules, and the largest ones are nearly the size of the particles in a suspension.

Colloidal particles may be removed from the dispersion medium by forcing the fluid, under pressure, through an appropriate membrane. This is termed *ultrafiltration.* By using membranes of varying porosity, it is possible to separate different colloids from each other and to estimate the size of colloid particles. A colloid particle is often termed a *micelle.*

Ultracentrifugation is another method of removing colloid particles. By centrifuging at a very high speed, the dispersed phase may be separated from the dispersion medium. Substances in true solution cannot be separated from their solvents by these two methods. Still another procedure is electrophoresis (p. 903)

A simpler method than any of those described is dialysis. This will be discussed later in the chapter.

Types of colloids Colloids may be grouped into two main classes, depending on their ability to take up the dispersion medium. The *lyophilic colloids* (emulsoids) have a great attraction for the dispersion medium; in fact, each particle has a layer of the dispersion medium surrounding it. The *lyophobic colloids* (suspensoids) contain no such layer. The names are quite descriptive, "lyophilic" meaning solvent-loving and "lyophobic" meaning solvent-hating. The lyophilic colloids include starch, egg albumin, blood proteins, soap, and gelatin. This is the more important type physiologically. Examples of the lyophobic colloids are the colloidal metals, e.g., gold, silver, platinum, etc. Both types exist in the fluid state as *sols.* Many lyophilic colloids form semisolid *gels.* A well-known example is gelatin, which, when dilute, is fluid. When a moderately high concentration is allowed to stand, it sets into a jelly or gel. This gel may be converted to its sol by warming, and, on cooling, it may again gel; i.e., the change from a sol to a gel is frequently reversible. However, this is not always the case, as we shall see when we study coagulation and denaturation of proteins. When a gel forms, apparently long chains of molecules of the colloid interlace and entrap the fluid by capillary forces. The gel then is really a liquid dispersed in a solid.

Some sol-gel transformations take place without change of temperature. For instance, if a colloidal iron oxide sol is allowed to stand quietly, it sets into a gel. Upon shaking, a sol is re-formed. This phenomenon is known as *thixotropy.* Protoplasm is said to have thixotropic properties.

Gels possess the tendency to take up and retain water and swell. This is called *imbibition*. A considerable degree of pressure is needed to squeeze out the water that has been taken up by imbibition. This property of lyophilic colloids is of great importance as regards the state of protoplasm in health and disease. For example, in edema, large quantities of water are absorbed and held by certain tissues. Imbibition is also of importance as regards blood volume. Each gram of albumin in blood plasma holds 17 ml. of water, which aids in maintaining the normal volume of the circulating blood. If the blood volume is reduced because of shock or hemorrhage, the administration of physiologic salt solutions is usually of little value because the fluid leaves the circulation and enters the tissues or is excreted quite promptly. Some material that will hold an amount of water equal to that lost, and thus maintain normal blood volume, must be introduced. If whole blood or plasma is not available, some material that will hold water by imbibition must be used. Gels with this property, called plasma substitutes or *extenders*, are widely used for such purposes clinically (p. 636). Imbibition is affected by hydrogen ion concentration and by other electrolytes, which in some instances enhance the swelling produced by pure water. This differs with different ions. Non-electrolytes such as urea and glucose have little effect.

Preparation of colloidal solutions. Various organic compounds, e.g., gelatin, starch, soap, form sols or "colloidal solutions," as they are frequently called, simply when added to water. Other colloidal solutions may be formed by chemical reaction; e.g., the reduction of gold chloride yields the lyophobic, colloidal gold. Mechanical grinding in a colloid mill may also be used to reduce a substance to such a fine state that it may readily be dispersed in colloidal form. The dispersal of any solid into the colloidal state is called *peptization;* e.g., the dispersal of gelatin in water is known as the peptization of the gelatin, and the water is the peptizing agent; but of course other liquids or solutes may also be peptizing agents. However, it should be noted that substances may form colloidal solutions in one dispersion medium and true solutions in another; e.g., soap is colloidal in water but crystalloidal in ethyl alcohol.

Electric charges on colloids Dispersed colloidal particles carry electric charges, with the dispersion medium carrying the opposite charge. These charges arise chiefly in two ways: groups on the surface of the colloid may ionize, as is the case for proteins; or ions from the medium may be preferentially adsorbed on the surface of the colloid. Since bodies carrying like charges repel each other, this serves to keep the colloids dispersed and is one of the factors that make for the stability of a colloidal system. If an electric current is sent through a colloidal system, the colloid passes to the anode if it is electronegative or to the cathode if it is electropositive. This is called *cataphoresis* or *electrophoresis*. Furthermore, a colloid may be precipitated by adding a colloid of opposite charge, thereby neutralizing the charge and upsetting the stability of the dispersed substance. A few examples of positively and negatively charged colloids of both the lyophilic and lyophobic classes are given in Table A-3.

Under certain conditions the phenomenon of *coacervation* may be observed. When two lyophilic colloids of opposite electric charge are mixed, they may not precipitate or flocculate in the ordinary sense but, because of

Table A-3. Electric charges on colloids

Lyophilic	Lyophobic
Proteins in neutral or alkaline solution (−)	Gold (−)
Proteins in acid solution (+)	Platinum (−)
Starch (−)	Stannic oxide (dispersed by HCl) (+)
Soaps (−)	Sols of metallic oxides and hydroxides and
Aluminum hydroxide (+)	basic dyestuffs (usually +)
Gum acacia (−)	

the hydration shell on each, may form microscopic droplets. These droplets, after a while, may coalesce to form a viscous, fluid layer. This is a coacervate. It contains the two colloids, held apart by the hydration shells, and each colloid retains its own electric charge. Therefore, if the pH is changed or an electrolyte is added to a coacervate, it may again form a sol of the original lyophilic colloids. Many phases of protoplasm are believed to be coacervate in nature. Thus vacuole formation closely resembles a phenomenon seen when complex coacervates are permitted to age.

Tyndall effect. A colloidal solution, e.g., dilute starch, appears slightly cloudy or opalescent to the eye. If a beam of light is passed through it, the beam becomes visible as a much cloudier path, particularly if viewed against a dark background. This is the Tyndall phenomenon and is the same phenomenon observed when a beam of sunlight enters a darkened room. In this instance the minute (colloidal) particles of dust in the air deflect the light. In the case of the colloidal solution, it is the colloidal particles that partly diffract the light and diffuse it. By means of an ultramicroscope or a dark-field microscope, the Tyndall effect becomes visible in another way. In these instruments, light is sent through a drop of solution in a horizontal direction. Visible particles reflect light to the observer's eye and can be seen as shining objects. Invisible particles, e.g., colloids, may be seen as dancing bright specks. They dance and dart in *Brownian movement*, just as visible particles do. The reason is that they are under constant bombardment from molecules of the dispersion medium. A large particle is likely to be hit by about the same number of bombarding particles from each side at the same instant; therefore, it will move less. The smaller particle, with less chance of instantaneous and equal striking from all sides, will move whenever it receives an unequal number of blows from different directions.

The nephelometer is an instrument that measures the Tyndall effect. Substances that form extremely fine precipitates in suspension (colloidal particles) may be estimated quantitatively by means of it.

Stability of colloids. The constant movement of particles is one of the forces that tend to keep a colloid stable. It keeps the colloidal particles distributed throughout the system, rather than allowing them to settle or rise. The size of the colloidal particle is another factor, since the smaller the size, the more closely the particle approximates molecular dimensions and there-fore more nearly resembles a true solution. This is not always the case, how-ever; for the lyophobic colloids may have extremely small dimensions and are, in general, less stable than the lyophilic colloids. The reason for this is that the lyophobes have little or none of the dispersion medium attached, or adsorbed, to their surfaces, and therefore the particles can approach each other closely enough to permit mass attraction to overcome the repulsion due to the electric charge. The lyophilic colloids have a layer of the fluid adsorbed, which makes them more stable because this keeps them farther apart. The electric charge present on the colloid, as a stabilizing factor, has already been discussed.

Any procedure that tends to diminish the effect of one or more of the sta-bilizing factors tends also to precipitate the colloid. Thus, as said before, the addition of another colloid of opposite electric charge has this effect. In the case of the lyophobic colloids, a small amount of electrolyte accomplishes this by also neutralizing the charge. The effect does not occur in the case of lyophilic colloids, although large amounts of electrolytes will precipitate them. Probably this "salting out" occurs as the result of dehydrating the sur-face layer of fluid. Furthermore, violent agitation, freezing and thawing, or heating, can "break" colloidal solutions by modifying one or more of the sta-bilizing factors.

Although lyophobic colloids may be precipitated by the addition of small amounts of electrolytes, this may be hindered by the presence of small quan-tities of a lyophilic colloid. Such "protective" action is believed to be ac-complished by the adsorption of the lyophilic colloid onto the surface of the lyophobic colloid, thereby preventing the electrolyte from easily reaching it. The protective action of colloids present in bile and urine may be a major reason for the prevention of the precipitation of almost insoluble constituents of these fluids. Conversely, when the protective colloidal action is not effec-tive, gallstones and kidney stones result. Lange's colloidal gold test is based on this protective colloidal action. Colloidal gold is a bright orange-red sol. The addition of normal cerebrospinal fluid does not precipitate it. Abnormal cerebrospinal fluid may do so, however, the result showing in various shades, depending on the degree of precipitation. The test is performed under exact quantitative conditions, and curves that are indicative of pathologic states are obtained.

Surface reactions of colloids The dispersed phase of a colloid differs from a suspension of solid matter in that the colloid is subdivided into much smaller particles. Each suspended particle has a surface. Similarly, each colloidal particle has a surface, and al-though the colloidal particle is far smaller than the suspension particle, the number of particles is much greater for the same weight and therefore the total area of surface is greater. This can be illustrated by a simple example. A cube of any material 1 cm. on a side has a surface area of 6×1 cm.^{2}, or 6 cm.^{2} If it is divided into eight cubes, each edge measuring $\frac{1}{2}$ cm., the total area will be $\frac{1}{2}$ cm. $\times \frac{1}{2}$ cm. $\times$ 6 sides $\times$ 8 cubes = 12 cm.^{2} The subdivision of each small cube is continued, and the amount of surface is doubled each time each cube is cut into eight smaller ones. Eventually, when the cubes are down to a size comparable with colloidal dimensions, i.e., 100 mμ on a side, the total of all the tiny cubes will be 600,000 cm.^{2}, i.e., 100,000 times the original surface area, produced by simply subdividing the cube. This indicates the enormous area presented by the surfaces of colloid particles. On these surfaces, substances present in solution may be adsorbed and become concentrated. Adsorption is the phenomenon in which there is condensed on a surface a layer of ions, molecules, or aggregates of molecules that are present in the medium with which the surface is in contact. The amount of adsorption depends on the extent of surface exposed and the specific nature of the surface and of the substance adsorbed upon it. Furthermore, the degree of adsorption is increased by a rise in pressure and is diminished by a rise in temperature. Many physiologic phenomena are surface reactions. The enzymes, which catalyze so many reactions of the body, probably act through surface forces. They are colloids and the substances they act on are probably adsorbed by them as a first step in the chemical action that is brought about.

Emulsions   Emulsions are dispersions of one liquid in another. If olive oil is shaken vigorously in water, it breaks up into small droplets and a yellow milky fluid results. An emulsion is a heterogeneous system comprising two phases, but the dispersed phase usually consists of particles larger than colloidal particles. An emulsion of olive oil and water does not last very long; the oil droplets coalesce and soon there is a layer of oil floating on the water. Certain substances—among others, soaps, gums, proteins—when added to the system, stabilize the emulsion. The stabilizing substance, an emulsifier, may form a protective layer around the oil droplets and so prevent them from coalescing. This is similar to the *protective colloidal action* just described. With any pair of nonmiscible liquids, two sets of emulsions are possible. Thus, with oil and water we may have (1) oil-in-water and (2) water-in-oil. In a general way, any emulsifying agent that stabilizes an oil-in-water emulsion is unsatisfactory for the corresponding water-in-oil emulsion, and vice versa.

Emulsions occur widely in nature. In fact, protoplasm is probably a mixture of emulsions, containing colloids in one or both phases of many of them. Emulsification, of course, increases the surface of the substance emulsified. This permits biologic reactions, which, as said, are frequently surface reactions, to take place more readily. For example, one of the functions of bile is to aid in the emulsification of fats in the small intestine. By doing so, it breaks up these water-insoluble substances into such tiny droplets that the digestive agent can readily attack them. If this were not done, the digestion of the mass of fat would take place extremely slowly.

SURFACE TENSION

The surface of a liquid behaves as if it were a stretched elastic film. This tension is due to the unbalanced attraction of the molecules to each other. According to Laplace, the molecules of a solution are strongly attracted to each other but only over a very short distance. The attraction is probably greatest at a distance equal to about the diameter of a molecule. Fig. A-1 illustrates and explains this phenomenon. Molecules *C*, *D*, *E*, and *F* are not at the surface and are attracted equally in all directions. They are, therefore, able

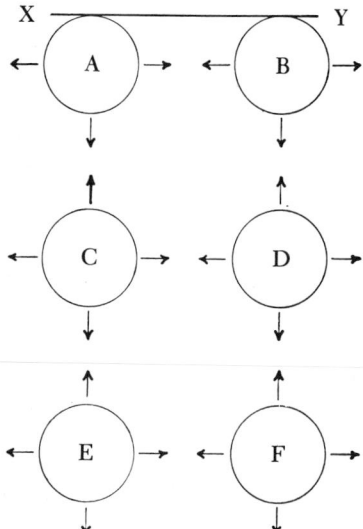

Fig. A-1. Diagram to explain surface tension. Molecules A and B are at the surface, X−Y, and are not attracted upward because of the absence of molecules above them. Consequently, they tend to be drawn downward and sideward, and the layer of molecules at the surface is thus stretched. Molecules C, D, E, and F are not at the surface and are attracted equally in all directions.

to move freely in all directions. Molecules A and B, however, are at the surface (XY) and are not attracted upward because of the absence of molecules of the fluid above the surface. Consequently, they tend to be drawn downward and pulled sideward, and the layer of surface molecules is thereby stretched. The effect of this "film" is seen in the tendency of drops of water and mercury and soap bubbles to assume a spheric form because of the cohesive pull sideward and inward. This phenomenon occurs at any surface or *interface* that separates a liquid from air or other gases or that separates one liquid from another. This explanation is a simplification of the phenomenon; other forces are involved besides that of attraction.

Surface tension may be measured in a number of ways, perhaps most conveniently with a stalagmometer. This is a pipette of special design with a capillary tube ending, permitting a measured amount of fluid to flow out drop by drop. The number of drops depends on the size of the drops, which, in turn, varies with the surface tension. A comparison with the number of drops of pure water permits one to calculate the surface tension of the solution. Surface tension is expressed as ergs per square centimeter or dynes per centimeter. For accurate work, great precautions of cleanliness must be taken, since small amounts of some substances alter the surface tension materially. Soaps, oils, proteins, and salts of the bile acids reduce the surface tension of water, whereas sodium chloride tends to increase it. These and similar effects aid in explaining some physiologic actions, e.g., fat digestion and absorption. Substances that reduce surface tension accumulate in the surface film and are said to be adsorbed, whereas the reverse is true of those that increase surface tension. There is a stalagmometric method for the determination of bile acids in bile that has been used as a liver function test, based on the fact that an important function of the liver is the secretion of bile acids. The du Noüy tensiometer is another device for determining surface tension. In this, a light metal ring is set on the surface of the fluid under examination. As the ring is raised, a film of the fluid clings to it. The amount of force required to pull the ring off and break this film is a measure of the surface tension and can be exactly and conveniently measured.

DIFFUSION, OSMOSIS, AND DIALYSIS

Diffusion. If a strong solution of a salt, e.g., copper sulfate, is placed in a glass vessel and a layer of distilled water is carefully poured over it, the blue copper sulfate rises gradually into the colorless water until finally the entire body of fluid has the same color. This process is called diffusion. The velocity with which it occurs depends on the size of the particles of the substance in solution. Thus Prussian blue, being composed of large particles, diffuses more slowly than copper sulfate. Higher temperatures also speed up the process. It should be observed that diffusion involves the passage of substances, in true solution or in colloidal solution, through the fluid in which they are suspended. In the many fluids of the body, within cells, during secretory activity, diffusion must be constantly occurring.

Osmosis. Osmosis is the passage of a solvent through a semipermeable membrane. Such a membrane is permeable only to the solvent, not to the solute, i.e., the substance in solution. The classic experiment of Pfeffer illustrates the point. He precipitated copper ferrocyanide in the walls of an unglazed porcelain jar by filling the jar with potassium ferrocyanide solution after immersing it in a solution of copper sulfate. Such a film of copper ferrocyanide permits water to pass through but does not allow certain soluble substances, e.g., sugars, to do so. Consequently, when such a jar, fitted with a glass tube into which the liquid can rise, and filled with sugar solution, is placed in distilled water, the water passes through the semipermeable membrane into the sugar solution until the column of diluted sugar solution is no longer increased. The pressure that would have to be exerted on the solution to prevent passage into it of solvent, namely, water, when separated from it by a perfectly semipermeable membrane is called the osmotic pressure. Osmotic pressure is evidenced only if there is a semipermeable membrane separating one solution from another. However, in biochemical and physiologic literature, it has become customary to allude to the osmotic pressure of a solution even when no membrane is present. Furthermore, in biologic systems the membranes are not "perfect" semipermeable membranes, but they permit solutes consisting of small particles or ions to pass through. There is, of course, some osmotic influence even under these circumstances. The student should have these facts in mind when, on the following pages, and especially on pp. 580 and 582, the osmotic pressure of certain solutions is discussed.

The osmotic pressure of a solution is directly proportional to the concentration of the solute. More concentrated solutions give rise to higher osmotic pressures than weak ones. Therefore, 1 gm. of salt dissolved in 100 ml. has twice the potential osmotic pressure of 1 gm. of salt dissolved in 200 ml. In other words, the osmotic pressure is *inversely* proportional to the volume, showing that Boyle's law is applicable to solutions. Similarly, it has been found that the osmotic pressure increases $1/273$ for each rise of 1° C. (Gay-Lussac's law). Avogadro's law also applies to osmotic pressure since all solutions containing the same number of dissolved particles exert the same osmotic pressure at a constant temperature; i.e., the osmotic pressure depends on the number of particles dispersed in the fluid. This pressure is independent of the nature of the particles. Consequently, a given number of ions, undissociated molecules, and aggregates of molecules (colloidal particles) in identical volumes of fluid all exert the same effect. Since each ion has the same effect as a molecule, evidently an electrolyte like sodium chloride, which furnishes two ions, will produce twice as high an osmotic pressure when completely dissociated as will a non-ionized substance of the same molecular weight. Also, since large aggregates of molecules have the same effect as ions or small molecules, colloidal "solutions" will exert low osmotic pressures because of the comparatively small *number* of such particles present.

Although osmotic pressure can be determined by such an apparatus as illustrated in Fig. A-2, in practice it is measured by indirect means. The boiling point of a solvent is raised by the addition of a solute, and the freezing point is lowered similarly. The amount of either change is proportional to the concentration of the particles of the solute and, as we have seen, the same holds true for osmotic pressure.

Solutions that exert the same osmotic pressure are said to be *isosmotic*. If a cell is in contact with a solution having the same osmotic pressure as the cell contents, the amount of water passing into the cell is balanced by that passing out, provided the cell membrane is impermeable to the solutes. In this case, the solution is not only isosmotic but also *isotonic;* i.e., the cell volume is unchanged; its tone is maintained. If the osmotic pressure of a solution of the same solutes is greater than that of the cell, the solution is hyperosmotic and is said to be *hypertonic*, and water will pass from the cell to the solution. If it is lower, the solution is hypo-osmotic and is *hypotonic*, and water will flow into the cell. In a hypertonic solution the cell shrinks, and in a hypotonic solution it swells. We have presupposed in each case that the solutes do not permeate the membrane. If, however, one or more of the solutes can pass through the membrane and are not present in the same concentration within the cell, an isosmotic solution may not be isotonic. Osmotic pressure is not the same as tonicity. However, physiologically the terms are almost interchangeable and are found to usually parallel each other rather closely.

Thus 0.9% NaCl solutions are isotonic to human erythrocytes, and if the two are in contact, the amount of water passing into the cell is balanced by that passing out. A solution of lower salt concentration has lower osmotic pressure than the cell. It is hypotonic. If erythrocytes are immersed in hypotonic solutions, water passes from the more dilute to the more concentrated solution (i.e., from the lower to the higher osmotic pressure) in so great an amount that the erythrocytes swell and may even burst. Hypertonic solutions cause water to pass out of the cells and the cells to become shriveled or *cre-*

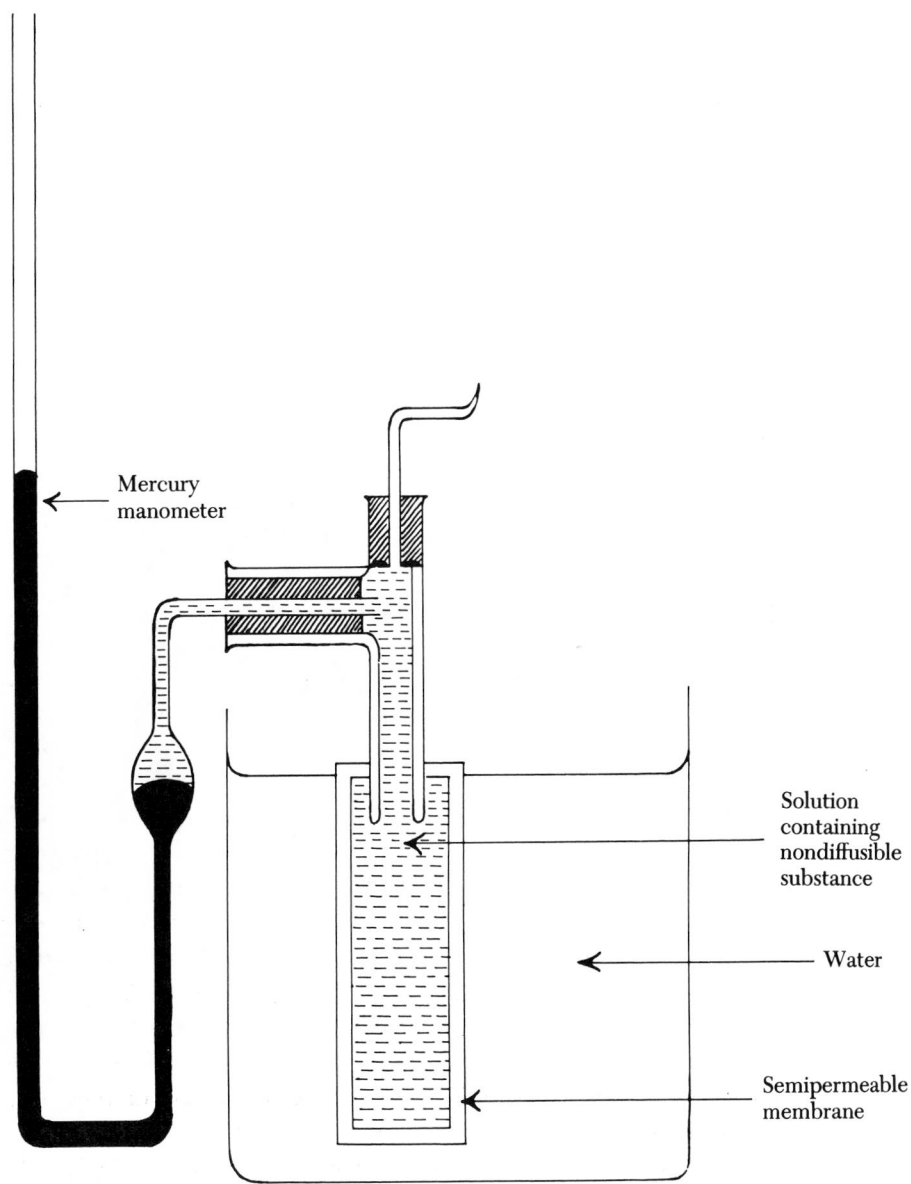

Fig. A-2. Osmometer.

nated. Therefore, solutions used for injection are made up to be isotonic; otherwise unphysiologic effects would be produced on the corpuscles. Similarly, whenever cut tissues or viscera are bathed with fluid, isotonic solutions are used since they cause less change in the cells with which they come in contact. The body adjusts its various fluids to approximately the same osmotic pressure. For example, the osmotic pressures of such extremely divergent types of fluids as blood, hepatic bile, pancreatic juice, and lymph collected simultaneously have been found to be practically the same.

Dialysis. As just explained, osmosis requires a membrane that is permeable to the solvent, not to substances dissolved or dispersed in it. Membranes of varying porosity that permit smaller particles of varying sizes to pass through but are impermeable to larger particles exist or can be prepared. In general, membranes such as parchment, collodion, or cellophane allow crystalloids to pass but prevent colloids from doing so. The process involved is termed *dialysis*. Thus, if a mixture of crystalloids and colloids is placed in a dialyzing bag that is then immersed in distilled water, the colloids remain behind while the crystalloids dialyze out. By changing the outside fluid frequently, the colloids may be completely freed of crystalloids. It is easily seen, however, that since colloids themselves vary in size some membranes will permit colloids of smaller dimensions to pass.

Membranes in the animal body Since all cells — plant and animal — are enclosed by membranes, the question naturally arises: Are these membranes semipermeable or permeable, or do they behave like filter paper? This cannot be answered categorically since the wall of a living cell cannot be compared with an artificial membrane or even with a dead biologic membrane. Animal membranes (see also p. 10) do not have the simple structure of artificial membranes. It is probable that cell membranes in different tissues vary in their permeability. Certainly the cells lining different parts of the kidney permit different ions and compounds to pass. Indeed, adjacent portions of the kidney tubules exhibit varying properties of this nature. It is also probable that the same cell wall changes from hour to hour, depending on respiratory and metabolic conditions. Therefore the idea formerly held, that living membranes are impermeable to colloids but are permeable to electrolytes, must be modified.

A remarkable degree of selectivity sometimes is seen in these biologic migrations. The erythrocyte membrane, for example, allows cations to pass through less easily but is quite permeable to anions — a fact important in explaining respiratory phenomena. Furthermore, some fat-soluble as well as some water-soluble substances pass through the erythrocyte wall. The membrane is believed to be composed of at least three layers, two outer layers of protein and an inner lipid core, that are permeable to certain fat-soluble and water-soluble materials. However, all the phenomena pertaining to membranes cannot be explained on the basis of porosity, i.e., sieve action, or on the theory of solubility. In some cases, the electric charge of the membrane must be taken into account. For example, if the charge on erythrocytes is reversed, the cells become impermeable to anions and permeable to cations.

Gibbs-Donnan equilibrium If a membrane that permits the passage of crystalloids but not colloids is placed between two solutions of a simple electrolyte such as sodium chloride, the sodium and chloride ions pass through the membrane until, at equilibrium, the product of the concentrations of these two ions on one side equals the product of their concentrations on the other side. Concentrations such as gram molecules per liter are again represented by bracketed symbols. The conditions stated may be represented thus:

$$[Na^+]_1 \times [Cl^-]_1 = [Na^+]_2 \times [Cl^-]_2$$

$[Na^+]_1$ means, of course, the concentration of sodium ions on side 1, $[Na^+]_2$ its concentration on side 2, etc. Moreover, not only are the products of the concentrations the same, but under these conditions the concentrations of the cations are the same, and also those of anions:

$$[Na^+]_1 = [Na^+]_2$$
$$[Cl^-]_1 = [Cl^-]_2$$

Let us assume that, in addition to a simple electrolyte, we have on side 1 the sodium salt of a colloid, NaR, which can ionize to $[Na^+]$ and $[R^-]$ but the colloid ion is too large to pass through the membrane. Now the additional Na^+ may pass through but not the R^-.

As before, chloride ions may pass back and forth. Finally, equilibrium will occur and the question arises as to how this will affect the distribution of the diffusible ions. As in the first instance, the product of the concentrations of the diffusible cation-anion pair on one side will equal the product of the concentrations of the same pair on the other side. (This is derived from thermodynamics.)

$$(1) \quad [Na^+]_3 \times [Cl^-]_3 = [Na^+]_4 \times [Cl^-]_4$$

But

$$[Na^+]_4 = [Cl^-]_4$$

This is evident since there is only sodium chloride present on side 4 and there can be no more of one ion than the other. If we remember that on side 3 there is a nondiffusible ion R^- balancing electrically some of the Na^+, it is evident that

$$[Na^+]_3 > [Cl^-]_3$$

Now, referring to the equation (1), if the members of the left side are unequal, we can see that the larger value on the left must be larger than either of the two on the right (which are equal to each other) and the smaller value on the left must be smaller than either one on the right or:

$$[Na^+]_3 > [Na^+]_4$$
$$[Cl^-]_3 < [Cl^-]_4$$

We can therefore see how the presence of a colloidal ion may cause an inequality in the distribution of ions on the opposite sides of a membrane. If there are several colloidal ions and many noncolloidal ions present, the state of affairs becomes exceedingly complex. This is what happens in animal tissues, where different types of cells, bathed by the same or different body fluids, under varying conditions, differ fundamentally in the chemical makeup of their contents. This unequal balance of ions also leads to a difference in potential between the solutions on the two sides of the membrane. The phenomenon is known as the Gibbs-Donnan equilibrium, after Willard Gibbs and F. G. Donnan, who first studied and explained it.

Membrane potentials. One of the most interesting physicochemical phenomena in living matter is the existence of potentials, of as much as 60 or more millivolts, across cell membranes. These are manifested as the clinically important electroencephalogram (EEG), the electrocardiogram (EKG), and the action current in the conduction of nerve impulses.

The phenomenon has been studied extensively for many years and a number of theoretic explanations have been proposed, none of which is universally accepted. For a complete discussion of these hypotheses, consult the general references listed at the end of the chapter. Only a brief summary will be presented here. The fundamental reason for the potential appears to be a different net charge on the two sides of the membrane due to differing ionic concentrations. The latter may result from a selective permeability of the membrane, a sieve action, a pump mechanism, or some sorption or association-induction effect, or a combination of these. The Donnan effect just described is undoubtedly involved in at least some instances. Important in biochemistry is the fact that the membrane potential changes with the transfer of ions across the cell membrane in varying metabolic and physiologic situations.

VISCOSITY

Viscosity is the resistance offered by a fluid to flow. It is due to the internal friction of the molecules of a liquid. A solvent is almost always less viscid than a solution and considerably less viscid than a colloidal system. Viscosity ordinarily is not expressed in absolute units but is referred to the viscosity of water. It is measured by allowing a definite amount of the fluid under consideration to flow through a capillary tube at a definite temperature. The time required is compared with that taken by an equal volume of water. With water as unity, the normal viscosity of blood serum is about 1.5 to 2.0, whereas that of plasma, which has a higher protein content, is about 20% greater, and whole blood has a viscosity of 2.5 to 4.0. These are approximate values for the viscosity of normal human blood. When dehydration occurs, as it does in some pathologic states, the viscosity of whole blood may be three or four times the normal value.

General references

Clark, W. M.: Topics in physical chemistry, ed. 2, Baltimore, 1952, The Williams & Wilkins Co.

Montgomery, R., and Swenson, C. A.: Quantitative problems in the biochemical sciences, San Francisco, 1969, W. H. Freeman & Co., Publishers.

Williams, V. R., and Williams, H. B.: Basic physical chemistry for the life sciences, San Francisco, 1967, W. H. Freeman & Co., Publishers.

ANALYTIC TECHNIQUES FREQUENTLY USED IN BIOCHEMISTRY

CHROMATOGRAPHY

Experience with chromatography goes back to 1850, when Runge described a method for the analysis of mixtures of dyes by applying drops of dye solutions to blotting paper and noting the separation of the different colors. In 1897, Day used a column of limestone for the fractionation of crude petroleum. However, the credit for discovering chromatography is usually given to Tswett, a botanist, who, in 1906, effected the separation of plant pigments by filtering a solution of the mixed pigments through a tube containing finely divided, solid adsorbing material. The individual pigments settled in separate bands and thus formed a *chromatogram* or pattern of pigments. Each substance adsorbed, called *adsorbate,* could be removed or *eluted* from the *adsorbent.* The term "chromatography" is still used for this type of separation, despite the fact that the process is no longer limited to colored substances. It has now been greatly extended and is widely used in biochemistry as well as in other branches of chemistry. Many different adsorbents are used and are selected for their affinity for the adsorbates. They include talc, asbestos, clays, charcoal, starches, and filter paper.

Paper chromatography differs somewhat, although the principle is the same. A large sheet of filter paper is treated in one corner with a small amount of the solution to be studied. It is then draped over a glass rod, with the edge containing the sample dipping into a tray of the desired solvent. As the solvent travels up the paper, it takes with it the unknown substances, which are deposited in spots. These spots can be "developed" as colors by suitable chemical treatment. They are identified by running controls in which known substances are used. Sometimes there is a second run, using a different solvent, at right angles—a two-dimensional chromatogram, which separates spots placed too closely together by the first run for easy identification.

Within the past few years, many modifications and improvements in chromatographic procedures have been made, increasing the resolving power and applicability of the procedures. For example, thin-layer chromatography utilizes the same principles as those for paper chromatography. Such supports as silica gel or cellulose are dried onto a glass or plastic sheet as very thin layers. In this process the chromatographic separation is quite rapid.

Molecular sieve chromatography takes advantage of differences in molecular size and shape. Protein solutions are passed through columns of synthetic polyacrylamide gels or polysaccharide gels called *dextrans*. These substances function by virtue of differences in pore sizes in the particles. Small molecules pass through the pores and enter the particles whereas larger ones or macromolecules are unable to do so readily. In this way the larger molecules pass through the column whereas the smaller ones are retained with the particles.

Gas chromatography is also a valuable tool for the separation of volatile substances or volatile derivatives of otherwise nonvolatile substances. The sample molecules are volatilized and separated by passing, with the help of a carrier gas, through a long column of narrow diameter containing a suitable stationary support.

ION-EXCHANGE CHROMATOGRAPHY

Ion exchange is a reversible interchange of ions between a liquid and a solid, involving no radical alteration in the structure of the solid. Natural products such as certain sands, peat, and coal, operating on this principle, have been used to soften water for many years; but not until 1935 were synthetic resins employed for this purpose. The English scientists Adams and Holmes reasoned that acidic and basic groups that are not involved in the condensation of the constituents of synthetic resins should be free to ionize. If so, they should permit cation and anion exchange processes. Ion exchangers consist, therefore, of insoluble resins or supports, $\textcircled{R}$, to which are attached a variety of acidic or basic groups. These substances are often packed into columns and the solutions containing the exchangeable ions are percolated through the column.

Resins bearing anionic components of the type $\textcircled{R}\text{-}SO_3^-H^+$ or $\textcircled{R}\text{-}CO_2^-H^+$ are called *cation exchangers*. For example the proton may be exchanged by sodium ion so that:

$$\textcircled{R}\text{-}SO_3^-H^+ + NaCl \rightarrow \textcircled{R}\text{-}SO_3^-Na^+ + HCl$$

In the separation of amino acids:

$$\textcircled{R}\text{-}SO_3^-NH_4^+ + \text{Amino acid-}NH_3^+Cl^- \rightarrow \textcircled{R}\text{-}SO_3^-\text{-amino acid-}NH_3^+ + NH_4^+Cl^-$$

The exchanged cation may then be removed from the column by a regenerating process:

$$\textcircled{R}\text{-}SO_3^-\text{-amino acid-}NH_3^+ + HCl \rightarrow \textcircled{R}\text{-}SO_3^-H^+ + \text{Amino acid-}NH_3^+Cl^-$$

Anion exchangers may possess amino groups, $\textcircled{R}\text{-}NH_2$, that form an ammonium salt with HCl:

$$\textcircled{R}\text{-}NH_2 + HCl \rightarrow \textcircled{R}\text{-}NH_3^+Cl^-$$

The chloride may be replaced by another anion in the exchange process:

$$\textcircled{R}\text{-}NH_3^+Cl^- + \text{Amino acid-}CO_2^- \xrightarrow{Na^+} \textcircled{R}\text{-}NH_3^+\text{-amino acid-}CO_2^- + NaCl$$

The amino acid may be removed by regenerating with HCl.

Proteins are commonly isolated and purified by ion-exchange chromatography. The now standard procedure is to use columns of cellulose derivatives such as diethylaminoethyl- and triethylaminoethylcellulose (DEAE and TEAE) as anion exchangers. Carboxymethylcellulose (CM) is often used as a cation exchanger for this purpose.

ELECTROPHORESIS

The movement of a charged particle in an external electric field toward the oppositely charged electrode is called electrophoresis. The electrophoresis of biocolloids, for the most part proteins, has been commonly performed in the apparatus developed by Tiselius, in Sweden. Current is applied to the ends of a U-tube, which is filled with a protein solution overlaid by a buffer solution of the same ionic strength, pH, and conductivity. The buffer solution is stratified carefully over the protein layer so that the boundary between the two solutions is sharp. During the electrophoresis period, the various proteins migrate towards the electrode of opposite charge. The degree of migration depends on the magnitude of the protein charges. New boundaries may be formed if more than one protein is present, and their locations in the limbs of the tube (and therefore the distances traveled from the starting position), as well as their relative concentrations, may be determined by an optic process. Light, refracted by the various boundaries, is converted by an optic system into a pattern of peaks, each peak representing a boundary between protein molecules and the buffer. The type of profile obtained is shown in Figs. 7-15 and 19-2.

The Tiselius apparatus is used to determine the isoelectric point and electrophoretic mobility of proteins. The method is also frequently employed to study the homogeneity of protein preparations.

A highly simplified modification of the Tiselius electrophoretic system is called *zone electrophoresis*. In this procedure the electrophoretic separation is performed on an inert support soaked in the buffer to be used. Such supports are usually paper, starch, agar, certain plastics, and cellulose acetate. The paper support, wet with buffer, serves as a bridge between the two electrode vessels. The sample is applied to the support as a narrow strip. Separation of molecules is in the form of zones of proteins that migrate in accord with their charge densities. After the separation is complete, the paper strip is dried to fix the separate molecules on the paper. The sample molecules are rendered visible by a suitable dye. Their relative concentrations may be estimated by the use of a densitometer.

ULTRACENTRIFUGATION

The ultracentrifuge produces sufficiently high speeds to cause the sedimentation of macromolecules in solutions. The rate at which sedimentation occurs depends on such parameters as molecular weight and shape. Under carefully controlled conditions, the macromolecules sediment at a characteristic velocity, which can be measured as the movement of the boundary between molecules and solvents.

In the apparatus developed by Svedberg (the analytic ultracentrifuge) an optic system converts the sedimenting boundary of molecules into a peak, which actually represents changes in refractive index. The rate of movement of this peak, dx/dt, is used to calculate the sedimentation coefficient, s.

$$s = \frac{v}{\omega^2 x}$$

In this equation, v is velocity (dx/dt) of sedimentation, ω is angular rotor velocity in radians per second, and x is the distance of the boundary to the center of the rotor in centimeters. The sedimentation constant, s, has the magnitude of 10^{-13} second. The constant, however, is usually given in *Svedberg units*, S, which is $10^{13} \times s$.

Svedberg then used this constant to develop the equation for molecular weight, M.

$$M = \frac{s\,RT}{D\,(1 - V\rho)}$$

Here R is the gas constant, T the absolute temperature, and D the diffusion constant. $(1 - V\rho)$ is a buoyancy correction in which ρ is the solvent density, and V the partial specific volume of the solute molecules.

DENSITY GRADIENT CENTRIFUGATION

A relatively recent development in the area of ultracentrifugation utilizes density gradients and a preparative ultracentrifuge. In this method a continuous linear gradient of sucrose, varying, for example, from 20% at the bottom to 5% at the top, is formed in a plastic centrifuge tube. The sucrose gradient is often produced automatically with a controlled mixing device, the gradient maker. The sample is carefully layered on top of the gradient and the tubes are then spun at high speed in a "swinging-bucket" rotor. During the centrifugation, the molecules migrate through the gradient at characteristic velocities. At the termination of the centrifugation, the tubes are pierced with a hypodermic needle and equal fractions are collected for various assays.

Salts such as CsCl form gradients of high density and low viscosity. Such gradients are used in isopyknic or equilibrium sedimentation because the sample molecules migrate to zones of equal density. This technique was used in the separation of ^{14}N-, ^{15}N-, and ^{14,15}N-DNA's in the studies of Meselson and Stahl (p. 50).

Density gradient methods are popular because they allow both analytic and preparative studies. They may also be used in the determination of molecular weight by the method of Martin and Ames.

X-RAY DIFFRACTION

When a beam of X rays enters a crystalline substance, the waves are deflected from their course, i.e., diffracted, by the various planes of atoms. In this situation the angle of incidence equals the angle of diffraction. In 1912, Bragg showed that this diffraction of X rays obeys the expression:

$$n\lambda = 2d \sin \theta$$

This equation says, in effect, that when the path difference for waves diffracted by successive sheets of atoms is a whole number of wavelengths the waves will be in phase, resulting in a summation of intensity and a diffraction maximum. The location of these diffracted beams and their relative intensities are evaluated by a photographic procedure. Since in a crystalline substance, atoms are arranged in an orderly manner, the characteristic diffraction pattern can be used to determine the relative positions in space of these atoms. In a crystal of protein, the X rays are diffracted by the electron fields of C, O_2, and N_2. This phenomenon is evaluated mathematically and an electron-density map, called the *Fourier pattern*, is produced. The electron densities of successive sheets of atoms in the crystal are reproduced in such maps. In the final model each successive electron-density contour map is placed one on top of the other until a three-dimensional model of the protein is produced. Since a hemoglobin molecule contains 10,000 atoms and many thousands of measurements must be performed, the complexity of the procedure is obvious.

References

Bier, M., editor: Electrophoresis: theory, methods, and applications, New York, 1959, 1967, Academic Press, Inc.

Bragg, L.: X-ray crystallography, Sci. Amer. **219**:58, 1968.

Epstein, H. T.: Elementary biophysics, selected topics, Reading, Mass., 1963, Addison-Wesley Publishing Co., Inc.

Giddings, J. C., and Keller, R. A., editors: Advances in chromatography, vols. 1–8, New York, 1966–1969, Marcel Dekker, Inc.

Heftmann, E.: Chromatography, New York, 1961, Reinhold Publishing Corp.

Williams, V. R., and Williams, H. B.: Basic physical chemistry for the life sciences, San Francisco, 1967, W. H. Freeman & Co., Publishers.

INDEX

907